Dementia
Third edition

Edited by

Alistair Burns MPhil, MD, FRCP, FRCPsych
Professor of Old Age Psychiatry,
Wythenshawe Hospital,
Manchester, UK

John O'Brien MA, DM, FRCPsych
Professor of Old Age Psychiatry,
Institute for Ageing and Health,
University of Newcastle upon Tyne,
Newcastle upon Tyne, UK

David Ames BA, MD, FRCPsych, FRANZCP
Professor of Psychiatry of Old Age,
University of Melbourne, St George's Hospital, Melbourne,
Victoria, Australia

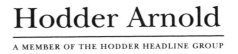

Hodder Arnold

A MEMBER OF THE HODDER HEADLINE GROUP

First published in Great Britain in 1994 by Chapman & Hall
Second edition published in 2000 by Arnold
This third edition published in 2005 by
Hodder Arnold, an imprint of Hodder Education and a member of the Hodder Headline Group,
338 Euston Road, London NW1 3BH

http://www.hoddereducation.com

Distributed in the United States of America by
Oxford University Press Inc.,
198 Madison Avenue, New York, NY10016
Oxford is a registered trademark of Oxford University Press

Whilst the advice and information in this book are believed to be true and
accurate at the date of going to press, neither the author[s] nor the publisher
can accept any legal responsibility or liability for any errors or omissions
that may be made. In particular (but without limiting the generality of the
preceding disclaimer) every effort has been made to check drug dosages;
however, it is still possible that errors have been missed. Furthermore,
dosage schedules are constantly being revised and new side effects
recognized. For these reasons the reader is strongly urged to consult the
drug companies' printed instructions before administering any of the drugs
recommended in this book.

British Library Cataloguing in Publication Data
A catalogue record for this book is available from the British Library

Library of Congress Cataloging-in-Publication Data
A catalog record for this book is available from the Library of Congress

ISBN-10 0 340 812 036
ISBN-13 978 0 340 812 037

1 2 3 4 5 6 7 8 9 10

Commissioning Editor: Clare Christian
Project Editor: Layla Vandenbergh/Clare Patterson
Production Controller: Jane Lawrence
Cover Designer: Nichola Smith
Copy-editor: Michèle Clarke
Proofreader: Lotika Singha
Editorial Assistant: Clare Weber
Index: Indexing Specialists (UK) Ltd

Typeset in 10/12 pt Minion by Charon Tec Pvt. Ltd, Chennai, India
www.charontec.com
Printed and bound in Great Britain by CPI Bath.

What do you think about this book? Or any other Hodder Arnold title?
Please send your comments to www.hoddereducation.com

Contents

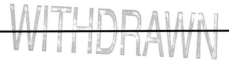

List of contributors

Dag Aarsland MD, PhD
Head of Research,
Psychiatry Centre for Clinical Neuroscience Research,
Stavanger University Hospital,
Stavanger, Norway

Kirsten Abelskov MD
Consultant, Psychiatrist,
Psychogeriatric Department,
Aarhus University Hospitals,
Denmark

George Alexopoulos MD
Professor of Psychiatry,
Weill Medical College,
Cornell University,
New York, USA

Osvaldo P Almeida MD, PhD, FRANZCP
Professor of Geriatric Psychiatry,
School of Psychiatry and Clinical Neurosciences,
University of Western Australia,
Australia

David Ames BA, MD, FRCPsych, FRANZCP
Professor of Psychiatry of Old Age,
University of Melbourne,
St George's Hospital, Melbourne,
Victoria, Australia

Sylvaine Artero
Institut National de la Santé et de la Recherche
Médicale (INSERM),
Hôpital La Colombière,
Montpellier, France

Olusegun Baiyewu MBBS, FMC(Psych), FWACP
Professor of Psychiatry,
College of Medicine,
University of Ibadan,
Ibadan, Nigeria

Robert C Baldwin DM, FRCP, FRCPsych
Consultant Old Age Psychiatrist and
Honorary Professor of Psychiatry,
Institute for the Health of the Elderly,
Wolfson Research Centre,
Newcastle City Health NHS Trust,
Newcastle upon Tyne, UK

Clive Ballard MD, MB ChB, M MedSci, MRCPsych
Professor and Research Director of the Alzheimer's Society,
Wolfson Research Centre for Age-Related Diseases,
King's College London,
London, UK

Carol Bannister MB ChB, MRCPsych
Consultant in Old Age Psychiatry,
The Fiennes Centre,
Banbury, UK

Robert Barber MRCPsych, MD
Consultant Old Age Psychiatrist,
Institute for the Health of the Elderly,
Wolfson Research Centre,
Newcastle General Hospital,
Newcastle upon Tyne, UK

German Berrios BA (OXFORD), MD, DM H.C. HEIDELBERG, FRCPsych, FBPSS
Professor,
University of Cambridge Department of Psychiatry,
Cambridge, UK

Konrad Beyreuther Dr rer nat, Dr med hc
Professor of Molecular Biology and
Head of the Laboratory of Molecular Neuropathology,
Centre for Molecular Biology,
University of Heidelberg,
Heidelberg, Germany

Angelo Bianchetti MD
Head of Department of Internal Medicine and
Alzheimer Evaluation Unit,
Instituto Clinico S. Anna
Brescia, Italy

Michael Bird BA, MPsych, PhD
Senior Clinical Psychologist for the Aged and
Co-ordinator of Aged Mental Health,
Southern Area Health Service,
Queanbeyan, Australia

Betty S Black PhD
Assistant Professor,
Department of Psychiatry and Behavioral Sciences,
John Hopkins School of Medicine,
Baltimore, Maryland, USA

Andrew D Blackwell MA (hons), PhD
Research Associate,
University of Cambridge Department of Psychiatry,
Addenbrooke's Hospital,
Cambridge, UK

B Bos
ARH, Agence Regionale d'Hospitalisation,
Toulouse, France

Stephen C Bowden PhD
Head of Neuropsychology,
St Vincent's Hospital, Melbourne, and
Department of Psychology, University of Melbourne,
Australia

Henry Brodaty AO, MBBS, MD, FRACP, FRANZCP
Professor,
School of Psychiatry,
University of New South Wales,
Australia

Simon P Brooks PhD
Senior Post Doctoral Researcher,
Brain Repair Group,
Cardiff University,
Cardiff, UK

Martin Brown DM, MRCPsych
Consultant in Old Age Psychiatry,
St James Hospital,
Portsmouth, UK

Roger Bullock MA MRCPsych
Consultant in Old Age Psychiatry,
Kingshill Research Centre,
Victoria Hosptial,
Swindon, UK

Alistair Burns MPhil, MD, FRCP, FRCPsych
Professor of Old Age Psychiatry,
Wythenshawe Hospital,
Manchester, UK

E Jane Byrne MB ChB, FRCPsych
Senior Lecturer and Honorary Consultant Psychiatrist,
School of Psychiatry and Behavioural Sciences,
Wythenshawe Hospital,
Manchester, UK

Robin Casten PhD
Assistant Professor,
Department of Psychiatry and Human Behavior,
Jefferson Medical College,
Philadelphia, USA

David Challis
Professor of Community Care Research and
Director, PSSRU,
University of Manchester, Manchester, UK

Edmond Chiu AM, MBBS, DPM, FRANZCP
Professor and Director,
Huntington's Disease Clinic,
University of Melbourne, Australia

Helen Chiu FRCPsych
Chair and Professor of Psychiatry,
Department of Psychiatry,
The Chinese University of Hong Kong,
Tai Po, Hong Kong

Phyllis Chua MB BS, MMed, FRANZCP
Senior Lecturer,
University of Melbourne and
Consultant Psychiatrist,
Department of Neuropsychiatry,
The Royal Melbourne Hospital, Australia

Nicholas A Clarke MD, MRCPsych
Consultant in Old Age Psychiatry,
West Kent NHS and Social Care Trust,
and King's Hill Kent and Honorary Research Associate,
Wolfson Centre for Age-Related Diseases,
King's College London,
London, UK

John Collinge MD, FRCP, FRCPath, FMedSci
Professor,
MRC Prion Unit and
Department of Neurodegenerative Disease,
Institute of Neurology,
National Hospital for Neurology and Neurosurgery,
London, UK

Jody Corey-Bloom MD, PhD
Professor of Neurosciences,
Department of Neurosciences,
University of California, La Jolla,
San Diego, USA

Bernard M Dickens PhD, LLD, FRS(C)
Professor Emeritus of Health Law and Policy,
University of Toronto,
Canada

Nadine J Dougall BSc, MSc Grad. Stat.
Research Fellow,
Division of Psychiatry,
School of Molecular and Clinical Medicine,
University of Edinburgh,
Edinburgh, UK

Barnaby D Dunn MA, PhD, DClinPsy
Post-doctoral Scientist at the MRC Cognition and
Brain Sciences Unit
Cambridge, UK

Stephen B Dunnett DSc
Professor and Head,
Brain Repair Group,
Cardiff University,
Cardiff, UK

Rebecca Eastley MRCPsych
Consultant in Psychiatry of Old Age,
Avon and Western Wiltshire Mental Health Care NHS Trust,
Avonmead, Southmead Hospital,
Bristol, UK

Klaus P Ebmeier MD
Professor,
Gordon Small Centre for Research in Old Age Psychiatry,
University of Edinburgh,
Edinburgh, UK

Timo Erkinjuntti MD, PhD
Chief, Memory Research Unit,
Department of Neurology,
Helsinki University Central Hospital,
Helsinki, Finland

Ian Paul Everall PhD, MRCPsych, FRCPath
Professor of Psychiatry,
University of California,
San Diego, USA

Adam S Fleisher MD
Medical Director of Alzheimer's Disease
Co-operative Study,
University of California,
San Diego, USA

Leon Flicker MBBS, GDipEpid, PhD, FRACP
Professor,
School of Medicine and Pharmacology,
University of Western Australia,
Australia

Eleanor Flynn MBBS, BEd, BTheol, Dip Ger Med, FRACGP, FRACMA, AFACHSE
Senior Lecturer in Medical Education,
Faculty of Medicine, Dentistry and Health Science,
University of Melbourne, Australia

Stephen Foli MB ChB, MRCPsych
Consultant Psychiatrist,
West London Mental Health NHS Trust,
London, UK

Hans Förstl FRANZCP
Professor and Director,
Department of Psychiatry and Psychotherapy,
Technical University of Munich,
Munich, Germany

Paul T Francis PhD
Senior Lecturer in Biochemistry,
Wolfson Centre for Age-Related Diseases,
King's College London,
London, UK

Serge Gauthier MD, FRCPC
Director,
Alzheimer Disease Research Unit,
McGill Centre for Studies in Aging,
Verdun, QC, Canada

Yonas Endale Geda MD
Neuropsychiatrist,
Assistant Professor of Psychiatry,
Alzheimer's Disease Research Center,
Mayo Clinic College of Medicine,
Rochester, USA

Colin Godber FRCPsych, FRCP, MPhil, OBE
Consultant in Old Age Psychiatry,
Moorgreen Hospital,
Southampton, UK

Andrew Graham MRCP
Wellcome Research Training Fellow and
Honorary Senior Clinical Fellow in Neurology,
MRC Cognition and Brain Sciences Unit,
Cambridge, UK

Nori Graham BM BCh, FRCPsych, D Univ
Chairman of Alzheimer's Disease International,
Consultant in Old Age Psychiatry,
Department of Psychiatry,
Royal Free Hospital,
London, UK

Alisa Green BSc(Psych)(Hons)
Research Psychologist,
Academic Department of Old Age Psychiatry,
Prince of Wales Hospital,
New South Wales, Australia

L Gregoire
DHOS, Ministry of Health,
Paris, France

Joanne M Hamilton PhD
Assistant Project Neuroscientist,
Department of Neurosciences,
University of California,
San Diego, USA

Richard J Harvey MD, MRCPsych, FRANZCP
Associate Professor and
Consultant Psychiatrist for Older People,
Aged Psychiatry Service,
The Geelong Hospital,
Victoria, Australia

Thea J Heeren MD
Professor of Old Age Psychiatry,
Medical Director of the Department of Old Age Psychiatry,
Altrecht Mental Health Care,
The Netherlands

John Hodges FMedSci
Professor of Behavioural Neurology,
MRC Cognition and Brain Sciences Unit and
University of Cambridge Department of Neurology,
Cambridge, UK

Akira Homma MD
Senior Research Scientist,
Tokyo Metropolitan Institute of Gerontology,
Tokyo, Japan

Robert Howard MD, MRCPsych
Professor of Old Age Psychiatry,
Section of Old Age Psychiatry,
Institute of Psychiatry,
University of London, UK

Jane Hughes MSc, BA(Econ), DSW, CQSW
Lecturer in Community Care Research,
PSSRU,
University of Manchester, UK

Julian C Hughes MA, MB ChD, PhD, MRCPsych
Consultant in Old Age Psychiatry and
Honorary Clinical Senior Lecturer,
University of Newcastle upon Tyne,
Newcastle upon Tyne, UK

Paul G Ince MD, FRCPath
Professor of Neuropathology,
University of Sheffield,
Sheffield, UK

Domenico Inzitari MD
Staff Neurologist,
Department of Neurological and Psychiatric Sciences,
University of Florence,
Florence, Italy

Saleem Ismail MD
Department of Neurology,
University of Rochester Medical Center,
Rochester, New York, USA

Robin Jacoby DM, FRCP, FRCPsych
Professor of Old Age Psychiatry,
University of Oxford,
Oxford, UK

Carmen Janvin MPsych
Psychologist,
Section for Geriatric Psychiatry,
Stavanger University Hospital,
Stavanger, Norway

Anthony F Jorm PhD, DSc
Director and Professor,
Centre for Mental Health Research,
Australian National University,
Canberra, Australia

Raj N Kalaria FRCPath
Professor of Cerebrovascular Pathology,
Wolfson Research Centre, CBV Group,
Institute for the Health of the Elderly,
Newcastle General Hospital,
Newcastle upon Tyne, UK

Kalyanasundaram S MD
Principal and Professor of Psychiatry,
The Richmond Fellowship Society (India),
Jayangar, Bangalore, India

Apsara Kandanearatchi PhD
Postdoctoral Research Worker,
Section of Experimental Neuropathology and Psychiatry,
Institute of Psychiatry,
King's College London,
London, UK

Göran Karlsson PhD
Health Economist,
AstraZeneca,
Stockholm, Sweden

Benoit Lavallart MD
Direction Generale de la Santé,
Ministry of Health,
Paris, France

Iracema Leroi MD, FRCP, MRCPsych
Consultant/Honorary Lecturer in Old Age Psychiatry,
University of Manchester,
Manchester, UK

James Lindesay DM, MRCPsych
Professor of Psychiatry for the Elderly,
University of Leicester,
Leicester General Hospital,
Leicester, UK

Dina LoGiudice MB BS, PhD, FRACP
Geriatrician,
Melbourne Extended Care and Rehabilitation Service,
Victoria, Australia

Michael Loh BAppSc (Occupational Therapy), BSc, Grad Dip Gerontology
Clinical Manager,
Mobile Aged Psychiatry Services,
Caulfield General Medical Centre,
Caulfield, Victoria, Australia

Stephen J Louw MB ChB, MD, FCP(SA), FRCP(Lond), FRCP(Edin)
Consultant Physician and
Clinical Director of Internal Medicine and
Geriatric Medicine,
Freeman Hospital,
Newcastle upon Tyne, UK

Lee-Fay Low BSc
Centre for Mental Health Research,
The Australian National University,
Canberra, Australia

Rebekah Loy PhD
Department of Neurology,
University of Rochester Medical Center,
Rochester, New York, USA

Constantine G Lyketsos MD, MhS
Professor of Psychiatry and Behavioral Sciences,
Co-Director, Division of Geriatric Psychiatry and
Neuropsychiatry,
The Johns Hopkins Hospital,
Baltimore, Maryland, USA

Ian G McKeith MD, BS, FRCPsych, FMedSci
Professor, Department of Old Age Psychiatry,
Wolfson Research Centre,
Newcastle upon Tyne, UK

Catriona McLean BSc, MBBS, FRCPA, MD
Associate Professor and Consultant Pathologist,
The Alfred Hospital,
Prahran, Australia

João Carlos Barbosa Machado
Director,
Aurus IEPE,
Institute of Research and Education on Ageing,
Belo Horizonte, Brazil

David M A Mann BSc, PhD, FRCPath
Professor of Neuropathology,
University of Manchester,
Hope Hospital,
Salford, UK

Mary Marshall MA, DSA, DASS
Professor and Director,
Dementia Services Development Centre,
University of Stirling,
Stirling, UK

Colin L Masters BMedSci, MBBS, MD, FRACP
Professor and Head,
Department of Pathology,
University of Melbourne, Parkville,
Victoria, Australia

Manuel Martín-Carrasco MD, PhD
Clinical Director,
Clínica Psiquiàtrica Padre Menni, and
Associate Professor,
Universidad de Navarra School of Medicine,
Pamplona, Spain

Raimundo Mateos MD, PhD
Professor of Psychiatry,
Department of Psychiatry,
Universidad de Santiago de Compostela (USC),
Coordinator of the Psychogeriatric Unit,
Conxo Psychiatric Hospital,
Complejo Hospitalario Universitario de Santiago de
Compostela,
Santiago, Spain

Pamela S Melding MB ChB, FFARCS, FRANZCP, Dip.HSM
Clinical Senior Lecturer,
Department of Psychological Medicine,
University of Auckland,
New Zealand

Bronwyn Moorhouse BAppSci (Speech Path), MPhil, PhD
Speech Pathologist,
Acquired Brain Injury Unit,
Royal Talbot Rehabilitation Centre,
Victoria, Australia

Emerson Moran
Writer,
Florida, USA

Elizabeta B Mukaetova-Ladinska MD, MMedSci, PhD, MRCPsych
Senior Lecturer/Honorary Consultant in Old Age Psychiatry,
Department of Old Age Psychiatry,
University of Newcastle,
Newcastle upon Tyne, UK

Michelle Murray RMN
Specialist Development Nurse,
Young Onset Dementia Service,
Manchester Royal Infirmary,
Manchester, UK

David Neary MD, FRCP
Professor, Department of Neurology,
Greater Manchester Neuroscience Centre,
Hope Hospital,
Salford, UK

Selam Negash PhD
Cognitive Neuroscience Fellow,
Alzheimer's Disease Research Center,
Mayo Clinic College of Medicine,
Rochester, New York, USA

Ian O Nnatu MB ChB, MRCPsych
Specialist Registrar in Old Age Psychiatry and
General Adult Psychiatry,
West London Mental Health NHS Trust,
Middlesex, UK

John O'Brien MA, DM, FRCPsych
Professor of Old Age Psychiatry,
Institute for Ageing and Health,
University of Newcastle upon Tyne,
Newcastle upon Tyne, UK

Daniel W O'Connor MD, FRANZCP
Professor of Psychiatry of Old Age,
Department of Psychological Medicine,
Monash University,
Victoria, Australia

Adesola O Ogunniyi MB ChB, FMCP, FWACP
Professor of Medicine,
College of Medicine,
University of Ibadan,
Ibadan, Nigeria

Desmond O'Neill
Senior Lecturer in Geriatrics,
Trinity College,
Dublin, Ireland

Adrian M Owen PhD
MRC Senior Scientist,
MRC Cognition and Brain Sciences Unit,
Cambridge, UK

Leonardo Pantoni MD, PhD
Staff Neurologist,
Department of Neurological and Psychiatric Sciences,
University of Florence,
Florence, Italy

Elaine K Perry BSc, PhD, DSc
Professor of Neurochemical Pathology,
MRC Neurochemical Pathology Unit,
Newcastle General Hospital,
Newcastle upon Tyne, UK

Ronald C Petersen PhD, MD
Professor of Neurology and Director,
Alzheimer's Disease Research Center,
Mayo Clinic College of Medicine,
Rochester, New York, USA

Bill Pettit MB ChB, FRCGP
General Practitioner,
Wythenshawe,
Manchester, UK

Michael Philpot BSc, MB BS, FRCPsych
Consultant in Old Age Psychiatry,
Mental Health of Older Adults,
South London and Maudsley NHS Trust,
London, UK

Louis Profenno MD, PhD
Department of Psychiatry and Neurology,
University of Rochester Medical Center,
Rochester, New York, USA

Nitin B Purandare MBBS, DPM MD, DGM MRCPsych
Senior Lecturer and
Honorary Consultant in Old Age Psychiatry,
Wythenshawe Hospital,
Manchester, UK

Peter V Rabins MD, MPH
Professor,
Department of Psychiatry and Behavioral Sciences,
John Hopkins Medical Institutions,
Baltimore, Maryland, USA

David Resnikoff MD
Psychogeriatrician,
Instituto Mexicano De Neurociencias,
Estado de Mexico, Mexico

Alonso Riestra
Behavioural Neurologist and Educational Resources Chairman,
Instituto Mexicano De Neurociencias,
Estado de Mexico, and Consultant Neurologist,
Hospital Angeles Lomas,
Mexico

Craig W Ritchie MB ChB, MRCPsych
Lecturer in Psychiatry,
Royal Free Hospital School of Medicine,
London, UK

Karen Ritchie MPsych, PhD
Research Director,
Institut National de la Santé et de la Recherche Médicale,
Hôpital la Colombière,
Montpellier, France

Alison J Ritter PhD
Turning Point Alcohol and Drug Centre,
Victoria, Australia

Gustavo Román MD, FACP, FRSM (Lond)
Professor of Medicine/Neurology,
Director, Memory Disorders and Dementia Clinic,
University of Texas Health Sciences Center at
San Antonio,
San Antonio, Texas, USA

Martin N Rossor MA, MD, FRCP, FMedSci
Professor of Clinical Neurology,
Director of Dementia Research Centre,
Institute of Neurology,
London, UK

Barry W Rovner MD
Professor, Departments of Psychiatry and Neurology,
Director, Division of Geriatric Psychiatry and
Director, Clinical Alzheimer's Disease Research,
Jefferson Medical College/Thomas Jefferson University,
Philadelphia, USA

Barbara J Sahakian BA, PhD, DipClinPsych
Professor of Clinical Neuropsychology,
University of Cambridge and Donders Chair of
Psychopharmacology, Utrecht University,
The Netherlands

David P Salmon PhD
Professor in Residence,
Helen A. Jarrett Chair in Alzheimer's Disease Research,
Department of Neurosciences,
University of California,
San Diego, USA

Manuel Sánchez-Pérez MD
Coordinator of the Pscyhogeriatric Unit,
Sagrat Cor, Serveis de Salut Mental,
Martorell,
Management Coordinator of the Master in
Psychogeriatrics,
Universidad Autonoma de Barcelona (UAB),
Barcelona, Spain

Martina Schäufele MD
Clinical Psychologist and Senior Researcher,
Psychogeriatric Research Unit,
Central Institute of Mental Health,
Mannheim, Germany

Lon S Schneider MD
Professor of Psychiatry, Neurology, and Gerontology,
Keck School of Medicine,
University of Southern California,
Los Angeles, USA

Ajit Shah MB ChB, MRCPsych
Consultant Psychiatrist and
Honorary Senior Lecturer in Psychiatry of Old Age,
West London Mental Health NHS Trust and
Imperial College School of Medicine,
London, UK

Bindu Shanmugham MD, MPH
Weill Medical College,
Cornell University,
New York, USA

Masahiro Shigeta MD
Professor of Psychiatry and Mental Health,
Tokyo Metropolitan University of Health Science,
Japan

Margie Smith BSc, PhD
Senior Scientist of Molecular Pathology,
Royal Melbourne Hospital,
Melbourne, Australia

Irene Smith Lassen BSc
Chief Physiotherapist,
Psychogeriatric Department,
Aarhus University Hospitals,
Risskov, Denmark

Julie S Snowden PhD
Consultant Neuropsychologist,
Cerebral Function Unit,
Greater Manchester Neuroscience Centre,
Hope Hospital,
Manchester, UK

Robert Stewart MD
Senior Lecturer,
Institute of Psychiatry,
London, UK

Elsdon Storey MBBS, DPhil, FRACP
Director,
Van Cleef Roet Centre for Nervous Diseases,
Monash University,
Prahran, Australia

Caroline Sutcliffe BSc, MSc
Research Associate,
PSSRU,
University of Manchester, UK

Jane K Sutherland MB ChB, MRCPsych
Specialist Registrar in Psychiatry,
Royal Edinburgh Hospital,
Edinburgh, UK

Peggy A Szwabo PhD
Consultant in Aging and Family Matters,
Szwabo and Associates,
St Louis, Missouri, USA

Pierre Tariot MD
Department of Psychiatry, Medicine, Neurology and
Center for Aging and Developmental Biology,
University of Rochester Medical Center,
Rochester, New York, USA

Nicoleta Tătaru MD
Senior Consultant Psychiatrist,
Ambulatory Psychiatric Clinic Oradea,
President of Romanian Association of Geriatric Psychiatry,
Romania

Jennifer Torr MBBS, MMed (Psychiatry), FRANZCP
Senior Lecturer,
Centre for Developmental Disability Health Victoria,
Monash University,
Victoria, Australia

Marco Trabucchi
President of Italian Society of Gerontology and Geriatrics,
Brescia, Italy

Anne Unkenstein MA, MAPS
Neuropsychologist,
Cognitive, Dementia and Memory Service,
Melbourne Extended Care and Rehabilitation Service,
Victoria, Australia

Mathew Varghese MBBS, MD
Additional Professor of Psychiatry,
National Institute of Mental Health and Neurosciences,
Bangalore, India

Anoop Varma DM, FRCP, MD
Consultant Neurologist,
Cerebral Function Unit,
Greater Manchester Neurosciences Centre,
Hope Hospital,
Salford, Manchester, UK

Bruno Vellas
Alzheimer Disease Clinical and Research Centre (CMRR),
Department of Internal Medicine and Geriatrics,
Toulouse University Hospital,
Toulouse, France

James P Warner BSc, MBBS, MD, MRCP, MRCPsych
Senior Lecturer in Old Age Psychiatry,
Imperial College London,
London, UK

Jason D Warren PhD, FRACP
Honorary Consultant Neurologist,
Dementia Research Centre,
Institute of Neurology,
London, UK

Siegfried Weyerer PhD
Professor of Epidemiology,
Head of the Psychogeriatric Research Unit,
Central Institute of Mental Health,
Mannheim, Germany

Gordon K Wilcock DM (Oxon), FRCP
Professor, Department of Care of the Elderly,
University of Bristol,
Bristol, UK

David G Wilkinson MB ChB, MRCGP, FRCPsych
Consultant in Old Age Psychiatry and
Honorary Clinical Senior Lecturer,
University of Southampton and
Memory Assessment and Research Centre,
Moorgreen Hospital,
Southampton, UK

Anders Wimo MD, PhD
Associate Professor,
Department of Clinical Neuroscience and Family Medicine,
Division of Geriatric Medicine,
Karolinska Institute,
Stockholm and Department of Family Medicine,
Umeå University,
Umeå, Sweden

Bengt Winblad MD, PhD
Department of Clinical Neuroscience and Family Medicine,
Division of Geriatric Medicine,
Karolinska Institute,
Stockholm

Yu Xin MD
Geriatric Psychiatrist, Executive Director,
Institute of Mental Health,
Peking University,
Beijing, PR China

Foreword

When Raymond Levy and Alistair Burns conceptualized and delivered the first edition of *Dementia* it was a very significant event in the worldwide dissemination of knowledge about dementia. At that time dementia research was already in full flight and workers in the field were finding it increasingly difficult to keep up to date with the rapid advances achieved by dedicated and creative researchers. It was not too long before a second edition was required to add to the knowledge base. No sooner was this edition published, than a further edition was required, such was the speed of knowledge acquisition in fundamental science, clinical practice and service delivery around the world.

This, the third edition, under the charge of Alistair Burns, John O'Brien and David Ames, has set a benchmark that is nigh impossible to surpass. Its content of 65 chapters characterized by breadth, depth, comprehensiveness, thoroughness and relevance has been a Herculean labour of commitment to the essential and necessary education of all who are involved in caring for the elderly.

In addition to the 'usual suspects' of epidemiology, biology, fundamental science and therapeutics underpinning the text, it has comprehensive service reports from a global perspective ranging from Australia, China, many parts of Asia, Africa, East and Western Europe to Latin America, the Caribbean and North America. These chapters remind us that service to the people with dementia is central to all our endeavours and the core of our commitment to this field. The chapter on services to younger people with dementia is very welcome and reminds us that not all people with dementia are elderly and that younger people also require us to attend to their plight.

Chapters on topics such as sexuality, quality of life, moral and legal issues alert and challenge all readers to look at the personhood and humanity of all people with dementia in a deep and searching analysis of our own attitude towards them. A chapter on trial designs fills a gap in most workers' knowledge and instructs on the backdrop to the development of therapeutics, thus enabling readers to understand how efficacy and safety are established and how the published data may be interpreted. Psychosocial approaches continue to be explored and updated as well as the advances in vascular contributions to dementia, which have gained more relevance between the second and third editions. Other dementias continue to be included to inform the readers that Alzheimer's disease is not the only dementia confronting us all.

No text on dementia is satisfactory without reference to the roles of carers, without whom all systems including fundamental scientific research will not thrive. The moving chapter by Emerson Moran serves to give a very touching practical, human and humorous face to this book. 'And we laugh. Always' – the final four words of this chapter should keep us all warmed and humbled.

Any medical school, hospital and health service to the elderly, which does not have a copy of this book, should not be considered to have any level of quality in their educational and training programme. Indeed, Key Performance Indicators in these clinical environments should include the possession of, or ready access to, this third edition of *Dementia*.

Alistair, John and David, thank you for your continuing contribution to the dissemination of knowledge to the world.

Edmond Chiu
Melbourne, March 2005

Preface to the Third Edition

It is a pleasure to present the Third Edition of our textbook *Dementia*. We have found the success of the first and second edition very gratifying but were conscious of the need to justify the publication of a textbook of this size and scope in a field that is developing very rapidly. It is easy to imagine that such a potential dinosaur may quickly become outdated, will sit on shelves, be thought of affectionately but not be of much practical use to anyone.

However, we became convinced by a number of people, fuelled by our own determination, that we could not let a brand name die, and that a third edition was not only possible but might actually be appreciated by some people.

It is trite to say that the field has moved on since the last edition – of course it has. This is not just in the usual areas where one would expect it, i.e. basic science and treatment, but also, reassuringly in areas such as service development and carer research.

We have kept the format as it was because it seems to work, but have introduced briefer overviews of services in areas throughout the world.

We owe a great thanks to the contributors who, in the main, have kept to time – we know and they know who they are! The publishers at Hodder Arnold, particularly Layla Vandenbergh, have been helpful and we are grateful to Ed Chiu for such a generous foreword. Most of all, our secretaries, Norma Welsh in Newcastle, Marilyn Kemp in Melbourne and particularly Barbara Dignan in Manchester, deserve the biggest thanks. Without their dedication the project would not have been completed.

AB
Manchester, UK

JO'B
Newcastle upon Tyne, UK

DA
Melbourne, Australia

Preface to the Second Edition

In the 6 years since the first edition of *Dementia* was published in 1994, advances in our knowledge and understanding of the disorder and its subtypes have proceeded at a truly breathtaking pace. Clearly we have a greater appreciation of the importance of genetic factors in dementia, whilst molecular biology has provided novel insights into possible pathogenic mechanisms. However, great advances have also been made in several other areas that, unfortunately, often receive less prominence than they deserve. For example, major progress has been made in the nosology, classification and diagnosis of the many subtypes of dementia and there are now several important sets of clinical and neuropathological diagnostic criteria published, many of which have already been the subject of prospective validation studies. Several subtypes of dementia that were of arguable significance when the first edition was published, such as dementia with Lewy bodies and frontotemporal dementia, have been recognized as important conditions with great clinical relevance. Concepts of vascular dementia have changed and the notion of multi-infarct dementia has now been replaced by more sophisticated models that recognize the fact that several different types of vascular pathology, not just cortical infarction, can cause dementia. In parallel with better understanding of the many conditions that cause dementia, there is also increasing recognition of the importance of heterogeneity and overlap at clinical, neurochemical and neuropathological levels between different disorders. This particularly applies to the overlap between vascular dementia and Alzheimer's disease. The advent in the last few years of cholinesterase inhibitors has for the first time allowed rational and, at least in some patients, moderately effective treatment of cognitive as well as non-cognitive features of Alzheimer's disease. These drugs may also prove helpful in treating some other subtypes of dementia. Services have improved considerably in many countries, allowing research advances to be directly applied to what must be the main goal, that of improving patient care.

However, we cannot at any level be complacent and clearly there is still a long way to go. Statistics regarding demographic changes abound, though it is a sobering thought that in Western society life expectancy has increased from 45 years in 1901 to 80 years in 2001. Such longevity, combined with the well-recognized increase in prevalence and incidence of dementia with age, will continue to lead to a huge increase in dementia cases over the next 30 years, especially in the developing world. Many problems remain. We still lack sufficiently accurate *in vivo* diagnostic markers to replace the 'gold standard' of neuropathology. We still need to learn more about aetiological factors and the definitive neurobiological mechanisms that ultimately cause neuronal loss remain elusive. Current therapeutic approaches remain limited and effective disease-modifying and preventive strategies still have to be determined. Despite progress, services in many countries remain underdeveloped and too fragmented to cope with the increase in cases which lies ahead. The socioeconomic burden of dementia remains enormous and will continue to increase. Dementia is one of the major challenges facing all societies in the new millennium and will remain so for the foreseeable future.

This combination of exciting recent progress combined with continued challenges ahead was the major driving force for producing this second edition of *Dementia*, which has been radically restructured and updated. Several changes will be immediately apparent. First, the layout of the book reflects the richness and diversity of the different subtypes of dementia and, instead of a simple division between Alzheimer's disease and other dementias, there are now separate sections on each of the main causes of dementia. Second, a number of new chapters are included to provide comprehensive coverage of topics such as new diagnostic criteria, rating scales, investigations, neurobiological mechanisms, as well as all aspects of management including psychosocial and psychological approaches. There are too many new chapters to mention them all, but other important topics, such as moral, ethical and legal aspects of dementia, sexuality and current and new therapeutic options, are included. The section on services has been expanded to include more contributions from Europe as well as from China, South and Central America, the former Soviet Union and services for younger people with dementia. The inclusion of a chapter on Alzheimer's Disease Societies and Associations is a measure of the influence that these have had world wide in supporting patients, carers and researchers. Dementia with Lewy bodies, increasingly recognized as the second main cause of degenerative dementia, is given prominent coverage with four new chapters. The section on focal dementias includes frontotemporal dementia, Pick's disease, semantic dementia and progressive aphasia and allows readers to observe the different approaches that can be used to define and understand such disorders. Over all, 17 new chapters are included whilst other chapters have been updated and, in most cases, entirely rewritten.

In choosing our authors, we have deliberately sought to try to achieve a balance between retaining sufficient authors from the first edition to provide some continuity whilst including some new contributors. We have also deliberately sought an authorship to reflect a mixture of those who are already internationally renowned experts and those whom we consider to be the rising stars of the future.

This second edition was commissioned by Chapman and Hall, who published the first edition, and has subsequently been published by Arnold, a member of the Hodder Headline Group. We are indebted to all who have been involved in the production of this book, including Peter Altman of Chapman and Hall, who was responsible for the first edition, Georgina Bentliff, Catherine Barnes and Sarah De Souza of Arnold and to our secretaries (Norma Welsh, Yvonne Liddicoat, Barbara Dignan) for their great efforts and help. We are also deeply grateful to Edmond Chiu for his generous Foreword and to Professor Elaine Murphy for providing the Epilogue. Most of all, we thank all our authors who found the time to produce such excellent chapters and upon whose efforts the success of this book will ultimately rely. Our aim was to produce fully comprehensive and up-to-date coverage of all aspects of dementia within a single text, which would prove accessible to clinicians, researchers and allied professional groups. As before, we leave you, our readers and reviewers, to judge the extent to which this aim has been achieved.

John O'Brien, David Ames, Alistair Burns
Newcastle upon Tyne, Melbourne,
Manchester, April 2000

Preface to the First Edition

It was with some trepidation that we decided to edit a large textbook on dementia. There are, and will continue to be, many texts on dementia and one has to consider critically the need for another. Dementia is one of the major challenges to face society in the twentieth century, numerically dwarfing other disorders which have caught the public's imagination. The attraction of being involved in this venture is that it attempts to encompass, in a single volume, all aspects of all types of dementia. However hard we have tried we could obviously not succeed in this and someone somewhere will complain we have omitted something important. In addition, this is a field which is expanding rapidly and we have tried therefore to concentrate on a solid core of information, which although requiring some updating in the future is likely to remain part of the mainstream view of the field.

We have divided the book into two parts, the first dealing with Alzheimer's disease and the second with other dementias. We recognize that this will be considered by many to be a false dichotomy and we accept that criticism. However, from an organizational point of view some form of order was necessary and we hope this makes sense. Overlap between chapters is a difficult issue and while we have exercised the editorial Tippex to the best of our ability, some duplication remains. However, much of this is intentional and some chapters would have been denuded unnecessarily and could not have stood alone. Areas where we have unashamedly fostered such overlap include Chapters 7 and 8, Chapters 12 and 13 and Chapters 46 and 51. We feel this is a way of encouraging debate about contentious subjects as well as avoiding undue artistic tantrums.

We have been lucky in our choice of authors, the vast majority of whom have delivered their manuscripts on time and without much persuasion. To them, we give thanks, and to our recalcitrant contributors we heave a sigh of relief that we received their submissions at all. We are indebted to Annelisa Page and Peter Altman of Chapman & Hall for their tireless support and to our secretaries for their help. We also thank Professor Alwyn Lishman for his generous foreword.

We hope that our efforts have not been wasted and will leave you, the readers and reviewers, to judge.

AB
Manchester

RL
London

Acknowledgements

CHAPTER 5

ADB is funded by a Wellcome Trust Programme Grant (RN 019407). Portions of the work described in this chapter were supported by an MRC LINK grant and carried out within the MRC Centre for Behavioural and Clinical Neuroscience. BJS is a consultant for Cambridge Cognition Ltd.

CHAPTER 23

The authors gratefully acknowledge the thoughts and comments of Jacques Touchon that helped form the basis for this chapter.

CHAPTER 24

We should like to thank Ms Donna Asleson for her superb secretarial assistance. Preparation of this chapter was supported by UO1 AG06786, P50 AG16574, U01 AG10483 and KO1 MH68351.

CHAPTER 31

I am most grateful to Dr Charles R Harrington for his, as always, knowledgeable comments and suggestions and thorough reading of the text. His red pen changed its colour to blue on this occasion, and found out hidden 'gran chasing bears'. I would also like to thank Mrs Caroline Kirk for editing the text and secretarial support, Mr Stephen Lloyd for IT support and Dr Vladimir B Ladinski for help with graphic presentation and constructive discussions during various stages of writing the manuscript. The text is based on a review of the published literature up to and including 31 January 2004.

CHAPTER 39

The author gratefully acknowledges, first, the support of the Australian Government Department of Health and Ageing, Office for Older Australians, who funded some of the research reported in this chapter. Second, profound thanks are due to all the people with dementia, their families, and residential aged care nursing staff, who participated in the clinical interventions described and so generously assisted in providing research data. Finally, thanks to Tanya Caldwell, who assisted in preparation of this paper.

CHAPTER 45

Our work has been supported by grants from the Medical Research Council (UK), Alzheimer's Association (Chicago, USA) and the Alzheimer's Research Trust (UK).

CHAPTER 49

Preparation of this chapter was supported by funds from NIA grants AG-05131 and AG-12963 to the University of California, San Diego.

CHAPTER 53

AG is supported by the Wellcome Trust.

CHAPTER 57

The authors thank Professor Elizabeth Warrington for helpful discussion and Dr Nick Fox for permission to reproduce the brain images.

Abbreviations

α2M	α2-macroglobulin
Aβ$_{42}$	amyloid beta protein 42
AAAD	Alzheimer's disease affective disorder
AAC	augmentative and alternative communication
AACD	ageing-associated cognitive decline
AAMI	age-associated memory impairment
ABC	abacavir
ABCD	Arizona Battery for Communication Disorders of Dementia
ACA	anterior cerebral artery
ACASs	Aged Care Assessment Services
ACE	angiotensin-converting enzyme
ACh	acetylcholine
AChEIs	acetylcholinesterase inhibitors
AD	Alzheimer's disease
ADAPT	Alzheimer's Disease Anti-Inflammatory Prevention Trial
ADAS-cog	Alzheimer's Disease Assessment Scale – cognitive Scale
ADAS-noncog	Alzheimer's Disease Assessment Scale – non-cognitive subscale
ADC	AIDS dementia complex
ADCAs	autosomal dominant cerebellar ataxias
ADCS	Alzheimer's Disease Cooperative Study
ADFACS	Alzheimer's Disease Functional Assessment and Change Scale
ADI	Alzheimer's Disease International
ADL	activities of daily living
ADRQL	Alzheimer's disease related quality of life
AEP	auditory evoked potential
AEUs	Alzheimer Evaluation Units
AGD	argyrophilic grain disease
AHEAD	assessment of health economics in Alzheimer'sdisease
AIHW	Australian Institute of Health and Welfare
AIMA	Italian Association for Alzheimer Disease
ALD	adrenoleukodystrophy
a-MCI	amnestic mild cognitive impairment
AMPA	amino-3-hydroxy-5-methyl-4-isoxazolepropionic acid
AMPS	Assessment of Motor and Process Skills
AMT	Abbreviated Mental Test Score
APATTs	aged psychiatry assessment and treatment teams
aPc	activating potential for communication
ApoE	apolipoprotein E
APP	amyloid precursor protein
ARCD	age-related cognitive decline
ARDSI	Alzheimer's and Related Disorders Society of India
AS	Alzheimer's Society (UK)
AT1	angiotensin II type 1
ATA	atmospheres absolute
ATR	assessment treatment and rehabilitation
AWARE	Aricept Withdrawal and Rechallenge Study
AZT	azidothymidine
BADS	Behavioural Assessment of the Dysexecutive Syndrome
BAS	Body Awareness Scale
BAT	body awareness therapy
BBB	blood–brain barrier
BCR	bicaudate ratio
BD	Binswanger's disease
BDNF	brain-derived neurotrophic factor
BEHAVE-AD	Behavioral Pathology in Alzheimer's Disease Rating Scale
BIMC	Blessed Information-Memory-Concentration
BLA	Barnes Language Assessment
BLT	bright light therapy
BOLD	blood oxygen level dependent
BPRS	Brief Psychiatric Rating Scale
BPSD	behavioural and psychological symptoms of dementia
BRSD	Behavioural Rating Scale for Dementia
BSE	bovine spongiform encephalopathy
BSF	benign senescent forgetfulness
BuChE	butyryl-cholinesterase
C	cognition
CA	conversational analysis
CA	cost analysis
CAA	cerebral amyloid angiopathy
CADASIL	cerebral autosomal dominant arteriopathy with subcortical infarcts and leukoencephalopathy
CAMCOG	Cambridge Cognitive Examination

CAMDEX	Cambridge Examination for Mental Disorders in the Elderly		CSI-D	Community Screening Interview for Dementia
CANDID	Counselling and Diagnosis in Dementia		CST	cognitive stimulation therapy
CANTAB	Cambridge Neuropsychological Test Automated Battery		CT	computed tomography
			CTX	cerebrotendinous xanthomatosis
CARASIL	cerebral autosomal recessive arteriopathy with subcortical infarcts and leukoencephalopathy		CUA	cost utility analysis
			CVD	cerebrovascular disease
			DACSA	Domestic and Community Skills Assessment
CARE	Comprehensive Assessment and Referral Evaluation		DAD	Disability Assessment in Dementia
CAS	Caregiver Activity Survey		DALYs	disability adjusted life years
CATIE	Clinical Antipsychotic Trials of Intervention Effectiveness		DASH	Dietary Approaches to Stop Hypertension
			DAT	dementia of the Alzheimer's type *see* Alzheimer's disease (AD)
CATS	Caregiver Activities Time Survey			
CBA	cost benefit analysis		DB	double blind
CBD	corticobasal degeneration		DCLB	dementia associated with cortical Lewy bodies
CBF	cerebral blood flow			
CBS	Cornell–Brown Scale		DCM	dementia care mapping
CCA	cost-consequence analysis		DDDS	Dementia Differential Diagnostic Schedule
CCOHTA	Canadian Health Technology Assessment Guidelines for Pharmaco-economics		DDMS	Depression in Dementia Mood Scale
			DDPAC	disinhibition-dementia-parkinsonism-amyotrophy complex
CCSMA	Cache County Study of Memory in Aging			
CD	cost description		DECO	Deterioration Cognitive Observée
CDAMSs	Cognitive, Dementia and Memory Services		DED	depression-executive dysfunction syndrome
CDC	Centers for Disease Control		DHEA	dehydroepiandrosterone
CDR	Clinical Dementia Rating		DHEAS	dehydroepiandrosterone sulphate
CDR-SB	Clinical Dementia Rating – Sum of Boxes		DIADS-2	Depression in AD Study-2
CEA	cost effectiveness analysis		DLB	dementia with Lewy bodies
CENSIS	Centre for Social Studies (Italy)		DLBD	diffuse LB disease
CERAD	Consortium to Establish a Registry for Dementia (or Alzheimer's disease)		DLDH	dementia lacking distinctive histology
			DMR	dementia in mental retardation
CGI	Clinical Global Impression		DqoL	dementia quality of life instrument
ChAT	choline acetyltransferase		DRS	Dementia Rating Scale
ChEIs	cholinesterase inhibitors		DS	Down's syndrome
CHS	Cardiovascular Health Study		DSDS	Down Syndrome Dementia Scale
CIBIC-plus	Clinicians' Interview-Based Impression of Change – plus caregiver input		DSM-IIIR	*Diagnostic and Statistical Manual of Mental Disorders*, revised 3rd edition
CILQ	Cognitively Impaired Life Quality Scale		DSM-IV	*Diagnostic and Statistical Manual of Mental Disorders*, 4th edition
CIND	cognitive impairment no dementia			
CJD	Creutzfeldt–Jakob disease (vCJD: variant CJD)		DSS	Depressive Signs Scale
			DTI	diffusion tensor imaging
CMA	cost minimization analysis		DWI	diffusion-weighted imaging
CMAI	Cohen–Mansfield Agitation Inventory		DWMH	deep white matter hyperintensities
CMPs	Centres Memoire de Proximité		e	extension
CMRR	Centre Memoire de Recherche et de Resources		EADC	European Alzheimer's Disease Consortium
CNS	central nervous system		EE	expressed emotion
COI	cost of illness		EEG	electroencephalogram (qEEG quantitative analysis of the electroencephelogram)
CPI	consumer price index			
CPMC	Commission for Medicinal and Pharmaceutical Compounds		EGF	epidermal growth factor
			EOAD	early-onset AD
CPN	community psychiatric nurse		EOFAD	early-onset familial AD
CQLI	caregiver quality of life index		EP	evoked potential
CRF	corticotrophin releasing factor		EPI	Eysenck Personality Inventory
CRP	C-reactive protein		EPS	extrapyramidal signs
CSF	cerebrospinal fluid		ERP	event-related potential

ESTs	expressed sequence tags
FA	Friedreich's ataxia
FAST	Functional Assessment Staging
FBD	familial British dementia
F-CMRR-SF	Federation of the Alzheimer's Centres from the South of France
FDA	Food and Drug Administration
FFI	fatal familial insomnia
FGF	fibroblast growth factor
FGF1	fibroblast growth factor 1
FIRDA	frontal intermittent rhythmic delta activity
FLAIR	fluid attenuated inversion recovery
fMRI	functional magnetic resonance imaging
FTD	frontotemporal dementia
FTD-MND	frontotemporal dementia with motor neurone disease
FTDP-17	frontotemporal dementia with parkinsonism linked to chromosome 17
FTLD	frontotemporal lobar degeneration
FvFTD	frontal variant frontotemporal dementia
GABA	gamma aminobutyric acid
GBS Scale	Gottfries–Bråne–Steen Scale
GDS	Geriatric Depression Scale
GDS	Global Deterioration Scale
GI	gastrointestinal
GMSS	Geriatric Mental State Schedule
GP	general practitioner
GPCOG	General Practitioner Assessment of Cognition
GSK-3	glycogen synthase kinase-3
GSS	Gerstmann–Sträussler syndrome (also known as Gerstmann–Sträussler–Scheinker disease)
HAART	highly active antiretroviral therapy
HAD	HIV-associated dementia complex
HC	homocysteine
HCHWA-D	hereditary cerebral haemorrhage with amyloidosis – Dutch type
HCHWA-I	hereditary cerebral haemorrhage with amyloidosis – Icelandic type
Hcy	homocysteine (total Hcy 5 tHcy)
HD	Huntington's disease
HDL	high density lipoproteins
HE	Hashimoto's encephalopathy
HELP	heparin-mediated extracorporeal LDL/fibrinogen precipitation
HERNS	hereditary endotheliopathy, retinopathy, nephropathy and stroke
HIV	human immunodeficiency virus
HIVE	HIV encephalitis
HIVL	HIV leukoencephalopathy
HMG-CoA	3-hydroxy-3-methylglutaryl coenzyme A
HNRC	HIV Neurobehavioural Research Center
HOT	hyperbaric oxygen treatment
HRQoL	health-related quality of life
HSG	Huntington Study Group
5HT	5-hydroxytryptamine
HUI	Health Utilities Index
HYE	Healthy Years Equivalents
I	intellectual capability
IADL	instrumental activities of daily living
ICC	immunocytochemistry
ID	intellectual disability
IDE	insulin degrading enzyme
IGF	insulin-like growth factor
IHA	International Huntington Association
IHD	ischaemic heart disease
IL	interleukin
ILSA	Italian Longitudinal Study on Aging
IMC	Information Memory Concentration
iNOs	inducible nitric oxide synthase
IPA	International Psychogeriatric Association
IQ	Intelligence Quotient
IQCODE	Informant Questionnaire for Cognitive Decline in the Elderly
IQLS	Italian QoL Scale
IT	interesting transcript
ITT	intent to treat
KI	knock-in [mice]
KSS	Kearns–Sayre syndrome
LA	leukoaraiosis
LADIS	leukoaraiosis and disability
LAI	Latin American Initiative
LB	Lewy body
LBD	Lewy body disease/dementia (see DLB: dementia with Lewy bodies)
LBVAD	LB variant of Alzheimer's disease
LDL	low density lipoprotein
LDL-R	low density lipoprotein receptor
LLAs	lipid lowering agents
LLF	late-life forgetfulness
LOAD	late-onset AD
LOCF	last observation carried forward
LRP	lipoprotein receptor-related protein
LRP1	low-density lipoprotein receptor-related protein
LSBs	life story books
LTCI	Long-Term Care Insurance (Japan)
LTD	long-term depression
LTP	long-term potentiation
MAC	macroangiopathic
MACS	Multicentre AIDS Cohort Study
MAO	monoamine oxidase
MAP	microtubule-associated proteins
MC	mitochondrial cytopathy
MC	multicentre
MCD	mild cognitive disorder
MCI	mild cognitive impairment
MCMD	minor cognitive/motor disorder
MDS	European Movement Disorder Society
MEG	magnetoencephalography

MELAS	mitochondrial encephalomyopathy with lactic acidosis and stroke-like episodes		NPV	negative predictive value
MERRF	myoclonic epilepsy with ragged red fibres		NR	not reported
MHC	major histocompatibility complex		NSAID	non-steroidal anti-inflammatory drug
MIC	micro		NSE	neuronal specific enolase
MID	multi-infarct dementia		NT	neurotrophin
MLD	metachromatic leukodystrophy		OAS	Overt Aggression Scale
MMN	mismatch negativity		OBS	Organic Brain Scale
MMSE	Mini-Mental State Examination		OC	observed cases
MNCD	mild neurocognitive disorder		OPCA	olivopontocerebellar atrophy
MND	motor neurone disease		OT	occupational therapy
MNDID	motor neurone disease inclusion dementia		PA	progressive aphasia
MNGIE	mitochondrial myopathy, peripheral neuropathy, encephalopathy and gastrointestinal disease		PAF	platelet-activating factor
			PAHO	Pan American Health Association
			PAS	periodic-acid-Schiff
MOSES	Multidimensional Observation Scale for Elderly Subjects		PASAT	Paced Serial Addition Test
			PAX	progressive apraxia
MQ	Memory Quotient		PBS	Pharmaceutical Benefits Scheme
MRI	magnetic resonance imaging		PC	placebo-controlled
MRS	magnetic resonance spectroscopy		PCA	posterior cerebral artery
MRT	magnetic resonance tomography		PCO	primary care organization
MSA	multisystem atrophy (parkinsonian [MSA-P] and ataxic [MSA-C] variants)		PCR	polymerase chain reaction
			PCT	primary care trust
			PD	Parkinson's disease
MSQ	Mental Status Questionnaire		PDD	Parkinson's disease with dementia
MT	microtubule		PDGF	platelet derived growth factor
MTA	medial temporal lobe atrophy		PD	personal detractor
MTHFR	methylenetetrahydrofolate reductase		PDS	Progressive Deterioration Scale
MTI	magnetization transfer imaging		PEG	percutaneous endoscopic gastrostomy
N/A	not available		PEO	progressive external ophthalmoplegia
NA	noradrenaline		PES-AD	Pleasant Events Schedule-AD (also PES-Elderly and Short PES-AD)
NAA	N-acetylaspartate			
NAPDC	National Action Plan for Dementia Care		PET	positron emission tomography
NASC	Need Assessment Service Coordinators (NZ)		PGDRS	Psychogeriatric Dependency Rating Scale
nbM	nucleus basalis of Meynert		PHF	paired helical filament
NCL	neuronal ceroid lipofuscinosis		PHRC	Programme Hospitalier de Recherche Clinique
NFT	neurofibrillary tangle			
NGF	nerve growth factor		PiD	Pick's disease
NGO	non-governmental organization		Pin1	peptidyl prolyl cis/trans isomerase
NGT	nasogastric tube		PKB	protein kinase B
NICAM	National Institute for Complementary and Alternative Medication		PL	plaques
			PLE	paraneoplastic limbic encephalitis
NICE	National Institute for Clinical Excellence		PNFA	progressive non-fluent aphasia
NIMH	National Institute of Mental Health		PP2A	protein phosphatase 2A
NMDA	N-methyl-D-aspartate		PPA	primary progressive aphasia
NMS	neuroleptic malignant syndrome		PPF	propentofylline
NO	nitric oxide		PPP	purchase power parity
NOS	[dementia] not otherwise specified		PPV	positive predictive value
NOs	nitric oxide synthase		PRN	pro re nata (as needed)
NOSGER	Nurses' Observation Scale for Geriatric Patients		PROSPER	placebo-controlled trial of pravastatin
			PS1 [2]	presenilin 1 [2]
NPD-C	Niemann–Pick disease type C		PSE	Present State Exam
NPI	Neuropsychiatric Inventory		PSMS	Physical Self-Maintenance Scale
NPI	neuropsychological impairment		PSP	progressive supranuclear palsy
NPI-NH	Neuropsychiatric Inventory – Nursing Home version		PSWC	periodic sharp wave complexes
			PVH	periventricular hyperintensities

PWB-CIP	Psychological Wellbeing in Cognitively Impaired Persons
PWI	perfusion-weighted imaging
QALY	quality adjusted life year
QD	questionable dementia'
qEEG	quantitative analysis of EEG
QoL	quality of life
QoLAD	Quality of Life-Alzheimer's disease
QoLAS	Quality of Life Assessment Schedule
QoLASCA	Quality of Life Assessment by Construct Analysis
QUALID	Quality of Life in Late Stage Dementia Scale
QWB	quality of wellbeing
QWBS	Quality of Wellbeing Scale
RBD	REM-sleep behaviour disorder
RC	respiratory chain
RCT	randomized controlled trial
REM	rapid eye movement
ROI	region of interest
RPM	Raven's Progressive Matrices
RUD	Resource Utilization in Dementia
s	severity
SAP	serum amyloid P
SAP	single assessment process
SBD	sleep behaviour disorder
SBO	specified bovine offal
SCA	spinocerebellar ataxia
SCAG	Sandoz Clinical Assessment-Geriatric Scale
SCE	spontaneous cerebral micro-emboli
SCOPE	Study on Cognition and Prognosis in the Elderly
SCOPED	spending, cooking, operating automobiles, pill taking, everyday activities and decision-making
SCU	Special Care Unit
SD	semantic dementia
SDLT	senile dementia of Lewy body type
SEAC	Spongiform Encephalopathy Advisory Committee
SEGP	Sociedad Española de Gerontopsiquiatría y Psicogeriatría
SGRS	Stockton Geriatric Rating Scale
SHG	self-help group
SIB	Severe Impairment Battery
SIRS	Severe Impairment Rating Scale
SIVD	subcortical ischaemic vascular dementia
SKT	Syndrom Kurz Test
SLE	systemic lupus erythematosus
SLT	speech and language therapist
SNF	skilled nursing facility
SOAS	Staff Observation Aggression Scale
SPECT	single photon emission computed tomography
SPET	single photon emission tomography
SPM	statistical parametric mapping
SPMSQ	Short Portable Mental Status Questionnaire
SR	spaced retrieval
SSEP	somatosensory evoked potential
SSRI	selective serotonin reuptake inhibitor
STMS	Short Test of Mental Status
SWM	spatial working memory
Tg	transgenic
THA	tetrahydroaminoacridine [tacrine]
TIA	transient ischaemic attack
TIB	Trouble Indicating Behaviour
TICS	Telephone Interview for Cognitive Status
TMS	transcranial magnetic stimulation
TNF	tumour necrosis factor
ToM	theory of mind
tPA	tissue-type plasminogen activator
TRH	thyrotropin-releasing hormone
TROG	Test for Reception of Grammar
TTg	triple transgenic [mice]
UPDRS	United Parkinson's Disease Rating Scale
UPGS	ubiquitin-positive granular structures
VaD	vascular dementia
VBM	voxel-based morphometry
VCI	vascular cognitive impairment [mVCI, mild VCI]
VCIND	VCI without dementia
VEP	visual evoked potential (FVEP, flashes of light VEP; PRVEP, pattern reversal VEP)
VGLUT	vesicular glutamate transporters
VLCFA	very long chain fatty acids
VLDL-R	very low density lipoprotein receptor
VMCI	vascular mild cognitive decline
VOSP	Visual Object and Space Perception
VP	vascular parkinsonism
WFN	World Federation of Neurology for HD
WAIS-R	Wechsler Adult Intelligence Scale – revised
WISC-R	Wechsler Adult Intelligence Scale for Children – revised
WMH	white matter hyperintensities
WML	white matter lesions
WMS-R	Wechsler Memory Scale – revised
ZRP	zone of reduced penetrance

Dementia: general aspects

Dementia: historical overview

GERMAN BERRIOS

Since the second edition of this textbook, no ground-breaking scholarly work has been published that may challenge the historical hypotheses propounded therein on the development of the concept of dementia (Berrios, 2000a); indeed, the 'constructionist' view has gained support from the way in which the nosological surface of 'dementia' has been redrawn during the last 10 years.

All clinical categories, including those pertaining to the dementias, are the result of the coming together in the work of an author of selected behavioural markers, explanatory concepts and terms to refer to them. Complex social and economic variables will determine whether or not the ensuing 'convergence' will last. For reason that have to do with the rhetoric of science, these social acts are sold to the throng as pure 'scientific acts'. For example, it would be naïve to believe that the decision to consider a symptom-cluster such as, for example, 'Lewy body dementia' as a 'new disease' is solely based on the 'discovery' of powerful, ineluctable and replicable correlations (Perry *et al.*, 1996). Given that not all correlations are privileged in this way, and that there is no clear theory linking all the symptoms to each other and to the Lewy bodies themselves, it is not difficult to surmise that such consideration is also driven by social variables. The current model of science as a pure pursuit of truth, however, leaves no space for broader explanations and hence all manner of social variables remain understudied.

This is not a new phenomenon, for the same complex mechanisms operated at the time when Kraepelin constructed the concept of Alzheimer's disease (AD) (Berrios, 1990b). The crucial issue here is that there is nothing wrong with the fact that social forces shape 'scientific facts' and hence contribute to the construction of psychiatric diseases. Indeed, understanding such mechanisms would render psychiatry more complete, the psychiatrist wiser and doctoring more useful to patients. Hopefully, the time will come when denying social processes may be considered as unethical and offensive to patients.

Knowledge of the history of dementia as a word, a concept and a behavioural syndrome is a precondition for scientific research. Successive historical convergences have shaped the current notion of dementia. A full study should map the changes in the history of 'dementia' at least since Roman times. For the purposes of this chapter, however, it should suffice to study a shorter period, say, the one stretching from the work of Boissier de Sauvages (1771), who still offered a static view of disease to Marie (1906) whose great treatise would read as very modern to anachronistic eyes. The former defined 'dementia' as a generic term; the latter saw in dementia a 'syndrome', which could be enacted by a variety of 'diseases' each with its recognizable phenomenology and putative neuropathology.

1.1 TERMS

Up to the 1700s, states of cognitive and behavioural deterioration of whatever origin ending up in psychosocial incompetence were called amentia, dementia, imbecility, morosis, *fatuitas*, anoea, foolishness, stupidity, simplicity, carus, idiocy, dotage and senility. In Roman times, the word 'dementia' was also used to mean 'being out of one's mind, insanity, madness, folly' (Lewis and Short, 1969). For example, in the first century BC, Cicero (1969) (*Tusculanan disputations*, Book 3, para 10) and Lucretius (1975) (*De Rerum Natura*, Book 1, line 704) used 'dementia' as a synonym of madness.

The term dementia first appears in the European vernaculars after the seventeenth century. In Blancard's English dictionary (1726) it is used as an equivalent of *anoea* or 'extinction of the imagination and judgment' (p. 21). By 1644, according to the *Oxford English Dictionary*, an adjectival form ('demented') entered the English language. In his Spanish–French dictionary Sobrino (1791) wrote: 'demencia = démence, folie, extravagance, égarement, alienation d'esprit' (p. 300). Rey (1995), in turn, states that *démence* appeared in French in 1381 to refer to 'madness, extravagancy' but that the adjective *dément* came into currency only from 1700. It would seem, therefore, that between the seventeenth and eighteenth centuries the Latin stem *demens* (without mind) had found a home in most European vernaculars. As we shall see presently the full medicalization of 'dementia' started after the 1750s.

1.2 MEDICAL USAGE

Evidence for an early medical usage of the term dementia is found in the French Encyclopaedia (Diderot and d'Alembert, 1765):

> Dementia is a disease consisting in a paralysis of the spirit characterized by abolition of the reasoning faculty. It differs from *fatuitas*, morosis, *stultitia* and *stoliditas* in that in the latter there is a weakening of understanding and memory; and from delirium which is a temporary impairment in the exercise of the said functions. Some modern writers confuse dementia with mania, which is a delusional state accompanied by disturbed behaviour (*audace*); these symptoms are not present in subject[s] with dementia who exhibit foolish behaviour and cannot understand what they are told, cannot remember anything, have no judgment, are sluggish, and retarded … Physiology teaches that the vividness of our understanding depends on the intensity of external stimuli … in pathological states these may be excessive, distorted or abolished; dementia results from abolition of stimuli which may follow: 1. damage to the brain caused by excessive usage, congenital causes or old age, 2. failure of the spirit, 3. small volume of the brain, 4. violent blows to the head causing brain damage, 5. incurable diseases such as epilepsy, or exposure to venoms (Charles Bonnet reports of a girl who developed dementia after being bitten by a bat) or other substances such as opiates and mandragora.

> Dementia is difficult to cure as it is related to damage of brain fibres and nervous fluids; it becomes incurable in cases of congenital defect or old age … [otherwise] treatment must follow the cause …

> [The legal definition of dementia reads]: Those in a state of dementia are incapable of informed consent, cannot enter into contracts, sign wills, or be members of a jury. This is why they are declared incapable of managing their own affairs. Actions carried out before the declaration of incapacity are valid unless it is demonstrated that dementia predated the action.

> Ascertainment of dementia is based on examination of handwriting, interviews by magistrates and doctors, and testimony from informants. Declarations made by notaries that the individual was of sane mind whilst signing a will are not always valid as they may be deceived by appearances, or the subject might have been in a lucid period. In regards to matrimonial rights, démence is not a sufficient cause for separation, unless it is accompanied by aggression (*furour*). It is, however, sufficient for a separation of property, so that the wife is no longer under the guardianship of her husband. Those suffering from dementia cannot be appointed to public positions or receive privileges. If they became demented after any has been granted, a coadjutor should be appointed …

Although modern-sounding, the above definition must be read with caution: its clinical description depends on contrasts and differences with delirium and a list of disorders which are no more; its legal meaning is based on the old Roman accounts, and its mechanisms make use of the camera obscura metaphor and assume the passive definition of the mind that Condillac (who inspired the author of the article) had borrowed from John Locke.

1.3 BEHAVIOURS REDOLENT OF CURRENT DEMENTIA DURING THIS PERIOD

In the literature of the seventeenth and eighteenth centuries (and indeed of earlier periods), it is possible to recognize behaviours that nowadays we may wish to refer as dementia being reported under different rubrics. For example, in relation to 'Stupidity or Foolishness', Thomas Willis (1684) wrote:

> although it chiefly belongs to the rational soul, and signifies a defect of the intellect and judgement, yet it is not improperly reckoned among the diseases of the head or brain; for as much as this eclipse of the superior soul proceeds from the imagination and the memory being hurt, and the failing of these depends upon the faults of the animal spirits, and the brain itself (p. 209).

Willis suggested that stupidity might be genetic ('original', as when 'fools beget fools') or caused by ageing ('Some at first crafty and ingenious, become by degrees dull, and at length foolish, by the mere declining of age, without any great errors in living') (p. 211), or other causes such as 'strokes or bruising upon the head', 'drunkenness and surfeiting', 'violent and sudden passions' and 'cruel diseases of the head' such as epilepsy.

The same is the case with Boissier de Sauvages (1771), one of the great classificators of the eighteenth century. Order 3rd (8th class) of his *Nosographie Methodique* encompasses delirium, paraphrosyne, imbecility, melancholia, demonomania and mania. Synonyms of 'Imbecility are *Bêtise* (stupidity, foolishness), *Niaiserie* (silliness), and *Démence*; in Greek *paranoia*, and in Latin *Dementia, Fatuitas, Vecordia*. The term is used to refer to patients who are fools, (*fous*), imbeciles (*imbécilles*), mentally weak (*foibles d'esprit*), mad (*insensés*)' (p. 723). Boissier lists 12 subtypes of imbecility of which the first one is the imbecility of the elderly (*L'imbécillite de vieillard*), also known as puerile state, drivelling or senile madness, and which he explains thus: 'Because of the stiffness of their nervous fibres, old people are less sensitive to external impressions …' (p. 724).

In the *Nosographie* (1818; first published 1798), Pinel dealt with cognitive impairment under amentia and morosis, which he explains as a failure in the association of ideas leading to disordered activity, extravagant behaviour, superficial emotions, memory loss, difficulty in the perception of objects, obliteration of judgement, aimless activity, automatic existence, and forgetting of words or signs to convey ideas. He also referred to *démence senile* (para 116). Pinel did not emphasize the difference between congenital and acquired dementia (Pinel 1806).

The above entries summarize well views on dementia before the nineteenth century. There was, first of all, a 'legal' meaning according to which dementia was a state of non-imputability. In France, this was enshrined in Article 10 of the Napoleonic Code: 'There is no crime when the accused is in a state of dementia at the time of the alleged act' (Code Napoléon, 1808). Second, there was a clinical meaning. This could be very general (i.e. a synonym of madness) or specific, i.e. a clinical condition that was differentiable from mania (which, at the time, described any state of acute excitement, be it schizophrenic, hypomanic, or organic) and delirium (which referred, more or less, to what goes on nowadays under the same name). Although chronic, dementia could still be reversible, affect individuals of any age, and be a final common pathway, i.e. the end deficit for many other mental disorders. This created a template for the alienists of the nineteenth century.

1.4 DEMENTIA DURING THE NINETEENTH CENTURY

There is a major difference between eighteenth-century views on dementia and what the historian finds a century later when dementia starts to refer more or less specifically to states of cognitive impairment mostly affecting the elderly, and almost always irreversible. The word 'amentia' was no longer used in this context and started to name a 'psychosis, with sudden onset following severe, often acute physical illness or trauma' (Meynert, 1890). The syndromatic view of the dementias was still in use but mainly in regards to the 'vesanic dementias', i.e. terminal states for all manner of mental disorders. This section will explore such momentous changes.

In his doctoral thesis, Esquirol (1805) used the word dementia to refer to loss of reason, as in *démence accidental, démence mélancolique*; then, he distinguished between acute, chronic and senile dementia. Acute dementia was short-lived, reversible, and followed fever, haemorrhage and metastasis; chronic dementia was irreversible and caused by masturbation, melancholia, mania, hypochondria, epilepsy, paralysis and apoplexy; lastly, senile dementia resulted from ageing, and consisted in a loss of the faculties of the understanding (Esquirol, 1814). Esquirol's final thoughts on dementia were

influenced by his controversy with Bayle (1822) who via his concept of *chronic arachnoiditis* propounded an anatomical ('organic') view of all the insanities and scorned Pinel's views that some vesanias might develop in a psychological space (Bayle, 1826).

Together with his student Georget, Esquirol supported a 'descriptivist' approach, at least in relation to some forms of mental disorder. He reported 15 cases of dementia (seven males and eight females) with a mean age of 34 years (SD = 10.9), seven being, in fact, cases of general paralysis of the insane, showing grandiosity, disinhibition, motor symptoms, dysarthria and terminal cognitive failure. There also was included a 20-year-old girl who, in modern terms, suffered from a catatonic syndrome; and a 40-year-old woman with pica, cognitive impairment, and space-occupying lesions in her left hemisphere and cerebellum (Esquirol, 1838). Although the mean age of these samples and the absence of cases of senile dementia may simply reflect a short life expectancy in Esquirol's day, or that at the Charenton Hospital some selection bias was in operation, it is more likely to reflect the view that age was not an important variable. Together with irreversibility, age became a defining criterion only by the second half of the nineteenth century.

Like his teacher Esquirol, aware of the importance of clinical description, Calmeil wrote: 'It is not easy to describe dementia, its varieties, and nuances; because its complications are numerous … it is difficult to choose its distinctive symptoms' (p. 71). Dementia followed chronic insanity and brain disease, and was partial or general. Calmeil was less convinced than his co-student Georget that all dementias were associated with alterations in the brain.

In regards to senile dementia, Calmeil remarked: 'there is a constant involvement of the senses, elderly people can be deaf, and show disorders of taste, smell and touch; external stimuli are therefore less clear to them, they have little memory of recent events, live in the past, and repeat the same tale; their affect gradually wanes away …' (p. 77). Although a keen neuropathologist, Calmeil concluded that there was no sufficient information on the nature and range of anomalies found in the skull or brain to decide on the cause of dementia (pp. 82–83) (Calmeil, 1835).

A Ghent alienist, thinking in Flemish and writing in French, Guislain believed that in dementia:

All intellectual functions show a reduction in energy, external stimuli cause only minor impression on the intellect, imagination is weak and uncreative, memory absent, and reasoning pathological. There are two varieties of dementia … one affecting the elderly (senile dementia of Cullen) the other younger people. Although confused with dementia, idiocy must be considered as a separate group (p. 10). [In dementia,] 'the patient has no memory, or at least is unable to retain anything … impressions evaporate from his mind. He may remember names of people but cannot say whether he has seen them before. He does not know what time or day of the week it is, cannot tell morning from evening, or say what 2 and 2 add to … he has lost the instinct of preservation, cannot avoid fire or water, and is unable to recognize dangers; has also lost spontaneity, is incontinent of urine and faeces, and does not ask for anything, he cannot even recognize his wife or children ... (p. 311) (Guislain, 1852).

Because in the past the mentally ill: 'had been categorized only in terms of a [putative] impairment of their mental faculties ...' (p. 2), Morel (1860) endeavoured to develop a taxonomy that distinguished between occasional and determinant causes of mental disorder (p. 251) and suggested six clinical groups: hereditary, toxic, associated with the neuroses, idiopathic, sympathetic and dementia In regards to the latter, Morel (1860) believed that:

... if we examine dementia (amentia, progressive weakening of the faculties) we must accept that it constitutes a terminal state. There will, of course, be exceptional insane individuals who, until the end, preserve their intellectual faculties; the majority, however, are subject to the law of decline. This results from a loss of vitality in the brain ... Comparison of brain weights in the various forms of insanity shows that the heavier weights are found in cases of recent onset. Chronic cases show more often a general impairment of intelligence (dementia). Loss in brain weight – a constant feature of dementia – is also present in ageing, and is an expression of decadence in the human species. [There are] natural dementia and that dementia resulting from a pathological state of the brain ... some forms of insanity are more prone to end up in dementia (idiopathic) than others ... it could be argued that because dementia is a terminal state it should not be classified as a sixth form of mental illness ... I must confess I sympathize with this view, and it is one of the reasons why I have not described the dementias in any detail ... on the other hand from the legal and pathological viewpoints, dementia warrants separate treatment ... (pp. 837–838).

Morel's view is in keeping with his 'degenerationist' hypothesis, which he himself had developed three years earlier (Morel, 1857; Pick, 1989). One consequence of this view was that there were no specific brain alterations in dementia.

In spite of his early death, L. F. Marcé published a series of important articles on the neuropathology of senile dementia which challenged Morel's non-specificity hypothesis.

There is no space in this chapter to analyse with the same level of detail the evolution of the concept of dementia in other European countries, although it can be said that it followed similar lines. Views in England, for example, were mainly derivative from French ones. In a popular textbook, and following Pinel, Esquirol and Calmeil, Prichard included a category which he called 'incoherence or dementia':

[it] is a very peculiar and well-marked form of mental disorder. The mind in this state is occupied, without ceasing, by unconnected thoughts and evanescent emotions; it is incapable of continued attention and reflection, and at length loses the faculty of distinct perception or apprehension. Numerous examples of this disease, or decay of the mental powers are to be met within every receptacle containing a considerable assemblage

of deranged persons ... incoherence is either a primary disease, arising immediately from the agency of exciting causes on a constitution previously health, or it is a secondary affection, the result of other disorders of the brain and nervous system which, by their long duration or severity, give rise to disease in the structure of those organs ... secondary incoherence or dementia follows long-protracted mania, attacks of apoplexy, epilepsy or paralysis, or fevers attended with severe delirium. This decay of the faculties has been termed fatuity or imbecility, and it has been confounded with idiotism, which in all its degrees and modifications is a very different state ... (pp. 83–85) (Prichard, 1835).

The same can be said of the views expressed by Bucknill and Tuke in their popular textbook:

Dementia may be either primary or consecutive; acute or chronic. It may also be simple or complicated; it is occasionally remittent but rarely intermittent. It is primary when it is the first stage of the mental disease of the patient; and when this occurs, it is, perhaps, one of the most painful forms of insanity; the patient often being acutely sensible of a gradual loss of memory, power of attention, and executive ability. At this period, the distinction is often well marked between the strictly intellectual and affective disorder ... dementia is much more frequently consecutive, that is the consequence of other diseases of the mind. Thus during 44 years, while 277 cases of mania and 215 of melancholia were admitted at the Retreat, only 48 of dementia were admitted during the same period; yet, at the end of that term, there were remaining in the institution, 20 patients in a state of dementia out of 91 inmates. Mania very often degenerates into dementia; as also do melancholia and monomania ... it should be observed, that the term dementia may be, and sometimes is, too indiscriminately employed. All writers of authority agree in representing impairment of the memory as one of the earliest symptoms of dementia; but we believe cases are occasionally classed under incipient dementia, in which close observation would show that the memory is unimpaired ... It is often rather a torpid condition of the mind, falling under the division 'apathetic insanity, which ought not to be confounded with dementia ...' (pp. 117–119) (Bucknill and Tuke, 1858).

The same concepts are found in German-speaking nations and the views of Heinroth, Feuchtersleben, Griesinger and Kahlbaum were influential until the beginning of the second half of the nineteenth century. Heinroth (1818/1975) used the term dementia in a very broad sense to refer to a state of mind that might accompany or follow other mental disorders, i.e. 'vesanic dementia', a term that late in the century was to become very popular, particularly in France. This concept, which is not related to age, is redolent of the later notion of secondary dementia, i.e. the state of psychosocial and cognitive incompetence that might follow a functional psychosis. Feuchtersleben's usage (1845/1847) is even more general. In his work he uses dementia as a synonym of madness and may refer to forms of acute madness with and without accompanying idiocy. There is only one form of dementia, which he refers to as *moria* and considered as more or less chronic and more or less cognitive. Although possibly ending up in a state of idiocy, the patient can also show lucid intervals. Once again, age is of no relevance to moria and hence one must conclude that Feuchtersleben is referring to a form of vesanic dementia.

Griesinger's nosology is not altogether clear and has often been interpreted as being based on the belief that there is only one form of madness (*unitary psychoses concept*), which may go through at least three stages: depression (as in melancholia), exaltation (as in mania) and weakness (as in chronic madness and dementia). In the second edition of his great work, Griesinger (1861/1867) insists that the states of mental weakness 'do not constitute primary but consecutive forms of insanity' (p. 319). This suggests that he is also referring to a form of vesanic dementia, although he includes under this large class all the forms of mental handicap where no preliminary 'primary' forms of madness can be recognized. Under the heading 'dementia', Griesinger includes mental disorders fundamentally caused by a 'general weakness of the mental faculties' including loss of emotions. Age is not a factor in the development of dementia or apathetic dementia and hence it must also be concluded that Griesinger is referring to vesanic dementia.

The work of Kahlbaum, particularly his important book of 1863 on the definition and classification of mental disorders, mark the beginning of a new era in psychiatry. His incorporation of time as a variable in the analysis of madness (longitudinal definition) and his view that period of life is relevant to the form of the disease remain the pillars of psychiatric nosology to this day. The concept of 'Dementia' is dealt with in the third section of Kahlbaum's book (1863) under the name of *aphrenia*. This clinical category refers to states of mental impotence (*Zustand geistiger Impotenz*) (p. 153), which Kahlbaum equates to the old German notion of *Blödsinn*. After complaining that neither the Greeks nor Latin writers managed to specify a term for this condition, he insists that a word is needed to refer to states of cognitive and behavioural incompetence such as those seen in *dementia terminalis* (Berrios, 1996).

1.5 THE FRAGMENTATION OF DEMENTIA

During the second half of the nineteenth century, and based on the clinical observations and reconceptualization carried out by the French, German and English writers mentioned above, dementia starts to be considered as a syndrome and hence could be attached to a variety of disorders. The primary classification was to be between primary and secondary, the latter including all the vesanic dementias, i.e. states of defect that could follow any severe form of insanity. An increased use of light microscopy during the second half of the century led to the view that primary forms of dementia could be caused by degenerations of cerebral parenchyma or

by arteriosclerosis. By 1900, senile, arteriosclerotic, infectious and traumatic forms of dementia had been reported (Berrios and Freeman, 1991). 'Mixed forms', such as 'dementia praecox' were also suggested reflecting Kahlbaum's view that mental disorders appeared during specific biological transitions. The list of parenchymal forms became longer after the inclusion of states of degeneration from alcoholism, epilepsy, myxoedema and lead poisoning. The history of some of these forms will be discussed presently.

1.5.1 General paralysis of the insane

Bayle (1822) described under the name *arachnitis chronique* cases of what later was to be called 'general paralysis of the insane'. Whether this 'new phenomenon' resulted from 'a mutation in the syphilitic virus towards the end of the eighteenth century' is unclear (p. 623) (Hare, 1959). Equally dubious is the claim that its discovery reinforced the belief of alienists in the anatomoclinical view of mental disease (Zilboorg, 1941). In fact, it took more than 30 years for general paralysis to gain acceptance as a 'separate' disease. Bayle's 'discovery' was more important in another way, namely that it challenged the 'cross-sectional' view of disease; in the words of Bercherie (1980): 'for the first time in the history of psychiatry there was a morbid entity which presented itself as a sequential process unfolding itself into successive clinical syndromes' (p. 75).

By the 1850s, no agreement had yet been reached as to how symptoms were caused by the *periencephalite chronique diffuse* (as general paralysis was known at the time). Three clinical types were recognized: manic-ambitious, melancholic-hypochondriac, and dementia; according to the 'unitary view', all three constituted stages of a single disease, the order of their appearance depending on the progress of the cerebral lesions. Baillarger (1883), however, sponsored a 'dualist' view: 'paralytic insanity and paralytic dementia are different conditions'. It is clear that the debate had less to do with the nature of the brain lesions than with how mental symptoms and their contents were produced in general: how could the 'typical' content of paralytic delusions (grandiosity) be explained? Since the same mental symptoms could be seen in all manner of conditions, Baillarger believed that chronic periencephalitis could account only for the motor signs – mental symptoms 'therefore, having a different origin' (p. 389). The absence of a link between lesion and symptom also explained why some patients recovered.

The view that general paralysis might be related to syphilis (put forward by Fournier, 1875) was resisted. Indeed, the term 'pseudogeneral paralysis' was coined to refer to cases of infections causing psychotic symptoms (Baillarger, 1889). In general, there is little evidence that alienists considered general paralysis as a 'paradigm-disease', i.e. a model for all other mental diseases. It can even be said that the new 'disease' created more problems than it solved (for a discussion of this issue see Berrios, 1985a).

1.5.2 The vesanic dementias

The term 'vesanic dementia' began to be used after the 1840s to refer to the clinical states of cognitive disorganization following insanity (Berrios, 1987); its meaning has changed with equal speed alongside psychiatric theory. According to the unitary insanity notion, vesanic dementia was a terminal stage (after mania and melancholia); according to degeneration theory, it was the final expression of a corrupted pedigree; and according to post-1880s' nosology, a final common pathway to some insanities. Vesanic dementias were reversible, and could occur at any age; risk factors such as old age, lack of education, low social class, bad nutrition etc., accelerated the progression of the dementia or impeded recovery (p. 597) (Ball and Chambard, 1881).

The vesanic dementias included cases suffering from cognitive impairment associated with melancholia. Under the term *démence mélancolique* Mairet (1883) reported a series of cases of depressed patients with cognitive impairment who on post mortem showed changes in the temporal lobe; this led Mairet to hypothesize that the affected sites were related to feelings, and to suggest that nihilistic delusions appeared when the lesion spread to the cortex (Berrios, 1985a). Mairet's cases (some of which would now be called 'Cotard's syndrome') showed psychomotor retardation, refused food and died in stupor (Cotard, 1882; Berrios and Luque, 1995). Others, however, got better and these cases are redolent of what nowadays might be called 'depressive pseudodementia'.

Another contributor to the understanding of cognitive impairment in the affective disorders was George Dumas (1894) who suggested that it was 'mental fatigue that explained the psychological poverty and monotony of melancholic depressions' and that the problem was not 'an absence but a stagnation of ideas'; he was, therefore, the first to explain the disorder as a failure in performance.

The *word* 'pseudodementia', however, originated in a different clinical tradition. It was first used by Carl Wernicke to refer to 'a chronic hysterical state mimicking mental weakness' (Bulbena and Berrios, 1986). Not used until the 1950s, it was given a lease of life by writers such as Madden *et al.* (1952), Anderson *et al.* (1959) and Kiloh (1961). Current usage is ambiguous in that it relates to three clinical situations: a real (albeit reversible) cognitive impairment accompanying some psychoses, a parody of such impairment, and the cognitive deficit of delirium (Bulbena and Berrios, 1986).

1.5.3 Brain changes and ageing

Since the beginning of the nineteenth century, cases had been described of brain 'softening' followed by cognitive failure. Rostan (1823) reported 98 subjects thus affected, thought to be scorbutic in origin, and divided them into simple, abnormal and complicated (the latter two groups being accompanied by psychiatric changes). Mental symptoms might occur before, during and after the softening itself; thus, senile dementia

and insanity might precede the brain changes. When it accompanied stroke, Rostan described cognitive failure and attacks of insanity suggesting that these symptoms were 'a general feature … not a positive sign of localisation' (pp. 214–215). Durand-Fardel (1843) provided an account of the relationship between softening and insanity, warning that softening was used to refer both to a disease (stroke) and to a state of the brain. Psychiatric complications were acute and long term, the former including confusion, depression, irritability, acute insanity and loss of mental faculties (p. 139); the latter had gradual onset, and exhibited an impairment of memory, poverty of thinking, and a regression to infantile forms of behaviour, features which led to 'true dementia' (pp. 327–328).

Years later, Jackson (1875) reviewed the problem: 'softening … as a category for a rude clinical grouping was to be deprecated' (p. 335); he nonetheless, followed Durand-Fardel's classification, and suggested that, after stroke, mental symptoms might be immediate or occurring after a few hours or months; he recognized that major cognitive failure may ensue, and saw this as an instance of 'dissolution': emotional symptoms being release phenomena (for an analysis of this concept see Berrios, 1991). He believed that anxiety, stress and irritability might be harbingers of stroke.

1.5.4 The concept of arteriosclerotic dementia

Old age was considered an important factor in the development of arteriosclerosis (Berrios, 1994) and a risk factor in diseases such as melancholia (Berrios, 1991). By 1910, there was a trend to include all dementias under 'mental disorders of cerebral arteriosclerosis' (Barrett, 1913). Arteriosclerosis, might be generalized or cerebral, inherited or acquired, and caused by syphilis, alcohol, nicotine, high blood pressure or ageing. In those genetically predisposed, cerebral arteries were considered as thinner and less elastic. Arteriosclerosis caused mental changes by narrowing of arteries and/or reactive inflammation. The view that arteriosclerotic dementia resulted from a gradual strangulation of blood supply to the brain was also formed during this period; consequently, emphasis was given to prodromal symptoms, and strokes were but the culmination of a process started years before.

Some opposed this view from the beginning. For example, Marie (1906) claimed that such explanation was a vicious circle, as alienists claimed that: 'ageing was caused by arteriosclerosis and the latter by ageing' (p. 358), and Walton (1912) expressed serious doubts from the histopathological point of view. The frequent presence in post mortem of such changes also concerned pathologists who worried that they could not 'safely exclude cerebral arteriosclerosis of greater or lesser degree in any single case' of senile dementia (p. 677) (Southard, 1910). Based on a review of these arguments, Olah (1910) concluded that there was no such thing as 'arteriosclerotic psychoses'. However, the 'chronic global ischaemia' hypothesis won the day, and it was to continue well into the second half of the twentieth century. For some it became a general explanation; for example, North and Bostock (1925) reported a series of 568 general psychiatric cases in which around 40 per cent suffered from 'arterial disease', which – according to the authors – was even responsible for schizophrenia. The old idea of an apoplectic form of dementia, however, never disappeared.

1.5.5　Apoplectic dementia

'Apoplectic dementia' achieved its clearest enunciation in the work of Benjamin Ball (Ball and Chambard, 1881). 'Organic apoplexy' resulted from bleeding, softening or tumour and might be 'followed by a notable decline in cognition, and by a state of dementia which was progressive and incurable … of the three, localized softening (*ramollissement en foyer*) caused the more severe states of cognitive impairment' (p. 581). Ball believed that prodromal lapses of cognition (e.g. episodes of somnolence and confusion with automatic behaviour, for which there was no memory after the event) and sensory symptoms were caused by atheromatous lesions. Visual hallucinations, occasionally of a pleasant nature, were also common. After the stroke, persistent cognitive impairment was frequent. Post-mortem studies showed in these cases softening of 'ideational' areas of cortex and white matter. Ball also suggested a laterality effect (p. 582) in that right hemisphere strokes led more often to dementia whereas left hemisphere ones caused perplexity, apathy, unresponsiveness, and a tendency to talk to oneself (p. 583). Following Luys, he believed that some of these symptoms resulted from damage to corpus striatum, insular sulci and temporal lobe. During Ball's time, attention also shifted from white to red softening. Charcot (1881) wrote on cerebral haemorrhage (the new name for red softening): 'having eliminated all these cases, we find ourselves in the presence of a homogeneous group corresponding to the commonest form of cerebral haemorrhage. This is, par excellence, sanguineous apoplexy … as it attacks a great number of old people, I might call it senile haemorrhage' (p. 267).

1.5.6　Presbyophrenia and confabulation

The word 'presbyophrenia' was coined by Kahlbaum (1863) to name a subtype of the paraphrenias (insanities occurring during periods of biological change). Presbyophrenia was a form of paraphrenia senilis characterized by amnesia, disorientation, delusional misidentification and confabulation. Ignored for more than 30 years, the term reappeared in the work of Wernicke, Fischer and Kraepelin. Wernicke's classification of mental disorders was based on his theory of the three-partite relational structure consciousness (outside world, body and self) (Lanczik, 1988). Impairment of the link between consciousness and outside world led to presbyophrenia, delirium tremens, Korsakoff's psychosis, and hallucinoses. Amongst the features of presbyophrenia, Wernicke included confabulations, disorientation, hyperactivity, euphoria, and a fluctuating

course; acute forms resolved without trace, chronic ones merged with senile dementia (Berrios, 1986).

In France, Rouby (1911) conceived of presbyophrenia as a final common pathway for cases suffering from Korsakoff's psychosis, senile dementia or acute confusion. Truelle and Bessière (1911) suggested, in turn, that it might result from a toxic state caused by liver or kidney failure. Kraepelin (1910) lumped presbyophrenia together with the senile and presenile insanities, and (as compared with Korsakoff's patients) believed presbyophrenic patients to be older, free from polyneuritis and history of alcoholism, and showing hyperactivity and elevated mood. Ziehen (1911) wrote that 'their marked memory impairment contrasts with the relative sparing of thinking'. Fischer (1912) suggested that disseminated cerebral lesions were the essential anatomical substrate of presbyophrenia.

During the 1930s, two new hypotheses emerged. Bostroem (1933) concluded on phenomenological grounds that presbyophrenia could be identified with mania, suggesting an interplay between two factors: cerebral arteriosclerosis and cyclothymic premorbid personality. Lafora (1935) emphasized the role of cerebrovascular pathology, and claimed that disinhibition and presbyophrenic behaviour were caused by a combination of senile and atherosclerotic changes. Burger-Prinz and Jacob (1938), however, questioned the view that cyclothymic features were a necessary precondition. Bessière (1948) claimed that presbyophrenia was a syndrome found in conditions such as senile dementia, brain tumours, traumatic psychoses and confusional states. More recently, it has been suggested that presbyophrenia may be a subform of AD characterized by a severe atrophy of locus caeruleus (Berrios, 1985b).

One of the features of presbyophrenia was confabulation. This complex symptom has not quite found a place in psychopathology (Berrios, 2000b). Two phenomena are included under the name 'confabulation'. The *first type* concerns 'untrue' utterances of subjects with memory impairment; often provoked or elicited by the interviewer, these confabulations are accompanied by little conviction and are believed by most clinicians to be caused by the (conscious or unconscious) need to 'cover up' for some memory deficit. Researchers wanting to escape the 'intentionality' dilemma have made use of additional factors such as presence of frontal lobe pathology, dysexecutive syndrome, difficulty with the temporal dating of memories leading to an inability temporally to string out memory data, etc.

The *second type* concerns confabulations with fantastic content and great conviction as seen in subjects with functional psychoses and little or no memory deficit. Less is said in the neuropsychological literature about this group, although (at least in the case of schizophrenics) it has been correlated with a bad performance on frontal lobe tests. It is our belief that this group remains of crucial importance to psychiatrists. Little is known about the epidemiology of either type of confabulation.

In clinical practice, these two 'types' can be found in combination. It remains unclear why so many patients with

Korsakoff's psychosis or frontal lobe disorder, in spite of the fact that they do meet the putative conditions for confabulation (amnesia, frontal lobe damage, difficulty with the dating of memories, etc.) do not confabulate. Furthermore, confabulations have also been reported in subjects with lesions in the non-dominant hemisphere and in the thalamus.

Under different disguises, the 'covering up' or 'gap filling' hypothesis is still going strong. Although superficially plausible, it poses a serious conceptual problem in regard to the issue of 'awareness of purpose': if full awareness is presumed, then it is difficult to differentiate confabulations from lying; if no awareness is presumed, then the semantics of the concept of 'purpose' is severely stretched and confabulations cannot be differentiated from delusions.

The received view of confabulations also neglects the clinical observation that confabulations (particularly provoked ones!) do occur in dialogical situations: for example, the way in which the patient is asked questions may increase the probability of producing a confabulation. This suggests that the view that confabulations are a disorder of a putative narrative function found in normal human subjects must be taken seriously. It is hypothesized here that this trait is normally distributed in the population. In the absence of adequate epidemiological information, research efforts should be directed at mapping the distribution of this narrative (or confabulatory) capacity in the community at large. Only then will it be possible to understand the significance of its disorders. In the long term, this approach will prove more heuristic than unwarranted speculation based on a few anecdotal cases.

Reported in relation to clinical conditions other than memory deficit, 'confabulation-like' behaviours can already be found in the clinical literature of the second half of the nineteenth century. Sully (1885) suggested that such behaviours might be related to a psychological function whose role was filling gaps in the flow of our lives and explained why 'our image of the past is essentially one of an unbroken series of conscious experiences'. Sully believed that this function also intervened when memory failed: 'just as the eye sees no gap in its field of vision corresponding to the 'blind' spot of the retina, but carries the impression over this area, so memory sees no lacuna in the past, but carries its image of conscious life over each of the forgotten spaces' (p. 282).

Kraepelin (1886–1887) reported typical cases of confabulation associated with, among other things, general paralysis of the insane, melancholia and dementia; and later on suggested that 'pseudomemories' could be a symptom of paraphrenia (*without* cognitive impairment), and described a clinical variety called *paraphrenia confabulans* (Kraepelin, 1919). Under schizophrenic *akzessorischen Gedachtnisstörungen*, Bleuler (1911) discussed three related phenomena: *Gedächnisillusionen* (illusions or distortions of memory), *identifizierenden Erinnerungstäuschungen* (memory falsifications based on identification), and *Erinnerungshalluzinationen* (memory hallucinations). Of the former he wrote: 'memory illusions often constitute the main material for the construction of delusions in paranoids. The entire previous life of the patient may be changed in his memory in terms of this complex' (p. 115). On this definition, it is difficult, on the basis of their *intrinsic* features, to distinguish illusion of memory from confabulation. Indeed, symptom-naming is determined by whether schizophrenia or 'organic disorder' is the associated disease. Unsuccessfully, Bleuler (1911) tried to establish a differentiation on the basis of *mechanism*: 'until now, and in contrast to the views of some authors, I have not observed confabulation as it appears in organic cases; e.g. memory hallucinations which fill in memory gaps which at first appear at a (usually external) given moment and mostly adapt themselves to such an occasion' (p. 117). Kleist (1960) described patients with 'progressive confabulosis' as 'cheerful, expansive, and with little in the way of thought or speech disorder' (p. 211); and Leonhard (1957) redescribed the condition as 'confabulatory euphoria'.

1.5.7 Alzheimer's disease

AD has become the prototypical form of dementia. From this point of view, a study of its origins should throw light on the evolution of the concept of dementia. The writings of Alzheimer, Fischer, Fuller, Lafora, Bonfiglio, Perusini, Ziveri, Kraepelin and other protagonists are deceptively fresh, and this makes anachronistic reading inevitable. However, the psychiatry of the late nineteenth century is a remote country: concepts such as dementia, neurone, neurofibril and plaque were then still in process of construction and meant different things to different people. A discussion of these issues is beyond the scope of this chapter (for this see Berrios, 1990b).

1.5.7.1 THE NEUROPATHOLOGY OF DEMENTIA BEFORE ALZHEIMER

Enquiries into the brain changes accompanying dementia started during the 1830s but consisted in descriptions of external appearance (Wilks, 1865). The first important microscopic study was that of Marcé (1863) who described cortical atrophy, enlarged ventricles and 'softening'. The vascular origin of softening was soon ascertained (Parrot, 1873), but the distinction between vascular and parenchymal factors had to await until the 1880s. From then on, microscopic studies concentrated on cellular death, plaques and neurofibrils.

1.5.7.2 ALZHEIMER AND HIS DISEASE

Alzheimer (1907) reported the case of a 51-year-old woman, with cognitive impairment, delusions, hallucinations, focal symptoms, and whose brain showed plaques, tangles and arteriosclerotic changes. The existence of neurofibrils had been known for some time (DeFelipe and Jones, 1988); for example, that in senile dementia 'the destruction of the neurofibrils appears to be more extensive than in the brain of a paralytic subject' (Bianchi 1906, p. 846). Fuller (1907) had remarked in June 1906 (i.e. five months before Alzheimer's report) on the presence of neurofibrillar bundles in senile dementia (p. 450). Likewise, the association of plaques with dementia was not a novelty: Beljahow (1889) had reported them in 1887, and so had Redlich and Leri few years later (Simchowicz, 1924); in Prague, Fischer (1907) gave an important paper in June 1907 pointing out that miliary necrosis could be considered as a marker of senile dementia.

Nor was the syndrome described by Alzheimer new: states of persistent cognitive impairment affecting the elderly, accompanied by delusions and hallucinations were well known (Marcé, 1863; Krafft-Ebing, 1873; Crichton-Browne, 1874; Marie, 1906). As a leading neuropathologist Alzheimer was aware of this work. Did he then mean to describe a new disease? The answer is that it is most unlikely he did, his only intention having been to point out that such a syndrome could occur in younger people (Alzheimer, 1911). This is confirmed by commentaries from those who worked for him: Perusini (1911) wrote that for Alzheimer 'these morbid forms do not represent anything but atypical form of senile dementia' (p. 143).

1.5.7.3 THE NAMING OF THE DISEASE

Kraepelin (1910) coined the term in the 8th edition of his *Handbook*: at the end of the section on 'senile dementia' he wrote:

> the autopsy revels, according to Alzheimer's description, changes that represent the most serious form of senile dementia ... the *Drusen* were numerous and almost one third of the cortical cells had died off. In their place instead we found peculiar deeply stained fibrillary bundles that were closely packed to one another, and seemed to be remnants of degenerated cell bodies ... The clinical interpretation of this AD is still confused. Whilst the anatomical findings suggest that we are dealing with a particularly serious form of senile dementia, the fact that this disease sometimes starts already around the age of 40 does not allow this supposition. In such cases we should at least assume a 'senium praecox' if not perhaps a more or less age-independent unique disease process.

1.5.7.4 THE RECEPTION OF THE NEW DISEASE

Alzheimer (1911) showed surprise at Kraepelin's interpretation, and always referred to his 'disease' as *Erkrankungen* (in the medical language of the 1900s a term softer than *Krankheit*, the term used by Kraepelin). Others also expressed doubts. Fuller (1912), whose contribution to this field has been sadly neglected, asked 'why a special clinical designation – Alzheimer's disease – since, after all, they are but part of a general disorder' (p. 26). Hakkébousch and Geier (1913), in Russia, saw it as a variety of the involution psychosis. Simchowicz (1911) considered 'Alzheimer's disease' as only a severe form of senile dementia. Ziehen (1911) does not mention the disease in his major review of senile dementia. In a meeting of the New York Neurological Society, Ramsay Hunt (Lambert, 1916) asked Lambert, the presenter of a case of 'Alzheimer's disease' that 'he would like to understand clearly whether he made any distinction between the so-called Alzheimer's disease and senile dementia' other than ... in degree and point of age'. Lambert agreed suggesting that, as far as he was concerned, the underlying pathological mechanisms were the same (Lambert, 1916). Lugaro (1916) wrote: 'For a while it was believed that a certain agglutinative disorder of the neurofibril could be considered as the main "marker" (*contrassegno*) of a presenile form [of senile dementia], which was "hurriedly baptized" (*fretta battezzate*) as "Alzheimer's disease"' (p. 378). He went on to say that this state is only a variety of senile dementia. Simchowicz (1924), who had worked with Alzheimer, wrote 'Alzheimer and Perusini did not know at the time that the plaques were typical of senile dementia [in general] and believed that they might have discovered a new disease' (p. 221). These views, from men who lived in Alzheimer's and Kraepelin's time, must be taken seriously (for a detail discussion of these issues see Berrios, 1990a).

Of late there has been an attempt to rewrite the history of AD. After having been lost for years, the case notes of Auguste D., the first patient with AD, were found in the late 1990s (Maurer and Maurer, 1998). As mentioned above the original report by Alzheimer (1907) clearly stated that Auguste suffered from severe confusion, delusions, hallucinations, focal symptoms, and on post mortem her brain showed plaques, tangles and, most importantly, *arteriosclerotic* changes. As if to confirm the ontology of AD, Graeber *et al.* (1998) reported that in tissue sections belonging to this case they confirmed the presence of neurofibrillar tangles and amyloid plaques. Most interestingly, and given that vascular changes are currently not supposed to be a diagnostic criterion, these authors have put Alzheimer right by stating that Auguste's brain showed no arteriosclerotic lesions. Furthermore, they report that the apolipoprotein E (ApoE) genotype of Auguste was $\varepsilon3/\varepsilon3$, 'indicating that mutational screening of the tissue is feasible'.

On the basis of these findings, can one say that back in 1910 Kraepelin was, after all, right in claiming that Alzheimer had 'discovered' a new disease? The answer has to be that one must judge his decision in terms of what Kraepelin knew at the time and of the academic pressure he was under. He knew what Alzheimer's report stated in 1907, what the latter might have verbally added, and upon Kraepelin's perusal of Auguste's case notes, which were requested by him from Frankfurt (indeed this is the reason why they were lost for such a long time). In clinical terms, Auguste was not a 'typical' case. At 51 she had delusions, hallucinations and Alzheimer's reported arteriosclerotic changes. None of these features is mentioned in Kraepelin's original claim. The question is, why?

It is also interesting that the so-called 'second case' of Alzheimer's (Graeber *et al.*, 1997), Johann F., reported in 1911, is now considered to have suffered a 'plaques-only' form of AD. The same authors suggest that knowledge of this case may have encouraged Kraepelin to report the discovery by Alzheimer of a new disease. Unfortunately, there is no evidence that Kraepelin knew of this case when he was writing the relevant section of the 8th edition of his *Lehrbuch*. More to the point is that he knew of Perusini's review (1909) as he himself had asked the young Italian assistant to collect four cases. In addition to Auguste D. (which includes more information than that provided by Alzheimer in 1907), Perusini reviewed the cases of Mr. R.M., a 45-year-old basket maker who had epileptic seizures, of Mrs. B.A. a 65-year-old who had marked clinical features of myxoedema, and Schl. L, a 63-year-old who had suffered from syphilis since 1870, was Romberg-positive, had a pupillary syndrome and heard voices. Since these are likely to have been the cases on which Kraepelin based his decision to construct the new disease, it would be interesting if the neuropathology and neurogenetics of the other three cases (Auguste's has already been done) were to be investigated.

1.5.8 Pick's disease and the frontal dementias

Dementias believed to be related to frontal lobe pathology have once again become of interest, and authors often invoke the name of Arnold Pick (Niery *et al.*, 1988). However, when the great Prague neuropsychiatrist described the syndrome named after him, all he wanted was to draw attention to a form of localized (as opposed to diffuse) atrophy of the temporal lobe (Pick, 1892). This alteration was to give rise to a dysfunction of language and praxis, and be susceptible to diagnosis during life. Pick believed that lobar atrophies constituted a stage in the evolution of the senile dementias.

The story starts, as it should, before Pick. Louis Pierre Gratiolet (1854) was responsible for renaming the cerebral lobes after their overlying skull: thus 'anterior' became 'frontal' lobe. He made no assumption as to the function of the 'anterior extremity of the cerebral hemisphere'. 'Phrenologists', however, did and related reflective and perceptive functions (qualitatively defined) to the forehead (Anonymous, 1832) (for the science of phrenology see Combe, 1873; Lanteri-Laura, 1970). 'Modular' assumptions (i.e. a one-to-one correlation between mental function and brain site) involving the frontal lobes started only during the 1860s, following reports on dysfunction of language in lesions of the frontal lobes (Broca, 1861; Henderson, 1986). These claims ran parallel to those of Jackson's that the cerebral cortex was the general seat of personality and mind (Jackson, 1894). Meynert (1885) believed that 'the frontal lobes reach a high state of development in man' but still defined mental disorders as diseases of the 'fore-brain' (by which he meant 'prosencephalon' or human brain as a whole).

In his first report (the case of focal senile atrophy and aphasia in a man of 71) Pick (1892) did not inculpate the frontal lobes nor did he in his second case (Pick, 1901) (a woman of 59 with generalized cortical atrophy, particularly of the left hemisphere). The association with the frontal lobes appears only in his fourth case (Pick, 1906) (a 60-year-old man with 'bilateral frontal atrophy'). Which of these cases should, therefore, be considered as the first with Pick's disease? At the time, in fact, no one thought that Pick had described a new

disease; Barrett (1913) considered the two first cases of Pick's as atypical forms of AD, and Ziehen (1911) did not see anything special in them.

During the same period, Liepmann, Stransky, and Spielmeyer had described similar cases with aphasia and circumscribed cerebral atrophy (Mansvelt, 1954); so much so, that Urechia and Mihalescu felt tempted to name the syndrome 'Spielmeyer's disease' (Caron, 1934). This did not catch on, however, and in two classical papers on what he called 'Pick's disease', Carl Schneider (1927, 1929) constructed the new view of the condition by suggesting that it evolved in three stages – the first with a disturbance of judgement and behaviour, the second with localized symptoms (e.g. speech), and the third with generalized dementia. He recognized rapid and slow forms, the former with an akinetic and aphasic subtypes and a malignant course, and the latter with a predominance of plaques (probably indistinguishable from AD).

1.6 THE AFTERMATH

The history of the word 'dementia' must not be confused with that of the concepts or behaviours involved. By the year 1800, two definitions of dementia were recognized and both had psychosocial incompetence as their central concept: in addition to cognitive impairment, the clinical definition included other symptoms such as delusions and hallucinations; irreversibility and old age were not features of the condition, and in general dementia was considered to be a terminal state to all sorts of mental, neurological and physical conditions. The adoption of the anatomoclinical model by nineteenth century alienists changed this. Questions were asked as to the neuropathological basis of dementia and this, in turn, led to readjustments in its clinical description. The history of dementia during the nineteenth century is, therefore, the history of its gradual attrition. Stuporous states (then called acute dementia), vesanic dementias and localized memory impairments, were gradually reclassified, and by 1900 the cognitive paradigm, i.e. the view that the essential feature of dementia was intellectual impairment, was established. From then on, efforts were made to explain other symptoms, such as hallucinations, delusions, and mood and behavioural disorders, as epiphenomena and as unrelated to whatever the central mechanism of dementia was. There has also been a fluctuating acceptance of the parenchymal and vascular hypotheses, the latter leading to the description of arteriosclerotic dementia. The separation of the vesanic dementias and of the amnestic syndromes led to the realization that age and ageing mechanisms were important, and by 1900 senile dementia became the prototype of the dementias; by 1970, AD had become the flagship of the new approach. During the last few years, the cognitive paradigm has become an obstacle, and a gradual re-expansion of the symptomatology of dementia is fortunately taking place (Berrios, 1989, 1990a).

REFERENCES

Alzheimer A. (1907) Über eine eigenartige Erkrankung der Hirnrinde. *Allgemeine Zeitschrift für Psychiatrie und Psychisch-Gerichtlich Medizine* **64**: 146–148

Alzheimer A. (1911) Über eigenartige Krankheitsfälle des späteren Alters. *Zeitschrift für die gesamte Neurologie und Psychiatrie* **4**: 356–385

Anderson EW, Threthowan WH, Kenna JC. (1959) An experimental investigation of simulation and pseudodementia. *Acta Psychiatrica et Neurologica Scandinavica* **34** (Suppl. 132)

Anonymous (1832) An exposure of the unphilosophical and unchristian expedients adopted by antiphrenologists, for the purpose of obstructing the moral tendencies of phrenology. A review of John Wayte's book. *The Phrenological Journal and Miscellany* **7**: 615–622

Baillarger J. (1883) Sur la théorie de la paralysie générale. *Annales Médico-Psychologiques* **35**: 18–52; 191–218

Baillarger J. (1889) Doit-on dans la classification des maladies mentales assigner une place á part aux pseudo-paralysies générales? *Annales Médico-Psychologiques* **41**: 521–525

Ball B and Chambard E. (1881) Démence. In: A. Dechambre and L. Lereboullet (eds), *Dictionnaire Encyclopédique des Sciences Médicales*. Paris, Masson, pp. 559–605

Barrett AM. (1913) Presenile, arteriosclerotic and senile disorders of the brain and cord. In: WA White and SA Jelliffe (eds), *The Modern Treatment of Nervous and Mental Diseases*. London, Kimpton, pp. 675–709

Bayle ALJ. (1822) *Recherches Sur Les Maladies Mentales*. Paris, Thése de Médecine

Bayle ALJ. (1826) *Traité Des Maladies Du Cerveau*. Paris, Gabon et Compagnie

Beljahow S. (1889) Pathological changes in the brain in dementia senilis. *Journal of Mental Science* **35**: 261–262

Bercherie P. (1980) *Les Fondements De La Clinique*. Paris, La Bibliothéque d'Ornicar

Berrios GE. (1985a) 'Depressive pseudodementia' or 'melancholic dementia': a nineteenth century view. *Journal of Neurology, Neurosurgery, and Psychiatry* **48**: 393–400

Berrios GE. (1985b) Presbyophrenia: clinical aspects. *British Journal of Psychiatry* **147**: 76–79

Berrios GE. (1986) Presbyophrenia: the rise and fall of a concept. *Psychological Medicine* **16**: 267–275

Berrios GE. (1987) History of the functional psychoses. *British Medical Bulletin* **43**: 484–498

Berrios GE. (1989) Non-cognitive symptoms and the diagnosis of dementia. historical and clinical aspects. *British Journal of Psychiatry* **154** (Suppl. 4): 11–16

Berrios GE. (1990a) Memory and the cognitive paradigm of dementia during the nineteenth century: a conceptual history. In: R Murray and T Turner (eds), *Lectures on the History of Psychiatry*. London, Gaskell, pp. 194–211

Berrios GE. (1990b) Alzheimer's disease: a conceptual history. *International Journal of Geriatric Psychiatry* **5**: 355–365

Berrios GE. (1991) Affective disorders in old age: a conceptual history. *International Journal of Geriatric Psychiatry* **6**: 337–346

Berrios GE. (1994) The psychiatry of old age: a conceptual history. In: J Copeland, M Abou-Saleh and D Blazer (eds), *The Principles and Practice of Geriatric Psychiatry*. Chichester, Wiley, pp. 11–16

Berrios GE. (1996) The classification of mental disorders: Part III. *History of Psychiatry* **7**: 167–182

Berrios GE. (2000a) Dementia: A historical overview. In: O'Brien J, Ames D and Burns A (eds), *Dementia*, 2nd edition. London, Arnold, pp. 3–13

Berrios GE. (2000b) Confabulations. In: Berrios GE and Hodges JR (eds) *Memory Disorders in Clinical Practice*, Cambridge, Cambridge University Press, pp. 348–368

Berrios GE and Freeman H (eds) (1991) *Alzheimer and the Dementias*. London, Royal Society of Medicine

Berrios GE and Luque R. (1995) Cotard's delusion or syndrome? A conceptual history. *Comprehensive Psychiatry* **36**: 218–223

Bessière R. (1948) La presbyophrénie. *L'Encéphale* **37**: 313–342

Bianchi L. (1906) *A Texbook Of Psychiatry*. London, Baillière, Tindall and Cox

Blancard S. (1726) *The Physical Dictionary wherein the Terms of Anatomy, the Names and Causes of Diseases, Chirurgical Instruments, and their Use, are Accurately Described*. London, John and Benjamin Sprint

Bleuler E. (1911) *Dementia Praecox*. Leipzig, Deuticke (English Translation: *Dementia Praecox* (1950), New York, International Universities Press)

Boissier de Sauvages F. (1771) *Nosologie Methodique, Dans Laquelle les Maladies Sont Rangées par Classes, Suivant le Systême de Sydenham, et l'Order des Botanistes*. Paris, Hérissant le Fils

Bostroem A. (1933) Über Presbyophrenie. *Archiv für Psychiatrie und Nervenkrankenheiten* **99**: 339–354

Broca P. (1861) Perte de la parole, ramollissement chronique et destruction partielle du lobe anterieur gauche du cerveau. *Bulletin de la Société de Anthropologie* Paris **2**: 235–238

Bucknill JC and Tuke DH. (1858) *A Manual of Psychological Medicine*. London, John Churchill

Bulbena A and Berrios GE. (1986) Pseudodementia: facts and figures. *British Journal of Psychiatry* **148**: 87–94

Burger-Prinz H and Jacob H. (1938) Anatomische und klinische Studien zur senilen Demenz. *Zeitschrift für die gesamte Neurologie und Psychiatrie* **161**: 538–543

Calmeil LF. (1835) Démence. In: *Dictionnaire de Médicine on Repertoire General des Sciences Médicales*, 2nd edition. Paris, Bechet, pp. 70–85

Caron M. (1934) *Etude Clinique De La Maladie De Pick*, Paris, Vigot Fréres

Charcot JM. (1881) *Clinical Lectures on Senile and Chronic Diseases*. London, The New Sydenham Society

Cicero (1969) *Tusculanan disputations*. Translated by JE King. Vol XVIII, Cambridge, Loeb Classical Library

Code Napoléon (1808) *Edition Originale et Seule Officielle*. Paris, l'Imprimerie Impériale

Combe G. (1873) *Elements of Phrenology*, Edinburgh, MacLachlan and Stewart

Cotard J. (1882) Du délire des negations. *Archives de Neurologie* **4**: 152–170; 282–296

Crichton-Browne J. (1874) Senile dementia. *BMJ* i: 601–603; 640–643

DeFelipe J and Jones EG (eds) (1988) *Cajal on the Cerebral Cortex. An Annotated Translation of the Complete Writings*. Oxford, Oxford University Press

Diderot and d'Alembert (eds) (1765) *Encyclopédie ou Dictionnaire Raisonné des Sciences, des Arts et des Métieres, par une Societé de Gens de Lettres*. Vol 4, A Paris, Briasson, David, Le Breton, Durand, pp. 807–808

Dumas G. (1894) *Les États Intellectuels dans la mélancolie*. Paris, Alcan

Durand-Fardel M. (1843) *Traité du Ramollissement du Cerveau*. Paris, Baillière

Esquirol E. (1805) *Des Passions.* Paris, Didot Jeune

Esquirol E. (1814) Démence. In: *Dictionaire des Sciences Médicales, par une Societé de Médicins et de Chirurgiens.* Paris, Panckouke, pp. 280–293

Esquirol E. (1838) *Des Maladies Mentales.* Paris, Baillière

Feuchtersleben E. (first published in 1845, translated in 1847) *The Principles of Medical Psychology.* Translated by HE Lloyds and BG Babington. London, Sydenham Society.

Fischer O. (1907) Miliare Nekrosen mit drusigen Wucherungen der Neurofibrillen, eine regelmaessege Verandaerung der Hirnrinde bei seniler Demenz. *Monatsschrift für Psychiatrie und Neurologie* **22**: 361–372

Fischer O. (1912) Ein weiterer Beitrag zur Klinik und Pathologie der presbyophrenen Demenz. *Zeitschrift für die gesamte Neurologie und Psychiatrie* **12**: 99–135

Fournier A. (1875) *Syphilis du Cerveau.* Paris, Baillière

Fuller SC. (1907) A study of the neurofibrils in dementia paralytica, dementia senilis, chronic alcoholism, cerebral lues and microcephalic idiocy. *American Journal of Insanity* **63**: 415–468

Fuller SC. (1912) Alzheimer's disease (senium praecox): the report of a case and review of published cases. *Journal of Nervous and Mental Disease* **39**: 440–455; 536–557

Graeber MB, Kosel S, Egensperger R *et al.* (1997) Rediscovery of the case described by Alois Alzheimer in 1911: historical, histological and molecular genetic analysis. *Neurogenetics* **1**: 73–80

Graeber MB, Kosel S, Grasbon-Frodl E *et al.* (1998) Histopathology and APOE phenotype of the first Alzheimer's disease patient. *Neurogenetics* **1**: 223–238

Gratiolet LP. (1854) *Mémoires sur les Plis Cérébraux de l'homme et des Primates.* Paris, Bertrand

Griesinger W. (first published in 1861, translated in 1867) *Mental Pathology and Therapeutics.* Translated by CL Robertson and J Rutherford, London, Sydenham Society

Guislain J. (1852) *Leçons Orales sur les Phrénopathies.* Gand, L Hebbelynck

Hakkébousch BM and Geier TA. (1913) De la maladie d'Alzheimer. *Annales Médico-Psychologiques* **71**: 358

Hare E. (1959) The origin and spread of dementia paralytica. *Journal of Mental Science* **105**: 594–626

Heinroth JC. (first published 1818, translated in 1975) *Textbook of disturbances of mental life.* Baltimore, Johns Hopkins University Press

Henderson VH. (1986) Paul Broca's less heralded contributions to aphasia research. Historical perspective and contemporary relevance. *Archives of Neurology* **43**: 609–612

Jackson JH. (1875) A lecture on softening of the brain. *Lancet* **ii**: 335–339

Jackson JH. (1894) The factors of insanities. *Medical Press and Circular* **ii**: 615–625

Kahlbaum KL. (1863) *Die Gruppierung der psychischen Krankheiten,* Danzig, AW Kafemann

Kiloh LG. (1961) Pseudo-dementia. *Acta Psychiatrica Scandinavica* **37**: 336–351

Kleist K. (1960) Schizophrenic symptoms and cerebral pathology. *Journal of Mental Science* **106**: 246–255

Kraepelin E. (1886–1887) Über Erinnerungsfälschungen. *Archiv für Psychiatrie und Nervenkrankheiten* **17**: 830–843; **18**: 199–239, 395–436

Kraepelin E. (1910) *Psychiatrie: Ein Lehrbuch für Studierende und Ärzte.* Leipzig, Johann Ambrosius Barth

Kraepelin E. (1919) *Dementia Praecox.* Translated by RM Barclay and GM Robertson, Edinburgh, Livingstone

Krafft-Ebing R. (1873) De la démence sénile. *Annales Médico-Psychologiques* **34**: 306–307

Lafora GR. (1935) Sobre la presbiofrenia sin confabulaciones. *Archivos de Neurobiologia* **15**: 179–211

Lambert Cl. (1916) The clinical and anatomical features of Alzheimer's disease. *Journal of Mental and Nervous Disease* **44**: 169–170

Lanczik M. (1988) *Der Breslauer Psychiater Carl Wernicke.* Sigmaringen, Thorbecke

Lanteri-Laura G. (1970) *Histoire de la Phrenologie.* Paris, Presses Universitaires de France

Leonhard K. (1957) *Aufteilung der endogenen Psychosen.* Berlin, Akademie-Verlag

Lewis CT and Short C. (1969) *A Latin Dictionary.* Oxford, at the Clarendon Press (1st edition, 1879)

Lucretius (1975) *De Rerum Natura.* Translation by WHD Rouse. Cambridge. Harvard University Press.

Lugaro E. (1916) La psichiatria tedesca nella storia e nell'attualita. *Rivista di Patologia Nervosa e Mentale* **21**: 337–386

Madden JJ, Luhan JA, Kaplan LA *et al.* (1952) Non-dementing psychoses in older persons. *JAMA* **150**: 1567–1570

Mairet A. (1883) *De la Démence Mélancolique.* Paris, Masson

Mansvelt J. (1954) *Pick's Disease.* Enchede, Van der Loeff

Marcé LV. (1863) Recherches cliniques et anatomo-pathologiques sur la démence senile et sur les différences qui la separent de la paralysie générale. *Gazette Médicale de Paris* **34**: 433–435; 467–469; 497–502; 631–632; 761–764; 797–798; 831–833; 855–858

Marie A. (1906) *La Démence.* Paris, Doing

Maurer K and Maurer U. (1998) *Alzheimer. Das Leben eines Arztes und die Karriere einer Krankheiten.* Munich, Piper.

Meynert T. (1885) *Psychiatry. A Clinical Treatise on Diseases of the Fore-brain* (translated by B Sachs). New York, Putnam

Meynert T. (1890) Amentia. In: *Klinische Vorlesungen über Psychiatrie auf Wissenschaftlichen Grundlagen, für Studierende und Ärzte, Juristen und Psychologen.* Vienna, Braumüller

Morel BA. (1857) *Traité des Dégénérescences Physiques Intellectuelles et Morales de l'Espèce Humaine.* Paris, Baillière

Morel BA. (1860) *Traité des Maladies Mentales.* Paris, Masson

Niery D, Snowden JS, Northen B, Goulding P. (1988) Dementia of frontal lobe type. *Journal of Neurology, Neurosurgery, and Psychiatry* **51**: 353–361

North HM and Bostock F. (1925) Arteriosclerosis and mental disease. *Journal of Mental Science* **71**: 600–601

Olah G. (1910) Was kann man heute unter Arteriosklerotischen Psychosen verstehen? *Psych. Neur. Wochenschrift* **52**: 532–533

Parrot J. (1873) Cerveau. VIII Ramollissement. In: A Dechambre and L Lereboullet (eds), *Dictionnaire Encyclopédique des Sciences Médicales* Vol 14. Paris, Mason and Asselin, pp. 400–431

Perry R, McKeith I and Perry E (eds) (1996) *Dementia with Lewy Bodies,* Cambridge, Cambridge University Press

Perusini G. (1909) Über klinish und histologisch eigenartige psychische Erkrankungen des späteren Lebensalters. In: Nissl F and Alzheimer A (eds), *Histologische und histopatologische Arbeiten.* Vol **3**, 297–351

Perusini G. (1911) Sul valore nosografico di alcuni reperti istopatologici caratteristiche per la senilitá. *Rivista Italiana di Neuropatologia, Psichiatria ed Elettroterapia* **4**: 193–213

Pick A. (1892) Über die Beziehungen der senilen Hirnatrophie zur Aphasie. *Prager Medicinische Wochenschrift* **17**: 165–167 (Translated by Berrios GE and Girling DM (1994) Introduction to and translation of 'On the relationship between senile cerebral atrophy and aphasia' by Arnold Pick. *History of Psychiatry*, 1994, **5**: 539–549)

Pick A. (1901) Senile Hirnatrophie als Grundlage von Herderscheinungen. *Wiener Klinische Wochenschrift* **14**: 403–404

Pick A. (1906) Über einen weiterer Symptomenkomplex im Rahmen der Dementia senilis, bedingt durch umschriebene sträkere Hirnatrophie (gemische Apraxie). *Monatschrift für Psychiatrie und Neurologie* **19**: 97–108

Pick D. (1989) *Faces of Degeneration*. Cambridge, Cambridge University Press

Pinel Ph. (1806) *A Treatise On Insanity* (translated by DD Davis). Sheffield, Cadell and Davies

Pinel Ph. (1818) *Nosographie Philosophique*, 6th edition. Paris, Brosson (first published: 1798)

Prichard JC. (1835) *A Treatise on Insanity*. London, Sherwood, Gilbert and Piper

Rey A. (1995) *Dictionnaire Historique de la Langue Française*. 2 vols. Paris, Dictionnaire Le Robert

Rostan L. (1823) *Recherches sur le Ramollissement du Cerveau*, 2nd edition. Paris, Bechet

Rouby J. (1911) *Contribution á l'étude de la presbyophrénie*, Thèse de Médicine. Paris, E Nourris

Schneider C. (1927) Über Picksche Krankheit. *Monatschrift für Psychiatrie und Neurologie* **65**: 230–275

Schneider C. (1929) Weitere Beiträge zur Lehre von der Pickschen Krankheit. *Zeitschrift für the gesamte Neurologie und Psychiatrie*, **120**: 340–384

Simchowicz T. (1911) Histologische Studien über die Senile Demenz. *Histologische und histopathologischen Arbeiten über der Grosshirnrinde* **4**: 267–444

Simchowicz T. (1924) Sur la signification des plaques séniles et sur la formule sénile de l'écorce cérébrale. *Revue Neurologique* **31**: 221–227

Sobrino (1791) *Aumentado o Nuevo Diccionario de las Lenguas Española, Francesa Y Latina*. Leon de Francia, JB Delamollière

Southard EE. (1910) Anatomical findings in 'senile dementia': a diagnostic study bearing especially on the group of cerebral atrophies. *American Journal of Insanity* **61**: 673–708

Sully J. (1885) *Illusions. A psychological study*, 5th edition. London, Kegan Paul

Truelle V and Bessière R. (1911) Recherches sur la Presbyophrénie. *L'Encéphale* **6**: 505–520

Walton GL. (1912) Arteriosclerosis probably not an important factor in the etiology and prognosis of involution psychoses. *Boston Medical and Surgical Journal* **167**: 834–836

Wilks S. (1865) Clinical notes on atrophy of the brain. *Journal of Mental Science* **10**: 381–392

Willis T. (1684) *Practice of Physick* (translated by S Pordage). London, T Dring, C Harper and J Leigh, pp. 209–214

Ziehen T. (1911) Les démences. In: A. Marie (ed.) *Traité International de Psychologie Pathologique*, Vol 2, Paris, Alcan, pp. 281–381

Zilboorg G. (1941) *A History of Medical Psychology*. New York, Norton

Epidemiology

DANIEL W O'CONNOR

2.1 SCOPE OF EPIDEMIOLOGY

Epidemiology is the study of the distribution and determinants of disease in human populations. It maps the frequency of disease and identifies people at higher or lower risk of contracting particular conditions. Once risk factors are confirmed, their impact can be reduced. Studies linking cigarette smoking with lung cancer and hypertension with stroke have sparked successful campaigns to limit smoking and detect hypertension. These programmes have saved lives and extended life expectancy. Ideally, epidemiological studies will identify triggers to Alzheimer's disease (AD) and other causes of dementia.

Links between life experience and disease are identified by means of *observational, analytical* and *experimental* approaches (Jablensky, 2002). Observational studies entail large scale surveys to measure the frequency of dementia and note simple correlations with sociodemographic, biological and medical variables. Surveys, while costly and time-consuming, are essential in conditions like dementia, which go mostly unrecognized by primary and specialist health services, even in developed countries. In one UK study, in a town with well-developed aged psychiatry services, general practitioners recognized only 58 per cent of dementia cases and psychiatrists knew of only 20 per cent (O'Connor *et al.*, 1988, 1990).

Analytical studies contrast the backgrounds of people with dementia (drawn from community surveys or clinical practice) with those of matched controls to identify points of difference that might, on further study, prove to be risk factors. These could include past illnesses or injuries, occupational exposures, diet and lifestyle. Case–control studies are economical, but accurate matching is problematic and correlations may emerge by chance if questions cover many dozens of items. To complicate matters, people with advanced dementia cannot report accurately on their own social, occupational and medical histories. Information must therefore be sought from relatives whose knowledge is imperfect and subject to bias.

Both types of study, observational and analytical, generate hypotheses to be tested in randomized control trials (RCTs). These are essential as analytical studies are sometimes misleading. The finding in some (but not all) case–control studies that oestrogen replacement therapy conferred protection against dementia (e.g. Yaffe *et al.*, 1998) was not confirmed by RCTs (e.g. Shumaker *et al.*, 2003). Possible explanations for this anomaly include small study size and sample bias (e.g. women in the case–control series who took hormone therapy were often better educated and generally healthier) (Shumaker *et al.*, 2003).

Epidemiology, which is both an applied and theoretical science, also addresses healthcare requirements, carer burden, access to services and the larger-scale effectiveness of medical and social interventions. Practical questions regarding social burden, service use and the like are easily 'tacked on' to community surveys. More penetrating questions regarding the larger-scale effectiveness of medical and social interventions require independent study.

2.1.1 Scope of this chapter

Other chapters in this text address risk factors for AD (Chapter 27) and vascular dementia (Chapter 43); carer burden (Chapter 11); health economics (Chapter 12) and international service perspectives (Chapter 20). This chapter will focus instead on the prevalence and incidence of dementia, AD and vascular dementia (VaD).

2.2 METHODOLOGICAL ISSUES

The *prevalence* of dementia is the proportion of people within a defined population who meet investigators' diagnostic specifications (usually expressed as a per cent). *Incidence* refers to the proportion of people who develop dementia within a period of time (usually expressed as a rate per 1000 person-years at risk). Prevalence studies are simpler: people are divided into 'cases' of dementia and 'non-cases' at a single point in time. Some will have developed dementia recently: others will have had it for many years. A community might therefore have a higher than usual prevalence because residents with dementia live longer than usual. *Incidence* studies entail two surveys, a year or more apart, to determine annual conversion rates of former 'non-cases' to 'cases'. They are of greater scientific value since risk factors for conversion are not confounded by longevity.

The first surveys of mental disorder date from the 1950s. Lin (1953), who supplemented brief evaluations of the inhabitants of three Taiwanese communities with information from relatives, officials and hospitals, concluded that only 0.5 per cent of people aged 60+ had 'senile dementia'. By contrast, Essen-Möller (1956), who made a similar two-staged sweep of the entire population of adjoining Swedish parishes, diagnosed 19 per cent of people aged 70+ years with 'mild dementia' and another 9 per cent with 'severe dementia'.

This 30-fold discrepancy might reflect genuine differences between European and Asian communities or else discrepancies in contact procedures, refusal rates, assessment procedures and diagnostic criteria. Methodological factors were most probably to blame. Studies in which a low score on a simple cognitive test triggers a 'diagnosis' will generate more cases than studies that require evidence of cognitive and functional decline (Jorm *et al.*, 1987).

Even the simplest assessment procedures distinguish correctly between healthy old people and those with advanced dementia. Discrepancies arise mostly at the cleavage point between 'mild cognitive impairment' on the one hand and 'early dementia' on the other. Since most early dementias merge imperceptibly with age-related cognitive impairment, the dividing line is arbitrary.

Erkinjuntti *et al.* (1997) used data from a multistage survey of 10 000 older Canadians to illustrate how diagnostic criteria (and also assessment procedures) shape prevalence rates. Within the 19 per cent of respondents selected for further testing, 3.1 per cent met ICD-10 criteria for dementia compared with 29 per cent for DSM-IIIR. The more stringent ICD-10 requires impairment of long-term memory, activities of daily living and executive function. Had all respondents in this study been examined in detail, the discrepancy would certainly have been smaller but the point remains that results are influenced by assessment procedures, diagnostic criteria and cutpoints.

Despite decades of research, there is no commonly recognized procedure to identify, screen, assess and diagnose dementia in community populations. Table 2.1 summarizes the methods employed in three unusually large, well-documented reports from established researchers in Liverpool, UK (Copeland *et al.*, 1987); Shanghai, China (Zhang *et al.*, 1990) and Cache County, USA (Lyketsos *et al.*, 2000). Their diversity of approach, which makes it difficult to compare one study with another, stems from dementia's insidious onset and lack of distinct biological correlates. Other degenerative conditions

Table 2.1 *Comparison of methods in three dementia prevalence studies*

	Liverpool, UK (1987)	Shanghai, China (1990)	Cache County, USA (2000)
First author	Copeland	Zhang	Lyketsos
Respondents (N)	1070	5055	5092
Age range	65+	55+	65+
Contact mode	General practice sample	Household sample	Whole aged population
Institutions	Included	Excluded	Included
First screening test	None	MMSE	Modified MMSE or informant interview
Second screening test	None	None	Dementia Questionnaire
Diagnostic assessment	Structured interview	Clinical evaluation	Clinical evaluation
Other investigations	None	Neuropsychology, physical examination	Neuropsychology, physical examination, laboratory tests, brain MRI
Diagnostic criteria	AGECAT	DSM-III	DSM-IV
Dementia severity ratings	AGECAT	DSM-III	CDR scale
Dementia subtypes*	No	AD, VaD	AD, VaD, FTD, DLB, others
Research personnel	Trained interviewers	Trained interviewers, psychiatrist	Trained interviewers, psychiatrist, neurologist, neuropsychologist
Dementia prevalence 65+	5.2%	4.6%	6.6%

* Dementia subtypes: Alzheimer (AD), vascular (VaD), frontotemporal (FTD), dementia with Lewy bodies (DLB)

like arthritis and cataracts can be visualized and graded directly: dementia cannot, with the result that investigators persist in developing their own procedures and instruments. Despite this, prevalence rates in the three selected projects are remarkably similar.

2.2.1 Screening

Surveys are so expensive that most researchers use the Mini-Mental State Examination (MMSE) (Folstein *et al.*, 1975) or other brief cognitive tests to select respondents for more detailed evaluation (Fratiglioni *et al.*, 1999). The 30-point MMSE, which takes only 10 minutes or so to administer and requires no specialist equipment, is well-suited to this task, at least in developed countries. In a large British community survey, 86 per cent of people with dementia scored 23 points or less (sensitivity) and 92 per cent of 'normals' scored 24 and above (specificity) (O'Connor *et al.*, 1989a). However, only 55 per cent of persons scoring 23 points or less met criteria for an organic mental disorder (true positive ratio) so further investigation is mandatory.

Since the MMSE tests reading, writing and arithmetic, performance is shaped by education. In the same UK study, 11 per cent of 'normal' older people who left school before their fifteenth birthday scored 23 points or less compared with only 3 per cent of those with higher education. Conversely, the same cut-point missed 27 per cent of dementias in better educated people compared with only 12 per cent in those with limited educations (O'Connor *et al.*, 1989b). One strategy in two-phase studies is to evaluate all who fail the screening test and a proportion of 'high scorers' to limit the risk of missing early dementias.

The MMSE is not an appropriate screening tool in developing countries where older people are often illiterate and innumerate. It is better to combine tests less subject to educational bias (e.g. naming, praxis and recall) with reports from family members about cognitive and functional capacity. One such instrument, the Community Screening Instrument for Dementia (CSI-D), has high sensitivity and specificity in Native American, African American and Nigerian communities, particularly when scores are adjusted for years of education (Hall *et al.*, 1993). Further refinements emerged from a multinational study of older people in India, China, Asia, Latin America and the Caribbean (Prince *et al.*, 2003), but these instruments still tap skills acquired in the schoolroom. Computer-administered tests with a game-like interface have been developed for clinical purposes but have much to offer in community research (Sahakian and Owen, 1992; Darby *et al.*, 2002).

With respect to geographic scope, some investigators approach all eligible residents of a suburb or town. Others employ complex strategies to select representative residents of entire cities, states or countries. A narrower focus promotes compliance, reduces costs and makes follow up easier. Larger scale studies ensure that findings can be generalized to the whole of a region or nation (Jablenksy, 2002). The choice of method is driven by study resources and objectives.

2.2.2 Diagnosis

Diagnostic evaluations vary widely. Structured interviews administered by lay interviewers (e.g. the Geriatric Mental State: Copeland *et al.*, 1987) or trained clinicians (e.g. CAMDEX: Roth *et al.*, 1986) have been largely supplanted by combinations of a history, mental state examination, cognitive battery and informant interview. Interviews, which are conducted by a neurologist or psychiatrist with input from a neuropsychologist, are then supplemented by laboratory tests and neuroimaging. Most recent European and North American surveys have adopted the latter, more expensive approach (e.g. Fratiglioni *et al.*, 1999).

Informant interviews are essential. Dementia impairs memory, insight and understanding and so information must be sought from a relative or carer about the subject's personal details, cognitive and functional status, medical and psychiatric history and current medications. These details help to confirm the diagnosis of dementia, especially in its early stages, and to distinguish AD from other disorders. Informants' reports correlate highly with other markers of cognitive and functional capacity: underreporting and overreporting are remarkably uncommon (Jorm and Korten, 1988; O'Connor *et al.*, 1989c). Unfortunately, some respondents forbid contact with informants and a few have no surviving relatives.

If research findings are to carry weight, diagnostic criteria must be interpreted similarly in different centres (i.e. have high interrater reliability) and be accurate. In a study of five research centres in Australia, Germany, the Netherlands, UK and USA, in which clinicians were asked to apply DSM-IIIR and Clinical Dementia Rating (CDR) criteria to 100 vignettes of older people identified in clinics and community surveys, between-centre agreement rates were good (Kappa 0.74–0.83 for DSM-IIIR, and 0.50–0.69 for CDR). Rates were lower for people in the borderland between 'normal ageing' and 'mild dementia', and for those who were physically frail, deaf, anxious or depressed (O'Connor *et al.*, 1996), but not to a degree that jeopardized comparison of one study with another.

Community diagnoses based on thorough clinical evaluations and informant histories have acceptable validity. In a large British survey, only three of 56 people diagnosed with mild dementia by CAMDEX were passed as normal 2 years later (O'Connor *et al.*, 1991). Factors contributing to mistaken diagnoses included deafness, depression and unstable diabetes mellitus.

Validity is best confirmed by neuropathological examination but collecting post-mortem material in community populations is difficult. Holmes *et al.* (1999) succeeded in collecting brain tissue from 80 aged people with dementia recruited from psychiatric, medical and social services in London, UK. Initial assessments comprising a structured diagnostic and informant interview (CAMDEX), physical examination and CT brain scan were followed by yearly re-examinations until death. Clinical and neuropathological diagnoses were based on detailed, standardized criteria and protocols. Of the 38 people judged in life to have probable AD, 29 showed only neuritic plaques at autopsy, six had mixed pathologies and three had other conditions. Of the seven judged to have probable vascular dementia (VaD), three showed only infarcts and four had other conditions. Similarly, 41 per cent of people with dementia in a community autopsy series in Cambridge, UK had 'micro-infarcts', 14 per cent had 'macro-infarcts' and 23 per cent had cortical Lewy bodies (Xuereb et al., 2000). Multiple pathologies are the norm in advanced old age and simple attributions to AD or VaD must be interpreted cautiously.

2.3 DEMENTIA PREVALENCE

If dementia is truly commoner in one part of the world, or in people from a particular background, searches using finer-grained observational and analytical techniques will uncover the genetic, sociodemographic or environmental factors responsible. Unfortunately, the discrepancies reported to date most probably stem from the methodological vagaries noted already and there is little point, therefore, in listing every completed study. The following sections will focus instead on

- meta-analyses that pool the results of individual studies, and
- reports comparing prevalence rates in disparate communities using identical techniques.

The latter approach is of greater scientific interest since meta-analyses, which arrive at an average figure, might overlook genuinely novel observations.

In the first of several meta-analyses, Jorm et al. (1987) took findings from 22 reports to construct a statistical model relating dementia prevalence to age and study characteristics (Table 2.2). Rates varied widely but underlying all studies was a consistent trend for prevalence to rise exponentially with age with a doubling in rates with every 5.1 years. This was confirmed by Hofman et al. (1991) who reanalysed data from 12 European studies conducted between 1977 and 1989 in which dementia was defined using DSM-III or equivalent criteria. No major differences emerged between countries. Fratiglioni et al. (1999) drew similar conclusions with the proviso that rates from a new African study were strikingly low (see below). Broadly speaking, the prevalence of dementia as defined by DSM-III or its equivalent looks to be fairly uniform, at least in developed countries.

This makes it possible to map the likely numbers of people with dementia in coming decades. Since the growth in older age-groups is higher in developing countries than developed ones, half of all people with dementia currently live in Asia (Table 2.3). Wimo et al. (2003) anticipate that dementia cases will increase in number in less developed countries from 13 million in the year 2000 to 84 million in 2050 (646 per cent increase). Numbers in developed countries might grow from 12 million to 20 million (167 per cent increase). The implications for health and social services in all world areas are staggering.

Table 2.3 *Estimated numbers of people with dementia in 2000 (Source: Wimo et al., 2003)*

	Number of cases (millions)	% of total
Asia	11.87	46.5
Europe	7.43	29.1
North America	3.08	12.1
Latin America	1.69	6.6
Africa	1.25	4.9
Oceania	0.21	0.8
Total		100.0

Table 2.2 *Prevalence rates (%) for dementia in four meta-analyses*

	Jorm et al. (1987)	Hofman et al. (1991)	Ritchie and Kaldea (1995)	Fratiglioni et al. (1999)	
Number of studies	22	12	9	36	
Places	Europe, USA, Japan, Australia	Europe	Europe, Canada, Japan	Europe, USA, Canada, Asia, Africa	
Results					
Age					Mean
65–69	1.4	1.4	1.5	1.5	1.5
70–74	2.8	4.1	3.5	3	3.5
75–79	5.6	5.7	6.8	6	6.3
80–84	10.5	13.0	13.6	12	13.1
85–89	20.8	21.6	22.3		22.1
90–94	38.6	32.2	31.5		31.7
95–99		34.7	44.5		41.2

If it is true that prevalence increases exponentially with age, varying only in its time of onset, all of us will be affected at some point in our lives. This hypothesis, which has major public health implications, was tested by Ritchie and Kildea (1995), who constructed another statistical model derived from 12 studies with data for subjects over age 80 and with adequate sampling procedures and diagnostic methods. This modified logistic model differed slightly – but critically – from Jorm's, showing a flattening of growth at age 95 when prevalence is 40 per cent, suggesting that dementia is not inevitable.

2.4 ALZHEIMER'S DISEASE

2.4.1 Prevalence

While mapping the spread of dementia, irrespective of cause, has great practical value, pointers to risk factors are more likely to come from studies of specific dementing conditions. Unfortunately, 'yes-no' diagnoses of AD, VaD and the like are artificial constructs and epidemiological reports must be interpreted cautiously. Neuropathology in advanced old age, when most dementias arise, is so complex that many 'Alzheimer' cases also have cerebrovascular disease and *vice versa* (see above).

Table 2.4 presents findings from a meta-analysis of AD prevalence using data from 11 European studies conducted in the 1990s (Lobo *et al.*, 2000). Rates were similar to those in an earlier, overlapping analysis by Rocca *et al.* (1991). Differences exist between studies nonetheless. In the 11

reports considered by Lobo *et al.*, methods varied widely with prevalence at age 85–89 years, for example, ranging from 5 per cent to 25 per cent.

Rates were lower overall in the 17 Chinese reports summarized by Liu *et al.* (2003) but females were at higher risk than men on both continents. In China, for instance, about 5 per cent of men aged 80–84 years have AD compared with 13 per cent of women. In China, rates were also higher in urban areas than rural ones.

Corrada *et al.* (1995) applied logistic regression to identify methodological reasons for differences in 15 published papers from Europe, USA, Japan and China. After age had been adjusted for, higher rates occurred in studies that included mild cases and used laboratory tests to aid in diagnosis. Lower rates emerged from studies that used CT brain scans and cerebral ischaemia scores. This is not surprising. Studies that can afford laboratory tests are likely to be more thorough in other respects too, and studies using brain scans might attribute cases (rightly or wrongly) to vascular pathology.

2.4.2 Incidence

Differences between groups in the prevalence of AD could stem from differences in either its incidence or duration. Incidence studies, which entail a second sweep of a population to identify new cases, are better suited to identifying causative factors, but are expensive and relatively few in number.

Table 2.5 summarizes findings from four meta-analyses. Incidence rose with age in all four, just as expected. Rates were somewhat higher in two and lower in the others. Incidence levelled off in extreme old age in one study (Gao *et al.*, 1998) but not in another (Jorm and Jolley, 1998). (It also decreased in a recent, well-conducted study of 5000 older people in the USA (Miech *et al.*, 2002).) Women were at increased risk in all of the three studies that specified rates by gender. Possible explanations include women's lower levels of education and the premature onset of dementia in men owing to head trauma, occupational toxicity and smoking (Andersen *et al.*, 1999; Fratiglioni *et al.*, 2000). Rates were a little lower in Asian countries than the USA and Europe,

Table 2.4 *Prevalence rates (%) of Alzheimer's disease in a meta-analysis of 11 European studies (Source: Lobo et al., 2000)*

Age	Males	Females
65–69	0.6	0.7
70–74	1.5	2.3
75–79	1.8	4.3
80–84	6.3	84
85–89	8.8	14.2
90+	17.6	23.6

Table 2.5 *Incidence rates (cases per 1000 person years at risk) of Alzheimer's disease in four meta-analyses*

	Jorm and Jolley (1998)	Gao *et al.* (1998)	Fratiglioni *et al.* (2000)	Brookmeyer *et al.* (1998)
Number of studies	23	7	8	4
Places	Europe, USA, Asia	Europe, USA	Europe	USA
Age				
65–69	3.5	3.3	1.2	1.7
70–74	7.4	8.4	3.3	3.5
75–79	15.5	18.2	9.1	7.1
80–84	32.7	33.6	21.8	14.4
85–89	68.7	53.3	35.3	29.2
90–94	144.3	72.9		59.5
95+				121.0

perhaps because of the lower prevalence of the ApoE ε4 allele in Japan and environmental and lifestyle differences (Jorm and Jolley, 1998).

2.4.3 Comparative studies

Putative socio-environmental risk factors will be identified more confidently if identical case-finding tools are applied to groups with vastly different social, educational, dietary, occupational and medical exposures. Studies of North American Whites, Blacks and Latinos generally show higher dementia rates in socially disadvantaged groups (Hendrie, 1999) but their backgrounds overlap too much to draw straightforward conclusions.

More revealing findings have emerged from a direct comparison of dementia in elderly Nigerian Africans and African Americans. This decade-long study applied identical screening tests and diagnostic evaluations comprising neuropsychology, informant interviews, personal evaluations and CT brain scans to residents of Ibadan, Nigeria and Indianapolis, USA (Hendrie et al., 1995). Contrary to expectation, the age-standardized prevalence rate of AD was lower in Nigerians aged 65+ years than African Americans (1.4 per cent versus 6.2 per cent). Rates for dementia of all causes were lower too (2.3 per cent versus 8.2 per cent). This disparity was not due just to the longer survival of dementia cases in North America. In a 5-year follow up, age-standardized annual incidence rates of AD were still lower in Ibadan than Indianapolis (1.2 per cent versus 2.5 per cent) (Hendrie et al., 2001). Possible reasons include the marginally significant association in Africa between AD and possession of the ApoE ε4 allele (Osuntokun et al., 1995) and also lower cholesterol levels, lower body mass index, less hypertension and less diabetes mellitus (Hendrie et al., 2001). Other methodologically rigorous cross-cultural investigations will prove of great interest.

2.5 VASCULAR DEMENTIA

2.5.1 Prevalence

Estimating the prevalence of VaD is difficult: definitions and assessment methods vary too widely to give confidence in study findings. In a review by Rocca and Kokmen (1999), for example, prevalence rates were higher in studies that lumped 'mixed dementia' with 'vascular dementia' and that based diagnoses on neuroimaging reports rather than clinically evident stroke.

In a meta-analysis by Lobo et al. (2000), rates were lower than those for AD (Table 2.6). This fits well with findings from community autopsy series in the USA and UK showing the preponderance of Alzheimer's pathology with high admixtures of vascular abnormalities (Holmes et al., 1999; Lim et al., 1999).

Vascular dementia rates look to be higher, though, in Asian countries. When Fratiglioni et al. (1999) summarized findings from 25 European studies and five from Japan, Korea, India and China, the proportions of cases ascribed to VaD were 28 per cent in Europe and 38 per cent in Asia. It occurred twice as often than AD in a series of Japanese studies but exceptions exist: ratios were similar, for example, in two studies conducted in China with US collaborators (Graves et al., 1996).

Caucasian-Asian differences might be real, not artefactual. In one rigorous, 7-year Japanese study in which diagnoses were confirmed whenever possible by post-mortem examination, 61 per cent of dementias in men were attributed to vascular disease, a much higher rate than observed in equivalent studies in Europe and the USA (Yoshitake et al., 1995). Lifestyle is possibly more influential than genes: rates of VaD in elderly Japanese-American men in mainland USA were similar to those of other North Americans (Graves et al., 1996). By contrast, Japanese men in Hawaii, whose lifestyle is more authentically Asian, have VaD rates similar to those in Japan (White et al., 1996).

2.5.2 Incidence

Incidence rates vary widely from study to study for the reasons outlined above but are generally much lower than for AD (Table 2.7). Males are possibly at higher risk than females in 'younger' old age but at lower risk later (Rocca and Kokmen, 1999; Fratiglioni et al., 2000). Rates look to be higher too in Asian populations than North American ones (Fratiglioni et al., 2000), more in older studies perhaps than recent ones (Homma

Table 2.6 *Prevalence rates (%) of vascular dementia in a meta-analysis of 11 European studies (Source: Lobo et al., 2000)*

Age	Males	Females
65–69	0.5	0.1
70–74	0.8	0.6
75–79	1.9	0.9
80–84	2.4	2.3
85–89	2.4	3.5
90+	3.6	5.8

Table 2.7 *Incidence rates (cases per 1000 person years at risk) of vascular dementia in a meta-analysis of 8 European studies (Source: Fratiglioni et al., 2000)*

Age	Males	Females
65–69	1.2	0.3
70–74	1.6	0.8
75–79	3.9	3.2
80–84	8.3	4.5
85–89	6.2	6.1
90+	10.9	7.0

and Hasegawa, 2000). More definitive findings will emerge from the ongoing Ni-Hon-Sea dementia project which applies identical methodologies to longitudinal surveys in Japan, Hawaii and Seattle (Graves *et al.*, 1996).

2.6 OTHER DEMENTIAS

While most attention has been paid to AD and VaD, dementia due to other causes accounted for 11 per cent of cases in the 25 European prevalence surveys summarized by Fratiglioni *et al.* (1999) and 15 per cent of North American and Asian ones. Few studies have applied current diagnostic criteria for dementia with Lewy bodies (DLB) and frontotemporal dementia (FTD) to community populations, but more will do so in the future as study methods become more sophisticated.

The findings to hand are too variable to interpret. In Finland, 3.3 per cent of people aged 75 years and over were judged to have DLB (Rahkonen *et al.*, 2003). By contrast, only 0.1 per cent of Japanese people aged 65 years and over met identical criteria following a detailed personal evaluation (Yamada *et al.*, 2001). Dementias due to genuinely reversible causes (e.g. vitamin deficiency, cerebral tumours and normal pressure hydrocephalus) are rare (Clarfield, 2003).

2.7 CONCLUSIONS

Descriptive epidemiological surveys have failed to identify factors other than age and genetic endowment that cause dementia in community populations. The return for investment to date is very low.

Surveys of dementia prevalence and incidence provide widely varying rates, mostly because of differences in methodology.

Dementia might be commoner in certain places and cultures. It is important, therefore, to compare incidence (not prevalence) rates of AD, VaD, etc. in aged people from widely different genetic, social, occupational and medical backgrounds.

Future studies will rely greatly on culture-free cognitive tests and interviews with informants. Computerized tests with game-like interfaces offer great promise.

REFERENCES

Andersen K, Launer LJ, Dewey ME *et al.* (1999) Gender differences in the incidence of AD and vascular dementia: the Eurodem studies. *Neurology* **53**: 1992–1997

Brookmeyer R, Gray S, Kawas C. (1998) Projections of Alzheimer's disease in the United States and the public health impact of delaying disease onset. *American Journal of Public Health* **88**: 1337–1342

Clarfield AM. (2003) The decreasing prevalence of reversible dementias: an updated meta-analysis. *Archives of Internal Medicine* **163**: 2219–2229

Copeland JRM, Dewey ME, Wood N. (1987) Range of mental illness among the elderly in the community – prevalence in Liverpool using the GMS-AGECAT package. *British Journal of Psychiatry* **150**: 815–823

Corrada M, Brookmeyer R, Kawas C. (1995) Sources of variability in prevalence rates of Alzheimer's disease. *International Journal of Epidemiology* **24**: 1000–1005

Darby D, Maruff P, Collie A, McStephen M. (2002) Mild cognitive impairment can be detected by multiple assessments in a single day. *Neurology* 59: 1042–1046

Erkinjuntti T, Ostbye T, Steenhuis R, Hachinski V. (1997) The effect of different diagnostic criteria on the prevalence of dementia. *New England Journal of Medicine* **337**: 1667–1674

Essen-Möller E. (1956) Individual traits and morbidity in a Swedish rural population. *Acta Psychiatrica Scandanavica* **100** (Suppl.): 1–160

Folstein MF, Folstein SE, McHugh PR. (1975) Mini-mental State: a practical method for grading the cognitive state of patients for clinicians. *Journal of Psychiatric Research* **12**: 189–198

Fratiglioni L, De Ronchi D, Aguera-Torres H. (1999) Worldwide prevalence and incidence of dementia. *Drugs and Aging* **15**: 365–375

Fratiglioni L, Launer LJ, Anderson K *et al.* (2000) Incidence of dementia and major sub-types in Europe: a collaborative study of population-based cohorts. *Neurology* **54** (Suppl. 5), S10–15

Gao S, Hendrie HC, Hall KS, Hui S. (1998) The relationships between age, sex and the incidence of dementia and Alzheimer disease: a meta-analysis. *Archives of General Psychiatry* **55**: 809–815

Graves AB, Larson EB, Edland SD *et al.* (1996) Prevalence of dementia and its subtypes in the Japanese American population of King County, Washington State: the Kame project. *American Journal of Epidemiology* **144**: 760–771

Hall KS, Hendrie HC, Brittain HM *et al.* (1993) The development of a dementia screening interview in two distinct languages. *International Journal of Methods in Psychiatric Research* **3**: 1–28

Hendrie HC. (1999) Alzheimer's disease: a review of cross-cultural studies. In: R Mayeux and Y Christen (eds), *Epidemiology of Alzheimer's: from Gene to Prevention*. Berlin, Springer-Verlag, pp. 87–101

Hendrie HC, Osuntokun BO, Hall KS *et al.* (1995) Prevalence of Alzheimer's disease and dementia in two communities: Nigerian Africans and African Americans. *American Journal of Psychiatry* **152**: 1485–1492

Hendrie HC, Ogunniyi A, Hall KS *et al.* (2001) Incidence of dementia and Alzheimer's disease in 2 communities: Yoruba residing in Ibadan, Nigeria and African Americans residing in Indianapolis, Indiana. *JAMA* **285**: 739–747

Hofman A, Rocca WA, Brayne C *et al.* (1991) The prevalence of dementia in Europe: a collaborative study of 1980–1990 findings. *International Journal of Epidemiology* **20**: 736–748

Holmes C, Cairns N, Lantos P, Mann A. (1999) Validity of current clinical criteria for Alzheimer's disease, vascular dementia and dementia with Lewy bodies. *British Journal of Psychiatry* **174**: 45–50

Homma A and Hasegawa K. (2000) Epidemiology of vascular dementia in Japan. In: E Chiu, L Gustafson, D Ames and MF Folstein (eds), *Cerebrovascular Disease and Dementia: Pathology, Neuropsychiatry and Management*. London, Martin Dunitz, pp. 33–46

Jablenksy A. (2002) Research methods in psychiatric epidemiology: an overview. *Australian and New Zealand Journal of Psychiatry* **36**: 297–310

Jorm AF and Korten AE. (1988) Assessment of cognitive decline in the elderly by informant interview. *British Journal of Psychiatry* **152**: 209–213

Jorm AF and Jolley D. (1998) The incidence of dementia: a meta-analysis. *Neurology* **51**: 728–733

Jorm AF, Korten AE, Henderson AS. (1987) The prevalence of dementia: a quantitative integration of the literature. *Acta Psychiatrica Scandanavica* **76**: 465–479

Lin TY. (1953) A study of the incidence of mental disorder in Chinese and other cultures. *Psychiatry* **16**: 313–336

Lim A, Tsuang D, Kukull W *et al.* (1999) Clinico-neuropathological correlation of Alzheimer's disease in a community-based case series. *Journal of the American Geriatrics Society* **47**: 564–569

Liu L, Guo XE, Zhou YQ, Xia JL. (2003) Prevalence of dementia in China. *Dementia and Geriatric Cognitive Disorders* **15**: 226–230

Lobo A, Launer LJ, Fratiglioni L *et al.* (2000) Prevalence of dementia and major sub-types in Europe: a collaborative study of population-based cohorts. *Neurology* **54** (Suppl. 5), S4–9

Lyketsos CG, Steinberg M, Tschanz JT *et al.* (2000) Mental and behavioural disturbances in dementia: findings from the Cache County study on memory in aging. *American Journal of Psychiatry* **157**: 708–714

Miech RA, Breitner JCS, Zandi PP *et al.* (2002) Incidence of AD may decline in the early 90s for men, later for women. *Neurology* **58**: 209–218

O'Connor DW, Pollitt PA, Hyde JB *et al.* (1988) Do general practitioners miss dementia in elderly patients? *BMJ* **297**: 1107–1110

O'Connor DW, Pollitt PA, Hyde JB *et al.* (1989a) The reliability and validity of the Mini-mental State in a British community survey. *Journal of Psychiatric Research* **23**: 87–96

O'Connor DW, Pollitt PA, Treasure FP *et al.* (1989b) The influence of education, social class and sex on Mini-Mental State scores. *Psychological Medicine*: **19**: 771–776

O'Connor DW, Pollitt PA, Brook CPB, Reiss BB. (1989c) The validity of informant histories in a community study of dementia. *International Journal of Geriatric Psychiatry* **4**: 203–208

O'Connor DW, Pollitt PA, Roth M, Brook CPB, Reiss BB. (1990) Problems reported by relatives in a community study of dementia. *British Journal of Psychiatry* **156**: 835–841

O'Connor DW, Pollitt PA, Jones BJ *et al.* (1991) Continued clinical validation of dementia diagnosed in the community using the Cambridge Mental Disorders of the Elderly Examination. *Acta Psychiatrica Scandanavica* **83**: 41–45

O'Connor DW, Blessed G, Cooper B *et al.* (1996) Cross-national interrater reliability of dementia diagnosis in the elderly and factors associated with disagreement. *Neurology* **47**: 1194–1199

Osuntokun BO, Sahota A, Ogunniyi AO *et al.* (1995) Lack of an association between apolipoprotein E epsilon 4 and Alzheimer's disease in elderly Nigerians. *Annals of Neurology* **38**: 463–465

Prince M, Acosta D, Chiu H *et al.* (2003) Dementia diagnosis in developing countries: a cross-cultural validation study. *Lancet* **361**: 909–917

Rahkonen T, Eloniemi-Sulkava U, Rissanen S *et al.* (2003) Dementia with Lewy bodies according to the consensus criteria in a general population aged 75 years and older. *Journal of Neurology, Neurosurgery, and Psychiatry* **74**: 720–724

Ritchie K and Kildea D. (1995) Is senile dementia 'age-related' or 'ageing-related'? – Evidence from meta-analysis of dementia prevalence in the oldest old. *Lancet* **346**: 931–934

Rocca WA, Hofman A, Brayne C *et al.* (1991) Frequency and distribution of Alzheimer's disease in Europe: a collaborative study of 1980–1990 prevalence findings. *Annals of Neurology* **30**: 381–390

Rocca WA and Kokmen E. (1999) Frequency and distribution of vascular dementia. *Alzheimer's Disease and Associated Disorders* **13** (Suppl. 3), S9–14

Roth M, Tym E, Mountjoy CQ *et al.* (1986) CAMDEX: a standardized instrument for the diagnosis of mental disorder in the elderly with special reference to the early detection of dementia. *British Journal of Psychiatry* **149**: 648–709

Sahakian BJ and Owen AM. (1992) Computerised assessment in neuropsychiatry using CANTAB. *Journal of the Royal Society of Medicine* **85**: 399–402

Shumaker SA, Legault C, Rapp SR *et al.* (2003) Estrogen plus progestin and the incidence of dementia and mild cognitive impairment in postmenopausal women. *JAMA* **289**: 2651–2662

Wimo A, Winblad B, Aguero-Torres H, von Strauss E. (2003) The magnitude of dementia occurrence in the world. *Alzheimer's Disease and Associated Disorders* **17**: 63–67

White L, Petrovich H, Ross W *et al.* (1996) Prevalence of dementia in older Japanese-American men in Hawaii: the Honolulu-Asia Aging Study. *JAMA* **276**: 955–960

Xuereb JH, Brayne C, Dufouil C *et al.* (2000) Neuropathological findings in the very old: results from the first 101 brains of a population-based longitudinal study of dementing disorders. *Annals of New York Academy of Sciences* (Suppl.): *Vascular Factors in Alzheimer's Disease* **903**: 490–496

Yaffe K, Sawaya G, Lieberburg I, Grady D. (1998) Estrogen therapy in postmenopausal women: effects on cognitive function and dementia. *JAMA* **279**: 688–695

Yamada T, Hattori H, Miura A *et al.* (2001) Prevalence of Alzheimer's disease, vascular dementia and dementia with Lewy bodies in a Japanese population. *Psychiatry and Clinical Neurosciences* **55**: 21–25

Yoshitake T, Kiyohara Y, Kato I *et al.* (1995) Incidence and risk factors of vascular dementia and Alzheimer's disease in a defined elderly Japanese population: the Hisayama study. *Neurology* **45**: 1161–1168

Zhang M, Katzman R, Salmon D *et al.* (1990) The prevalence of dementia and Alzheimer's disease in Shanghai, China: impact of age, gender and education. *Annals of Neurology* **27**: 428–437

3

Criteria for the diagnosis of dementia

CLIVE BALLARD AND CAROL BANNISTER

There are two main diagnostic challenges within the dementia field, distinguishing patients with dementia from those without and the accurate differential diagnosis of dementia subtypes (Kaye, 1998). The diagnosis of dementia has always had enormous prognostic implications, however, with the availability of licensed treatments for dementia (O'Brien and Ballard, 2001) and with the likelihood of more effective treatments becoming available over the next decade, issues of differential diagnosis will become progressively more important. This chapter will initially review criteria and standardized approaches for the diagnosis of dementia, and then tackle the diagnosis of common specific subtypes of dementia.

3.1 DIAGNOSIS OF DEMENTIA

The concept of dementia has evolved from the rather non-specific notion of organic brain syndrome to a more specific operationalized concept. For example the ICD 10 criteria (World Health Organization, 1992) described dementia as:

> a syndrome due to disease of the brain, usually of a chronic or progressive nature in which there is disturbance of multiple higher cortical function including memory, thinking, orientation, comprehension, calculation, learning capacity, language and judgement. Consciousness is not clouded. The impairments of cognitive function are commonly accompanied, and occasionally preceded by deterioration in emotional controls, social behaviour or motivation.

The DSM-IV (American Psychiatric Association, 1994) definition incorporates similar elements, emphasizing the necessity for a detrimental influence upon activities of daily living. A number of key elements exist across all diagnostic criteria, mainly that dementia is a brain disease, tends to be progressive, and globally affects higher cognitive functions as well as emotional and social functioning. The DSM-IIIR criteria (American Psychiatric Association, 1987) (Box 3.1), attempted to operationalize these concepts and have been widely used as the basis for the diagnosis of dementia in research studies, with interrater reliability keeping scores of up to +0.7 (Baldereschi et al., 1994). Although the key elements within these definitions are based upon sound, commonsense principles, with much that most clinicians would agree upon, there are a number of subtle difficulties. For example, the majority of definitions suggest that disturbances of consciousness or delirium should be absent. We all, however, recognize that disturbances of consciousness are common in both vascular dementia (Hachinski et al., 1975) and dementia with Lewy bodies (Ballard et al., 1993) and occur in a minority of patients with Alzheimer's disease (AD) (Robertson et al., 1998). There are also well documented cases of patients suffering from a variety of different dementia syndromes where the early manifestations were relatively focal (e.g. Coen et al., 1994). In addition not all cases of dementia are progressive.

Despite these minor caveats, the majority of diagnostic criteria have good face validity, and are probably useful in clinical practice when applied flexibly. There are, however, greater difficulties when applying these criteria within research studies. Much research work published within the dementia domain has focused upon specific dementia subtypes, and has therefore avoided this issue. Within a research setting the operationalized format of the DSM-IIIR criteria have advantages of established interrater reliability. Validity is not, however, a straightforward issue. Unlike specific disease processes such as AD, dementia is ultimately a clinical diagnosis describing a syndrome, and neuropathology cannot be used as a gold standard.

Semistructured psychiatric interviews have been used as an alternative. The Cambridge Examinations for Mental Disorders in the Elderly (CAMDEX; Roth et al., 1986), for example,

Box 3.1   *DSM-IIIR criteria for dementia*

1. Demonstrable evidence of impairment in short- and long-term memory. Impairment in short-term memory (inability to learn new information) may be indicated by inability to remember three objects after 5 minutes. Long-term memory impairment (inability to remember information that was known in the past) may be indicated by inability to remember past personal information (e.g. what happened yesterday, birthplace, occupation) or facts of common knowledge (e.g. past presidents, well-known dates).

2. At least one of the following:
   (a) impairment in abstract thinking, as indicated by inability to find similarities and differences between related words, difficulty in defining words and concepts, and other similar tasks;
   (b) impaired judgement, as indicated by inability to make reasonable plans to deal with interpersonal, family, and job-related problems and issues;
   (c) other disturbances of higher cortical function, such as aphasia (disorder of language), apraxia (inability to carry out motor activities despite intact comprehension and motor function), agnosia (failure to recognize or identify objects despite intact sensory function), and 'constructional difficulty' (e.g. inability to copy three-dimensional figures, assemble blocks, or arrange sticks in specific designs);
   (d) personality change, i.e. alteration or accentuation of premorbid traits.

3. The disturbance in 1 and 2 significantly interferes with work or usual social activities or relationships with others.

4. Not occurring exclusively during the course of delirium.

5. Either (a) or (b):
   (a) There is evidence from the history, physical examination, or laboratory tests of a specific organic factor (or factors) judged to be aetiologically related to the disturbance.
   (b) In the absence of such evidence, an aetiological organic factor can be presumed if the disturbance cannot be accounted for by any non-organic mental disorder, e.g. major depression accounting for cognitive impairment.

includes an informant history, physical examination and standardized cognitive assessment, to which operationalized check spelling criteria can be applied. The technique provides a standardized information base that can discriminate controls from patients with dementia with adequate reliability and validity, and is hence useful in either a clinical or research setting. The Geriatric Mental State Schedule (GMSS; Copeland *et al.*, 1976) is a further semistructured psychiatric interview, which covers a range of psychiatric conditions and includes a brief cognitive screening section. It is applied directly as a patient interview and can be completed by medical or allied professionals with appropriate training. Diagnosis is based upon a diagnostic algorithm (Copeland *et al.*, 1986), which specifies the degree of certainty. The requirement for the computerized diagnostic system probably limits its value in clinical settings, although it has again been demonstrated to have adequate reliability and validity in discriminating controls from dementia patients.

A technique, used by many epidemiological studies, has been to use a standardized cognitive screening instrument, such as the Mini-Mental State Examination (Folstein *et al.*, 1975) or a brief semistructured interview, usually using a two stage design with a more detailed evaluation of patients scoring below a set cut-off score (Boothby *et al.*, 1994). Outside the context of a dual design, the cut-off score on a cognitive screening instrument is an unsatisfactory way of diagnosing dementia, given the great variability between individuals and the high level of impact that previous education, current psychiatric morbidity and motivation have upon test results.

The Clinical Dementia Rating Scale (Hughes *et al.*, 1982, updated by Morris, 1987) provides a mechanism for grading dementia severity in a relatively user-friendly manner. A description of typical performance for dementia patients with different severities of illness, in a number of different domains are provided, with the rater required to make a judgement as to which category of severity most appropriately matches the impairments of an individual patient. Whilst this is not intended as a method to diagnose dementia *per se*, it provides an excellent method in tandem with a standardized definition to characterize the severity of impairments either in a clinical or research setting. Although the method was designed predominantly to improve the sensitivity of clinical staging in people with more severe dementia, the Functional Assessment Staging tool of Auer and Reisberg (1997) could be used in the same way.

Any of the standardized clinical definitions, particularly when used in conjunction with a severity rating, are likely to be very successful in the diagnosis of patients with moderate or severe dementia. The study populations used to investigate the reliability and validity of instruments such as the CAMDEX and GMSS, have been rather polarized. This has avoided the much more difficult issue of whether these criteria can distinguish between patients with no dementia and those with minimal or questionable dementia. Various terms have been used to describe older patients with a mild degree of cognitive impairment, who are clearly functioning below their premorbid level, but who do not have dementia. Historically, labels such as benign senescent forgetfulness (Kral, 1978) and age-associated memory impairment (Crook *et al.*, 1986) have been employed. Currently, the most widely used concept for early cognitive deficits is Mild Cognitive Impairment (MCI; Petersen *et al.*, 1999, 2001), which focuses upon memory deficits to identify 'pre-AD'. To meet the criteria, people have to perform at a level of 1.5 standard deviations below the mean of an age-matched group on a standardized memory task. The criteria therefore achieve a form of 'thresholding', which identifies a cluster of people at increased risk of AD, together with a heterogeneous mix of individuals with mild memory deficits for a range of reasons. Other frequently used concepts include Aging-Associated Cognitive Decline (AACD; Ritchie et al., 2001), which again relies upon thresholding but can be applied to impairments in any cognitive domain; and Cognitive Impairment No Dementia (CIND; Tuokko et al., 2003), which relates to global cognitive performance in addition to operationalized clinical criteria. A detailed review of MCI or the related concepts is beyond the remit of the current chapter, although it would appear from numerous follow-up studies that between 4 and 12 per cent of people per year will develop dementia depending upon the population sampled (higher in clinic settings, lower in the community, e.g. O'Connor et al., 1990; O'Brien et al., 1992; Petersen et al., 1999, 2001; Ritchie et al., 2001; Tuokko et al., 2003). As there are no satisfactory methods for distinguishing patients with progressive decline from those who continue to exhibit a static degree of mild impairment or improve, it is difficult to see how any clinical diagnostic criteria could distinguish these patients accurately from those in the early stages of a dementia process, and in many ways this is an arbitrary distinction, as 'early cognitive impairment' is not a disease entity. Although some characteristics, such as the presence of hippocampal atrophy, may increase the risk of developing dementia (Jack et al., 2000), the only reliable diagnostic method at present is clinical follow up and re-evaluation. Combining clinical, neuropsychological and neuroimaging indices over time is probably the best method. Whilst this approach is prudent clinically, it is extremely difficult to employ in research studies without considerable resources for large scale prospective longitudinal studies, which probably explains the paucity of such studies in the literature.

A number of exciting recent studies highlight the potential utility of various biological markers such as phosphorylated tau in the cerebrospinal fluid (CSF) (Buerger et al., 2002), characteristic patterns of hypometabolism identified on positron emission tomography (PET) scanning (de Leon et al., 2001) and the identification of amyloid with specific PET ligands (Agdeppa et al., 2001). We hope that further understanding of these markers will enable us to progress to a point where we can make more meaningful diagnoses such as 'very early AD' rather than relying upon thresholding from coarse neuropsychological evaluations.

Concurrent psychiatric morbidity is a further major confounding factor in the diagnosis of dementia. Probably the most extreme example is so called 'depressive pseudodementia' (Kiloh, 1961; Caine, 1981), where a typical patient will experience an apparently rapid onset of cognitive impairment, in the context of a past history or family history of affective disorder, and will probably exhibit concurrent depressive symptoms (Caine, 1981). The overlap between depression and

cognitive impairment is, however, more complex (Feinberg and Goodman, 1984). It is well established that depression affects both motivation and attention, therefore detrimentally influencing performance on activities of daily living and cognitive assessments. In addition, however, there is growing evidence of subtle neuropsychological deficits which may be specific to patients with late onset depression, and which persist after treatment (Abas and Sahakian, 1990). This issue is further confounded by the fact the many psychotropic drugs detrimentally influence cognitive function, whilst some organic factors, such as diffuse microvascular pathology, may predispose to both cognitive impairment and depression (O'Brien et al., 1996). Other psychiatric conditions such as anxiety may also affect attention and performance on activities of daily living and formal cognitive assessments, while both depression and anxiety disorders are common in people with dementia, especially in the early stages of the illness. It is well known that a proportion of patients with late onset psychosis have a degree of cortical atrophy (Pearlson and Rabins, 1988), whilst a substantial minority of patients with early onset of psychotic disorders experience cognitive decline (Carpenter and Strauss, 1991). Again, except in patients with marked depressive pseudodementia who should be clinically diagnosed, it is unlikely that these factors will substantially affect misdiagnosis of patients with moderate or severe dementia, but they could have a substantial impact upon the diagnosis of minimal or mild dementia. Although well recognized by clinicians and described in a number of review articles, this is, however, an issue that has not received a great deal of research attention. In clinical practice a certain degree or pragmatism can be employed, while treating any concurrent psychiatric morbidity and evaluating the progress of any cognitive deficits over time. For research studies, however, these diagnostic issues could be a major confounding factor, which is why, for example, patients with concurrent psychiatric symptoms are often excluded from pharmacological trials pertaining to dementia.

The inclusion of statements pertaining to disturbances of consciousness in the standardized diagnostic definitions of dementia is clearly designed to distinguish dementia from delirium. Some of the difficulties with this approach have already been described, but in addition, although delirium is classically thought of as an acute condition, related to a treatable physical condition, a proportion of patients experience a subacute delirium, which can persist for some months (Lipowski, 1989) and those most vulnerable to delirium are patients with pre-existing dementia. As a consequence, in practice it is not always straightforward to make the diagnosis, particularly in patients with chronic physical conditions predisposing to repeated delirium. Certainly within the CAMDEX and GMSS validation studies, patients with delirium and dementia were distinguished with a good degree of interrater reliability and validity against expert clinical diagnosis and it is unlikely to apply to a large enough group of patients to make it a relevant issue in research studies. Within clinical services, however, this issue will occasionally arise and is probably best dealt with by clinical judgement rather than standardized diagnostic criteria.

In summary, standardized clinical definitions of dementia have good face validity and are probably useful in both clinical practice and research studies, particularly combined with a standardized rating of severity. There are, however, specific groups of patients where diagnostic difficulties might exist, particularly patients with concurrent psychiatric morbidity, those with very mild degrees of cognitive impairment and patients with persistent delirium. For these groups longitudinal follow up and clinical judgement are better methods of diagnosis than the standardized diagnostic criteria.

3.2 DIFFERENTIAL DIAGNOSIS OF DEMENTIA SUBTYPES

3.2.1 Alzheimer's disease

More than 50 per cent of dementia patients have AD (Cummings and Benson, 1992). It is most the common dementia condition and is therefore the most important to diagnose accurately, particularly as licensed pharmacological treatments are now available.

As with all types of dementia, a wide array of diagnostic criteria have been published, including various renditions of the DSM and ICD classifications. However, it was the introduction of the NINCDS ADRDA criteria in 1984 (McKhann et al., 1984) that represented a major landmark in dementia research, with the availability of reliable and valid operationalized criteria for AD. These criteria have been used far more widely than any other in research studies, and are also straightforward to use in a clinical setting. This section will therefore review the evidence pertaining to these criteria. The criteria themselves are shown in Box 3.2. Two degrees of certainty are described: probable AD and possible AD. Section 1 is the most important and contains the operationalized element of the diagnosis. First it is necessary to establish that the person has dementia. Although the same caveats exist as in the previous section where this problem was discussed, the criteria make sensible recommendations that standardized assessments of cognitive function and activities of daily living are completed as well as a detailed clinical examination, in order to establish the presence of dementia. It is also specifies that deficits are required in two or more areas of cognition, which should ensure that an individual is not suffering from a focal cognitive deficit. Note of progressive decline of memory and other cognitive functions is required. Disturbances of consciousness render patients unsuitable for a diagnosis of probable AD. Even though recent work does suggest that 20 per cent of AD patients do experience disturbances of consciousness (Robertson et al., 1998), this is probably a sensible exclusion and a diagnosis of possible AD can still be made. An upper age limit of 90 is set, which is sensible in some ways given the difficulties in determining the significance of

cognitive impairment in patients above this age, but renders the criteria inapplicable to an increasingly large section of the population who are at especially high risk of AD. In the final part of section 1, it is stated that the systemic disorders or other brain diseases that could account for the progressive cognitive deficits should be excluded. Although this is an appropriate recommendation, the lack of operationalization does permit variable interpretation.

Whilst application is clear cut when another significant brain disease is present, for example cerebrovascular disease, difficulties can arise in the presence of systemic disorders, such as hypothyroidism, which can result in cognitive deficits but are not necessarily the cause of cognitive impairment in a particular individual. In practice, the presence of a concurrent disorder, which may contribute to the dementia, does not preclude a diagnosis of possible AD, particularly if treatment has not resulted in an improvement of the dementia syndrome. Other typical clinical features and the results of investigations such as electroencephalogram (EEG) and CT scans, can be used in support of the diagnosis but are not a fundamental part of the operationalized criteria.

There are several advantages to applying these criteria in clinical practice. First, they require a standardized blood screen, detailed clinical evaluation and standardized cognitive assessment, but do not depend upon novel or expensive investigative techniques, which are unlikely to be available in many clinical centres. Second, they follow a logical diagnostic process similar to that adopted by most clinicians in the diagnosis of AD. Third, the criteria for probable AD would seem to be a suitably rigorous method for selecting patients with a clear-cut diagnosis in pharmacological interventions.

The NINCDS ADRDA criteria have been widely evaluated in a large number of research studies, with excellent interrater reliability (Kukull et al., 1990; Baldereschi et al., 1994; Farrer et al., 1994). In addition a number of clinicopathological correlative studies have been completed, demonstrating good agreement between clinical and neuropathological diagnosis (Morris et al., 1987; Martin et al., 1987; Tierney et al., 1988; Boller et al., 1989; Jellinger et al., 1989; Burns et al., 1990). Although 100 per cent diagnostic accuracy for probable AD has been reported in some studies, the overall specificity is approximately 80 per cent. Put in to context, this is substantially better than can be achieved by using a CT scan alone (Jacoby and Levy, 1980) and is better than has been achieved for the diagnosis of Parkinson's disease (PD) (Hughes et al., 1992). Despite the excellent overall performance of these criteria, a number of caveats must be considered.

First, the exact accuracy of clinical diagnostic criteria, depends to some degree upon the neuropathological criteria (Nagy et al., 1998) chosen for diagnosis. Second, the majority of studies have compared polarized groups of patients such as controls and those with moderate dementia, omitting many of the difficult-to-diagnose cases. This issue is not relevant if the study is aiming to recruit a group of patients with clear cut AD. However, if the objective is to differentially diagnose a representative epidemiological or clinical sample of patients,

Box 3.2   *Criteria for clinical diagnosis of Alzheimer's disease*

I   The criteria for the clinical diagnosis of PROBABLE Alzheimer's disease include:
  • dementia established by clinical examination and documented by the Mini-Mental test, Blessed Dementia Scale, or some similar examination, and confirmed by neuropsychological tests;
  • deficits in two or more areas of cognition;
  • progressive worsening memory and other cognitive functions;
  • no disturbance of consciousness;
  • onset between ages 40 and 90, most often after age 65; and absence of systemic disorders or other brain diseases that in and of themselves could account for the progressive deficits in memory and cognition.

II   The diagnosis of PROBABLE Alzheimer's disease is supported by:
  • progressive deterioration of specific cognitive functions such as language (aphasia), motor skills (apraxia) and perception (agnosia);
  • impaired activities of daily living and altered patterns of behaviour;
  • family history of similar disorders, particularly if confirmed neuropathologically; and
  • laboratory results of:
    – normal lumbar puncture as evaluated by standard techniques;
    – normal pattern or non-specific changes in EEG; such as increased slow-wave activity; and
    – evidence of cerebral atrophy on CT with progression documented by serial observation.

III   Other clinical features consistent with the diagnosis of PROBABLE Alzheimer's disease, after exclusion of causes of dementia other than Alzheimer's disease, include:
  • plateaus in the course of progression of the illness;
  • associated symptoms of depression, insomnia, incontinence, delusions, illusions, hallucinations, catastrophic verbal, emotional, or physical outbursts, sexual disorders, and weight loss;
  • other neurological abnormalities in some patients, especially with more advanced disease and including motor signs such as increased muscle tone, myoclonus, or gait disorder;
  • seizures in advanced disease; and
  • CT normal for age.

IV   Features that make the diagnosis of PROBABLE Alzheimer's disease uncertain or unlikely include:
  • sudden, apoplectic onset;
  • focal neurological findings such as hemiparesis, sensory loss, visual field deficits and incoordination early in the course of the illness; and
  • seizures or gait disturbances at the onset or very early in the course of the illness.

V   Clinical diagnosis of POSSIBLE Alzheimer's disease:
  • may be made on the basis of the dementia syndrome, in the absence of other neurological, psychiatric, or systemic disorder sufficient to cause dementia, and in the presence of variation in the onset, in the presentation, or in the clinical course;
  • may be made in the presence of a second systemic or brain disorder sufficient to produce dementia, which is not considered to be the cause of the dementia; and
  • should be used in research studies when a single, gradually progressive severe cognitive deficit is identified in the absence of other identifiable cause.

VI   Criteria for diagnosis of DEFINITE Alzheimer's disease are:
  • the clinical criteria for probable Alzheimer's disease and histopathological evidence obtained from a biopsy or autopsy.

VII   Classification of Alzheimer's disease for research purpose should specify features that may differentiate subtypes of the disorder, such as:
  • familial occurrence;
  • onset before age 65;
  • presence of trisomy-21; and
  • coexistence of other relevant conditions such as Parkinson's disease.

it does become more important. Third, many of these studies were completed before there was wide clinical awareness of dementia with Lewy bodies (DLB) as a major form of dementia, although most reports focusing on more diverse samples including patients with DLB suggest that the criteria still perform well. For example, McKeith *et al.* (2000) reported a sensitivity and specificity of around 80 per cent for probable AD, whereas Litvan *et al.* (1998), in an even more diverse sample, reported a sensitivity of 95 per cent and specificity of 79 per cent for probable AD; in a further study Lopez *et al.* (1999) reported a sensitivity of 95 per cent and a specificity of 79 per

cent for probable AD. Fourth, many people with dementia have a combination of different disease pathologies, for example a substantial number of patients with Alzheimer-type pathology will have some degree of concurrent cerebrovascular disease and a small number of cortical Lewy bodies, which are often seen in the amygdala in people with otherwise clear cut AD. Again the exact degree of diagnostic accuracy will depend upon whether mixed cases are considered separately or as a subtype of AD, but in general the presence of mixed pathologies reduces the level of diagnostic accuracy (Holmes *et al.*, 1999).

Box 3.3 *The Hachinski ischaemia score*

Abrupt onset	2
Stepwise progression	1
Fluctuating course	2
Nocturnal confusion	1
Relative preservation of personality	1
Depression	1
Somatic complaints	1
Emotional incontinence	1
History of hypertension	1
History of strokes	2
Evidence of associated atherosclerosis	1
Focal neurological symptoms	2
Focal neurological signs	2

3.2.2 Vascular dementia (VaD)

VaD is probably the second most common dementia illness, accounting for 10–20 per cent of people with late onset dementia (Rocca *et al.*, 1991), either on its own or in combination with neurodegenerative pathologies. There have been far fewer studies examining the diagnostic accuracy of criteria for VaD than for AD. The longest established criteria are based upon the Hachinski ischaemic score (Hachinski *et al.*, 1975; Box 3.3), originally derived on the basis of cerebral blood flow patterns in dementia patients. On the weighted scale, a score of 7 or more is taken to indicate VaD, whilst a score of 4 or less suggests that this is an unlikely diagnosis. Although the scale has been much criticized, either in its pure form, or in the modified form suggested by Rosen *et al.* (1980), sensitivities and specificities of approximately 80 per cent have been achieved for the diagnosis of 'pure' VaD cases (Loeb and Gandolfo, 1983; Small, 1985; Katzman *et al.*, 1988). The scale is, however, far less successful in identifying mixed cases (Katzman *et al.*, 1988). Items within the scale, such as abrupt onset, stepwise progression, fluctuation and focal neurological symptoms and signs, are geared much more to the identification of multiple infarctions than to other forms of VaD (Chui, 1989), such as the insidious development of microvascular pathology, hypoxia or haemorrhage. In addition, individual symptoms within the scale are poorly operationalized and are therefore open to variable interpretation. Despite this, rather like the concept of hysteria, this scale has yet to be bettered and is likely to outlive its obituarists.

More recently two sets of operationalized criteria (Boxes 3.4 and 3.5) have been proposed, the California criteria – ADDTC (Chui *et al.*, 1992) and the NINDS AIREN criteria (Roman *et al.*, 1993). Diagnostic criteria for VaD are also included within ICD 10 (World Health Organization, 1992), DSM-IV (American Psychiatric Association, 1994) and the CAMDEX (Roth *et al.*, 1986). A preliminary study examining the ICD 10 research criteria was rather disappointing, suggesting that only 25 per cent of patients with clear vascular lesions on a CT scan fulfilled ICD 10 criteria for VaD (Wallin, 1994). Baldereschi *et al.* (1994) did, however, demonstrate a good interrater reliability of +0.66 for the diagnosis of VaD using these criteria. Chui *et al.* (1998) compared several different diagnostic criteria for VaD in 25 case vignettes, examining interrater reliability as well as sensitivity and specificity against expert clinical judgement. The highest interrater reliability was achieved for the Hachinski scale, which performed better than the DSM-IV, the California criteria (ADDTC) and the NINDS AIREN criteria. Most of the criteria had poor sensitivity, but specificity was generally adequate. The DSM-IV criteria had the best sensitivity (50 per cent), and the best specificity was achieved by the NINDS AIREN criteria (97 per cent). In a more extensive study, the same group (Chui *et al.*, 2000) examined the interrater reliability for the NINDS AIREN, ADDTC, DSM-IV, modified Hachinski score and ICD 10 criteria, identifying only moderate agreement (κ values of 0.24–0.60) between the criteria; again the DSM-IV and the Hachinski score were the most liberal and the NINDS AIREN were the most conservative.

Gold *et al.* (1997) examined the diagnosis of VaD in a study of 113 autopsy-confirmed dementia cases. For a diagnosis of VaD, the Hachinski scale had the best specificity of 0.88, with the NINDS AIREN criteria achieving a specificity of 0.80. The ADDTC criteria had the best sensitivity (0.63). More recently Gold *et al.* (2002) examined the validity of various operationalized clinical criteria for VaD (NINDS AIREN, DSM-IV, ADDTC, ICD-10) against autopsy criteria. Eighty-nine patients (20 VaD, 23 mixed dementia, 46 AD) were included. Overall the NINDS AIREN criteria for possible VaD (sensitivity 0.55, specificity 0.84) and the possible ADDTC criteria (sensitivity 0.70, specificity 0.78) performed best. Consistent with previous studies the NINDS AIRENS criteria were the more conservative of the two. All of the criteria for probable VaD were too restrictive. A fuller breakdown is shown in Table 3.1. Across both of the Gold studies, none of the criteria performed well for mixed cases. There is, however, a slight caveat in interpreting these results as the neuropathological criteria were very weighted towards infarcts, and would not have labelled people with extensive small vessel disease but no infarcts or lacunae as having VaD. In practice this is likely to be a small proportion of individuals.

Given the current state of play, NINDS AIREN and ADDTC criteria for possible VaD appear to be the most useful instruments, although the Hachinski scale probably remains useful, particularly as a clinical instrument to help distinguish between VaD and other types of dementia in clinical practice.

The notoriously unreliable clinical diagnosis of 'mixed' Alzheimer and VaD, with no established clinical diagnostic criteria (Bowler, 2000), is, however, a considerable concern, particularly as at least 40 per cent of dementia patients have an overlap of vascular and neurodegenerative pathologies (Kalaria and Ballard, 1999). To give an indication of the scope of the problem, the Gold studies indicated that between 30 and 50 per cent of 'mixed dementia' cases are misclassified as VaD (Gold *et al.*, 1997, 2002). The potential overlap of

Box 3.4   *Criteria for the diagnosis of ischaemic vascular dementia (IVD)*

I   Dementia
Dementia is a deterioration from a known or estimated prior level of intellectual function sufficient to interfere broadly with the conduct of the patient's customary affairs of life, which is not isolated to a single narrow category of intellectual performance, and which is independent of level of consciousness.

This deterioration should be supported by historical evidence and documented either by bedside mental status testing or ideally by more detailed neuropsychological examination, using tests that are quantifiable, reproducible, and for which normative data are available.

II   Probable IVD
The criteria for the clinical diagnosis of PROBABLE IVD include ALL of the following:

- dementia;
- evidence of two or more ischaemic strokes by history, neurological signs, and/or neuroimaging studies (CT or T1-weighted MRI); or occurrence of a single stroke with a clearly documented temporal relationship to the onset of dementia;
- evidence of at least one infarct outside the cerebellum by CT or T1-weighted MRI.

The diagnosis of PROBABLE IVD is supported by:

- evidence of multiple infarcts in brain regions known to affect cognition;
- a history of multiple transient ischaemic attacks;
- history of vascular risk factors (e.g. hypertension, heart disease, diabetes mellitus);
- elevated Hachinski ischaemia scale (original or modified version).

Clinical features that are thought to be associated with IVD, but await further research include:

- relatively early appearance of gait disturbance and urinary incontinence;
- periventricular and deep white matter changes on T2-weighted MRI that are excessive for age;
- focal changes in electrophysiological studies (e.g. EEG, evoked potentials) or physiological neuroimaging studies (e.g. SPECT, PET, NMR spectroscopy).

Other clinical features that do not constitute strong evidence either for or against a diagnosis of PROBABLE IVD include:

- periods of slowly progressive symptoms;
- illusions, psychosis, hallucinations, delusions;
- seizures.

Clinical features that cast doubt on a diagnosis of PROBABLE IVD include:

- transcortical sensory aphasia in the absence of corresponding focal lesions on neuroimaging studies;
- absence of central neurological symptoms/signs, other than cognitive disturbance.

III   Possible IVD
A clinical diagnosis of POSSIBLE IVD may be made when there is dementia and one or more of the following:

- a history or evidence of a single stroke (but not multiple strokes) without a clearly documented temporal relationship to the onset of dementia; or
- Binswanger's syndrome (without multiple strokes) that includes all of the following:
  - early onset urinary incontinence not explained by urological disease, or gait disturbance (e.g. parkinsonian, magnetic, apraxic, or 'senile' gait) not explained by peripheral cause,
  - vascular risk factors, and
  - extensive white matter changes on neuroimaging.

IV   Definite IVD
A diagnosis of DEFINITE IVD requires histopathological examination of the brain, as well as:

- clinical evidence of dementia;
- pathological confirmation of multiple infarcts, some outside of the cerebellum.

(Note: if there is evidence of Alzheimer's disease or some other pathological disorder that is to have contributed to the dementia, a diagnosis of MIXED dementia should be made.)

V   Mixed dementia
A diagnosis of MIXED dementia should be made in the presence of one or more other systemic or brain disorders that are thought to be causally related to the dementia.

The degree of confidence in the diagnosis of IVD should be specified as possible, probable, or definite, and the other disorder(s) contributing to the dementia should be listed. For example: mixed dementia due to probable IVD and possible Alzheimer's disease or mixed dementia due to definite IVD and hypothyroidism.

VI   Research classification
Classification of IVD for RESEARCH purposes should specify features of the infarcts that may differentiate subtypes of the disorder, such as:

- location – cortical white matter, periventricular, basal ganglia, thalamus;
- size – volume;
- distribution – large, small or microvessel;
- severity – chronic ischaemia versus infarction;
- aetiology – atherosclerosis, embolism, arteriovenous malformation, hypoperfusion.

Box 3.5   *Criteria for clinical diagnosis of vascular dementia (VaD)*

I   The criteria for the clinical diagnosis of probable vascular dementia include all of the following:
   • dementia defined by cognitive decline from a previously higher level of functioning and manifested by impairment of memory and of two or more cognitive domains (orientation, attention, language, visuospatial functions, executive functions, motor control, and praxis), preferably established by clinical examination and documented by neuropsychological testing; deficits should be severe enough to interfere with activities of daily living not due to physical effects of stroke alone.
      Exclusion criteria: cases with disturbance of consciousness, delirium, psychosis, severe aphasia, or major sensorimotor impairment precluding neuropsychological testing. Also excluded are systemic disorders or other brain diseases (such as AD) that in and of themselves could account for deficits in memory and cognition.
   • cerebrovascular disease (CVD), defined by the presence of focal signs on neurological examination, such as hemiparesis, lower facial weakness, Babinski sign, sensory deficit, hemianopia, and dysarthria consistent with stroke (with or without history of stroke), and evidence of relevant CVD by brain imaging (CT or MRI) including multiple large-vessel infarcts or a single strategically placed infarct (angular gyrus, thalamus, basal forebrain, or PCA or ACA territories), as well as multiple basal ganglia and white matter lacunes or extensive periventricular white matter lesions, or combinations thereof.
   • a relationship between the above two disorders, manifested or inferred by the presence of one or more of the following:
      (a) onset of dementia within 3 months following a recognized stroke;
      (b) abrupt deterioration in cognitive functions; or fluctuating, stepwise progression of cognitive deficits.

II Clinical features consistent with the diagnosis of probable vascular dementia include the following:
   • early presence of a gait disturbance (small-step gait or marche à petits pas, or magnetic apraxic-ataxic or parkinsonian gait);
   • history of unsteadiness and frequent, unprovoked falls;
   • early urinary frequency, urgency, and other urinary symptoms not explained by urological disease;
   • pseudobulbar palsy; and

   • personality and mood changes, abulia, depression, emotional incontinence, or other subcortical deficits including psychomotor retardation and abnormal executive function.

III Features that make the diagnosis of vascular dementia uncertain or unlikely include:
   • early onset of memory deficit and progressive worsening of memory and other cognitive functions such as language (transcortical sensory aphasia), motor skills (apraxia), and perception (agnosia), in the absence of corresponding focal lesions on brain imaging;
   • absence of focal neurological signs, other than cognitive disturbance; and
   • absence of cerebrovascular lesions on brain CT or MRI.

IV Clinical diagnosis of possible vascular dementia may be made:
   • in the presence of dementia (Section I) with focal neurological signs in patients in whom brain imaging studies to confirm definite CVD are missing; or
   • in the absence of clear temporal relationship between dementia and stroke; or
   • in patients with subtle onset and variable course (plateau or improvement) of cognitive deficits and evidence of relevant CVD.

V   Criteria for diagnosis of definite vascular dementia are:
   • clinical criteria for probable vascular dementia;
   • histopathological evidence of CVD obtained from biopsy or autopsy;
   • absence of neurofibrillary tangles and neuritic plaques exceeding those expected for age; and
   • absence of other clinical or pathological disorder capable of producing dementia.

VI Classification of vascular dementia for research purposes may be made on the basis of clinical, radiological and neuropathological features, for subcategories or defined conditions such as cortical vascular dementia, subcortical vascular dementia, BD and thalamic dementia.

The term 'AD with CVD' should be reserved to classify patients fulfilling the clinical criteria for possible AD and who also present clinical or brain imaging evidence of relevant CVD. Traditionally, these patients have been included with VaD in epidemiological studies. The term 'mixed dementia', used hitherto, should be avoided.

pathologies is multifaceted and broadly classifying lesions as vascular or neurodegenerative may be inadequate; meaningful neuropathological classification of different types of vascular and neurodegenerative changes that reflect specific neurochemical and clinical symptom patterns that have prognostic value are required. Furthermore, these distinctions are arbitrary unless they are clinically useful and guide the clinician with respect to treatment approaches.

Table 3.1 *Clinicopathological validation of the major criteria for vascular dementia (numbers extracted from Gold et al., 2002)*

N = 89 (20 VaD, 23 Mixed, 46 AD) Criteria	Sensitivity	Specificity
DSM-IV	0.5	0.84
ICD 10	0.2	0.94
Possible ADDTC	0.7	0.78
Possible NINDS AIREN	0.55	0.84
Probable ADDTC	0.2	0.91
Probable NINDS AIREN	0.2	0.93

There are three main substrates of dementia in patients with VaD: localized areas of infarction (e.g. Tomlinson *et al.*, 1970), microvascular disease (e.g. Esiri *et al.*, 1997), and concurrent atrophy (e.g. Cordoliani-Mackowiak *et al.*, 2003). Focusing on specific substrates of VaD may help improve the diagnostic accuracy for both 'pure' and 'mixed' VaD cases. The best example of this approach so far has been the development of criteria for subcortical ischaemic vascular dementia (SIVD; Erkinjuntti *et al.*, 2000), which describes VaD related to small-vessel disease, combining the overlapping clinical syndromes of 'Binswanger's disease' and 'lacunar state' (Erkinjuntti *et al.*, 2000; Román *et al.*, 2002). SIVD is hypothesized to be caused by a loss of subcortical neurones or disconnection of cortical neurones from subcortical structures. The neuropsychological profile is described as characteristic of:

- a dysexecutive syndrome (difficulties in goal formulation, initiation, planning, organizing, sequencing, executing, set-shifting and abstracting);
- slowed cognitive and motor processing speed;
- other more general attentional impairments (Erkinjuntti *et al.*, 2000; Román *et al.*, 2002; O'Brien *et al.*, 2003);
- memory deficits with impaired recall but relatively intact recognition.

The concept appears useful, but has not yet been validated in a prospective clinicopathological study.

3.2.3 Dementia with Lewy bodies (DLB)

A number of representative, hospital-based post-mortem series and studies based upon clinical cohorts have suggested that DLB is a common form of dementia, accounting for 10–20 per cent of cases in clinical settings (Lennox *et al.*, 1989; Burns *et al.*, 1990; Hansen *et al.*, 1990; Kosaka, 1990; Perry *et al.*, 1990). Diagnostic criteria were proposed by Byrne *et al.* (1991) and McKeith *et al.* (1992), although they have been superseded by international consensus criteria (McKeith *et al.*, 1996; Box 3.6). A general description of the condition is given, followed by three operationalized criteria, two of which need to be present for diagnosis of probable DLB. A number of validation studies have now been reported (Table 3.2). The data do suggest that probable DLB can be diagnosed with a specificity better than 80 per cent, and Mega *et al.* (1996) suggested that this was

Box 3.6 *Consensus criteria for the clinical diagnosis of probable and possible DLB*

The central feature required for a diagnosis of DLB is progressive cognitive decline of sufficient magnitude to interfere with normal social or occupational function. Prominent or persistent memory impairment may not necessarily occur in the early stages but is usually evident with progression. Deficits on tests of attention and of frontal-subcortical skills and visuospatial ability may be especially prominent.

Two of the following core features are essential for a diagnosis of probable DLB, and one is essential for possible DLB:

- fluctuating cognition with pronounced variations in attention and alertness;
- recurrent visual hallucinations that are typically well formed and detailed;
- spontaneous motor features of parkinsonism.

Features supportive of the diagnosis are:

- repeated falls;
- syncope;
- transient loss of consciousness;
- neuroleptic sensitivity;
- systematized delusions;
- hallucinations and other modalities.

A diagnosis of DLB is less likely in the presence of:

- stroke disease, evident as focal neurological signs or on brain imaging;
- evidence on physical examination and investigation of any physical illness or other brain disorder sufficient to account for the clinical picture.

improved further if parkinsonism was present. Sensitivity has, however, been very variable across these studies. The McKeith *et al.* (2000) study reported a specificity >90 per cent and a sensitivity >80 per cent. Many of the other studies have, however, reported sensitivities <50 per cent (Table 3.2).

The majority have been retrospective, identifying clinical symptoms from a case-note review, which may well have reduced the accuracy of diagnosis. Fluctuating cognition appears to be particularly difficult to identify, with two inter-rater reliability studies suggesting very poor agreement between different expert raters (Mega *et al.*, 1996; Litvan *et al.*, 1998), problems that are likely to be compounded by a retrospective design. Patients with a combination of cerebrovascular disease and cortical Lewy bodies are also particularly difficult to diagnose accurately (McKeith *et al.*, 2000).

Importantly, diagnostic accuracy may also vary with dementia severity; for example, Lopez *et al.* (2000) compared 180 patients with AD alone to 60 patients with AD and concurrent DLB. In patients with mild dementia, there was no specific clinical syndrome associated with concurrent

Table 3.2   *Sensitivity, specificity, positive predictive value and negative predictive value of the consensus criteria fro probable DLB: diagnostic validation studies*

Reference	No. of cases	Diagnosis	Sensitivity	Specificity	PPV	NPV
Retrospective						
Mega *et al.*, 1996	24	AD, PD, PSP	0.4	1.0	1.0	0.93
Litvan *et al.*, 1998		DLB, PD, PSP, CBD, MSA, FTD, AD, CJD, VP	0.18	0.99	0.75	0.89
Luis *et al.*, 1999	56	DLB, AD, mixed DLB/AD	0.57	0.9	0.91	0.56
Lopez *et al.*, 1999	40	AD, PSP, FTD, DLB	0.34	0.94	/	/
Verghese *et al.*, 1999	18	DLB	0.61	0.84	0.48	0.96
Prospective						
Hohl *et al.*, 2000	10	AD, DLB, PSP	0.80	0.80	0.80	0.80
Holmes *et al.*, 1999	75	AD, VaD, DLB, mixed	0.22	1.0	1.0	0.91
McKeith *et al.*, 2000	50	DLB, AD, VaD	0.83	0.91	0.96	0.80
Lopez *et al.*, 2002	26	DLB, AD, mixed AD/VaD, PSP, CJD, FTD	38%	100%	/	/

AD, Alzheimer's disease; DLB, dementia with Lewy bodies; VaD, vascular dementia; PSP, progressive supranuclear palsy; CBD, corticobasal degeneration; MSA, multisystem atrophy; CJD, Creutzfeldt–Jacob disease; NPV, negative predictive value; PPV, positive predictive value; VP, vascular parkinsonism; PD, Parkinson's disease; FTD, frontotemporal dementia

Lewy bodies. However, as the disease progressed, patients with AD and concurrent DLB developed progressively more extrapyramidal signs. In the progression from mild to severe dementia, sensitivity of the DLB diagnosis rose from 62 per cent to 93 per cent, while specificity declined from 54 per cent to 16 per cent. The authors concluded that the relatively high sensitivity/low specificity of the DLB diagnosis, seen in more severe dementia, suggests that AD patients can also develop symptoms of DLB in the later stages of the dementia process.

In the clinical diagnosis of DLB, considerable attention has been paid to differentiating it from AD, PD and VaD. As the majority of DLB cases exhibit some pathological features of AD, the distinctions are in some ways arbitrary; although are useful as they are associated with different clinical and neurochemical phenotypes. Seventy five per cent of DLB patients have many of the neuropathological features of AD, particularly senile plaques (Hansen *et al.*, 1990). Although typically the density of neocortical plaques is similar to AD (Hansen *et al.*, 1990), the burden of tangles is less than in 'pure' AD (Hansen *et al.*, 1990; Del Ser *et al.*, 2001). For example, when Lewy bodies occur in conjunction with Alzheimer pathology sufficient to meet CERAD criteria for probable or definite AD, neocortical neurofibrillary tangles are usually rare or absent, and tangles in the entorhinal cortex and hippocampus are intermediate between elderly controls and AD patients (Hansen *et al.*, 1990; Del Ser *et al.*, 2001). Fewer than 40 per cent of DLB patients meet criteria for a Braak stage IV or higher, although importantly several recent studies indicate that these patients are less likely to present with a 'typical' DLB profile and are less likely to meet consensus criteria for probable DLB (Ballard *et al.*, 2004).

With regard to the relationship between PD and DLB, however, overlap in symptoms very probably reflects a common underlying molecular pathology. Lewy bodies are a common diagnostic feature for both conditions at autopsy. PD patients have severe loss of nigrostriatal dopaminergic neurones (Kuikka *et al.*, 1993; Ouchi *et al.*, 1999) and neocortical

cholinergic deficits, which are greatest in the context of cognitive impairment (e.g. Piggott and Marshall, 1996), although diffuse cortical Lewy bodies appear to be the main substrate of dementia (Apaydin *et al.*, 2002). Although for clinical diagnosis within the framework of the consensus criteria DLB and PD dementia are distinguished on the basis of whether the parkinsonism is present for more than a year prior to the dementia, this is not an evidence-based distinction.

The majority of people developing dementia in the context of longstanding parkinsonism meet the clinical criteria for a diagnosis of DLB, and the similarities in the neuropsychiatric (Aarsland *et al.*, 2001a), cognitive (Ballard *et al.*, 2002) and motor symptoms (Aarsland *et al.*, 2001b) of the two groups are becoming increasingly apparent. Following a recent consensus meeting, this is likely to change in a new revision of the criteria to stipulate that the differential diagnosis between PD dementia and DLB should be made upon the basis of whether the cognitive or motor symptoms present first. This, however, is clearly still a very arbitrary distinction and future studies need to clarify the similarities and differences in the underlying pathology, clinical syndromes and treatment response of DLB and PD dementia to determine whether there is clinical usefulness in distinguishing the syndromes, and if so where the boundaries lie. One of the diagnostic validation studies (Litvan *et al.*, 1998) did include a number of patients with other parkinsonian syndromes, and suggested that diagnostic discrimination is possible between patients with DLB and other parkinsonian syndromes using the current criteria.

The consensus criteria also describe a typical neuropsychological profile characterized by marked attention deficits, although these have no weighting in the actual diagnostic process. Comparative studies do confirm greater impairment of attention and fluctuating attention in DLB patients compared with people with AD (e.g. Ala *et al.*, 2001; Calderon *et al.*, 2001; Ballard *et al.*, 2002). In addition, visuospatial deficits are more severe in DLB (Walker *et al.*, 1997; Gnanalingham *et al.*, 1997; Ballard *et al.*, 1999a).

Neuropsychology may therefore also contribute to diagnosis in some instances.

Various neuroimaging techniques have been used to compare DLB and AD patients. From a point of view of potential differential diagnosis, studies using SPECT scans with dopaminergic ligands such as FP-CIT and other similar compounds are of particular interest. Clear differences are evident between DLB and AD patients in dopaminergic loss in the basal ganglia and subtle differences in the symmetry and rostrocaudal gradient have been identified between DLB and PD dementia (Walker *et al.*, 2002). The full clinical usefulness of this is not yet evident; for example, is this just a marker of the severity of parkinsonism or does it contribute something additional that is useful in the differential diagnosis?

Overall the consensus criteria for DLB work reasonably well in clinical practice, and certainly people who meet the criteria are very likely to actually have the condition. People with concurrent vascular pathology or marked concurrent neurofibrillary tangle pathology are, however, much more difficult to diagnose clinically. There are some useful clinical commonsense steps that can be adopted to try to improve the accuracy in everyday practice. For example, visual hallucinations are much more indicative of DLB if they initially arise in the relatively early stages of the dementia, and become more frequent in AD patients during the moderate stages of the disease (Ballard *et al.*, 1999b). Similarly parkinsonian symptoms are a less useful discriminator in the more severe stages of the disease where they become more frequent in the context of AD (Lopez *et al.*, 2000). In addition, better methods for evaluating fluctuating cognition may be useful, with three published standardized clinical rating methods (Walker *et al.*, 2000; Doubleday *et al.*, 2002).

The criteria also describe a list of features that are considered to be supportive of the diagnosis of DLB. These include:

- repeated falls
- syncope
- transient loss of consciousness
- neuroleptic sensitivity
- systematized delusions and
- hallucinations in modalities other than visual (auditory, olfactory, and tactile)

and are likely to also include REM sleep behaviour disorder (Boeve *et al.*, 2001) in the next revision of the criteria. Although these have no formal weighting in the operationalized diagnostic method, they may be useful in supporting a diagnosis of possible DLB (where only one of the three core features is present) as a primary clinical diagnosis.

3.2.4 Other dementias

Although much less common than AD, VaD or DLB, criteria for the clinical evaluation of frontal lobe dementias have been published (Lund and Manchester Groups, 1994). This includes a description of typical clinical symptoms, together with a SPECT profile. Several studies have confirmed the predominance of behavioural problems, language impairments and hypoprontality (Miller *et al.*, 1997; Lindau *et al.*, 1998) in these patients. Litvan *et al.* (1998) included several participants with frontotemporal dementia in their clinico-pathological study, reporting a sensitivity and specificity of 97 per cent for clinical diagnosis against autopsy confirmation. A further report has, however, suggested that the interrater agreement for the pathological diagnosis of frontotemporal dementia is poor (Halliday *et al.*, 2002), which makes interpretation of clinicopathological studies difficult. Further validation studies are clearly required.

The ICD-10 criteria (World Health Organization, 1992) include a description of dementia in Pick's disease, dementia in Creutzfeld–Jakob disease, dementia in Huntingdon's disease, dementia in human immunodeficiency virus (HIV) disease and dementia in other specified diseases classified elsewhere (which incorporates a list including a variety of conditions such as epilepsy, hypothyroidism, intoxications, multiple sclerosis, neurosyphilis, niacin deficiency, polyarthritis nodosa and vitamin B_{12} deficiency). For specific systemic diseases, diagnosis can be more difficult than it first appears, as often the severity of cognitive impairments can be exacerbated without the underlying condition being the predominant cause of the dementia. For many of these conditions, where an underlying cause or specific gene can be identified, the validity of clinical criteria is obviously redundant as long as the clinical profile indicates the appropriate investigation.

3.3 CONCLUSION

In the current chapter many of the potential difficulties in differential diagnosis have been highlighted. However, particularly for AD, the success of operationalized diagnostic criteria is considerable and they can be used with a degree of confidence for the diagnosis of most dementia patients. There are clearly a number of areas where further work is required, and for dementias other than AD further validation studies are needed to improve and establish accurate diagnostic methodology. The current chapter has not focused upon more detailed neuropsychological evaluation or biological markers, but it is likely in the future that more comprehensive research diagnostic criteria will include results from additional neuropsychological evaluation and more specialized investigation.

REFERENCES

Aarsland D, Ballard C, Larsen JP *et al.* (2001a) A comparative study of psychiatric symptoms in dementia with Lewy bodies and Parkinson's disease with and without dementia. *International Journal of Geriatric Psychiatry* **16**: 528–536

Aarsland D, Ballard C, McKeith I *et al.* (2001b) Comparison of extrapyramidal signs in dementia with Lewy bodies and Parkinson's disease. *Journal of Neuropsychiatry and Clinical Neuroscience* **13**: 374–379

Abas MA and Sahakian BJ. (1990) Neuropsychological deficits and CT scan changes in elderly depressives. *Psychological Medicine* **20**: 507–520

Agdeppa ED, Kepe V, Liu J *et al.* (2001) Binding characteristics of radiofluorinated 6-dialkylamino-2-naphthylethylidene derivatives as positron emission tomography imaging probes for beta-amyloid plaques in Alzheimer's disease. *Journal of Neuroscience* **21**: RC189

Ala TA, Hughes LF, Kyrouac GA *et al.* (2001) Pentagon copying is more impaired in dementia with Lewy bodies than in Alzheimer's disease. *Journal of Neurology, Neurosurgery, and Psychiatry* **70**: 483–488

American Psychiatric Association (1987) *Diagnostic and Statistical Manual of Mental Disorders*, 3rd edition revised. Washington DC, American Psychiatric Association

American Psychiatric Association (1994) *Diagnostic and Statistical Manual of Mental Disorders*, 4th edition. Washington DC, American Psychiatric Association

Apaydin H, Ahlskog JE, Parisi JE. (2002) Parkinson's disease neuropathology: later-developing dementia and loss of the levodopa response. *Archives of Neurology* **59**: 102–112

Auer S, Reisberg B. (1997) The GDS/FAST staging system. *International Psychogeriatrics* **9** (Suppl. 1): 167–171

Baldereschi M, Amato MP, Nencini P *et al.* (1994) Cross National Inter-Rater Agreement on the Clinical Diagnostic Criteria for Dementia. *Neurology* **42**: 239–242

Ballard CG, Mohan RWC, Patel A *et al.* (1993) Idiopathic clouding of consciousness – do the patients have cortical Lewy body disease. *International Journal of Geriatric Psychiatry* **8**: 571–576

Ballard CG, Ayre G, O'Brien J *et al.* (1999a) Simple standardised neuropsychological assessments aid in the differential diagnosis of dementia with Lewy bodies from Alzheimer's disease and vascular dementia. *Dementia and Geriatric Cognitive Disorders* **10**: 104–108

Ballard C, Holmes C, McKeith I *et al.* (1999b) Psychiatric morbidity in dementia with Lewy bodies: a prospective clinical and neuropathological comparative study with Alzheimer's disease. *American Journal of Psychiatry* **156**: 1039–1045

Ballard CG, Aarsland D, McKeith I *et al.* (2002) Fluctuations in attention: PD dementia vs DLB with parkinsonism. *Neurology* **59**: 1714–1720

Ballard C, Jacoby R, Del Ser T. (2004) Neuropathological substrates of psychiatric symptoms in autopsy confirmed prospectively studied patients with dementia with Lewy bodies (DLB). *American Journal of Psychiatry* **161**: 843–849

Boeve BF, Silber MH, Ferman TJ. (2001) Association of REM sleep behavior disorder and neurodegenerative disease may reflect an underlying synucleinopathy. *Movement Disorders* **16**: 622–630

Boller F, Lopez O, Moossy J *et al.* (1989) Diagnosis of dementia: clinico-pathologic correlations. *Neurology* **39**: 76–79

Boothby H, Blizard R, Livingston E *et al.* (1994) The Gospel Oak Study Stage III: the incidence of dementia. *Psychological Medicine* **24**: 89–95

Bowler JV. (2000) Criteria for vascular dementia: replacing dogma with data. *Archives of Neurology* **57**: 170–171

Buerger K, Teipel SJ, Zinkowski R *et al.* (2002) CSF tau protein phosphorylated at threonine 231 correlates with cognitive decline in MCI subjects. *Neurology* **59**: 627–629

Burns A, Luthert P, Levy R *et al.* (1990) Accuracy of clinical diagnosis of Alzheimer's disease. *BMJ* **301**: 1026

Byrne EJ, Lennox G, Goodwin-Austin LB. (1991) Dementia associated with cortical Lewy bodies: proposed diagnostic criteria. *Dementia* **2**: 283–284

Caine ED. (1981) Pseudodementia. *Archives of General Psychiatry* **38**: 1359–1364

Calderon J, Perry RJ, Erzinclioglu SW *et al.* (2001) Perception, attention, and working memory are disproportionately impaired in dementia with Lewy bodies compared with Alzheimer's disease. *Journal of Neurology, Neurosurgery, and Psychiatry* **70**: 157–164

Carpenter WT and Strauss JS. (1991) The prediction of outcome in schizophrenia IV: Eleven year follow-up of the Washington IPSS cohort. *Journal of Nervous and Mental Disease* **179**: 517–525

Chui HC. (1989) Dementia: A review emphasising clinico-pathologic correlations and brain behaviour relationships. *Archives of Neurology* **46**: 805–814

Chui HC, Victoroff JI, Margolin D *et al.* (1992) Criteria for the diagnosis of ischaemic vascular dementia proposed by the state of California Alzheimer's Disease Diagnostic and Treatment Centres. *Neurology* **42**: 473–480

Chui HC, Mack W, Jackson, E *et al.* (1998) Clinical criteria for the diagnosis of vascular dementia: a multi-centre study of reliability and validity (Abstract). *Neurology* **50**: (Suppl. 4), A337

Chui HC, Mack W, Jackson JE *et al.* (2000) Clinical criteria for the diagnosis of vascular dementia: a multicenter study of comparability and interrater reliability. *Archives of Neurology* **57**: 191–196

Coen RF, O'Mahoney D, Bruce I *et al.* (1994) Differential diagnosis of dementia: a prospective evaluation of the DAT inventory. *Journal of the American Geriatrics Society* **42**: 16–20

Copeland JRM, Kelleher MJ, Kellet JM *et al.* (1976) A semi-structured clinical interview for the assessment and diagnosis of mental state in the elderly. *Psychological Medicine* **6**: 439–449

Copeland JRM, Dewey ME, Griffiths-Jones HM. (1986) Psychiatric case nomenclature and a computerised diagnostic system for elderly subjects: GMS and AGECAT. *Psychological Medicine* **16**: 89–99

Cordoliani-Mackowiak MA, Henon H, Pruvo JP *et al.* (2003) Poststroke dementia: influence of hippocampal atrophy. *Archives of Neurology* **60**: 585–590

Crook T, Bartus RT, Ferris SH *et al.* (1986) Age associated memory impairment: Proposed diagnostic criteria and measures of clinical change – report of a National Institute of Mental Health Workgroup. *Developmental Neuropsychology* **2**: 261–276

Cummings JL and Benson DF. (1992) Dementia: definition, prevalence, classification and approach to diagnosis. In: Cummings JL, Benson DF (eds), *Dementia: a Clinical Approach*. Boston, Butterworth-Heinemann

de Leon MJ, Convit A, Wolf OT *et al.* (2001) Prediction of cognitive decline in normal elderly subjects with 2-[(18)F]fluoro-2-deoxy-D-glucose/positron-emission tomography (FDG/PET) *Proceedings of the National Academy of Sciences of the United States of America* **98**: 10966–10971

Del Ser T, Hachinski V, Merskey H *et al.* (2001) Clinical and pathologic features of two groups of patients with dementia with Lewy bodies: effect of coexisting Alzheimer-type lesion load. *Alzheimer Disease and Associated Disorders* **15**: 31–44

Doubleday EK, Snowden JS, Varma AR *et al.* (2002) Qualitative performance characteristics differentiate dementia with Lewy bodies and Alzheimer's disease. *Journal of Neurology, Neurosurgery, and Psychiatry* **72**: 602–607

Erkinjuntti T, Inzitari D, Pantoni L *et al.* (2000) Research criteria for subcortical vascular dementia in clinical trials. *Journal of Neural Transmission* **59** (Suppl.): 23–30

Esiri MM, Wilcock GK, Morris JH. (1997) Neuropathological assessment of the lesions of significance in vascular dementia. *Journal of Neurology, Neurosurgery, and Psychiatry* **63**: 749–753

Farrer LA, Cupples LA, Blackburn S et al. (1994) Inter-rater agreement for the diagnosing of Alzheimer's disease: The MIRAGE Study. *Neurology* **44**: 652–656

Feinberg T, Goodman B. (1984) Affective illness, dementia and pseudodementia. *Journal of Clinical Psychiatry* **45**: 99–103

Folstein MF, Folstein SE, McHugh PR. (1975) Mini-mental State. A practical method for grading the cognitive state of patients for the clinician. *Journal of Psychiatric Research* **12**: 189–198

Gnanalingham KK, Byrne EJ, Thornton A et al. (1997) Motor and cognitive function in Lewy body dementia: comparison with Alzheimer's and Parkinson's diseases. *Journal of Neurology, Neurosurgery, and Psychiatry* **62**: 243–252

Gold G, Giannakopoulos P, Motes-Paicao C et al. (1997) Sensitivity and specificity of newly proposed clinical criteria for possible vascular dementia. *Neurology* **49**: 690–694

Gold G, Bouras C, Canuto A et al. (2002) Clinicopathological validation study of four sets of clinical criteria for vascular dementia. *American Journal of Psychiatry* **159**: 82–87

Hachinski VC, Ilief LD, Zilhka E et al. (1975) Cerebral blood flow in dementia. *Archives of Neurology* **32**: 632–637

Halliday G, Ng T, Rodriguez M et al. (2002) Consensus neuropathological diagnosis of common dementia syndromes: testing and standardising the use of multiple diagnostic criteria. *Acta Neuropathologica* **104**: 72–78

Hansen L, Salmon D, Galasko D et al. (1990) The Lewy body variant of Alzheimer's disease: A clinical and pathological entity. *Neurology* **40**: 1–8

Holmes C, Cairns N, Lantos P et al. (1999) Validity of current clinical criteria for Alzheimer's disease, vascular dementia and dementia with Lewy bodies. *British Journal of Psychiatry* **174**: 45–50

Hughes CP, Berg L, Danziger WL et al. (1982) a new clinical scale for the staging of dementia. *British Journal of Psychiatry* **140**: 556–572

Hughes AJ, Daniel SE, Kilford L et al. (1992) Accuracy of clinical diagnosis of iiopathic Parkinson's disease: a clinico-pathological study of 100 cases. *Journal of Neurology, Neurosurgery, and Psychiatry* **55**: 181–184

Jack CR Jr, Petersen RC, Xu Y et al. (2000) Rates of hippocampal atrophy correlate with change in clinical status in aging and AD. *Neurology* **55**: 484–489

Jacoby R and Levy R. (1980) Computerised tomography in the elderly 2. Senile dementia: diagnosis and functional impairment. *British Journal of Psychiatry* **136**: 256–269

Jellinger K, Danielczyk W, Fischer P et al. (1989) Diagnosis of dementia in the aged: clinico-pathological analysis. *Clinical Neuropathology* **8**: 234–235

Kalaria RN and Ballard C. (1999) Overlap between pathology of Alzheimer disease and vascular dementia. *Alzheimer Disease and Associated Disorders* **13** (Suppl. 3): S115–123

Katzman R, Lacker B, Bernstein N. (1988) Advances in the diagnosis of dementia: accuracy of diagnosis and consequences of misdiagnosis of disorders causing dementia. In: RD Terry (ed.), *Ageing and the Brain*. New York, Raven Press, pp. 251–260

Kaye JA. (1998) Diagnostic challenges in dementia. *Neurology* **51** (Suppl. 1): 545–552

Kiloh LG. (1961) Pseudodementia. *Acta Psychiatrica Scandinavica* **37**: 336–351

Kosaka K. (1990) Diffuse Lewy body disease in Japan. *Neurology* **37**: 197–204

Kral AA. (1978) Benign senescent forgetfulness. In: R Katzman, RD Terry, KL Black (eds), *Alzheimer's Disease: Senile Dementia and Related Disorders*. New York, Raven Press

Kuikka JT, Bergstrom KA, Vanninen E et al. (1993) Initial experience with single-photon emission tomography using iodine-123-labelled 2 beta-carbomethoxy-3 beta-(4-iodophenyl) tropane in human brain. *European Journal of Nuclear Medicine* **20**: 783–786

Kukull WA, Larson E.B, Reifler BB et al. (1990) Inter-rater reliability of Alzheimer's disease diagnosis. *Neurology* **40**: 257–260

Lennox G, Lowe J, Morrell K et al. (1989) Antiubiquitin immunocytochemistry is more sensitive than conventional techniques in the detection of diffuse Lewy body disease. *Journal of Neurology, Neurosurgery, and Psychiatry* **52**: 67–71

Lindau M, Almkvist D, Johanssen SE et al. (1998) Cognitive and behavioural differences of frontal lobe degeneration of the non-Alzheimer type and Alzheimer's *disease*. *Dementia* **9**: 205–213

Lipowski ZJ. (1989) Delirium in the elderly patient. *New England Journal of Medicine* **320**: 578–582

Litvan I, MacIntyre A, Goetz CG et al. (1998) Accuracy of the clinical diagnoses of Lewy body disease, Parkinson disease, and dementia with Lewy bodies: a clinicopathologic study. *Archives of Neurology* **55**: 969–978

Loeb C and Gandolfo C. (1983) Diagnostic evaluation of degenerative and vascular dementia. *Stroke* **14**: 399–401

Lopez OL, Litvan I, Catt KE et al. (1999) Accuracy of four clinical diagnostic criteria for the diagnosis of neurodegenerative dementias. *Neurology* **53**: 1292–1299

Lopez OL, Hamilton RL, Becker JT et al. (2000) Severity of cognitive impairment and the clinical diagnosis of AD with Lewy bodies. *Neurology* **54**: 1780–1787

Lopez OL, Becker JT, Kaufer DI et al. (2002) Research evaluation and prospective diagnosis of dementia with Lewy bodies. *Archives of Neurology* **59**: 43–46

Luis CA, Barker WW, Gajaraj K et al. (1999) Sensitivity and specificity of three clinical criteria for dementia with Lewy bodies in an autopsy-verified sample. *International Journal of Geriatric Psychiatry* **14**: 526–533

Lund and Manchester Groups (1994) Clinical and neuropathological criteria for fronto-temporal dementia. *Journal of Neurology, Neurosurgery, and Psychiatry* **57**: 416–418

McKeith IG, Perry RH, Fairbairn AF et al. (1992) Operational criteria for senile dementia of Lewy body type. *Psychological Medicine* **22**: 911–922

McKeith IG, Galasko D, Kosaka K et al. (1996) Consensus guidelines for the clinical and pathologic diagnosis of dementia with Lewy bodies (DLB). *Neurology* **47**: 1113–1124

McKeith IG, Ballard CG, Perry RH et al. (2000) Prospective validation of consensus criteria for the diagnosis of dementia with Lewy bodies. *Neurology* **54**: 1050–1058

McKhann G, Drachman D, Folstein M et al. (1984) Clinical diagnosis of Alzheimer's disease. Report of the NINCDS ADRDA work group under the auspices of the Department of Health and Human Service Task forces on Alzheimer's disease. *Neurology* **34**: 939–944

Martin E, Wilson R, Penn R et al. (1987) Cortical biopsy results in Alzheimer's disease: correlation with cognitive deficits. *Neurology* **37**: 1201–1204

Mega M, Masterman DL, Benson F et al. (1996) Dementia with Lewy Bodies: reliability of clinical and pathologic criteria. *Neurology* **47**: 1403–1409

Miller BL, Ikonta C, Ponton M et al. (1997) A study of the Lund Manchester Criteria for fronto-temporal dementia: clinical and single photos emission computerised tomography correlations. *Neurology* **48**: 937–942

Morris J, McKeel D, Fulling K et al. (1987) Validation of clinical diagnostic criteria in senile. dementia of the Alzheimer type. *Annals of Neurology* **22**: 122

Nagy Z, Esiri M, Hindley N et al. (1998) Accuracy of clinical operational diagnostic criteria for Alzheimer's disease in relation to different pathological diagnostic protocols. *Dementia* **9**: 181–238

O'Brien J and Ballard C. (2001) Cholinesterase Inhibitors in the management of dementia: summary and appraisal of the NICE guidelines. *BMJ* **323**: 123–124

O'Brien J, Beats B, Hill K et al. (1992) Do subjective memory complaints precede dementia? A 3 year follow-up of patients with supposed benign senescent forgetfulness. *International Journal of Geriatric Psychiatry* **7**: 481–486

O'Brien J, Ames D, Schwietzer I. (1996) White matter changes in depression and Alzheimer's disease: a review of magnetic resonance imaging studies. *International Journal of Geriatric Psychiatry* **11**: 681–694

O'Brien JT, Erkinjuntti T, Reisberg B et al. (2003) Vascular cognitive impairment. *Lancet Neurology* **2**: 89–98

O'Connor DW, Pollit PA, Hyde JB et al. (1990) A follow-up study of dementia diagnosed in the community using the Cambridge Mental Disorders of the Elderly Examination (CAMDEX). *Acta Psychiatrica Scandinavica* **81**: 78–82

Ouchi Y, Yoshikawa E, Okada H et al. (1999) Alterations in binding site density of dopamine transporter in the striatum, orbitofrontal cortex, and amygdala in early Parkinson's disease: compartment analysis for beta-CFT binding with positron emission tomography. *Annals of Neurology* **45**: 601–610

Pearlson G and Rabins P. (1988) The late onset psychoses – possible risk factors. In: *Psychiatric Clinics of North America* Vol II, 1. (eds DV Jeste and S Zisook). Philadelphia, W Saunders, pp. 15–22

Perry RH, Irving D, Blessed G et al. (1990) A clinically and pathologically distinct form of Lewy body dementia in the elderly. *Journal of the Neurological Sciences* **95**: 119–139

Petersen RC, Smith GE, Waring SC et al. (1999) Mild cognitive impairment: clinical characterization and outcome. *Archives of Neurology* **56**: 303–308

Petersen RC, Doody R, Kurz A et al. (2001). Current concepts in mild cognitive impairment. *Archives of Neurology* **58**: 1985–1992

Piggott MA and Marshall EF. (1996) Neurochemical correlations of pathological and iatrogenicextrapyramidal symptoms. In: RH Perry, IG McKeith, EK Perry (eds), *Dementia with Lewy Bodies: Clinical, Pathological and Treatment Issues.* Cambridge, Cambridge University Press, pp. 449–467

Ritchie K, Artero S, Touchon J (2001) Classification criteria for mild cognitive impairment: a population-based validation study. *Neurology* **56**: 37–42

Robertson B, Blennow K, Gottfries CG et al. (1998) Delirium in dementia. *International Journal of Geriatric Psychiatry* **13**: 49–56

Rocca WA, Hofman A, Brayne C et al. (1991) The prevalence of vascular dementia in Europe: facts and fragments from 1980–1990 studies. EURODERM. *Annals of Neurology* **30**: 817–824

Rogers SL, Farlow MR, Doody RS et al. (1998) A 24-week, double-blind, placebo-controlled trial of donepezil in patients with Alzheimer's disease. *Neurology* **50**: 136–145

Román GC, Tatemichi T, Erkinjuntti T et al. (1993) Vascular dementia: diagnostic criteria for research studies. Report of the NINCDS AIRENS International Workshop. *Neurology* **43**: 250–260

Román GC, Erkinjuntti T, Wallin A et al. (2002) Subcortical ischaemic vascular dementia. *Lancet Neurology* **1**: 426–436

Rosen WG, Terry RD, Fuld PA et al. (1980) Pathological verification of ischaemic score in the differentiation of dementias. *Annals of Neurology* **7**: 485–488

Roth M, Tymm E, Mountjoy C et al. (1986) CAMDEX: A standardized instrument for the diagnosis of mental disorder in the elderly, with special reference to the early detection of dementia. *British Journal of Psychiatry* **149**: 698–709

Small GW. (1985) Revised ischaemic score for diagnosing multi-infarct dementia. *Journal of Clinical Psychiatry* **46**: 514–517

Tierney M, Fisher R, Lewis A et al. (1988) The NINCDS/ADRDA workgroup criteria for the clinical diagnosis of probable Alzheimer's disease: A clinico-pathologic study of 57 cases. *Neurology* **38**: 359–364

Tomlinson BE, Blessed G, Roth M (1970) Observations on the brains of demented old people. *Journal of the Neurological Sciences* **11**: 205–242

Tuokko H, Frerichs R, Graham J et al. (2003) Five-year follow-up of cognitive impairment with no dementia. *Archives of Neurology* **60**: 577–582

Verghese J, Crystal HA, Dickson DW et al. (1999) Validity of clinical criteria for the diagnosis of dementia with Lewy bodies. *Neurology* **53** (9): 1974–1982

Walker MP, Ayre GA, Cummings JL et al. (2000) The clinician assessment of fluctuation and the one day fluctuation assessment scale: two methods to assess fluctuating confusion in dementia. *British Journal of Psychiatry* **177**: 252–256

Walker Z, Allen RL, Shergill S et al. (1997) Neuropsychological performance in Lewy body dementia and Alzheimer's disease. *British Journal of Psychiatry* **170**: 156–158

Walker Z, Costa DC, Walker RW et al. (2002) Differentiation of dementia with Lewy bodies from Alzheimer's disease using a dopaminergic presynaptic ligand. *Journal of Neurology, Neurosurgery, and Psychiatry* **73**: 134–140

Wallin A. (1994) The clinical diagnosis of vascular dementia. *Dementia* **5**: 181–184

World Health Organization. (1992) *International Classification of Diseases and Health Related Problems*, 10th revision. Geneva, World Health Organization

4

Assessment of dementia

REBECCA EASTLEY AND GORDON K WILCOCK

4.1 CAUSES OF DEMENTIA AND COGNITIVE IMPAIRMENT

There are probably over a hundred different disorders that may cause dementia or chronic cognitive impairment. Box 4.1 lists the commonest causes.

Alzheimer's disease (AD) is the most frequently diagnosed cause of dementia but the majority of people with AD have concomitant cerebrovascular pathology including a third who have cerebral infarction (Kalaria, 2000). Although vascular pathology has been found in 29–41 per cent of dementia cases in post-mortem studies, pure vascular pathology was only identified as a cause for dementia in 9–10 per cent of cases (Holmes et al., 1999; Lim et al., 1999). VaD(VaD) is a syndrome that includes a number of heterogeneous subtypes such as dementia caused by 'strategic' infarction, cerebral haemorrhage, and conditions where there is diffuse ischaemic damage (Amar and Wilcock, 1996).

Dementia with Lewy bodies (DLB) accounts for 15–20 per cent cases in hospital post-mortem series (Weiner, 1999) and is the second commonest cause of neurodegenerative dementia after AD. Again, mixed pathological changes are the rule and cases of pure DLB without plaques, tangles or vascular changes are uncommon (Holmes et al., 1999).

Frontotemporal dementia is less common than AD, DLB or VaD overall but the second commonest form of primary neurodegenerative dementia in middle age, accounting for up to 20 per cent of presenile dementia cases (Snowden et al., 2002).

4.1.1 Potentially reversible dementia

In a study of 1000 memory clinic patients a potentially reversible primary underlying cause was found in 19 per cent

cases, and one or more potentially reversible concomitant conditions in 23 per cent (Hejl et al., 2002). Potentially reversible causes were more likely to be found in people who

- had no objective cognitive deficits, or
- had cognitive impairment but not dementia

compared to people with dementia. Potentially reversible causes were also found more frequently in those under the age of 60 years. Only 4 per cent of people who had dementia had a potentially reversible primary cause. Probably only about 1 per cent of potentially reversible cases of dementia actually do reverse with treatment (Walstra et al., 1997), but a higher proportion may show a partial response. The commonest causes of 'reversible or partially reversible dementia' found in Clarfield's (1988) review of 32 studies involving 2889 subjects were as shown in Box 4.2.

Some potential causes of cognitive impairment such as vitamin B_{12} deficiency appear to be most amenable to treatment before dementia is established (Eastley et al., 2000), and so people presenting with mild cognitive impairment should receive the same degree of assessment as those who present with a dementia syndrome.

4.1.2 Delirium

Delirium is an important differential diagnosis, and a common cause of the misdiagnosis of dementia (Ryan, 1994). Delirium is commonly superimposed on dementia and some causes of delirium may subsequently lead to the development of dementia if not treated. Almost any acute illness may cause delirium in an elderly person, but infections, particularly of the urinary tract or respiratory system, and iatrogenic causes are frequent culprits. Clinical features that help to distinguish delirium from dementia are given in Box 4.3.

Physical disorders that can cause cognitive impairment do not always present with delirium. An insidious onset and slow progressive deterioration may be observed in hypothyroidism and vitamin B_{12} deficiency for example.

4.1.3 Depression

The relationship between dementia and depression is complex. In a memory clinic setting depression was found to be the most common potential reversible cause of cognitive symptoms and the most common potentially reversible concomitant condition (Hejl *et al.*, 2002). However, elderly people with depression often show deficits on standard cognitive tests, which do not always resolve with treatment (Abas *et al.*, 1990). Poor performance on cognitive testing is sometimes related to lack of motivation and impaired concentration, and is typically characterized by 'I don't know' answers, or a similar response. In some cases the cognitive impairment does not appear to be directly related to 'lack of effort' but may still resolve with treatment of the depression. However, those patients with 'reversible dementia' presumed to be secondary to depression are at higher risk of subsequently developing dementia on follow up than those with depression alone (Alexopoulos *et al.*, 1993). Depression can also be a comorbid condition with dementia. The prevalence rate of comorbid depressive illness in people with dementia varies with the study population and definition of depression, but the mean is 20 per cent (Ballard *et al.*, 1996).

It may not be possible at the initial assessment to determine whether delirium, depression or other treatable disorder is a primary diagnosis or a comorbid condition. In either case appropriate treatment should be initiated and the patient reassessed. Depressive symptoms in the elderly and cognitive dysfunction may take several months to improve with treatment, so full neuropsychological testing should probably not be repeated until a minimum of 3 months have elapsed.

4.2   THE ASSESSMENT PROCESS

The assessment of the person with dementia or cognitive impairment usually requires a multidisciplinary approach and should be holistic rather than solely aimed at making a diagnosis. Functional ability, behaviour, the presence of psychiatric symptoms, and the psychosocial consequences of the illness on the person and their carer should also be assessed. Assessment should be a dynamic process. This chapter focuses on the diagnostic aspect of the assessment process. Obviously local service arrangements will determine where the patient is seen and by whom. The initial assessment process will involve history-taking, mental state and physical examination, blood tests and neuroimaging.

4.2.1 History

The history is the cornerstone of any assessment. The quality of information available from the patient will depend on the degree of cognitive impairment and the level of insight. Even when a patient has adequate insight into their difficulties, it is still essential to obtain supplementary information from other sources. Informants should be reliable, know the patient well and be in close contact with them. A review of the medical notes often provides important clues to the present problem.

4.2.2 Presenting complaint

The publicity generated by the launch of drug treatment for AD has done much to raise general awareness of this illness. Clinicians are increasingly likely to see patients who refer themselves with complaints of memory impairment. This requires the same degree of assessment as severe global cognitive impairment. Memory impairment in isolation is insufficient for a diagnosis of dementia but can represent the first symptom of a dementing illness. Potentially treatable causes of dementia are most likely to be amenable to reversal in the early stages of the illness, and initial symptoms of cognitive dysfunction may be quite subtle.

Subjective cognitive impairment is a common symptom of depression. Typically patients complain of thinking difficulties, poor concentration and memory impairment. There may be evidence of concentration and memory impairment on examination, but cortical symptoms such as dysphasia, dyspraxia or agnosia are rare in uncomplicated depression. Affective disorder is an important differential diagnosis for dementia, but also a common comorbid condition.

While patients may admit to mislaying things, or having to rely on written notes as *aides-memoire*, carers usually provide a better assessment of the severity of the impairment. Patients rarely offer information, which raises concern about their ability to function independently. It is invariably concerned friends or relatives who reveal that the patient forgets to lock their door or turn the gas off.

Much can be learnt about other areas of cognitive function from the history. Special attention should be given to symptoms of language impairment, dyspraxia, agnosia and visuospatial impairment. Direct enquiry may provide evidence of problems with orientation, initiating, planning and carrying through activities, reading, or handling money.

Non-cognitive symptoms, such as a change in personality, behavioural disturbance and psychiatric symptoms, are usually best elicited from a carer. Patients who have impaired insight into their dementia are less likely to admit to depressive symptoms for example (Ott and Fogel, 1992).

The importance of the assessment of non-cognitive symptoms is two-fold. First they provide essential information for the diagnostic process. Loss of drive, disinhibition, and poverty of speech are common symptoms of frontal lobe damage, and may be the first signs of frontal lobe dementia. Visual hallucinations may point to delirium or DLB, or prominent mood symptoms may suggest an affective disorder. Second, non-cognitive symptoms have an enormous impact on the day-to-day life of both patient and carer, and may require intervention in their own right.

4.2.2.1 HISTORY OF PRESENTING COMPLAINT

A sudden, acute onset of cognitive impairment, usually excludes a neurodegenerative condition. However, caution should be exercised when assessing this. Physical or psychiatric illness may exacerbate existing problems, which only become evident on careful enquiry. Social changes such as moving house or illness in the carer may suddenly reveal deficits that hitherto went unnoticed.

The onset of AD is typically insidious, and the decline in function occurs gradually. Memory impairment is followed by the development of dysphasia, dyspraxia and agnosia. The course of dementia after a stroke is usually like that of AD (Kokmen *et al.*, 1996). The sudden onset of cognitive impairment without subsequent deterioration might suggest a cerebrovascular infarct or other acute event. The classic description of a step-wise deterioration in vascular dementia is sometimes seen but not invariably so. The symptom profile in vascular dementia is variable and determined by the site and severity of the damage.

A relatively short history with fluctuations in the level of consciousness could suggest delirium, either as a primary cause or superimposed on a dementia, or subdural haematoma. Marked fluctuation in the degree of cognitive impairment is a hallmark characteristic of DLB.

4.2.3 Past medical history

Treatment decisions may be influenced by the medical history, and past medical conditions may be implicated in the aetiology of the cognitive impairment, or be responsible for an exacerbation of current problems. However, causality should not be inferred without supporting evidence. A close temporal relationship between recent medical problems and the onset of cognitive impairment rightly raises suspicion but could be coincidental. People also measure their lives by events, and not infrequently relate their history to medical landmarks.

A multitude of medical conditions may compromise brain function through a variety of pathological mechanisms, and only the more common can be considered here. Vascular risk factors such as hypertension, diabetes and hyperlipidaemia are risk factors for both VaD and AD (Stewart, 1998). Past myocardial infarction or episodes of dysrhythmias may suggest a vascular component. Any condition that could cause anoxic or hypoxic damage may be relevant, such as severe respiratory problems or anaemia.

Hypothyroidism can lead to cognitive impairment and should always be considered in an elderly person with a past history of thyroid disease. Liver and renal disease may impact on cognitive function but are rare causes of dementia.

Particular attention should be given to any history of head injury. Even minor head trauma can cause a subdural haematoma in elderly people, and this occasionally presents with deteriorating cognitive function. Head injury also increases the risk of normal pressure hydrocephalus and AD.

4.2.4 Systems review

A brief review of the major body systems should not be forgotten. Occasionally important symptoms are only elicited by direct questioning as the patient or carer may not have made any association between them and the cognitive dysfunction.

4.2.5 Psychiatric history

A specific enquiry about any past psychiatric illness is recommended as this information is often not volunteered. A history of depressive illness increases the risk of current affective disorder, whether this is the primary diagnosis or not. Details about the symptom profile of any past episodes of psychiatric disorder often prove extremely helpful. Occasionally a review of the psychiatric notes reveals that cognitive problems were prominent during a previous illness but resolved with treatment. More rarely younger patients with somatoform or dissociative disorders may present with complaints of cognitive impairment.

Alcoholism or alcohol abuse is more likely to be missed in elderly people than younger adults (Caracci and Miller, 1991). Alcohol is neurotoxic and the damage caused by long-term abuse can be irreversible. There is an association between alcoholism and thiamine deficiency although the exact relationship is not fully understood (Kopelman, 1995). Thiamine deficiency can cause Wernicke's encephalopathy and Korsakoff's psychosis. Wernicke's encephalopathy presents acutely with confusion, clouded consciousness, ophthalmoplegia, nystagmus and ataxia, and requires immediate treatment. Korsakoff's psychosis is an amnesic syndrome.

4.2.6 Medication and substance use/abuse

When you are taking the medication history, it is always worthwhile checking the length of time particular drugs have been prescribed. A new treatment or change in dosage coinciding with the onset or exacerbation of cognitive problems should alert the clinician to the possibility of an iatrogenic cause. However, longstanding prescriptions can sometimes be implicated. The development of a medical illness may change the bioavailability or metabolism of previously well-tolerated drugs. The possibility of non-prescription drug use, such as cough and cold remedies, or the use of relative's medications should not be forgotten.

Older people are particularly vulnerable to adverse effects from psychotropic medication for a variety of reasons. Age-related physiological factors can alter drug pharmacokinetics and dynamics. Additionally, elderly people are more likely to be suffering from physical illness and taking multiple medications. Special consideration should be given to the possible effects of tricyclic antidepressants, long-acting hypnotics, neuroleptics and the older anticonvulsants. Any medication with anticholinergic activity may impact cognitive function, and those individuals with reduced neuronal reserve are especially sensitive.

Sometimes the medication problems arise secondary to cognitive impairment, and exacerbate it further. People with impaired memory function may overdose because they forget they have taken their tablets, or else forget to take them at all. Non-compliance may account for poor diabetic control, or inadequate thyroid treatment, for example.

Illicit substance use is rare in current elderly cohorts but alcohol abuse is much commoner. Present and past alcohol intake should be assessed.

4.2.7 Family history

Family histories can aide the diagnostic process but need to be reliable. Reports of 'confusion' in elderly relatives adds little to the assessment, but a family history of formally diagnosed AD or Huntington's chorea, for example, can be all important. It is also necessary to ascertain the age at which first-degree relatives died as, especially for late-onset AD, relatives may have died before reaching the age of maximum risk.

Affective disorders in first-degree relatives may be relevant if depressive symptoms are prominent. Sometimes enquiries about general health problems in the family yield crucial information about possible aetiological causes, which would not otherwise be considered. Inherited clotting disorders or thrombophilias for example may come to light.

4.2.8 Social history

It is essential to assess the person's social circumstances in order to formulate a care plan. Living arrangements and support networks may be inadequate and this part of the history may reveal unmet needs for assistance with practical tasks such as shopping or food preparation. There may be issues involving the patient's financial situation that need to be addressed, such as their ability to manage their own finances or their entitlement to benefits. If not already covered at this point a specific enquiry should be made about whether the patient is still driving and, if they are, whether there have been any difficulties. Both patients and informants are often reluctant to admit to any problems with driving because of the potential consequences. If patients are driving, special attention should be given to the findings of the neuropsychological examination.

4.3　MENTAL STATE EXAMINATION

The mental state examination begins with the first contact with the patient whether this is at home or in a clinic setting. Untidiness, inappropriate clothing or poor personal hygiene may indicate dyspraxia or self-neglect from severe depression. A mood disorder may be suggested by a downcast or anxious expression. Disinhibition may be demonstrated by an inappropriate greeting.

Language function is assessed during the interview and by formal testing. Abnormalities in the rate and form of speech may be indicative of an affective disorder or underlying neurological dysfunction. Decreased rate or poverty of speech may be a feature of depression or frontotemporal dementia. Patients who repeat answers, phrases or words from preceding questions are perseverating, a sign of frontal lobe impairment. Dysarthria, the disorder of the articulation of speech, can be caused by lesions of the upper or lower motor neurones, extrapyramidal and cerebellar pathways. Paraphasias, which are slightly incorrect words, can be a feature of temporal lobe problems, but also can occur when the patient is particularly anxious. Expressive dysphasia occurs secondary to frontal lobe involvement, and receptive dysphasia is caused by a lesion in Wernicke's area.

The symptoms of mood disorders in people with mild to moderate cognitive impairment or dementia are the same as for anyone else. People who are more severely impaired may lack the ability to express their distress in cognitive terms, and then the diagnosis relies more on the biological symptoms, informant history and behavioural assessment. Suicide ideation should be assessed if there are any depressive symptoms whether the person has dementia or not. Dementia does not necessarily preclude a completed suicide (Cattell and Jolley, 1995). Lability of mood is classically seen in vascular dementia and cognitive impairment and, when extreme, is termed emotional incontinence.

Psychotic symptoms may arise secondary to functional psychiatric illness, in which case they are usually mood congruent. In delirium, delusions are often paranoid in flavour and not well systematized. Some abnormal beliefs occurring in a person with dementia can often be understood in terms of the person trying to make sense of their experiences. Family members may be accused of stealing things, or neighbours of coming into the house and moving things. Hallucinations can occur in any modality, but are commonly auditory or visual.

Detailed visual hallucinations of people or animals in particular are common symptoms in DLB.

The mental state examination should include basic cognitive testing, although a more detailed neuropsychological assessment by a psychologist may be required. The general interview will give an impression of the patient's attention and concentration. Formal tests of attention include asking them to repeat a series of digits forwards and backwards, giving the months of the year or days of the week backwards, or subtracting serial sevens from 100. Aspects of memory including registration and recall can be briefly assessed by asking the patient to repeat a name and address or a series of words immediately and after a delay. The inability to understand instructions may indicate receptive language problems. The presence of nominal dysphasia may not be apparent in social conversation as patients often compensate by using circumlocution. It is tested by asking the patient to name a series of objects. Visuospatial function can be assessed by a number of tests including drawing a clock face and copying an asymmetric design. Parietal lobe impairment may be evidenced by loss of the ability to distinguish right from left, finger agnosia (cannot name fingers), astereognosis (cannot recognize an item placed in the hand with eyes closed), dressing apraxia (cannot dress), topographical agnosia (cannot find way around) and sensory inattention. Perseveration in frontal lobe impairment can be demonstrated by card-sorting tests and repetition in motor tasks. The FAS word fluency test is a useful screening test for frontal impairment.

The person's degree of insight into their current difficulties can aid the diagnosis and of course has implications for further management.

4.4　PHYSICAL EXAMINATION

Like the mental state examination, the physical examination begins as soon as you meet the patient. Some conditions may be apparent from the patient's appearance alone.

There may be obvious discomfort when they get out of the chair in the waiting room, or unsteadiness on standing. Shaking hands when introduced may reveal the forced grasping seen in frontal lobe lesions. The gait can be observed when the patient is walking to the consulting room or through the house. Is there evidence of ataxia, the broad-based gait of normal pressure hydrocephalus, or the parkinsonian shuffling steps? Does the patient get out of breath with minimal exertion? Abnormal movements such as resting tremors or choreoathetoid movements may be obvious before a neurological examination is performed.

Noting the skin colour takes seconds and may reveal the paleness of anaemia, jaundice, cyanosis, or the plethoric appearance of polycythaemia.

Measure the patient's temperature if toxicity is suspected. The general examination should include a check of the thyroid gland, lymph nodes and breasts (in women).

4.4.1 Cardiorespiratory examination

A vascular cause for the cognitive impairment may be indicated by the rate and rhythm of the pulse, the presence of hypertension, heart murmurs, carotid bruits, or poor peripheral circulation. A slow regular pulse may suggest heart block, overtreatment with some drugs, e.g. β-blockers, or hypothyroidism. Sitting and standing blood pressure should be measured in the case of orthostatic hypotension.

Chest examination may reveal evidence of infection, cardiac failure, or occasionally pleural effusion.

4.4.2 Abdomen

Any abnormal findings may be important but liver disease stigmata, the presence of an aortic aneurysm or discomfort on bladder palpation may be directly relevant to the aetiology. Faecal loading in the large bowel sometimes accounts for new behavioural problems. Constipation can be caused by medications with anticholinergic activity and also opiate derivatives, which themselves may exacerbate cognitive impairment.

4.4.3 Musculoskeletal

Musculoskeletal disorders are only rarely associated with the aetiology of cognitive impairment, but require assessment in their own right. A few conditions such as rheumatoid arthritis can cause cognitive impairment through vascular pathology.

4.4.4 Nervous system

Any abnormalities in posture, gait and movement may already have been noted but should also be formally assessed. Intention and static tremors are found when there is a cerebellar disorder, and the pill-rolling tremor is characteristic of parkinsonism. Action tremors may be exaggerated in thyrotoxicosis, uraemia and liver disease.

Of particular importance in the cranial nerve examination is any sign of facial weakness, abnormal eye movements, nystagmus and visual field defects. Ophthalmoscopy should be performed routinely as it may reveal signs of systemic disease such as diabetic or hypertensive retinopathy as well as papilloedema secondary to raised intracranial pressure.

Abnormalities in the pyramidal and the extrapyramidal motor systems may help to confirm the diagnosis of VaD, DLB, Parkinson's disease, and amyotrophic lateral sclerosis. Myoclonus may be associated with epilepsy, or Creuztfeldt–Jakob disease.

The grasp, sucking and snout reflexes are examples of primitive reflexes which are normal in infants. People with frontal dementias usually acquire primitive reflexes in the early stages of their illness, otherwise their occurrence is usually associated with advanced dementia. The grasp reflex, a flexion of the thumb and fingers, can be elicited by stroking the patient's palm between their thumb and index finger. The sucking reflex can be provoked by touching the lips with a wooden spatula or other instrument and, as it name implies, involves contraction of the muscles used for sucking. A pout provoked by tapping the centre of closed lips is the snout reflex.

Sensation is particularly difficult to assess in a person with dementia and in addition an impairment of lower limb vibratory sense and proprioception is a common normal finding in many elderly people. However, sensory examination can still be useful and may reveal abnormalities suggestive of cerebrovascular lesions, peripheral neuropathy in diabetes or vitamin B_{12} deficiency and, more rarely these days, tabes dorsalis and subacute combined degeneration of the cord.

4.5 INVESTIGATIONS

Standard blood screening is a recommended part of the assessment, and serves several purposes. It may reveal potentially treatable causes of cognitive impairment and organic mood disorder, or coexistent medical disorders which were not suspected from the history or physical examination. Additionally impaired renal function or liver function tests for example may influence treatment decisions.

Standard blood investigations should include those in Box 4.4.

There are areas, such as parts of North America, where tertiary syphilis has become so rare that screening for syphilis is no longer recommended as a routine investigation (Knopman *et al.*, 2001). However, if there is a clinical suspicion or the patient resides in a high incidence area, screening should be performed.

Other investigations including an electrocardiogram may be arranged as indicated by the history and examination.

Unfortunately clinical rules for predicting which patients should have standard structural neuroimaging introduce the risk of missing clinically significant structural lesions (Gifford *et al.*, 2000). Where neuroimaging is possible as part of the initial evaluation, this should be with either non-contrast computed tomography (CT) or magnetic resonance imaging (Knopman *et al.*, 2001).

Although it is not widely available, there is evidence that using a dopaminergic presynaptic ligand, ^{123}I-labelled

---

Box 4.4   *Standard blood investigations*

- Full blood count
- Viscosity or ESR
- Urea, creatinine and electrolytes
- Vitamin B_{12}
- Liver function tests
- Folate
- Thyroid function tests
- Blood glucose
- Calcium
- Cholesterol

2β-carbomethoxy-3β-(4-iodophenyl)-N-(3-fluoropropyl) nortropane (FP-CIT) and single photon emission tomography (SPET) can distinguish DLB from AD during life (Walker *et al.*, 2002). Further evaluation is required to determine whether this will be useful as a routine investigation.

Lumbar puncture is only indicated as an investigation if an infective or inflammatory cause is suspected.

There has been a lot of interest in cerebrospinal fluid (CSF) markers but to date only the CSF 14-3-3 protein assay for Creutzfeld–Jakob disease has clinical usefulness, although the ratio of phosphorylated τ to β-amyloid peptide in the CSF looks promising as an aid to diagnosing AD (Galasko, 2003).

4.6 CONCLUSION

The clinical features of the history, mental state, physical examination and the findings of investigations must all be considered when making a diagnosis of dementia. Many causes of dementia or cognitive impairment are potentially reversible, and comorbid conditions may require therapeutic intervention. For those causes that are irreversible, there are treatment options that may offer symptomatic improvement and alter the course of the illness.

REFERENCES

Abas MA, Sahakian BJ, Levy R. (1990) Neuropsychological deficits and CT scan changes in elderly depressives. *Psychological Medicine* **20**: 507–520

Alexopoulos GS, Meyers BS, Young RC *et al.* (1993) The course of geriatric depression with 'reversible dementia': a controlled study. *American Journal of Psychiatry* **150**: 1693–1699

Amar K and Wilcock GK. (1996) Vascular dementia. *BMJ* **312**: 227–312

Ballard CG, Bannister C, Oyebode F. (1996) Depression in dementia sufferers. *International Journal of Geriatric Psychiatry* **11**: 507–515

Caracci G and Miller NS. (1991) Epidemiology and diagnosis of alcoholism in the elderly (a review). *International Journal of Geriatric Psychiatry* **6**: 511–515

Cattell H and Jolley DJ. (1995) One hundred cases of suicide in elderly people. *British Journal of Psychiatry* **166**: 451–457

Clarfield AM. (1988) The reversible dementias: do they reverse? *Annals of Internal Medicine* **109**: 476–486

Eastley R, Wilcock GK, Bucks RS. (2000) Vitamin B_{12} deficiency in dementia and cognitive impairment: the effect of treatment on neuropsychological function. *International Journal of Geriatric Psychiatry* **15**: 226–233

Galasko D. (2003) Cerebrospinal fluid biomarkers in Alzheimer's disease. *Archives of Neurology* **60**: 1195–1196

Gifford DR, Holloway RG, Vickrey BG. (2000) Systematic review of clinical prediction rules for neuroimaging in the evaluation of dementia. *Archives of Internal Medicine* **160**: 2855–2862

Hejl A, Hogh P, Waldemar G. (2002) Potentially reversible conditions in 1000 consecutive memory clinic patients. *Journal of Neurology, Neurosurgery, and Psychiatry* **73**: 390–394

Holmes C, Cairns N, Lantos P, Mann A. (1999) Validity of current clinical criteria for Alzheimer's disease, vascular dementia and dementia with Lewy bodies. *British Journal of Psychiatry* **174**: 45–50

Kalaria RN. (2000) The role of cerebral ischaemia in Alzheimer's disease. *Neurobiology of Aging* **21**: 321–330

Knopman DS, DeKosky ST, Cummings JL *et al.* (2001) Practice parameter: diagnosis of dementia (an evidence-based review). Report of the Quality Standards Subcommittee of the American Academy of Neurology. *Neurology* **56**: 1143–1153

Kokmen E, Whistman JP, O'Fallon WM *et al.* (1996) Dementia after ischemic stroke: a population-based study in Rochester, Minnesota (1960–1984). *Neurology* **19**: 154–159

Kopelman MD. (1995) The Korsakoff syndrome. *British Journal of Psychiatry* **166**: 154–173

Lim A, Tsuang D, Kukull W *et al.* (1999) Clinico-neuropathological correlation of Alzheimer's disease in a community-based case series. *Journal of the American Geriatrics Society* **47**: 564–569

Ott BR and Fogel BS. (1992) Measurement of depression in dementia: Self vs clinical rating. *International Journal of Geriatric Psychiatry* **7**: 899–904

Ryan DH. (1994) Misdiagnosis in dementia: comparisons of diagnostic error rate and range of hospital investigations according to medical speciality. *International Journal of Geriatric Psychiatry* **9**: 141–147

Snowden JS, Neary D, Mann DMA. (2002) Frontotemporal dementia. *British Journal of Psychiatry* **180**: 140–143

Stewart R. (1998) Cardiovascular factors in Alzheimer's disease. *Journal of Neurology, Neurosurgery, and Psychiatry* **65**: 143–147

Walker Z, Costa DC, Walker RWH *et al.* (2002) Differentiation of dementia with Lewy bodies from Alzheimer's disease using a dopaminergic presynaptic ligand. *Journal of Neurology, Neurosurgery, and Psychiatry* **73**: 134–140

Walstra GJM, Teunisse S, van Gool WA, van Crevel H. (1997) Reversible dementia in elderly patients referred to a memory clinic. *Journal of Neurology* **244**: 17–22

Weiner MF. (1999) Dementia associated with Lewy bodies. *Archives of Neurology* **56**: 1441–1442

Neuropsychological assessment of dementia

ANDREW D BLACKWELL, BARNABY D DUNN, ADRIAN M OWEN AND BARBARA J SAHAKIAN

It is estimated that dementia currently affects approximately 37 million people worldwide, with an estimated 775 200 cases in the United Kingdom (World Health Organization, 2001; Alzheimer's Society Demography Policy Position, 2004). As the population ages these prevalence rates can be expected to increase substantially, especially in industrialized nations (Hebert et al., 2003). Dementia can have a devastating personal impact upon the lives of patients and their carers, and may also be associated with substantial financial costs; the total cost of Alzheimer's disease (AD) alone in the US for the year 2000 has been estimated to be US$1.75 billion (World Health Organization, 2001).

Over the past two decades, the concept of dementia as a 'progressive global cognitive decline in clear consciousness' has been revised. It is increasingly apparent that each form of dementia has a distinct cognitive profile, at least in the mild stages of the disease, and that this reflects the pattern of underlying neuropathological change (Hodges, 1998; Rahman et al., 1999a; Lee et al., 2003). The advent of potentially disease-modifying therapies has reinforced the immediate need for reliable, sensitive and specific in vivo markers for each form of dementia. Significant recent advances in our understanding of the cognitive neuropsychology of the dementias (coupled with an absence of accurate biomarkers) have emphasized the importance of neuropsychological assessment in the early and differential diagnosis of the dementias, in objective monitoring of changes in cognitive function across disease course or as a function of treatment, and in estimating functional status.

In this chapter a brief outline of the rationale for neuropsychological assessment will be given, together with a description of what a detailed neuropsychological assessment can offer a clinician over and above simple rating scales such as the Mini-Mental State Examination (MMSE) (Folstein et al., 1975) and Alzheimer's Disease Assessment Scale (ADAS-cog) (Rosen et al., 1984). The chapter will focus on Alzheimer's disease (AD), since this is the most prevalent and probably the best understood dementia from a neuropsychological perspective, but will also refer to frontotemporal dementia, dementia with Lewy bodies (DLB) and vascular dementia (VaD) in the section on differential diagnosis. In describing the neurocognitive profile of these conditions, an emphasis will be placed on neuropsychological tests that are of use in the early detection and differential diagnosis of the dementias.

5.1 NEUROPSYCHOLOGICAL ASSESSMENT: BACKGROUND AND GENERAL CONSIDERATIONS

5.1.1 What is neuropsychological assessment and how is it relevant to dementia?

Clinical neuropsychology is an applied science concerned with the behavioural expression of brain dysfunction (Lezak, 1995). In general, the aim of neuropsychological assessment in cases of dementia is to provide a clinician with a profile of the patient's performance demonstrating specific areas of cognitive impairment and cognitive sparing. The acquired information can be used for several purposes. These include aiding diagnosis, informing management, care and planning, evaluating the efficacy of a treatment, providing information about competency for legal matters, or for research.

5.1.2 How should I choose which tests to use?

The neuropsychological tests used in a particular clinical assessment must be tailored to the individual needs of the patient and the reason for the referral. Nevertheless, it is also important to include 'benchmark' tests in order that the neuropsychologist can compare between patients within the same group, across patient groups and for use in longitudinal follow up. On a very general level, the assessment of a patient should involve an evaluation of their cognitive function in the major domains afflicted by the dementia, an assessment of mood (e.g. Beck Depression Inventory [Beck *et al.*, 1961], Hamilton Depression Rating Scale [Hamilton, 1960]), an estimate of premorbid intelligence level together with years of education to compare results to, and a measure of how much the deficits in cognitive function affect the patient's functioning in everyday life. The test battery chosen should ideally be sensitive to even subtle deficits in patients, be relatively easy and quick to administer and have been validated longitudinally (including equivalent forms and characterization of any practice effects) (Ferris and Kluger, 1997).

The quality of a neuropsychological test is measured by how well its psychometric properties conform to theoretical notions of reliability and validity (Kline, 1986). Good validity means that the test actually measures what it is purported to measure. Good reliability means that the test's measurements are accurate and consistent across different clinicians, locations and times. So that the test can be used reliably for diagnosis at a single case level, the key qualities required are specificity (any deficit found on a test is unique to one patient group and not a range of conditions) and sensitivity (the test should be sensitive to the earliest stages of a neurodegenerative disease and even subtle changes in a patient's condition).

Exactly which test to use depends on the precise hypothesis being tested. For example, different tests are sensitive to different levels of severity of dementia. A test like the CANTAB Paired Associate Learning task (Sahakian *et al.*, 1988) is excellent for early detection of AD (see below), but owing to its sensitivity it may not be ideal for measuring disease progression in more advanced stages of disease progression. Other CANTAB tests, such as the Delayed Matching To Sample Test, the Attentional Shift Test and the Visual Search Test may be more suitable for assessing stage and severity of dementia (see Sahakian *et al.*, 1988, 1990; Sahgal *et al.*, 1992a). Further, a lengthy battery may be useful for the detailed assessment of cognitive function in the mild stages of dementia but may not be appropriate or feasible in more moderately/severely demented patients with major attentional difficulties. It is important to include verbal and non-verbal stimuli, to examine both recognition and recall, and to assess performance at both immediate and delayed memory. The CANTAB non-verbal tests may be combined with tests of verbal function,

together with measures of premorbid or current intelligence level (e.g. National Adult Reading Test [NART], Wechsler Adult Intelligence Scale – Revised [WAIS-R], respectively). For those without access to computerized assessment, an example of a 'pencil and paper' battery may include measures of premorbid and current intellectual function (e.g. NART, WAIS-R, respectively), episodic memory (e.g. Wechsler Logical Memory, Kendrick Object Learning Task, Warrington Recognition Memory for words and faces), working memory (e.g. Corsi block tapping task, forward and backwards digit span), semantic memory (e.g. Graded Naming Test, category fluency, Boston Naming Test, Pyramids and Palm Trees Test), attention (e.g. the Stroop test, symbol digit substitution, Test of Everyday Attention), visuospatial perception and construction (e.g. drawing a clock face, Ray–Oesterreich figure, the Visual Object and Space Perception Battery [VOSP]), language comprehension and expression (e.g. Test for Reception of Grammar [TROG], Token Test) and executive functions (e.g. Wisconson Card Sorting Test, Behavioural Assessment of the Dysexecutive Syndrome [BADS]). An alternative to combining individual tests is to use an already constructed battery. Some batteries commonly used in memory clinics are described briefly below.

- The Consortium to Establish a Registry for Dementia of the Alzheimer's type (CERAD; Morris, 1997; Welch *et al.*, 1992) battery includes the Boston Naming Test, verbal fluency, the MMSE and two other subtests, covering memory, language, constructional praxis and intellectual status.
- The Wechsler Memory Scale revised (WMS-R; Kaplan *et al.*, 1991) is made up of 13 subtests that take about 45 minutes to administer. The areas tested include orientation, attention, verbal memory, visual memory and delayed recall.
- The Halstead–Reitan battery (Reitan and Wolfson, 1993) consists of 10 tests that tap sensory, perceptual, motor, attention, language and problem solving abilities.
- The Cambridge Neuropsychological Test Automated Battery (CANTAB; Robbins and Sahakian, 1994) is a set of computerized neuropsychological tests that tap visual memory, attention, and working memory and planning. Computerized batteries have number of distinct advantages over more traditional 'paper and pencil' tests and this has been discussed in detail elsewhere (see Robbins *et al.*, 1994b, 1998; Fray *et al.*, 1996).

5.1.3 What is the merit in using a battery of tests versus a short screening tool?

A neuropsychological assessment involving a battery of tests is almost always preferable to short screening measures where resources and time permit. This is because short mental status tests are suitable for some aspects of performance assessment (e.g. some forms of screening, gross staging of severity), but neglect others. For example, the MMSE (Folstein *et al.*, 1975) is one of the most widely used brief measures of global cognitive function. Its strengths are that it is inexpensive, rapid, highly portable, and can be interpreted and administered with little training. It is standardized and has been successfully applied in cross-national studies. However, the MMSE has poor sensitivity to very mild dementia, is sensitive to age and educational level, and demonstrates ethnicity biases (Tombaugh and McIntyre, 1992; Nadler et al., 1994; Wilder et al., 1995). It is also limited in that it provides only a global index of cognitive performance; a full neuropsychological battery taps more cognitive domains and has greater sensitivity, increasing the usefulness of the assessment in terms of early and differential diagnosis within the dementias. In addition, a comprehensive assessment can provide information from which to measure change in multiple cognitive domains as a result of the progression of the disease or the administration of a new treatment and, in some cases, may aid in the management decisions regarding individual patients.

5.1.4 Feedback of test results

Neuropsychological reports should be informative and useful and should highlight, where possible, the practical implications for improving the patient's quality of life (e.g. use of memory aids, carer support and training). These reports should also include observations of the behaviour of the client during testing (e.g. distractability, motivation, anxiety), as such observations can usefully complement the results of objective neuropsychological tests (see Lezak, 1995).

In all cases, neuropsychology should be viewed as contributing to a diagnosis along with other forms of assessment (e.g. structured clinical interview, neuroimaging, etc.). The most accurate diagnosis and treatment recommendations will always be made by combining converging forms of clinical, neuropsychological and neuroimaging evidence.

5.2 NEUROPSYCHOLOGICAL ASSESSMENT IN THE EARLY DETECTION OF DEMENTIA

Current criteria for the diagnosis of probable AD stipulates deterioration in two or more areas of cognition including memory and this to be of sufficient magnitude to interfere with work or social function (McKhann et al., 1984; see also Small et al., 1997). Clinically, the presenting problem in probable AD patients is often difficulty in new learning and memory (Sahakian et al., 1988). In particular, AD is characterized by deficits in episodic memory (i.e. memory for specific events or experiences that can be defined in terms of time and space) (Welch et al., 1992). Critically, however, substantial neuropathological change may have occurred before clinically significant symptoms appear (Jack et al.,1999; Killiany et al., 2002; Visser et al., 2002). Thus, commencing treatment of AD at the time of clinical diagnosis may be suboptimal or

even ineffective owing to the advanced stage of neurodegeneration at that time. The identification of cognitive tests that are sensitive to early pathological changes would facilitate the diagnosis of patients in a 'prodromal' state (i.e. those in whom the pathological process is present but whose symptoms are currently subclinical).

Until relatively recently, the early detection of dementia has been neglected, partly due to the absence of effective treatments and also because sufficiently sensitive neuropsychological tests were not available. The emergence of drugs to treat the symptoms of AD (e.g. rivastigmine, donepezil, galantamine) brings an end to the therapeutic nihilism previously seen in the dementias and, excitingly, several drugs are currently in development that are hoped will modify disease progression. However, it is widely believed that if neuroprotective agents that modify the disease process are to be effective (or indeed for their efficacy to be evaluated), then it is vital that clinicians are able to detect a dementia early and accurately, before the emergence of global cognitive impairment and substantial and irreversible atrophic damage (Fox et al., 1999; Blackwell et al., 2004). Early detection of dementias can also offer patients and their families more time to come to terms with the diagnosis of dementia, to make the necessary personal and financial arrangements, and to reduce the anxiety patients may feel when they are unsure of their diagnosis (Morgan and Baade, 1997; see also Holroyd et al., 1996, 2002; Geldmacher et al., 2003). Thus, early detection would serve to maximize the potential therapeutic benefit of treatment, enhance patient quality of life and, in so doing, reduce the burden on residential and nursing care services. Consequently, a very high therapeutic and economic premium is placed on the early detection and diagnosis of AD.

Over the past few years, attempts to identify individuals in the prodrome of AD (and other dementias) have largely focused upon patients who report memory problems but who do not fulfil criteria for clinically probable AD, in that activities of daily living and non-memory cognitive faculties are intact. This condition has been given several labels, including 'questionable dementia' (see e.g. Swainson et al., 2001; Blackwell et al., 2004) and 'mild cognitive impairment' (MCI) (Petersen et al., 1999).

According to Petersen (2003), 'the concept of MCI represents the earliest point in the cognitive decline of an individual who is destined to develop AD' and approximately 7–15 per cent per annum of a sample meeting criteria for MCI will 'convert' to meet criteria for probable AD, several fold the conversion rate expected in a general population (Celsis, 2000; Bennett et al., 2002; Petersen, 2003). There is, however, controversy regarding the prognostic utility of MCI as it has been currently defined (see Box 5.1). In particular, the usefulness of the subjective memory complaint (Jorm et al., 1997; Busse et al., 2003), the stability of MCI diagnosis over time, and the optimal operationalization of the objective memory criteria (e.g. the choice of a particular test and criteria to deem a deficit clinically significant) have all been questioned (Ritchie et al., 2001; Larrieu et al., 2002; see also Collie et al., 2002; Petersen,

Box 5.1   *(Amnestic*) mild cognitive impairment criteria*

- Memory complaint, preferably corroborated by a collateral source
- Objective memory impairment for age and education
- Normal general cognition
- Preserved activities of daily living
- Non-demented

*Other clinical subtypes of MCI have recently been proposed. It has been suggested that 'single non-memory cognitive domain MCI' and 'multiple-domain MCI' may have a different aetiology and outcome (Petersen, 2003). Further research is needed to evaluate the validity/utility of these subtypes

2003). Identifying appropriate tests with which to objectively quantify memory impairment is likely to improve the prognostic utility of MCI as a nosological entity and represents a crucial step in identifying patients who may benefit from disease-modifying treatments, while avoiding exposure of those who do not have prodromal AD to potential side effects of these drugs (and unnecessary costs).

In attempting to identify neuropsychological tests that are sensitive to the cognitive markers of prodromal AD (and thus appropriate indices of memory function in MCI), it is crucial to ensure that performance on such tests is not deleteriously affected by other neuropsychiatric complaints that may confuse diagnosis. Furthermore, in order for maximum diagnostic sensitivity to be achieved, it is important to test those cognitive functions that are subserved by brain areas directly implicated in AD neuropathogenesis. The earliest pathological markers of AD, neurofibrillary tangles and neuropil threads, are first seen in the transentorhinal cortex, before neuropathology later spreads to the entorhinal cortex and hippocampus proper (Braak and Braak, 1991). Converging evidence from lesion studies in humans (Smith and Milner, 1981) and experimental animals (McDonald and White, 1993; Miyashita et al., 1998) and functional neuroimaging studies in normal volunteers (Owen et al., 1996; Maguire et al., 1998) suggests that these brain areas are necessarily involved in visuospatial associative learning. Accordingly, it is likely that a decline in visuospatial associative learning ability may be a good candidate marker of early neuropathological abnormality.

A number of longitudinal studies have investigated the relative merits of various neuropsychological tests of memory for announcing AD in its prodromal phase. Fox et al. (1998) followed 63 asymptomatic individuals at risk of autosomal dominant AD over a 6-year period. The 10 subjects who developed dementia during this time could be identified at first assessment (when they were ostensibly unaffected) by significantly lower verbal memory and performance IQ on cognitive testing. These subjects were initially no different in terms of age, family history and initial MMSE scores. First assessment was typically 2–3 years before symptoms were manifest and 4–5 years before a diagnosis of probable AD was made, a result which clearly illustrates the potential sensitivity

of cognitive testing. Blinded assessment of serial MRI imaging showed that diffuse cerebral and medial temporal lobe atrophy was found in subjects only after they were clinically affected, suggesting that a patient's neuropsychological profile may be a more sensitive early indicator than structural brain imaging data (see also Laakso et al., 2000). These results support the notion that the earliest cognitive deficits seen in AD include objective episodic memory impairments that may even precede the onset of subjective memory complaints.

Other longitudinal studies in elderly subjects generally concur with these results. In the Framingham study 'preclinical' deficits in verbal recall (as indexed by the per cent retained in the Logical Memory Test and Paired Associate Learning Test) preceded clinical diagnosis of AD in some cases by more than 6 years (Linn et al., 1995; Elias et al., 2000). Similarly, in the Bronx ageing study, two tests of verbal memory, the Fuld Object Memory Evaluation and the Bushke Selective Reminding Test, predicted many subjects who would go on to develop AD (Masur et al., 1995) (see also Albert et al., 2001; Artero et al., 2003).

Fowler et al. (1995, 1997, 2002) used the Cambridge Neuropsychological Test Automated Battery (CANTAB) to ascertain whether early AD could be detected in a group of individuals with 'questionable dementia' (QD). As discussed above, these are people who present with subjective memory complaints, may or may not show some degree of impairment on standard neuropsychological tests (this differentiates QD from MCI criteria), but do not fulfil NINCDS-ADRDA criteria for dementia (McKhann et al., 1984). Fowler et al. (1997) demonstrated that the CANTAB PAL scores of the QD group fell into two clusters: follow-up longitudinal data revealed that individuals in one cluster (characterized by declining PAL performance) had a poor prognosis and an increased likelihood of a diagnosis of AD, whereas those in the other cluster (characterized by stable PAL performance) had a good prognosis and remained unimpaired. A later study (Swainson et al., 2001; Blackwell et al., 2004) found that PAL performance could be used to accurately predict incident probable AD diagnosis in a QD group based on assessment at a one-time point alone (see below).

The CANTAB PAL requires subjects to learn and remember abstract visual patterns associated with various locations on a touch-sensitive computer screen. Patterns are presented in one of six or eight boxes around the edge of the screen (Figure 5.1). After a brief delay, the same patterns are presented in the middle of the screen and the subject is required to touch the box in which they saw that pattern appear. If this is not completed correctly the subject is reminded where each pattern belonged and tested again. This process continues until the task is satisfactorily completed or 10 trials have been attempted.

Further studies using CANTAB PAL have confirmed it to be useful in early and differential diagnosis in AD on a case-by-case basis. The CANTAB PAL performance of patients with mild AD was impaired relative to both demographically-matched healthy controls (Sahakian et al., 1988) and to

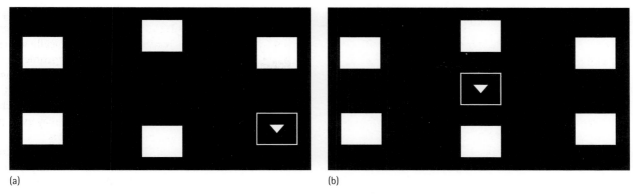

(a)   (b)

Figure 5.1 (a, b) *CANTAB paired associates learning task – 1, 2, 3, 6 or 8 patterns are displayed sequentially in the available boxes (in the 8-pattern stage two more boxes are added). Each pattern is then presented in the centre of the display and the subject is required to touch the box in which the pattern was previously seen. If all the responses are correct the test moves on to the next stage; an incorrect response results in all the patterns being redisplayed in their original locations, followed by another recall phase. The task terminates after 10 presentations and recall phases if all patterns have not been placed correctly. Reproduced by kind permission of CANTAB, Cambridge Cognition Ltd.*

individuals with frontal variant frontotemporal dementia (Lee *et al.*, 2003). Of critical importance, CANTAB PAL was also found to be relatively insensitive to major unipolar depression (only 7 per cent of scores of patients with depression and AD fell within an overlapping range) (Swainson *et al.*, 2001) (see Figure 5.2). This result suggests that PAL is of use in the differential diagnosis of early AD and depression (unlike word recall tests – see O'Carroll *et al.*, 1997). Unlike on ADAS-cog, performance on PAL was also found to correlate significantly with subsequent deterioration in global cognitive function. Furthermore, in a group of individuals with QD, baseline PAL results revealed an apparent subgroup of patients who performed like AD patients. In a follow-up study, Blackwell *et al.* (2004) showed that by taking into account age and performance on one other neuropsychological test (the Graded Naming Test [McKenna and Warrington, 1980]), CANTAB PAL gave a 100 per cent distinction between subjects with QD who either did or did not convert to probable AD (NINCDS-ADRDA criteria) 32 months after baseline testing (see also De Jager *et al.*, 2002). These studies also revealed that the sensitivity (in detecting prodromal AD in a QD group) and specificity (in differentiating AD from depression) of CANTAB PAL was considerably better than that of all other frequently used tests included in the study (including ADAS-cog and Wechsler Logical Memory Delayed Passage Recall).

The accumulating evidence demonstrating the sensitivity and specificity of CANTAB PAL for the early and differential diagnosis of AD suggest that this test represents a potential tool for operationalizing the criteria for objective memory impairment in MCI along with other candidate tests (see Petersen, 2003). CANTAB PAL has the additional advantage of existing in a form that can be used in experimental animals (Taffe *et al.*, 2002), facilitating translational medicine phases of treatment development, and may be less sensitive than other tests to the effects of depression (Swainson *et al.*, 2001). Further research into the usefulness and operationalization of each of the MCI criteria will doubtless improve their prognostic use.

Ultimately, however, the results of neuropsychological tests that are found to be sensitive and specific for early AD should be incorporated into AD diagnostic criteria, rather than invoking amnestic MCI as an intermediary state.

5.3 NEUROPSYCHOLOGICAL ASSESSMENT IN THE DIFFERENTIAL DIAGNOSIS OF THE DEMENTIAS

The need for early and accurate detection of AD is paralleled by the need to accurately differentiate the dementias. Accurate differential diagnosis is important because it allows clinicians to make appropriate treatment decisions and to provide appropriate advice to patients and relatives regarding the likely nature and course of decline. Over the last decade our understanding of the neurocognitive profiles of various dementias has advanced significantly; this knowledge can be used to facilitate accurate differential diagnosis.

5.3.1 Frontotemporal dementias and AD

The prevalence of frontotemporal dementia equals that of AD in individuals aged 45–64 (Ratnavalli *et al.*, 2002). The term frontotemporal dementia is used to refer to a group of non-Alzheimer's conditions most frequently characterized by a predominant pathology of either the frontal lobes (frontal variant frontotemporal dementia: FvFTD) or of the temporal lobes (often referred to as semantic dementia: SD). In SD there is a selective impairment of semantic memory, which causes severe anomia, single word comprehension, reduced exemplar production in category fluency tests, and an impaired general knowledge. Other components of speech production, perceptual and non-verbal problem-solving abilities, and episodic memory are relatively spared (Snowden *et al.*, 1989; Hodges *et al.*, 1992; Breddin *et al.*, 1994; Saffran and Schwartz, 1994).

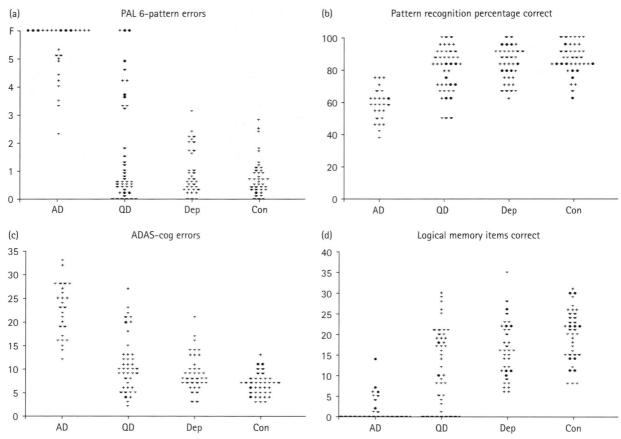

Figure 5.2 (a–d)   *Scores of individual subjects on PAL, ADAS-cog, pattern recognition and logical memory recall (i.e. the four tests best able to classify Alzheimer's disease (AD) and depressed/control (Dep/Con) subjects). NB. PAL and ADAS-cog are scored in terms of errors so a high score indicates poor performance, whereas pattern recognition and logical memory recall are scored in terms of items correct, so a low score indicates poor performance. 'F' indicates that the subjects failed to reach the 6-pattern stage. In the 'questionable dementia' (QD) group, baseline PAL results revealed an apparent subgroup of patients who performed like AD patients. PAL performance of individuals with depression did not differ significantly from that of matched control subjects (Swainson et al., 2001). Reproduced with permission from Karger, Basel.*

FvFTD is usually associated with failure on frontal lobe tests in the absence of severe amnesia, aphasia, perceptual or spatial disorders. However, there are frequently marked behavioural changes including lack of insight, disinhibition, loss of personal and social awareness, mental rigidity and inflexibility, perseverative behaviour, and emotional lability (Gregory and Hodges, 1996). Recent studies by Rahman, Sahakian and colleagues (Rahman *et al.*, 1999a, b) indicate that performance neuropsychological tests of decision-making that are sensitive to orbitofrontal/ventromedial cortex could be used to differentiate mild FvFTD patients from IQ-matched control subjects. By contrast, patients and controls did not show performance differences on tasks thought to be sensitive to dorsolateral prefrontal cortex function.

Hodges *et al.* (1999) directly compared the neuropsychological profiles of FTD (both frontal and temporal variants) and early AD. AD patients showed a substantial deficit in episodic memory (as indexed by the logical memory subtest of Wechsler Memory Scale – Revised [Wechsler, 1987] and 45

minute recall of the Rey complex figure drawing [Rey, 1941]) accompanied by more modest deficits in semantic memory (memory for meaning and facts) and visuospatial skills; SD was associated with major isolated deficits in semantic memory and anomia. The FvFTD group were, overall, the least impaired group, and showed mild deficits in episodic memory and verbal fluency with relatively preserved semantic memory. A follow up with the same diagnostic groups examining attention, executive function and semantic memory has recently complemented these findings. SD patients showed a preservation of attention and executive function with severe deficits in semantic memory; FvFTD patients showed the opposite pattern (Perry and Hodges, 2000). A study by Lee *et al.* (2003) has further reinforced the value of CANTAB PAL in the differentiation of SD, FvFTD and AD. Analysis revealed that relative to patients with AD, the PAL performance (as indexed by stages completed, and errors at the six pattern stage) of patients with FvFTD and SD was generally spared. By contrast, the PAL 'memory score' measure was impaired in both SD and AD but not FvFTD.

5.3.2 VaD versus AD

Vascular dementia (VaD) is the second most common form of dementia comprising approximately 20 per cent of dementia cases in the United Kingdom (Alzheimer's Society Demography Policy Position Report, 2004).

A number of studies have investigated the cognitive profile associated with VaD and its differentiation from AD. Cross-study comparison has been impeded by problems such as differing diagnostic criteria and failure to match adequately for demographic factors and disease severity but some consensus is now forming. In general, when compared with patients with probable AD, VaD patients appear to show relatively preserved episodic memory but impaired executive and attentional function. Both AD and VaD show deficits of a comparable severity in the domains of language, constructional abilities, and working memory (see Looi and Sachdev, 1999).

In contrast to episodic memory and executive function, there is a paucity of data in the literature relating to the semantic memory in VaD. One recent study (Graham et al., 2004) has addressed this issue by examining neurocognitive performance in groups of patients with subcortical vascular dementia and probable AD (groups matched for age, education, global cognitive and everyday function), and included assessment of semantic memory in the testing battery. In accordance with previous literature, AD was associated with more impairment in episodic memory, whereas VaD was associated with more deficient executive/attentional functioning and visuospatial skills. Importantly semantic memory was also found to be generally more impaired in the VaD group. Logistic regression analysis indicated that the most useful discriminator of VaD and AD in this study was a combination of delayed passage recall and performance of a test of naming silhouetted objects at various rotations (a test that can be considered to measure both visuospatial processing and semantic processing).

5.3.3 Dementia with Lewy bodies versus AD

It is estimated that dementia with Lewy bodies (DLB) is the third most prevalent form of dementia, representing approximately 15 per cent of all dementia cases (Alzheimer's Society Demography Policy Position Report, 2004). DLB is characterized by progressive cognitive decline, hallucinations, fluctuating course, spontaneous parkinsonism and heightened sensitivity to neuroleptic drugs (McKeith et al., 1992, 2000). The neurocognitive profile of DLB is less well understood than that of AD and VaD, but some important studies have been conducted.

Sahgal et al. (1992b) investigated matching-to-sample visual recognition memory in DLB and AD patients. The results revealed that, although the performance of both DLB and AD patients was impaired relative to controls, the DLB patients performed most poorly, particularly when a delay was introduced between stimulus presentation and recognition. In a follow-up study of mnemonic processing (Saghal et al., 1995) AD and DLB patients were compared on a self-ordered test of spatial working memory (CANTAB Spatial Working Memory: SWM). The results revealed that SWM was more impaired in the DLB group than in the AD group, but the authors suggest that, since the two groups did not differ from each other in the performance of a different test of spatial span, the SWM deficit may not reflect a specific impairment per se, but rather reflect the failure of a non-mnemonic cognitive process subserved by frontostriatal circuitry (i.e. attention or planning).

Shimomura et al. (1998) compared the performance of age-, MMSE-, sex-, and education-matched DLB and AD patients on standard neuropsychological tests from the Alzheimer's Disease Assessment Scale – Cognitive Scale (ADAS-cog), Raven's Progressive Matrices (RPM) (Raven, 1965), and the Wechsler Adult Intelligence Scale – Revised (WAIS-R; Wechsler, 1981). Relative to AD, DLB was associated with a greater degree of impairment on the ADAS construction score, WAIS-R picture arrangement, Block Design, Object Assembly, and Picture Substitution scales. RPM score was also significantly worse in the DLB group. By contrast, ADAS word recall performance was generally spared in the DLB relative to the AD group.

More recently, Calderon et al. (2001) found that DLB was associated with deficits in visual object and space perception relative to AD and controls. DLB subjects also showed deficits in tests of attention and executive function greater than those seen in AD at a similar stage of global cognitive decline, but were significantly less impaired on tests of episodic memory. Additionally, DLB, but not AD subjects, showed impaired performance in a test of divided attention.

In summary, although more research is needed, studies to date suggest that DLB is characterized, in neurocognitive terms, by a relative sparing of episodic memory but marked attentional and visuospatial deficits when compared to AD.

5.4 NEUROPSYCHOLOGICAL ASSESSMENT FOR THE PURPOSES OF MONITORING CHANGE IN COGNITIVE FUNCTION

Another role for neuropsychological testing is to measure the rate of progression of disease, achieved by giving an identical assessment (usually in parallel forms) at a number of different time intervals. This is important because it can help the clinician assess the efficacy of any pharmacological intervention. At the moment the ADAS-cog (Rosen et al., 1984; Mohs et al., 1997) is a test commonly used clinical tool for this purpose. However, as discussed above, other objective measures of cognitive function have been shown to be more sensitive and specific in the early stages of AD and therefore may provide more appropriate indices of change at these early stages. Furthermore, other tests (e.g. CANTAB Rapid Visual Information Processing Task, CANTAB Simple and Choice Reaction

Time Task) are also likely to prove to be effective in monitoring change later in the disease course (see Sahakian *et al.*, 1989, 1993; Eagger *et al.*, 1992).

5.5 CONCLUSIONS

Neuropsychological assessment can make an important contribution to the early and differential diagnosis of the dementias, including for the identification of 'enriched samples' for clinical trials, and is also vital for the objective monitoring of changes in cognitive function across disease course or as a function of treatment.

Key challenges for neuropsychologists over the next decade include decomposing the cognitive and neural substrates of task performance in order to more accurately characterize the neuropsycho-endophenotype of each form of dementia. It will be particularly important to examine the relationship between neuropsychological function and specific neuropathological features using novel *in vivo* neurochemical techniques (Shoghi-Jadid *et al.*, 2002; Klunk *et al.*, 2004). Improved neuropsychological characterization will be translated into more sensitive and specific diagnostic tools, which in turn should lead to earlier intervention with psychological and pharmacological therapies, potentially even prior to the onset of disabling cognitive impairments.

REFERENCES

Albert MS, Moss MB, Tanzi R, Jones K. (2001) Preclinical prediction of AD using neuropsychological tests. *Journal of the International Neuropsychology Society* 7: 631–639

Alzheimer's Society Demography Policy Position Report. (2004) http://www.alzheimers.org.uk/News_and_Campaigns/Policy_Watch/demography.htm

Artero S, Tierney MC, Touchon J, Ritchie K. (2003) Prediction of transition from cognitive impairment to senile dementia: a prospective, longitudinal study. *Acta Psychiatrica Scandinavica* 107: 390–393

Beck AT, Ward C H, Mendelson M, Mock J, Erbaugh J. (1961) An inventory for measuring depression. *Archives of General Psychiatry* 4: 561–571

Bennett DA, Wilson RS, Schneider JA et al. (2002) Natural history of mild cognitive impairment in older persons. *Neurology* 59: 198–205.

Blackwell AD, Sahakian BJ, Vesey R, Semple JM, Robbins TW, Hodges JR. (2004) Detecting dementia: novel neuropsychological markers of preclinical Alzheimer's disease. *Dementia and Geriatric Cognitive Disorders* 17: 42–48

Braak H and Braak E. (1991) Neuropathological staging of Alzheimer-related changes. *Acta Neuropathologica* 82: 239–259

Breddin SD, Saffran FM, Coslett HB. (1994) Reversal of the concreteness effect in a patient with semantic dementia. *Cognitive Neuropsychology* 2: 617–661

Busse A, Bischkopf J, Riedel-Heller SG, Angermeyer MC. (2003) Subclassifications for mild cognitive impairment: prevalence and predictive validity. *Psychological Medicine* 33: 1029–1038

Calderon J, Perry RJ, Erzinclioglu SW, Berrios GE, Dening TR, Hodges JR. (2001) Perception, attention, and working memory are disproportionately impaired in dementia with Lewy bodies compared with Alzheimer's disease. *Journal of Neurology, Neurosurgery, and Psychiatry* 70: 157–164

Celsis P. (2000) Age-related cognitive decline, mild cognitive impairment or preclinical Alzheimer's disease? *Annals of Medicine* 32: 6–14

Collie A, Maruff P, Currie J. (2002) Behavioral characterization of mild cognitive impairment. *Journal of Clinical and Experimental Neuropsychology* 24: 720–733

De Jager CA, Milwain E, Budge M. (2002) Early detection of isolated memory deficits in the elderly: the need for more sensitive neuropsychological tests. *Psychological Medicine* 32: 483–491

Eagger SA, Levy R, Sahakian BJ. (1992) Tacrine in Alzheimer's disease. *Acta Neurologica Scandinavica* 139 (Suppl.): 75–80

Elias MF, Beiser A, Wolf PA, Au R, White RF, D'Agostino RB. (2000) The preclinical phase of Alzheimer disease: a 22-year prospective study of the Framingham Cohort. *Archives of Neurology* 57: 808–813

Ferris SH and Kluger A. (1997) Assessing cognition in Alzheimer disease research. *Alzheimer Disease and Associated Disorders.* 11 (Suppl. 6): 45–49

Folstein MF, Folstein SE, McHugh PR. (1975) Mini-mental state: a practical method for grading the cognitive state of patient for clinician. *Journal of Psychiatric Research* 12: 189–198

Fowler KS, Saling MM, Conway EL, Semple JS, Louis WJ. (1995) Computerized delayed matching-to-sample and paired associate performance in the early detection of dementia. *Applied Neuropsychology* 2: 72–78

Fowler KS, Saling MM, Conway EL, Semple JM, Louis WJ. (1997) Computerised neuropsychological tests in the early detection of dementia: prospective findings. *Journal of the International Neuropsychological Society* 3: 139–146

Fowler KS, Saling MM, Conway EL, Semple JM, Louis WJ. (2002) Paired associate performance in the early detection of DAT. *Journal of the International Neuropsychology Society* 8: 58–71

Fox NC, Warrington EK, Seiffer AL, Agnew SK, Rossor MN. (1998) Presymptomatic cognitive deficits in individuals at risk of familial Alzheimer's disease: a longitudinal prospective study. *Brain* 121: 1631–1639

Fox NC, Warrington EK, Rossor MN. (1999) Serial magnetic resonance imaging of cerebral atrophy in preclinical Alzheimer's disease. *Lancet* 353: 2125

Fray PJ, Robbins TW, Sahakian BJ. (1996) Neuropsychiatric applications of CANTAB. *International Journal of Geriatric Psychiatry* 11: 329–336

Geldmacher DS, Provenzano G, McRae T, Mastey V, Ieni JR (2003) Donepezil is associated with delayed nursing home placement in patients with Alzheimer's disease. *Journal of the American Geriatrics Society* 51: 937–944

Graham NL, Emery T, Hodges JR. (2004) Distinctive cognitive profiles in Alzheimer's disease and subcortical vascular dementia. *Journal of Neurology, Neurosurgery, and Psychiatry* 75: 61–71

Gregory CA and Hodges JR. (1996) Clinical features of frontal lobe dementia in comparison to Alzheimer's disease. *Journal of Neural Transmission* 47 (Suppl.): 103–123

Hamilton M. (1960) A rating scale for depression. *Journal of Neurology, Neurosurgery, and Psychiatry* 23: 56–62

Hebert LE, Scherr PA, Bienias JL, Bennett DA, Evans DA. (2003) Alzheimer disease in the U.S. population: prevalence estimates using the 2000 census. *Archives of Neurology* 60: 1119–1122

Hodges JR. (1998) The amnestic prodrome of Alzheimer's disease. *Brain* **121**: 1601–1602

Hodges JR, Patterson K, Oxbury S, Funnell E. (1992) Semantic dementia: progressive fluent aphasia with temporal lobe atrophy. *Brain* **115**: 1783–1806

Hodges JR, Patterson K, Ward R et al. (1999) The differentiation of semantic dementia and frontal lobe dementia (temporal and frontal variants of frontotemporal dementia) from early Alzheimer's disease: a comparative neuropsychological study. *Neuropsychology* **13**: 31–40

Holroyd S, Snustad DG, Chalifoux ZL. (1996) Attitudes of older adults on being told the diagnosis of Alzheimer's disease. *Journal of the American Geriatric Society* **44**: 400–403

Holroyd S, Turnbull Q, Wolf AM. (2002) What are patients and their families told about the diagnosis of dementia? Results of a family survey. *International Journal of Geriatric Psychiatry* **17**: 218–221

Jack CR Jr, Petersen RC, Xu YC et al. (1999) Prediction of AD with MRI-based hippocampal volume in mild cognitive impairment. *Neurology* **52**: 1397–1403

Jorm AF, Christensen H, Korten AE, Henderson AS, Jacomb PA, Mackinnon A. (1997) Do cognitive complaints either predict future cognitive decline or reflect past cognitive decline? A longitudinal study of an elderly community sample. *Psychological Medicine* **27**: 91–98

Kaplan E, Fein D, Morris R et al. (1991) *WAIS-R as a neuropsychological instrument.* San Antonio, Psychological Corporation

Killiany RJ, Hyman BT, Gomez-Isla T et al. (2002) MRI measures of entorhinal cortex vs hippocampus in preclinical AD. *Neurology* **58**: 1188–1196

Kline P. (1986) *A Handbook of Test Construction.* London, Metheun and Co, Ltd

Klunk WE, Engler H, Nordberg A et al. (2004) Imaging brain amyloid in Alzheimer's disease with Pittsburgh Compound-B. *Annals of Neurology* **55**: 306–19

Laakso MP, Hallikainen M, Hanninen T, Partanen K, Soininen H. (2000) Diagnosis of Alzheimer's disease: MRI of the hippocampus vs delayed recall. *Neuropsychologia* **38**: 579–584

Larrieu S, Letenneur L, Orgogozo JM et al. (2002) Incidence and outcome of mild cognitive impairment in a population-based prospective cohort. *Neurology* **59**: 1594–1599

Lee AC, Rahman S, Hodges JR, Sahakian BJ, Graham KS. (2003) Associative and recognition memory for novel objects in dementia: implications for diagnosis. *European Journal of Neuroscience* **18**: 1660–1670

Lezak MD. (1995). *Neuropsychological Assessment* (3rd edition). New York, Oxford University Press

Linn RT, Wolf PA, Bachman DL et al. (1995) The 'preclinical phase' of probable Alzheimer's disease: A 13 year prospective study of the Framingham cohort. *Archives of Neurology* **52**: 485–490

Looi JC and Sachdev PS. (1999) Differentiation of vascular dementia from AD on neuropsychological tests. *Neurology* **53**: 670–678

McDonald RJ and White NM. (1993) A triple dissociation of memory systems: hippocampus, amygdala, and dorsal striatum. *Behavioural Neuroscience* **107**: 3–22

McKeith I, Fairbairn A, Perry R, Thompson P, Perry E. (1992). Neuroleptic sensitivity in patients with senile dementia of Lewy body type. *BMJ* **305**: 673–678

McKeith IG, Ballard CG, Perry RH et al. (2000). Prospective validation of consensus criteria for the diagnosis of dementia with Lewy bodies. *Neurology* **54**: 1050–1058

McKenna P and Warrington EK. (1980) Testing for nominal dysphasia. *Journal of Neurology, Neurosurgery, and Psychiatry* **43**: 781–788

McKhann G, Drachman D, Folstein M, Katzman R, Price D, Stadlan EM. (1984). Clinical diagnosis of Alzheimer's disease: report of the NINCDS-ADRDA Work Group under the auspices of the Department of Health and Human Services Task Force on Alzheimer's Disease. *Neurology* **34**: 939–944

Maguire EA, Frith CD, Burgess N, Donnett JG, O'Keefe J. (1998) Knowing where things are parahippocampal involvement in encoding object locations in virtual large-scale space. *Journal of Cognitive Neuroscience* **10**: 61–76

Masur DM, Sliwinski M, Lipton RB, Blau AD, Crystal HA. (1995) Neuropsychological prediction of dementia and the absence of dementia in healthy elderly persons. *Neurology* **45**: 2112–2113

Miyashita Y, Kameyama M, Hasegawa I, Fukushima T. (1998) Consolidation of visual associative long-term memory in the temporal cortex of primates. *Neurobiology of Learning and Memory* **70**: 197–211

Mohs RC, Knopman D, Petersen RC et al. (1997) Development of cognitive instruments for use in clinical trials of antidementia drugs: additions to the Alzheimer's Disease Assessment Scale that broaden its scope. The Alzheimer's Disease Cooperative Study. *Alzheimer Disease and Associated Disorders* **11** (Suppl. 2): S13–S21

Morgan CD and Baade LE. (1997) Neuropsychological testing and assessment scales for dementia of the Alzheimer's type. *Geriatric Psychiatry, The Psychiatric Clinics of North America* **20**: 25–43

Morris JC. (1997) Clinical assessment of DAT. *Neurology* **49** (Suppl.): 1–6

Nadler JD, Richardson ED, Malloy PF. (1994) Detection of impairment with the mini-mental state examination. *Neuropsychiatry, Neuropsychology, and Behavioural Neurology* **7**: 109–113

O'Carroll RE, Prentice N, Conway S, Ryman A. (1997) Performance on the delayed word recall test (DWL) fails to clearly differentiate between depression and Alzheimer's disease in the elderly. *Psychological Medicine* **27**: 967–971

Owen AM, Milner B, Petrides M, Evans A. (1996) A specific role for the right parahippocampal region in the retrieval of object-location: a positron emission tomography study. *Journal of Cognitive Neuroscience* **8**: 588–602

Perry RJ and Hodges JR. (2000) Differentiating frontal and temporal variant frontotemporal dementia from Alzheimer's disease. *Neurology* **54**: 2277–2284

Petersen RC. (2003) Mild cognitive impairment clinical trials. *Nature Reviews. Drug Discovery* **2**: 646–653

Petersen RC, Smith GE, Waring SC, Ivnik RJ, Tangalos EG, Kokmen E. (1999) Mild cognitive impairment: clinical characterization and outcome. *Archives of Neurology* **56**: 303–308

Raven JC. *RCPM: Guide to Using the Colored Progressive Matrices.* New York, Psychological Corporation

Rahman S, Sahakian BJ, Hodges JR, Rogers RD, Robbins TW. (1999a) Specific cognitive deficits in frontal variant frontotemporal dementia. *Brain* **122**: 1469–1493

Rahman S, Robbins TW, Sahakian BJ. (1999b) Comparative cognitive neuropsychological studies of frontal lobe function: implications for therapeutic strategies in frontal variant frontotemporal dementia. *Dementia and Geriatric Cognitive Disorders* **10** (Suppl. 1): 15–28

Ratnavalli E, Brayne C, Dawson K, Hodges JR. (2002) The prevalence of frontotemporal dementia. *Neurology* **58**: 1615–1621

Reitan RM and Wolfson D. (1993) *The Halstead-Reitan Neuropsychological Test Battery: Theory and Clinical Interpretation*, 2nd edition. Tuscon, Neuropsychology Press

Rey A. (1941) L'examen psychologique dans les cas d'encephalopathie traumatique [The psychological examination of traumatic encephalopathy]. *Archives de Psychologie* **28**: 286–340

Ritchie K, Artero S, Touchon J. (2001) Classification criteria for mild cognitive impairment: a population-based validation study. *Neurology* **56**: 37–42

Robbins TW and Sahakian BJ. (1994a) Computer methods of assessment of cognitive function. In: JRM Copeland, MT Abou-Selah and DG Blazer (eds), *Principles and Practice of Geriatric Psychiatry.* Chichester, John Wiley and Sons Ltd

Robbins TW, James M, Owen AM *et al.* (1994b) Cognitive deficits in progressive supranuclear palsy, Parkinson's disease and multiple system atrophy in tests sensitive to frontal lobe dysfunction. *Journal of Neurology, Neurosurgery, and Psychiatry* **57**: 79–88

Robbins TW, James M, Owen A, Sahakian BJ, McInnes L, Rabbit PM. (1994c) Cambridge Neuropsychological Test Automated Battery (CANTAB) a factor analytical study of a large sample of normal elderly volunteers. *Dementia* **5**: 266–281

Robbins TW, James M, Owen A, Sahakian BJ, McInnes L, Rabbit PM. (1998) A study of performance on tests from the CANTAB battery sensitive to frontal lobe dysfunction in a large sample of normal volunteers: implications for theories of executive function and cognitive ageing. *Journal of the International Neuropsychological Society* **4**: 474–490

Rosen WG, Mohs RC, Davis KL. (1984) A new rating scale for Alzheimer's disease. *American Journal of Psychiatry* **141**: 1356–1364

Saffran EM and Schwartz MF. (1994) Of cabbages and things: semantic memory from a neuropsychological perspective – a tutorial review. In: C Umita and M Moscovitch (eds), *Attention and Performance*, vol 15. Cambridge Massachusetts, MIT Press, pp. 507–535

Sahakian BJ, Morris RG, Evenden JL *et al.* (1988) A comparative study of the visuospatial memory and learning in Alzheimer-type dementia and Parkinson's disease. *Brain* **111**: 695–718

Sahakian B, Jones G, Levy R, Gray J, Warburton D. (1989) The effects of nicotine on attention, information processing, and short-term memory in patients with dementia of the Alzheimer type. *British Journal of Psychiatry* **154**: 797–800

Sahakian BJ, Downes JJ, Eagger S *et al.* (1990) Sparing of attentional relative to mnemonic function in a subgroup of patients with dementia of the Alzheimer type. *Neuropsychologia* **28**: 1197–1213

Sahakian BJ, Owen AM, Morant NJ *et al.* (1993) Further analysis of the cognitive effects of tetrahydroaminoacridine (THA) in Alzheimer's disease: assessment of attentional and mnemonic function using CANTAB. *Psychopharmacology* (Berl) **110**: 395–401

Sahgal A, Lloyd S, Wray CJ *et al.* (1992a) Does visuospatial memory in senile dementia of the Alzheimer type depend on the severity of the disorder? *International Journal of Geriatric Psychiatry* **7**: 427–436

Sahgal A, Galloway PH, McKeith IG *et al.* (1992b) Matching to sample deficits in patients with senile dementias of the Alzheimer and Lewy body types. *Archives of Neurology* **49**: 1043–1046

Sahgal A, McKeith IG, Galloway PH, Tasker N, Steckler T. (1995) Do differences in visuospatial ability between senile dementias of the Alzheimer and Lewy body types reflect differences solely in mnemonic function. *Journal of Clinical and Experimental Neuropsychology* **17**: 35–43

Shimomura T, Mori E, Yamashita H *et al.* (1998) Cognitive loss in dementia with Lewy bodies and Alzheimer disease. *Archives of Neurology* **55**: 1547–1552

Shoghi-Jadid K, Small GW, Agdeppa ED *et al.* (2002) Localization of neurofibrillary tangles and beta-amyloid plaques in the brains of living patients with Alzheimer disease. *American Journal of Geriatric Psychiatry* **10**: 24–35

Small GW, Rabins PV, Barry PP *et al.* (1997) Diagnosis and treatment of Alzheimer disease and related disorders. Consensus statement of the American Association for Geriatric Psychiatry, the Alzheimer's Association, and the American Geriatrics Society. *JAMA* **278**: 1363–1371

Smith ML and Milner B. (1981) The role of the right hippocampus in recall of spatial location. *Neuropsychologia* **19**: 781–793

Snowden JS, Goulding PJ, Neary D. (1989) Semantic dementia: a form of circumscribed cerebral atrophy. *Behavioural Neurology* **2**: 167–182

Swainson R, Hodges JR, Galton CJ *et al.* (2001) Early detection and differential diagnosis of Alzheimer's disease and depression with neuropsychological tasks. *Dementia and Geriatric Cognitive Disorders* **12**: 265–280

Taffe MA, Weed MR, Gutierrez T, Davis SA, Gold LH. (2002) Differential muscarinic and NMDA contributions to visuo-spatial paired-associate learning in rhesus monkeys. *Psychopharmacology (Berl)* **160**: 253–262

Tombaugh TM and McIntyre NJ. (1992) The Mini-Mental State Examination: A comprehensive review. *Journal of the American Geriatrics Society* **40**: 922–935

Visser PJ, Verhey FR, Hofman PA, Scheltens P, Jolles J. (2002) Medial temporal lobe atrophy predicts Alzheimer's disease in patients with minor cognitive impairment. *Journal of Neurology, Neurosurgery, and Psychiatry* **72**: 491–497

Wechsler D. (1981) *Wechsler Adult Intelligence Scale – Revised.* San Antonio, TX, The Psychological Corporation

Wechsler D. (1987) *Wechsler Adult Intelligence Scale – Revised.* San Antonio, TX, The Psychological Corporation

Welch K, Butters N, Hughes JP, Mohs RC, Heyman A. (1992) Detection and staging of dementia in Alzheimer's disease: use of the neuropsychological measures developed for the Consortium to Establish a Register For Alzheimer's Disease (CERAD). *Archives of Neurology* **49**: 448–452

Wilder D, Cross P, Chen J *et al.* (1995) Operating characteristics of brief screens for dementia in a multicultural population. *American Journal of Geriatric Psychiatry* **3**: 96–107

World Health Organization. (2001) Mental Health: New understanding, New Hope. World Health Reports. Geneva, The World Health Organization. http://www.who.int/whr2001/2001/

6

Neuropsychiatric aspects of dementia

IRACEMA LEROI AND CONSTANTINE G LYKETSOS

The neuropsychiatric changes in dementia are nearly universal and may result in extremely challenging management problems. This is in spite of the definition of dementia being based on the cognitive and functional changes alone. These symptoms include personality changes, mood deterioration, perceptual abnormalities, psychomotor disturbances (such as agitation, aggression, wandering and purposeless behaviour), and neurovegetative changes (alterations in sleep and appetite). Collectively, these manifestations in dementia syndromes can be regarded under the recently adopted rubric of 'behavioural and psychological symptoms of dementia' (BPSD) (Finkel et al., 1996); however, they have been variously termed as 'neuropsychiatric symptoms', 'behavioural disturbances', 'non-cognitive changes' and 'challenging behaviours'. Here we will refer to them as the neuropsychiatric symptoms of dementia. The importance and ubiquity of these symptoms is highlighted by Alois Alzheimer's first clinical description of Alzheimer's disease (AD) in 1907. In this case study, he stated:

> The first noticeable symptom of illness shown by this 51-year-old woman was suspiciousness of her husband. Soon, a rapidly increasing memory impairment became evident; she could no longer orient herself in her own dwelling, dragged objects here and there and hid them, and at times, believing that people were out to murder her, started to scream loudly (Alzheimer, translated by Jarvik and Greenson, 1987).

The impact of these disturbances on both patients with dementia and their families and caregivers has been well documented. The burden on caregivers is significant and is most often the primary reason for admission to long-term care (Sanford, 1975; Rabins et al., 1982; Victoroff et al., 1998).

Furthermore, patients suffering with the disturbances require more medication and physical restraints (Teri et al., 1989; Bianchetti et al., 1997).

6.1 EPIDEMIOLOGY AND SPECTRUM OF NEUROPSYCHIATRIC SYMPTOMS OF DEMENTIA

Neuropsychiatric symptoms are extremely common in the dementias; however, a given symptom or syndrome may not reliably appear in any one dementia diagnosis. Unlike the inexorable decline seen in cognitive and functional abilities of patients with dementia, the neuropsychiatric symptoms may fluctuate in their presence and intensity. It has been suggested that early detection of such symptoms, even in the absence of cognitive impairment, might be a harbinger of dementia. Such a diagnosis of 'mild neuropsychiatric syndrome' later in life might be an early marker of dementia, in much in the same way as the syndrome of 'mild cognitive impairment' predicts later cognitive decline (Assal and Cummings, 2002). Indeed, there is evidence that the first onset of a depressive episode in older age, which is associated with a transient dementia syndrome ('pseudodementia'), may predict the later development of dementia (Alexopoulos and Chester, 1992). The risk for development of later dementia in this group is so great that it appears that the risk for developing AD increases for each depressive symptom suffered by those over the age of 65 (Wilson et al., 2002). These findings underscore the necessity for early detection of neuropsychiatric symptoms in the non-demented elderly population.

In AD, the most common form of dementia, several studies have examined incidence and prevalence rates of neuropsychiatric symptoms. The most robust epidemiological studies are population based. Burns *et al.* (1990a–d) examined 178 patients with AD from a defined area in the United Kingdom. They found the following cumulative prevalences of neuropsychiatric disturbances ranging from 3.5 per cent for mania to 41 per cent for apathy (see Table 6.1).

To date, the largest population based study of neuropsychiatric disturbances in dementia is from the Cache County Study of Memory in Aging (CCSMA): 5092 participants, constituting 90 per cent of the elderly resident population of a particular county in the United States, were enrolled and thoroughly screened for dementia (Breitner *et al.*, 1999); 329 people were diagnosed with a prevalent dementia syndrome, of which 214 (65 per cent) had AD, 62 (19 per cent) had vascular dementia (VaD), and 53 (16 per cent) had another DSM-IV dementia diagnosis. Using the Neuropsychiatric Inventory (NPI)(Cummings *et al.*, 1994), a widely used method for ascertainment and classification of dementia-associated mental and behavioural disturbances, 201 (61 per cent) of the participants with dementia were reported by their caregivers to have had one or more mental or behavioural disturbances in the past month. Apathy, depression and agitation/aggression were the most common (see Table 6.1) (Lyketsos *et al.*, 2000). In participants specifically with AD, delusions were reported in 23 per cent and hallucinations in 13 per cent, whereas for those with VaD, 8 per cent had delusions and 13 per cent had hallucinations (Leroi *et al.*, 2003). The delusions seen in AD are usually quite simple and most often do include the bizarre and complex delusions seen in schizophrenia. Misidentification phenomena and jealous delusions are more common in dementia compared to schizophrenia. Likewise, Schneiderian first-rank symptoms such as voices commenting, commanding or conversing are not commonly seen in dementia. The most common form of hallucinations in AD are visual hallucinations (80 per cent), which far exceed auditory hallucinations in frequency (20 per cent) (Leroi *et al.*, 2003).

Increasing attention is being focused on the syndrome of mild cognitive impairment (MCI), which involves impairment in memory and possibly other areas of cognition in elderly individuals whose day-to-day functioning is relatively preserved. MCI may be a precursor to AD (Morris *et al.*, 2001) and appears to have, like AD, neuropsychiatric manifestations. As part of the analysis of data from the recent Cardiovascular Health Study (CHS)(Fried *et al.*, 1991), prevalence estimates of neuropsychiatric symptoms of MCI were sought. Of the 320 individuals who were identified as having MCI, 43 per cent (138) exhibited neuropsychiatric symptoms with depression, apathy and irritability being the most common (see Table 6.1) (Lyketsos *et al.*, 2002). Almost 30 per cent of those with symptoms were rated as clinically significant. Almost 75 per cent of those with a full diagnosis of dementia (n = 362) had at least one neuropsychiatric symptom.

In the frontotemporal dementias, unlike AD or vascular dementia (VaD), the behavioural and psychological disturbances are embedded in the diagnostic consensus criteria (McKhann *et al.*, 2001). Earlier diagnostic criteria for the frontal lobe dementias as a group, proposed by Neary *et al.* (1998), outlined one specific behavioural subtype or 'prototypic neurobehavioral syndrome', which is marked by profound personality and behavioural changes. This presentation, namely, frontotemporal dementia (FTD), is distinct from the progressive non-fluent aphasia (PNFA) and semantic dementia (SD) presentations, which constitute other manifestations of the frontal lobe dementias. In FTD, the core changes are characterized by an insidious onset and gradual decline in social functioning, and regulation of personal conduct,

Table 6.1 *Population-based prevalence of neuropsychiatric symptoms in dementia*

Study	Camberwell Health Authority, UK (Burns *et al.*, 1990a–d)	Cache County Study of Memory in Aging, USA (Lyketsos *et al.*, 2000)	Cardiovascular Health Study, USA (Lyketsos *et al.*, 2002)	
Condition	Alzheimer's disease (n = 178)	Dementia (n = 329)	Mild cognitive impairment (n = 320)	Dementia (n = 362)
Delusions (%)	16	23	3	18
Hallucination (%)	17	13	1	11
Depression (%)	24 (Major depression)	24	20	32
Mania/ euphoria (%)	3.5	1	0.6	3
Agitation/aggression (%)	20	24	11	30
Wandering/aberrant motor activity (%)	19	27	4	16
Apathy (%)	41	27	15	37
Irritability (%)		20	15	27
Disinhibition (%)		9	3	13
Anxiety (%)		17	10	27
Any neuropsychiatric symptom (%)		61	43	75

accompanied by emotional blunting, and loss of insight. Supportive diagnostic features include a decline in personal care, hyperorality, perseverative and stereotyped behaviours, and utilization behaviours. Speech and language changes and executive dysfunction can also be seen.

In the frontal lobe dementias, the presentation of associated neuropsychiatric symptoms can be used to distinguish SD, which involves temporal lobe dysfunction primarily on the left, from FTD presenting with temporal lobe dysfunction primarily on the right. In the former, compulsive behaviours are more common, whereas in the latter, aberrant social behaviour, hyperorality, hypersexuality and changes in self-defining functions such as dress, religious or ideological beliefs are typical (Miller et al., 2001; Mychack et al., 2001).

As with the frontal lobe dementias, neuropsychiatric symptoms are part of the defining characteristics of dementia with Lewy bodies (DLB). Visual hallucinations, fluctuating cognition and parkinsonism, together with progressive cognitive decline, form the core features of the consensus criteria for the clinical diagnosis of DLB (McKeith et al., 1996). The prevalence of visual hallucinations in DLB can be as high as 93 per cent compared to 27 per cent in AD, depending on the sample (Ballard et al., 1997). Phenomenologically, these hallucinations have similarities to those in Parkinson's disease (PD) or Charles Bonnet syndrome, but are usually more complex and involved compared to those see in AD (Cummings, 1992; Howard and Levy, 1994; Ballard et al., 1997). Delusions, misidentification phenomena and auditory hallucinations are also commonly present in DLB and also occur at higher prevalence rates than in AD patients (Ballard et al., 1995). Depression has been reported in up to 50 per cent of DLB patients and it may be associated with greater severity of parkinsonism (Klatka et al., 1996). Finally, an increasingly recognized syndrome, which may be a harbinger of DLB and other neurodegenerative synucleopathies, is rapid eye-movement (REM)-sleep behaviour disorder (RBD) (Ferman et al., 2002). RBD involves movements associated with dreaming and may involve potentially harmful sleep behaviour, acting out of dreams, and behaviour that continually interrupts sleep.

The degenerative diseases of the basal ganglia, such as Huntington's disease (HD), progressive supranuclear palsy (PSP) and Wilson's disease, have traditionally been classified as movement disorders, with associated cognitive and psychiatric manifestations. However, the confluence of symptoms (the three Ds: dyskinesia, dementia, and depression) seen in these disorders has led to the rubric of 'triadic syndromes' (McHugh, 1989) and underscores the high prevalence of neuropsychiatric manifestations in neurodegenerative movement disorders (Rosenblatt and Leroi, 2000). In particular, the prevalence of major depression in these disorders is high: up to 38 per cent in HD (Folstein et al., 1987) and 20 per cent in Wilson's disease (Denning and Berrios, 1989). Mania is less common and has been reported in up to 10 per cent of HD patients (Folstein, 1989), and even less in PD. There are few reports of mania or hypomania in other basal ganglia disorders, although emotional lability and irritability have been reported in

Wilson's disease and PSP (Denning and Berrios, 1989; Litvan et al., 1996). Psychotic symptoms have been reported in 3–12 per cent of HD patients (Mendez, 1994) but less than 2 per cent of patients with Wilson's disease (Denning and Berrios, 1989). Behavioural disturbances such as obsession and compulsions, sexual disorders, aggression, irritability and apathy are also well-recognized in neurodegenerative disorders involving the basal ganglia (Rosenblatt and Leroi, 2000).

PD, also considered a 'triadic disorder', shares neuropsychiatric features with the other disorders as well as an underlying pathophysiology involving protein abnormalities of α-synuclein. These synucleopathies, which include PD, DLB, multiple system atrophy (MSA) and striatonigral degeneration, appear to share vulnerabilities to a cluster of symptoms including hallucinations, delusions and RBD (Cummings, 2002).

In PD specifically, most patients develop a certain degree of cognitive impairment, which usually manifests as a dysexecutive syndrome (Gabrieli et al., 1996). Depression in PD, with an average prevalence across studies of 31 per cent (Slaughter et al., 2001) can significantly exacerbate this cognitive impairment (Starkstein et al., 1990). Neuropsychiatric symptoms are more common in those with some degree of cognitive impairment, and in the 30–40 per cent of PD patients who develop dementia (PDD) (Aarsland, 1996b), the vulnerability to neuropsychiatric symptoms is even greater (Holroyd et al., 2001; Goetz et al., 2001). The profile of neuropsychiatric symptoms in PDD and DLB is increasingly recognized as being similar, suggesting that these disease processes might exist on a continuum. The symptoms that predominate in PDD and DLB include delusions and hallucinations which may be varyingly related to antiparkinsonian medications (Aarsland et al., 2001).

6.2 CLASSIFICATION OF SYMPTOMS

There have been various classification schemes for the neuropsychiatric symptoms in dementia. These symptoms have been considered as monosymptomatic phenomena, as DSM-IV categories (1994), as separate phenomena based on unique criteria (Jeste and Finkel, 2000; Lyketsos et al., 2001a, b; Olin et al., 2002), and as part of specific behavioural syndromes (Reisberg et al., 1987; Absher and Cumming, 1994; Lyketsos et al., 2001a, b). This rather fragmented approach to the field has hampered efforts at investigation, particularly in the fields of epidemiology and pathophysiology.

The simplest approach is a monosymptomatic consideration of the neuropsychiatric symptoms of dementia. An example of such an approach was adopted by the landmark AD epidemiological study of Burns et al., 1990. In this study, the prevalence of symptoms derived from the Geriatric Mental State Schedule (GMSS; Copeland et al., 1976) – an interview schedule based on the Present State Exam (PSE; Wing et al., 1974) – was examined. These symptoms included: delusions of thought (including delusions of theft, suspicion, persecutory ideation and 'any disorder of thought'); disorders of perception (auditory hallucinations, visual hallucinations and misidentification syndromes); and disorders of mood (depressed and elevated mood). The final category of examination was disorders of behaviour in which 33 behaviour items from the Stockton Geriatric Rating Scale (SGRS; Meer and Baker, 1966) were sought.

The risk of such a monosymptomatic approach is that it is contrary to current data supporting the frequent co-occurrence of several neuropsychiatric symptoms in a given patient (Lyketsos et al., 2001a, b). This approach also limits treatment to a hypothesis-driven, phenomenological approach rather than moving towards an evidence-driven approach based on disorders, syndromes and frequently co-occurring symptoms.

An alternative, and more widely adopted, approach to categorization is to use the American Psychiatric Association's *Diagnostic and Statistical Manual of Mental Disorders*, 4th edition (DSM-IV) (1994). This is a heuristically useful approach and has the advantage of reliability, which enables cross-centre comparability. The disadvantage of this approach is that disturbances in AD and the other dementias are frequently phenotypically distinct from primary psychiatric disturbances. Hence, depression in AD severe enough to warrant treatment, may not meet all the criteria for a 'major depressive disorder' in the DSM-IV. In particular, the depression of dementia more commonly presents with anhedonia, irritability, agitation, apathy and non-specific worry, whereas the symptoms of guilty feelings, self-blame, frank sadness, crying and suicidality are relatively rare (Zubenko et al., 2003). Neurovegetative changes are common in both primary and dementia-related depression. Likewise, the psychosis in dementia presents differently from the psychotic syndrome of schizophrenia and primary mood disorders.

The syndromal approach attempts to address several of the methodological liabilities of the monosymptomatic approach. This approach is based on the observation of co-occurrence of several behavioural symptoms in individual patients (Baker et al., 1991; Cohen et al., 1993). In particular, the co-occurrence of aggression and verbal outbursts with hallucinations and delusions has frequently been reported. (Deutsch et al., 1991; Kotrla et al., 1995; Aarsland et al., 1996a). One of the earlier mentions of a behavioural syndrome in dementia was recognition of the Kluver–Bucy syndrome (visual agnosia, hyperphagia, stimulus bound behaviour, hypersexuality and emotional lability) in AD (Sourander and Sjogren, 1970) and in Pick's disease (Cummings and Duchen, 1981). Burns et al. (1990a) found the full syndrome to be relatively rare; however, individual items associated with the syndrome appeared to be interrelated. Other syndromes identified include a three-syndrome classification: overactivity (walking more, walking aimlessly, trailing the carer, checking where the carer was); aggressive behaviour (physical aggression, aggressive resistance, verbal aggression); and psychosis (anxiety, persecutory ideas and hallucinations) (Hope et al., 1997).

Several authors have employed a factor-analytical approach to explore the issue of co-occurrence of symptoms and some have found correlations of factor scores to clinical variables and functional imaging patterns (Devanand et al., 1992; Sultzer et al., 1995). A factor analysis of neuropsychiatric disturbances in an AD clinic population in Italy found three syndromes occurring in isolation in different patients. These were, a 'psychotic' syndrome (high factor loads of agitation; hallucinations, delusions and irritability); a 'mood' syndrome (high loads of anxiety and depression); and a 'frontal' syndrome (high loads of disinhibition and euphoria) (Frisoni et al., 1999). Each syndrome had unique risk factors and associations. The 'psychotic' group tended to be older, of male sex and with poorer cognitive performance and more rapid decline, whereas the 'frontal' group tended to be more educated, have longer disease duration and slower progression. The existence of a 'psychotic' syndrome of delusions, hallucinations, aggression, agitation and disruptive behaviour is supported by the findings of several other groups of researchers (Flynn et al., 1991; Rockwell et al., 1994; Gilley et al., 1997). This syndrome has been shown to be a significant factor in nursing home placement of AD patients (Steele et al., 1990). Finally, factor analysis of a large cross-sectional sample of patients with HD found that the neuropsychiatric symptoms clustered into three groups: irritability, depression and apathy (Craufurd et al., 2001).

A more recent attempt at classifying symptoms based clusters is using a latent class analysis in a population-based study of 198 individuals with AD (Lyketsos et al., 2001a). Latent class analysis differs from factor analysis in that it examines whether *individuals* tend to cluster into groups (classes) based on their clinical profile, as opposed to factor analysis, which examines the grouping of clinical *characteristics* across individuals. Results revealed that, based on analysis of NPI symptom profiles, three groups (classes) of AD patients were evident. The largest class included AD cases with no neuropsychiatric symptoms (40 per cent) or with a monosymptomatic disturbance (19 per cent). A second class (28 per cent) exhibited a predominantly affective syndrome, while a third class (13 per cent) had a psychotic syndrome. This last group presented with hallucinations all of the time, delusions often, and occasionally, apathy, agitation, depression, irritability, aberrant motor behaviour and anxiety.

Unfortunately, investigations of the underlying pathophysiological and neuroimaging correlates have tended to use the monosymptomatic, rather than the syndromic, approach. Hence, we are only in the nascent phases of a deeper understanding of the aetiology of such behavioural syndromes in the dementias. Quantitative neuropsychiatry is one approach that attempts to examine clusters of neuropsychiatric symptoms based on the underlying molecular biology of the type of neurodegenerative disorder.

As described in a recent review of 'quantitative neuropsychiatry' by Cummings (2003), neuropsychiatric phenotypes may be due to regional differences in cell vulnerability to abnormalities of protein metabolism. Most of the neurodegenerative disorders involve abnormalities of protein metabolism, such as the accumulation of α-synuclein protein underlying the *synucleopathies* (e.g. LBD, PD, MSA), hyperphosphorylated τ protein in the *tauopathies* (e.g. FTD, progressive supranuclear palsy), and β-amyloid protein accumulation in AD (*amyloidosis*). Each proteinopathy appears to be associated with particular neuropsychiatric phenotypes that transcend the actual disease diagnosis. For example, hallucinations, delusions and RBD are commonly seen in the synucleopathies, whereas the tauopathies present more often with disinhibition, apathy and compulsions. AD has a more mixed underlying proteinopathy, including abnormalities of β-amyloid, τ- and α-synuclein, suggesting a neuropsychiatric phenotype that incorporates elements of all three neuropathological categories.

6.3 DIAGNOSTIC CRITERIA FOR THE NEUROPSYCHIATRIC SYMPTOMS OF DEMENTIA

Several authors have recently proposed the need for unique, validated diagnostic criteria for the neuropsychiatric phenomena of dementia (Jeste and Finkel, 2000; Olin *et al.*, 2002). This would provide the reliability endowed by a DSM-IV-type approach, facilitate hypothesis-driven and evidence-based research, and provide a consistent treatment target. Proposed criteria, whose validation is underway, include: 'psychosis of AD' (Jeste and Finkel, 2000); 'depression of AD' (Olin *et al.*, 2002); and 'AD-associated affective disorder' or 'AD-associated psychotic disorder' (Lyketsos *et al.*, 2001b).

Jeste and Finkel (2000) make the case for 'psychosis of AD' being a phenomenon distinct from the psychosis seen in elderly people with schizophrenia. Compared to schizophrenia, in AD, the duration of psychosis is shorter, the dosages of antipsychotic medications required for successful treatment are much lower, the phenomenology is distinct, and the neuropathological basis of the psychosis is different. The DSM-IV provides no specific criteria for this subcategory while proposing additional coding if delusions are a predominant feature of the dementia. The proposed criteria for 'psychosis of AD' (Box 6.1) have reliability and face validity and have been accepted by the United States Federal Drug Administration (FDA) as a specific target for treatment intervention. With further field trials, this classification may eventually be extrapolated to become 'psychosis of dementia' and apply to other dementia types such as DLB, vascular dementia and mixed dementia.

The criteria for 'depression of AD' were proposed in 2002 by a group of investigators with extensive research and clinical experience in late-life depression and AD (Olin *et al.*, 2002). These criteria (Table 6.2) differ from the DSM-IV criteria for a 'major depressive episode' in four ways:

- only three or more symptoms (rather than five or more) of depression are required;
- symptoms do not have to occur on a daily basis;
- criteria for irritability, social isolation and withdrawal have been added; and

Box 6.1 *Diagnostic criteria for psychosis of Alzheimer's disease (Jeste and Finkel, 2000, reproduced with permission)*

A Characteristic symptoms
Presence of one (or more) of the following symptoms
- Visual or auditory hallucinations
- Delusions

B Primary diagnosis
All the criteria for dementia of the Alzheimer-type are met

C Chronology of the onset of symptoms psychosis versus onset of symptoms of dementia
There is evidence from the history that the symptoms in criterion A have not been present continuously since prior to the onset of the symptoms of dementia

D Duration and severity
The symptom(s) in criterion A have been present, at least intermittently, for 1 month or longer. Symptoms are severe enough to cause some disruption in patients' and/or others' functioning.

E Exclusion of schizophrenia and related psychotic disorders
Criteria for schizophrenia, schizoaffective disorder, delusional disorder, or mood disorder with psychotic features have never been met

F Relationship to delirium
The disturbance does not occur exclusively during the course of a delirium

G Exclusion of other causes of psychotic symptoms
The disturbance is not better accounted for by another general-medical condition or direct physiological effects of a substance (e.g. a drug of abuse, a medication) Associated features: *specify* if associated

- with agitation
- with negative symptoms
- with depression

- the 'loss of interest' criterion has been modified to include a diminished positive response to social interaction.

These criteria are designed to be broad and to rely on clinical judgement.

An alternative set of criteria for Alzheimer's disease affective disorder (AAAD) (Table 6.2) has been proposed by Lyketsos *et al.* (2001b). Both sets of criteria are in the process of being validated as part of the DIADS-2 (Depression in AD Study-2) and the Cache County-Dementia Progression Study in the USA.

One of the most extensive studies of the clinical features of depression in AD was that of Zubenko and colleagues (2003). They derived data from structured diagnostic assessments of 243 patients with AD. In the most severely demented patients, major depressive episodes were diagnosed in nearly 50 per cent. The validity of a major depressive syndrome of

Table 6.2 *Provisional diagnostic criteria for depression of Alzheimer's disease and Alzheimer-associated affective disorder*

Olin *et al.*, 2002	Lyketsos *et al.*, 2001b (adapted)

A Three (or more) of the following symptoms have been present during the same 2-week period of functioning: at least one of the symptoms is either
 	
• depressed mood or
• decreased positive affect or pleasure.
 	
Note: Do not include symptoms that, in your judgment are clearly due to a medical condition or the result of a non-mood-related dementia syndrome (e.g. loss of weight owing to difficulties with food intake).
 	
  1 Clinically significant depressed mood (e.g. depressed, sad, hopeless, discouraged, tearful)
  2 Decreased positive affect or pleasure in response to social contacts and usual activities
  3 Social isolation or withdrawal
  4 Disruption in appetite
  5 Disruption in sleep
  6 Psychomotor changes (e.g. agitation or retardation)
  7 Irritability
  8 Fatigue or loss of energy
  9 Feelings of worthlessness, hopelessness, or excessive or inappropriate guilt
 10 Recurrent thoughts of death, suicidal ideation, plan or attempt
 	
B All criteria are met for dementia of the Alzheimer-type (DSM-IV-TR)
C The symptoms cause clinically significant distress or disruption in functioning
D The symptoms do not occur exclusively during the course of a delirium
E The symptoms are not due to the direct physiological effects of a substance (e.g. drug or a medication)
F The symptoms are not better accounted for by other conditions such as major depression, schizophrenia, schizoaffective disorder, psychosis of Alzheimer's disease, anxiety disorder or substance-related disorder
 	
Specify if:
• Co-occurring onset: if onset antedates or co-occurs with the AD symptoms
• Post-AD onset: if onset occurs after AD symptoms
 	
Specify:
• with psychosis of Alzheimer's disease
• with other significant behavioural signs or symptoms
• with past history of mood disorder
	A1 A prominent disturbance of affect, disruptive to the patient or the care environment and representing a change from the patient's baseline, as evidenced by the presence of one or more of the following symptoms:
	
	• depression
	• irritability
	• anxiety
	
	A2 Associated symptoms, also representing a change from baseline, that are less prominent than the disturbance of affect. One or more of the following must be present:
	
	• aggression
	• psychomotor agitation
	• delusions
	• hallucinations
	• sleep disturbance
	• appetite disturbance
	
	B Alzheimer's disease by NINCDS/ADRDA criteria
	C The symptoms from 'A1' and 'A2' above cluster together in time and occur most days, and the disturbance has a duration of two weeks or longer
	D The disturbance has its first onset after (or within 2 years before) the onset of cognitive symptoms that eventually progressed into dementia
	E The disturbance cannot be explained in its entirety by another cause such as a general medical condition, medication, caregiver approach, environmental precipitant, or life stressor (such as relocation of residence or death of a spouse)
	
	Specify:
	• with or without psychotic symptoms

AD was supported by the finding that the majority of patients who developed depression had no premorbid history of depression. In addition, the depression tended to appear after the onset of cognitive decline, and the clinical presentation differed from that seen in depressed elderly without dementia. Neuropathological and neurochemical changes in depressed AD patients differ from those of their non-depressed counterparts by demonstrating greater loss of aminergic nuclei, particularly in the locus caeruleus, thus supporting the notion of a distinct depressive entity (Zweig *et al.*, 1988; Zubenko *et al.*, 1990; Förstl *et al.*, 1992).

6.4 PATHOPHYSIOLOGY OF NEUROPSYCHIATRIC SYMPTOMS OF DEMENTIA

Examining the underlying neurophysiology of neuropsychiatric symptoms may lead to the eventual validation of observations of given symptoms and syndromes. Increasingly, newer modalities of investigation, such as functional imaging and behavioural neurogenetics, will aid in the understanding of these symptom clusters (Assal and Cummings, 2002).

Post-mortem neuropathological and neurochemical studies have shown that, compared with those with no psychosis in AD, those with psychosis have more extensive neurodegenerative changes in the cortex, decreased cortical and subcortical serotonin/5-HIAA and increased subcortical norepinephrine (Zubenko et al., 1991). They also have increased muscarinic M2 receptor density in the orbitofrontal cortex (Lai et al., 2001). Furthermore, psychosis in AD is associated with a significantly increased level of abnormal paired helical filament (PHF)-τ protein in the temporal and entorhinal cortices (Mukaetova-Ladinska et al. (1995).

Depression in AD is associated with damage to the locus caeruleus resulting in disturbances in norepinephrine (Reifler et al., 1989; Petracca et al., 1996) and cholinergic deficiency may underlie neuropsychiatric disturbances in PDD and DLB (Kaufer et al., 1998; Kaufer et al., 1996). Agitation in dementia is associated with increased density of tangles in the anterior cingulate and orbitofrontal regions (Assal and Cummings, 2002). Aggression in AD specifically appears to be associated with degeneration of serotinergic areas in the brain accompanied by retained integrity of dopaminergic areas (Katz et al., 1999; Street et al., 1999). Finally, apathy results from deterioration in medial prefrontal, anterior cingulate, and anterior temporal paralimbic structures (Marin, 1996) and may involve disruption in dopaminergic circuits (Marin et al., 1995).

In functional neuroimaging studies, depression in AD has been associated with frontal hypometabolism (Hirono et al., 1998). Depression in PD has been associated with hypometabolism in the caudate and inferior orbital-frontal regions (Mayberg et al., 1990) and medial frontal lobes (Ring et al., 1994). Apathy in AD has been associated with single photon emission computed tomography hypoperfusion in the anterior cingulate (Migneco et al., 2001). Neuroimaging studies in AD with delusions have revealed various findings, including greater dysfunction in the paralimbic areas of the frontotemporal cortex (Seltzer, 1996), and marked right medial posterior parietal hypoperfusion (Fukuhara et al., 2001). In those with hallucinations in AD, hypoperfusion was seen in the right parietal, left medial temporal and left dorsolateral prefrontal cortex (Lopez et al., 2001).

6.5 CONCLUSIONS

The neuropsychiatric complications of dementia syndromes are common and nearly universal. It is becoming increasingly evident that certain neuropsychiatric phenotypes are linked with the underlying pathophysiology of the dementia type. These neuropsychiatric symptoms, which may appear even before the cognitive and functional decline has become evident, have significant consequences, not only for the patients themselves but also for their caregivers. On an optimistic note, while therapeutic approaches to the cognitive and functional decline remain limited, the neuropsychiatric symptoms remain the most treatment responsive aspects of dementia.

REFERENCES

Aarsland D, Cummings JL, Yenner G, Miller BL. (1996a) Relationship of aggressive behavior to other neuropsychiatric symptoms in patients with Alzheimer's disease. *American Journal of Psychiatry* **153**: 243–247

Aarsland D, Tandberg E, Larsen JP, Cummings J. (1996b) Frequency of dementia in Parkinson disease. *Archives of Neurology* **53**: 538–542

Aarsland D, Ballard C, Larsen JP, McKeith I. (2001) A comparative study of psychiatric symptoms in dementia with Lewy bodies and Parkinson's disease with and without dementia. *International Journal of Geriatric Psychiatry* **16**: 528–536

Absher JR and Cummings JL. (1994) Cognitive and noncognitive aspects of dementia syndromes: an overview. In: A Burns and R Levy (eds), *Dementia*. London, Chapman and Hall

Alexopoulos GS and Chester JS. (1992) Outcomes of geriatric depression. *Clinics in Geriatric Medicine* **8**: 363–376

Alzheimer A (translated by Jarvik L and Greenson H). (1987) About a peculiar disease of the cerebral cortex. *Alzheimer Disease and Associated Disorders* **1**: 7–8

American Psychiatric Association. (1994) *Diagnostic and Statistical Manual of Mental Disorders, 4th edition (DSM-IV)*. Washington DC: American Psychiatric Association

Assal F and Cummings JL. (2002) Neuropsychiatric symptoms in the dementias. *Current Opinion in Neurology* **15**: 445–450

Baker FM, Kokmen E, Chandra V, Schoenberg BS. (1991) Psychiatric symptoms in cases of clinically diagnosed Alzheimer's disease. *Journal of Geriatric Psychiatry and Neurology* **4**: 71–78

Ballard C, O'Brian J, Coope B et al. (1995) Associations of psychotic symptoms in dementia sufferers. *British Journal of Psychiatry* **167**: 537–540

Ballard C, Bannister C, Graham C et al. (1997) A prospective study of psychotic symptoms in dementia sufferers: psychosis in dementia. *International Psychogeriatrics* **9**: 57–64

Bianchetti A, Benvenuti P, Ghisla KM, Frisoni GB, Trabucchi M. (1997) An Italian model of dementia Special Care Units: results of a preliminary study. *Alzheimer Disease and Associated Disorders* **11**: 53–56

Breitner JCS, Wyse BW, Anthony JC et al. (1999) APOE epsilon-4 count predicts age when prevalence of Alzheimer's disease increases then declines: the Cache County Study. *Neurology* **53**: 321–331

Burns A, Jacoby R, Levy R. (1990a). Psychiatric phenomena in Alzheimer's disease. I: Disorders of thought content. *British Journal of Psychiatry* **157**: 72–76

Burns A, Jacoby R, Levy R. (1990b) Psychiatric phenomena in Alzheimer's disease. II: Disorders of perception. *British Journal of Psychiatry* **157**: 76–81

Burns A, Jacoby R, Levy R. (1990c) Psychiatric phenomena in Alzheimer's disease. III: Disorders of mood. *British Journal of Psychiatry* **157**: 81–86

Burns A, Jacoby R, Levy R. (1990d) Psychiatric phenomena in Alzheimer's disease. IV: Disorders of behaviour. *British Journal of Psychiatry* **157**: 86–94

Cohen D, Eisdorfer C, Gorelick P et al. (1993) Psychopathology associated with Alzheimer's disease and related disorders. *Journal of Gerontology* **48**: M255–M260

Copeland J, Kelleher M, Kellett J et al. (1976) The Geriatric Mental State Schedule: 1 Development and reliability. Psychological Medicine 6: 439–449

Craufurd D, Thompson JC, Snowden JS. (2001) Behavioral changes in Huntington disease. Neuropsychiatry Neuropsychology and Behavioral Neurology 14: 19–226

Cummings JL. (1992) Neuropsychiatric complications of drug treatment of Parkinson's disease. In: SJ Huber, JL Cummings, C Frith (eds), The Cognitive Neuropsychology of Schizophrenia. Hove, Lawrence Eribaum Associates, pp. 313–327

Cummings JL. (2002) The Neuropsychiatry of Alzheimer's Disease and Related Dementias. London, Martin Dunitz

Cummings JL. (2003) Toward a molecular neuropsychiatry of neurodegenerative diseases. Annals of Neurology 54: 147–154

Cummings JL and Duchen L. (1981) Kluver-Bucy syndrome in Pick disease: clinical and pathologic condition. Neurology 31: 1415–1422

Cummings JL, Mega M, Gray K et al. (1994) The Neuropsychiatric Inventory: comprehensive assessment of psychopathology in dementia. Neurology 44: 2308–2314

Denning TR and Berrios GE. (1989) Wilson's disease: psychiatric symptoms of 195 cases. Archives of General Psychiatry 46: 1126–1134

Deutsch LH, Bylsma FW, Rovner BW, Steele C, Folstein MF. (1991) Psychosis and physical aggression in probable Alzheimer's disease. American Journal of Psychiatry 148: 1159–1163

Devanand DP, Brockington CD, Moody BJ, Brown RP, Mayeux R, Endicott J. (1992) Behavioral syndromes in Alzheimer's disease. International Psychogeriatrics 4 (Suppl. 2): 161–184

Ferman TJ, Boeve BF, Smith GE et al. (2002) Dementia with Lewy bodies may present as dementia and REM sleep behavior disorder without parkinsonism or hallucinations. Journal of the International Neuropsychological Society 8: 907–914

Finkel SI, Costa e Silva J, Cohen G et al. (1996) Behavioral and psychological signs and symptoms of dementia: a consensus statement on current knowledge and implications for research and treatment. International Psychogeriatrics 8 (Suppl. 3): 497–500

Flynn FG, Cummings FL, Gornbein J. (1991) Delusions in dementia syndromes: investigations of behavioural and neuropsychological correlates. Journal of Neuropsychiatry and Clinical Neuroscience 3: 364–370

Folstein SE. (1989) Huntington's Disease: A Disorder of Families. Baltimore, MD, Johns Hopkins University Press

Folstein SE, Chase G, Wahl W et al. (1987) Huntington's disease in Maryland: clinical aspects of racial variation. American Journal of Human Genetics 41: 168–179

Förstl H, Burns A, Luthert P, Cairns N, Lantos P, Levy R. (1992) Clinical and neuropathological correlates of depression in Alzheimer's disease. Dementia 22: 877–884

Fried LP, Borhani NO, Enright P et al. for the CHS Study Group. (1991) The Cardiovascular Health Study: design and rationale. Annals of Epidemiology 1: 263–276

Frisoni GB, Rozzini L, Gozzetti A et al. (1999) Behavioral syndromes in Alzheimer's disease: Description and correlates. Dementia and Geriatric Cognitive Disorders 10: 130–139

Fukuhara R, Ikeda M, Nebu A et al. (2001) Alteration of rCBF in Alzheimer's disease patients with delusion of theft. NeuroReport 12: 2473–2476

Gabrieli JDE, Singh J, Strebbins GT, Goetz CG. (1996) Reduced working memory span in Parkinson's disease: evidence for the role of a frontostriatal system in working and strategic memory. Neuropsychology 10: 322–332

Gilley DW, Wilson RS, Beckett LA et al. (1997) Psychotic symptoms and physically aggressive behavior in Alzheimer's disease. Journal of the American Geriatrics Society 45: 1074–1079

Goetz CG, Leurgans S, Pappert EJ et al. (2001) Prospective longitudinal assessment of hallucinations in Parkinson's disease. Neurology 57: 2078–2082

Hirono N, Mori E, Ishii K et al. (1998) Frontal lobe hypometabolism and depression in Alzheimer's disease. Neurology 50: 380–383

Holroyd S, Currie L, Wooten GF. (2001) Prospective study of hallucinations and delusions in Parkinson's disease. Journal of Neurology, Neurosurgery, and Psychiatry 70: 734–738

Hope T, Keene J, Fairburn C, McShane R, Jacoby R. (1997) Behaviour changes in dementia. 2: Are there behavioural syndromes? International Journal of Geriatric Psychiatry 12: 1074–1078

Howard R and Levy R. (1994) Charles Bonnet Syndrome plus complex visual hallucinations of Charles Bonnet type in late paraphrenia. International Journal of Geriatric Psychiatry 9: 399–404

Jeste DV and Finkel SI. (2000) Psychosis of Alzheimer's disease and related dementias: diagnostic criteria for a distinct syndrome. American Journal of Geriatric Psychiatry 8: 29–34

Katz IR, Jeste DV, Mintzer JE, Clyde C, Napolitano J, Brecher M (Risperidone Study Group). (1999) Comparison of risperidone and placebo for psychosis and behavioural disturbances associated with dementia: a randomized, double-blind trial. Journal of Clinical Psychiatry 60: 107–115

Kaufer D. (1998) Beyond the cholinergic hypothesis: the effect of metrifonate and other cholinesterase inhibitors on neuropsychiatric symptoms in Alzheimer's disease. Dementia and Geriatric Cognitive Disorders 9 (Suppl. 2): 8–14

Kaufer DI, Cummings JL, Christine D. (1996) Effect of tacrine on behavioural symptoms in Alzheimer's disease: an open-label study. Journal of Geriatric Psychiatry and Neurology 9: 1–6

Klatka LA, Louis ED, Schiffer RB. (1996) Psychiatric features in diffuse Lewy body disease: a clinicopathologic study using Alzheimer's disease and Parkinson's disease comparison groups. Neurology 47: 1148–1152

Kotrla KJ, Chacko RC, Harper RG, Doody R. (1995) Clinical variables associated with psychosis in Alzheimer's disease. American Journal of Psychiatry 152: 1377–1379

Lai MK, Lai OF, Keene J et al. (2001) Psychosis of Alzheimer's disease is associated with elevated muscarinic M2 binding in the cortex. Neurology 57: 805–811

Leroi I, Voulgari A, Breitner JCS, Lyketsos CG. (2003) The epidemiology of psychosis in dementia. American Journal of Geriatric Psychiatry 11: 83–91

Litvan I, Mega MS, Cummings JL et al. (1996) Neuropsychiatric aspects of progressive supranuclear palsy. Neurology 47: 1184–1189

Lopez OL, Smith G, Becker JT et al. (2001) The psychotic phenomenon in probable Alzheimer's disease. Journal of Neuropsychiatry and Clinical Neuroscience 13: 50–55

Lyketsos CG, Steinberg M, Tschanz JT et al. (2000) Mental and behavioural disturbances in dementia: findings from the Cache County study on memory in aging. American Journal of Psychiatry 157: 708–714

Lyketsos CG, Sheppard JM, Steinberg M et al. (2001a). Neuropsychiatric disturbance in Alzheimer disease clusters into three groups: the Cache County study. International Journal of Geriatric Psychiatry 16: 1028–1029

Lyketsos CG, Breitner J, Rabins PV. (2001b). An evidence-based proposal for the classification of neuropsychiatric disturbance in Alzheimer's disease. The International Journal of Geriatric Psychiatry 16: 1037–1042

Lyketsos CG, Lopez O, Jones B, Fitzpatrick AL, Breitner J, DeKosky S. (2002) Prevalence of neuropsychiatric symptoms in dementia and mild cognitive impairment. Results from the Cardiovascular Health Study. JAMA 288: 1475–1483

McHugh PR. (1989) The neuropsychiatry of basal ganglia disorders: a triadic syndrome and its explanation. *Neuropsychiatry, Neuropsychology and Behavioral Neurology* **2**: 239–247

McKeith IG, Galasko D, Kosaka K *et al.* (1996) Consensus guidelines for the clinical and pathologic diagnosis of dementia with Lewy bodies (DLB) report of the consortium of DLB international workshop. *Neurology* **47**: 1113–1124

McKhann GM, Albert MS, Grossman M *et al.* (2001) Clinical and pathological diagnosis of frontotemporal dementia: report of the Work Group on Frontotemporal Dementia and Pick's Disease. *Archives of Neurology* **58**: 1803–1809

Marin RS. (1996) Apathy: concept, syndrome, neural mechanisms, and treatment. *Seminars in Clinical Neuropsychiatry* **1**: 304–314

Marin RS, Fogel BS, Hawkins J *et al.* (1995) Apathy: a treatable syndrome. *Journal of Neuropsychiatry and Clinical Neuroscience* **7**: 23–30

Mayberg HS, Starkstein SE, Sadzot B *et al.* (1990) Selective hypometabolism in the inferior frontal lobe in depressed patients with Parkinson's disease. *Annals of Neurology* **28**: 57–64

Meer B and Baker J. (1966) Stockton Geriatric Rating Scale. *Journal of Gerontology* **21**: 392–403

Mendez MG. (1994) Huntington's disease: update and review of neuropsychiatric aspects. *International Journal of Psychiatry and Medicine* **24**: 189–208

Migneco O, Benoit M, Koulibaly PM *et al.* (2001) Perfusion brain SPECT and statistical parametric mapping analysis indicate that apathy is a cingulate syndrome: a study in Alzheimer's disease and nondemented patients. *Neuroimage* **13**: 896–902

Miller BL, Seeley WW, Mychack P *et al.* (2001) Neuroanatomy of the self. Evidence from patients with frontotemporal dementia. *Neurology* **57**: 817–821

Morris JC, Storandt M, Miller JP *et al.* (2001) Mild cognitive impairment represents early-stage Alzheimer disease. *Archives of Neurology* **58**: 397–405

Mukaetova-Ladinska EB, Harrington CR, Xuereb J *et al.* (1995) Treating Alzheimer's and other dementias. In: M Bergener, S Finkel (eds), *Treating Alzheimer's and Other Dementias*. New York, Springer, pp. 57–80

Mychack P, Kramer JH, Boone KB, Miller BL. (2001) The influence of right frontotemporal dysfunction on social behavior in frontotemporal dementia. *Neurology* **56** (Suppl. 4): S11–S15

Neary D, Snowden JS, Gustafson L *et al.* (1998) Frontotemporal lobar degeneration: a consensus on clinical diagnostic criteria. *Neurology* **51**: 1546–1554

Olin JT, Schneider LS, Katz IR *et al.* (2002) Provisional diagnostic criteria for depression of Alzheimer disease. *American Journal of Geriatric Psychiatry* **10**: 125–128

Petracca G, Teson A, Chemerinski E, Leiguarda R, Starkstein SE. (1996) A double-blind placebo-controlled study of clomipramine in depressed patients with Alzheimer's disease. *Journal of Neuropsychiatry and Clinical Neuroscience* **8**: 270–275

Rabins P, Mace M, Lucas M. (1982) The impact of dementia on the family. *JAMA* **248**: 333–335

Reifler BV, Teri L, Raskind M *et al.* (1989) Double-blind trial of imipramine in Alzheimer's disease patients with and without depression. *American Journal of Psychiatry* **146**: 45–49

Reisberg B, Borenstein J, Salob SP, Ferris SH, Franssen E, Gerogotas A. (1987) Behavioral symptoms in Alzheimer's disease: phenomenology and treatment. *Journal of Clinical Psychiatry* **48** (Suppl.): 9–15

Ring HA, Bench CJ, Trimble MR *et al.* (1994) Depression in Parkinson's disease: a positron emission study. *British Journal of Psychiatry* **165**: 333–339

Rockwell E, Jackson E, Vilke G *et al.* (1994) A study of delusions in a large cohort of Alzheimer's disease patients. *American Journal of Geriatric Psychiatry* **2**: 157–164

Rosenblatt A and Leroi I. (2000) Neuropsychiatry of Huntington's disease and other basal ganglia disorders. *Psychosomatics* **41**: 24–30

Sanford J. (1975) Tolerance of disability in elderly dependents by supporters at home: its significance for hospital practice. *BMJ* **3**: 471–473

Seltzer DL. (1996) Neuroimaging and the origin of psychiatric symptoms in dementia. *International Psychogeriatrics* **8** (Suppl. 3): 239–243

Slaughter JR, Slaughter KA, Nichols D *et al.* (2001) Prevalence, clinical manifestations, etiology, and treatment of depression in Parkinson's disease. *Journal of Neuropsychiatry and Clinical Neuroscience* **13**: 187–196

Sourander P and Sjogren H. (1970) The concept of Alzheimer's disease and its clinical implications. In: G Wolstenholme and M O'Connor (eds), *Alzheimer's Disease and Related Conditions*. London, Churchill, 11–32

Starkstein SE, Preziosi TJ, Bolduc PL. Robinson RG. (1990) Depression in Parkinson's disease. *Journal of Nervous and Mental Disease* **178**: 27–31

Steele C, Rovner B, Chase GA *et al.* (1990) Psychiatric symptoms and nursing home placement of patients with Alzheimer's disease. *American Journal of Psychiatry* **147**: 1049–1051

Street J, Clark WS, Cannon KS, Miran S, Sanger T, Tollefson GD. (1999) Olanzapine in the treatment of psychosis and behavioral disturbances associated with Alzheimer's disease. *APA Annual Meeting New Research Program and Abstracts*. Washington DC, American Psychiatric Association, pp. 225–226

Sultzer DL, Mahler ME, Mandelkem MA *et al.* (1995) The relationship between psychiatric symptoms and regional cortical metabolism in Alzheimer's disease. *Journal of Neuropsychiatry and Clinical Neuroscience* **7**: 476–484

Teri L, Borson S, Kijak A, Yamagishi M. (1989) Behavioral disturbance, cognitive dysfunction, and functional skill. *Journal of the American Geriatrics Society* **109**: 109–116

Victoroff J, Mack WJ, Nielson KA. (1998) Psychiatric complications of dementia: impact on caregivers. *Dementia and Geriatric Cognitive Disorders* **9**: 50–55

Wilson RS, Barnes LL, Mendes de Leon CF *et al.* (2002) Depressive symptoms, cognitive decline, and risk of Alzheimer disease in older persons. *Neurology* **59**: 364–370

Wing JK, Cooper JE, Sartorius N. (1974) *The Measurement and Classification of Psychiatric Symptoms*. London, Cambridge University Press

Zubenko GS, Moossy J, Kopp U. (1990) Neurochemical correlates of major depression in primary dementia. *Archives of Neurology* **47**: 209–214

Zubenko GS, Moossy J, Martinez AJ *et al.* (1991) Neuropathological and neurochemical correlates of psychosis in primary dementia. *Archives of Neurology* **48**: 619–624

Zubenko GS, Zubenko WN, McPherson S *et al.* (2003) A collaborative study of the emergence and clinical features of the major depressive syndrome of Alzheimer's disease. *American Journal of Psychiatry* **160**: 857–876

Zweig RM, Ross CA, Hedreen JC *et al.* (1988) The neuropathology of aminergic nuclei in Alzheimer's disease. *Annals of Neurology* **24**: 233–242

7

Rating scales in dementia

7a

Screening instruments for the detection of cognitive impairment

LEON FLICKER

A frequently used method in the ascertainment of dementia in older people is the performance of a short cognitive test to determine the need to perform further testing to establish the diagnosis. At the time of writing, the case for detection of milder forms of cognitive impairment has not been established, mainly because therapeutic strategies for patients with conditions such as mild cognitive impairment (MCI) (Petersen *et al.*, 2001) have not been proven. Thus, the focus of this chapter remains on the use of short cognitive tests to aid in the detection of older people with dementia. These short cognitive tests are commonly described as 'screening instruments', but this is in fact a misnomer. Screening has been defined as 'an organized attempt to detect, among apparently healthy people in the community, disorders or risk factors of which they are unaware' (Cadman *et al.*, 1984). In reality, these short cognitive tests are used as a means of case-finding in certain clinical situations for which there is a high prior probability of finding individuals with cognitive impairment, usually associated with dementia or, in those individuals who are medically unwell, delirium.

7.1 DESCRIPTION OF TESTS

The type of cognitive testing has varied a little over the last 45 years. A minor change that has occurred in the more recently developed tests is the use of lengthier delayed recall tasks, both cued and non-cued. One of the earliest instruments was the Mental Status Questionnaire (MSQ) (Kahn *et al.*, 1960). In, 1968, Blessed *et al.* described the Information Memory Concentration (IMC) test, which was validated against the criterion of neuropathology. Hodkinson (1972) described a shortened version of the IMC test and called this the Abbreviated Mental Test Score (AMT). In North America, Pfeiffer (1975) described the Short Portable Mental Status Questionnaire (SPMSQ) and Folstein *et al.* (1975) devised the Mini-Mental Status Examination (MMSE), which has undergone standardization (Molloy *et al.*, 1991). Other short tests that have been developed include Kokmen's Short Test of Mental Status (STMS) (Kokmen *et al.*, 1991), and the General Practitioner Assessment of Cognition (GPCOG) (Brodaty *et al.*, 2002) both of which include the clock drawing test. All these instruments have in common their brevity, taking 10 minutes or less to administer with relatively little training.

One of the main problems with these cognitive tests is the fact that they exhibit both floor and ceiling effects. There have been attempts to develop tests that would be more suitable for testing impaired patients (Plutchik *et al.*, 1971; Albert and Cohen,1992). Longer tests and word lists have the advantage that they are less prone to ceiling effects. Word list instruments generally require some training. These include the seven minute screen (Solomon *et al.*, 1998), which is a test that comprises a cued recall task, verbal fluency, an orientation test and a clock drawing task. Similarly the Syndrome Kurz Test (SKT) (Lehfeld and Erzigkeit, 1997) has nine subtests, which include naming, memory, attention, cued recall and visuospatial functioning. A very short version of delayed free and cued recall tests has been developed called the Memory Impairment Screen (Buschke *et al.*, 1999), which consists of just four items.

Several other survey instruments have been developed which have incorporated both cognitive screening instruments and diagnostic schedules. These include the Cambridge Diagnostic Examination for the Elderly (Roth *et al.*, 1986), Consortium to Establish a Registry for Alzheimer's Disease (Morris *et al.*, 1989), Geriatric Mental State schedule (Copeland *et al.*, 1976) and a Structured Interview for the Diagnoses of Dementia of the Alzheimer's type, multi-infarct dementia and dementias of other aetiology according to ICD-10 and DSM-IIIR (SIDAM) (Zaudig *et al.*, 1991). The cognitive components of the Cambridge Diagnostic Examination for the Elderly (Roth *et al.,* 1986), the Alzheimer's' Disease Assessment Scale (ADAS-cog) (Rosen *et al.*, 1984) and the Mental Deterioration Battery (Carlesimo *et al.*,1996) take longer to administer and are not usually performed as initial brief tests, although the Organic Brain Scale (OBS) from the Geriatric Mental State has been used as a stand alone test (Ames *et al.*, 1992).

7.2 USE FOR THESE TESTS

The need for these 'screening' instruments has arisen because there is good evidence that clinicians will commonly miss dementia in their routine practice without the assistance of formal cognitive assessment (Williamson *et al.*, 1964; Mant *et al.*, 1988).

Even before the arrival of specific symptomatic treatments for the symptoms of Alzheimer's disease (AD), the presence or absence of significant cognitive impairment had major implications for the management of patients. In particular, older individuals with multiple medical problems requiring medications could not be managed appropriately without an assessment for the presence of cognitive impairment and some idea of its severity. Also, there is some evidence that the earlier identification of people with dementia and appropriate referral to support services and counselling can alleviate some of the stresses associated with caring for people with dementia and delay institutionalization (Green and Brodaty, 2002).

These short cognitive tests have limited domains of measurement. Table 7.1 refers to the domains of measurement of the common assessment tools. Orientation figures prominently in most of these tools and is a reflection of recent memory

acquisition. In a longitudinal study of cognitive function in people with AD, it was demonstrated that this dementing process particularly affects remote memory, immediate memory and language function (Flicker *et al.*, 1993). Since memory impairment is a *sine qua non* in the categorization of dementia in both the DSM-IV and ICD-10 criteria, it is hardly surprising that the short cognitive tests focus on this domain. It is also clear that these tests are highly correlated with each other. For example, Stuss *et al.* (1996) observed that the proportion of variance accounted for by a single common component was in excess of 0.80 for the Mattis Dementia Rating Scale, an abbreviated six-item version of the Orientation Memory Concentration Test adapted from Blessed *et al.* (1968), a Mental State Questionnaire and an Ottawa Mental State Examination. Also in this study there was no added benefit from longer tests and the shorter cognitive tests performed as well as longer tests with multiple domains. In another study the correlation between the AMTS and MMSE was greater than 0.85 (Flicker *et al.*, 1997). Similarly correlations between the MMSE and the ADAS-cog have been found to be strong, -0.9 (Burch and Andrews, 1987), although the correlation between the MMSE and the STMS may only be 0.74 (Kokmen *et al.*, 1991).

These short cognitive scales appear robust in many settings. The IMCT has been validated on telephone interview (Kawas *et al.*,1995) as has the Telephone Cognitive Assessment Battery (Debanne *et al.*,1997), and the Telephone Version of the MMSE (Roccaforte *et al.*, 1992). The OBS has been found to have good validity in three separate countries (Ames *et al.*, 1992). Some attempt has been made to develop self-administered tests, such as the Early Assessment Self Inventory (EASI) (Horn *et al.*, 1989). There is evidence that the place of testing can cause significant changes in the test score, with testing in a patient's own residence being associated with a higher score (Ward *et al.*, 1990).

These short cognitive screens obviously have their limitations, the most obvious being that they test only limited domains of cognition. Besides the use of full neuropsychological assessment, attempts have been made to develop other short tests of specific functions. An example of this is the Executive Interview (Royall *et al.*, 1992), which attempts to assess executive cognitive function. Also, the ability to draw a

Table 7.1 *Cognitive domains in commonly used short cognitive tests*

Test	Personal Information	Orientation	Short-term memory	Long-term memory	Attention	Other
MSQ	◆	◆		◆		
Blessed IMC Test	◆	◆	◆	◆	◆	
AMT	◆	◆	◆	◆	◆	◆
MMSE		◆	◆		◆	◆
SPMSQ	◆	◆		◆	◆	
OBS	◆	◆	◆	◆		◆
STMS		◆	◆	◆	◆	◆
GPCOG		◆	◆			◆

clock has been extensively studied as a short test that examines other cognitive domains. It has been used by itself in conjunction with other cognitive tests such as the SPMSQ or MMSE, or as part of the 7-minute screen, GPCOG or STMS. Clock drawing may miss a quarter of cognitively impaired individuals (Gruber *et al.*, 1997). Clock drawing may be able to detect cognitive alterations not related to delirium or dementia, with abnormal clock drawing being associated with other psychiatric disorders (Gruber *et al.*, 1997). Also it may provide additional information to the MMSE as suggested by Ferrucci *et al.* (1996), where the clock drawing test predicted cognitive decline in older people independently of the MMSE.

Short cognitive tests are known to be sensitive to bias associated with education, but adjustment for this effect does not necessarily improve test performance (Belle *et al.*, 1996). Another consideration is that these tests may not be sensitive to all stages of the disease. Stern *et al.* (1994) demonstrated that there was a quadratic relationship with dementia severity showing that the ADAS-Cog and IMCT show greater deterioration for patients with moderate dementia and that the deterioration is slower for mildly and severely demented patients. This may represent the relative insensitivity of the tests for patients with the least and greatest impairment, or may reveal true patterns of progressive cognitive decline at different parts of the disease process.

Attempts have also been made to shorten these tests even further – for example the 10-item AMT has been further shortened to four items (Swain and Nightingale, 1997) but it does seem to lose some predictive efficiency at this length. The potential problem of inadequate specificity of short cognitive tests for population screening has been revealed in a community study: the Canadian Study of Health in Ageing (Graham *et al.*, 1996). In this study the modified MMSE (3MS Exam) (Teng and Chui, 1987) was used as a community screen before a diagnostic battery. Cognitive impairment, not dementia, was found to be more common than dementing processes, with the prevalence of cognitive impairment not dementia found to be 16.8 per cent, whereas the prevalence of all types of dementia combined was 8 per cent (Graham *et al.*, 1997). The conditions identified within this category of cognitive impairment included delirium, alcohol use, drug intoxication, depression, psychiatric disorders, memory impairment associated with the ageing process and intellectual disability.

7.3 USING INFORMANT-BASED TESTS

Perhaps the most exciting development in the detection of cognitive impairment in older people in recent years has been the refinement and validation of structured tests administered to informants. Examples of this type of test include the DECO Test – Deterioration Cognitive Observée (Ritchie and Fuhrer, 1992) and the Informant Questionnaire for Cognitive Decline in the Elderly (IQCODE) (Jorm and Korten, 1988).

Important advantages of these tests is that they correlate relatively poorly with premorbid function and are relatively insensitive to the effects of education. The other consideration about informant questionnaires is that they have shown lower correlations with the cognitive tests: somewhere in the order of 0.6 (Flicker *et al.*, 1997). The work by Ritchie and Fuhrer (1992) would suggest that they seem to be better able to discriminate mild dementia from normality as opposed to cognitive screens such as the MMSE, although this was not replicated by others (Flicker *et al.*, 1997). This may represent a difference in the choice of informants as much of the sample described by Ritchie and Fuhrer (1992) were recruited through 'France Alzheimer' and may have represented carers who were well attuned to the problems associated with dementia, while the Flicker *et al.* (1997) patients were drawn from attendees at a memory clinic.

A meta-analysis (Jorm, 1997) suggests that informant tests may perform better than short cognitive tests, but it is important to emphasize that there was great heterogeneity within this meta-analysis and clearly the test results were dependent on the subject samples and the samples of informants. Nevertheless Harwood *et al.* (1997) demonstrated a remarkably similar result for both the AMT and the IQCODE in a sample of medical inpatients over the age of 65 admitted to a general medical unit. In that study, the 16-item version of the IQCODE was used with good effect. The IQCODE has been validated by longitudinal changes of cognitive tests (Jorm *et al.*, 1996) and also has been validated retrospectively against post-mortem diagnosis (Thomas *et al.*, 1994).

One of the important considerations for the use of combinations of tests or additional items is that the correlation between individual tests should not be too great. The importance of asymmetry of associations between tests to increase the positive predictive value of combinations of tests has been highlighted (Marshall, 1989). Hooijer *et al.* (1993) found some improvement in diagnosis in using pairs of short screening tests. This was not the case in work by Little *et al.* (1987) where a short AMT score was found to have better predictive value than longer combined tests.

To date, most work has focused on using either informant tests or short cognitive tests separately as a screen for further investigations and management, but clearly the tests can be combined. This was raised by Flicker *et al.* (1997) where the lower correlations and asymmetry of the test properties within different populations could be used so that the combined tests' sensitivity and specificity would be improved. This is quite different to the use of the alteration of cut points, where a trade-off occurs between sensitivity and specificity. The judicious use of the combination of informant and short cognitive tests potentially may result in an increase in both sensitivity and specificity.

This has been demonstrated by Gallo and Breitner (1995) where a telephone administered cognitive status was used as a first screen followed by an informant test. The informant test was falsely described as being more specific, but in fact it was the combination of using the two tests in series that

Table 7.2 *Positive predictive values in different clinical situations**

		Positive predictive value	
Clinical situation	Prevalence	AMT 7/8	AMT 8/9 in series with IQCODE 3.79/3.80
1 General population age group 80–84	11%	45%	63%
2 Patients seen through Aged Care Assessment Teams or in geriatric hospitals	44%	84%	92%
3 General patients over the age of 75 years admitted to acute teaching hospitals	26%	70%	83%

*Based on data from Ames and Tuckwell 1994; LoGiudice *et al.*, 1995; Ames *et al.*, 1994. Reprinted with permission from Flicker L, LoGiudice D, Carlin JB, Ames D. (1997) The predictive value of dementia screening instruments in clinical populations. *International Journal of Geriatric Psychiatry* 12: 203–9. Copyright John Wiley & Sons Limited.

resulted in the increased specificity needed for this two-stage screen. Another example of this approach being used in challenging population research is the work of Hall *et al.* (1993, 1996). In these studies a combination of short cognitive tests and informant testing was used in cross-cultural studies of African American, Cree Indian and Nigerian populations, and the relative insensitivity of the informant tests to the effects of culture and education improved the performance of these combinations. The combination of the MMSE and IQCODE has now been evaluated extensively in three separate studies (Mackinnon and Mulligan, 1998; Knafelc *et al.*, 2003; Mackinnon *et al.*, 2003) with the total evidence suggesting that the combination of tests performed better than either test alone, and that the tests could be combined usefully by either a requirement for both or either test to be positive or calculating a new score using a weighted sum rule.

Besides the characteristics of the population being assessed, it is important to realize that the absolute prevalence of the condition will also cause a need for an adjustment in the cut points. Very low prevalence will increase the need for specificity, otherwise there will be a large number of patients to investigate further. This could of course occur in either research or clinical practice. Some illustrative extrapolations have been provided where the positive predictive value of combinations of tests have been calculated across different population groups (see Table 7.2). It is important to emphasize that the cut points used in the combination of these tests in either series or parallel may be quite different from the ones normally employed by the tests in isolation.

7.4 CONCLUSIONS

There is now available a number of short cognitive tests that appear useful in helping clinicians to determine whether individuals require further assessment for the presence of a cognitive disorder. The tests seem to perform in a fairly similar fashion and it is difficult to predict the performance of these tests, either singly, or in combination with informant tests, from one population to the next. This depends on the asymmetry of test results in cases and normals within that

population, and is very much dependent on the characteristics of the population studied. There is now evidence that an improvement in the efficacy of cognitive assessments can be most easily achieved by combining informant and short cognitive tests to a single summative score, or using informant and cognitive tests with specific cut points and rules of combination. Alternative cut points will need to be used when the tests cannot be used together – for example, when there is no caregiver or informant to provide information on a particular subject, or alternatively, where a subject is delirious or dysphasic and is unable to perform cognitive testing to their potential ability.

REFERENCES

Albert M and Cohen C. (1992) The test for severe impairment: an instrument for the assessment of patients with severe cognitive dysfunction. *Journal of the American Geriatrics Society* 40: 449–453

Ames D and Tuckwell V. (1994) Psychiatric disorders among elderly patients in a general hospital. *Medical Journal of Australia* 160: 671–674

Ames D, Ashby D, Flicker L, Snowdon J, West C, Weyerer S. (1992) Jim Who? Recall of national leaders by elderly people in three countries. *International Journal of Geriatric Psychiatry* 7: 437–442

Ames D, Flynn E, Harrigan S. (1994) Prevalence of psychiatric disorders among inpatients of an acute geriatric hospital. *Australian Journal of Ageing* 13: 8–11

Belle SH, Seaberg EC, Ganguli M, Ratcliff G, DeKosky S, Kuller LH. (1996) Effect of education and gender adjustment on the sensitivity and specificity of a cognitive screening battery for dementia: results from the MoVIES project. *Neuroepidemiology* 15: 321–329

Blessed G, Tomlinson BE, Roth M. (1968) The association between quantitative measures of dementia and of senile change in the cerebral grey matter of elderly subjects. *British Journal of Psychiatry* 114: 797–811

Brodaty H, Pond D, Kemp NM *et al.* (2002) The GPCOG: a new screening test for dementia designed for general practice. *Journal of the American Geriatrics Society* 50: 530–534

Burch EA Jr and Andrews SR. (1987) Comparison of two cognitive rating scales in medically ill patients. *International Journal of Psychiatry in Medicine* 17: 193–200

Buschke H, Kuslansky G, Katz M et al. (1999) Screening for dementia with the Memory Impairment Screen. *Neurology* **52**: 231–238

Cadman D, Chambers L, Feldman W, Sackett D. (1984) Assessing the effectiveness of community screening programs. *JAMA* **251**: 1580–1585

Carlesimo A, Caltagirone C, Gainotti G et al. (1996) The mental deterioration battery: normative data, diagnostic reliability and qualitative analyses of cognitive impairment. *European Neurology* **36**: 378–384

Copeland JRM, Kelleher MJ, Kellett JM et al. (1976) A semi-structured interview for the assessment of diagnosis and mental state in the elderly. The Geriatric Mental State 1. Development and reliability. *Psychological Medicine* **6**: 439–449

Debanne SM, Patterson MB, Dick R et al. (1997) Validation of a telephone cognitive assessment battery. *Journal of the American Geriatrics Society* **45**: 1352–1359

Ferrucci L, Cecchi F, Guralnik JM et al. (1996) Does the clock drawing test predict cognitive decline in older persons independent of the Mini-mental State Examination? The FINE study group, Finland, Italy, The Netherlands Elderly. *Journal of the American Geriatrics Society* **44**: 1326–1331

Flicker C, Ferris SH, Reisberg B. (1993) A two year longitudinal study of cognitive function in normal ageing and Alzheimer's disease. *Journal of Geriatric Psychiatry and Neurology* **6**: 84–96

Flicker L, Logiudice D, Carlin JB, Ames D. (1997) The predictive value of dementia screening instruments in clinical populations. *International Journal of Geriatric Psychiatry* **12**: 203–209

Folstein MF, Folstein SE, McHugh PR. (1975) Mini-mental state: a practical method for grading the cognitive state of patients for the clinician. *Journal of Psychiatric Research* **12**: 189–198

Gallo JJ and Breitner JC. (1995) Alzheimer's disease in the NAS-NRC Registry of aging twin veterans, IV. Performance characteristics of a two-stage telephone screening procedure for Alzheimer's dementia. *Psychological Medicine* **25**: 1211–1219

Graham JE, Rockwood K, Beattie BL, Eastwood R, McDowell I, Gauthier S. (1996) Standardization of the diagnosis of dementia in the Canadian study of health and ageing. *Neuroepedimiology*, **15**: 246–256

Graham JE, Rockwood K, Beattie BL et al. (1997) Prevalence and severity of cognitive impairment with and without dementia in an elderly population. *Lancet* **349**: 1793–1796

Green A and Brodaty H. (2002) Care-giver interventions. In: N Qizilbash (ed.), *Evidence Based Dementia Practice*. Oxford, Blackwell Science, pp. 764–794

Gruber NP, Varner RV, Chen YW, Lesser JM. (1997) A comparison of the clock drawing test and the Pfeiffer short portable mental status questionnaire in a geropsychiatry clinic. *International Journal of Geriatric Psychiatry* **12**: 526–532

Hall KS, Hugh C, Hendrie HC, Brittain HM, Norton JA. (1993) The development of a dementia screening interview in two distinct languages. *International Journal of Methods in Psychiatric Research* **3**: 1–28

Hall KS, Ogunniyi AO, Hendrie HC et al. (1996) A cross-cultural community based study of dementias: methods and performance of the survey instrument Indianapolis, USA, and Ibadan, Nigeria. *International Journal of Methods in Psychiatric Research* **6**: 129–142

Harwood DM, Hope T, Jacoby R. (1997) Cognitive impairment in medical inpatients. 1: Screening for dementia – is history better than mental state? *Age and Ageing* **26**: 31–35

Hodkinson HM. (1972) Evaluation of a mental test score for the assessment of mental impairment in the elderly. *Age and Ageing* **1**: 233–238

Hooijer C, Jonker C, Lindeboom J. (1993) Cases of mild dementia in the community: improving efficacy of case finding by concurrent use of pairs of screening tests. *International Journal of Geriatric Psychiatry* **8**: 561–564

Horn L, Cohen CI, Teresi J. (1989). The EASI: a self-administered screening test for cognitive impairment in the elderly. *Journal of the American Geriatrics Society* **37**: 848–855

Jorm AF. (1997) Methods of screening for dementia: a meta-analysis of studies comparing an informant questionnaire with a brief cognitive test. *Alzheimer Disease and Associated Disorders* **11**: 58–62

Jorm AF and Korten AE. (1988) Assessment of cognitive decline in the elderly by informant interview. *British Journal of Psychiatry* **152**: 209–213

Jorm AF, Christiansen H, Henderson AS, Jacomb PA, Korten AE, Mackinnon A. (1996) Informant ratings of cognitive decline of elderly people: relationship to longitudinal change on cognitive tests. *Age and Ageing* **25**: 125–129

Kahn R, Goldfarb A, Pollack M, Peck A. (1960) Brief objective measures of mental status in the aged. *American Journal of Psychiatry* **117**: 326–328

Kawas C, Karagiozis H, Resau L, Corrada M, Brookmeyer R. (1995) Reliability of the Blessed telephone Information-Memory-Concentration Test. *Journal of Geriatric Psychiatry and Neurology* **8**: 238–242

Knafelc R, LoGiudice D, Harrigan S et al. (2003) The combination of cognitive testing and an informant questionnaire in screening for dementia. *Age and Ageing* **32**: 541–547

Kokmen E, Smith GE, Petersen RC, Tangalos E, Ivnik RC. (1991) The short test of mental status. Correlations with standardized psychometric testing. *Archives of Neurology* **48**: 725–728

Lehfeld H and Erzigkeit H. (1997) The SKT – a short cognitive performance test for assessing deficits of memory and attention. *International Psychogeriatrics* **9** (Suppl. 1): 115–121

Little A, Hemsley D, Bergmann K, Volans J, Levy R. (1987) Comparison of the sensitivity of three instruments for the detection of cognitive decline in elderly living at home. *British Journal of Psychiatry* **150**: 808–814

LoGiudice D, Waltrowicz W, McKenzie S, Ames D, Flicker L. (1995) Dementia in patients referred to an aged care assessment team and stress in their carers. *Australian Journal of Public Health* **19**: 275–280

Mackinnon A and Mulligan R. (1998) Combining cognitive testing and informant report to increase accuracy in screening for dementia. *American Journal of Psychiatry* **155**: 1529–1535

Mackinnon A, Khalilian A, Jorm AF, Korten AE, Christensen H, Mulligan R. (2003) Improving screening accuracy for dementia in a community sample by augmenting cognitive testing with informant report. *Journal of Clinical Epidemiology* **56**: 358–366

Mant A, Eyland EA, Pond DC, Saunders NA, Chancellor AH. (1988) Recognition of dementia in general practice: comparison of general practitioners' opinions with assessments using the Mini-mental State Examination and the Blessed Dementia Rating Scale. *Family Practice* **5**: 184–188

Marshall RJ. (1989) The predictive value of simple rules for combining two diagnostic tests. *Biometrics* **45**: 1213–1222

Molloy DW, Alemayehu E, Roberts R. (1991) Reliability of a standardized Mini-mental State Examination compared with the traditional Mini-mental State Examination. *American Journal of Psychiatry* **148**: 102–105

Morris JC, Heymann A, Mohs RC *et al.* (1989) The consortium to establish a registry for Alzheimer's disease (CERAD). Part 1. Clinical and neuropsychological assessment of Alzheimer's disease. *Neurology* **39**: 1159–1165

Petersen RC, Doody R, Kurz A *et al.* (2001) Current concepts in mild cognitive impairment. *Archives of Neurology* **58**: 1985–1992

Pfeiffer E. (1975) A short portable mental status questionnaire for the assessment of organic brain deficiency in elderly patients. *Journal of the American Geriatrics Society* **23**: 433–441

Plutchik R, Conte H, Lieberman M. (1971) Development of a scale (GIES) for assessment of cognitive and perceptual functioning in geriatric patients. *Journal of the American Geriatrics Society,* **19**: 614–623

Ritchie K and Fuhrer R. (1992) A comparative study of the performance of screening tests for senile dementia using receiver operating characteristics analysis. *Journal of Clinical Epidemiology* **45**: 627–637

Roccaforte WH, Burke WJ, Bayer BL, Wengel SP. (1992) Validation of a telephone version of the Mini-mental State Examination. *Journal of the American Geriatrics Society* **40**: 697–702

Rosen WG, Mohs RC, Davis KL. (1984) A new rating scale for Alzheimer's disease. *American Journal of Psychiatry* **141**: 1356–1364

Roth M, Tym E, Mountjoy CQ *et al.* (1986) CAMDEX: a standardised instrument for the diagnosis of mental disorder in the elderly with special reference to the early detection of dementia. *British Journal of Psychiatry* **149**: 698–709

Royall DR, Mahurin RK, Gray KF. (1992) Bedside assessment of executive cognitive impairment: the executive interview. *Journal of the American Geriatrics Society* **40**: 1221–1226

Solomon PR, Hirschoff A, Kelly B *et al.* (1998) A 7 minute neurocognitive screening battery highly sensitive to Alzheimer's disease. *Archives of Neurology* **55**: 349–355

Stern RG, Mohs RC, Davidson M *et al.* (1994) A longitudinal study of Alzheimer's disease: measurement, rate and predictors of cognitive deterioration: *American Journal of Psychiatry* **151**: 390–396

Stuss DT, Meiran N, Guzman DA, Lafleche G, Willmer J. (1996) Do long tests yield a more accurate diagnosis of dementia than short tests? A comparison of 5 neuropsychological tests. *Archives of Neurology* **53**: 1033–1039

Swain DG and Nightingale PG. (1997) Evaluation of a shortened version of the abbreviated mental test in a series of elderly patients. *Clinical Rehabilitation* **11**: 243–248

Teng EL and Chui HC. (1987) The Modified Mini-Mental State (3MS) examination. *Journal of Clinical Psychiatry* **48**: 314–318

Thomas LD, Gonzales MF, Chamberlain A, Beyreuther K, Masters CL, Flicker L. (1994) Comparison of clinical state, retrospective informant interview and the neuropathologic diagnosis of Alzheimer's Disease. *International Journal of Geriatric Psychiatry* **9**: 233–236

Ward HW, Ramsdell JW, Jackson JE, Renvall M, Swart JA, Rockwell E. (1990) Cognitive function testing in comprehensive geriatric assessment: a comparison of cognitive test performance in residential and clinic settings. *Journal of the American Geriatrics Society* **38**: 1088–1092

Williamson J, Stokoe IH, Gray S *et al.* (1964) Old people at home: their unreported needs. *Lancet* **1**: 1117–1120

Zaudig M, Mitelhammer J, Pauls A, Thora C, Morinizo A, Momboun W. (1991) SIDAM – A structured interview for the diagnoses of dementia of the Alzheimer's type, multi-infarct dementia and dementias of other aetiology according to ICD-10 and DSM III R. *Psychological Medicine* **21**: 225–236

7b

Measurement of behavioural disturbance, non-cognitive symptoms and quality of life

AJIT SHAH, STEPHEN FOLI AND IAN O NNATU

7.5 BPSD: DEFINITION

Burns and colleagues (1990a–d) originally classified non-cognitive symptoms in dementia into disorders of behaviour, mood, thought content and perception. The International Psychogeriatric Association labelled these as behavioural and psychological signs and symptoms of dementia (BPSD) and defined them as 'a heterogeneous range of psychological reactions, psychiatric symptoms, and behaviours occurring in people with dementia of any aetiology' (Finkel and Burns, 2000). We have added a further domain of disorders of personality alteration. The definition of any individual BPSD should be hierarchical and allow discrimination between the cognitive and non-cognitive (BPSD) domains, different BPSD domains, and individual signs and symptoms within a given BPSD domain (Shah, 2000).

7.6 DISORDERS OF BEHAVIOUR DISTURBANCE

7.6.1 Definition

Aggressive behaviour is described as a typical example of disturbed behaviour, but similar arguments can be rehearsed for other disorders of behaviour. There is no generally agreed definition of aggressive behaviour (Shah, 1999a). Varying definitions of aggressive behaviour have been used. The best definition of aggressive behaviour in the elderly is: 'Aggressive behaviour is an overt act, involving the delivery of noxious stimuli to (but not necessarily aimed) at another organism, object or self, which clearly is not accidental' (Patel and Hope, 1992a).

7.6.2 Samples, settings, methods of data collection and measurement instruments

Box 7.1 illustrates the samples studied in several settings including the community, outpatient clinics, residential and nursing homes, acute admission and continuing care geriatric and psychogeriatric wards (Shah, 1999a). More recent studies have largely been prospective and some include a longitudinal component. Methods of data collection are listed in Box 7.2. Essential properties of instruments measuring any BPSD, including aggressive behaviour, are illustrated in Box 7.3.

Box 7.1 *Samples (with references) studied for aggressive behaviour*

- Undifferentiated dementias   Shah, 1995
- Alzheimer's disease   Reisberg *et al.*, 1987; Burns *et al.*, 1990a, e, f; Devanand *et al.*, 1992a; Lyketsos *et al.*, 2001a
- Vascular dementia   Sultzer *et al.*, 1992, 1993
- Huntington's chorea   Burns *et al.*, 1990f

Box 7.2   *Methods of data collection (with references) for aggressive behaviour in dementia*

• Case-notes	Reisberg *et al.*, 1987
• Semistructured telephone interviews	Devanand *et al.*, 1992a
• Postal questionnaires directed at staff	Luckovits and McDaniel, 1992
• Postal questionnaires directed at informal carers	Luckovits and McDaniel, 1992
• Staff completed incident forms	Shah, 1995
• Informal staff reports	Hallberg *et al.*, 1993
• Specially designed forms completed by staff	Winger *et al.*, 1987
• Staff completed formal rating scales	Patel and Hope, 1992b
• Informal carer completed formal rating scales	Ryden, 1988
• Semistructured interviews	Devanand *et al.*, 1992b
• Direct observations	Hallberg *et al.*, 1993
• Voice recordings	Hallberg *et al.*, 1990
• Mechanical body movements	Rindlisbacher and Hopkins, 1992

Box 7.3   *Psychometric and other properties of instruments measuring non-cognitive symptoms in dementia (reprinted from Zaudig, 1996)*

• Patient characteristic
• User characteristic
• Type of instrument
• Setting for administration
• Data source
• Output of the instrument
• Psychometric properties
  – reliability
  – test-retest
  – interrater
  – intrarater
  – internal consistency
  – validity
  – face
  – content
  – concurrent
  – construct
  – predictive
  – incremental
  – sensitivity to change
• Time frame for symptoms
• Training needs
• Duration of symptoms
• Method of administration
• Qualification of users
• Costs
• Acceptability to raters

An important characteristic of some instruments measuring aggressive behaviour is the spontaneous tendency for aggressive behaviour to decline during a period of serial measurement. This has been observed with the Staff Observation Aggression Scale (SOAS) (Palmsteirna and Wistedt, 1987) on psychogeriatric wards (Nilsson *et al.*, 1988; Shah, 1999b). Therefore, a 'run in' period of up to 4 weeks has been recommended in intervention studies (Nilsson *et al.*, 1988; Shah, 1999b).

7.6.3 Comment

Many instruments measure aggressive behaviour, but not all the psychometric and other properties have been adequately evaluated. Individual instruments have been developed for use in specific settings or specific diagnostic groups. One example of this difficulty is the RAGE scale. It was developed for use by the nursing staff on psychogeriatric inpatients with dementia (Patel and Hope, 1992a), but it has also been used in nursing homes (Shah *et al.*, 1997) and psychogeriatric wards (Shah and De, 1997) for all diagnostic groups. Generalizability of instruments to other settings, diagnostic groups and different category of raters is unclear. Given the large number of instruments, with varying properties, there should be a moratorium on the development of new instruments. Research should be directed at comparing different instruments with each other, generating data on all of their properties, refining these instruments to improve their properties, adapting them for use in parallel settings, and developing guidelines and protocols for their use in research and clinical practice (Shah and Allen, 1999). This would ultimately allow measurement of aggression across settings, diagnostic groups and with different modes of data collection in a comparable common currency.

7.7 DISORDERS OF PERSONALITY ALTERATION

7.7.1 Definition

Personality changes in dementia include emergence of new features (Petry *et al.*, 1988; Dian *et al.*, 1990; Siegler *et al.*, 1991; Chatterjee *et al.*, 1992) or an exaggeration of premorbid personality traits.

7.7.2 Samples, settings and methods of data collection

Box 7.4 illustrates the samples and the settings in which personality change has been examined. Studies have included a comparison group of normal aged individuals (Rubins *et al.*, 1987a, b; Petry *et al.*, 1988; Cummings *et al.*, 1990; Dian *et al.*, 1990; Jacoub and Jorm, 1996), Parkinson's disease (Meins and Dammast, 2000), vascular dementia (Sultzer *et al.*, 1993) and frontotemporal dementia (Miller *et al.*, 1997), and compared Alzheimer's disease (AD) with norms for inpatients (Meins and Dammast, 2000). Comparison with the premorbid personality allows identification of personality changes (Siegler *et al.*, 1991; Chatterjee *et al.*, 1992); and, comparison with normal aged individuals allows exclusion of personality changes as an artefact of ageing (Rubins *et al.*, 1987a, b; Petry *et al.*, 1988; Cummings *et al.*, 1990; Dian *et al.*, 1990). Difficulties in measuring the type, nature and severity of personality change include: reduced insight, judgement and memory preclude use of self-reports (Petry *et al.*, 1988; Meins and Dammast, 2000); accounts from relatives may be biased by their emotional feelings (Dian *et al.*, 1990; Jacoub *et al.*, 1994; Meins and Dammast, 2000) and personality (Meins, 2000); and, a clear retrospective account of premorbid personality may not always be available. Methods of data collection are listed in Box 7.5.

7.7.3 Instruments used to measure personality alteration

The items of irritability and disinhibition on the Neuropsychiatric Inventory (NPI) (Cummings *et al.*, 1994) coupled with case-notes review was used to examine socially disruptive and antisocial behaviour in a comparative study of AD and frontotemporal dementia (Miller *et al.*, 1997). The Brooks and McKinlay (1983) personality inventory, originally used in brain injury patients, with 18 pairs of adjectives, measured on a five-point scale, has been administered to relatives of people with dementia (Petry *et al.*, 1988, 1989; Cummings *et al.*, 1990). The 11 personality items on the Blessed Dementia Rating Scale (Blessed *et al.*, 1968) has been used alone (Bozzola *et al.*, 1992) or in combination with six items from open-ended questions (Rubins *et al.*, 1987a, b). The Eysenck Personality Inventory (EPI) has been used to show that, among elderly psychiatric inpatients and day patients with organic disorder, impulsiveness correlates with extraversion but not psychoticism (Pearson, 1990, 1992). Subjects with mild-moderate dementia and neurotic disorders scored highly on the neuroticism component of the EPI in a community sample (Nilsson, 1983). 'Troublesome behaviour' has been reported to be associated with higher scores on the premorbid trait of neuroticism in Alzheimer's subjects (Meins *et al.*, 1998). Instruments measuring personality changes have been developed from the 'personality change' and impaired judgement of impulse control' components of DSM-IIIR and ICD-10 descriptions of dementias (Jacoub *et al.*, 1994) and asking clinicians to complete personality inventories on the basis of their experience (Jacoub and Jorm, 1996).

7.7.4 Clinical features

Changes in personality features include coarsening of affect, disinhibition, increase in passivity, apathy, aspontaneity, irritability, belligerence, demanding attention, indifference, egocentricity, less conscientiousness, lower extraversion, higher neuroticism and lower openness (Seltzer and Sherwin, 1983; Ishii *et al.*, 1986; Petry *et al.*, 1988, 1989; Cummings *et al.*, 1990; Siegler *et al.*, 1991; Bozzola *et al.*, 1992; Chatterjee *et al.*, 1992; Jacoub and Jorm, 1996; Meins and Dammast, 2000). Patients with AD, compared to normal elderly, have greater changes on 12 personality traits of being more out of touch, less self-reliant, less mature, less enthusiastic, less stable, more unreasonable, more lifeless, more unhappy, less affectionate, less kind, more irritable and less generous after the onset of the dementia (Petry *et al.*, 1988); similar results were observed in vascular dementia (Dian *et al.*, 1990). Subjects with frontotemporal dementias are more likely to demonstrate forensic behaviour like indecent exposure and shoplifting than those with AD (Miller *et al.*, 1997). Four patterns of personality alteration in AD emerge at 3-year follow up: change at onset with little change as the disease continues; ongoing change as the disease progressed; no change at all; and, regression of previously altered personality characteristics (Petry *et al.*, 1989).

7.7.5 Comment

Some BPSD may be secondary to personality change. However, the relationship between personality changes and other BPSD domains is unclear. They may be part of the same phenomenon, aetiologically linked or discrete entities. Many of the personality change features listed above overlap with features of frontal lobe dysfunction (Dian *et al.*, 1990) and depression (Sultzer *et al.*, 1993). Paucity of data on psychometric and other properties of instruments used to measure personality suggests that research efforts should be directed at rigorous evaluation of existing and new instruments (Strauss and Pasupathi, 1994). There is a clear need to develop instruments that measure personality features in individuals with dementia that are sensitive from the premorbid to the illness state and that allow for personality change as an artefact of ageing alone (Strauss *et al.*, 1997). They should be applicable across different diagnostic categories, settings and informants to measure personality change in a comparable common currency.

7.8 DISORDERS OF MOOD

7.8.1 Definition

These two disorders are common in old age and may occur together by chance. Patients with depression may demonstrate cognitive deficits (Verhey and Visser, 2000), including depressive pseudodementia. Depression may precede the onset of dementia either as an early presentation of incipient dementia or act as a risk factors for dementia (Verhey and Visser, 2000). Furthermore, depressive symptoms and illness in dementia require careful definition due to overlap with features of personality changes and cognitive impairment, especially frontal lobe features (Weiner *et al.*, 1997). Ideally this definition should be identical to that for primary depression.

7.8.2 Samples, settings and methods of data collection

Boxes 7.6 and 7.7 illustrate the diagnostic categories and settings, and methods of data collection used in studies of depression in dementia, respectively. Although no clear gold standard for diagnosis of depression in dementia has been established (Verhey and Visser, 2000), these instruments have mainly been validated against gold standard definitions of depression according to DSM-III (Reifler *et al.*, 1986; Cummings *et al.*, 1987; MacKenzie *et al.*, 1989), DSM-IIIR (Burns *et al.*, 1990d; Skoog, 1993; Weiner *et al.*, 1997), DSM-IV (Brodaty and Luscombe, 1996), Research Diagnostic (Alexopoulos *et al.*, 1988) and ICD-10 (Burns *et al.*, 1990b)

Box 7.6 *Sample or settings (and references) in studies of depression in dementia*

Sample

• Undifferentiated dementias	Skoog, 1993
• Vascular dementia	Cummings *et al.*, 1987; Brodaty and Luscombe, 1996
• Alzheimer's disease	Burns *et al.*, 1990b; Lyketsos *et al.*, 2001

Setting

• Community	Skoog, 1993; Lyketsos *et al.*, 2001
• Outpatient clinic	Cummings *et al.*, 1987; Brodaty and Luscombe, 1996
• Nursing homes	Brodaty *et al.*, 2001
• Mixed settings	Alexopoulos *et al.*, 1988; Burns *et al.*, 1990b
• Acute and Continuing care	Shah and Gray , 1997; Akoo and Shah, 1998; Elanchenny and Shah, 2001
• Psychogeriatric wards	

Box 7.7 *Methods of data collection (and references) for depression in dementia*

• Self-rating scales	Ott and Fogel, 1992; Espiritu *et al.*, 2001
• Interviewer-rated scales directed at patients	Cummings *et al.*, 1987; Ott and Fogel, 1992; Brodaty and Luscombe, 1996
• Interviewer-rated scales directed at care-givers as surrogates	Brodaty and Luscombe, 1996
• Combination of interviewer and observer rating	Sunderland *et al.*, 1988; Ott and Fogel, 1992
• Combination of interview and collateral sources	Katona and Aldridge, 1985; Alexopoulos *et al.*, 1988
• Pure observer scales	Shah and Gray, 1997; Akoo and Shah, 1998; Elanchenny and Shah, 2001

---

criteria for major depressive disorder. Some studies have also included dysthymia (Alexopoulos *et al.*, 1988; Skoog, 1993).

7.8.3 Instruments used to measure depression

Box 7.7 illustrates the self-rated and interviewer-rated scales used for measuring depression in dementia. Data on psychometric and other properties for most of these instruments are limited. These scales are generally less accurate as cognitive impairment increases and insight decreases (Ott and Fogel, 1992) because good attention, concentration, memory and judgement are required for their completion (Burke *et al.*, 1989). Furthermore, as cognitive impairment increases and insight decreases, the discrepancy between depression reported by patients and carers increases (Ott and Fogel, 1992). The recognition of this problem has led to development of instruments specially designed to measure depression in dementia using collateral sources of information (e.g. family members or nursing staff) in addition to clinical examination. Three such scales exist: the Depressive Signs Scale (DSS) (Katona and Aldridge, 1985); the Cornell Scale (Alexopoulous *et al.*, 1988); and, the Depression in Dementia Mood Scale (DDMS) (Sunderland *et al.*, 1988).

7.8.4 Comment

The prevalence of depressive symptoms and depressive illness in AD are 0–87 per cent (median 41 per cent) and 0–86 per cent (median, 19 per cent) respectively (Wragg and Jeste, 1989; Verhey and Visser, 2000). There are various methodological reasons for the variability in these rates. Instruments used to measure depression may be insensitive in severe dementia or patients with severe dementia may not be able to experience complex emotions like depression (Burns *et al.*, 1990b). Furthermore, depression may not present with the classical symptoms in dementia (Verhey and Visser, 2000), particularly in severe dementia (Burns *et al.*, 1990b). There should be a moratorium on developing new depression scales for use in dementia until all the properties of existing scales are thoroughly evaluated. Moreover, refining these instruments will also allow discrimination from other cognitive and personality features and allow examination of the relationship between depression and functional disability in dementia (Espiritu *et al.*, 2001). Efforts need to concentrate on scales that can measure depression across different groups of dementias, settings and informants at varying degrees of cognitive impairment in a comparable common currency.

7.9 DISORDERS OF THOUGHT CONTENT AND PERCEPTION

7.9.1 Definition and classification

Hallucinations and delusions in dementia have the same classical definition as in other psychiatric disorders (Cummings *et al.*, 1987). Presence for at least 7 days is an added requirement to exclude delirium as a cause of these phenomena. Auditory (Cummings *et al.*, 1987; Burns *et al.*, 1990d), visual (Cummings *et al.*, 1987; Reisberg *et al.*, 1987; Burns *et al.*, 1990d) and olfactory (Rubins *et al.*, 1989) hallucinations have been studied. Delusions were divided into four categories by Cummings (1985): simple persecutory; complex

---

Box 7.8 *Samples, settings and methods of data collection (and references) for study of psychotic symptoms in dementia*

Sample

• All nursing home residents	Brodaty *et al.*, 2001
• Undifferentiated dementia	Skoog, 1993
• Vascular dementia	Cummings *et al.*, 1987
• Lewy body dementia	Ballard *et al.*, 1995
• Alzheimer's disease	Cummings *et al.*, 1987; Reisberg *et al.*, 1987; Burns *et al.*, 1990c, d; Lyketsos *et al.*, 2001
• Huntingdon's chorea	Dewhurst *et al.*, 1969

Setting

• Community	Skoog, 1993; Lyketsos *et al.*, 2001
• Memory clinics	Ballard *et al.*, 1995
• Outpatient clinic	Cummings *et al.*, 1987; Reisberg *et al.*, 1987
• Referrals to a psychogeriatric service	Ballard *et al.*, 1995
• Inpatients	Trabucchi and Bianchetti, 1996
• Nursing homes	Brodaty *et al.*, 2001
• Mixed	Burns *et al.*, 1990c, d; Whitehouse *et al.*, 1996

Method of data collection

• Patient interview	Cummings *et al.*, 1987; Skoog, 1993
• Interview with caregiver	Cummings *et al.*, 1987; Burns *et al.*, 1990c, d; Brodaty *et al.*, 2001; Lyketsos *et al.*, 2001
• Case-notes	Cummings *et al.*, 1987

---

persecutory; grandiose; and those associated with specific neurological deficits. An alternative classification is of delusions of theft, delusions of suspicion and systematized delusions (Burns *et al.*, 1990c). Four types of misidentification syndromes have been described (Burns *et al.*, 1990d): people in the house, misidentification of mirror image, misidentification of television and misidentification of people.

7.9.2 Samples, settings, methods of data collection and measurement instruments

Box 7.8 illustrates the samples, settings and methods of data collection used. Box 7.9 illustrates common instruments used to measure psychotic symptoms. Several semistructured interviews and specially designed scales measure psychotic symptoms along with several other non-cognitive symptoms and thus produce diluted data on pure psychotic features (Ballard *et al.*, 1995).

> **Box 7.9** *Instruments used (and references) to measure psychotic symptoms in dementia*
>
> - *BEHAVE-AD   Reisberg *et al.,* 1987
> - *MOUSEPAD   Allen *et al.,* 1996
> - Columbia University   Devanand *et al.,* 1992b
>   Schedule for
>   Psychopathology in
>   Alzheimer's Disease
> - Neuropsychiatric Inventory   Cummings *et al.,* 1994
> - Burns symptom checklist   Ballard *et al.,* 1995
>
> *BEHAVE-AD, Behavioural Pathology in Alzheimer's Disease Rating Scale; MOUSEPAD, Manchester and Oxford Universities Scale for Psychopathological Assessment of Dementia

7.9.3 Comment

The prevalence of delusions (Cummings *et al.,* 1987; Reisberg *et al.,* 1987; Burns *et al.,* 1990c), hallucinations (Ballard *et al.,* 1995; Burns *et al.,* 1990d) and misidentification syndromes (Ballard *et al.,* 1995; Burns *et al.,* 1990d) in AD and vascular dementia varies from 20 to 50 per cent, 17 to 36 per cent and 11 to 34 per cent respectively. Methodological reasons primarily explain the variability in the rates. The boundaries between hallucinations, delusions and misidentification syndromes are often blurred (Whitehouse *et al.,* 1996) and delusions are difficult to differentiate from confabulations (Cummings *et al.,* 1987). The definitions and descriptions of the psychopathology require refinement and clarity (Trabucchi and Bianchetti, 1996). Psychometric and other important properties of measurement instruments have been poorly studied. A systematized check list of 17 categories of psychotic symptoms is the only pure instrument designed to measure psychotic symptoms, but has been poorly evaluated (Ballard *et al.,* 1995). This and similar instruments should be rigorously evaluated and refined to allow measurement of psychotic symptoms across different diagnosis, settings and informants in a common comparable currency. None of the extant instruments measures the degree of distress to the patient and potential for harm to others or self. Measurement of these two variables is important because clinicians will generally only treat psychotic symptoms if the patient is distressed or there is risk of harm to self or others.

7.10 BPSD: CONCLUSIONS AND A WAY FORWARD

Interrelationships between individual BPSD symptoms within and across BPSD domains has been examined by simple univariate correlations (Brodaty *et al.,* 2001), latent class analysis (Lyketsos *et al.,* 2001) and factor analysis (Hope *et al.,* 1997). Ultimately, such analysis will allow identification of the nosological validity of the empirically derived five domains of BPSD by establishing symptom and syndromal clusters

(Lyketsos *et al.,* 2001) and, in turn, facilitate a greater understanding of the demographic, clinical, genetic, biochemical, neuroimaging, neurophysiological and neuroanatomical correlates of BPSD, and their longitudinal course and prognosis.

These developments should be coupled with a moratorium on development of new BPSD rating instruments in order to allow researchers simultaneously to concentrate on comparing different extant BPSD instruments with each other, generate data on their psychometric and other properties, refine these instruments and improve their properties, adapt them for use in parallel settings, and develop detailed glossary, guidelines and protocols for use in audit, research and clinical practice. The ultimate objective should be to measure BPSD accurately by means of the same instrument across settings and diagnostic groups, using different modes of data collection and differing categories of raters. Using the same scale is important because patients move from different settings in different directions.

7.11 QUALITY OF LIFE

7.11.1 Definition

Quality of life (QoL) has several definitions with variable content and weighting given to different domains (Ready *et al.,* 2002). The problem of definition and quantification lies in the different perspectives of this concept and the individual differences in the perception of QoL (Calman, 1984). This perception has cultural-, subcultural-, social-, societal-, personal- and personality-based facets (Whitehouse *et al.,* 1997). The most comprehensive definition of QoL is from the World Health Organization (WHO): 'as individuals' perception of their position in life in the context of the culture and value system in which they live, and in relation to their goals, expectations, standards and concerns' (WHOQOL, 1995). The International Working Group on the Harmonisation of Dementia Drug Guidelines, defined QoL in dementia as 'the integration of cognitive functioning, activities of daily living, social interactions and psychological wellbeing' (Whitehouse *et al.,* 1997). A simpler definition of health-related quality of life in dementia is: 'the individual's subjective perception of the impact of a health condition on life' (Smith *et al.,* 2000; Banerjee *et al.,* 2002). They proposed examining domains of daily activities and looking after self, health and wellbeing, cognitive functioning, social relationships and self concept. Lawton (1994) proposed examining domains of cognitive function, competence in activities of daily living, socially appropriate behaviour, engagement in positive activities, and the presence of positive affect and absence of negative affect in AD.

7.11.2 Measurement of QoL

Measurement instruments can be generic or specific to dementia. Generic instruments have the advantage of allowing comparison across different disorders and are appealing to policy makers because comparisons across diagnostic categories can inform allocation of funds. Disease-specific instruments, by measuring items relevant to the disorder, allow measurement of the impact of treatment on the disease.

QoL instruments, specific for dementia, are required because a unique set of symptoms cluster in dementia (Rabins and Kasper, 1997). However, the measurement of QoL in dementia is difficult because cognitive impairment can compromise the subject's understanding of QoL, ability to recall relevant recent events, ability to make comparisons across complex QoL domains and insight (Banerjee et al., 2002; Smith et al., 2003). Moreover, the measurement of validity poses difficulties owing to lack of universally accepted definition and an absence of a 'gold standard' measure. Furthermore, subjects in the early stages of dementia give overtly optimistic ratings (Lawton, 1994). These issues raise the question of whether measurement instruments should be self-rated, proxy-rated or use both rating methods (Banerjee et al., 2002; Smith et al., 2003). Proxy measures, by informal or professional carers, may partly address these issues, and may also be necessary in severe dementia when subjects have poor comprehension and communication skills (Smith et al., 2003). However, it not clear at what severity of dementia should self-reports be replaced by proxy reports (Fletcher et al., 1992). Moreover, objective ratings of QoL by caregivers and health professionals are often inconsistent with subjective self-reports by people with dementia (Albert et al., 1996).

7.11.2.1 EXISTING SCALES

Many existing scales were developed in the field of oncology and chronic physical disorders and used in the evaluation of pharmacotherapeutic agents and other treatment interventions, and development of health economics. They are unsatisfactory for measuring QoL in dementia.

Several scales have been evaluated in dementia including Quality of Well Being Scale in AD (Kerner et al., 1998), Quality of Life in AD (Logsdon et al., 1998), AD-Related QoL (Rabins and Kasper, 1997), Cornell-Brown Scale for Quality of Life in Dementia (Ready et al., 2002), and Health-Related Quality of Life in Dementia (Banerjee et al., 2002; Smith et al., 2003). The later new measure of Health-Related Quality of Life in Dementia with satisfactory psychometric properties, has two separate and autonomous components: self-report by people with dementia (DEMQoL) and proxy report by carers (DEMQoL-Proxy) (Banerjee et al., 2002; Smith et al., 2003). These two measures give different but complementary perspectives on the quality of life in dementia. In most cases both measures would be used; however, in severe dementia, owing to the large amount of missing data on self-reports, DEMQoL-Proxy would be useful, and there may not be a need for DEMQoL-Proxy in those with mild cognitive impairment.

7.11.3 Comment

QoL instruments can be useful in screening and monitoring of psychosocial problems in individual patients, population surveys of perceived health problems, clinical audit, measuring outcome in health services and evaluation research, clinical trials, and conducting cost-utility analysis. However, most existing QoL measures in dementia cannot be considered satisfactory in the absence of an agreed definition of QoL, operational criteria and gold standard, lack of satisfactory data on psychometric and other properties (see Box 7.3), and absence of normative data on the subjective perception of QoL. In dementia, impaired judgement, reduced insight, cognitive impairment, personality changes, affective and psychotic symptoms, physical morbidity and temporary fluctuations may make subjective assessment of QoL difficult. There needs to be a moratorium on developing new QoL instruments for dementia. Existing QoL instruments in dementia should be further developed to measure QoL across different dementias, settings and raters, and for use directly with subject, by proxy or by observational ratings in a comparable common currency. Individual instruments measuring QoL should be compared with each other, and theoretically this can lead to further refinement of these instruments.

REFERENCES

Akoo S and Shah AK. (1998) Screening for depression by the nursing staff in an acute psychogeriatric unit. *Australasian Journal on Ageing* **17**: 81–84

Albert SM, Castillo-Castaneda C, Sano M et al. (1996) Quality of life in Alzheimer's disease is reported by patient proxies. *Journal of the American Geriatrics Society* **44**: 1342–1347

Alexopoulos GS, Abrams RC, Young RC, Shamoian CA. (1988) Cornell Scale for depression in dementia. *Biological Psychiatry* **23**: 271–284

Allen NHP, Gordon S, Hope T, Burns A. (1996) Manchester and Oxford Universities Scale for the Psychopathological Assessment of Dementia (MOUSEPAD). *British Journal of Psychiatry* **169**: 293–307

Ballard CG, Saad K, Patel A et al. (1995) The prevalence and phenomenology of psychotic symptoms in dementia sufferers. *International Journal of Geriatric Psychiatry* **10**: 477–485

Banerjee S, Smith S, Murray J et al. (2002) DEMQOL: a new measure of health related quality of life in dementia. *Neurobiology of Ageing* **23** (Suppl.1): S154

Bozzola FG, Gorelick PB, Freels S. (1992) Personality changes in Alzheimer's disease. *Archives of Neurology* **49**: 297–300

Brodaty H and Luscombe G. (1996) Studies on affective symptoms and disorders: depression in persons with dementia. *International Psychogeriatrics* **8**: 609–622

Brodaty H, Draper B, Saab D et al. (2001) Psychosis and behaviour disturbance in Sydney nursing home residents: prevalence and predictors. *International Journal of Geriatric Psychiatry* **16**: 504–512

Brooks DN and McKinlay W. (1983) Personality and behavioural change after severe blunt head injury: a relatives' view. *Journal of Neurology, Neurosurgery, and Psychiatry* **46**: 336–344

References 79

Burke WJ, Houston MJ, Boust SJ, Roccaforte WH. (1989) Use of the Geriatric Depression Scale in dementia of the Alzheimer type. *Journal of the American Geriatrics Society* 37: 856–860

Burns A, Jacoby R, Levy R. (1990a) Psychiatric phenomena in Alzheimer's disease. IV: disorders of behaviour. *British Journal of Psychiatry* 157: 86–94

Burns A, Jacoby R, Levy R. (1990b) Psychiatric phenomena in Alzheimer's disease. III: Disorders of mood. *British Journal of Psychiatry* 157: 81–86

Burns A, Jacoby R, Levy R. (1990c) Psychiatric phenomena in Alzheimer's disease. I: Disorders of thought content. *British Journal of Psychiatry* 15: 72–76

Burns A, Jacoby R, Levy R. (1990d) Psychiatric phenomena in Alzheimer's disease. II: Disorders of perception. *British Journal of Psychiatry* 157: 76–81

Burns A, Jacoby R, Levy R. (1990e) Behavioural abnormalities and psychiatric symptoms in Alzheimer's disease: preliminary findings. *International Psychogeriatrics* 2: 25–36

Burns A, Folstein S, Brandt J, Folstein M. (1990f) Clinical assessment of irritability aggression and apathy in Huntington and Alzheimer's disease. *Journal of Nervous and Mental Disease* 178: 20–26

Calman KC. (1984) Quality of life in cancer patients – an hypothesis. *Journal of Medical Ethics* 10: 124–127

Chatterjee A, Strauss ME, Smyth KA, Whitehouse PJ. (1992) Personality changes in Alzheimer's disease. *Archives of Neurology* 49: 486–491

Cummings J. (1985) Organic delusions: phenomenology anatomical correlations and review. *British Journal of Psychiatry* 146: 184–197

Cummings JF, Petry S, Dian L, Shapira J, Hill MA. (1990) Organic personality disorder in dementia syndromes: an inventory approach. *Journal of Neuropsychiatry* 2: 261–267

Cummings JL, Miller B, Hill MA, Neshkes R. (1987) Neuropsychiatric aspects of multiinfarct dementia and dementia of the Alzheimer's type. *Archives of Neurology* 44: 389–393

Cummings JL, Mega M, Gray K et al. (1994) The Neuropsychiatric inventory: comprehensive assessment of psychopathology in dementia. *Neurology* 44: 2308–2314

Devanand DP, Brockington CD, Moody BJ et al. (1992a) Behaviour syndromes in Alzheimer's disease. *International Psychogeriatrics* 4 (Suppl. 2): 161–184

Devanand DP, Miller L, Richards M et al. (1992b) The Columbia University scale for psychopathology in Alzheimer's disease. *Archives of Neurology* 49: 371–376

Dewhurst K, Oliver J, Trick K et al. (1969) Neuropsychiatric aspects of Huntington's disease. *Confinia Neurologica* 31: 258–268

Dian L, Cummings JL, Petry S, Hill MA. (1990) Personality alterations in multi-infarct dementia. *Psychosomatics* 4: 415–419

Ellanchenny N and Shah AK. (2001) Evaluation of three nurse-administered depression rating scales on acute and continuing care psychogeriatic wards. *International Journal of Methods in Psychiatric Research* 10: 43–51

Espiritu DAV, Rashid H, Mast BT, Fitzgerald J, Steinberg J, Lictenberg PA. (2001) Depression cognitive impairment and function in Alzheimer's disease. *International Journal of Geriatric Psychiatry* 16: 1098–1103

Finkel SI and Burns A. (2000) Introduction to behavioural and psychological symptoms of dementia (BPSD) a clinical and research update. *International Psychogeriatrics* 12 (Suppl. 1): 9–12

Fletcher AE, Dickinson EJ, Philp I. (1992) Review. Audit measures: quality of life instruments for everyday use with elderly patients. *Age and Ageing* 21: 142–150

Hallberg IR, Norberg A, Ericckson A. (1990) Functional impairment and behaviour disturbances in vocally disruptive patients in psychogeriatric wards compared with controls. *International Journal of Geriatric Psychiatry* 5: 53–61

Hallberg IR, Edberg A, Nordmark A, Johnsson K, Norberg A. (1993) Daytime vocal activity in institutionalised severely demented patients identified as vocally disruptive by nurses. *International Journal of Geriatric Psychiatry* 8: 155–164

Hope T, Keene J, Fairburn C, McShane R, Jacoby R. (1997) Behaviour changes in dementia. II: Are there behavioural syndromes? *International Journal of Geriatric Psychiatry* 12: 1074–1078

Ishii N, Nishihara Y, Imamura T. (1986) Why do frontal lobe symptoms predominate in vascular dementia syndrome? *Neurology* 36: 340–345

Jacoub P and Jorm A. (1996) Personality change in dementia of Alzheimer's type. *International Journal of Geriatric Psychiatry* 11: 201–207

Jacoub P, Jorm A, Christensen H, MacKinnon A et al. (1994) Personality changes in normal and cognitively impaired elderly: informant reports in a community sample. *International Journal of Geriatric Psychiatry* 9: 313–320

Katona CLE and Aldridge CR. (1985) The dexamethasone test and depressive signs in dementia. *Journal of Affective Disorders* 8: 83–89

Kerner DN, Patterson DL, Grant J et al. (1998) Validity of the Quality of Well-Being Scale for patients with Alzheimer's disease. *Journal of Ageing and Health* 10: 44–61

Lawton MP. (1994) Quality of life in Alzheimer's disease. *Alzheimer Disease and Associated Disorders* 5: 138–150

Logsdon RG, Gibbons LE, McCurry SM, Teri L. (1998) Quality of life in Alzheimer's disease: patient and carer reports (QOL-AD). *Journal of Mental Health and Ageing* 5: 21–32

Lukovits TG and McDaniel KD. (1992) Behavioural disturbance in severe Alzheimer's disease: a comparison of family member and nursing staff reporting. *Journal of the American Geriatrics Society* 40: 891–895

Lyketsos CG, Sheppard JME, Steinberg M et al. (2001) Neuropsychiatric disturbance in Alzheimer's disease clusters into three groups: the Cache County study. *International Journal of Geriatric Psychiatry* 16: 1043–1053

MacKenzie TB, Robiner WN, Knopman DS. (1989) Differences between patient and family assessments of depression in Alzheimer's disease. *American Journal of Psychiatry* 146: 1174–1178

Meins W. (2000) Impact of personality on behavioural and psychological symptoms of dementia. *International Psychogeriatrics* 12 (Suppl. 1): 107–109

Meins W and Dammast J. (2000) Do personality traits predict the occurrence of Alzheimer's disease? *International Journal of Geriatric Psychiatry* 15: 120–124

Meins W, Frey A, Thiesemann R. (1998) Premorbid personality traits in Alzheimer's disease: do they predispose to non-cognitive behavioural symptoms? *International Psychogeriatrics* 10: 369–378

Miller BL, Darby A, Benson DF, Cummings JL, Miller MH. (1997) Aggressive socially disruptive and antisocial behaviour associated with fronto-temporal dementia. *British Journal of Psychiatry* 170: 150–155

Nilsson LV. (1983) Personality changes in the aged. A transectional and longitudinal study with Eysenk personality inventory. *Acta Psychiatrica Scandinavica* 68: 202–211

Nilsson K, Palmsteirna T, Wistedt B. (1988) Aggressive behaviour in hospitalised psychogeriatric patients. *Acta Psychiatrica Scandinavica* 78: 172–175

O'Connor DW. (2000) Epidemiology of behavioral psychological symptoms of dementia. *International Psychogeriatrics* 12: 41–45

Ott BR and Fogel BS. (1992) Measurement of depression in dementia: self v clinician rating. *International Journal of Geriatric Psychiatry* 7: 899–904

Palmsteirna B and Wistedt B. (1987) Staff observation aggression scale: presentation and evaluation. *Acta Psychiatrica Scandinavica* **76**: 657–663

Patel V and Hope RA. (1992a) A rating scale for aggressive behaviour in the elderly- the RAGE. *Psychological Medicine* **22**: 211–221

Patel V and Hope RA. (1992b) Aggressive behaviour in elderly psychiatric inpatients. *Acta Psychiatrica Scandinavica* **85**: 131–135

Pearson PR. (1990) Impulsiveness and spiral maze performance in elderly psychiatric patients. *The Personality and Individual Differences* **11**: 1309–1310

Pearson PR. (1992) The relationship of impulsiveness to psychoticism and extraversion in elderly psychiatric patients. *Journal of Psychology* **126**: 443–444

Petry S, Cummings J, Hill M, Shapira J. (1988) Personality alterations in dementia of Alzheimer's type. *Archives of Neurology* **45**: 1187–1190

Petry S, Cummings J, Hill M, Shapira J. (1989) Personality alterations in dementia of the Alzheimer type: a three year follow-up study. *Journal of Geriatric Psychiatry and Neurology* **2**: 203–207

Rabins P and Kasper JD. (1997) Measuring quality of life in dementia: conceptual and practical issues. *Alzheimer Disease and Related Disorders* **11** (Suppl. 6): 100–104

Ready RE, Ott BR, Grace J, Fernandez I. (2002) The Cornell-Brown Scale for quality of life in dementia. *Alzheimer Disease and Related Disorders* **16**: 109–115

Reifler BV, Larson E, Teri L, Poulsen M. (1986) Dementia of the Alzheimer's type and depression. *Journal of the American Geriatrics Society* **34**: 855–859

Reisberg B, Borensteen J, Sabb S et al. (1987) Behavioural symptoms in Alzheimer's disease: phenomenology and treatment. *Journal of Clinical Psychiatry* **48** (Suppl.): 9–15

Rindlisbacher P and Hopkins RW. (1992) An investigation of the sundowning syndrome. *International Journal of Geriatric Psychiatry* **7**: 15–23

Rubins EH and Kinscherf DA. (1989) Psychopathology of very mild dementia of Alzheimer's type. *American Journal of Psychiatry* **146**: 1017–1021

Rubins EH, Morris JC, Storandt M, Berg L. (1987a) Behavioural changes in patients with mild senile dementia of Alzheimer's type. *Psychiatric Research* **21**: 55–62

Rubins EH, Morris JC, Berg L. (1987b) The progression of personality change in senile dementia of Alzheimer's type. *Journal of the American Geriatrics Society* **35**: 721–725

Ryden M. (1988) Aggressive behaviour in persons with dementia who live in the community. *Alzheimer Disease and Associated Disorders* **2**: 345–355

Seltzer B and Sherwin I. (1983) A comparison of clinical features in early onset and late onset primary degenerative dementia. *Archives of Neurology* **40**: 143–146

Shah AK. (1995) Violence among psychogeriatric inpatients with dementia. *International Journal of Geriatric Psychiatry* **10**: 887–891

Shah AK. (1999a) Aggressive behaviour in the elderly. *International Journal of Psychiatry in Clinical Practice* **3**: 85–103

Shah AK. (1999b) Some methodological issues in using aggression rating scales in intervention studies among institutionalised elderly. *International Psychogeriatrics* **11**: 439–444

Shah AK. (2000) What are the necessary characteristics of a behavioural and psychological symptoms of dementia rating scale? *International Psychogeriatrics* **12** (Suppl. 1): 205–209

Shah AK and Allen H. (1999) Is improvement possible in the measurement of behaviour disturbance in dementia? *International Journal of Geriatric Psychiatry* **14**: 512–519

Shah AK and De T. (1997) The relationship between two scales measuring aggressive behaviour amongst continuing care psychogeriatric inpatients. *International Psychogeriatrics* **9**: 471–477

Shah AK and Gray T. (1997) Screening for depression on continuing care psychogeriatric wards. *International Journal of Geriatric Psychiatry* **12**: 125–127

Shah AK, Chiu E, Ames D. (1997) The relationship between two aggression used in nursing homes for the elderly. *International Journal of Geriatric Psychiatry* **12**: 628–631

Siegler IC, Welsh KA, Fillenbaum GG, Earl NL, Kaplan EB, Clark CM. (1991) Ratings of personality change in patients being evaluated for memory disorders. *Alzheimer Disease and Associated Disorders* **4**: 240–250

Skoog I. (1993) The prevalence of psychotic depressive and anxiety syndromes in demented and non-demented 85-year olds. *International Journal of Geriatric Psychiatry* **8**: 247–253

Smith S, Lamping D, Banerjee S et al. (2003) DEMQOL: Measurement off health-related quality of life with dementia the development of a new instrument and an evaluation of current methodology. *Health Technology Assessment Monograph* (in press)

Strauss ME and Pasupathi M. (1994) Primary caregivers' descriptions of Alzheimer patients' personality traits: temporal stability and sensitivity to change. *Alzheimer Disease and Associated Disorders* **8**: 166–176

Strauss ME, Lee MM, DiFilippo JM. (1997) Premorbid personality and behavioural symptoms in Alzheimer's disease. Some cautions. *Archives of Neurology* **54**: 257–259

Sultzer DL, Levin HS, Mahler ME, High WM, Cummings JL (1992) Assessment of cognitive psychiatric and behavioural disturbance in patients with dementia: the neurobehavioural rating scale. *Journal of the American Geriatrics Society* **40**: 549–550

Sultzer DL, Levin HS, Mahler ME, High WM, Cumming JL. (1993) A comparison of psychiatric symptoms in vascular dementia and Alzheimer's disease. *American Journal of Psychiatry* **150**: 1806–1812

Sunderland T, Alterman IS, Yount D et al. (1988) A new scale for the assessment of depressed mood in dementia patients. *American Journal of Psychiatry* **145**: 955–959

Trabucchi M and Bianchetti A. (1996) Clinical perspectives: what should we be studying? Delusions. *International Psychogeriatrics* **8** (Suppl. 3): 383–385

Verhey FRJ and Visser PJ. (2000) Phenomenology of depression in dementia. *International Psychogeriatrics* **12** (Suppl. 1): 129–134

Weiner MF, Svetlik D, Risser RC. (1997) What depressive symptoms are reported in Alzheimer's patients. *International Journal of Geriatric Psychiatry* **12**: 648–652

Whitehouse P, Patterson MB, Strauss ME et al. (1996) Hallucinations. *International Psychogeriatrics* **8** (Suppl. 3): 387–392

Whitehouse PJ, Orgogozo JM, Becker RE et al. (1997) Quality of life assessment in dementia drug development. *Alzheimer Disease and Associated Disorders* **11** (Suppl. 3): 56–60

Winger J, Schirm V, Stewart D. (1987) Aggressive behaviour in long-term care. *Journal of Psychosocial Nursing and Mental Health Services* **25**: 28–33

WHOQOL Group. (1995) The World Health Organization Quality of Life Assessment (WHOQOL) Position Paper from the WHO. *Social Science and Medicine* **41**: 1403–1409

Wragg RE and Jeste D. (1989) Overview of depression and psychosis in Alzheimer's disease. *American Journal of Psychiatry* **146**: 577–587

Zaudig M. (1996) Assessing behavioural symptoms of dementia of Alzheimer's type: categorical and quantitative approaches. *International Psychogeriatrics* **8** (Suppl. 2): 183–200

8

Structural brain imaging

ROBERT BARBER AND JOHN O'BRIEN

This chapter focuses on the clinical and research uses of structural magnetic resonance imaging (MRI) in the study of dementia.

Traditionally, structural neuroimaging in dementia has been used to exclude intracranial lesions that may be responsible for cognitive impairment, especially so-called treatable or reversible causes. Although these causes are relatively uncommon and the cost-benefit of using neuroimaging for their detection continues to be debated, MRI and computed tomography (CT) have an unassailable role in their diagnosis because no combination of first line clinical and laboratory findings (which exclude imaging) can identify all treatable causes (Frisoni, 2001).

In addition, imaging is increasingly used to identify neuro-radiological features that characterize specific dementias. This has become possible because of improvements in image quality allowing subtle anatomical differences to be detected and measured. It also reflects a conceptual shift towards diagnosing dementia using both exclusion and inclusion criteria, and recognition that existing diagnostic criteria have finite sensitivity and specificity. Investigations that improve diagnostic accuracy should also help ensure that new treatments are targeted to patients most likely to benefit. In this way, MRI is being used to optimize diagnostic confidence by detecting the presence, and not solely the absence, of biological features specific to certain dementias. Conceivably, even if findings do not redirect the clinician to alternative diagnoses or treatment strategies, they will facilitate provision of accurate information to patients and their families about diagnosis and prognosis. Indeed, the significance of neuroimaging to patients and families should not be underestimated: the result of a scan often has a pivotal role in helping individuals understand and adjust to the diagnosis of dementia.

In a research context, cross-sectional and longitudinal MRI studies have been conducted to detect bioradiological markers that could aid presymptomatic diagnosis of dementia. MRI also offers new insights into the biology of dementia. These include understanding the links between pathology and symptoms, how dementia subtypes progress over time, whether pharmacotherapies modify these changes, and the identification of predictors to treatments.

Although the first human MR images were generated in the 1970s, the first systematic study of MRI in dementia dates from as recently as the late 1980s. Indeed, MRI remained niched as a research tool until 1990s, by which time it was recognized as a powerful, versatile and safe imaging modality with a central role in medical diagnostics. By 2002 approximately 22 000 MRI scanners were in operation worldwide, performing more than 60 million investigations per annum. The all-round significance of MRI to medical diagnostic and research was underlined in 2003 when two of the pioneers of MRI, Sir Peter Mansfield from the UK and Paul Lauterbur from the USA, were awarded Nobel Laureates in Medicine. The last Nobel Prize in Medicine in the field of diagnostics was awarded to Alan Cormack and Sir Godfrey Hounsfield for the development of CT in 1979.

8.1 MECHANISM OF MAGNETIC RESONANCE IMAGING

In essence, MRI is a non-invasive chemical probe capable of generating high-resolution three-dimensional images of the body's internal structures. It uses the electromagnetic properties of hydrogen nuclei (or protons) to construct a spatial representation of tissue. Under the controlled environment of the MR scanner, hydrogen nuclei act like microscopic radiotransmitters and a macroscopic impression of tissue structure is obtained by detecting their signal. Analogies have been drawn comparing the way MR images are assimilated from these multiple signals with how an impression of the structure of a city can be obtained from observing the pattern of street lights at night. MRI scanners use very powerful magnetic fields that are approximately 30 000 times greater than the earth's magnetic field. Alterations in water (or, in effect, proton) content and the molecular motion of water molecules provide a basis for detecting pathological change.

Box 8.1   *Main types of MRI sequences*

Conventional sequences
- *T1-weighted:* provides good definition of anatomy
- *T2-weighted:* provides high contrast and definition of soft tissue pathology
- *Proton density:* provides good brain/CSF contrast

Newer sequences
- Fluid attenuated inversion recovery (FLAIR): sensitive to changes in white matter
- Magnetization transfer imaging (MTI): sensitive to changes in structural integrity of tissue
- Diffusion-weighted imaging (DWI): provides information about the microscopic diffusion of water molecules and integrity of axons
- Perfusion-weighted imaging (PWI): provides information about the status of brain tissue perfusion
- Diffusion tensor imaging (DTI): identifies white matter tracts

---

A difference in water content of <1 one per cent is enough to distinguish normal and abnormal tissue.

One of the strengths of MRI is its versatility, and there are a number of imaging sequences which can be used to optimize anatomical and pathological differentiation. These standard or conventional sequences are summarized in Box 8.1 and illustrated in Figure 8.1. In addition, newer MRI sequences have been developed to enable a more detailed examination of white matter tracts, also summarized in Box 8.1. Importantly, they provide higher lesion contrast and can detect and quantify changes that may go undetected by conventional sequences. To date, the vast majority of MRI studies in dementia have used conventional imaging sequences, and only a small number of studies have explored the potential benefits of combining different MR modalities, or indeed structural and functional imaging.

8.1.1 Comparison between MRI and CT

MRI and CT have different advantages and disadvantages as summarized in Box 8.2. The availability of MRI scanners varies considerably from country to country, and by locality. In reality, local service issues such as access, cost and availability often affect the choice to use MRI or CT more than adherence to clinical or scientific considerations.

8.2 INDICATIONS FOR MAGNETIC RESONANCE IMAGING

MRI provides a sensitive method to study atrophy, cerebrovascular disease, white matter abnormalities and certain specific diseases associated with cognitive impairment, such as Creutzfeld–Jakob disease (CJD). High spatial resolution (<1 mm) and superior soft tissue contrast also provides greater

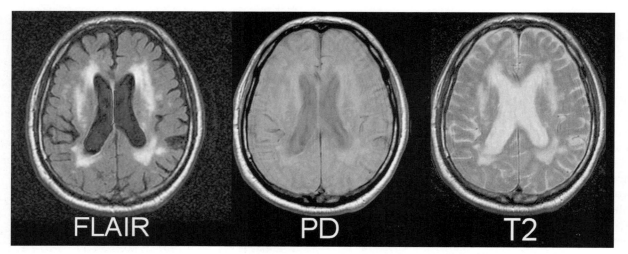

Figure 8.1   *Comparison of FLAIR, proton density (PD) and T2-weighted images from the same individual: note differences in appearance of white matter hyperintensities.*

potential for early diagnosis. Moreover, brain structure can be examined in any plane and detailed volumetric quantification of regional and global morphology obtained. Contraindications of MRI are summarized in Box 8.3.

Few studies have directly compared the diagnostic usefulness of MRI and CT. Frisoni (2001) suggested, that in the absence of suitable evidence-based guidelines, CT is sufficient (and necessary) to detect most reversible or treatable causes, particularly those liable to surgical intervention (e.g. brain tumours, subdural haematoma or normal pressure hydrocephalus). MRI, on the other hand, because of the superior image quality, may be more helpful in the differential diagnosis of dementia subtypes and in early/presymptomatic diagnosis. Which format is best suited to detect vascular disease is unresolved, but MRI is probably more sensitive, and CT more specific (especially when the disease process is more advanced).

Box 8.2 *Comparison between MRI and CT*

MRI
- Higher spatial and anatomical resolution
- Superior soft tissue definition and contrast
- Image in multiple planes; therefore superior views of middle and posterior fossa, pituitary, brain stem, and spinal cord
- Uses non-ionizing radiation
- Wide application for quantitative analysis
- Greater sensitivity to detect white matter pathology and lesions causing epilepsy

CT
- Shorter scan times
- Widely available
- Lower cost
- Better tolerated
- Good for bone abnormalities
- Better for lesions with little or no water content (e.g. meningiomas) and detection of acute intracerebral haemorrhage

---

Box 8.3 *Contraindications to MRI*

- Claustrophobia/poorly tolerated (5–10%): MRI scanners can be noisy and feel confined
- Ferromagnetic implants, e.g. pacemakers, intracranial aneurysm clips, cochlear implants, neurostimulators: cardiac pacemakers can de-program and misfire – under these circumstances, structural imaging with CT is the only option
- Ferromagnetic objects in eyes
- Orthopaedic implants are not contraindicated but may introduce local artefacts

---

8.3 CHOOSING A RATING SCALE AND MEASURING BRAIN ATROPHY

There are a plethora of tools to evaluate the extent and progression of atrophy and white matter pathology. Methods range from very basic visual rating scales to sophisticated computerized programs, requiring back-up from medical physics. Very few studies have compared the clinical usefulness of different tools, leaving the clinician uncertain about which tool to use. As a result they are rarely used routinely outside research clinics.

Nevertheless, tools that assess atrophy have a sensitivity and specificity for distinguishing Alzheimer's disease (AD) from controls of between 70 and 90 per cent, and perhaps in a counterintuitive way, there is little evidence that any method, simple or complex, performs better (Scheltens et al., 2002; Frisoni et al., 2003). The Consensus statement produced by the Neuroimaging Working Group of the European Alzheimer's Disease Consortium (EADC) could find only one MRI tool with evidence showing it had 'added diagnostic value' (Frisoni et al., 2003). This was a visual rating scale of medial temporal lobe atrophy (MTA). In terms of everyday clinical practice, Frisoni (2001) suggested that a visual rating scale (at least) of MTA on MRI (such as Scheltens et al., 1992) (or a linear measure of MTA on CT) should be used in each patient with cognitive impairment. Visual rating scales have the general advantage of being simple and quick to use, and can provide clinically relevant information that correlates sufficiently well with quantitative *in vivo* analysis and post-mortem neuropathology. Limitations include lack of detail and issues of subjectivity, with variable interobserver and intraobserver reliability.

Most research studies now use volumetric analysis for detailed quantification of even small amounts of atrophy. This is, however, time consuming, requires trained operators, high resolution images and, by definition, cannot be obtained from the direct visualization of radiological films. This level of analysis is not currently used in clinical settings, though some automated methods have been developed but require wider validation.

Voxel-based morphometry (VBM) is a new method to evaluate structural change. It combines data from individuals to estimate differences in the pattern and extent of atrophy between the specific groups under investigation. It achieves this by a voxel-based comparison of the local concentration of grey matter between two groups of subjects (Ashburner and Friston, 2000). It is particularly useful at exploring the entire brain without bias and in assessing anatomical differences in areas that would otherwise be difficult to quantify, e.g. total grey matter. However, comparison of individual subjects is not yet developed and VBM lacks the anatomical precision of detailed region of interest (ROI) volumetric studies. VBM has been used to map grey matter density reduction in degenerative dementias, as outlined below.

8.4 CROSS-SECTIONAL AND LONGITUDINAL STUDIES

Brain morphology can be assessed using cross-sectional or longitudinal study designs. The majority of neuroimaging studies so far have been cross-sectional. This design is widely used to compare atrophy in a diseased group with age-related change in an appropriately selected control group. In addition, by the study of age-stratified non-demented healthy individuals, morphological changes across the human life span can be defined in a relatively short time frame.

Longitudinal studies, in contrast, measure the same structure in the same individual at two time points. Differences in volumes between scans is then calculated and used to assess rate of change. Serial scans can be compared using a range of methods, most commonly repeated manual tracing or coregistration, subtraction techniques. Serial scans reduce the variance due to intersubject differences, with each subject acting as their own control, allowing individual changes over time to be precisely assessed. This approach is sufficiently sensitive to detect very small volume changes in the order of a few millilitres or less. There are a number of methodological challenges; atrophy rates can vary considerably between subjects, and serial scanning of patients with advancing dementia can, understandably, be problematic.

Serial MRI was initially used to evaluate whether atrophy rates could improve diagnostic accuracy. The premise, drawn from initial work from CT scanning, was that progressive atrophy over time in an individual patient may be a more sensitive and specific diagnostic marker than a cross-sectional measure obtained from only one scan. Wide variation in normal brain morphology means that within-subject change may discriminate patients with dementia from normal subjects with greater accuracy and at an earlier stage than absolute or group mean volumes. However, results from studies have so far been mixed, and looking ahead, the most exciting role for serial imaging in disease detection is likely to be during the presymptomatic stage of a dementia.

Progression of atrophy in different dementia subtypes can also be explored using serial MRI. Preliminary findings indicate that subjects with degenerative and vascular dementia are losing brain volume at a similar albeit greater rate than normal controls, suggesting serial measurement of global atrophy is unlikely to differentiate the main types of dementia, although, conceivably, measures of regional atrophy rates (such as the hippocampus) could prove to be more discriminating.

Serial MRI also provides a potential paradigm to evaluate the effects of new therapies in dementia. Although evidence is limited, initial studies indicate that this approach is feasible and can provide useful surrogate biomarkers in evaluating the outcome (Jack *et al.*, 2003; Krishnan *et al.*, 2003). Measures of the rate of atrophy have now been incorporated into several trials in MCI and AD.

Box 8.4 *Differences between cerebral infarcts and deep white matter hyperintensities on MRI*

Infarcts
- Hypointense on T1 and proton density weighted images
- Hyperintense on T2-weighted images
- Well-defined; wedge shape if peripheral
- Often single or low numbers
- Often evidence of cortical extension
- May be associated with focal enlargement of ventricles and sulci

Deep white matter hyperintensities
- Hyperintense on T2 and proton density weighted images
- No change/invisible on T1-weighted images
- Range from punctuate to diffuse confluent lesions
- Often multiple
- Restricted to white matter with no cortical extension
- Ventricles and sulci unchanged

8.5 WHITE MATTER LESIONS

MRI has had a leading role in characterizing white matter abnormalities. The nature and significance of such changes, however, remains an area of uncertainty and controversy, and is perhaps one of the most widely misunderstood and misinterpreted neuroimaging changes.

White matter lesions (WML) that appear as areas of reduced attenuation or leukoaraiosis on CT scanning are hyperintense on proton density and T2-weighted MR images. WML can be divided into those immediately adjacent to the ventricles (periventricular hyperintensities, PVH) and those located in the deep white matter (deep white matter hyperintensities, DWMH). As shown in Figure 8.2, PVH can be further subdivided into caps (frontal and occipital) and bands, and DWMH into punctate foci, early confluent foci and large confluent areas (Fazekas *et al.*, 1987). Box 8.4 summarizes the radiological differences between DWMH and established infarcts (see also Figure 8.3). WML on conventional MRI sequences can be assessed using simple rating scales, semi-quantitative scales and volumetric analysis, although there is currently no universally accepted standardized approach.

WML are clinically and pathologically heterogeneous (see Table 8.1, p. 87). They become more common with advancing age, and can be found in all major forms of dementias as well a host of other conditions, including multiple sclerosis, hydrocephalus, various leukodystrophies, cerebral oedema, neurosarcoid, and conditions such as late life depression. Given the variety of pathologies known to underlie white matter change, it is important not to overinterpret imaging changes (particularly on proton density and T2-weighted MRI) with regard to the vascular contribution to dementia.

The clinical significance of WML continues to be debated. As a general statement, more severe DWMH are more closely

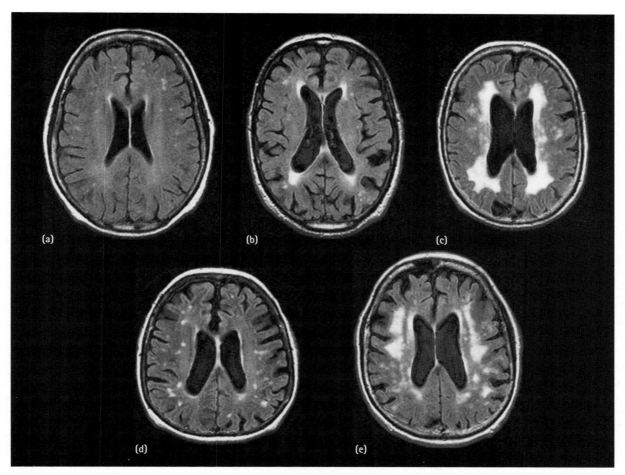

Figure 8.2   *Examples of white matter lesions on FLAIR. (a) No periventricular hyperintensities (PVH); (b) mild PVH (frontal and occipital caps); (c) moderate to severe PVH (frontal and occipital caps); (d) punctate deep white matter hyperintensities (DWMH) (in frontal and parietal lobes); (e) large, early confluent DWMH.*

coupled to both significant pathologic change (notably ischaemia) and clinical outcome, such as dementia and depression. The 'disconnection' of key cortical-subcortical circuits could mediate their effect on brain function. PVH, on the other hand, may have little impact on the clinical outcome. However, uncertainties remain, and the application of newer MRI sequences to this area of study may find links between lesions and symptoms that currently go undetected.

Looking ahead, should WML prove to be clinically significant, then this would have implications for treatment, either directly by opening up new therapeutic options (for example, whether treatment for vascular risk factors modifies ischaemic WML), or indirectly by understanding how WML may modify response to other treatments.

8.6   NORMAL AGEING

With maturity we lose approximately 0.5 per cent of our brain volume every year, and, as our brains become smaller, our ventricles become larger, often at a faster rate. The pace of this change accelerates with advancing age, particularly after 70 years of age. These age-related changes are common but not inevitable, and there is considerable variation between individuals. Atrophy is observed in most cortical and subcortical structures.

For reasons not yet understood, the hippocampus appears to be particularly sensitive to the effects of ageing, and atrophies at a faster rate than other structures (Scahill *et al.*, 2003). MTA in normal ageing could clinically be linked to mild cognitive impairment (MCI), as discussed in more detail later, and pathologically to AD-type pathology. Preliminary reports have found that increased levels of homocysteine are associated with hippocampal volume loss in non-demented subjects (den Heijer *et al.*, 2003).

Changes in white matter also occur. Indeed, WML are common in late life with a prevalence of between 8 and 92 per cent depending on the study. Across a life span it seems that white matter is in a constant state of change, with processes of maturation continuing into middle age, followed by progressive loss of myelin integrity (Bartzokis *et al.*, 2003).

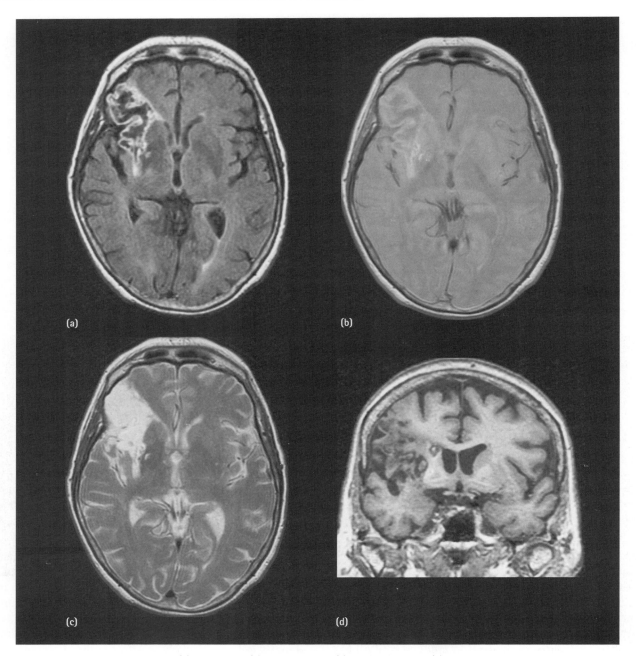

Figure 8.3   *Example of frontal stroke on (a) axial FLAIR, (b) proton density, (c) T2-weighted and (d) Coronal T1-weighted.*

8.7 ALZHEIMER'S DISEASE

Earlier MRI studies in AD compared atrophy between patients with established AD and age-matched non-demented controls. Although these studies continue, MRI now has a broader and arguably a more searching role. It is used to see whether subjects with presymptomatic AD, MCI or very early AD can be accurately detected, and in the differentiation of dementias. MRI can also detect biomarkers to track disease progression and predict response to treatment.

8.7.1 Early and established Alzheimer's disease

MTA is the most consistent and recognized structural difference in AD compared with age-matched controls, as illustrated in Figures 8.4 and 8.5. Patients with AD have significantly smaller (by up to 40–50 per cent) amygdalae, hippocampi and parahippocampi, which includes the entorhinal cortex. Lesser degrees of atrophy have also been observed in other temporal structures, including the fusiform gyrus and

Table 8.1   *Histopathology associated with white matter lesions in dementias*

Pathology	Possible mechanisms
PVH	
Less extensive PVH: loss of ependymal lining, increased interstitial fluid and gliosis, myelin pallor	In part secondary to atrophy processes
More extensive irregular PVH which extend into the deep white matter: likely to correspond to areas of reactive gliosis, lacunar infarction, loss of myelin, perivascular spaces and arteriolar thickening	Frontal caps extremely common in late life – could be considered 'normal' and secondary to age-related changes More extensive PVH probably linked to vascular risk factors
DWMH	
Punctuate WMH: reduced myelination and perivenous damage	Punctate lesions are probably not associated with ischaemia/infarction
Early confluent areas: show evidence of perivascular rarefaction of myelin, fibre loss and gliosis	Ischaemic damage implicated as lesions become larger and more confluent
Confluent WMH: have a similar histopathology as irregular PVH, including microcystic infarcts	Other possible causes of white matter change include focal cerebral oedema, hypoxia, acidosis, chronic perfusion changes, wallerian degeneration of axons secondary to neuronal loss in neocortex

DWMH, deep white matter hyperintensities; PVH, periventricular hyperintensities

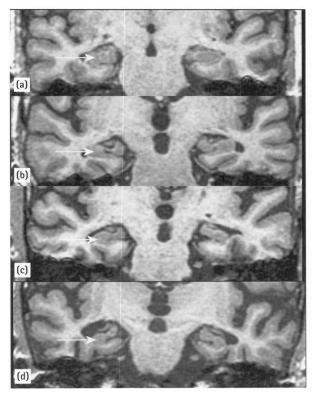

Figure 8.4 (a–d)   *Examples of graded medial temporal atrophy (MTA): arrows point to hippocampi.*

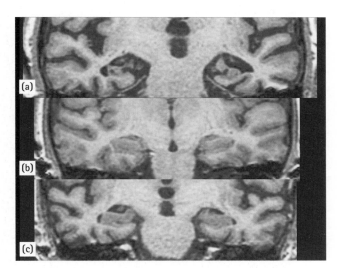

Figure 8.5   *Comparison of medial temporal atrophy in (a) AD, (b) DLB and (c) normal controls.*

lateral temporal gyri. Indeed, as AD progresses, nearly all limbic structures atrophy. Overall, the distribution of atrophy is symmetrical and more prominent in medial and posterior brain structures than anterior structures. By comparison, there is less atrophy in the frontal lobe, hypothalamus, thalamus, caudate and putamen, and relative sparing of the primary

motor and sensory cortex, inferior occipitotemporal region and cerebellum (Baron *et al.*, 2001). Generalized brain atrophy and ventricular enlargement is common but relatively nonspecific.

The pattern of *in vivo* atrophy is consistent with the topographical model of disease progression for AD postulated by Braak and Braak (1991). In this model AD pathology, particularly neurofibrillary tangles, are initially localized to the medial temporal lobe (entorhinal cortex then hippocampus), then extend to other temporal lobe structures, and ultimately beyond to multiple neocortical association areas, finally involving the primary neocortex.

MTA, notably atrophy of the hippocampus and entorhinal cortex, provides the greatest discrimination between AD and normal subjects with a sensitivity and specificity of 85–90 per cent. Results appear equally good when only very mild subjects are considered (Mini-Mental State Examination [MMSE] >21). This is perhaps not surprising given the extensive loss of neurones in this area of the brain. When measures of MTA are further combined with measures of atrophy involving other brain regions, differentiation is even greater.

Patients with AD are losing brain volume at a faster rate than normal controls. The highest levels of accelerated atrophy are again seen within those structures intimately associated with the disease, particularly the hippocampus (3.98 v 1.55 per cent in controls) and entorhinal cortex (6.5 per cent v 1.4 per cent) (Jack et al., 1998; Du et al., 2003). Increased rates of global atrophy also occur.

MTA is also a biologically relevant measurement, as hippocampal volume loss correlates with symptoms of cognitive impairment, particular memory loss, as well as functional decline and AD-type pathology. However, although MTA provides good discrimination between patients with AD and controls and is a relatively sensitive marker of AD pathology, it is not specific to AD. To lesser degrees MTA is seen in other dementias (as discussed below), Parkinson disease, temporal lobe epilepsy, schizophrenia, depression and certain medical conditions, such as type 2 diabetes (den Heijer et al., 2003).

Studies examining the relationship between measures of regional or global atrophy and variables such as ApoE ε4 allele status, oestrogen replacement and vascular risk factors, have not yielded consistent results. From a limited evidence base, the specificity of MTA as a biomarker for AD appears to decline with age.

In terms of WML, AD tends to have more extensive PVH (prevalence 44–100 per cent) than controls, but findings in relation to DWMH (prevalence 60–100 per cent) are less consistent. Recent evidence indicates a loss of integrity of white matter tracts that is not randomly distributed (Rose et al., 2000). It appears to selectively affect tracts linked to the association cortices (with relative sparing of other tracts), leading to a hypothesis that white matter changes are a downstream consequence to cortical pathology (Bozzali et al., 2002).

In summary, MTA occurs early in the course of AD, and the extent of the atrophy increases with increasing severity of dementia to involve other structures in a way that mirrors the Braak and Braak staging of AD. Indeed, although MTA appears to be necessary for the development of AD, without more extensive atrophy it may be insufficient to cause widespread cognitive impairment (Kaye et al., 1997). Thus, as Jack et al. (2002) speculate, MTA is a good marker for early AD, but. as the disease progresses beyond the limbic areas, measures of neocortical atrophy may be better markers of advanced disease. Overall, the diagnostic accuracy of MR volumetry of the hippocampus for distinguishing patients with AD from healthy elderly individuals is comparable to the accuracy of a pathologically confirmed clinical diagnosis (Kantarci and Jack, 2003).

8.7.2 Prognostic significance of medial temporal atrophy in individuals at risk of Alzheimer's disease

The pathogenesis of AD is thought to occur years or possibly even decades before clinical symptoms emerge. Given the expected topographical evolution of pathology, most presymptomatic studies have focused on measuring either the hippocampus or entorhinal cortex. Indeed, there is good evidence that atrophy of these structures occurs early in the natural history of the illness, and often before symptoms emerge (Killiany et al., 2002; Scahill et al., 2002). By the time mild symptoms are apparent hippocampal volume reductions exceeding 25 per cent have been reported (Fox and Rossor, 1999).

The prognostic relevance of MTA in predicting cognitive decline and eventual dementia in individuals at risk of AD has been studied in two main groups: subjects with a familial, dominantly inherited form of AD and subjects with MCI.

8.7.2.1 PRESYMPTOMATIC DETECTION OF INDIVIDUALS WITH FAMILIAL AD

Serial MRI studies of families with autosomal dominant forms of AD have shown that atrophy of the hippocampus and entorhinal cortex develops in parallel with the appearance of symptoms and progresses more rapidly in subjects who develop dementia (Fox et al., 1996a, b). Interestingly, by extrapolating back in time, Schott et al. (2003) estimated pathological atrophy started at least 3.5 years (95 per cent CI, 0.7–7.5) before symptoms emerged. This raises the exciting and realistic prospect that there are changes that could be detected in due course and enable subjects 'at risk' to be detected. Indeed, this transitional phase from pathology to emerging symptoms may be associated with the most aggressive phase of MTA, raising the exciting prospect that subjects 'at risk' of AD can be detected using serial MRI.

8.7.2.2 SUBJECTS WITH AGE–RELATED MINIMAL COGNITIVE IMPAIRMENT

Subjects with MCI are at increased risk of developing dementia (see Chapter 24). Detection of MCI is therefore important, and the role of neuroimaging in MCI has been extensively reviewed (Kantarci and Jack, 2003; Wolf et al., 2003).

As with presymptomatic studies, significant hippocampal (7–15 per cent) and entorhinal cortex volume (5–32 per cent) reductions are the most consistently described difference between subjects with MCI and cognitively unimpaired controls. Subjects who are moving along the trajectory from normal to MCI are losing more of their hippocampus than those who remain stable. Overall, the results from visual rating of atrophy and cross-sectional and longitudinal volumetric studies have found the changes in MCI are intermediate between normal subjects and AD. The intermediate nature of these results is reflected in the relatively lower sensitivity (60 per cent) and specificity (80 per cent) of measures of MTA in discriminating MCI and controls compared with their discrimination of AD (Xu *et al.*, 2000).

Currently, opinion is divided as to whether atrophy of the hippocampus or entorhinal cortex best predict conversion from MCI to AD. However, even though atrophy in both structures in MCI is a well-established risk factor for the development of AD, these measures cannot be regarded as being of high predictive value in an individual case (Wolf *et al.*, 2003).

8.8 DEMENTIA WITH LEWY BODIES

Standard ROI and VBM studies consistently find that dementia with Lewy bodies (DLB) and AD have a different pattern of temporal lobe atrophy. The most striking differences relate to medial rather than lateral temporal lobe structures. As shown in Figure 8.5, subjects with DLB have greater preservation of hippocampal, amygdala, and parahippocampal volumes (Barber *et al.*, 2000, 2001). Post-mortem studies back up these findings, and these differences may help explain differences in the profile of cognitive deficits between these disorders. Annual rates of global atrophy in DLB are similar to those in AD and VaD, but greater than normal controls (O'Brien *et al.*, 2001).

Although DLB is associated with visual hallucinations and occipital changes in blood flow and metabolism on single photon emission computed tomography (SPECT), there are no gross structural changes in the occipital lobe on MRI (Middelkoop *et al.*, 2001). Preliminary findings suggest a possible association between DLB and atrophy of the putamen,

but not the caudate nucleus, though there is no link between volumetry and symptoms (Barber *et al.*, 2002; Cousins *et al.*, 2003). Subjects with DLB shares a similar distribution, prevalence and severity of WML to AD on MRI, intermediate in severity between those with VaD and normal controls (Barber *et al.*, 1999).

8.9 FRONTOTEMPORAL DEMENTIA

Frontotemporal dementia (FTD) is characterized by a specific pattern of moderate to severe atrophy of the frontal and temporal lobes. Compared to AD and VaD, atrophy is more severe and has a high specificity for distinguishing FTD from other dementias. The atrophy is also more asymmetrical, and is particularly prominent in the left temporal lobes.

Hippocampal atrophy also occurs but tends to be less severe than in AD, although atrophy of the entorhinal cortex can be equally severe (Frisoni *et al.*, 1999; Boccardi *et al.*, 2003). FTD has increased rates of whole-brain atrophy compared with controls (3.2 per cent v 0.5 per cent per year) but overlaps with AD (2.4 per cent) (Chan *et al.*, 2001a).

The temporal lobe variants of this syndrome include progressive non-fluent aphasia (PNFA) and semantic dementia (SD). PNFA is characterized by asymmetrical, left-sided perisylvian atrophy. Atrophy in semantic dementia tends to be more bilateral, though can be asymmetrical, as shown in Figure 8.6. There is an anteroposterior gradient in the distribution of temporal lobe atrophy (Chan *et al.*, 2001b).

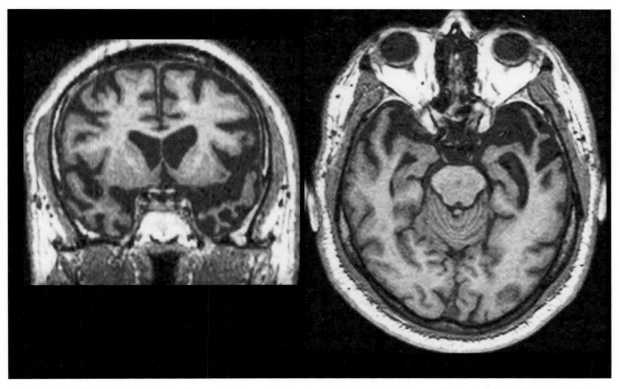

Figure 8.6 *Patient with clinical diagnosis of semantic dementia showing bilateral anterior temporal lobe atrophy, Left > right side: coronal and axial T1-weighted images (courtesy of Dr T Griffiths).*

Table 8.2 *Structural imaging requirements for current diagnostic systems for dementia*

Diagnosis	DSM-V	ICD-10	Specific diagnostic criteria	Comments
AD	Generalised brain atrophy and enlarged ventricles > normal ageing process	Not specified	NINCDS-ADRDA criteria (McKhann et al., 1984): ↑ ventricles, sulci are narrowed; general patterns may not be useful as diagnostic criteria in individual cases	All the major diagnostic criteria for AD focus on neuroimaging *excluding* competing causes of cognitive impairment and lack reference to possible neuroimaging *inclusion* criteria for AD, such as medial temporal lobe atrophy
DLB	Not specified	Not specified	Consensus criteria for DLB (McKeith et al., 1996): recognized lack of definitive evidence about specific abnormalities on imaging (at time of publication); CT or MRI might show generalized cortical atrophy	Growing evidence to suggest neuroimaging criteria should include the relative preservation of medial temporal lobe structures in subjects with DLB compared with those with AD
FTD	Prominent frontal and/or temporal atrophy on structural brain imaging, and localized frontotemporal hypometabolism on functional brain imaging, even in the absence of clear structural atrophy	Not specified	Consensus clinical criteria for fronto-temporal dementia (Neary et al., 1998): abnormalities (structural and/or functional imaging) may be bilaterally symmetrical or asymmetric, affecting the left or right hemisphere disproportionately, although failure to demonstrate these prototypic appearances need not exclude diagnosis	In addition, two neuroimaging exclusion features are described: the presence of multifocal lesions and predominant postcentral structural or functional deficits
VaD	Criteria require 'laboratory evidence of cerebrovascular disease', which may include laboratory evidence such as imaging. Structural imaging 'usually' demonstrates multiple vascular lesions	Not mandatory for the diagnosis, though in some cases it will be needed.	California criteria for ischaemic VaD (IVD) (Chui et al., 1992): 'Probable' IVD – requires at least one infarct outside the cerebellum. 'Possible' IVD – does not require neuroimaging evidence of infarction. The NINDS-AIREN criteria (Román et al., 1993): Need to define the extent, topography and severity of vascular lesions. 'Probable VaD' – multiple infarcts or strategic single infarcts or multiple subcortical or white matter lesions (at least 25% of total white matter)	The NINDS-AIREN criteria have the most rigorous neuroimaging criteria. Specifically state that the absence of cerebrovascular lesions on brain CT or MRI makes the diagnosis of vascular dementia unlikely. **NINDS-AIREN v California criteria:** NINDS-AIREN criteria recognize that a single lesion may cause VaD; radiological lesions regardless of location may be taken as evidence of cerebrovascular disease (excluding 'trivial' infarcts); require vascular change to fulfil criteria for both location and severity

AD, Alzheimer's disease; DLB, dementia with Lewy bodies; DSM: *Diagnostic and Statistical Manual* (American Psychiatric Association, 1994); FTD, frontotemporal dementia; ICD: International Classification of Diseases (World Health Organization, 1992); VaD, vascular dementia.

Provisional findings indicate WML in FTD are common, but as in AD and DLB are less severe than in vascular dementia (VaD) (Varma *et al.*, 2002).

8.10 VASCULAR DEMENTIA

VaD is associated with a wide variety of brain lesions including cortical infarcts, infarcts in strategic brain areas (basal ganglia and thalamus), multiple lacunes, extensive white matter change or combinations thereof. There may be evidence of focal atrophy, either cortical or ventricular, corresponding to focal infarction and subsequent local atrophy. In addition, VaD like AD is associated with relatively nonspecific changes such as generalized cerebral atrophy and ventricular dilatation. Hippocampal atrophy can occur but is less severe than in AD.

On MRI, VaD is associated with evidence of infarction and an increased severity of PVH (prevalence 70–100 per cent) and DWMH (prevalence up to 100 per cent) compared with AD, DLB and age-matched normal controls. Large irregular PVH, confluent DWMH and basal ganglia hyperintensities are characteristic of VaD, representing a greater burden of ischaemia.

Several neuroimaging studies have investigated the relationship between dementia and vascular change. The total number and location of infarcts appears to be important, especially left-sided or bilateral lesions and those located in strategic areas such as thalamus and anterior capsule. However, in addition to a 'lesion-based' view of VaD, generalized changes, such as cortical and central atrophy, as well as variables, such as age and level of education, may play an important role in the development of post-stroke dementia.

Table 8.2 summarizes the different neuroimaging criteria for main diagnostic classifications of dementias. Table 8.3 summarizes MRI findings in other conditions.

8.11 FINAL COMMENTS

From a clinical perspective, a key question remains: 'When should a MRI scan be requested?'. There is, however, no consensus about the threshold or indications for scanning. Instead, there is a spectrum of opinions from the selective to the wholly inclusive, as exemplified in Box 8.5 (see page 92).

Nevertheless, there is a general shift towards the view that all patients with dementia should be scanned at least once during their illness. This position recognizes that there can never be a comprehensive list of all indications for any investigation and, if scanning is combined with accurate clinical information, it offers the highest standard of diagnostic accuracy currently available. Perhaps an alternative question would be: 'If I need to make a diagnosis using a certain set of diagnostic criteria, what sort of imaging do I need to perform?'. A CT will, for cost and practical reasons, usually be the imaging modality of first choice, although an MRI, if accessible, would almost always be the superior imaging modality.

In clinical practice, imaging is not an end in itself but an investigation that contributes information about the biology of the brain, which needs to be interpreted as part of the overall clinical assessment. As with any test or investigation, imaging in dementia is neither perfectly sensitive nor specific, and false negative and positive results will occur. Inevitably, the clinician will need to interpret both the nature and significance of any radiological finding in weighing up its potential contribution to the clinical picture. This is a point of convergence between the art of clinical medicine and science that makes that practice more revealing.

Looking ahead, a more sophisticated blending of MR sequences and measurements could enhance the overall usefulness of MR technology. Indeed, the specific mix of MR tests for optimal diagnostic accuracy could well differ as diseases progress.

Table 8.3 *MRI findings in other disease associated with cognitive impairment*

Disorder	MRI findings
Variant Creutzfeldt-Jakob disease (nvCJD)	Symmetrical hyperintensity in the pulvinar (posterior) nuclei of the thalamus (pulvinar sign). Other features are hyperintensity of the dorsomedial thalamic nuclei, caudate head and periaqueductal grey matter (Collie *et al.*, 2003). FLAIR more sensitive than other sequences
Sporadic Creutzfeldt–Jakob disease	High signal changes in the putamen and caudate head
Huntington chorea (HC)	Bilateral caudate atrophy – may also have reduce volume of other basal ganglia structures and frontal lobes
Progressive supranuclear palsy (PSP)	Non-specific mild atrophy
Multisystem atrophy (MSA)	Olivopontocerebellar atrophy, pontocerebellar and putamenal hyperintensities on T2-weighted images
Normal pressure hydrocephalus (NPH)	Marked ventricular enlargement, with rounding of anterior horns of lateral ventricles. The enlargement is disproportionate to any sulcal widening (i.e. cortical atrophy not usually present), and there is no significant focal pathology or white matter change.)

Box 8.5 *Examples of guidelines for imaging in dementia*

Selective criteria: example from guidelines

Canadian Consensus Conference on Dementia (Patterson *et al.*, 2001) Recommendations for neuroimaging. Cranial CT scan is recommended if one or more of the following criteria are present:

A   Age less than 60 years

B   Rapid, (e.g. over 1–2 months) unexplained decline in cognition or function

C   Short duration of dementia (<2 years)

D   Recent and significant head trauma

E   Unexplained neurological symptoms, e.g. new onset of severe headache or seizures

F   History of cancer (especially in sites and types that metastasize to the brain)

G   Use of anticoagulants or history of a bleeding disorder

H   History of urinary incontinence and gait disorder early in the course of dementia (as may be found in normopressure hydrocephalus)

I   Any new localizing sign (e.g. hemiparesis or Babinski's reflex)

J   Unusual or atypical cognitive symptoms or presentation (e.g. progressive aphasia, gait disturbance)

All-inclusive criteria: examples of statements from opinion leaders and guidelines

- In elderly demented patients routine neuroimaging with CT or MR is the ideal that should be sought (Rossor, 1994) Practice parameters: diagnosis of dementia (evidence-based guidelines) from the American Academy of Neurology. Recommend:

- Structural neuroimaging with either a non-contrast CT or MR scan in the routine initial evaluation of patients with dementia is appropriate (Knopman *et al.*, 2001)

- Neuroimaging, and MRI in particular, is increasingly regarded as an essential part of the investigation of a patient with dementia (Scheltens *et al.*, 2002)

REFERENCES

American Psychiatric Association. (1994) *Diagnostic and Statistical Manual of Mental Disorders.* Washington, DC, American Psychiatric Association

Ashburner J and Friston KJ. (2000) Voxel-based morphometry – the methods. *Neuroimage* 11: 805–821

Barber R, Scheltens P, Gholkar A *et al.* (1999) White matter lesions on magnetic resonance imaging in dementia with Lewy bodies, Alzheimer's disease, vascular dementia, and normal aging. *Journal of Neurology, Neurosurgery, and Psychiatry* 67: 66–72

Barber R, Ballard C, McKeith IG *et al.* (2000) MRI volumetric study of dementia with Lewy bodies: A comparison with Alzheimer's disease and vascular dementia. *Neurology* 54: 1304–1309

Barber R, McKeith IG, Ballard C *et al.* (2001) A comparison of medial and lateral temporal lobe atrophy in dementia with Lewy bodies and Alzheimer's Disease: MRI volumetric study. *Dementia and Geriatric Cognitive Disorders* 12: 198–205

Barber R, McKeith IG, Ballard C, O'Brien JT. (2002) Volumetric MRI study of the caudate nucleus in patients with dementia with Lewy bodies, Alzheimer's disease and Vascular dementia. *Journal of Neurology Neurosurgery, and Psychiatry* 72: 406–407

Baron JC, Chetelat G, Desgranges B *et al.* (2001) In vivo mapping of gray matter loss with voxel-based morphometry in mild Alzheimer's disease. *Neuroimage* 14: 298–309

Bartzokis G, Cummings JL, Sultzer D *et al.* (2003) White matter structural integrity in healthy aging adults and patients with Alzheimer disease: a magnetic resonance imaging study. *Archives of Neurology* 60: 393–398

Boccardi M, Laakso MP, Bresciani L *et al.* (2003) The MRI pattern of frontal and temporal brain atrophy in fronto-temporal dementia. *Neurobiological Aging* 24: 95–103

Bozzali M, Falini A, Franceschi M *et al.* (2002) White matter damage in Alzheimer's disease assessed in vivo using diffusion tensor magnetic resonance imaging. *Journal of Neurology, Neurosurgery, and Psychiatry* 72: 742–746

Braak H and Braak E. (1991) Neuropathological staging of Alzheimer related changes. *Acta Neuropathologica* 82: 239–259

Chan D, Fox NC, Jenkins R *et al.* (2001a) Rates of global and regional cerebral atrophy in AD and frontotemporal dementia. *Neurology* 57: 1756–1763

Chan D, Fox NC, Scahill RI *et al.* (2001b) Patterns of temporal lobe atrophy in semantic dementia and Alzheimer's disease. *Annals of Neurology* 49: 433–442

Chui HC, Victoroff JI, Margolin D *et al.* (1992) Criteria for the diagnosis of ischaemic vascular dementia proposed by the State of California Alzheimer's Disease Diagnostic and Treatment Centres. *Neurology* 42: 473–480

Collie DA, Summers DM, Sellar RJ *et al.* (2003) Diagnosing variant Creutzfeld–Jakob disease with the pulvinar sign: MR imaging findings in 86 neuropathologically confirmed cases. *American Journal of Neuroradiology* 24: 1560–1569

Cousins DA, Burton EJ, Burn D *et al.* (2003). Atrophy of the putamen in dementia with Lewy bodies but not Alzheimer's disease: an MRI study. *Neurology* 61: 1191–1195

den Heijer T, Vermeer SE, van Dijk EJ *et al.* (2003) Type 2 diabetes and atrophy of medial temporal lobe structures on brain MRI. *Diabetologia* 46: 1604–1610

Du AT, Schuff N, Zhu XP *et al.* (2003) Atrophy rates of entorhinal cortex in AD and normal aging. *Neurology* 60: 481–486

Fazekas F, Chawluk JB, Alavi A *et al.* (1987) MR signal abnormalities at 1.5T in Alzheimer's disease and normal ageing. *American Journal of Roentgenology* 149: 351–356

Fox NC and Rossor MN. (1999) Diagnosis of early Alzheimer's disease. *Review of Neurology* 155 (Suppl. 4): S33–S37

Fox NC, Warrington EK, Freeborough PA *et al.* (1996a) Presymptomatic hippocampal atrophy in Alzheimer's disease. A longitudinal MRI study. *Brain* 119: 2001–2007

Fox NC, Warrington EK, Stevens JM *et al.* (1996b) Atrophy of the hippocampal formation in early Alzheimer's disease. A longitudinal MRI study of at-risk members of a family with an amyloid precursor protein 717$_{VAL-GLY}$ mutation. *Annals of the New York Academy of Sciences* **777**: 226–232

Frisoni GB. (2001) Structural imaging in the clinical diagnosis of Alzheimer's disease: problems and tools. *Journal of Neurology, Neurosurgery, and Psychiatry* **70**: 711–718. Erratum in: *Journal of Neurology, Neurosurgery, and Psychiatry* (2001) **71**: 418

Frisoni G, Laakso MP, Beltramello A *et al.* (1999) Hippocampal and entorhinal cortex atrophy in frontotemporal dementia and Alzheimer's disease. *Neurology* **52**: 91–100

Frisoni GB, Scheltens P, Galluzzi S *et al.* (2003) Neuroimaging tools to rate regional atrophy, subcortical cerebrovascular disease, and regional cerebral blood flow and metabolism: consensus paper of the EADC. *Journal of Neurology, Neurosurgery, and Psychiatry* **74**: 1371–1381

Jack CR Jr, Peterson RC, Xu YC *et al.* (1998) Rate of medial temporal lobe atrophy in typical aging and Alzheimer's disease. *Neurology* **51**: 993–999

Jack CR Jr, Dickson DW, Parisi JE *et al.* (2002) Antemortem MRI findings correlate with hippocampal neuropathology in typical aging and dementia. *Neurology* **58**: 750–757

Jack CR Jr, Slomkowski M, Gracon S *et al.* (2003) MRI as a biomarker of disease progression in a therapeutic trial of milameline for AD. *Neurology* **60**: 253–260

Kantarci K, Jack CR Jr. (2003) Neuroimaging in Alzheimer disease: an evidence-based review. *Neuroimaging Clinics of North America* **13**: 197–209

Kaye JA, Swihart T, Hovieson D *et al.* (1997) Volume loss of hippocampus and temporal lobe in healthy elderly persons destined to develop dementia. *Neurology* **48**: 1297–1304.

Killiany RJ, Hyman BT, Gomez-Isla T. (2002) MRI measures of entorhinal cortex vs hippocampus in preclinical AD. *Neurology* **58**: 1188–1196

Knopman DS, DeKosky ST, Cummings JL *et al.* (2001) Practice parameters: diagnosis of dementia (an evidence-based review). Report of the Quality Standards Subcommittee of the American Academy of Neurology. *Neurology* **56**: 1143–1153

Krishnan KR, Charles HC, Doraiswamy PM *et al.* (2003) Randomized, placebo-controlled trial of the effects of donepezil on neuronal markers and hippocampal volumes in Alzheimer's disease. *American Journal of Psychiatry* **160**: 2003–2011

McKeith IG, Galasko D, Kosaka K *et al.* (1996) Consensus guidelines for the clinical and pathological diagnosis of dementia with Lewy bodies (DLB): report of the Consortium on Dementia with Lewy Bodies International Workshop. *Neurology* **47**: 1113–1124

McKhann G, Drachman D, Folstein M *et al.* (1984) Clinical diagnosis of Alzheimer's disease: report of the NINCDS-ADRDA Work Group under the auspices of Department of Health and Human Service Task Force on Alzheimer's disease. *Neurology* **34**: 939–944

Middelkoop HA, van der Flier WM, Burton EJ *et al.* (2001) Dementia with Lewy bodies and AD are not associated with occipital lobe atrophy on MRI. *Neurology* **57**: 2117–2120

Neary D, Snowden JS, Gustafson L *et al.* (1998) Frontotemporal lobar degeneration: a consensus on clinical diagnostic criteria. *Neurology* **51**: 1546–1554

O'Brien JT, Paling S, Barber R *et al.* (2001) Progressive brain atrophy on serial MRI in dementia with Lewy bodies, AD, and vascular dementia. *Neurology* **56**: 1386–1388

Patterson C, Gauthier S, Bergman H *et al.* (2001) The recognition, assessment and management of dementing disorders: conclusions from the Canadian Consensus Conference on Dementia. *Canadian Journal of Neurological Sciences* **28** (Suppl. 1): S3–16

Román GC, Tatemichi T, Erkinjuntti T *et al.* (1993) Vascular dementia: diagnostic criteria for research studies. Report of the NINDS-AIRENS international workshop. *Neurology* **43**: 250–260

Rose SE, Chen F, Chalk JB *et al.* (2000) Loss of connectivity in Alzheimer's disease: an evaluation of white matter tract integrity with colour coded MR diffusion tensor imaging. *Journal of Neurology, Neurosurgery, and Psychiatry* **69**: 528–530

Rossor MN. (1994) Management of neurological disorders: dementia. *Journal of Neurology, Neurosurgery, and Psychiatry* **57**: 1451–1456

Scahill RI, Schott JM, Stevens JM *et al.* (2002) Mapping the evolution of regional atrophy in Alzheimer's disease: unbiased analysis of fluid-registered serial MRI. *Proceedings of the National Academy of Sciences of the United States of America.* **99**: 4703–4707

Scahill RI, Frost C, Jenkins R *et al.* (2003) A longitudinal study of brain volume changes in normal aging using serial registered magnetic resonance imaging. *Archives of Neurology* **60**: 989–994

Scheltens P, Leys D, Barkhof F *et al.* (1992) Atrophy of medial temporal lobes on MRI in 'probable' Alzheimer's disease and normal ageing: diagnostic value and neuropsychological correlates. *Journal of Neurology, Neurosurgery, and Psychiatry* **55**: 967–972

Scheltens P, Fox N, Barkhof F, De Carli C, (2002) Structural magnetic resonance imaging in the practical assessment of dementia: beyond exclusion. *Lancet Neurology* **1**: 13–21

Schott JM, Fox NC, Frost C *et al.* (2003) Assessing the onset of structural change in familial Alzheimer's disease. *Annals of Neurology* 2003 **53**: 181–188

Varma AR, Laitt R, Lloyd JJ *et al.* (2002) Diagnostic value of high signal abnormalities on T2 weighted MRI in the differentiation of Alzheimer's, frontotemporal and vascular dementias. *Acta Neurologica Scandinavica* **105**: 355–364

Wolf H, Jelic V, Gertz HJ *et al.* (2003) A critical discussion of the role of neuroimaging in mild cognitive impairment. *Acta Neurologica Scandinavica* **109** (Suppl.): 52–76. Erratum in: *Acta Neurologica Scandinavica* (Suppl.): 2003 **108**: 68

World Health Organization. (1992). *International Classification of Disease and Health Related Problems.* Geneva, WHO

Xu Y, Jack CR Jr, O'Brien PC *et al.* (2000) Usefulness of MRI measures of entorhinal cortex versus hippocampus in AD. *Neurology* **56**: 820–821

9

Functional imaging

KLAUS P EBMEIER, JANE K SUTHERLAND AND NADINE J DOUGALL

Functional brain imaging offers a window into the living brain, an organ that is, of course, not usually accessible to direct scrutiny and investigation. Observing functional activity also anticipates any irreversible structural changes and therefore implies treatability of the abnormalities detected. Both aspects make functional imaging of dementing illnesses a fascinating topic.

Radionuclide-based imaging modes, such as single photon emission computed tomography (SPECT) and positron emission tomography (PET) have been available for several decades now, but their impact on daily diagnostic practice has been minimal. The reasons for this will require exploring. Much emphasis will be placed in this chapter on clinical usefulness of imaging, but other aspects of functional neuroimaging, such as the brain–behaviour correlations observed during illness will be equally explored. These themes will be introduced by a short description of the imaging techniques used in dementia research.

9.1 IMAGING METHODS

9.1.1 Single photon emission computed tomography (SPECT)

SPECT uses gamma emitting radioisotopes, which are attached to biologically relevant molecules and injected intravenously to be distributed amongst others to the brain. The three-dimensional reconstruction of the tracer distribution in the brain gives a biologically meaningful map of, for example, blood flow, receptor binding capacity or similar measures. In order to focus the signal on the gamma camera, collimators are used. These collimators only admit photons coming from a defined direction to the photosensitive crystal (Figure 9.1). By implication, this method of directional filtering only allows for a small proportion of emitted photons to be detected, which limits the sensitivity of SPECT. In addition, scattered photons lose a certain amount of energy, and are therefore excluded with energy filters. The attenuation of gamma rays during their path through brain matter is usually modelled making assumptions of homogeneous attenuation across the brain and head. Some common applications of SPECT are listed in Table 9.1. Gamma emitters with half-lives of 6–12 hours are usually employed, as the tracers tend to be produced some distance from the scanner. Because of this, limited numbers of exposures are possible. The gamma-emitting nuclei employed (^{123}I and ^{99m}Tc) are relatively large and tend to change the pharmacology of the substituted molecule. The extensive pharmacological development work necessary for such tracers may therefore be one of the explanations for the relatively limited number of gamma (SPECT)-ligands available today.

9.1.2 Positron emission tomography (PET)

Positron emission tomography (PET), as the name implies, uses positron emitters to label physiological brain processes. Positrons (positively charged electrons) are not stable elementary particles; within millimetres of travel they react with an electron to generate two photons with a defined energy moving at approximately 180° away from each other. The detection of such coincidence signals with a detector ring thus makes it

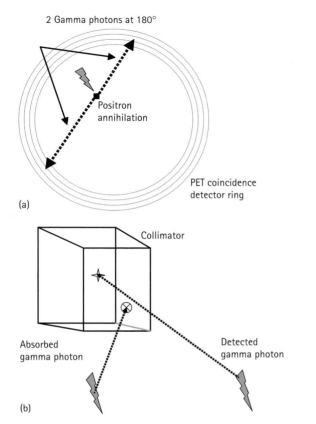

2 Gamma photons at 180°

Positron
annihilation

PET coincidence
detector ring

(a)

Collimator

Absorbed
gamma photon

Detected
gamma photon

(b)

Figure 9.1 (a, b) *Localization of photon source with PET and SPECT.*

Table 9.1 *Some common applications of SPECT and PET*

Tracer	Isotope–mode	Physiology	Clinical use
HMPAO	^{99m}T- SPECT	Perfusion	Yes
EDT	^{99m}Tc-SPECT	Perfusion	Yes
FP-CIT	^{123}I-SPECT	Dopamine transporter	Yes
Iomazenil	^{123}I-SPECT	Benzodiazepine receptor	No
Iodobenzamide	^{123}I-SPECT	Dopamine D2 receptor	No
Iodo-QNB	^{123}I-SPECT	Muscarinic receptor	No
5-I-A-85380	^{123}I-SPECT	Nicotinic receptor	No
MK-801	^{123}I-SPECT	NMDA receptor	No
Water	^{15}O-PET	Blood flow	Yes
Oxygen	^{15}O-PET	Oxygen uptake	No
FDG	^{18}F-PET	Glucose uptake (aerobic + anaerobic)	Yes
Glucose	^{11}C-PET	Glucose uptake (aerobic)	No
Nicotine	^{11}C-PET	Nicotinic receptor	No
MP4A	^{11}C-PET	AChE activity	No
6-OH-BTA-1	^{11}C-PET	Distribution of Aβ plaques	No
FDDNP	^{18}F-PET	NFTs and Aβ plaques	No
Altanserin	^{18}F-PET	5HT-2A receptor	No
WAY-100635	^{18}F-PET	5HT-1A receptor	No

possible to identify spatial as well as intensity information (Figure 9.1). Collimators are thus not necessary and signal detection is more sensitive. Positron-emitting nuclei, particularly ^{11}C, are easily incorporated into biological molecules, without changing their chemical characteristics. Positron emission is relatively energetic – only short exposure to radiation is possible, the short decay half-lives require on-site radiochemistry to incorporate the nuclei into physiologically active compounds. In turn, short half-lives allow for repeated application of tracers. Usually transmission scans with a gamma source in the detector rings are used to quantify the attenuation across the brain. Table 9.1 lists a number of commonly used PET-ligands.

9.1.3 Functional magnetic resonance imaging (fMRI)

Functional magnetic resonance imaging (fMRI) uses physical principles completely different from emission tomographies, both for the constitution and the spatial encoding of images (see Chapter 8). The most frequently used, and here the only described principle, is blood oxygen level dependent (BOLD) imaging. Haemoglobin and deoxyhaemoglobin behave differentially within the MRI magnetic field, so that a signal difference of a few per cent can be observed between brain areas

that are active and those that are not. Paradoxically, the concentration of deoxyhaemoglobin *decreases* in active brain areas, as blood flow *increases* disproportionately to oxygen extraction. The advantage of fMRI over nuclear medicine imaging is that repeated examinations are possible, and within each subject high signal-to-noise ratios can be achieved by repeating scans many times. To identify brain areas associated with a particular function, tasks are compared, which differ only with respect to the function of interest. Alternatively, the variability of behaviour over time can be correlated with the MRI signal of the parallel time series of scans, taking account of the delay equivalent to the 'haemodynamic response function'. Brain lesions are likely sources of error for fMRI, others are head movement and susceptibility artefacts owing to air and boundary effects. For obvious reasons, such artefacts are more likely to occur in older age and in psychiatric patients. The methods of fMRI have only recently been developed, are by no means standardized and have mainly been used in the research context. The clinical use of fMRI in dementia remains to be established.

9.2 ARE THERE DIAGNOSTIC PATTERNS?

As the macroscopic anatomy and natural history of brain changes in the dementias are variable, it is not surprising that there are no generally applicable 'rules' for diagnostic imaging patterns. Alzheimer-like pathology can be found in a substantial proportion of the brains of non-demented patient (Ince, 2001). In addition, the diagnoses of Alzheimer's disease (AD) and vascular dementia (VaD) are not mutually exclusive so that mixed patterns are likely to occur in a significant proportion of patients. Finally, at an advanced stage all dementias tend to involve large portions of the brain, preferentially (and in all likelihood) association cortex, so any differential features will disappear.

AD is said to initially present with posterior cingulate (Minoshima *et al.*, 1997a) or medial temporal (Callen *et al.*, 2002) reductions in brain activity, but soon after bilateral posterior temporoparietal reductions in brain activity intervene (Holman *et al.*, 1992; see Plate 1). During later stages, prefrontal activity reductions are added, so that some authors have suggested computing a ratio of association cortex over primary sensory-motor cortex as a diagnostic index for AD (Herholz *et al.*, 1999). Frontotemporal dementias, i.e. those that initially present with functional impairment of anterior parts of the brain, have a variety of underlying pathologies, from Pick's to AD. VaD is likely to result in patchy lesions of brain perfusion, often asymmetrical in distribution, or localized in 'watershed' regions of the brain (see Plate 1).

Experience with imaging of patients with dementia with Lewy bodies so far suggests little difference in perfusion patterns from Alzheimer's disease, although occipito-temporal changes have been described (Ishii *et al.*, 1999a; Minoshima *et al.*, 2001). More specific pharmacological probes are just now becoming available. Ligands binding to the dopamine transporter (β-CIT, FP-CIT) can be used as markers for dopaminergic cell loss. These radioligands may consequently prove useful in the differential diagnosis of AD and Lewy-body dementia (Walker *et al.*, 2002).

9.3 WHAT IS THE 'GOLD STANDARD'?

As hinted at above and described in more detail in Chapters 1 and 3, the clinical and pathological diagnoses of dementia are not congruent. The question about the true 'gold standard' for the evaluation of imaging studies, therefore, arises: should functional imaging reflect the distribution and severity of brain cell loss, or should it be representative of patients' functional impairment or their symptoms and signs? Either association would be of interest, but the most important purpose of imaging is, of course, the facilitation of effective treatment. Often the predictive validity of imaging methods is not known, but it should be ascertainable using standard empirical methods. This is in contrast to studies trying to validate imaging data with post-mortem results. By the time the brain comes to histology, a large number of confounding factors will have had a role to play: the time interval and natural history intervening between scan and post mortem examination; additional illness and treatment; the selection bias resulting from low uptake of post-mortem examinations. In the absence of really effective treatments, predictive validity more usually entails follow up within 2–3 years to confirm that the 'gold standard' clinical diagnosis was in fact reliable and that (hopefully) imaging results at baseline predict the observed clinical outcome.

9.4 DIAGNOSTIC ACCURACY OF FUNCTIONAL IMAGING

9.4.1 Guidelines and consensus statements

The role of functional imaging in the diagnosis of the dementias is controversial. Although the characteristic parietal and temporal deficits in AD and the widespread irregular deficits in VaD described above have been acknowledged and confirmed by consensus statement (Small *et al.*, 1997), guidelines have generally not recommended the routine clinical use of PET or SPECT in the diagnostic evaluation of dementia for *all* individuals. This is mainly justified by the lack of sufficient data on validity (Patterson *et al.*, 1999; Knopman *et al.*, 2001). For this reason, the American College of Radiology recommends using SPECT for clinically and diagnostically difficult cases only (Braffman *et al.*, 2000). Similarly, one of the more methodologically stringent systematic reviews recently suggested that there is little evidence to support a role for PET in the clinical evaluation of patients with suspected or established dementia (Gill *et al.*, 2003). In a more positive resumé, an international working group recommended that imaging techniques have an important role to play in the diagnosis and assessment of dementia and specifically AD (Reisberg *et al.*, 1997).

9.4.2 Alzheimer's disease

Bilateral temporoparietal hypometabolism has been frequently reported for AD compared with normal volunteers (Hoffman *et al.*, 2000; Okamura *et al.*, 2001; Alexander *et al.*, 2002a; Herholz *et al.*, 2002a; Volkow *et al.*, 2002). Although a temporoparietal deficit pattern is indicative of AD, it cannot be regarded as specific, but it does discriminate between demented and non-demented individuals (Masterman *et al.*, 1997). A systematic review and meta-analysis of literature in SPECT and dementia (Dougall *et al.*, 2003) found that using data pooled from 27 studies, SPECT successfully discriminated between healthy elderly controls and AD with a pooled sensitivity of 77 per cent against a pooled specificity of 89 per cent.

Additional significant abnormalities have been reported for AD in *posterior cingulate* (Rossor *et al.*, 1996; Minoshima *et al.*, 1997b) and *hippocampus* (Villa *et al.*, 1995; Ishii *et al.*, 1998; Elgh *et al.*, 2002; Lee *et al.*, 2003). For very early AD, reductions in posterior cingulate tend to be greater than in parietotemporal and frontal association cortices (Minoshima *et al.*, 1997a). Functional imaging in AD increases diagnostic sensitivity at least compared with structural imaging, with blood flow and metabolism first reduced in posterior cingulate gyrus and precuneus, before advancing to medial temporal structures and parietotemporal association cortex (Zakzanis *et al.*, 2003).

Entorhinal cortex and hippocampal metabolic reductions have been successfully used as a classifier in the discrimination of cognitively normal controls from mild cognitive impairment (MCI; De Santi *et al.*, 2001) with a diagnostic accuracy of 81 per cent and from AD using the temporal neocortex with a diagnostic accuracy of 100 per cent (De Santi *et al.*, 2001).

Neocortical metabolic reductions for AD are widely reported (Kumar *et al.*, 1991; Smith *et al.*, 1992; De Santi *et al.*, 2001). In a prospective longitudinal analysis using the ratio of deoxyglucose uptake in association cortex over primary sensory-motor cortex for classification, initial metabolic impairment was significantly associated with subsequent clinical deterioration, thus predicting for patients with mild cognitive deficits the progression to AD (Herholz *et al.*, 1999).

In advanced AD, bilateral parietotemporal perfusion deficits are reported to be more frequent and severe (Nitrini *et al.*, 2000) with a reported odds ratio (OR) of 17.0 (95 per cent CI 3.1–94.2) for severe AD (MMSE <10) and an OR of 5.2 (95 per cent CI 1.1–24.4) for moderate AD (MMSE 0–17). Finally, in a study of 68 AD subjects, metabolism in the cerebellum of a severe AD group was found to be significantly reduced (Ishii *et al.*, 1997) compared with 13 age-matched controls, which is of relevance as cerebellar activity is often taken as a 'normal' reference region (see below).

9.4.2.1 PATHOLOGICALLY CONFIRMED STUDIES

A multicentre study of PET in dementia with diagnostic verification by 3-year clinical follow up (Silverman *et al.*, 2001) concluded that regional brain metabolism was a sensitive indicator of AD. In the same study, a pathologically confirmed diagnosis of AD was predicted by PET with a sensitivity of 94 per cent (91 out of 97 subjects) against a specificity of 73 per cent (30 out of 41 subjects) against other patients presenting with symptoms of dementia. An overall diagnostic accuracy of 89 per cent was achieved for a subset of 55 patients who presented at the time of PET with questionable or mild dementia.

A PET study in a group considered 'diagnostically challenging or difficult to characterize by clinical criteria' (Hoffman *et al.*, 2000) produced sensitivity and specificity values of PET against a histological diagnosis at autopsy of AD of 93 per cent and 63 per cent, respectively. For comparison, clinical diagnosis of probable AD had sensitivity and specificity values of 63 per cent and 100 per cent, respectively, concluding that the overall diagnostic accuracy of PET at 82 per cent was better than clinical diagnosis at 73 per cent.

Two comparable SPECT studies with pathological verification of AD reported sensitivities of 86 per cent and 63 per cent (43 dementia patients v 11 healthy elderly controls) against specificities of 73 per cent and 93 per cent (70 dementia patients v 85 healthy elderly controls), respectively (Bonte *et al.*, 1997; Jagust *et al.*, 2001).

9.4.3 Vascular dementia (VaD)

Typical findings in VD are multiple small areas of reduced perfusion and metabolism extending over cortical and subcortical structures and a high diagnostic accuracy has been reported for the discrimination of probable AD and VD using this characteristic metabolic pattern (Mielke and Heiss, 1998). In addition, frontal lobes including cingulate and superior frontal gyri have been reported to be more affected in VD than in AD (Nagata *et al.*, 2000; Lee *et al.*, 2001). On the other hand, temporoparietal brain regions have been said best to discriminate AD from VD with sensitivities reported as high as 90 per cent and 82 per cent against 80 per cent and 82 per cent specificity, respectively (Butler *et al.*, 1995; deFigueiredo *et al.*, 1995). SPECT has been reported to differentiate AD from multi-infarct dementia in a study with a 77 per cent correct classification rate, compared with structural MRI, which correctly classified only 50 per cent in the same subject group (Butler *et al.*, 1995).

9.4.4 Frontotemporal dementia (FTD)

Highly significant metabolic abnormalities have been reported for PET in frontotemporoparietal association cortex, limbic area, basal ganglia and thalamus in FTD compared with normal volunteers (Ishii *et al.*, 1998). In particular, bilateral frontal hypoperfusion is a strong predictor of FTD versus AD in SPECT (Pickut *et al.*, 1997), with sensitivity and specificity estimated at 88 per cent and 79 per cent, respectively (Sjogren *et al.*, 2000). Medial temporal lobe reduction has been suggested as a marker to separate AD from FTD (Sjogren *et al.*, 2000).

9.4.5 Dementia with Lewy bodies (DLB)

An autopsy-confirmed PET study of the differential diagnosis of DLB and AD subjects found occipital metabolic reductions as a potential ante-mortem marker to distinguish DLB from AD, with sensitivity and specificity values determined at 90 per cent and 80 per cent respectively (Minoshima *et al.*, 2001). SPECT studies have confirmed occipital reduction in perfusion as an indicator of DLB (Ishii *et al.*, 1999b; Lobotesis *et al.*, 2001). Medial temporal and cingulate reductions in metabolism have been found to be significantly more pronounced in AD compared to DLB (Imamura *et al.*, 1997), while the occipital deficit in DLB appears irrespective of clinical severity (Okamura *et al.*, 2001).

9.4.6 Depression

SPECT has been reported to be a useful tool for the differential diagnosis of AD and depression, with perfusion deficits in depression lying between those of controls and AD and a reported sensitivity of 52 per cent (against 94 per cent in controls) using parieto-occipital perfusion as a marker (Stoppe et al., 1995).

9.4.7 SPECT v PET

A direct comparison (Herholz et al., 2002b) of SPECT and PET produced an overall significant correlation of abnormal tracer uptake between PET and SPECT across the entire brain ($r = 0.43$) with better correspondence achieved in the temporoparietal and posterior cingulate association cortices. Using quantitative statistical parametric mapping (SPM), the same study reported that PET discriminated between healthy volunteers and AD with greater reliability than SPECT, since PET was less sensitive to threshold effects in SPM. Another study of PET and SPECT compared patients with probable AD and normal controls using temporoparietal reductions as diagnostic criterion and determined a sensitivity for PET of 100 per cent and SPECT of 90 per cent, with the presence of abnormalities in associative cortex outside temporoparietal areas being better evaluated with PET (Messa et al., 1994).

9.5 METHODS OF IMAGE ASSESSMENT – PET AND SPECT

PET and SPECT images can be analysed qualitatively using visual inspection methods or quantitatively using a variety of semiautomated methods. The variability of visual interpretations has been reported as minimal for PET, with a good intraobserver ($\kappa = 0.56$, $P < 0.0005$) and interobserver ($\kappa = 0.51$, $P < 0.0005$) agreement (Hoffman et al., 1996). Good agreement has also been found for qualitative inspection of SPECT (Hellman et al., 1994; Pasquier et al., 1997). Attempts have been made to develop classification criteria according to perfusion deficit patterns on visual assessment (Holman et al., 1992; Sloan et al., 1995).

For quantitative region of interest (ROI) analysis, the brain is divided into areas often approximating underlying structural anatomy. Mean values of functional activity are then averaged within these regions and compared with a dataset of controls (Defebvre et al., 1999). More objective methods have been developed recently, such as statistical parametric mapping (Friston et al., 1995; Soonawala et al., 2002), discriminant function analysis (Mahony et al., 1994; O'Brien et al., 2001; Volkow et al., 2002) and neural network analysis (Chan et al., 1994; Dawson et al., 1994; Kippenhan et al., 1994; deFigueiredo et al., 1995; Page et al., 1996). Three-dimensional stereotactic surface projection images have been found to improve the accuracy of visually detecting AD with PET (Burdette et al., 1996). Finally,

a combination of structural MRI or CT and functional imaging has been found to improve the accuracy of diagnostic classification (Mattman et al., 1997; Scheltens et al., 1997; O'Brien et al., 2001; Callen et al., 2002; Varma et al., 2002).

9.6 IMAGING NEUROTRANSMITTER SYSTEMS

9.6.1 SPECT

Although FP-CIT is now licensed in the UK for the investigation of parkinsonism, its use in DLB is still experimental (Walker et al., 2002). The same applies to all other receptor ligands – be it because of limits in the validation and validity of the imaging protocol or because of doubts about the involvement of the receptor concerned in the pathophysiology of the respective dementia. However, there are now a number of SPECT ligands that can be used as probes into specific transmitter system deficits in dementia: Iodo-QNB and 5-IA-85380 for muscarinic and nicotinic receptors, respectively; FP-CIT and iodobenzamide for dopamine transporter and D2-receptor, respectively; iomazenil for the benzodiazepine/ GABA receptor complex and ^{123}I-MK-801 for the NMDA receptor (Pimlott et al., 2003).

9.6.2 PET

The greater flexibility of PET-ligand creation has made it possible to generate all the above and additional receptor ligands, e.g. for 5HT-2A receptors (altanserin; Meltzer et al., 1999), acetylcholinesterase activity (MP. 4A; Iyo et al., 1997) and, of particular interest in AD, ligands for neurofibrillary tangles and Aβ-plaques (FDDNP; Shoghi-Jadid et al., 2002). The latter are especially exciting, as the focus of dementia treatment may be shifting away from the selective enhancement of transmitter systems thought to be involved in the Alzheimer pathology, towards the biochemical entities, presumably more at the origin of the pathophysiological cascade leading to cell death and brain atrophy. Such markers could be used both for the diagnosis and 'purification' of patient samples for treatment research, as well as the follow-through of patients in treatment, using ligand binding as a proxy measure of treatment success. On a more fundamental level, if treatment should change ligand binding, the association of changes in ligand binding and clinical improvement could provide causal in vivo evidence for the active principle of the treatment concerned.

9.7 BRAIN–BEHAVIOUR CORRELATES IN DEMENTIA

Information from functional imaging modes, such as PET, SPECT and fMRI can be combined with neuropsychological information and be used to investigate the neural correlates of cognitive and behavioural processes. The use of imaging techniques has led to improvements in understanding of the dementias and their longitudinal course and may lead to further developments for example in evaluating potential treatments.

PET was first used in 1981 to show a global reduction in cerebral blood flow (CBF) in patients with degenerative dementia, which correlated with clinical measures of disease severity (Frackowiak *et al.*, 1981). Since then there have been many studies demonstrating the typical reductions in metabolism and blood flow. These are most consistent and severe in the temporal and parietal association cortices. As the disease advances, the occipital and frontal association cortices are progressively affected (Alexander *et al.*, 2002b). On neuropsychological examination, the typical pattern of AD begins with memory impairment followed by semantic and executive deficits, then deficits in praxis, behavioural problems and so on. These neuropsychological deficits have been correlated with regional metabolic deficits, though as with all 'lesion paradigms' the correspondence between specific cognitive functions and certain brain regions can only be an approximation since it is likely that multiple brain areas are involved in even simple functions. Despite these limitations, functional imaging has been able to add to the understanding of brain–behaviour correlates in dementia.

Neuropsychological testing has shown that the first deficit in AD is episodic memory loss. The first reduction in rCBF has been shown to be in the area of the posterior cingulate gyrus and precuneus which is known to be important in memory (Desgranges *et al.*, 1998). Supporting this correlation, a PET study revealed activation of the retrosplenial area of the cingulate cortex during an episodic memory encoding task, which is also backed by the clinical picture subsequent to other lesions of the retrosplenial cingulate cortex, such as tumours, in this area (Fletcher *et al.*, 1995).

The next area of functioning to show impairment is semantic memory and it is thought that this occurs when neurodegenerative changes extend to the adjacent temporal neocortex (Jobst *et al.*, 1992). It is possible that initial involvement of the transentorhinal region, as indicated by the first histological changes, then leads to disconnection of the hippocampus followed by the limbic structures and isocortical association areas (Hodges and Patterson, 1995). This disconnection hypothesis can also help to account for the variety and progression of symptoms in AD, as different areas become disconnected.

Short-term memory generally has been shown consistently to correlate with metabolism in the temporoparietal association cortex, with the left hemisphere for verbal and right for spatial memory (Trollor and Valenzuela, 2001). Asymmetries in hemisphere metabolism correlate with neuropsychological 'asymmetries' defined by the traditional verbal/non-verbal dichotomy (Haxby *et al.*, 1990). If there is 'asymmetrical' involvement, the left hemisphere is often the more affected side, although reasons for this are unknown. Bilateral parietotemporal hypoperfusion appears to be more frequent in

male patients, those with early onset and patients with severe AD (Nitrini *et al.*, 2000).

Following memory, attention is the next domain to be affected in AD. The anterior cingulate is thought to be involved in attentional function and a particular correlation has been shown between divided attention and anterior cingulate activity (Perry *et al.*, 2000; Matsuda, 2001). This is consistent with the clinical picture – it is thought that impairment of divided attention is responsible for problems in activities of daily living, which occur in AD at a relatively early stage. With regard to psychiatric phenomena, functional imaging has shown that psychotic symptoms in AD correlate with reduced frontal and temporal metabolism (Mega *et al.*, 2000); negative symptoms have been linked to decreased perfusion in the frontal cortex (Galynker *et al.*, 2000), and apathy has been associated with significantly decreased blood flow in anterior temporal, orbitofrontal, anterior cingulate and dorsolateral prefrontal regions (Benoit *et al.*, 1999; Cummings, 2000). With regard to depressive symptoms in AD, there is some evidence of correlation with reduced temporal lobe perfusion (Ebmeier *et al.*, 1998).

9.7.1 Cognitive activation studies

More recently, functional activation studies have demonstrated that in mild to moderately severe AD, a cognitive or sensory challenge task can cause nearly normal levels of activation in areas that are hypometabolic or hypoperfused at rest. However, with increased disease severity the degree of activation declines (Devous, 2002) Furthermore, increased activation may be required in AD patients who perform a task, or indeed activation of additional brain areas which are not activated by healthy controls (Cardebat *et al.*, 1998). It has been hypothesized that functional plasticity may be responsible for such a recruitment of new brain regions in patients. An fMRI activation study compared patients with early AD and FTD during a working memory task in order to try to differentiate between the groups. During performance of the task, there was reduced activation in the frontal, temporal and cingulate cortices in the FTD group compared with the AD group. There was, however, the opposite effect in the cerebellum, a region less consistently activated in functional working memory imaging studies. This cerebellar activation in FTD may reflect successful working memory specific compensation, since test performance of FTD patients were not different from the AD group (Rombouts *et al.*, 2003). Activation studies may, therefore, be useful in helping to reveal subtle changes in brain functioning in the early stages of dementia, as well as improving our understanding of the neural circuits involved in the tasks.

9.7.2 Longitudinal studies

A number of functional imaging studies have investigated cognitive functioning over time. These have shown that patients with more severe perfusion or metabolic deficits in the temporoparietal cortex at initial evaluation show a more rapid cognitive decline over time (Devous, 2002). In particular a strong correlation has been found between reduction in right parietal rCBF and patient survival (Jagust, 1994). With regard to mild cognitive impairment, significant bilateral rCBF decreases are seen in the posterior cingulate, parietal and precuneus regions of those who later meet criteria for AD. Subsequently, at the stage of a clinical diagnosis of AD, additional rCBF abnormalities are seen in the hippocampus and parahippocampus (Minoshima *et al.*, 1997b; Kogure *et al.*, 2000).

For individual patients, the particular neuropsychological pattern that develops during the progression of AD can be predicted by early metabolic asymmetries in the association cortices (Haxby *et al.*, 1990). This would indicate that there is a functional reserve in the brain, so that neuropsychological dysfunction is likely to follow rather than co-occur with rCBF changes. Similarly, greater premorbid ability is hypothesized to be linked with a cognitive reserve that can reduce the clinical expression of AD. Premorbid IQ and word reading ability have been shown to be inversely correlated with metabolism in AD (Mentis, 2000).

More recently, longitudinal functional imaging studies have been proposed to assess the response to treatments for AD (Alexander *et al.*, 2002b). Such activation studies are of particular interest, as they can help in identifying potentially reversible tissue damage.

9.8 CONCLUSION

One of the authors' central tenets is that the 'gold standard' of all imaging work has to be the patient's clinical state. By implication, 'predictive validity' is the concept of greatest interest: imaging results should *predict* a patient's prognosis and in particular whether they are going to respond to a treatment. This does not contradict the basic notion that diagnosis has to be at the beginning of effective treatment, but it reflects the observation that brain pathological changes are not always specific to a particular illness; that there is a substantial overlap of pathological changes even with health, and that pathological illness 'entities' are likely to be caused by a varying admixture of genotype–environment interactions: AD is really a collective term for a number of condition resulting in dementia, plaques and tangles. Histological diagnoses merely reflect recognizable final common pathways for a collection of pathological conditions and therefore do not necessarily predict treatment response or prognosis. In evaluating the usefulness of imaging methods, direct comparisons should be made with clinical outcome measures – histopathological follow-through studies are of interest, but will always be confounded by selection bias, intervening illness and other artefacts. The validation of neuroimaging in the dementias is clearly still in its infancy and clinically relevant research if few and far between (Dougall

et al., 2003). One of the binds we encounter is that useful data on sensitivity and specificity, and more particularly positive and negative predictive value, require representative clinical cohorts. If the introduction of a new imaging method is to be evidence based in a national health service and good evidence is only available after the establishment of a service, the creation of pilot services is necessary that are not technology driven, i.e. that are centred in a normal clinical set-up that will generate results transferable to the service in general. The theoretical appeal of imaging methods, after all we believe that the dementias are brain diseases, holds out the promise of visualizing brain changes that are relevant to illness outcome and treatment response.

REFERENCES

Alexander G, Chen K, Pietrini P, Rapoport S, Reiman E. (2002a) Longitudinal PET evaluation of cerebral metabolic decline in dementia: a potential outcome measure in Alzheimer's disease treatment studies. *American Journal of Psychiatry* **159**: 738–745

Alexander GE, Chen K, Pietrini P, Rapoport S, Reiman E. (2002b) Longitudinal PET evaluation of cerebral metabolic decline in dementia: a potential outcome measure in Alzheimer's disease treatment studies. *American Journal of Psychiatry* **159**: 738–745

Benoit M, Dygai I, Migneco O, Robert P *et al.* (1999) Behavioral and psychological symptoms in Alzheimer's disease. Relation between apathy and regional cerebral perfusion. *Dementia and Geriatric Cognitive Disorders* **10**: 511–517

Bonte F, Weiner M, Bigio E, White C. (1997) Brain blood flow in the dementias: SPECT with histopathologic correlation in 54 patients. *Radiology* **202**: 793–797

Braffman B, Drayer B, Anderson R *et al.* (2000) Dementia. American College of Radiology ACR Appropriateness Criteria. *Radiology* **215** (Suppl.): 525–533

Burdette J, Minoshima S, Vander Borght T, Tran D, Kuhl D. (1996) Alzheimer disease: improved visual interpretation of PET images by using three-dimensional stereotaxic surface projections. *Radiology* **198**: 837–843

Butler R.E, Costa D, Greco A ELL P, Katona C. (1995) Differentiation between Alzheimer's disease and multi-infarct dementia: SPECT vs MR imaging. *International Journal of Geriatric Psychiatry* **10**: 121–128

Callen D, Black S, Caldwell C. (2002) Limbic system perfusion in Alzheimer's disease measured by MRI- coregistered HMPAO SPET. *European Journal of Nuclear Medicine and Molecular Imaging* **29**: 899–906

Cardebat D, Demonet J, Puel M, Agniel A, Viallard G, Celsis P. (1998) Brain correlates of memory processes in patients with dementia of Alzheimer's type: a SPECT activation study. *Journal of Cerebral Blood Flow and Metabolism* **18**: 457–462

Chan K, Johnson K, Becker J, Satlin A, Mendelson J, Garada B, Holman B. (1994) A neural network classifier for cerebral perfusion imaging. *Journal of Nuclear Medicine* **35**: 771–774

Cummings J. (2000) Cognitive and behavioural heterogeneity in Alzheimer's disease: seeking the neurobiological basis. *Neurobiology of Aging* **21**: 845–861

Dawson M, Dobbs A, Hooper H, McEwan A, Triscott J, Cooney J. (1994) Artificial neural networks that use single-photon emission tomography to identify patients with probable Alzheimer's disease. *European Journal of Nuclear Medicine* **21**: 1303–1311

De Santi S, de Leon M, Rusinek H *et al.* (2001) Hippocampal formation glucose metabolism and volume losses in MCI and AD. *Neurobiology of Aging* **22**: 529–539

Defebvre L, Leduc V, Duhamel A *et al.* (1999) Technetium HMPAO SPECT study in dementia with Lewy bodies Alzheimer's disease and idiopathic Parkinson's disease. *Journal of Nuclear Medicine* **40**: 956–962

deFigueiredo R, Shankle W, Maccato A *et al.* (1995) Neural-network-based classification of cognitively normal demented Alzheimer disease and vascular dementia from single photon emission with computed tomography image data from brain. *Proceedings of the National Academy of Sciences of the United States of America* **92**: 5530–5534

Desgranges B, Baron J, de la Sayette V *et al.* (1998) The neural substrates of memory systems impairment in Alzheimer's disease PET study of resting brain glucose utilization. *Brain* **121**: 611–631

Devous M. (2002) Functional brain imaging in the dementias: role in early detection differential diagnosis and longitudinal studies. *European Journal of Nuclear Medicine and Molecular Imaging* **29**: 1685–1696

Dougall N, Bruggink S, Ebmeier K. (2003) Clinical use of SPECT in dementia – a quantitative review. In: KP Ebmeier (ed.), *Advances in Biological Psychiatry – Volume 22 SPECT in Dementia*. Basel, Karger Verlag, pp. 4–37

Ebmeier K, Glabus M, Prentice N, Ryman A, Goodwin G. (1998) A voxel-based analysis of cerebral perfusion in dementia and depression of old age. *Neuroimage* **7**: 199–208

Elgh E, Sundstrom T, Nasman B, Ahlstrom R, Nyberg L. (2002) Memory functions and rCBF (99m)Tc-HMPAO SPET: developing diagnostics in Alzheimer's disease. *European Journal of Nuclear Medicine and Molecular Imaging* **29**: 1140–1148

Fletcher P, Frith C, Grasby P, Shallice T, Frackowiak R, Dolan R. (1995) Brain systems for encoding and retrieval of auditory-verbal memory. An in vivo study in humans. *Brain* **118**: 401–416

Frackowiak R, Pozzilli C, Legg N *et al.* (1981) Regional cerebral oxygen supply and utilization in dementia clinical and physiological study with oxygen-15 and positron emission tomography. *Brain* **104**: 753–758

Friston K, Holmes A, Worsley K, Poline J-P, Frith C, Frackowiak R. (1995) Statistical parametric maps in functional imaging: a general linear approach. *Human Brain Mapping* **2**: 189–210

Galynker I, Dutta E, Vilkas N *et al.* (2000) Hypofrontality and negative symptoms in patients with dementia of Alzheimer type. *Neuropsychiatry, Neuropsychology and Behavior Neurology* **13**: 53–59

Gill S, Rochon P, Guttman M, Laupacis A. (2003) The value of positron emission tomography in the clinical evaluation of dementia. *Journal of the American Geriatrics Society* **51**: 258–264

Haxby J, Grady C, KOSS E, Horwitz B, Heston L, Schapiro M, Friedland R, Rapoport S. (1990) Longitudinal study of cerebral metabolic asymmetries and associated neuropsychological patterns in early dementia of the Alzheimer type. *Archives of Neurology* **47**: 753–760

Hellman R, Tikofsky R, Van H, Coade G, Carretta R, Hoffmann R. (1994) A multi-institutional study of interobserver agreement in the evaluation of dementia with rCBF/SPET technetium-99m exametazime (HMPAO). *European Journal of Nuclear Medicine* **21**: 306–313

Herholz K, Nordberg A, Salmon E *et al.* (1999) Impairment of neocortical metabolism predicts progression in Alzheimer's disease. *Dementia and Geriatric Cognitive Disorders* **10**: 494–504

Herholz K, Salmon E, Perani D. (2002a) Discrimination between Alzheimer dementia and controls by automated analysis of multicenter FDG PET. *Neuroimage* **17**: 302–316

Herholz K, Schopphoff H, Schmidt M *et al.* (2002b) Direct comparison of spatially normalized PET and SPECT scans in Alzheimer's disease. *Journal of Nuclear Medicine* **43**: 21–26

Hodges J and Patterson PK. (1995) Is semantic memory consistently impaired early in the course of Alzheimer's disease? Neuroanatomical and diagnostic implications. *Neuropsychologia* **33**: 441–459

Hoffman J, Hanson M, Welsh K *et al.* (1996) Interpretation variability of (18)FDG-positron emission tomography studies in dementia. *Investigative Radiology* **31**: 316–322

Hoffman J, Welsh-Bohmer K, Hanson M *et al.* (2000) FDG PET imaging in patients with pathologically verified dementia. *Journal of Nuclear Medicine* **41**: 1920–1928

Holman B, Johnson K, Gerada B, Carvalho P, Satlin A. (1992) The scintigraphic appearance of Disease-disease – a prospective-study using technetium-99m-HMPAO SPECT. *Journal of Nuclear Medicine* **33**: 181–185

Imamura T, Ishii K, Sasaki M *et al.* (1997) Regional cerebral glucose metabolism in dementia with Lewy bodies and Alzheimer's disease: a comparative study using positron emission tomography. *Neuroscience Letters* **235**: 49–52

Ince P. (2001) Pathological correlates of late-onset dementia in a multicentre community-based population in England and Wales: Neuropathology Group of the Medical Research Council Cognitive Function and Ageing Study (MRC CFAS)1. *Lancet* **357**: 169–175

Ishii K, Sasaki M, Kitagaki H *et al.* (1997) Reduction of cerebellar glucose metabolism in advanced Alzheimer's disease. *Journal of Nuclear Medicine* **38**: 925–928

Ishii K, Sakamoto S, Sasaki M *et al.* (1998) Cerebral glucose metabolism in patients with frontotemporal dementia. *Journal of Nuclear Medicine* **39**: 1875–1878

Ishii K, Yamaji S, Kitagaki H, Imamura T, Hirono N, Mori E. (1999a) Regional cerebral blood flow difference between dementia with Lewy bodies and AD. *Neurology* **53**: 413–416

Ishii K, Yamaji S, Kitagaki H, Imamura T, Hirono N, Mori E. (1999b) Regional cerebral blood flow difference between dementia with Lewy bodies and Alzheimer's disease. *Journal of Nuclear Medicine* **40**: 1185

Iyo M, Namba H, Fukushi K *et al.* (1997) Measurement of acetylcholinesterase by positron emission tomography in the brains of healthy controls and patients with Alzheimer's disease. *Lancet* **349**: 1805–1809

Jagust W. (1994) Functional imaging in dementia – an overview. *Journal of Clinical Psychiatry* **55**: 5–11

Jagust W, Thisted R, Devous M *et al.* (2001) SPECT perfusion imaging in the diagnosis of Alzheimer's disease – A clinical-pathologic study. *Neurology* **56**: 950–956

Jobst K, Smith A, Barker C *et al.* (1992) Association of atrophy of the medial temporal-lobe with reduced blood-flow in the posterior parietotemporal cortex in patients with a clinical and pathological diagnosis of Alzheimer's disease. *Journal of Neurology, Neurosurgery, and Psychiatry* **55**: 190–194

Kippenhan J, Barker W, Nagel J, Grady C, Duara R. (1994) Neural-network classification of normal and Alzheimer's disease subjects using high-resolution and low-resolution PET cameras. *Journal of Nuclear Medicine* **35**: 7–15

Knopman D, DeKosky S, Cummings J *et al.* (2001) Practice parameter: Diagnosis of dementia (an evidence-based review) – Report of the Quality Standards Subcommittee of the American Academy of Neurology. *Neurology* **56**: 1143–1153

Kogure D, Matsuda H, Ohnishi T et al. (2000) Longitudinal evaluation of early Alzheimer's disease using brain perfusion SPECT. Journal of Nuclear Medicine 41: 1155–1162

Kumar A, Schapiro M, Grady C et al. (1991) High-resolution PET studies in Alzheimer's disease. Neuropsychopharmacology 4: 35–46

Lee B, Liu C, Tai C et al. (2001) Alzheimer's disease: scintigraphic appearance of Tc-99m HMPAO brain SPECT. Kaohsiung Journal of Medical Science 17: 394–400

Lee Y, Liu R, Liao Y et al. (2003) Statistical parametric mapping of brain SPECT perfusion abnormalities in patients with Alzheimer's disease. European Neurology 49: 142–145

Lobotesis K, Fenwick J, Phipps A et al. (2001) Occipital hypoperfusion on SPECT in dementia with Lewy bodies but not AD. Neurology 56: 643–649

Mahony D, Coffey J, Murphy J et al. (1994) The discriminant value of semiquantitative SPECT data in mild Alzheimer's disease. Journal of Nuclear Medicine 35: 1450–1455

Masterman D, Mendez M, Fairbanks L, Cummings J. (1997) Sensitivity specificity and positive predictive value of technetium 99–HMPAO SPECT in discriminating Alzheimer's disease from other dementias. Journal of Geriatric Psychiatry and Neurology 10: 15–21

Matsuda H. (2001) Cerebral blood flow and metabolic abnormalities in Alzheimer's disease. Annals of Nuclear Medicine 15: 85–92

Mattman A, Feldman H, Forster B, Li D, Szasz I, Beattie B, Schulzer M. (1997) Regional HmPAO SPECT and CT measurements in the diagnosis of Alzheimer's disease. Canadian Journal of Neurological Sciences 24: 22–28

Mega M, Lee L, Dinov I, Mishkin F, Toga A, Cummings J. (2000) Cerebral correlates of psychotic symptoms in Alzheimer's disease. Journal of Neurology, Neurosurgery, and Psychiatry 69: 167–171

Meltzer C, Price J, Mathis C et al. (1999) PET Imaging of serotonin type 2A receptors in late-life neuropsychiatric disorders. American Journal of Psychiatry 156: 1871–1878

Mentis M. (2000) Positron emission tomography and single photon emission computed tomography imaging in Alzheimer's disease. Neurologist 6: 28–43

Messa C, Perani D, Lucignani G et al. (1994) High-resolution technetium-99m-HMPAO SPECT in patients with probable Alzheimer's-disease – comparison with fluorine-18-FDG PET. Journal of Nuclear Medicine 35: 210–216

Mielke RND and Heiss W. (1998) Positron emission tomography for diagnosis of Alzheimer's disease and vascular dementia. Journal of Neural Transmission (Suppl.) 53: 237–250

Minoshima S, Giordani B, Berent S, Frey K, Foster N, Kuhl D. (1997a) Metabolic reduction in the posterior cingulate cortex in very early Alzheimer's disease. Annals of Neurology 42: 85–94

Minoshima S, Giordani B, Berent S, Frey K, Foster N, Kuhl D. (1997b) Metabolic reduction in the posterior cingulate cortex in very early Alzheimer's disease. Annals of Neurology 42: 85–94

Minoshima S, Foster N, Sima A, Frey K, Albin R, Kuhl D. (2001) Alzheimer's disease versus dementia with Lewy bodies: Cerebral metabolic distinction with autopsy confirmation. Annals of Neurology 50: 358–365

Nagata K, Maruya H, Yuya H et al. (2000) Can PET data differentiate Alzheimer's disease from vascular dementia?. Annals of New York Academy of Sciences 903: 252–261

Nitrini R, Buchpiguel C, Caramelli P et al. (2000) SPECT in Alzheimer's disease: features associated with bilateral parietotemporal hypoperfusion. Acta Neurologica Scandinavica 101: 172–176

O'Brien J, Ames D, Desmond P et al. (2001) Combined magnetic resonance imaging and single-photon emission tomography scanning in the discrimination of Alzheimer's disease from age-matched controls. International Psychogeriatrics 13: 149–161

Okamura N, Arai H, Higuchi M et al. (2001) [18F]FDG-PET study in dementia with Lewy bodies and Alzheimer's disease. Progress in Neuropsychopharmacology, Biology and Psychiatry 25: 447–456

Page M, Howard R, Brien J, Buxton T, Pickering A. (1996) Use of neural networks in brain SPECT to diagnose Alzheimer's disease. Journal of Nuclear Medicine 37: 195–200

Pasquier F, Lavenu I, Lebert F, Jacob B, Steinling M, Petit H. (1997) The use of SPECT in a multidisciplinary memory clinic. Dementia and Geriatric Cognitive Disorders 8: 85–91

Patterson C, Gauthier S, Bergman H et al. (1999) The recognition assessment and management of dementing disorders: conclusions from the Canadian Consensus Conference on Dementia. CMAJ 160 (Suppl.): 1–15

Perry R, Watson P, Hodges J. (2000) The nature and staging of attention dysfunction in early (minimal and mild) Alzheimer's disease: relationship to episodic and semantic memory impairment. Neuropsychologia 38: 252–271

Pickut B, Saerens J, Marien P et al. (1997) Discriminative use of SPECT in frontal lobe-type dementia versus (senile) dementia of the Alzheimer's type. Journal of Nuclear Medicine 38: 929–934

Pimlott S, Owens J, Brown D, Wyper D. (2003) Novel SPECT receptor ligands for the investigation of dementia. In: K Ebmeier (ed.) Advances in Biological Psychiatry Vol. 22 – SPECT in Dementia. Basel, Karger Verlag, pp. 95–114

Reisberg B, Burns A, Brodaty H et al. (1997) Diagnosis of Alzheimer's disease. Report of an International Psychogeriatric Association Special Meeting Work Group under the cosponsorship of Alzheimer's Disease International the European Federation of Neurological Societies the World Health Organization and the World Psychiatric Association. International Psychogeriatrics 9 (Suppl. 1): 11–38

Rombouts S, van Swieten J, Pijnenburg Y, Goekoop R, Barkhof F, Scheltens P. (2003) Loss of frontal fMRI activation in early frontotemporal dementia compared to early AD. Neurology 60: 1904–1908

Rossor M, Kennedy A, Frackowiak R. (1996) Clinical and neuroimaging features of familial Alzheimer's disease. Neurobiology of Alzheimer's Disease 777: 49–56

Scheltens P, Launer L, Barkhof F, Weinstein H, Jonker C. (1997) The diagnostic value of magnetic resonance imaging and technetium 99m-HMPAO single-photon-emission computed tomography for the diagnosis of Alzheimer disease in a community-dwelling elderly population. Alzheimer Disease and Associated Disorders 11: 63–70

Shoghi-Jadid K, Small G, Agdeppa E et al. (2002) Localization of neurofibrillary tangles and beta-amyloid plaques in the brains of living patients with Alzheimer disease. American Journal of Geriatric Psychiatry 10: 24–35

Silverman D, Small G, Chang C et al. (2001) Positron emission tomography in evaluation of dementia – Regional brain metabolism and long-term outcome. JAMA 286: 2120–2127

Sjogren M, Gustafson L, Wikkelso C, Wallin A. (2000) Frontotemporal dementia can be distinguished from Alzheimer's disease and subcortical white matter dementia by an anterior-to-posterior rCBF-SPET ratio. Dementia and Geriatric Cognitive Disorders 11: 275–285

Sloan E, Fenton G, Kennedy N, MacLennan J. (1995) Electroencephalography and single photon emission computed tomography in dementia: a comparative study. Psychological Medicine 25: 631–638

Small G, Rabins P, Barry P *et al.* (1997) Diagnosis and treatment of Alzheimer disease and related disorders. Consensus statement of the American Association for Geriatric Psychiatry the Alzheimer's Association and the American Geriatrics Society. *JAMA* **278**: 1363–1371

Smith G, deLeon M, George A *et al.* (1992) Topography of cross-sectional and longitudinal glucose metabolic deficits in disease – pathophysiologic implications. *Archives of Neurology* **49**: 1142–1150

Soonawala D, Amin T, Ebmeier K *et al.* (2002) Statistical parametric mapping of 99mTc-HMPAO-SPECT images for the diagnosis of Alzheimer's disease: normalizing to cerebellar tracer uptake. *Neuroimage* **17**: 1193–1202

Stoppe G, Staedt J, Kogler A *et al.* (1995) 99mTc-HMPAO-SPECT in the diagnosis of senile dementia of Alzheimer's type – a study under clinical routine conditions. *Journal of Neural Transmission (Genetic Section)* **99**: 195–211

Trollor J and Valenzuela M. (2001) Brain ageing in the new millennium. *Australian and New Zealand Journal of Psychiatry* **35**: 788–805

Varma A, Adams W, Lloyd J *et al.* (2002) Diagnostic patterns of regional atrophy on MRI and regional cerebral blood flow change on SPECT in young onset patients with Alzheimer's disease frontotemporal dementia and vascular dementia. *Acta Neurologica Scandinavica* **105**: 261–269

Villa G, Cappa A, Tavolozza M *et al.* (1995) Neuropsychological tests and [99mTc]-HM PAO SPECT in the diagnosis of Alzheimer's dementia. *Journal of Neurology* **242**: 359–366

Volkow N, Zhu W, Felder C *et al.* (2002) Changes in brain functional homogeneity in subjects with Alzheimer's disease. *Psychiatry Research – Neuroimaging* **114**: 39–50

Walker Z, Costa D, Walker R *et al.* (2002) Differentiation of dementia with Lewy bodies from Alzheimer's disease using a dopaminergic presynaptic ligand. *Journal of Neurology, Neurosurgery, and Psychiatry* **73**: 134–140

Zakzanis K, Graham S, Campbell Z. (2003) A meta-analysis of structural and functional brain imaging in dementia of the Alzheimer's type: a neuroimaging profile. *Neuropsychology Review* **13**: 1–18

10

The neurophysiology of dementia

MICHAEL PHILPOT

During the last 80 years a number of advances have been made in the development of techniques for demonstrating the electrical activity of the brain. Conventional electroencephalography (EEG) was effectively 'founded' in the 1920s when it became possible to record such activity from the scalp. The techniques of evoked potentials were first developed in the 1950s and 'event-related' potentials became available in the 1960s. Quantitative analysis of the electroencephalogram (qEEG) has been possible since the 1970s and recording of the magnetic fields induced by electrical brain activity since the 1980s.

This chapter will deal with clinical and applied research in neurophysiology with regard to ageing and dementia. Technical details are beyond the scope of this review and the interested reader is referred a general text such as Osselton et al. (2002).

10.1 THE ELECTROENCEPHALOGRAM

10.1.1 EEG in healthy older people

The prevalence of EEG abnormalities increases with age with an emphasis in the temporal regions (Busse and Obrist, 1965). Using traditional visual methods, there appears to be a progressive slowing of the mean frequency and a reduction in α activity. There is an increase in the frequency and amount of β activity as well as an increase in θ and δ activity (Torres et al., 1983).

Studies employing qEEG have also shown some consistency, in spite of the large number of variables available for measurement. An increase in β activity combined with a reduction in θ and δ power with age has been demonstrated (Polich, 1997; Dustman et al., 1999). Recently, more complex methods of analysis have examined aspects of the organization of brain activity. These include the following changes with age: a reduction in interhemispheric coherence at rest but an increase in coherence to photic stimulation (Kikuchi et al., 2000), an increase in the complexity of spatial distribution of EEG activity (Pierce et al., 2003), and an increase in slow wave variability (Dustman et al., 1999).

Most studies have been cross-sectional, comparing results in different age groups, but the few longitudinal studies carried out have produced conflicting results. Coben et al. (1985) found no change in α or θ frequency over 3 years (or the ratio of δ to θ), although there were significant reductions in β and δ frequency. No changes in any power band were found by Förstl et al. (1996) over a 4-year period. Elmståhl and Rosén (1997) performed EEGs 5 years apart in a group of initially healthy elderly women. Those who remained cognitively unimpaired showed an increase in absolute α and θ power, together with a reduction in relative posterior β power.

10.1.2 Mild cognitive impairment (MCI)

Williamson et al. (1990) found that healthy elderly subjects who had MCI also had markedly reduced β power in all brain regions. Stevens and Kircher (1998) used a form of temporo-spatial analysis and found that the duration of stable voltage patterns (known as EEG microstates) was reduced in people with MCI, as was EEG reactivity to eye opening. Grunwald et al. (2001) reported that θ activity increased as a function of reducing hippocampal volume. Jelic et al. (2000) found that MCI patients who later developed obvious dementia had abnormalities of EEG coherence, α and θ power when compared with MCI patients who remained stable.

10.1.3 Alzheimer's disease (AD)

10.1.3.1 FEATURES AND ASSOCIATIONS OF EEG

Berger (1932) first described the general slowing of the EEG in a patient with dementia. The changes in AD can be summarized as follows: a slowing of the α frequency, amplitude and relative power with a shift towards the anterior frontal regions; a decrease in relative and absolute β power; and, an increasing predominance of diffuse and symmetrical θ and δ waves in posterior regions, reflected by an increase in δ and θ power (Knott et al., 2001). Other changes include a reduction in general reactivity (Visser et al., 1985), and reduced EEG coherence (Stevens et al., 2001; Hogan et al., 2003). These quantitative changes are associated with degree of cognitive impairment (Grunwald et al., 2001; Stam et al., 2003), reduced cerebral blood flow (Ihl et al., 1989a; Rodriguez et al., 1999b; Claus et al., 2000; Mattia et al., 2003) and hypometabolism (Dierks et al., 2000). Abnormalities may also be associated with early onset (Pucci et al., 1999) and psychotic symptoms (Edwards-Lee et al., 2000). Riekkinen et al. (1991) reported that reduction in acetylcholinesterase activity in the cerebrospinal fluid (CSF) of AD patients was associated with increased δ power. The same group later reported that patients with the most marked slowing of the EEG had the lowest choline acetyltransferase levels in the frontal cortex post mortem (Soininen et al., 1992). Jelic et al. (1998a) found a strong association between CSF τ protein and EEG activity.

Genetic risk factors may also influence EEG activity. Jelic et al. (1997) compared EEG coherence in AD patients homozygous for the ε4 allele of apolipoprotein E (ApoE) with patients carrying either one or no ε4 allele. Coherence was reduced in the temporoparietal regions of the homozygotes. Lehtovirta et al. (2000) reported pronounced slow-wave activity in AD patients carrying the σ4 allele but this did not carry any prognostic significance.

Epileptic seizures and related EEG abnormalities occur in 10–20 per cent of AD patients, usually >6 years into the course of the disease. They are more likely in early onset dementia and may be mistaken for symptoms of the dementia itself (Mendez and Lim, 2003).

10.1.3.2 EEG AND CHOLINERGIC DRUGS

A number of studies have used qEEG as a marker to assess the effects of cholinergic drugs. Modest reductions in δ and θ power and an increase in fast activity (i.e. a shift to more normal EEG) have been reported following the long-term use of tacrine (Riekkinen et al., 1991; Jelic et al., 1998b) and donepezil (Kogan et al., 2001; Reeves et al., 2002; Rodriguez et al., 2002). Changes in the mean frequency of each waveband mirror brain perfusion in the parietal lobe (Rodriguez et al., 2004). Acute administration of nicotine (Knott et al., 2000a) and rivastigmine (Adler and Brassen, 2001) have broadly the same effect. EEG may also be used to identify possible responders to cholinesterase inhibitors after a single drug dose (Knott et al., 2000b; Almkvist et al., 2001). Similarly, a decrease in θ power after a week of rivastigmine treatment identified those who responded in the longer term (Adler et al., 2004).

10.1.3.3 EEG CHANGES WITH DISEASE PROGRESSION

Patients with EEG abnormalities on visual inspection at the time of diagnosis may have a shorter survival than those whose EEGs are normal when diagnosed (Kaszniak et al., 1978; Soininen et al., 1991). The presence of qEEG abnormalities at diagnosis also has been associated with a more rapid progression of the disorder (Lopez et al., 1997; Nobili et al., 1999) and earlier death (Claus et al., 1998). As the disease progresses there is a gradual reduction in α power and an increase in θ power, or reduction in the α/θ ratio (Coben et al., 1985; Soininen et al., 1991; Förstl et al., 1996; Rodriguez et al., 1999a). Fast activity shifts from a predominance in posterior regions to the frontal region (Ihl et al., 1989b). Mean EEG frequency, θ and δ power correlate with global dementia severity (Penttilä et al., 1985) and more specifically parietal dysfunction (Edman et al., 1998; Matousek et al., 2001). The precise relationship between qEEG markers and disease progression is inconsistent and Förstl et al. (1996) have pointed out that EEG measures are so variable that they are less useful in predicting the course of AD than the actual cognitive performance of the patient.

10.1.3.4 DIAGNOSTIC USE OF EEG IN AD

The EEG may be 'visually' normal in the early stages of AD and Robinson et al. (1994) reported that a 'normal' EEG ruled out the diagnosis in 83 per cent of cases. Claus et al. (1999) used a method of scoring the visual appearance of the EEG and at the optimal cut-point this had positive predictive value of 88 per cent, although it had a relatively modest negative predictive value. Many studies have attempted to use qEEG to discriminate between AD patients and healthy elderly subjects but there has been little overall agreement about the best variables to use. Jonkman (1997) reviewed studies up to 1994 and found a reported accuracy of diagnosis ranging between 54 and 100 per cent. However, sensitivity was low when qEEG was being used as a screening tool in populations with a low prevalence of AD. In general, the diagnostic performance of these measures is reduced in early or mild cases. Table 10.1 shows a selection of studies from 1996 indicating the variability of diagnostic usefulness and discriminator variables.

Nott and Fleminger (1975) found that visual inspection of the EEG did not reliably differentiate between dementia and depression, although this view has been contested (Ron et al., 1979). Non-specific abnormalities of the EEG may be found in up to 40 per cent of patients with affective disorders (Wright et al., 1986). Adler et al. (1999) found increased δ and θ power in depressed patients with cognitive impairment when compared with those without, and Dahabra et al. (1998) demonstrated that these abnormalities persisted after recovery.

Table 10.1   *Performance of quantitative EEG as a diagnostic test (studies from 1996): patients with Alzheimer's disease (AD) versus healthy older people*

Study	Year of publication	No. of AD patients (mean age in years)	No. of controls	Positive predictive value (%)	Negative predictive value (%)	Optimal discriminating variables
Jelic *et al.*	1996	18 (61)	16	100	80	Relative $\alpha + \theta$ power + temporoparietal coherence
Wada *et al.*	1997	9 (57)	9	80	90	Occipital α power to 10 Hz photic stimulation
Strijers *et al.*	1997	9 (81)	49	50	93	Absolute θ power
Besthorn *et al.*	1997	50 (69)	42	95	83	Age + 7 groups of variables (including coherence and α blocking)
Rodriguez *et al.*	1998	42 (72)	18	94	57	Right temporoparietal relative $\alpha + \beta + \theta$ power
Huang *et al.*	2000	38 (63)	24	89	80	Relative θ power
Ihl *et al.*	2000	36 (69)	44	89	93	Topography of β and δ activity + δ power

10.1.4 Vascular dementias (VaD)

Mild cerebrovascular disease is associated with appearance of slow and sharp waves in the temporal region (Inui *et al.*, 2001). The EEG of multi-infarct dementia (MID) is similar to that of AD, but focal and paroxysmal abnormalities are more prominent and there is greater asymmetry of activity (Sloan and Fenton, 1992; d'Onofrio *et al.*, 1996). Slow wave activity correlates with cerebral metabolism (Szelies *et al.*, 1999). Despite this the EEG is likely to be normal, particularly in the early stages (Sloan *et al.*, 1995).

Leuchter *et al.* (1994) found that patients with periventricular white matter hyperintensities had lower EEG coherence in the pre- and post-Rolandic areas. This effect was present in areas connected by fibres crossing the periventricular region, but not in those connected by long corticocortical tracts suggesting that vascular lesions might bring about different types of neurophysiological disconnection depending on their distribution. Indeed, studies of EEG coherence suggest that this may be a useful way of distinguishing between MID and AD (Leuchter *et al.*, 1992).

10.1.5 Parkinson's disease (PD) and dementia with Lewy bodies (DLB)

In cognitively intact PD patients, the EEG is essentially normal, but abnormalities such as slowing of the occipital α frequency and an increase in diffuse fast activity age are present in approximately 30 per cent of patients (Neufeldt *et al.*, 1994). It is now thought that dementia in PD is part of spectrum that also includes DLB (McKeith *et al.*, 2004). The appearance of transient slow waves in the temporal region (Briel *et al.*, 1999) or bilateral frontal intermittent rhythmic δ activity (FIRDA) (Calzetti *et al.*, 2002) may be useful diagnostic markers, although this has been disputed by others (Barber *et al.*, 2000; Londos *et al.*, 2003). Walker *et al.* (2000b) reported the successful use of a battery of attentional and cognitive measures including mean EEG frequency to distinguish between DLB,

AD and VaD. A greater variation of slow wave activity was characteristic of DLB and this correlated with fluctuations in cognition (Walker *et al.*, 2000a).

10.1.6 Creutzfeldt–Jakob disease (CJD)

The characteristic EEG changes of biphasic or triphasic periodic sharp wave complexes (PSWC) occurring at 1–2 Hz appear within the first 3 months of the condition in nearly 90 per cent of cases (Levy *et al.*, 1986). However, runs of frontal δ activity often precede the onset of PSWC (Hansen *et al.*, 1998) and PSWC tend to disappear in the terminal stages of the disease in many cases. The timing of the EEG can therefore be crucial and a study involving serial EEG recordings suggested that PSWC appear in conjunction with the motor symptoms of CJD (Hansen *et al.*, 1998). A large international study has reported that PSWC were present on EEG in 66 per cent of pathologically confirmed cases. The positive predictive value of this marker was 93 per cent (Zerr *et al.*, 2000).

10.1.7 Other dementias

The EEG in Pick's disease is usually normal until the dementia is fairly well established (Gordon and Sim, 1967). Likewise, no specific abnormalities are associated with frontotemporal dementia (FTD). Indeed, a 'normal' EEG is one of the core diagnostic features (Lund and Manchester Groups, 1994). However, qEEG may be useful in distinguishing between FTD and AD (Lindau *et al.*, 2003). In Huntington's disease there is a general poverty of rhythmic activity but an irregular low-voltage slow waveform emerges, which correlates with the severity of cognitive impairment (Bylsma *et al.*, 1994) and the degree of cortical atrophy found at autopsy (Scott *et al.*, 1972).

10.1.8 Delirium

It is sometimes necessary to distinguish between 'organic' and non-organic causes of acute onset mental dysfunction, the latter being associated with severe depression, mania or acute psychosis. An abnormal EEG generally indicates an organic cause, but the abnormalities identifiable by visual inspection can depend on the underlying cause of the delirium. Generalized slowing may indicate a diffuse encephalopathy, excessive fast activity delirium tremens or a tranquillizer overdose (Binnie and Prior, 1994). Koponen *et al.* (1989) compared elderly delirious patients with healthy subjects and found that the former showed reductions in α power. The mean EEG frequency correlated with the severity of cognitive impairment. The presence of EEG changes during delirium may predict subsequent deterioration in cognitive state (Katz *et al.*, 2001). θ power may be the most sensitive discriminator between delirious and non-delirious patients (Jacobson *et al.*, 1993).

10.2 SLEEP EEG

There is a gradual reduction in total night-time sleep throughout adult life, although much of this occurs before the age of 30. The duration of slow wave or 'deep' sleep (stages 3 and 4) falls and there is an increase in the number of periods of wakefulness (Prinz *et al.*, 1990). The latter occur more frequently in non-REM sleep, particularly stages 1 and 2 (Boselli *et al.*, 1998). There is also a reduction in both amplitude and quantity of δ waves even in healthy adults not troubled by insomnia, but other waveforms and REM sleep are less affected. Sleep spindles and K-complexes fall in number with age (Crowley *et al.*, 2002) and in addition to the relative lightening of night-time sleep there is an increase in day-time napping (Prinz *et al.*, 1990). Overall the changes suggest an increase in cortical activation during sleep (Carrier *et al.*, 2001).

The changes associated with ageing are more pronounced in dementia. There is a reduction in the period spent in deep sleep (stage 4 is often absent), very little REM sleep and frequent awakenings. Sleep spindles and K-complexes are poorly formed and often are absent (Prinz *et al.*, 1982). Montplaisir *et al.* (1998) suggested that the degree of REM sleep EEG slowing mirrored the topographical pattern of cortical abnormalities found in AD. Grace *et al.* (2000) found that sleep disturbances were more severe in DLB than in AD and that treatment with rivastigmine helped normalize sleep in some patients. Indeed, more severe behavioural or motor disturbance during REM sleep may be particularly associated with DLB (Boeve *et al.*, 1998), although disordered sleep is also common in Huntington's disease (Wiegand *et al.*, 1991).

The slowing of the mean frequency seen in the conventional EEG is more prominent in REM sleep and has been used to discriminate between patients with mild AD and healthy subjects (Prinz *et al.*, 1992; Montplaisir *et al.*, 1995). These changes contrast with those found in elderly depressed patients to the extent that measures, such as REM latency or density have been used to discriminate between the two groups (Reynolds *et al.*, 1988; Moe *et al.*, 1993; Dykierek *et al.*, 1998). Reynolds

et al. (1988) did include a comparison of patients with depressive 'pseudodementia' and those with progressive dementia complicated by depressive features. The combination of four sleep EEG measures enabled correct classification of 64 per cent of patients. It is doubtful, however, whether the sleep EEG has much to offer in clinical practice. A diagnosis of dementia would not necessarily rule out a good response to antidepressants in an individual patient.

10.3 EVOKED POTENTIALS

An evoked potential (EP) is the sequence of EEG changes following a sensory stimulus. If the stimulus is repeated, the specific EEG pattern related to it can be discerned by 'averaging' the responses and removing the effects of spontaneous background activity. EPs are made up of a number of wave forms or components representing electrical activity at different levels in the central nervous system usually occurring within 300 ms of the stimulus. They are numbered by convention or by reference to their latency. EPs are essentially passive responses, requiring no special effort on the part of the subject. This distinguishes them from 'event-related' potentials, discussed below. The topographical distribution of the responses can be 'mapped'.

10.3.1 Visual evoked potentials (VEPs)

Visual potentials are commonly evoked either by flashes of light (FVEP) or pattern reversal, as in checkerboard shifts or multifocal stimulation (PRVEP). These techniques are used to assess the integrity of the optic tract (Aminoff and Goodin, 1994). Potential latency and amplitude may be altered by a great number of factors including gender, head size, systemic disease, visual acuity, accommodation and attention.

10.3.1.1 VEPS IN AGEING AND DEMENTIA

Age is an important factor accounting for the variability of VEPs (Pitt and Daldry, 1988). The change is likely to be due to physical attributes within the eye (Crow *et al.*, 2003). There is an exaggerated or augmented response to increasing the intensity of the stimulus reflecting a reduction in cortical inhibition (Dustman *et al.*, 1981).

A number of studies report the increased latency of components of FVEPs in AD, particularly the P2 wave, which arises in the visual association cortex (Table 10.2). The latency delay of the P2 correlates with dementia severity (Coburn *et al.*, 2003). The early positive peak of the PRVEP (the P1 or P100), which arises in the visual cortex, is usually within normal limits, although later components may also be delayed (Visser *et al.*, 1985; Philpot *et al.*, 1990). A significant P2–P100 latency difference was initially thought to be a specific marker for AD (Harding *et al.*, 1985) but later was shown to be non-specific (Wright and Furlong, 1988; Sloan and Fenton, 1992). The

Table 10.2 *Abnormalities reported in visual evoked responses: patients with Alzheimer's disease (AD) versus healthy older people*

Study	Year of publication	No. of AD patients (mean age in years)	No. of controls	PR P100 latency delay	Flash P2 latency delay	P2–P100 difference
Harding *et al.*	1985	20 (64)	20	X	✓	✓
Visser *et al.*	1985	39 (76)	48	✓	n/d	n/d
Wright *et al.*	1986	41 (64)	30	X	✓	✓
Pollock *et al.*	1989	16 (67)	16	✓	X	n/d
Philpot *et al.*	1990	25 (75)	13	X	✓	✓
Coburn *et al.*	1991	23 (75)	12	X	✓	✓
Sloan and Fenton	1992	40 (74)	30	X	✓	✓
Swanwick *et al.*	1996b	16 (71)	15	n/d	✓	n/d
Coburn *et al.*	2003	45 (73)	60	X	✓	✓

n/d, not done; X, no difference between AD patients and controls; ✓, significant difference between AD patients and controls

diagnostic accuracy of the P2–P100 measure in studies of AD patients compared with healthy subjects is reported as between 60 and 80 per cent though the P2 latency may be a more effective diagnostic measure on its own (Coburn *et al.*, 2003).

Longitudinal studies of VEPs in AD fail to demonstrate progressive delay of components (Sloan and Fenton, 1992; Swanwick *et al.*, 1996a). Consequently, the clinical use VEPs may be restricted to early diagnosis although Moore *et al.* (1996) demonstrated that subjects with mild cognitive impairment also had delayed flash P2 latency. The long-held view that the peripheral visual pathway is unaffected in AD has been challenged. Using electroretinography, an EP technique that records electrical activity in the ganglion cells of the retina, a significant reduction in response amplitude was found in AD patients (Trick *et al.*, 1989; Katz *et al.*, 1989).

PRVEPs are delayed in PD (Nightingale *et al.*, 1986; Calzetti *et al.*, 1990), especially in patients with PD and dementia (Okuda *et al.*, 1996). The PR P100 delay in PD can be reversed by dopaminergic drugs and induced or worsened by antipsychotic drugs (Onofrj *et al.*, 1986).

10.3.2 Auditory evoked potentials (AEPs)

Repeated clicks or tones are used as the stimulus in AEPs and the major waveforms are generated in the auditory brain stem and the auditory association areas. AEPs are also used in the assessment of demyelinating diseases, acoustic neuroma and coma. Transmission delays are frequently caused by ageing changes in the peripheral auditory apparatus or the brain stem (Amenedo and Diaz, 1998). Delays in major peaks have been reported in dementia (Hendrickson *et al.*, 1979), although the variability of later peaks may be so great that significant delays are not found (Knott *et al.*, 1999). Electrodes may be placed so as to record activity in the brain stem. Green *et al.* (1997) found that the P1 component of this response was missing in about half AD patients tested. These patients also had a delay in the contralateral blink reflex response suggesting that there was a dysfunction of the reticular formation. Tachibana *et al.* (1989a) found increased interpeak latencies in both AD and MID and significant delays were also found in patients with Parkinson's disease and dementia (Tachibana *et al.*, 1989b).

Similar abnormalities have been found in patients with CJD (Pollak *et al.*, 1996) and Huntington's disease (Uc *et al.*, 2003).

10.3.3 Somatosensory evoked potentials (SSEPs)

SSEPs are used in the functional assessment of spinal cord lesions as well as the detection of subclinical lesions in multiple sclerosis. Levy *et al.* (1971) employed ulnar nerve stimulation and showed delayed N35 (or N2) in patients with dementia as compared with those with depression. Amplitudes were also reduced. Huisman *et al.* (1985) confirmed the delay of all peaks after P25 using the more frequently employed median nerve stimulation. Kato *et al.* (1990) reported that SSEP peak latency correlated with the degree of white matter low attenuation in MID, and Okuda *et al.* (1996) found delayed SSEPs in patients with Binswanger's disease but not with PD. Shiga *et al.* (2001) found a reduction in amplitude of N20 in patients with CJD.

10.4 EVENT-RELATED POTENTIALS

Event-related potentials (ERPs) require some 'active' cognitive participation from the subject and therefore demonstrate the integrity of information processing pathways. The most commonly investigated waveform component is the positive peak occurring at around 300 ms after the stimulus or task, the P300 or P3. The subject has to differentiate between two stimuli; for example a frequently presented low tone and an infrequently presented high tone. This is known as the 'oddball' paradigm. The order of stimuli is semirandom so as to increase the unpredictability of the high or 'target' tone. To ensure attention, subjects usually have to register their awareness of the target by pressing a button. Reaction time can thus be measured.

The requirement that the task has to be attended to can be a problem in older, cognitively impaired or unmotivated individuals. Mismatch negativity (MMN) forms part of the negative N2 peak arising at around 200 ms after stimulus offset and is elicited whether or not the subject makes a discriminative response. The 'mismatch' in question occurs between the sensory memory trace of the frequent stimulus and the target.

10.4.1 Auditory ERPs

In cross-sectional studies of different age groups P3 latency increases with age and amplitude reduces (Ford et al., 1997; Anderer et al., 2003). The effect on latency may be more pronounced in men (Hirayasu et al., 2000). The distribution of the reduction has been reported as maximal in the temporoparietal region (Frodl et al., 2000) and the frontal region (Anderer et al., 2003). However, latency, amplitude and distribution all are affected by the nature of task involved (Fein and Turetsky, 1989; Fjell and Walhovd, 2001), the type of auditory stimulus employed and whether effort is required in processing (Squires and Ollo, 1999; Federmeier et al., 2002). MMN amplitudes are reduced in older adults (Kazmerski et al., 1997; Bertoli et al., 2002). In longitudinal studies, P3 latency and amplitude are relatively consistent over periods up to 3 years (Sandman and Patterson, 2000; Walhovd and Fjell, 2002).

Many studies have reported the P3 latency delay and reduced amplitude in AD patients (Goodin, 1990; Williams et al., 1991; Swanwick et al., 1996b; Ford et al., 1997) but others have failed to do so (St. Clair et al., 1985; Kraiuhin et al., 1990; Ruessman et al., 1990). MMN amplitudes are smaller in patients with mild AD than in healthy older people suggesting a degraded sensory memory trace in the early stages of the disease (Kazmerski et al., 1997). P3 abnormalities correlate with the degree of cognitive impairment (Blackwood et al., 1987) and worsen along with intellectual deterioration (St. Clair et al., 1988; Ball et al., 1989; Swanwick et al., 1997). Treatment with cholinesterase inhibitors reduced P3 latency but not amplitude in two recent open studies (Katada et al., 2003; Werber et al., 2003).

Goodin (1990) reviewed 12 studies published up until 1988 and found that the average sensitivity of the P3 latency as a marker of dementia was just 51 per cent, ranging from 7 to 83 per cent. Results of more recent studies, which have included comparisons with depressed patients (Kraiuhin et al., 1990; Polich et al., 1990; Attias et al., 1995; Swanwick et al., 1996b) report sensitivities ranging from 82 to 100 per cent but the positive predictive value of an abnormal result is still relatively modest. Pfefferbaum et al. (1990) have cast doubt on the clinical utility of AERPs given the wide range of sensitivity and the fact that abnormalities of latency and amplitude occur in many other neurological and psychiatric disorders, such as PD (Tanaka et al., 2000; Wang et al., 2002). Filipovic et al. (1990) were unable to distinguish between patients with AD, Huntington's chorea and PD with or without dementia using AERPs. Patients in this study had been carefully matched for dementia severity and a delayed P3 occurred in two-thirds irrespective of diagnosis. Similarly, the utility of the P3 in distinguishing between MID and AD is contested (Neshige et al., 1988; Yamaguchi et al., 2000).

10.4.2 Visual ERPs

The 'oddball' paradigm can be adapted to the visual modality. Here, a frequently presented pattern, letter or word is displayed with an infrequently presented one, or words may be paired with pictures (Ford et al., 2001). Increased latency and reduced amplitude of the P3 component (Saito et al., 2001) and attenuation of the error response (Mathalon et al., 2003) have been reported. The visual modality has been used less than the auditory one to investigate AD but Pfefferbaum et al. (1984) found that reaction time to the visual stimuli was the best measure for discriminating between demented and depressed patients.

P3 latency and reaction time were significantly longer in a group of non-demented PD patients but the degree of slowing was unrelated to clinical features (Tachibana et al., 1997). Similar abnormalities have been reported in cognitively impaired patients with supranuclear palsy (Johnson, 1995) and Huntington's disease (Münte et al., 1997).

10.4.3 Olfactory ERPs

The sense of smell is particularly prone to the effects of ageing (Doty et al., 1984). It has recently become possible to study olfactory ERPs using measured doses of volatile substances such as amyl acetate. Olfactory neurones take up to 90 s to recover from responding to a single stimulus, making it technically difficult to record responses. However, the major components of olfactory ERPs are delayed in latency and reduced in amplitude in older people (Hummel et al., 1998; Murphy et al., 2000). Initial studies indicate that peak latencies are further delayed in AD and that this correlates with dementia severity (Morgan and Murphy, 2002; Peters et al., 2003).

10.5 OTHER TECHNOLOGIES

10.5.1 Magnetoencephalography (MEG)

During the last 20 years techniques to measure the magnetic fields generated by electrical activity within the brain have been developed. 'Whole-head' MEG can capture magnetic field information from up to 100 locations on the scalp enabling the mapping of the sources of abnormal fields or waveform frequencies and amplitudes (Roberts et al., 1998). The technique has a higher temporal resolution than EEG, despite the tiny fields generated, that may be improved by combination with other imaging methods such as magnetic source imaging or functional magnetic resonance (Roberts et al., 1998). Early studies of AD patients have confirmed the decreased fast wave power, increased slow wave activity and decreased coherence found using conventional EEG techniques (Berendse et al., 2000; Stam et al., 2002; Fernandez et al., 2003). MEG activity correlates with volumetric measures of brain structures, such as the hippocampus (Maestu et al., 2003).

10.5.2 Transcranial magnetic stimulation (TMS)

Traditionally, electrical stimuli have been used to excite cortical areas, either via intracerebral electrodes or during the course of neurosurgical procedures. TMS employs powerful, rapidly alternating magnetic fields and allows a non-invasive method of electrically stimulating the cortex (George *et al.*, 1996). It has also been used in the treatment of depression (Grunhaus *et al.*, 2003). In AD, interest has centred on the use of TMS to determine motor cortex excitability. When magnetic stimulation is applied to the appropriate parts of the motor cortex, movements of upper or lower limbs can be induced. The threshold (or 'dose' of magnetic field) at which this happens is reduced in AD (De Carvalho *et al.*, 1997; Ferreri *et al.*, 2003). This change correlates with dementia severity (Alagona *et al.*, 2001) and may worsen as the disease progresses (Pennisi *et al.*, 2002). Cholinesterase inhibitors such as donepezil (Liepert *et al.*, 2001) and rivastigmine (Di Lazzaro *et al.*, 2002) have been shown to reverse this abnormality in the short term.

10.6 SUMMARY

Before the advent of brain CT the EEG had a prominent role in clinical practice and probably still does in centres where neuroimaging is not readily available. The conventional EEG remains the most reliable and cost-effective method of neurophysiological investigation in dementia. Its main clinical uses remain the differentiation of organic disorders (including delirium) from non-organic disorders and to support the diagnosis of epilepsy (Binnie and Prior, 1994).

Clinicians have been criticized for their injudicious requests for EEGs in the assessment of dementia, and the low yield of results that affect the patient's management is well known (Binnie and Prior, 1994; Philpot and Pereira, 2002). Nearly all the studies referred to in this chapter have compared well-characterized groups of subjects with each other, rather than including cases in which there have been real uncertainties about the diagnosis. Very few have confirmed diagnosis at autopsy. Perhaps as a result, the technologically attractive techniques such as evoked and event-related potentials, and MEG, do not yet have a place in routine clinical practice and, because of their lack of specificity, do not present the hoped-for short cut to diagnosis. Indeed, neurophysiological methods no longer figure in the latest practice guidelines for the diagnosis of dementia (Royal College of Psychiatrists, 1995; Knopman *et al.*, 2001). However, as research methods they clearly have continuing potential in augmenting knowledge derived from other approaches.

REFERENCES

Adler G and Brassen S. (2001) Short-term rivastigmine treatment reduces EEG slow-wave power in Alzheimer's patients. *Neuropsychobiology* **43**: 273–276

Adler G, Bramesfield A, Jajcevic A. (1999) Mild cognitive impairment in old-age depression is associated with increased EEG slow-wave power. *Neuropsychobiology* **40**: 218–222

Adler G, Brassen S, Chwalek K *et al.* (2004) Prediction of treatment response to rivastigmine in Alzheimer's disease. *Journal of Neurology, Neurosurgery, and Psychiatry* **75**: 292–294

Alagona G, Bella R, Ferri R *et al.* (2001) Transcranial magnetic stimulation in Alzheimer's disease: motor cortex excitability and cognitive severity. *Neuroscience Letters* **314**: 57–60

Almkvist O, Jelic V, Amberla K *et al.* (2001) Responder characteristics to a single oral dose of cholinesterase inhibitor: a double-blind placebo-controlled study with tacrine in Alzheimer's patients. *Dementia and Geriatric Cognitive Disorders* **12**: 22–32

Amenedo E and Diaz F. (1998) Effects of aging on middle latency auditory evoked potentials: a cross-sectional study. *Biological Psychiatry* **43**: 210–299

Aminoff MJ and Goodin DS. (1994) Visual evoked potentials. *Journal of Clinical Neurophysiology* **11**: 493–499

Anderer P, Saletu B, Semlitsch HV, Pascual-Marqui RD. (2003) Non-invasive localization of P300 sources in normal aging and age-associated memory impairment. *Neurobiology of Aging* **24**: 463–479

Attias J, Huberman M, Cott E, Pratt H. (1995) Improved detection of auditory P3 abnormality in dementia using a variety of stimuli. *Acta Neurologica Scandinavica* **92**: 96–101

Ball SS, Marsh JT, Scubarth G *et al.* (1989) Longitudinal P300 latency changes in Alzheimer's disease. *Journal of Gerontology* **44**: M195–200

Barber PA, Varma AR, Lloyd JJ *et al.* (2000) The electroencephalogram in dementia with Lewy bodies. *Acta Neurologica Scandinavica* **101**: 53–56

Berendse HW, Verbrunt JP, Scheltens P *et al.* (2000) Magneto-encephalographic analysis of cortical activity in Alzheimer's disease: a pilot study. *Clinical Neurophysiology* **111**: 604–612

Berger H. (1932) Uber das Elektrencephalogramm des Menschen V. English translation by Gloor P. (1969) Hans Berger and the electroencephalogram. *Electroencephalography and Clinical Neurophysiology* **28**(Suppl.): 151–171

Bertoli S, Smuzynski J, Probst R. (2002) Temporal resolution in young and elderly subjects as measured by mismatch negativity and a psychoacoustic gap detection task. *Clinical Neurophysiology* **113**: 396–406

Besthorn C, Zerfass R, Geiger-Kabisch C *et al.* (1997) Discrimination of Alzheimer's disease and normal aging by EEG data. *Electroencephalography and Clinical Neurophysiology* **103**: 241–248

Binnie CD and Prior PF. (1994) Electroencephalography. *Journal of Neurology, Neurosurgery, and Psychiatry* **57**: 1308–1319

Blackwood DHR, St Clair DM, Blackburn IM, Tyrer GMB. (1987) Cognitive brain potentials and psychological deficits in Alzheimer's dementia and Korsakoff's amnesic syndrome. *Psychological Medicine* **17**: 349–358

Boeve BF, Silber MH, Ferman TJ *et al.* (1998) REM sleep behaviour disorder and degenerative dementia. *Neurology* **51**: 363–70

Boselli M, Parrino L, Smerieri A, Terzano MG. (1998) Effects of age on EEG arousal in normal sleep. *Sleep* **21**: 351–358

Briel RC, McKeith IG, Barker QA *et al.* (1999) EEG findings in dementia with Lewy bodies and Alzheimer's disease. *Journal of Neurology, Neurosurgery, and Psychiatry* **66**: 401–403

Busse EW and Obrist WD. (1965) Pre-senescent electro-encephalographic changes in normal subjects. *Journal of Gerontology* **20**: 315–320

Bylsma FW, Peyser CE, Folstein SE *et al.* (1994) EEG power spectra in Huntington's disease: clinical and neuropsychological correlates. *Neuropsychologia* **32**: 137–150

Calzetti S, Franchi A, Taratufolo G, Groppi E. (1990) Simultaneous VEP and PERG investigations in early Parkinson's disease. *Journal of Neurology, Neurosurgery, and Psychiatry* **53**: 114–147

Calzetti S, Bortone E, Negrotti A *et al.* (2002) Frontal intermittent rhythmic delta activity (FIRDA) in patients with dementia with Lewy bodies: a diagnostic tool? *Neurological Sciences* **23** (Suppl. 2): S65–S66

Carrier J, Land S, Buysse DJ *et al.* (2001) The effects of age and gender on sleep EEG power spectral density in the middle years of life (ages 20–60 years old). *Psychophysiology* **38**: 232–242

Claus JJ, van Gool WA, Teunisse S *et al.* (1998) Predicting survival in patients with early Alzheimer's disease. *Dementia and Geriatric Cognitive Disorders* **9**: 284–293

Claus JJ, Strijers RLM, Jonkman EJ *et al.* (1999) The diagnostic value of electroencephalography in mild senile Alzheimer's disease. *Clinical Neurophysiology* **110**: 825–832

Claus JJ, Ongerboer De Visser BW, Bour LJ *et al.* (2000) Determinants of quantitative spectral electroencephalography in early Alzheimer's disease: cognitive function, regional cerebral blood flow, and computed tomography. *Dementia and Geriatric Cognitive Disorders* **11**: 81–89

Coben LA, Danziger W, Storandt M. (1985) A longitudinal EEG study of mild senile dementia of Alzheimer type: changes at 1 year and at 2.5 years. *Electroencephalography and Clinical Neurophysiology* **61**: 101–112

Coburn KL, Ashford JW, Moreno MA. (1991) Visual evoked potentials in dementia: selective delay of flash P2 in probable Alzheimer's disease. *Journal of Neuropsychiatry and Clinical Neurosciences* **3**: 431–435

Coburn KL, Arruda JE, Estes KM, Amoss RT. (2003) Diagnostic utility of visual evoked potential changes in Alzheimer's disease. *Journal of Neuropsychiatry and Clinical Neurosciences* **15**: 175–179

Crow RW, Levin LB, LaBree L, Rubin R, Feldon SE. (2003) Sweep visual potential evaluation of contrast sensitivity in Alzheimer's dementia. *Investigations in Ophthalmology and Vision Science* **44**: 875–878

Crowley K, Trinder J, Kim Y *et al.* (2002) The effects of normal aging on sleep spindle and K-complex production. *Clinical Neurophysiology* **113**: 1615–1622

Dahabra S, Ashton CH, Bahrainian M *et al.* (1998) Structural and functional abnormalities in elderly patients clinically recovered from early- and late-onset depression. *Biological Psychiatry* **44**: 34–46

De Carvalho M, de Mendonca A, Miranda PC *et al.* (1997) Magnetic stimulation in Alzheimer's disease. *Journal of Neurology* **244**: 304–307

Di Lazzaro V, Oliviero A, Tonali PA *et al.* (2002) Noninvasive in vivo assessment of cholinergic cortical circuits in AD using transcranial magnetic stimulation. *Neurology* **59**: 392–397

Dierks T, Jelic V, Pasqual-Marqui RD *et al.* (2000) Spatial pattern of cerebral glucose metabolism (PET) correlates with localization of intracerebral EEG-generators in Alzheimer's disease. *Clinical Neurophysiology* **111**: 1817–1824

d'Onofrio F, Salvia S, Petretta V *et al.* (1996) Quantified-EEG in normal aging and dementias. *Acta Neurologica Scandinavica* **93**: 336–345

Doty RL, Shaman P, Applebaum SL *et al.* (1984) Smell identification ability: changes with age. *Science* **226**: 1441–1443

Dustman RE, Snyder EW, Schlehuber CJ. (1981) Life-span alterations in visually evoked potentials and inhibitory function. *Neurobiology of Aging* **2**: 187–192

Dustman RE, Shearer DE, Emmerson RY. (1999) Life-span changes in EEG spectral amplitude, amplitude variability and mean frequency. *Clinical Neurophysiology* **110**: 1399–1409

Dykiererk P, Stadmuller G, Schramm P *et al.* (1998) The value of REM sleep parameters in differentiating Alzheimer's disease from old-age depression and normal aging. *Journal of Psychiatric Research* **32**: 1–9

Edman Å, Matousek M, Sjögren M, Wallin A. (1998) Longitudinal EEG findings in dementia related to the parietal brain syndrome and the degree of dementia. *Dementia and Geriatric Cognitive Disorders* **9**: 199–204

Edwards-Lee T, Cook I, Fairbanks L *et al.* (2000) Quantitative electroencephalographic correlates of psychosis in Alzheimer's disease. *Neuropsychiatry, Neuropsychology and Behavioural Neurology* **13**: 163–170

Elmståhl S and Rosén I. (1997) Postural hypotension and EEG variables predict cognitive decline: results from a 5-year follow up of healthy elderly women. *Dementia and Geriatric Cognitive Disorders* **8**: 180–187

Federmeier KD, McLennan DB, De Ochoa E, Kutas M. (2002) The impact of semantic memory organization and sentence context information on spoken language processing by younger and older adults: an ERP study. *Psychophysiology* **39**: 133–146

Fein G and Turetsky B. (1989) P300 latency variability in normal elderly: effects of paradigm and measurement technique. *Electroencephalography and Clinical Neurophysiology* **72**: 384–394

Fernandez A, Arrazola J, Maestu F *et al.* (2003) Correlation of hippocampal atrophy and focal low-frequency magnetic activity in Alzheimer's disease: volumetric MR imaging-magnetoencephalographic study. *American Journal of Neuroradiology* **24**: 481–487

Ferreri F, Pauri F, Pasqualetti P *et al.* (2003) Motor cortex excitability in Alzheimer's disease: a transcranial magnetic stimulation study. *Annals of Neurology* **53**: 102–108

Filipovic S, Kostic VS, Sternic N *et al.* (1990) Auditory event-related potentials in different types of dementia. *European Neurology* **30**: 189–193

Fjell AM and Walhovd KB. (2001) P300 and neuropsychological tests as measures of aging: scalp topography and cognitive changes. *Brain Topography* **14**: 25–40

Ford JM, Roth WT, Isaacks BG *et al.* (1997) Automatic and effortful processing in aging and dementia: event-related brain potentials. *Neurobiology of Aging* **18**: 169–180

Ford JM, Askari N, Mathalon DH *et al.* (2001) Event-related brain potential evidence of spared knowledge in Alzheimer's disease. *Psychology of Aging* **16**: 161–176

Förstl H, Sattel H, Besthorn C *et al.* (1996) Longitudinal cognitive, electroencephalographic and morphological brain changes in ageing and Alzheimer's disease. *British Journal of Psychiatry* **168**: 280–286

Frodl T, Juckel G, Gallinat J *et al.* (2000) Dipole localization of P300 and normal aging. *Brain Topography* **13**: 3–9

George MS, Wasserman EM, Post RM. (1996) Transcranial magnetic stimulation: a neuropsychiatric tool for the 21st century. *Journal of Neuropsychiatry and Clinical Neuroscience* **8**: 373–382

Goodin DS. (1990) Clinical utility of long latency 'cognitive' event-related potentials (P3): the pros. *Electroencephalography and Clinical Neurophysiology* **76**: 2–5

Gordon EB and Sim M. (1967) The E.E.G. in presenile dementia. *Journal of Neurology, Neurosurgery, and Psychiatry* **30**: 285–291

Grace JB, Walker MP, McKeith IG. (2000) A comparison of sleep profiles in patients with dementia with Lewy bodies and Alzheimer's disease. *International Journal of Geriatric Psychiatry* **15**: 1028–1033

Green JB, Burba A, Freed DM *et al.* (1997) The P1 component of the middle latency auditory potential may differentiate a brainstem subgroup of Alzheimer disease. *Alzheimer Disease and Associated Disorders* **11**: 153–157

Grunhaus L, Schreiber S, Dolberg OT *et al.* (2003) A randomised controlled comparison of electroconvulsive therapy and repetitive transcranial magnetic stimulation in severe and resistant non-psychotic major depression. *Biological Psychiatry* **53**: 324–331

Grunwald M, Busse F, Hensel A *et al.* (2001) Correlation between cortical theta activity and hippocampal volumes in health, mild cognitive impairment and mild dementia. *Journal of Clinical Neurophysiology* **18**: 178–184

Hansen H-C, Zschocke S, Stürenburg H-J, Kunze K. (1998) Clinical changes and EEG patterns preceding the onset of periodic sharp wave complexes in Creutzfeldt–Jakob disease. *Acta Neurologica Scandinavica* **97**: 99–106

Harding GFA, Wright CE, Orwin A. (1985) Primary presenile dementia: the use of the visual evoked potential as a diagnostic indicator. *British Journal of Psychiatry* **147**: 532–539

Hendrickson E, Levy R, Post F. (1979) Averaged evoked responses in relation to cognitive and affective state of elderly psychiatric patients. *British Journal of Psychiatry* **134**: 494–501

Hirayasu Y, Samura M, Ohta H, Ogura C. (2000) Sex effects of rate of change of P300 latency with age. *Clinical Neurophysiology* **111**: 187–194

Hogan MJ, Swanwick GR, Kaiser J *et al.* (2003) Memory-related EEG power and coherence reductions in mild Alzheimer's disease. *International Journal of Psychophysiology* **49**: 147–163

Huang C, Wahlund L-O, Dierks T *et al.* (2000) Discrimination of Alzheimer's disease and mild cognitive impairment by equivalent EEG sources: a cross-sectional and longitudinal study. *Clinical Neurophysiology* **111**: 1961–1967

Huisman UW, Posthuma J, Hooijer V *et al.* (1985) Somatosensory evoked potentials in healthy volunteers and patients with dementia. *Clinical Neurology and Neurosurgery* **87**: 11–16

Hummel T, Barz S, Pauli E, Kobal G. (1998) Chemosensory event-related potentials change with age. *Electroencephalography and Clinical Neurophysiology* **108**: 208–217

Ihl R, Eilles C, Frolich F *et al.* (1989a) Electrical brain activity and cerebral blood flow in dementia of the Alzheimer type. *Psychiatry Research* **29**: 449–452

Ihl R, Maurer K, Dierks T *et al.* (1989b) Staging in dementia of the Alzheimer type: topography of electrical brain activity reflects the severity of the disease. *Psychiatry Research* **29**: 399–401

Ihl R, Brinkmeyer J, Janner M, Kerdar MS. (2000) A comparison of ADAS and EEG in the discrimination of patients with dementia of the Alzheimer type from healthy controls. *Neuropsychobiology* **41**: 102–107

Inui K, Motomura E, Kaige H, Nomura S. (2001) Temporal slow waves and cerebrovascular diseases. *Psychiatry and Clinical Neurosciences* **55**: 525–531

Jacobson SA, Leuchter AF, Walter DO. (1993) Conventional and quantitative EEG in the diagnosis of delirium among the elderly. *Journal of Neurology, Neurosurgery, and Psychiatry* **56**: 153–158

Jelic V, Shigeta M, Julin P *et al.* (1996) Quantitative electroencephalography power and coherence in Alzheimer's disease and mild cognitive impairment. *Dementia and Geriatric Cognitive Disorders* **7**: 314–323

Jelic V, Julin P, Shigeta M *et al.* (1997) Apolipoprotein E 4 allele decreases functional connectivity in Alzheimer's disease as measured by EEG coherence. *Journal of Neurology, Neurosurgery, and Psychiatry* **63**: 59–65

Jelic V, Blomberg M, Dierks T *et al.* (1998a) EEG slowing and cerebrospinal fluid tau levels in patients with cognitive decline. *NeuroReport* **9**: 157–60

Jelic V, Dierks T, Amberla K *et al.* (1998b) Longitudinal changes in quantitative EEG during long-term tacrine treatment of patients with Alzheimer's disease. *Neuroscience Letters* **254**: 85–88

Jelic V, Johansson SE, Almkvist O *et al.* (2000) Quantitative electroencephalography in mild cognitive impairment: longitudinal changes and possible prediction of Alzheimer's disease. *Neurobiology of Aging* **21**: 533–540

Johnson R. (1995) On the relation between exogenous and endogenous ERP component activity: evidence from patients with a subcortical dementia. *Electroencephalography and Clinical Neurophysiology* **44** (Suppl.): 414–427

Jonkman EJ. (1997) The role of the electroencephalogram in the diagnosis of dementia of the Alzheimer type: an attempt at technology assessment. *Neurophysiology Clinics* **27**: 211–219

Kaszniak AW, Fox J, Gandell JL *et al.* (1978) Predictors of mortality in presenile and senile dementia. *Annals of Neurology* **3**: 246–252

Katada E, Sato K, Sawaki A *et al.* (2003) Long-term effects of donepezil on P300 auditory event-related potentials in patients with Alzheimer's disease. *Journal of Geriatric Psychiatry and Neurology* **16**: 39–43

Kato H, Sugawara Y, Ito H, Kogure K. (1990) White matter lucencies in multi-infarct dementia: a somatosensory evoked potentials and CT study. *Acta Neurologica Scandinavica* **81**: 181–183

Katz B, Rimmer S, Iragui V, Katzman R. (1989) Abnormal pattern electroretinogram in Alzheimer's disease: evidence for retinal ganglion cell degeneration? *Annals of Neurology* **26**: 221–225

Katz IR, Curyton KJ, TenHave T *et al.* (2001) Validating the diagnosis of delirium and evaluating its association with deterioration over a one-year period. *American Journal of Geriatric Psychiatry* **9**: 148–159

Kazmerski VA, Friedman D, Ritter W. (1997) Mismatch negativity during attend and ignore conditions in Alzheimer's disease. *Biological Psychiatry* **42**: 382–402

Kikuchi M, Wada Y, Koshino Y *et al.* (2000) Effects of normal aging upon interhemispheric EEG coherence: analysis during rest and photic stimulation. *Clinical Electroencephalography* **31**: 170–174

Knopman DS, DeKosky ST, Cummings JL *et al.* (2001) Practice parameter: diagnosis of dementia (an evidence based review). Report of the Quality Standards Subcommittee of the American Academy of Neurology. *Neurology* **56**: 1143–1153

Knott V, Mohr E, Hache N *et al.* (1999) EEG and the passive P300 in dementia of the Alzheimer type. *Clinical Electroencephalography* **30**: 64–72

Knott V, Engeland C, Mohr E *et al.* (2000a) Acute nicotine administration in Alzheimer's disease: an exploratory EEG study. *Neuropsychobiology* **41**: 210–220

Knott V, Mohr E, Mahoney C, Ilivitsky V. (2000b) Pharmaco-EEG test dose response predicts cholinesterase inhibitor treatment outcome in Alzheimer's disease. *Methods in Experimental Clinical Pharmacology* **22**: 115–122

Knott V, Mohr E, Mahoney C, Ilivitsky V. (2001) Quantitative electroencephalography in Alzheimer's disease: comparison with a control group, population norms and mental status. *Journal of Psychiatry and Neuroscience* **26**: 106–116

Kogan EA, Korczyn AD, Virchgovsky RG *et al.* (2001) EEG changes during long-term treatment with donepezil in Alzheimer's disease patients. *Journal of Neural Transmission* **108**: 1167–1173

Koponen H, Partanen J, Paakkonen A et al. (1989) EEG spectral analysis in delirium. *Journal of Neurology, Neurosurgery, and Psychiatry* **52**: 980–985

Kraiuhin C, Gordon E, Coyle S et al. (1990) Normal latency of the P300 event-related potential in mild-to-moderate Alzheimer's disease and depression. *Biological Psychiatry* **28**: 372–386

Lehtovirta M, Partanen J, Kononen M et al. (2000) A longitudinal quantitative EEG study of Alzheimer's disease: relation to apolipoprotein E polymorphism. *Dementia and Geriatric Cognitive Disorders* **11**: 29–35

Leuchter AF, Newton TF, Cook IA et al. (1992) Changes in brain functional connectivity in Alzheimer-type and multi-infarct dementia. *Brain* **115**: 1543–1561

Leuchter AF, Dunjun JJ, Kufkin RB et al. (1994) Effect of white matter disease on functional connections in the aging brain. *Journal of Neurology, Neurosurgery, and Psychiatry* **57**: 1347–1354

Levy R, Isaacs A, Behrman J. (1971) Neurophysiological correlates of senile dementia. II. The somatosensory evoked response. *Psychological Medicine* **1**: 159–165

Levy S, Chiappa K, Burke C, Young R. (1986) Early evolution and incidence of electro-encephalographic abnormalities in Creutzfeldt–Jakob disease. *Journal of Clinical Neurophysiology* **3**: 1–21

Liepert J, Bar KJ, Meske U, Weiller C. (2001) Motor cortex disinhibition in Alzheimer's disease. *Clinical Neurophysiology* **112**: 1436–1441

Lindau M, Jelic V, Johansson SE et al. (2003) Quantitative EEG abnormalities and cognitive dysfunction in fronto-temporal dementia and Alzheimer's disease. *Dementia and Geriatric Cognitive Disorders* **15**: 106–114

Londos E, Passant U, Brun A et al. (2003) Regional cerebral blood flow and EEG in clinically diagnosed dementia with Lewy bodies and Alzheimer's disease. *Archives of Gerontology and Geriatrics* **36**: 231–245

Lopez OL, Brenner RP, Becker JT et al. (1997) EEG spectral abnormalities and psychosis as predictors of cognitive and functional decline in probable Alzheimer's disease. *Neurology* **48**: 1521–1525

Lund and Manchester Groups. (1994) Clinical and neuropathological criteria for frontotemporal dementia. *Journal of Neurology, Neurosurgery, and Psychiatry* **57**: 416–418

McKeith I, Mintzer J, Aarsland D et al. (2004) Dementia with Lewy bodies. *Lancet Neurology* **3**: 19–28

Maestu F, Arrazola J, Fernandez A et al. (2003) Do cognitive patterns of brain magnetic activity correlate with hippocampal atrophy in Alzheimer's disease? *Journal of Neurology, Neurosurgery, and Psychiatry* **74**: 208–212

Mathalon DH, Bennett A, Askari N et al. (2003) Response-monitoring dysfunction in aging and Alzheimer's disease: an event-related potential study. *Neurobiology of Aging* **24**: 675–685

Matousek M, Brunovsky M, Edman A, Wallin A. (2001) EEG abnormalities in dementia reflect the parietal lobe syndrome. *Clinical Neurophysiology* **112**: 1001–1005

Mattia D, Babiloni F, Romigi A et al. (2003) Quantitative EEG and dynamic susceptibility contrast MRI in Alzheimer's disease: a correlative study. *Clinical Neurophysiology* **114**: 1210–1216

Mendez M and Lim G. (2003) Seizures in elderly patients with dementia: epidemiology and management. *Drugs and Aging* **20**: 791–803

Moe K, Larsen L, Prinz P, Vitiello M. (1993) Major unipolar depression and mild Alzheimer's disease. *Electroencephalography and Clinical Neurophysiology* **86**: 238–246

Montplaisir J, Petit D, Larrain D et al. (1995) Sleep in Alzheimer's disease: further considerations on the role of brainstem and forebrain cholinergic populations in sleep-wake mechanisms. *Sleep* **18**: 145–148

Montplaisir J, Petit D, Gauthier S et al. (1998) Sleep disturbances and EEG slowing in Alzheimer's disease. *Sleep Research Online* **1**: 147–151

Moore NC, Vogel RL, Tucker KA et al. (1996) P2 Flash visual evoked response delay may be a marker of cognitive dysfunction in healthy elderly volunteers. *International Psychogeriatrics* **8**: 549–859

Morgan CD and Murphy C. (2002) Olfactory event-related potentials in Alzheimer's disease. *Journal of the International Neuropsychology Society* **8**: 753–763

Münte TF, Ridao-Alonso ME, Preinfalk J et al. (1997) An electrophysiological analysis of altered cognitive functions in Huntington disease. *Archives of Neurology* **54**: 1089–1098

Murphy C, Morgan CD, Geisler MW et al. (2000) Olfactory event-related potentials and aging: normative data. *International Journal of Psychophysiology* **36**: 133–145

Neshige R, Barrett G, Shibasaki H. (1988) Auditory long latency event-related potentials in Alzheimer's disease and multi-infarct dementia. *Journal of Neurology, Neurosurgery, and Psychiatry* **51**: 1120–1125

Neufeldt M, Blumen S, Aitkin I et al. (1994) EEG frequency analysis in demented and non-demented parkinsonian patients. *Dementia and Geriatric Cognitive Disorders* **5**: 23–28

Nightingale S, Mitchell KW, Howe JW. (1986) Visual evoked cortical potentials and pattern electroretinograms in Parkinson's disease and control subjects. *Journal of Neurology, Neurosurgery, and Psychiatry* **49**: 1280–1287

Nobili F, Copello F, Vitali P et al. (1999) Timing of disease progression by quantitative EEG in Alzheimer's patients. *Journal of Clinical Neurophysiology* **16**: 566–573

Nott PN and Fleminger JJ. (1975) Presenile dementia: the difficulties of early diagnosis. *Acta Psychiatrica Scandinavica* **52**: 210–217

Okuda B, Tachibana H, Takeda M et al. (1996) Visual and somatosensory evoked potentials in Parkinson's and Binswanger's disease. *Dementia and Geriatric Cognitive Disorders* **7**: 53–58

Onofrj M, Ghilardi MF, Basciani M, Gambi D. (1986) Visual evoked potentials in Parkinsonism and dopamine blockade reveal a stimulus-dependent dopamine function in humans. *Journal of Neurology, Neurosurgery, and Psychiatry* **49**: 1150–1159

Osselton JW, Binnie CD, Cooper R et al. (eds) (2002) *Clinical Neurophysiology: Electroencephalography, Paediatric Neurophysiology, Special Techniques and Applications.* Oxford, Butterworth-Heinemann Medical

Pennisi G, Alagona G, Ferri R et al. (2002) Motor cortex excitability in Alzheimer's disease: one year follow-up study. *Neuroscience Letters* **329**: 293–296

Penttilä M, Partanen JV, Soininen H, Riekkinen PJ. (1985) Quantitative analysis of occipital EEG in different stages of Alzheimer's disease. *Electroencephalography and Clinical Neurophysiology* **60**: 1–6

Peters JM, Hummel T, Kratzsch T et al. (2003) Olfactory function in mild cognitive impairment and Alzheimer's disease: an investigation using psychophysical and electrophysiological techniques. *American Journal of Psychiatry* **160**: 1995–2002

Pfefferbaum A, Wenegrat BG, Ford JM et al. (1984) Clinical application of the P3 component of event-related potentials. II. Dementia, depression and schizophrenia. *Electroencephalography and Clinical Neurophysiology* **59**: 104–124

Pfefferbaum A, Ford JM, Kraemer HC. (1990) Clinical utility of long latency 'cognitive' event-related potentials (P3): the cons. *Electroencephalography and Clinical Neurophysiology* **76**: 6–12

Philpot MP, Amin D, Levy R. (1990) Visual evoked potentials in Alzheimer's disease: correlations with age and severity. *Electroencephalography and Clinical Neurophysiology* 77: 323–329

Philpot M and Pereira J. (2002) Reversible dementias. In: Copeland J *et al.* (eds), *The Principles and Practice of Geriatric Psychiatry*, 2nd edition. Chichester, John Wiley

Pierce TW, Watson TD, King JS *et al.* (2003) Age differences in factor analysis of EEG. *Brain Topography* 16: 19–27

Pitt MC and Daldry SJ. (1988) The use of weighted quadratic regression for the study of latencies of the P100 component of the visual evoked potential. *Electroencephalography and Clinical Neurophysiology* 71: 150–152

Polich J. (1997) EEG and ERP assessment of normal aging. *Electroencephalography and Clinical Neurophysiology* 104: 244–256

Polich J, Ladish C, Bloom FE. (1990) P300 assessment of early Alzheimer's disease. *Electroencephalography and Clinical Neurophysiology* 77: 179–189

Pollak L, Klein C, Giladi R *et al.* (1996) Progressive deterioration of brainstem auditory evoked potentials in Creutzfeldt–Jakob disease: clinical and electroencephalographic correlation. *Clinical Electroencephalography* 24: 95–99

Pollock VE, Schneider LS, Chui HC *et al.* (1989) Visual evoked potentials in dementia: a meta-analysis and empirical study of Alzheimer's disease patients. *Biological Psychiatry* 25: 1003–1013

Prinz PN, Peskind ER, Vitaliano PP *et al.* (1982) Changes in the sleep and waking EEGs of non-demented and demented elderly subjects. *Journal of the American Geriatrics Society* 30: 86–93

Prinz PN, Dustman RE, Emmerson R. (1990) Electrophysiology and aging. In: Birren JE and Schaie KW. (eds), *The Handbook of the Psychology of Aging*, 3rd edition. San Diego, Academic Press

Prinz PN, Larsen LH, Moe KE, Vitiello MV. (1992) EEG markers of early Alzheimer's disease in computer tonic REM sleep. *Electroencephalography and Clinical Neurophysiology* 83: 36–43

Pucci E, Belardinelli N, Cacchio G. (1999) EEG power spectrum differences in early and late onset forms of Alzheimer's disease. *Clinical Neurophysiology* 110: 621–631

Reeves RR, Struve FA, Patrick G. (2002) The effects of donepezil on quantitative EEG in patients with Alzheimer's disease. *Clinical Electroencephalography* 33: 93–96

Reynolds CF, Kupfer DJ, Houck PR *et al.* (1988) Reliable discrimination of elderly depressed and demented patients by electroencephalographic sleep data. *Archives of General Psychiatry* 45: 258–264

Riekkinen P, Buzsaki G, Riekkinen P *et al.* (1991) The cholinergic system and EEG slow waves. *Electroencephalography and Clinical Neurophysiology* 78: 89–96

Roberts TPL, Poeppel D, Rowley HA. (1998) Magnetoencephalography and magnetic source imaging. *Neuropsychiatry, Neuropsychology and Behavioural Neurology* 11: 49–64

Robinson D, Merskey H, Blume W *et al.* (1994) Electroencephalography as an aid in the exclusion of Alzheimer's disease. *Archives of Neurology* 51: 280–284

Rodriguez G, Nobili F, Rocca G *et al.* (1998) Quantitative electroencephalography and regional cerebral blood flow: discriminant analysis between Alzheimer's patients and healthy controls. *Dementia and Geriatric Cognitive Disorders* 9: 274–283

Rodriguez G, Copello F, Vitali P *et al.* (1999a) EEG spectral profile to stage Alzheimer's disease. *Clinical Neurophysiology* 110: 1831–1837

Rodriguez G, Nobili F, Copello F *et al.* (1999b) 99mTc-HMPAO regional cerebral blood flow and quantitative electroencephalography in Alzheimer's disease: a correlative study. *Journal of Nuclear Medicine* 40: 522–529

Rodriguez G, Vitali P, De Leo C *et al.* (2002) Quantitative EEG changes in Alzheimer's patients during long-term donepezil therapy. *Neuropsychobiology* 46: 49–56

Rodriguez G, Vitali P, Canfora M *et al.* (2004) Quantitative EEG and perfusional single photon emission computed tomography correlation during long-term donepezil therapy in Alzheimer's disease. *Clinical Neurophysiology* 115: 39–49

Ron MA, Toone BK, Garralda ME, Lishman WA. (1979) Diagnostic accuracy in presenile dementia. *British Journal of Psychiatry* 134: 161–168

Royal College of Psychiatrists. (1995) *Consensus Statement on the Assessment and Investigation of an Elderly Person with Suspected Cognitive Impairment by a Specialist Old Age Psychiatry Service.* Council Report CR49. London, Royal College of Psychiatrists

Ruessman K, Sondag HD, Beneicke U. (1990) P300 latency of the auditory evoked potential in dementia. *International Journal of Neuroscience* 54: 291–296

St Clair DM, Blackwood DHR, Christie JE. (1985) P3 and other long latency auditory evoked potentials in presenile dementia Alzheimer type and Korsakoff's syndrome. *British Journal of Psychiatry* 147: 702–706

St Clair D, Blackburn I, Blackwood D, Tyrer G. (1988) Measuring the course of Alzheimer's disease. A longitudinal study of neurophysiological function and changes in P3 event-related potential. *British Journal of Psychiatry* 152: 48–54

Saito H, Yamazaki H, Matsouka H *et al.* (2001) Visual event-related potential in mild dementia of the Alzheimer's type. *Psychiatry and Clinical Neurosciences* 55: 365–371

Sandman CA and Patterson JV. (2000) The auditory event-related potential is a stable and reliable measure in elderly subjects over a 3 year period. *Clinical Neurophysiology* 111: 1427–1437

Scott DF, Heathfield KWG, Toone B, Margerison JH. (1972) The EEG in Huntington's chorea: a clinical and neuropathological study. *Journal of Neurology, Neurosurgery, and Psychiatry* 35: 97–102

Shiga Y, Seki H, Onuma A *et al.* (2001) Decrement of N20 amplitude of the median nerve somatosensory evoked potential in Creutzfeldt–Jakob disease patients. *Journal of Clinical Neurophysiology* 18: 576–582

Sloan EP and Fenton GW. (1992) Serial visual evoked potential recordings in geriatric psychiatry. *Electroencephalography and Clinical Neurophysiology* 84: 325–331

Sloan EP, Fenton GW, Kennedy NS, MacLennan JM. (1995) Electroencephalography and single photon emission computed tomography in dementia: a comparative study. *Psychological Medicine* 25: 631–638

Soininen H, Partanen J, Paakkonen A *et al.* (1991) Changes in absolute power values of EEG spectra in the follow-up of Alzheimer's disease. *Acta Neurologica Scandinavica* 83: 133–136

Soininen H, Reinikainen K, Partanen J *et al.* (1992) Slowing of electroencephalogram and choline acetyl-transferase activity in definitive Alzheimer's disease. *Neuroscience* 49: 529–535

Squires NK and Ollo C. (1999) Comparison of endogenous event-related potentials in attend and non-attend conditions: latency changes with normal aging. *Clinical Neurophysiology* 110: 564–574

Stam CJ, van Cappellen van Walsum AM, Pijnenburg YA *et al.* (2002) Generalized synchronization of MEG recordings in Alzheimer's disease: evidence for involvement of the gamma band. *Journal of Clinical Neurophysiology* 19: 562–574

Stam CJ, van der Made Y, Pijnenburg YA, Scheltens P. (2003) EEG synchronization in mild cognitive impairment and Alzheimer's disease. *Acta Neurologica Scandinavica* **108**: 90–96

Stevens A and Kircher T. (1998) Cognitive decline unlike normal aging is associated with alternations of EEG temporo-spatial characteristics. *European Archives of Psychiatry and Clinical Neuroscience* **248**: 259–266

Stevens A, Kircher T, Nickola M *et al.* (2001) Dynamic regulation of EEG power and coherence is lost early and globally in probable DAT. *European Archives of Psychiatry and Clinical Neuroscience* **251**: 199–204

Strijers RLM, Scheltens P, Jonkman EJ *et al.* (1997) Diagnosing Alzheimer's disease in community-dwelling elderly: a comparison of EEG and MRI. *Dementia and Geriatric Cognitive Disorders* **8**: 198–202

Swanwick GRJ, Rowan M, Coen RF *et al.* (1996a) Longitudinal visual evoked potentials in Alzheimer's disease: a preliminary study. *Biological Psychiatry* **39**: 455–457

Swanwick GRJ, Rowan M, Coen RF *et al.* (1996b) Clinical application of electrophysiological markers in the differential diagnosis of depression and very mild Alzheimer's disease. *Journal of Neurology, Neurosurgery, and Psychiatry* **60**: 82–86

Swanwick GRJ, Rowan MJ, Coen RF *et al.* (1997) Measuring cognitive deterioration in Alzheimer's disease. *British Journal of Psychiatry* **170**: 580

Szelies B, Mielke R, Kessler J, Heiss WD. (1999) EEG power changes are related to regional cerebral glucose metabolism in vascular dementia. *Clinical Neurophysiology* **110**: 615–620

Tachibana H, Takeda M, Sugita M. (1989a). Brainstem auditory evoked potentials in patients with multi-infarct dementia and dementia of the Alzheimer type. *International Journal of Neuroscience* **48**: 325–331

Tachibana H, Takeda M, Sugita M. (1989b). Short-latency somatosensory and brainstem auditory evoked potentials in patients with Parkinson's disease. *International Journal of Neuroscience* **48**: 321–326

Tachibana H, Aragane K, Kawabata K, Sugita M. (1997) P3 latency change in aging and Parkinson's disease. *Archives of Neurology* **54**: 296–302

Tanaka H, Koenig T, Pascuel-Marqui RD *et al.* (2000) Event-related potential and EEG measures in Parkinson's disease without and with dementia. *Dementia and Geriatric Cognitive Disorders* **11**: 39–45

Torres F, Fauro A, Loewenson R, Johnson E. (1983) The electroencephalogram of elderly subjects revisited. *Electroencephalography and Clinical Neurophysiology* **56**: 391–398

Trick GL, Barris MC, Bickler-Bluth M. (1989) Abnormal pattern electroretinograms in patients with senile dementia of the Alzheimer type. *Annals of Neurology* **26**: 226–231

Uc EY, Skinner RD, Rodnitzky RL, Garcia-Rill E. (2003) The mid-latency auditory evoked potential P50 is abnormal in Huntington's disease. *Journal of the Neurological Sciences* **15**: 1–5

Visser SL, Van Tilburg W, Hooijer C *et al.* (1985) Visual evoked potentials (VEPs) in senile dementia (Alzheimer type) and in non-organic behavioural disorders in the elderly: comparison with EEG parameters. *Electroencephalography and Clinical Neurophysiology* **60**: 115–121

Wada Y, Nanbu Y, Jiang Z-Y *et al.* (1997) Electroencephalographic abnormalities in patients with presenile dementia of the Alzheimer type: quantitative analysis at rest and during photic stimulation. *Biological Psychiatry* **41**: 217–225

Walhovd KB and Fjell AM. (2002) One-year test-retest reliability of auditory ERPs in young and old adults. *International Journal of Psychophysiology* **46**: 29–40

Walker MP, Ayre GA, Cummings JL *et al.* (2000a) Quantifying fluctuations in dementia with Lewy bodies, Alzheimer's disease, and vascular dementia. *Neurology* **54**: 1616–1625

Walker MP, Ayre GA, Perry EK *et al.* (2000b) Quantification and characteristics of fluctuating cognition in dementia with Lewy bodies and Alzheimer's disease. *Dementia and Geriatric Cognitive Disorders* **11**: 327–335

Wang H, Wang Y, Wang D *et al.* (2002) Cognitive impairment in Parkinson's disease revealed by event-related potential N270. *Journal of the Neurological Sciences* **194**: 49–53

Werber EA, Gandelman-Marton R, Klein C, Rabey JM. (2003) The clinical use of P300 event related potentials for the evaluation of cholinesterase inhibitors treatment in demented patients. *Journal of Neural Transmission* **110**: 659–669

Wiegand M, Moller AA, Lauer CJ *et al.* (1991) Nocturnal sleep in Huntington's disease. *Journal of Neurology* **238**: 203–208

Williams PA, Jones GH, Briscoe M *et al.* (1991) P300 and reaction-time measures in senile dementia of the Alzheimer type. *British Journal of Psychiatry* **159**: 410–414

Williamson PC, Merskey H, Morrison S *et al.* (1990) Quantitative electroencephalographic correlates of cognitive decline in normal elderly subjects. *Archives of Neurology* **47**: 1185–1188

Wright CE and Furlong PL. (1988) Visual evoked potentials in elderly patients with primary or multi-infarct dementia. *British Journal of Psychiatry* **152**: 679–682

Wright CE, Harding GFA, Orwin A. (1986) The flash and pattern VEP as a diagnostic indicator of dementia. *Documenta Ophthalmologica* **62**: 89–96

Yamaguchi S, Tsuchiya H, Yamagata S *et al.* (2000) Event-related brain potentials in response to novel sounds in dementia. *Clinical Neurophysiology* **111**: 195–203

Zerr I, Pocchiari M and Collins S *et al.* (2000) Analysis of EEG and CSF 14-3-3 proteins as aids to the diagnosis of Creutzfeldt–Jakob disease. *Neurology* **55**: 811–815

11

Caring for people with dementia

Family carers for people with dementia

HENRY BRODATY, ALISA GREEN AND LEE-FAY LOW

There is a maxim that when a person is diagnosed with dementia, there is (almost) always a second patient. Dementia is not just one person's illness. The stone cast sends ripples through families, friends and society. This chapter focuses on informal carers, usually family, sometimes friends.

11.1 WHO ARE INFORMAL CARERS?

There are many definitions of a carer. It may be defined by the:

- relationship – spouse, child, professional;
- primacy – primary or secondary carer;
- living arrangement – with the patient or separately;
- style of care – routine, regular, occasional;
- by job description – unpaid or paid; or
- as formal or informal (Barer and Johnson, 1990).

In the UK and Australia the term carer is used, whereas in North America caregiver is more usual. In India and some other countries, caretaker is a more common term. Pearlin *et al.* (1990) differentiate between caring (the affective part of a relationship), and caregiving (the behavioural component). Both are intrinsic to any close relationship but, with impairment, there is increasing dependency and the restructuring of the relationship so that caregiving becomes dominant and overrides other aspects of the relationship, resulting in a loss of reciprocity. A definition of a caregiver proffered by Zarit and Edwards (1996, p. 334) is 'a family member (or friend), helping someone on a regular (usually daily) basis with tasks necessary for independent living'. The care-recipients, or

patients for the purposes of this chapter, are dependent, disabled and mentally-impaired persons with dementia, most commonly Alzheimer's disease (AD).

The majority of carers, from 33 to over 60 per cent, are spouses (US Congress Office of Technology Assessment, 1987; Brodaty and Hadzi-Pavlovic, 1990; Wells *et al.*, 1990) of whom about 75 per cent are women (Stone *et al.*, 1987; Brodaty and Hadzi-Pavlovic, 1990; Dwyer and Seccombe, 1991; Dwyer and Coward, 1992; Cohen *et al.*, 1997; Tsien and Cheng, 1999), although the proportion does vary according to both the sampling techniques and the country surveyed. Adult children and their partners make up about a third of informal carers, but in Asian countries, such as China, Hong Kong and India, adult children are more often the carers than spouses (Patterson *et al.*, 1998; Tsien and Cheng, 1999; Shaji *et al.*, 2003). Moreover, daughters are far more likely to be primary carers than sons (Horowitz, 1985; Coward and Dwyer, 1990; Dwyer and Coward, 1991; Lee *et al.*, 1993), outnumbering them in a ratio of about 4:1 (Brody, 1990). Likewise, daughters-in-law often inherit the burden of care, particularly in certain cultures such as in Korea, Hong-Kong and India (Choi, 1993; Lee and Sung, 1997, 1998; Patterson *et al.*, 1998; Tsien and Cheng, 1999; Shaji *et al.*, 2003).

About 4 per cent of people with dementia live alone (US Congress Office of Technology Assessment, 1987). Persons living alone are less likely to have a carer, and likely to be institutionalized earlier (Brody, 1981; Mace and Rabins, 1982). There is an enormous difference between living with a person and caring from a distance. Spouses almost always live with the person with dementia, whereas adult children who are carers often live separately.

There are cultural differences as to who in the family will take on the care. The USA being a more mobile society makes it less likely that offspring will be close at hand to provide care when a parent starts to dement, yet moving the person with dementia to another city can be quite disorientating. There are differences in the ways Caucasian, African American and Hispanic carers cope (see below). In Japan, the tradition is that the wife of the eldest son is responsible for the care of ageing parents. In developing countries and in many rural settings there is more likely to be an extended family network who can provide care. Economic conditions in many rural economies have meant that many of the adult children have migrated internally to cities, leaving older parents stranded. Further, many older people have significant assets, such as a house, but little income, and incur financial hardship when facing the need to provide care for a person with dementia.

11.2 WHY DO FAMILY CARERS CARE?

Eisdorfer (1991) posited that family carers are motivated to provide care for several reasons. It may be out of a sense of love or reciprocity: the bonds of 50 years, the credit points accumulated over a lifetime together, and the recognition that the other partner would provide care were the situation reversed. Caregiving may be seen as spiritually fulfilling. Other carers do it out of a sense of duty because they feel guilt, or in response to social pressure or cultural mores. These latter carers are more likely to resent their role and suffer greater psychological distress than the former carers in the first two groups. Rarely, the motivation is greed: the prospect of financial gain as a result of caring.

11.3 HOW DO FAMILY CARERS CARE?

The concept of care providers and care managers (Archbold, 1981) is useful. The former provide hands-on care – dressing the person with dementia, providing daily supervision, managing finances, or doing whatever else is required. Care managers, on the other hand, arrange for others to provide care: a nurse to attend daily to assist with medications and personal care; an accountant to look after financial matters; personal care assistants to provide companionship. Spouses tend to be care providers; adult children, friends and other relatives tend to be care managers. Care providers are generally more stressed than care managers (Archbold, 1981).

While the negative aspects of caring have received most attention, caring has been associated with benefits and positive feelings, such as a feeling of satisfaction, a feeling that the carer has helped the patient and a sense of meaning (Archbold, 1983; Miller, 1988; Sheehan and Nuthall, 1988; Walker et al., 1989; Cohen et al., 2002).

Recent research has indicated that differences in cultural or ethnic affiliation can influence the way that family carers approach and view their caring role and responsibilities. For instance, it is quite common in African American communities for the extended family to take on the care of persons with dementia, especially in lower socioeconomic groups (Gelfand, 1982; Cantor, 1983; Wood and Parham, 1990). Similarly, in American-Hispanic communities, the extended family typically care for elderly relatives with dementia (Valle, 1988; Mintzer et al., 1992). For some minority groups, such as African American and Asian-American communities, placing an elderly relative in a nursing home is considered abandonment and therefore unthinkable, even in cases of extreme stress and burden to the carer (Wood and Parham, 1990; Yeo, 1996; Wallsten, 1997).

The caregiving role is perceived more positively by African American carers compared with Caucasian carers (Smith, 1996). African American carers tend to report less subjective burden, fewer difficulties in accepting restrictions on recreational activities, and lower levels of depression than Caucasian carers (Gibson, 1982; Lawton et al., 1992; Roth et al., 2001). It was suggested that this is because of greater caregiving support by members of minority extended families but a recent review concluded that minority group caregivers do not have more support than white people (Janevic and Connell, 2001). In developing countries, where levels of caregiver strain appear at least as high as in the developed world despite the extended family structure of care, there appears to be less coresident caregiver burden in larger households (Prince et al., 2004). African American carers appraise caregiving tasks as less subjectively stressful and themselves as having higher effectiveness than Caucasian carers (Haley et al., 1996). Additionally, African American carers tend to use religion and prayer as coping strategies, and view God as an essential part of their support system (Wood and Parnham, 1990).

The beliefs and values of different ethnic groups can furthermore affect the way in which family members appraise and understand dementia, and therefore manage it. For instance, in some cultures there is the belief that behaviours related to dementia are part of normal ageing, rather than a disease process, and therefore may evoke little concern until symptoms are quite advanced (Valle, 1989). Similarly, in some cultures, confusion, disorientation, and memory loss may be viewed as signs of 'craziness' (Yeo, 1996). A cross-national European study found that 2 per cent of overall carer burden was explained by perceived negative social reactions (Schneider et al., 1999).

11.4 EFFECTS OF DEMENTIA ON CARERS

Dementia is an 'unremitting burden' on the family (Anderson, 1987). Caring for a person with a chronic mental condition is more stressful than caring for a person with a physical disorder or disability (Lezak, 1978; Gilleard, 1984; Poulshock

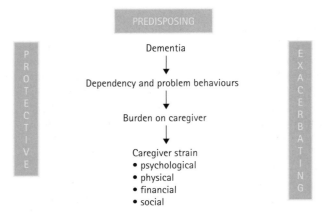

Figure 11.1 *Dementia leads to dependency and problem behaviours, which impose an objective burden on the carer. (Adapted from Poulshock and Deimling, 1984).*

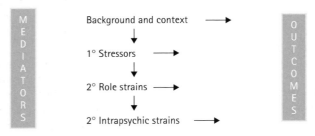

Figure 11.2 *Background and context lead to primary stresses, secondary role strains, and secondary intrapsychic strains (Pearlin et al., 1990, reprinted with permission).*

and Deimling, 1984; Mohide *et al.*, 1988). The effects on family carers are diverse and complex and there are many other factors that may exacerbate or ameliorate how carers react and feel as a result of their role.

Two models of the effects of caregiving are shown in Figures 11.1 and 11.2. In the first, adapted from the work of Poulshock and Deimling (1984), dementia leads to dependency and problem behaviours, which impose an objective burden on the carer. Objective burden results in strain, which varies in how it is manifested in carers. Strain may be psychological, physical, financial or social, or may lead to increased use of health services. Carer strain may be influenced by patient, carer, protective and exacerbating variables.

In the second model from Pearlin *et al.* (1990), which overlaps with the first, there are a background and context which lead to primary stresses, secondary role strains, and secondary intrapsychic strains. Several variables can mediate the results of these leading to different outcomes.

11.4.1 Objective burden

Objective burden reflects the dependency of the patient, as evidenced by the loss of activities of daily living, instrumental activities, cognition, other abilities, companionship and communication. Problem behaviours and psychiatric disorders

that commonly accompany dementia are further types of objective burden.

11.4.2 Subjective strain

Subjective burden is the appraisal by the carer. It includes feelings of entrapment, resentment, stress, overload, inability to cope and exhaustion. Activities become restricted, outside relationships diminish.

11.4.3 Psychological morbidity

Numerous studies have demonstrated increased psychological morbidity in carers (Gilleard *et al.*, 1982, 1984; Poulshock and Deimling, 1984; George and Gwyther, 1986; Morris *et al.*, 1988; Brodaty and Hadzi-Pavlovic, 1990; Grafström and Winblad, 1995). Depression levels and rates are also high (Haley *et al.*, 1987; Morris *et al.*, 1988; Gallagher *et al.*, 1989; Schulz and Williamson, 1991; Baumgarten *et al.*, 1992; Pearson *et al.*, 1993; Rosenthal *et al.*, 1993; Mittelman *et al.*, 1995). For example, Gallagher *et al.* (1989) found that amongst carers seeking help, 26 per cent met Research Diagnostic Criteria (RDC) for major depression and 18 per cent for minor depression. Rates among non-help-seekers were 10 per cent and 8 per cent respectively. In a study by Coope *et al.* (1995) of 109 carers of research subjects, 29.4 per cent met GMS-AGECAT criteria for case level depression and 11.9 per cent had sub-case symptoms of depression. Mittelman *et al.* (1995) reported that over 41.7 per cent of carers had a Geriatric Depression Scale score of 11 or greater, the rate being higher amongst women (50 per cent) than men (30 per cent).

A recent meta-analysis of 84 studies comparing caregivers of elderly to non-caregivers found that there were significantly higher levels of depression and stress and significantly lower levels of self-efficacy, general subjective wellbeing and physical health in caregivers. This difference was larger when dementia caregivers were compared with non-carers than with heterogeneous samples of caregivers of elderly patients (Pinquart and Sorensen, 2003).

11.4.4 Physical morbidity

Carers have poorer physical health than non-carer controls (Schulz *et al.*, 1990), higher levels of chronic conditions, prescription medications and doctor visits (Haley *et al.*, 1987) and more physical symptoms and poorer self-rated health (Baumgarten *et al.*, 1992). Those with poor psychological health are even more likely to have physical morbidity (Brodaty and Hadzi-Pavlovic, 1990). The findings of decreased immunological competence in carers of Alzheimer's disease patients (Kiecolt-Glaser *et al.*, 1987) has been supported in an elegant study of response to influenza vaccine. Vedhara *et al.* (1999; 2003) reported that elderly carers of spouses with dementia have increased activation of the hypothalamopituitary axis and a poorer antibody response to the influenza vaccine, which could be enhanced by cognitive behavioural intervention (see below). They concluded that carers may be vulnerable to infectious disease. A meta-analysis of 23 studies of dementia caregivers found that caregiving was associated with a slightly greater risk for health problems and that this risk was moderated by measure of health (e.g. self-rated global health, medication use, antibodies, cardiovascular measures) and greater in females (Vitaliano et al., 2003).

Other indicators of poorer physical health are increased service use – hospitalization, physician visits, drug use, aggregate use of health service; and less healthy behaviours – increased alcohol intake, smoking more and poorer sleep patterns, eating behaviour and nutrition (Schulz and Williamson, 1997). Further, pre-existing conditions such as hypertension are more likely to be exacerbated by the caregiving role (Schulz and Williamson, 1997). Caregiving has also been associated with a higher mortality rate (Schulz and Beach, 1999).

11.4.5 Social isolation

Dementia is a very isolating condition. At the very time that families need more support, friends feel unsure about what to say on the taboo topic of dementia, are disconcerted by their friend's lack of communicativeness and feel embarrassed by the displays of disinhibition (Brodaty, 1998a). They may feel uncomfortable about the carer's distress and tend to avoid paying visits. Simultaneously, carers abandon their leisure pursuits and hobbies, stop seeing friends and discontinue employment. Their lives become focused on the caregiving role, which takes up most of their time (Brodaty, 1998a). In a survey of Australian carers, we found that half of them had seen a person from outside their home only once a week or less often (Brodaty and Hadzi-Pavlovic, 1990).

11.4.6 Financial

There are considerable financial costs to families looking after persons with dementia. The direct costs are those of medical consultations, investigations, pharmaceuticals, provision of personal and nursing care and later, residential care. Indirect costs comprise loss of earnings by the patient and by family carers if they have to relinquish employment.

Max et al. (1995) estimated that the informal care provided to patients with Alzheimer's disease living at home is substantial, averaging 286 hours per month. Even after patients were placed in a nursing home, the number of monthly informal caregiving hours was reported to be 36. For patients at home, primary carers had been caring for an average of 3.7 years; for institutionalized patients, the average length of time carers had been caring was 6.3 years.

Most of the care for patients at home is provided informally by family members and friends (Max, 1999). While the cost of caring for an institutionalized patient is twice the cost of caring for a patient at home (Hu et al., 1986), the total social costs of care per person were nearly the same in two settings where both paid and unpaid informal care were included (Rice et al., 1993). However, most of the expenses for patients living at home are borne by their families (Gray and Fenn, 1993; Rice et al., 1993; Stommel et al., 1994). As the disease progresses, the cost of care increases. Hu et al. (1986) found that severely demented patients required more than twice as many hours of informal care as mildly demented ones. Others have found rates of 1.28–1.63 times greater costs for severely demented patients compared with mildly demented ones living at home (Rice et al., 1993; Souetre et al., 1995). Max (1999) went on to conclude that 'Alzheimer's disease is extremely costly, no matter how it is measured and what cost is included ... for patients cared for at home, most of the care is provided informally by family members and friends and most of the burden of care for patients at home is borne by their families, in the form of out-of-pocket payments for services or in the form of hours of time spent caring for the patients without reimbursement'(p. 367).

In a US survey, families spent the equivalent of $US18 200 annually (Stommel et al., 1994). Four out of five families in Stommel's sample reported out-of-pocket expenditures averaging $US2088 (14 per cent of total) but the lion's share ($US11 560 or 59 per cent) was accounted for by the primary carer's time spent providing care. The US National Longitudinal Caregiver Study estimated the annual cost of providing informal care to elderly community-dwelling veterans with dementia to be $US18 385 in 1998. The majority of this cost comprised caregiving time ($US6295) and caregiver's lost earnings ($US10 709) (Moore et al., 2001).

In Australia in 2002 with a population of 19 million including 165 000 with dementia, the direct health costs for dementia (residential care, hospitals, GPs and specialists, outpatients, research, pharmaceutical and other services) was $A3236 million, and indirect costs (loss of earnings, absenteeism and mortality burden) were estimated as $A365 million (Access Economics, 2003). The value of informal care for people with dementia was $A1713 million, or 32 per cent of the total cost of care (Access Economics, 2003).

11.5 PREDICTORS OF CARER DISTRESS

11.5.1 Demographic variables

Carers who are women, and those who are spouses, have higher rates of psychological morbidity than their counterparts (Fitting et al., 1986; Baumgarten et al., 1992; Collins, 1992; Gallicchio et al., 2002). The spouses of younger patients may have higher rates of psychological morbidity, perhaps because of the high stresses inherent in being married to a younger person with dementia, and the high likelihood of having younger children at home (Luscombe et al., 1998).

Carers who cohabit with patients are more likely to be depressed or psychologically stressed than those living apart (Gilhooley, 1984; George and Gwyther, 1986; Wells and Jorm, 1987; Brodaty and Hadzi-Pavlovic, 1990; Harper and Lund, 1990). The gender of the patient does not appear to affect carer wellbeing once allowance is made for the increased likelihood of behavioural disturbances in men (Brodaty and Hadzi-Pavlovic, 1990).

There have been no consistent associations found between carer age and psychological distress, with higher levels having been reported in older (Fiore et al., 1986) and younger supporters (Gilleard et al., 1984). Such comparisons need to control for the effects of relationship.

11.5.2 Dementia variables

11.5.2.1 TYPE

There is little evidence to suggest that one type of dementia is associated with more psychological stress in carers than another. Similar levels have been reported in carers of patients with vascular dementia and AD (Draper et al., 1992, 1996) and dementia with Lewy bodies and AD (Lowery et al., 2000). On theoretical grounds, one might expect that the increased likelihood of behavioural disturbances and personality changes in frontotemporal dementias might be associated with more carer distress.

11.5.2.2 DURATION

Two possibilities have been hypothesized to account for the lack of consistent link between duration of dementia and carer outcome. The adaptation hypothesis proposes that some carers adapt to the stress of providing care. The sequestration theory hypothesizes that carers experiencing greater stress are more likely to arrange admission of the patient to a nursing home, thus removing these dyads from cross-sectional surveys correlating duration and psychological morbidity.

In support of the adaptation hypothesis, several researchers have found that carers experience less burden over time (Gilhooley, 1984; Zarit et al., 1986; Novak and Guest, 1989; Townsend et al., 1989; Rabins et al., 1990; Brodaty et al., 1997). For example, Grafström and Winblad (1995), in a study limited by a large number of drop-outs and few subjects, reported that, over 2.5 years, spouses and adult children caring for elderly people with dementia reported less burden, decreased behavioural problems in the demented elderly, less conflict with other relatives and close friends, less social limitation and less affective limitations. Additionally, self-rated health improved and the number of visits to a physician decreased. The mean use of psychotropic drugs increased slightly. These effects were still present when analyses were repeated for carers of elderly still living at home. For the relatives of non-dementing elderly, there were no significant differences over time. This is consistent with the findings of Bond and Buck (1998), who found that there were no significant

changes in the General Health Questionnaire (GHQ) scores (a measure of psychological morbidity) of carers over a 2-year follow-up period, and Roth and colleagues (2001) who found that depression scores of caregivers remained constant over a 2-year period. By comparison, the GHQ scores of carers in the control group of an intervention study gradually rose over 12 months (Brodaty and Gresham, 1989). Also, Pot and colleagues (1997) found that over a 2-year period, the psychological wellbeing of carers actually declined and psychological distress increased in terms of depression and anxiety.

11.5.2.3 SEVERITY

The association between dementia severity and carer health is complex (Baumgarten, 1989). Carers may respond quite differently to three manifestations of dementia: cognitive, functional and behavioural decline. Most studies have found no significant correlation between cognitive status and carer psychological health. Functional decline is significantly correlated with restriction in carer activity (Deimling and Bass, 1986) but not with depressive symptoms (Deimling and Bass, 1986; Haley et al., 1987). Functional decline has been linked to increased burden on carers. Haley et al. (1987) found that the patient's ability to perform instrumental activities of daily living was highly correlated with the carer's depression score, but not with life satisfaction or self-rated health problems. The difficulty in interpreting the association between patient functional status and carer health, which in any case is not strong, is that patients who have declined functionally are more likely to exhibit behavioural disturbances. Analyses have not allowed for the strong effect of behavioural disturbances on carer health (see below).

The most consistent finding is the strong association between behavioural disturbance and carer distress. Despite differences in outcome measures, methods of assessing behavioural disturbances, populations and countries from which studies are reported, a robust and consistent finding emerges: behavioural disturbances account for about 25 per cent of the variance in carer psychological distress (Mangone et al., 1993; Brodaty, 1996; Cohen et al., 1997; Bond and Buck, 1998). Certain types of behaviour are particularly likely to be associated with distress – incontinence, immobility, nocturnal wandering, proneness to fall, inability to engage in meaningful activities, difficulties with communication, sleep disturbance, loss of companionship, disruptiveness, constant demands and aggression (Gilleard et al., 1982; Greene et al., 1982; Morris et al., 1988; Brodaty and Hadzi-Pavlovic, 1990).

11.5.3 Carer variables

Effective coping strategies can mitigate carer distress (Pruchno and Resch, 1989) and possibly enhance the quality of life for the dementing person. Problem-focused strategies – reframing, problem-solving, developing more social support or a greater social network – are associated with positive effects such as greater satisfaction with life, decreased feelings of burden and lower depression levels (Pruchno and Resch, 1989). Emotion-based responses (Lazarus and Folkman, 1984) – wishfulness, acceptance and fantasy (e.g. 'I wish I was a stronger person to deal with it all better', 'accept the situation', 'fantasies about how things might end out') are associated with more distress. The more immature the coping strategies and the more neurotic the personality style (Gallant and Connell, 2003), the greater the likelihood of increased burden, decreased satisfaction with life, and increased depression. Of course it may be possible that depression in carers leads to regression and to the adoption of less effective types of coping, which then perpetuates the depression. An association has been found between expressed emotion (EE) and distress in the daughters of people with dementia (Bledin et al., 1990) and carers in general (Fearon et al., 1998).

11.5.4 Relationship factors

Premorbid unsatisfactory relationships are more likely to be associated with carer distress (Brodaty and Hadzi-Pavlovic, 1990). This may accompany the fragmentation of communication between couples, the increase in tension, the loss of companionship, the loss of a confidante, the increase in economic and household responsibilities and the waning of sexual intimacy (Chenoweth and Spencer, 1986; Fitting et al., 1986; Wright, 1991).

11.6 SUPPORT

The relationship between support and carer outcome is extremely complex. There are differences between actual and perceived support, formal (from professionals) and informal (from friends and relatives) support, between psychological and instrumental support, and between how males and females use support (Brodaty, 1994). Enright (1991) reported that husbands were more likely to receive help than wives. There is also the potential for negative effects from so-called supportive figures, i.e. visits from other family members may be more stressful than helpful (Fiore et al., 1986; Edwards and Cooper, 1988).

An association between the number of supports and carer distress might merely reflect an increased likelihood of distressed carers seeking help; while a negative correlation could suggest that support has an ameliorating effect (Brodaty, 1994). A lack of either a positive or a negative correlation might result where both effects occur in the one population being sampled. Also carers who use more informal services may need less professional help and make fewer demands on community services (Fitting et al., 1986; Chesterman et al., 1987). Finally, gender and culture influence the use of informal supports. For example, men, who are more likely than female carers to seek help, and African American carers, who are more likely than Caucasian carers to engage with larger extended networks of family and friends, both have lower levels of psychological distress than their counterparts (see above).

In summary, there is support for a relationship between informal supports and lower psychological distress, but it may be that happier people are more inclined to seek contact in the first place or that lack of happiness and social support are independently related to disturbing behaviours. Carer satisfaction with social support is generally associated with better health (Gilhooley, 1984; Fiore et al., 1986). It may be that unhappy carers perceive the world negatively in general and so rate the satisfaction with their supports in the same way, thus contaminating the results. On the other hand, social support may provide a protective buffer against stress but have little effect on those who are not exposed to stress (Baumgarten, 1989). For instance, it has been shown that paid help buffers the relationship between caregiver stress and burden while perceived availability of social support buffers the relationship between caregiver stress and depression (Majerovitz, 2001).

11.7 PROTECTORS FROM CARER DISTRESS

The corollary to the above studies is that carers who are care managers are able to distance themselves physically or emotionally from the patient, use problem-focused coping strategies, are able to use supports to buffer stress and are able to deal more competently with the care recipient's behavioural disturbances or have them treated well (e.g. Hinchliffe et al., 1995) are less likely to experience psychological distress. Membership of a support group, such as the Alzheimer's Association may also be helpful (see Chapter 22).

11.8 NURSING HOME ADMISSION AND CARERS

In general, carer factors are more potent predictors of institutionalization than patient or dementia variables. Having a coresident carer has a 20-fold protective effect against institutionalization (Banerjee et al., 2003). Carer psychological distress has been consistently associated with institutionalization (Colerick and George, 1986; Lieberman and Kramer, 1991; Brodaty et al., 1993; Yaffe et al., 2002). Older carers are more likely to institutionalize (Yaffe et al., 2002). Paradoxically, spouses are less likely to institutionalize dementing partners than children, and carers who express a stronger 'desire to institutionalize' are more likely to follow though (Morycz, 1985). Some studies have found that severity of dementia and rate of progression – how 'far' and how 'fast' – significantly increased the likelihood of institutionalization (Drachman et al., 1990; Brodaty et al., 1993). Institutionalization has also been associated with financial and psychological problems in the carer and family problems (Lieberman and Kramer, 1991). A 3-year study found that caregivers who experience a gradual entry into caregiving (providing care and recognizing symptoms before obtaining a diagnosis) were less likely to institutionalize their relatives (Gaugler *et al.*, 2003).

11.9 THE FAMILY AND THE MANAGEMENT OF DEMENTIA

The management of the family will evolve and change throughout the course of the illness (Steele, 1994). It is convenient to consider three stages.

11.9.1 Early stage

After assessment, the first opportunity to intervene is when the diagnosis is communicated – a crucial time in the career of caregiving (Fortinsky and Hathaway, 1990). When dementia caregivers were asked what topics they would have liked to learn more about, 25 per cent said they wanted to know about disease progression and 19 per cent said they wanted more information on the disease (Thomas *et al.*, 2002). A routine family diagnostic conference to communicate the diagnosis to the family can allow for clarification of behaviour, explanations of prognosis, and a discussion of current and future needs so that the family can be organized into an effective system of carers and the burden shared (Steele, 1994). We have found than when the family is seen separately to the patient, they are more likely to raise sensitive issues, such as genetic risk, time to nursing home admission and general prognosis. It is also useful to have a large family conference following discussion with the primary family carers, in order to enlist the support and help of other family members and friends.

For the many family carers who resist obtaining help for themselves, it is useful to emphasize that they are the most important element in the continuing management of the patient, and that the carer's wellbeing is critical to the patient's quality of life. In this way, requests for help from family and friends, use of family supports and later use of respite care are seen as positive therapeutic moves rather than admissions of inadequacy and failure.

Carers should be made aware of support groups through the local Alzheimer's Association and encouraged to make use of them, although it is recognized that they are not suitable for all carers. The commonest reason for carers not to access services or support groups is lack of knowledge or failure of health professionals to make a referral (Molinari *et al.*, 1994; Thomson *et al.*, 1997). The local Alzheimer's Association can provide educational materials, counselling, access to a support group or specific training courses. With the arrival of medications for Alzheimer's disease, patients are being diagnosed earlier and more services are being offered for them in tandem with those for carers. For example, there is a computer-based support group for people with dementia (Dementia Advocacy and Support Network; http://www.dasninternational.com), support groups for people with early stage dementia (Yale, 1995) and in Australia, the Living with Memory Loss

Program, a 7-week course for people with early stage dementia and their partner, that has been reported by attendees to be extremely helpful.

Another useful concept is the family carer as therapist (Brodaty *et al.*, 1997). This underscores the importance of the carer obtaining as much knowledge as possible about what is happening with the patient, and what to expect and how to manage. Brochures, books and videotapes are available through the Alzheimer's Association. Books such as *The 36 Hour Day* (Mace and Rabins, 1991) have been a boon to families. Carers can be taught behavioural management strategies and how to supervise exercise programmes for patients, which can be beneficial to the physical health and level of depression of the person with dementia (Teri *et al.*, 2003).

Sensitive issues arise: when should the patient discontinue driving, when should the patient stop working (if still doing so) and what are the hereditary risks to relatives of the patient? Financial management, enduring or durable power of attorney, enduring guardianship, advance directives and wills should be considered while the patient still retains competency. The possibility that the carer may suddenly take ill or even predecease the patient should be canvassed. For example, many couples have mirror wills and should the carer die suddenly, the patient, if named as the executor, would be unable to act in this capacity later in the illness. Obtaining durable power of attorney earlier avoids subsequent lengthy court proceedings required to obtain legal guardianship. In many jurisdictions it is possible to arrange enduring guardianship and to provide for advance directives, which only come into effect once the patient loses capacity. These important topics should be discussed with the patient and family separately and together to enable harmonious decisions to be reached.

Drugs are now available for the treatment of AD and other medications may be of assistance in ameliorating some risk factors for vascular dementia. Families are usually well aware of these and are desperate for information and prescriptions. Medications for AD appear to be of benefit for caregivers, as well as for patients. Cholinesterase inhibitors have been reported to reduce the time required for caregiving by about 1 hour per day and to decrease carer burden (Brodaty and Green, 2000). Even so, carers should be appraised of what to expect realistically from drug treatments (Brodaty, 1998a).

Family carers should be advised of their increased risk for depression and psychological stress. As the disease progresses the family carer appears to suffer more than the patient. Carers should be encouraged to meet regularly with their general practitioner, primary care physician or other aged care workers in order to ventilate concerns and seek advice on management. Our own practice is to advise general practitioners to meet with families at least quarterly to review the situation as well as to consult as necessary.

11.9.2 Middle stages

In the middle stage of the illness there is increasing memory loss, language difficulties, agnosia and apraxia, and loss of planning and other executive functions. Personality changes, apparent from the beginning, now become more prominent and the most common complaint of carers is the loss of companionship and lack of communicativeness (Brodaty et al., 1990). Carers can be taught practical strategies to assist the patient to compensate for cognitive deficits: establishing a routine, keeping a diary, having a whiteboard by the telephone, using visual prompts if verbal memory is more severely affected, capitalizing on old memories (e.g. rereading books from the past, playing familiar music, watching classical movies on television) and pursuing activities that do not rely on memory, such as physical exercise, craft hobbies or games.

Behavioural and psychiatric problems come to the fore as the disease progresses (Carrier and Brodaty, 1999). Behaviours such as wandering, aggression, sexual disinhibition, repeated questioning, 'shadowing' and disrupted sleep patterns, can be quite distressing to the carer. Depression, hallucinations, delusions and misidentification syndromes occur more commonly in the middle and later stages. Their management is discussed in Chapters 38 and 39. Often an explanation about these phenomena and their cause can be very helpful to the carer. For example, it may be that hallucinations are more distressing to the family than they are to the patient, and that once this is explained, carers become more accepting and less stressed.

Carers can be taught behavioural management strategies (e.g. Teri et al., 1997, see below) given practical advice (e.g. using identity bracelets for wandering patients, establishing routines for daytime naps so as to encourage the patient to stay up longer and establish a more normal sleeping rhythm), use of distraction when agitation occurs (e.g. music, physical activity), and establishment of a daily routine to achieve a sense of stability in the patient's life and compensate for memory deficits.

As the dementia progresses, patients become more functionally dependent, requiring assistance with instrumental activities of daily living and supervision with self-care. Carers are more likely to use support services in the middle stages of dementia: day centre; in-home respite; residential respite care; other relatives taking over for short periods of time. It is important that appropriate and timely referral be made to services, as caregivers have reported that general practitioners only referred them to community care services after they had experienced difficulties for a considerable time period (Bruce and Paterson, 2000).

Throughout the course of the disease, regular counselling to discuss problems as they arise and assistance with their management can help carers. Patients have usually lost competency by this stage, and treatment interventions and use of medication require informed consent from the carer. Legal requirements for this consent will vary according to the jurisdiction.

11.9.3 Late stage

In the later stages the patient becomes completely dependent in activities of daily living and requires assistance with bathing, toileting, dressing and eating. Paradoxically for many carers this stage may become somewhat easier. The demands are purely physical and labour intensive and the emotional strain is less.

At some stage, in most developed countries, institutionalization is considered. Each family has its own threshold for nursing home placement and for many families the answer is never. The financial costs of nursing home care can be a powerful disincentive to admission. Typically, carers decide to institutionalize their dependant when the patient requires more nursing care than one person can provide, when the patient can no longer recognize the carer as someone meaningful, when the patient develops urinary and/or faecal incontinence, when behavioural disturbances become unmanageable, or when the carer becomes physically ill, experiences excessive psychological stress or breaks down. The decision to institutionalize a loved one can induce in family carers powerful feelings of guilt and anguish, which may be mitigated by open discussion. For example, admission can be 'reframed' as an opportunity to provide 'quality time' with the patient and free the carer from the drudgery of physical care and household chores. Sometimes the decision to institutionalize precipitates intense family disagreement. If an extended family interview fails to resolve the issue, usually having the dissenting family member care for the patient over a weekend succeeds.

A study comparing home social services, day centres, expert centres, group living and respite hospitalization in seven different centres in the European Union found that caregivers of AD patients in group living arrangements experienced the lowest level of burden followed by caregivers of patients receiving home social services (Colvez et al., 2002).

Ethical issues arise in the terminal stages of dementia. The family must be consulted about decisions when to withhold treatment or when to institute feeding devices when patients are no longer able to swallow.

11.9.4 After the death of the patient

'The funeral that never ends' finally does so. However, carers do not feel a sense of relief that their ordeal is now over. Often the care of the patient has become the entire focus of the carer's life and the death heralds a black void rather than a new freedom. The grief can be 'remarkably intense' (Steele, 1994). For those considering autopsy, usually for scientific reasons to determine hereditary risk, decisions about postmortem examination should be made well before death so that these can be arranged expeditiously.

11.10 CARER INTERVENTIONS

While education, support groups and provision of information alone have limited efficacy in reducing carer distress (although they have been demonstrated to result in carer satisfaction with the training and increase in knowledge [Brodaty, 1992]), other carer interventions can reduce carer stress or burden

(Kahan *et al.*, 1985; Zarit *et al.*, 1987; Lovett and Gallagher, 1988; Brodaty and Gresham, 1989; Brodaty and Peters, 1991; Mittelman *et al.*, 1993, 1995; Hinchcliffe *et al.*, 1995), improve physical activity levels (Castro *et al.*, 2002) and increase immune response (Vedhara *et al.*, 2003).

A meta-analysis of 30 studies of psychosocial interventions for caregivers of people with dementia found that there were significant benefits for caregiver psychological distress, caregiver knowledge, any main caregiver outcome measure, and patient mood, but not caregiver burden (Brodaty *et al.*, 2003). Interventions were more likely to be successful if they involved both patients and caregivers (Brodaty *et al.*, 2003). Another meta-analysis, of 78 studies of interventions for caregivers of older adults, found that intervention effects for dementia caregivers (61 per cent of studies) were smaller than for carers of other groups (Sorensen *et al.*, 2002)

Carer interventions can delay nursing home admission (Brodaty *et al.*, 2003). A 10-day intensive, residential, comprehensive and extensive training programme, consisting of counselling, provision of information, practical advice, role plays and skills training for groups of up to four carers and their charges, delayed nursing home admission by almost a year (Brodaty and Gresham, 1989; Brodaty *et al.*, 1997). For the following year the groups of carers were linked by telephone conference calls second-weekly, then fourth-weekly and sixth-weekly. The programme was part of a randomized controlled trial with one group of carers receiving training immediately, a second group receiving training after 6 months' delay and a third group receiving no training at all. For the third or control group, patients were admitted for 10 days and participated in a memory-retraining programme while their carers had 10 days respite. All groups of carers had similar telephone conference links over 12 months (Brodaty and Gresham, 1989). At the end of the 12 months, patients declined uniformly on tests of cognition and function regardless of which group they were in. However, the carers in the immediate training programme had a significant decline in their (GHQ) scores, (a measure of psychological morbidity), over the 12 months, while the GHQ scores of control carers rose. The GHQ score of the delayed training carers remained steady. Rates of institutionalization were significantly lower for both carer training groups over 8 years' follow up. For example, at 4 years 55 per cent of patients in the immediate dementia caregiving training programme, and 40 per cent of those in the delayed programme, were still at home, whereas, only 8 per cent of patients whose carers were in the control group were still at home (Brodaty *et al.*, 1997). Although the programme was more costly than necessary, as it was residential and within a hospital setting, it still resulted in savings of about (in 1987) \$US6000 per couple over 39 months, because of the delay in nursing home admission (Brodaty and Peters, 1991). Over 8 years the odds ratio of surviving patients staying at home was 5.03 (95 per cent CI 1.73–14.7) greater if the carer had participated in training.

Mittelman and colleagues demonstrated almost identical findings using a different modality of intervention (Mittelman *et al.*, 1993, 1995, 1996). Carers were randomly assigned to receive counselling or standard management. The counselling condition consisted of four family sessions and two individual sessions but *ad libitum* contact and the availability of weekly support group meetings. The counselling programme was effective in reducing depression scores (Mittelman *et al.*, 1995) and delaying nursing home admission (Mittelman *et al.*, 1996). Over 8 years, there was a delay in nursing home admission in the counselling condition by a median 327 days (Mittelman *et al.*, 1996).

Eloniemi-Sulkava *et al.* (1999) and Riordan and Bennett (1998) (and Chu *et al.*, 2000 for more impaired patients) demonstrated a longer median time of home care with interventions. Qualitatively, factors associated with interventions delaying nursing home placement were a continuing relationship between helper and carer, flexibility of the intervention, and a variety of interventions tailored to meet the varied needs of the carer (Brodaty *et al.*, 2003).

The potential for carers to be effective therapists was demonstrated by two elegant multicentre US studies by Teri *et al.* (1997, 2003). The first study (Teri *et al.*, 1997) selected patients with AD who had coexisting depression and were living with a carer. The aim of the study was to investigate whether training carers in behavioural techniques could alleviate patients' depression. Carers were allocated to one of two behavioural interventions: training in problem-solving techniques or training in the use of pleasurable activity schedules; or one of two control conditions, typical care or wait-list. Patients whose carers had participated in the behavioural interventions had significantly reduced levels and rates of depression compared with patients whose carers were in the control conditions. There was no difference in outcome between the two behavioural or between the two control conditions. The benefits were retained at 6 months' follow up. Moreover, the depression scores of the carers fell significantly. In the second study, a randomized controlled trial, behavioural management strategies combined with supervision of a home-based exercise programme for people with dementia improved physical health and depression in patients with AD (Teri *et al.*, 2003). An important lesson emerging from these studies is the ability of carers to be effective therapists, given training and support.

11.11　SPECIAL CATEGORIES OF CARERS

Certain groups of carers face extra levels of isolation beyond that usually experienced by others in this role (Brodaty, 1998b). Migrants are doubly isolated by culture and language and are less likely to use services. Patients tend to lose their acquired languages first, making integration into mainstream care more difficult. Indigenous people tend to have poorer health, inferior health services and more difficulty with access to services. Younger people with dementia encounter special problems as they are more likely to be still working, have school-age children at home, have heavier financial commitments, have greater concern about heritability, have more difficulty obtaining a diagnosis and have greater difficulty integrating with mainstream services (Luscombe et al., 1997). Patients who are professionals or prominent citizens, often find it difficult to accept community and residential services. Persuading such patients that they are no longer able to continue working can be a particular problem. Where couples dement, problems are more than doubled because of the lack of an informant to obtain a history, a carer to assist in management or anyone to compensate for the patient's cognitive losses. Finally, feelings of obligation and reciprocity in a relationship are not as well developed in second marriages. There is more likely to be resentment and more difficulties and disagreements amongst children from previous marriages with different viewpoints about management, especially about finances.

11.12 CONCLUSION

The management of the carers is integral to good care of a person with dementia. Carers should be regarded as partners, alongside patients, doctors, and other health professionals in the long haul that is the tragedy of dementia. Psychosocial interventions have the capacity to reduce carer distress and delay nursing home admission. They are also cost-effective. Prescription of psychosocial interventions should be made with the same rigour and specificity as in prescribing medications. Doctors recognize that for drugs there are indications and contraindications, side effects, latency periods for onset of action, limited duration of need for the medication and need for constant review of continuing medication. These same considerations apply to psychosocial interventions (Brodaty and Gresham, 1992).

REFERENCES

Access Economics. (2003) The Dementia Epidemic: Economic Impact and Positive Solutions for Australia. Canberra, Alzheimer's Australia

Anderson R. (1987) The unremitting burden on carers. BMJ 204: 73

Archbold PG. (1981) Impact of parent caring on women. Paper presented at the XII International Congress of Gerontology, Hamburg, West Germany, July 1981

Archbold PG. (1983) Impact of parent-caring on women. Family Relations 32: 39–45

Banerjee S, Murray J, Foley B et al. (2003) Predictors of institutionalisation in people with dementia. Journal of Neurology, Neurosurgery, and Psychiatry 74: 1315–1316

Baumgarten M. (1989) The health of persons giving care to the demented elderly: a critical review of the literature. Epidemiology 42: 1137–1148

Baumgarten M, Battista RN, Infante-Rivard C et al. (1992) The psychological and physical health of family members caring for an elderly person with dementia. Journal of Clinical Epidemiology 45: 61–70

Barer BM, Johnson CL. (1990) A critique of the caregiving literature. The Gerontologist 30: 26–29

Bledin K, Kuipers L, MacCarthy B, Woods R. (1990) Daughters of people with dementia. Expressed emotion, strain and coping. British Journal of Psychiatry 157: 221–227

Bond J and Buck D. (1998) Long-term psychological distress among informal caregivers of frail older people in England: A longitudinal study. Paper presented at the 6th International Conference on Alzheimer's Disease and Related Disorders, 18–23 July, 1998

Brodaty H. (1992) Carers: training informal carers. In: T Arie (ed.), Recent Advances in Psychogeriatrics 2. Singapore, Churchill Livingstone

Brodaty H. (1994) Dementia and the family. In: S Bloch, J Hafner, E Harari, GI Szmukler (eds), The Family in Clinical Psychiatry. Oxford, Oxford University Press, pp. 224–246

Brodaty H. (1996) Caregivers and behavioural disturbances: effects and interventions. International Psychogeriatrics 8: 455–458

Brodaty H. (1998a) The family and drug treatments for Alzheimer's disease. In: S Gauthier (ed.), Pharmacotherapy of Alzheimer's Disease. London, Martin Dunitz

Brodaty H. (1998b) Managing Alzheimer's Disease in Primary Care. London, Science Press

Brodaty H and Gresham M. (1989) Effects of a training programme to reduce stress in carers of patients with dementia. BMJ 299: 1375–1379

Brodaty H and Gresham M. (1992) Prescribing residential respite care for dementia – effects, side-effects, indications and dosage. International Journal of Geriatric Psychiatry 7: 357–362

Brodaty H and Hadzi-Pavlovic D. (1990) Psychosocial effects on carers of living with persons with dementia. Australian and New Zealand Journal of Psychiatry 24: 351–361

Brodaty H and Peters KE. (1991) Cost effectiveness of a training program for dementia carers. International Psychogeriatrics 3: 11–22

Brodaty H and Green A. (2000) Family caregivers for people with dementia, In: J O'Brien, D Ames, A Burns (eds), Dementia, 2nd edition. London, Arnold, pp. 193–206

Brodaty H, Griffin D, Hadzi-Pavlovic D. (1990) A survey of dementia carers: doctors' communications, problem behaviours and institutional care. Australian and New Zealand Journal of Psychiatry 24: 362–367

Brodaty H, McGilchrist C, Harris L, Peters K. (1993) Time until institutionalization and death in patients with dementia: role of caregiver training and risk factors. Archives of Neurology 50: 643–650

Brodaty H, Gresham M, Luscombec G. (1997) The Prince Henry Hospital Dementia Caregivers' Training Programme. International Journal of Geriatric Psychiatry 12: 183–192

Brodaty H, Green A, Koschera A. (2003) Meta-analysis of psychosocial interventions of caregivers of people with dementia. Journal of the American Geriatrics Society 51: 657–664

Brody EM. (1981) The formal support network: congregate treatment settings for residents with senescent brain dysfunction. In: NE Miller, GD Cohen (eds), Clinical Aspects of Alzheimer's Disease and Senile Dementia, Aging, vol. 15. New York, Raven Press

Brody EM. (1990) Women in the Middle: Their Parent-Care Years. New York, Springer

Bruce DG and Paterson A. (2000) Barriers to community support for the dementia carer: a qualitative study. International Journal of Geriatric Psychiatry 15: 451–457

Cantor MH. (1983) Strain among caregivers: a study of experience in the United States. The Gerontologist 23: 597–604

Carrier L and Brodaty H. (1999) Mood and behaviour management. In: S Gauthier (ed.), *Clinical Diagnosis and Management of Alzheimer's Disease*, 2nd edition. London, Martin Dunitz

Castro CM, Wilcox S, O'Sullivan P *et al.* (2002) An exercise program for women who are caring for relatives with dementia. *Psychosomatic Medicine* **64**: 458–468

Chenoweth B and Spencer B. (1986) Dementia: the experience of family caregivers. *The Gerontologist* **26**: 267–272

Chesterman J, Challis D, Davies B. (1987) Long-term care at home for the elderly: a four-year follow-up. *British Journal of Social Work* **18**: 43–53

Choi H. (1993) Cultural and noncultural factors as determinants of caregiver burden for the impaired elderly in South Korea. *The Gerontologist* **33**: 8–15

Chu P, Edwards J, Levin R, Thomson J. (2000) The use of clinical case management for early stage Alzheimer's patients and their families. *American Journal of Alzheimer's Disease and Other Dementias* **15**: 284–290

Cohen RF, Swanwick GRJ, O'Boyle CA, Coakley D. (1997) Behaviour disturbance and other predictors of carer burden in Alzheimer's disease. *International Journal of Geriatric Psychiatry* **12**: 331–336

Cohen CA, Colantonio A, Vernich L. (2002) Positive aspects of caregiving: rounding out the caregiver experience. *International Journal of Geriatric Psychiatry* **17**: 184–188

Collins C. (1992) Carers: gender and caring for dementia. In: T Arie (ed.), *Recent Advances in Psychogeriatrics 2*. Edinburgh, Churchill Livingstone, pp. 173–186

Colerick EJ, George LK. (1986) Predictors of institutionalization among caregivers of patients with Alzheimer's disease. *Journal of the American Geriatrics Society* **34**: 493–498

Colvez A, Joel M-E, Ponton-Sanchez A, Anne-Charlotte R. (2002) Health status and work burden of Alzheimer patients' informal caregivers: comparisons of five different care programs in the European Union. *Health Policy* **60**: 219–233

Coope B, Ballard C, Saad K *et al.* (1995) The prevalence of depression in the carers of dementia sufferers. *International Journal of Geriatric Psychiatry* **10**: 237–242

Coward RT and Dwyer JW. (1990) The association of gender, sibling network composition, and patterns of parent care by adult children. *Research on Aging* **12**: 158–181

Deimling GT and Bass DM. (1986) Symptoms of mental impairment among elderly adults and their effects on family caregivers. *Journal of Gerontology* **41**: 778–784

Drachman DA, O'Donnell BF, Lew RA, Swearer JM. (1990) The prognosis in Alzheimer's disease. *Archives of Neurology* **47**: 851–856

Draper B, Poulos CJ, Cole AMD *et al.* (1992) A comparison of caregivers for elderly stroke and dementia victims. *Journal of the American Geriatrics Society* **40**: 896–901

Draper B, Poulos R, Poulos CJ *et al.* (1996) Risk factors for stress in elderly caregivers. *International Journal of Geriatric Psychiatry* **11**: 227–231

Dwyer JW and Coward RT. (1991) A multivariate comparison of the involvement of adult sons versus adult daughters in the care of impaired parents. *Journal of Gerontology: Social Sciences* **46**: S259–S269

Dwyer JW and Coward RT. (1992) *Gender, Families, and Elder Care*. Newbury Park, California, Sage Publications

Dwyer JW and Seccombe K. (1991) Elder care as family labor: the influence of gender and family position. *Journal of Family Issues* **12**: 229–247

Edwards JR and Cooper CL. (1988) Research in stress, coping and health: theoretical and methodological issues. *Psychological Medicine* **18**: 15–20

Eisdorfer C. (1991) Caregiving: an emerging risk factor for emotional and physical pathology. *Bulletin of the Menninger Clinic* **55**: 238–247

Eloniemi-Sulkava U, Sivenius J, Sulkava R. (1999) Support program for demented patients and their carers: the role of dementia family care coordinator is crucial. In: K Iqbal, DF Swaab, B Winblad, HM Wisinewski (eds), *Alzheimer's Disease and Related Disorders*. Chichester, John Wiley and Sons, pp. 795–802

Enright RB. (1991) Time spent caring and help received by spouses and adult children of brain-impaired adults. *The Gerontologist* **31**: 375–383

Fearon M, Donaldson C, Burns A, Tarrier N. (1998) Intimacy as a determinant of expressed emotion in carers of people with Alzheimer's disease. *Psychological Medicine* **28**: 1085–1090

Fiore J, Coppel DB, Becker J *et al.* (1986) Social support as a multi-faceted concept: examination of important dimensions for adjustment. *American Journal of Community Psychology* **14**: 93–111

Fitting M, Rabins P, Lucas J, Eastham J. (1986) Caregivers for dementia patients: a comparison of husbands and wives. *The Gerontologist* **26**: 248–252

Fortinsky RH and Hathaway TJ. (1990) Information and service needs among active and former family caregivers of persons with Alzheimer's disease. *The Gerontologist* **30**: 604–609

Gallagher D, Rose J, Rivera P *et al.* (1989) Prevalence of depression in family caregivers. *The Gerontologist* **29**: 449–456

Gallant MP and Connell CM. (2003) Neuroticism and depressive symptoms among spouse caregivers: do health behaviors mediate this relationship? *Psychology and Ageing* **18**: 587–592

Gallicchio L, Siddiqi N, Langenberg P, Baumgarten M. (2002) Gender differences in burden and depression among informal caregivers of demented elders in the community. *International Journal of Geriatric Psychiatry* **18**: 154–163

Gaugler JE, Zarit SH, Pearlin LI. (2003) The onset of dementia caregiving and its longitudinal implications. *Psychology and Ageing* **18**: 171–180

Gelfand D. (1982) *Aging: The Ethnic Factor*. Boston, Little and Brown

George LK and Gwyther LP. (1986) Caregiver well-being: a multidimensional examination of family caregivers of demented adults. *The Gerontologist* **26**: 253–259

Gibson RC. (1982) Blacks in the middle and late life: resources and coping. *Annals of the American Academy of Political and Social Sciences* **464**: 79–90

Gilhooley MLM. (1984) The impact of care-giving on care-givers: factors associated with the psychological well-being of people supporting a demented relative in the community. *British Journal of Medical Psychology* **57**: 35–44

Gilleard CJ. (1984) Problems posed for supporting relatives of geriatric and psychogeriatric day patients. *Acta Psychiatrica Scandinavica* **70**: 198–208

Gilleard CJ, Belford H, Gilleard E *et al.* (1982) Problems in caring for the elderly mentally infirm at home. *Archives of Gerontology and Geriatrics* **1**: 151–158

Gilleard CJ, Belford H, Gilleard E *et al.* (1984) Emotional distress amongst the supporters of the elderly mentally infirm. *British Journal of Psychiatry* **145**: 172–177

Gray A and Fenn P. (1993) Alzheimer's disease: the burden of the illness in England. *Health Trends* **25**: 31–37

Grafström M and Winblad B. (1995) Family burden in the care of the demented and nondemented elderly – a longitudinal study. *Alzheimer Disease and Associated Disorders* **9**: 78–86

Greene JG, Smith R, Gardiner M *et al.* (1982) Measuring behavioural disturbance of elderly demented patients in the community and its effects on relatives: a factor analytic study. *Age and Ageing* **11**: 121–126

Haley WE, Levine EG, Brown SL et al. (1987) Stress, appraisal, coping and social support as predictors of adaptational outcome among dementia caregivers. *Psychological Aging* **2**: 323–230

Haley WE, Roth DL, Coleton MI et al. (1996) Appraisal, coping, and social support as mediators of well-being in black and white Alzheimer's family caregivers. *Journal of Consulting and Clinical Psychology* **64**: 121–129

Harper S and Lund DA. (1990) Wives, husbands, and daughters caring for institutionalised and noninstitutionalised dementia patients: toward a model of caregiver burden. *International Journal of Aging and Human Development* **30**: 241–262

Hinchliffe AC, Hyman I, Blizard B et al. (1995) Behavioural complications of dementia – can they be treated? *International Journal of Geriatric Psychiatry* **10**: 839–847

Horowitz A. (1985) Sons and daughter as caregivers to older parents: differences in role performance and consequences. *The Gerontologist* **25**: 612–617

Hu T, Huang L, Cartwright W. (1986) Evaluation of the costs of caring for the senile demented elderly: a pilot study. *The Gerontologist* **26**: 158–163

Janevic MK and Connell CM. (2001) Racial, ethnic, and cultural differences in the dementia caregiving experience: recent findings. *The Gerontologist* **41**: 334–347

Kahan J, Kemp B, Staples FR, Brummel-Smith K. (1985) Decreasing the burden in families caring for a relative with a dementing illness: a controlled study. *Journal of the American Geriatrics Society* **33**: 664–670

Kiecolt-Glaser JK, Glaser R, Shuttleworth EC et al. (1987) Chronic stress and immunity in family caregivers of Alzheimer's disease victims. *Psychosomatic Medicine* **49**: 523–535

Lawton MP, Rajagopal D, Brody E et al. (1992) The dynamics of caregiving for demented elderly among black and white families. *Journals of Gerontology: Social Sciences* **47**: S156–S164

Lazarus RS and Folkman S. (1984) *Stress, Appraisal and Coping.* New York, Springer

Lee GR, Dwyer JW, Coward RT. (1993) Gender differences in parent care: demographic factors and same-gender preferences. *Journal of Gerontology: Social Sciences* **48**: S9–S16

Lee YR and Sung KT. (1997) Cultural differences in caregiving motivations for demented parents: Korean caregivers versus American caregivers. *International Journal of Aging and Human Development* **44**: 115–127

Lee YR and Sung KT. (1998) Cultural influences on caregiver burden: case of Koreans and Americans. *International Journal of Aging and Human Development* **46**: 125–141

Lezak MD. (1978) Living with the characterologically altered brain injured patient. *Journal of Clinical Psychiatry* **39**: 592–598

Lieberman MA and Kramer JH. (1991) Factors affecting decisions to institutionalise demented elderly. *The Gerontologist* **31**: 371–374

Lovett S and Gallagher D. (1988) Psychosocial interventions for family caregivers: preliminary efficacy data. *Behavior Therapy* **19**: 321–330

Lowery K, Mynt P, Aisbett J et al. (2000) Depression in the carers of dementia sufferers: a comparison of the carers of patients suffering from dementia with Lewy Bodies and the carers of patients with Alzheimer's disease. *Journal of Affective Disorders* **59**: 61–65

Luscombe G, Brodaty H, Freeth S. (1998) Younger people with dementia: diagnostic issues, effects on carers and use of services. *International Journal of Geriatric Psychiatry* **13**: 323–330

Mace NL and Rabins PV. (1982) Areas of stress on families of dementia patients: a two year follow up. Paper presented at the Gerontological Society of America meeting, Boston, 21 November, 1982

Mace NL and Rabins PV. (1991) *The 36 Hour Day: A Family Guide to Caring for Persons with Alzheimer's Disease, Related Dementing Illnesses, and Memory Loss in Later Life.* Baltimore, Johns Hopkins University Press

Majerovitz DS. (2001) Formal versus informal support: stress buffering among dementia caregivers. *Journal of Mental Health and Aging* **7**: 413–423

Mangone CA, Sanguinetti RM, Baumann PD et al. (1993) Influence of feelings of burden on the caregiver's perception of the patient's functional status. *Dementia* **4**: 287–293

Max W. (1999) Drug treatments for Alzheimer's disease. Shifting the burden of care. *CNS Drugs* **11**: 363–372

Max W, Webber PA, Fox PJ. (1995) Alzheimer's disease: the unpaid burden of caring. *Journal of Aging Health* **7**: 179–199

Miller B. (1988) Adult children's perceptions of caregiving stress and satisfaction. Paper presented at the Annual Scientific Meeting of the Gerontological Society of America, San francisco

Mintzer JE, Rupert MP, Loewenstein D et al. (1992) Daughters caregiving for Hispanic and non-Hispanic Alzheimer patients: does ethnicity make a difference? *Community Mental Health Journal* **28**: 293–303

Mittelman MS, Ferris SH, Steinberg G et al. (1993) An intervention that delays institutionalisation of Alzheimer's Disease patients: treatment of spouse-caregivers. *The Gerontologist* **33**: 730–740

Mittelman MS, Ferris SH, Shulman E et al. (1995) A comprehensive support group program: effect on depression in spouse-caregivers of AD patients. *The Gerontologist* **35**: 792–802

Mittelman MS, Ferris SH, Shulman E et al. (1996) A family intervention to delay nursing home placement of patient's with Alzheimer's Disease. A randomized controlled trial. *JAMA* **276**: 1725–1731

Mohide EA, Torrance GW, Streiner DL et al. (1998) Measuring the wellbeing of family caregivers using the time trade-off technique. *Journal of Clinical Epidemiology* **41**: 475–482

Molinari V, Nelson N, Shekelle S, Crothers MK. (1994) Family support groups of the Alzheimer's association: an analysis of attendees and non-attendees. *Journal of Applied Gerontology* **13**: 86–98

Moore MJ, Zhu CW, Clipp EC. (2001) Informal costs of dementia care: estimates from the national longitudinal caregiver study. *Journal of Gerontology: Social Sciences* **56B**: S19–S28

Morris RG, Morris LW, Britton PG. (1988) Factors affecting the emotional wellbeing of the caregivers of dementia sufferers. *British Journal of Psychiatry* **153**: 147–156

Morycz RK. (1985) Caregiving strain and the desire to institutionalise family members with Alzheimer's disease. *Research on Aging* **7**: 329–361

Novak M and Guest C. (1989) Caregiver responses to Alzheimer's disease. *International Journal of Aging and Human Development* **28**: 67–77

Patterson TL, Semple SJ, Shaw WS et al. (1998) The cultural context of caregiving: a comparison of Alzheimer's caregivers in Shanghai, China and San Diego, California. *Psychological Medicine* **28**: 1071–1084

Pearlin LI, Mullan JT, Semple SJ et al. (1990) Caregiving and the stress process: an overview of concepts and their measures. *The Gerontologist* **30**: 583–594

Pearson JL, Teri L, Wagner A et al. (1993) The relationship of problem behaviours in dementia patients to the depression and burden of caregiving spouse. *American Journal of Alzheimer's Disease* (Jan/Feb): 15–22

Pinquart M and Sorensen S. (2003) Differences between caregivers and noncaregivers in psychological health and physical health: a meta-analysis. *Psychology and Aging* **18**: 250–267

Pot AM, Deeg DJH, Van Dyck R. (1997) Psychological well-being of informal caregivers of elderly people with dementia: changes over time. *Aging and Mental Health* **1**: 261–268

Poulshock SW and Deimling GT. (1984) Families caring for elders in residence: issues in the measurement of burden. *Journal of Gerontology* **39**: 230–239

Prince M, Acosta D, Chiu H *et al.* (2004) Care arrangements for people with dementia in developing countries. *International Journal of Geriatric Psychiatry* **19**: 170–177

Pruchno RA and Resch NL. (1989) Aberrant behaviors and Alzheimer's disease: mental health effects on spouse caregivers. *Journal of Gerontology* **44**: S177–S182

Rabins PV, Fitting MD, Eastham J *et al.* (1990) Emotional adaptation over time in care-givers for chronically ill elderly people. *Age and Ageing* **19**: 185–190

Rice DR, Fox PJ, Max W *et al.* (1993) The economic burden of Alzheimer's disease care. *Health Affairs* **12**: 165–176

Riordan J and Bennett A. (1998) An evaluation of an augmented domiciliary service to older people with dementia and their carers. *Aging and Mental Health* **2**: 137–143

Rosenthal CJ, Sulman J, Marshall VW. (1993) Depressive symptoms in family caregivers of long-stay patients. *The Gerontologist* **33**: 249–257

Roth DL, Haley WE, Owen JE *et al.* (2001) Latent growth models of the longitudinal effects of dementia caregiving: a comparison of African American and White family caregivers. *Psychology and Aging* **16**: 427–436

Schneider J, Murray J, Banerjee S, Mann A on behalf of the EUROCARE Consortium. (1999) EUROCARE: a cross-national study of co-resident spouse carers for people with Alzheimer's disease: I – factors associated with carer burden. *International Journal of Geriatric Psychiatry* **14**: 61

Schulz R and Williamson GM. (1991) A 2-year longitudinal study of depression among Alzheimer's caregivers. *Psychology and Aging* **6**: 569–578

Schulz R and Williamson GM. (1997) The measurement of caregiver outcomes in Alzheimer disease research. *Alzheimer Disease and Associated Disorders* **11**: 117–124

Schulz R and Beach S. (1999) Caregiving as a risk factor for mortality: The Caregiver Health Effects Study. *JAMA* **282**: 2215–2219

Schulz R, Vistainer P, Williamson GM. (1990) Psychiatric and physical morbidity effects of caregiving. *Journal of Gerontology: Psychological Sciences* **45**: P181–P191

Shaji KS, Smitha K, Praveen Lal K, Prince MJ. (2003) Caregivers of people with Alzheimer's disease: a qualitative study from the Indian 10/66 dementia research network. *International Journal of Geriatric Psychiatry* **18**: 1–6

Sheehan NW and Nuthall P. (1988) Conflict, emotion, and personal strain among family caregivers. *Family Relations* **37**: 92–98

Smith A. (1996) Cross-cultural research on Alzheimer's disease: a critical review. *Transcultural Psychiatric Research Review* **33**: 247–276

Sorensen S, Pinquart M, Duberstein P. (2002) How effective are interventions with caregivers? An updated meta-analysis. *The Gerontologist* **42**: 356–372

Souetre EJ, Qing W, Vigoureux I *et al.* (1995) Economic analysis of Alzheimer's disease in outpatients: impact of symptom severity. *International Psychogeriatrics* **7**: 115–122

Steele CD. (1994) Management of the family. In: A Burns and R Levy (eds), *Dementia.* London, Arnold, p. 546

Stommel N, Collins CE, Given BA. (1994) The costs of family contributions to the care of persons with dementia. *The Gerontologist* **34**: 199–205

Stone R, Cafferata G, Sangl J. (1987) Caregivers of the frail elderly: a national profile. *The Gerontologist* **27**: 616–626

Teri L, Logsdon RB, Uomoto J *et al.* (1997) Behavioural treatment of depression in dementia patients: a controlled clinical trial. *Journal of Gerontology: Psychological Sciences* **52B**, P159–P166

Teri L, Gibbons LE, McCurry SM *et al.* (2003) Exercise plus behavioral management in patients with Alzheimer disease: a randomized controlled trial. *JAMA* **290**: 2015–2022

Thomas P, Chantoin-Merlet S, Hazif-Thomas C *et al.* (2002) Complaints of informal caregivers providing home care for dementia patients: the Pixel study. *International Journal of Geriatric Psychiatry* **17**: 1034–1047

Thomson C, Fine M, Brodaty H. (1997) *Carers Support Needs Project: Dementia Carers and the Non-Use of Community Services: Report on the Literature Review.* Commissioned by the Ageing and Disability Department, University of New South Wales. Sydney, Social Policy Research Centre

Townsend A, Noelker L, Deimling G *et al.* (1989) Longitudinal impact of inter-household caregiving on adult children's mental health. *Psychological Aging* **4**, 393–401

Tsien TBK and Cheng W. (1999) Caregiving impacts and needs of Chinese demented elderly families in Hong Kong. Paper presented at the *Asia-Pacific Regional Conference for the International Year of Older Persons*, April 26–29, 1999, Hong Kong

US Congress Office of Technology Assessment. (1987) *Losing a Million Minds: Confronting the Tragedy of Alzheimer's Disease and Other Dementias.* Washington, DC, US Government Printing Office

Valle R. (1988) Outreach to ethnic minorities with Alzheimer's disease: the challenge to the community. *Health Matrix* **6**: 13–27

Valle R. (1989) Cultural and ethnic issues in Alzheimer's disease family research. In: E Light and BD Leibowitz (eds), *Alzheimer's Disease and Family Stress: Directions for Research.* Rockville, MD, National Institute of Mental Health, pp. 122–154

Vedhara K, Cox NKM, Wilcock GK *et al.* (1999) Chronic stress in elderly carers of dementia patients and antibody response to influenza vaccination. *Lancet* **3531**: 627–631

Vedhara K, Bennett PD, Clark S *et al.* (2003) Enhancement of antibody responses to influenza vaccination in the elderly following a cognitive-behavioural stress management intervention. *Psychotherapy and Psychosomatics* **72**: 245–252

Vitaliano PP, Zhang J, Scanlan JM. (2003) Is caregiving hazardous to one's physical health? A meta-analysis. *Psychological Bulletin* **129**: 946–972

Walker AJ, Jones LL, Martin SK. (1989) Relationship quality and the benefits and costs of caregiving. Paper presented at the Meeting of the National Council on Family Relations, New Orleans

Wallsten SM. (1997) Elderly caregivers and care receivers. Facts and gaps in the literature. In: PD Nussbaum (ed.), *Handbook of Neuropsychology and Aging.* New York, Plenum Press, pp. 467–482

Wells Y and Jorm AF. (1987) Evaluation of a special nursing home unit for dementia sufferers: a randomised controlled comparison with community care. *Australian and New Zealand Journal of Psychiatry* **21**: 524–531

Wells YD, Jorm AF, Jordan F, Lefroy R. (1990) Effects on care-giver of special daycare programmes for dementia sufferers. *Australian and New Zealand Journal of Psychiatry* **24**: 82–90

Wood J and Parham IA. (1990) Coping with perceived burden: ethnic and cultural issues in Alzheimer's family caregiving. *Journal of Applied Gerontology* **9**: 325–339

Wright LK. (1991) The impact of Alzheimer's disease on the marital relationship. *The Gerontologist* **31**: 224–237

Yaffe K, Fox P, Newcomer R *et al.* (2002) Patient and caregiver characteristics and nursing home placement in patients with dementia. *JAMA* **187**: 2090–2097

Yale R. (1995) *Developing Support Groups for Individuals with Early-Stage Alzheimer's Disease.* Baltimore, Health Professions Press

Yeo G. (1996) Background. In: G Yeo and D Gallagher-Thompson (eds), *Ethnicity and the Dementias.* Bristol, Taylor and Francis, pp. 3–7

Zarit SH and Edwards AB. (1996) Family caregiving: research and clinical intervention. In: RT Woods (ed.), *Handbook of the Clinical Psychology of Aging.* Chichester, John Wiley and Sons

Zarit SH, Todd PA, Zarit JM. (1986) Subjective burden of husbands and wives as caregivers: a longitudinal study. *The Gerontologist* **26**: 260–266

Zarit SH, Anthony CR, Boutselis M. (1987) Interventions with caregivers of dementia patients: comparison of two approaches. *Psychology and Aging* **2**: 225–232

One caregiver's view

EMERSON MORAN

Emerson Moran is a writer in Florida. Pat, his wife, was diagnosed with early onset Alzheimer's disease in 1999. Previously, Mr Moran was a communications executive with the American Medical Association. This article is adapted from his remarks at an AMA scientific news briefing in New York City in January 2004.

The first time Pat didn't know who I was felt like we'd each been kidnapped.

Her early onset Alzheimer's had been at the centre of our life for several years, but I never expected our connection to fracture so soon. After all, I'd just quit a 10-year job to better manage our living with the disease by moving from Washington, DC, to South Florida, where Pat loved the warmth, water, bright flowers and the exotic birds.

That evening, after supper, we'd gone to the ocean to visit Pat's pelicans – when they fly low, she waves and calls them to come 'over here, over here'. At sunset, we headed home, about 15 minutes away. I remember the big thunderheads ahead of us, out over the Everglades, the wind shearing off their tops like anvils. It was like a Frederic Edward Church painting.

Halfway home, Pat was distressed and frightened. She asked who I was, what was I doing to her, where was I taking her. She tried to open the car door to escape. I was scared. Shortness of breath, dry mouth, jumbled thoughts. It was hard to look calm, talk and drive calmly at the same time.

At home, we looked at photos of our Philadelphia Quaker wedding, of trips to Tuscany and Cape May Point, of family and friends. She couldn't recognize the facts of our history, but she cried over our emotional memories. She didn't know my name, but knew we'd loved each other a long time. That was good enough for me then, and still is.

When I first saw Pat 20 years ago it was like in those movies when they freeze the frame. My frame froze. I've been with her in that frame ever since. What I didn't know for years and years was that Alzheimer's was in our frame, too.

Pat's Alzheimer's was diagnosed 5 years ago, but had already been controlling our life for a long time. We just didn't deal with it. Denial is a powerful force.

We had a very tough time at first. After all, a diagnosis of Alzheimer's is a death sentence, isn't it? And that's the first thing I felt: death, despair, deep depression, grief and fear – gripping, chilling, stunning fear. When CS Lewis lost his wife – she was the love of his life, too – he wrote that no one ever told him how much grief feels like fear. Well, yes it does.

We got through that, and, gradually and gratefully, and with a lot of help, we found ways to cope. We also discovered that our ability to deal with Alzheimer's progressed right along with the disease's progression. What we never expected was how far we'd end up going, geographically and spiritually, to manage our living with Alzheimer's before Alzheimer's totally managed us.

We tried to perpetuate our old way of life for a long time, and then reached a point where it made no sense, where our old 'normal' didn't work any more. In the landscape of our life, normal had moved. We had to move with it, by creating a new landscape and a new normal, and by building a new life frame, with Alzheimer's now the biggest figure in our picture.

We began our new way of life Labor Day weekend 2002 when we moved 985 miles from Washington to Florida, leaving behind old job, old home, old normal. It felt like jumping off a cliff. The 2-day drive was easier than I thought it would be. We could never do it today. But, back then, Pat could still handle herself alone in a strange bathroom; eat without help in a crowded, noisy restaurant; feel safe in an unfamiliar motel room. She was happy in the car. She munched M&Ms, and sang along to the Beatles and Sarah Brightman. We stopped in St Augustine – the oldest permanent European settlement in North America – and took the horse and carriage ride to the Fountain of Youth, of all places.

A week later, she didn't know who I was. I'd read the Alzheimer's books, like *The 36 Hour Day*, and knew intellectually that this moment was certain to arrive. But, Lord, I thought, not this day! Please, not this day!

Later, I had one of those dreams where I'm trying to get some place. This time I was struggling to get to the airport in some desolate, desert-like place. I had to climb up a steep incline, crawl down a deep depression, and back up over rocks and through dust. The airline check-in desk was up above me, to the right, on the edge of a cliff. Out of nowhere, a pickup truck blocked my way, machine gun in the back, like those 'technicals' the Somalian war lords drove in *Black Hawk Down*. There was shooting, confusion. Then I woke up, full of dread and apprehension.

Yes, changing our life was like jumping off a cliff. But we had to jump. It was the only way to break away from our old way of life. I took a family leave from the job I'd had for 10 years. That, plus accumulated vacation, bought 4 months to sort things out, and to just be together. We decided that I'd quit my job. We'd move to Florida, where we had family and friends. Cost of living was going to be much lower, and we figured I could earn enough freelancing to get by. What we hoped to do was carve out a way of living that would:

- keep us together as many hours in each day as possible;
- embrace Pat with care and comfort and laughter;
- allow me to work from home;
- prop me up with enough emotional and physical support to keep us going.

Looking back, I can see how we actually changed the equation of what had been a pretty conventional career-driven middle-class American existence. In our old formula, work was cemented solidly at the centre, with everything else in orbit, around the edges. In our new formula, we put Pat and Alzheimer's in the centre, with work kicked out into an orbit of its own, not quite on the edge, but not in the centre, either.

This is pretty easy to articulate after the fact. But at the time it felt like radical, uprooting, life-altering, mind-boggling, heart-thumping, cliff-jumping change. Some simple things have helped a lot. Here are six that seem real clear to me from where we sit today:

1. Family: **there is a higher power in a loving family** – we feel it and it fuels us every day. When we met, Pat was a widow, I was divorced. She never had the chance to have her own kids. Then along came my crowd. Now it's up to three married sons (one, a Marine Corp F-18 fighter pilot, serving twice in Iraq), six grandchildren, plus three step-grandchildren, my sister, brother, nieces, nephews, cousins and their kids, my own ancient parents – we now live 2 minutes away – and they all love Pat. Even my first wife loves Pat!

2. Early on, in those darkest weeks after 'The Diagnosis', a colleague told me: '**This is not the end of the world**. You still have years ahead of quality and value and love together'. That stuck like glue. It's my creed.

3. A friend reminded me: 'This is that rainy day they tell you about. **The future is now**'. Whatever you have now, use it for what you need to do now.

4. To best care for Pat I had to **take care of myself** – physically, mentally and emotionally. Early on, I was mad as hell and didn't even know it until I exploded in front of a co-worker and kicked a door so hard that they tell me it's still dented. By 3.00 pm the next day I was sitting in front of a psychologist with a lot of experience dealing with Alzheimer's families. We made a deal. I'd stick with Dr Jacobek's counselling, and she would help me stay as 'whole' as possible, no matter what happened, all the way to the end, and beyond. That was almost 5 years ago, and we're still at it, 1200 miles apart, over the phone, every 10 days. **Therapy is my gut check**, my outlet of last resort. I'm not sure how Pat and I could carry on without it.

   Working out – physical exercise – is therapeutic, too. I'm not a jock, but today, working out is actually a refuge for me. Neighborhood power walks; the gym's monthly 'geezer discount'; free weights in the garage. The cadence, the repetitions, the breathing are meditative. The endorphins fight depression.

5. **Get Pat all the help we can find**. We've been blessed with skilled, attentive doctors, and we learned that it's a good idea to have the same internist. He treats us as individuals and as a couple. Pat can't be left alone while I work. Handling this defines how we function. A sign on Dixie Highway in our new hometown led us to a local day programme for Alzheimer's. It was a big factor in deciding where to live.

   The programme is 10 minutes from home, in a church, next to our local high school. Pat's there from 8.00 am to 4:00 pm Monday through Friday. The morning roundtrip is my commute to work and Pat's time there gives me a chance to get my own job done.

   The programme's home is a 40-year-old Lutheran church hall, across a vacant lot from our local high school ('Home of the Gators'). More therapeutic than just day care, it's staffed by professionals, small enough for lots of gentle attention, and full of fun.

   At Christmas, one registered nurse brought her kids' pet goat, wearing reindeer antlers. Pat still remembers the 'rein-goat,' a remarkable memory for a woman whose only moment of meaning usually is the one she is in.

   One patient, a former golf pro, taught Pat how to putt. Some days, I wouldn't mind being there myself. Then there's Stacia, a crusty, no-nonsense, loving 70-something Polish angel who couldn't stand retirement and seems to find great satisfaction helping people just like us. Stacia brings Pat home in the afternoon, helps around the house, takes Pat to get her hair and nails done, and stays with her when my work takes me away. Stacia's parting words usually are, 'I'll take care of Pat. You take care of yourself'.

6. **Medication to manage and modify Pat's behaviour** is the final factor that holds the whole thing together. Pat has exploded with all the agitation, rage and aggression that can accompany Alzheimer's. It's terrifying when it erupts. I learned the hard way to keep a table between us for protection.

   A wise geriatric psychiatrist prescribed a strong antipsychotic that many people with schizophrenia use to help keep their lives in order. This little pill calms the rage, quiets the aggression and takes away the agitation, without taking away anything else. I don't know how we would get through the day, much less live at home together, without it.

With or without medication, though, Rule Number One is this: You will never win an argument with someone with Alzheimer's. Never. Don't even try.

Rule Number Two is old and golden: Do unto Pat as I would have Pat do unto me. Pat can't bathe herself, choose between red or blue blouse, put on earrings, shave her legs, read the paper, chew steak or pizza, pour herself a cup of coffee, or find our bathroom on her own and in time. She can, however, always find the chocolate chip cookies. We joke about putting the cookies in the bathroom. Thankfully, 'Depends' have taken the crises out of incontinence.

The Pat I fell in love with had a wonderful artistic talent (sketches and watercolours mostly), but the Alzheimer's blocked the path to her creativity years ago. Passion for her art once consumed her. Today she won't even pick up a crayon. We still have her rough drawings and pencilled story line for a children's book on meerkats in the Kalahari Desert, a cherished, unfinished work, frozen in time by her disease, an artefact of Alzheimer's.

Her brain blocks other forms of communications. Most times, she can't find the words to ask for what she wants, tell me about her day, or name who's talking to her on the phone. She says 'Thank me', instead of 'Thank you' – then giggles at the odd sound of it.

What she can do is whistle, as she never did before. It's the first sound she makes in the morning and the last at night. I tell her she's in 'full pucker'. Old movie tunes from the 1940s are favourites. Over Christmas, she was stuck on 'Easter Parade'. Sometimes I whistle with her; it's one of the few things we can still do in harmony; intimacy, redefined.

We've always loved movies, and our own critique afterwards. But now Pat can't follow a movie or TV shows with complex story lines. However, she really likes 'Sponge Bob', and belly-laughs at 'Seinfeld'. We joke a lot. I tell her that, with Alzheimer's, there's no such thing as TV reruns.

Except for 9/11. We lived in DC, on Connecticut Avenue, close enough to hear sirens and see smoke from the Pentagon. Pat experienced 9/11 on TV over and over, each time the first time, each time brand new, on September 11 and September 12: right up to today. She still gets scared when she sees the images. But then, so do I. I'm pretty sure that my own post-9/11 priorities propelled how and when we changed our life so profoundly.

What we are doing has a high cost. Nearly 45 per cent of our income goes for health insurance, medications, the day programme, Stacia helping at home. Just like hundreds of thousands of other American families, we do this on our own.

Much has changed. The kids up North have to pay their own airfare when they come down to see us. We've ended our week-long family vacations at Cape May Point. But then, where we live now sure removes the urge for a mid-winter get-away in the sun. There's no more eating out several nights a week, but my home cooking is improving. I roasted the Thanksgiving turkey over charcoal, with cornbread stuffing and a maple syrup glaze. A pot of chilli is on the stove as I write this.

Shopping is more Sears than Bloomingdales, eBay and web discounts. I clip coupons. I've discovered warehouse shopping – toilet paper in 35-roll bundles, 300-ounce Tide. Plus, a perk of paradise, $19 orchids in full bloom.

Our favourite time of the day is bedtime, which is earlier and earlier. Pat starts shutting down when the sun starts going down. She seems to settle into her own private peace in bed, curled up, eyes closed, covers pulled into a tight cocoon. She'll lay awake for 2 or 3 hours while I read, watch TV, talk to my family on the phone. We listen to music; New Age Celtic tunes strike her Irish chords. I ask, but she can't tell me, what goes on behind her closed eyes, except to say, 'I'm working on things'.

She doesn't pay much attention to the TV, unless it's the Chicago Cubs baseball team. When we lived in Chicago in the 1990s, Pat loved taking the elevated train to Wrigley Field. One night, the broadcasters cut from the playing field to the cheering fans. Pat seemed sound asleep. It was loud, it was late, I turned off the TV. In the darkness Pat said, 'Put it back. It's fun'.

Pat and I are the lucky ones. Somehow, so far, we are pulling this off, a day at a time and we do have fun. We laugh a lot, and we play a lot.

The great irony is that they tell us that Alzheimer's is a catastrophic disease but, on any given day, we don't feel like we're in the middle of a catastrophe. In many ways, we are happier now than ever before. We talk about it. We agree that surrender, acceptance, and loving each other no matter what are big reasons why.

I've been to the support groups and I've seen that not all Alzheimer's families are as fortunate. There's terrible pain and fierce anger out there. It hurts just to be near it.

I read a terrible news story maybe four years ago, from Washington. Just up 16th Street from the White House, in front of the Capital Hilton, a woman driving a Ford Taurus stopped at the light. Her father was sitting beside her. The paper said he had Alzheimer's, that she took care of him. Before the light could turn green, she pulled a gun, killed him and turned it on herself. The light changed to green, the traffic moved around them, and there they sat, at the bloody end of their own sad road.

I worry how close many other families have gotten to that point. I bet more than we'd like to think, not the point of violence, certainly, but maybe, secretly, wishing the end would come sooner rather than later.

This disease really is different, you know. There is no real treatment yet. Drugs can briefly slow down the clock, but there will be no remission, no cure, not for Pat and not, yet, for the 4 or 5 million others in the USA just like her.

We hope our 'together' lasts a long time, but, like many Alzheimer's patients, Pat's body has not been kind to her. Doctors call it 'comorbidity' – coronary artery disease, breast cancer, diverticulitis, fibromyalgia, depression – and she's only in her mid-60s. In a medical crisis, do we treat or not treat? What's moral, what's ethical? Do we risk the distress of heart surgery, colostomy, chemotherapy? Or do we let nature take its course? Where's the right and wrong?

Nothing prepared us for issues like these. Pat can't decide for herself. It's up to me. Some nights, when answers don't come, the loneliness of Alzheimer's can be worse than the certainty of how it's all going to end, no matter what we do.

Alzheimer's is a medical Mount Everest that no one has figured out how to conquer. When they do, when they break through to the summit, it'll be too late for us, but not for many of the others. I guess that's the best hope there is with Alzheimer's: that money, hard work, luck and genius will pry loose the mystery of this disease that is so slowly being unlocked from inside this human genome of ours.

Pat and I work hard every day to just live life on life's terms. One melody Pat whistles is an old Irving Berlin tune called 'Always'. I have no idea where she gets it from. I 'Googled' the lyrics. They're up on our refrigerator door, held there by a tacky magnet from the boardwalk at the New Jersey seashore. This is the refrain:

The days may not be fair – always.
That's when I'll be there – always.
Not for just an hour,
Not for just a day,
Not for just a year – but always.

I can't bear to think of the silence in my life when the whistling stops.

Pat sometimes looks at me, startled, and asks, 'Where's Emerson?' I tell her, 'I don't know, but if you see him, tell him I'm looking for him, too'. And we laugh. Always.

12

Health economic aspects of dementia

ANDERS WIMO, GÖRAN KARLSSON AND BENGT WINBLAD

A highly prevalent group of disorders such as dementia presents a challenge for any healthcare and social support system. The combination of a costly care (Ernst and Hay, 1994; Winblad *et al.*, 1997), difficulties in funding health care and an important contribution by informal caregivers focus on the basics in any health economic analysis and has indeed put the costs of dementia and cost effectiveness of dementia care into focus. It has been debated whether 'the welfare state' will be able to care for the increasing number of elderly people in general (OECD, 1996), and with dementia in particular (Lovestone, 2002). However, in the light of the enormous economic impact of dementia, it is surprising that the health economics of dementia has such a small scientific base (Jonsson *et al.*, 2000; Gray, 2002). The first (and still the only) basic textbook in this field (Wimo *et al.*, 1998a) was published in 1998 and reviewers have stressed the need for further studies (Salek *et al.*, 1998; Walker *et al.*, 1998; Jonsson *et al.*, 2000; Shukla *et al.*, 2000; Grutzendler and Morris, 2001; Lamb and Goa, 2001; NICE, 2001; Clegg *et al.*, 2002; Gray, 2002; Lyseng-Williamson and Plosker, 2002; Wolfson *et al.*, 2002; Birks and Harvey, 2003; Jonsson, 2003; Leung *et al.*, 2003; Lyseng-Williamson and Plosker, 2003; Olin and Schneider, 2003).

12.1 PERSPECTIVE

An important purpose of economic evaluation is that it should serve as a tool for decision-making regarding allocating of scarce resources (Drummond *et al.*, 1997). There are many 'players and payers' involved in delivery and financing of dementia care. Therefore it is essential to define the perspective of any pharmaco-economical analysis. The viewpoint may be a county council, a municipality, the public sector in general, an insurance company, a family member or a patient. The main cost drivers are costs for living (in its wide context, including also care in nursing homes) and informal caring (Wimo and Winblad, 2003b). There is a complex interaction on one hand between those who finance the care and on the other hand those who may benefit from the results of interventions (such as drugs or caregiver support programmes). Therefore, the detection of inoptimal incentives is an essential part of the economic analysis. Limiting the economic analysis only to the healthcare sector or the public sector exclude substantial components from the analysis. Thus, a societal perspective where all relevant costs are included regardless of where they occur and regardless of who pays is often to be preferred.

12.2 TYPES OF STUDIES AND DESIGN ASPECTS

Different types of analyses are presented in Box 12.1.

12.2.1 Descriptive studies

Cost description (CD) describes only the costs (no outcome) of a single treatment/care, without making any comparison between alternative treatments. Thus, CD cannot give any support in priority discussions but presents a framework for how costs are calculated.

Cost of illness (COI) studies are also descriptive. The COI is equal to what these resources would have been used for if there had been no case of illness (the opportunity cost). Two approaches can be used: an incidence approach or a prevalence approach. With the incidence approach the costs for new cases are estimated where both the annual costs and future (discounted) costs are included. In the prevalence approach the costs for all cases during, for example, a year are estimated – both for those already suffering from dementia and for new cases occurring during the year in question (Lindgren, 1981; Rice *et al.*, 1985). Only exceptionally have both approaches shown the same results. The choice of approach depends on the purpose of the study; if the aim is to illustrate the economic consequences of interventions, the incidence approach is preferable. If the idea is to estimate the economic burden during a defined year the prevalence approach is the option.

Another issue is whether to use a top-down or a bottom-up approach. In the 'top-down' approach the total national cost for a specific resource is distributed on different diseases. The 'bottom-up' method starts from a defined subgroup with, for example, dementia, and registers all cost of illness related to it, followed by an extrapolation to the total dementia population. The problem is that to compensate for comorbidity and net costs may be difficult to estimate. It is also important to specify the included cost categories (e.g. cost of informal care). It is obvious that dementia care is costly, but the great range in cost figures in Table 12.1 illustrates that the costing approaches vary.

12.2.2 Economical evaluations

In a cost analysis (CA), only the costs of different therapies are compared (not outcomes). Thus a CA is an incomplete economical evaluation. A complete economical evaluation includes the incremental costs and outcomes, and comparisons between different treatment alternatives.

In a cost minimization analysis (CMA), the effects of different treatments are assumed to be equivalent and the analysis is focused on identifying the cheapest therapy. The value of CMA is questioned, since the assumption of similar treatment effects is problematic (Briggs and O'Brien, 2001).

In a cost effectiveness analysis (CEA), the effect is expressed as a non-monetary quantified unit such as the cost per nursing home admission averted.

A cost benefit analysis (CBA) expresses all costs and outcomes in monetary units, e.g. dollars or euros. Few attempts have been made to apply CBA to dementia. It has, however, been argued that CBA-approaches such as 'willingness to pay' could be of value (Wimo *et al.*, 2002).

Box 12.1   *Different kinds of health economical studies*

Descriptive studies
- CD   Cost description
- COI   Cost of illness

Evaluation studies
- CA   Cost analysis (incomplete evaluation)
- CBA   Cost benefit analysis
- CEA   Cost effectiveness analysis
- CMA   Cost minimization analysis
- CUA   Cost utility analysis
- (CCA   Cost consequence analysis)

Table 12.1   *Cost of illness studies expressed as US$ 2003 (currency conversions to US$ by PPPs [purchasing power parities], time transformations by CPI [consumer price index])*

Country	Annual costs per patient US$ 2003	Cost categories included	Source
USA	57 000	D, IC	Ernst and Hay, 1994
England	6600	D	Smith and Shah, 1995
Canada	14 300	D, IC	Ostbye and Crosse, 1994
Sweden	24 400	D	Wimo *et al.*, 1997b (gross costs)
Sweden	16 500	D	Wimo *et al.*, 1997b (net costs)
Germany	12 800	D	Schulenberg and Schulenberg, 1998
Denmark	10 400	D	Kronborg Andersen *et al.*, 1999
Italy	64 400	D, IC	Cavallo and Fattore, 1997
The Netherlands	10 800	D	Koopmanschap *et al.*, 1998
Ireland	13 900	DC, IC	O'Shea and O'Reilly, 2000

Source for PPP and CPI: OECD, data on file: www.oecd.org. Figures are rounded off.
D, direct costs; IC, informal care

In a cost utility analysis (CUA), the effect is expressed as utilities, such as QALYs (Quality Adjusted Life Years) (Torrance, 1997).

It is important to include a discussion of uncertainty in economical evaluations (Briggs and O'Brien, 2001) and important factors should be varied in a sensitivity analysis.

In a cost consequence analysis (CCA), cost and outcomes are analysed and presented separately. The value of CCA is under discussion (Winblad et al., 1997), since results may be difficult to interpret and the selection of outcomes may be biased.

12.3 THE NEED FOR MODELLING

An intervention in dementia may influence the course of the disease (e.g. the deterioration rate in functional ability, the position in a care organization and perhaps survival). Therefore, an economic evaluation has to take into account impacts on costs and outcomes during the whole lifespan. Most clinical studies last for 6–12 months. Owing to practical and ethical issues, single studies covering the whole disease period will probably never be undertaken. One option to determine long-term effects is to extend ongoing studies. In randomized controlled trials (RCTs) it is difficult to maintain the original design for many years, but open follow-up studies have been used on tacrine (Knopman et al., 1996) and donepezil (Geldmacher et al., 2003). However, there are several drawbacks, such as selection bias, patients lost to follow up and problems in defining controls.

Therefore, there is a need for modelling approaches (Buxton et al., 1997). The basic idea is that results from a short core period are extrapolated to a longer period. Inputs from several sources, e.g. efficacy, costing and progression, are used. Markov models are frequently used for this purpose (Sonnenberg and Leventhal, 1998). Other approaches, such as decision tree models (Weinstein and Fineberg, 1980) and survival models (Fenn and Gray, 1999) can also be used. Discounting of costs (and perhaps outcomes) is recommended. The discount rate is often 3–5 per cent (Siegel et al., 1997), but it can be varied in a sensitivity analysis.

Models are controversial. Long-term effects, such as exhaustion of carers and staff, which do not occur in the core period, and symptoms that do not have a linear progressive course, such as BPSDs (Behavioural and Psychological Symptoms in Dementia) (Ferris and Mittelman, 1996), are difficult to model. A model is also linked, implicitly or explicitly, to a specific organization of care. The drug authorities are often sceptical to models, since such studies are not 'empirical'.

12.4 FAMILY MEMBERS AND INFORMAL CARE

Informal carers (mostly spouses or children of demented patients) are of great importance in dementia care. An informal carer is often part of a 'dementia family'. In that sense, their situation can be analysed in terms of, for example, burden, quality of life, coping, stress, social network and morbidity (Max et al., 1995; Jansson et al., 1998; Schulz and Beach, 1999; Wimo et al., 1999b; Almberg et al., 2000).

They are also often producers of an extensive amount of unpaid informal care (Rice et al., 1993; Stommel et al., 1994; Langa et al., 2001; Moore et al., 2001; Wimo et al., 2002), which constitute a great part of the societal costs.

Measuring caregiver time is problematic. Support in personal activities of daily living (ADL) and instrumental activities of daily living (IADL) are rather well-defined activities. However, a substantial part of caregiver activities is linked to supervision to manage behavioural symptoms or to prevent dangerous events (Wimo et al., 2002). The assessments of supervision and surveillance in terms of minutes and hours may, however, be difficult.

Two other important factors are care productivity and joint production. A formal caregiver is probably more efficient and takes less time to support ADL tasks than an informal caregiver. This must be considered if a replacement approach is used (see below). Joint production means that the patient and the caregiver are doing things together, for example shopping.

Costing informal care is a complicated and controversial issue (Koopmanschap, 1998; Jonsson et al., 2000). There are two frequently used methods: the opportunity cost approach and the replacement cost approach.

Whether the caregiver is paid or not is not of interest for the economic valuation. Payment has an impact on the distribution of the economic burden but not on the total societal cost. The relevant cost is the opportunity cost, i.e. the benefits that are forgone because a resource – in this case caregiver time – is not put to its best alternative use. Thus, the question is to identify the alternative use of the caregiver's time. If the alternative is working on the labour market, the cost for informal care should be valued to the production loss owing to absence from work.

However, more problematic is the costing of leisure time and caregiver time during retirement. There is no consensus on how this should be performed. The cost for the caregiver's time may the value of the time used as leisure time (Karlsson et al., 1998). However, there is no such market price available. Survey methods (for example the contingent valuation method – Johannesson et al., 1992) is an option.

With the replacement cost approach it is assumed that the informal carer should be replaced with a professional carer on a 1:1 ratio. The informal caregiver's time and the professional caregiver's time are regarded as perfect substitutes. However, we do not know if there actually will be a complete replacement with a professional carer.

12.5 OUTCOME MEASURES

Cognition is considered as the mandatory primary efficacy outcome in most dementia trials. There are, however, other outcomes that are probably more important for the patients and the caregivers. Quality of life, ADL-capacity, mood-depression or BPSDs may be of greater interest than cognition in the long run. ADL-capacity and BPSDs are also essential in care planning.

Surrogate end points are inappropriate to use in CEA (Johannesson et al., 1996). Mini-Mental State Examination (MMSE) (Folstein et al., 1975) is often used in dementia studies as well as other measures of cognitive capacity such as the ADAS-cog (Alzheimer's Disease Assessment Scale – cognitive subscale) (Rosen et al., 1984). However, in our view, they should be regarded as surrogate end points. Since MMSE is highly correlated to costs (Ernst et al., 1997; Hux et al., 1998; Wimo et al., 1998c; Jonsson et al., 1999b), and also to other, more relevant outcomes, such as ADL-capacity, position in care organization and severity of dementia, it has frequently been used in economic evaluations of dementia. MMSE is also used in most longitudinal population based studies and thus it may be useful as a link between clinical studies and population studies in the discussions of efficacy versus clinical effectiveness.

However, delay in progression in terms of severity presents a broader outcome than cognition and severity scales such as clinical dementia rating (CDR) (Berg, 1988) and the global deterioration scale (GDS) (Reisberg et al., 1988) or multidimensional instruments such as Gottfries–Brane–Steen scale (GBS) (Brane et al., 2001) are therefore more relevant to use than cognition.

Postponing or preventing nursing home placement has also been suggested. A study by Knopman et al. (1996) indicated that nursing home care can be postponed about by about 1 year with tacrine treatment. Sano et al. (1997) showed similar effects with vitamin E/selegeline treatment. A study on donepezil indicated an even longer postponing of institutionalization (Geldmacher et al., 2003). However, the situation is more complex regarding caregivers. On the one hand, it may be an advantage that spouses can go on living together, but on the other hand, a prolonged period at home may be more stressful for the caregiver (Max, 1996). This potential risk was, however, not confirmed in the two published RCTs where the amount of informal care has been measured (Wimo et al., 2003a, b).

Quality of Life (QoL) of both patients and caregivers is considered as a relevant outcome. Health-related QoL includes several dimensions, such as ADL, social interaction, perception, pain, anxiety, economic status, etc. One potential problem in QoL assessments is the patient's difficulties in evaluating his or her own health state (Stewart and Brod, 1996). Thus, proxies (mostly caregivers) are often used. Proxies per se is not necessarily a problem. The US Panel for Cost-Effectiveness recommends that the general public should value the health states and, in that sense, an indirect measurement is not disqualified (Siegel et al., 1997). If the proxy is a family member, the answers partly may reflect the situation and interests of the proxy, which must be considered. Some attributes may be difficult for proxies, such as 'pain', whereas others, such as

'mobility' are less problematic. Interestingly, in a project where proxy-rated and self-rated QoL were used simultaneously, great differences between the two approaches occurred (Jönsson, 2003).

In principle, two kinds of instruments can be used: diagnostic specific or generic instruments (Bowling, 1995; Spilker, 1996; Salek et al., 1998; Walker et al., 1998).

More or less dementia-specific instruments such as DQoL (the Dementia Quality of Life instrument) (Brod et al., 1999), QoLAD (Quality of life-Alzheimer's disease) (Selai et al., 2001; Logsdon et al., 2002) and Quality of Life Assessment Schedule (QoLAS) (Selai et al., 2000; Elstner et al., 2001) may be useful in CCA-trials but are inappropriate for complete economic evaluations since these instruments not are preference based (Torrance et al., 1996; Siegel et al., 1997).

There are a great number of generic QoL scales, such as the Sickness Impact Profile (Bergner et al., 1981), the Short Form 36 (SF-36) (Ware and Sherbourne, 1992), the QLA-scale (Blau, 1977), the Health Utilities Index (HUI) (Torrance et al., 1996; Neumann et al., 2000), the EuroQoL/EQ-5D (Coucill et al., 2001) or the Quality of Wellbeing Scale (QWBS) (Kerner et al., 1998). HUI, EQ-5D, QWBS and the caregiver quality of life index (CQLI) (Mohide et al., 1988) can be used to calculate QALYs (Torrance, 1997).

QALYs are used in CUA and reflect both quantity and quality of life (Torrance, 1996; Torrance et al., 1996) and give opportunities for comparisons with other diseases. Utilities are expressed as a figure between 0 (death) and 1 (perfect health). QALYs are not uncontroversial (Tsuchiya et al., 2003). Chronic incurable progressive disorders may be disfavoured when compared with, for example, curative surgical treatment, such as cataract surgery or hip replacement surgery.

There are also other approaches, such as DALYs (Disability Adjusted Life Years) (Allotey et al., 2003) and HYE (Healthy Years Equivalents) (Dolan, 2000). However, DALYs focus on productivity more than quality of life and HYEs require a great number of health scenarios (Torrance, 1996).

Burden scales, such as the Burden Interview (Zarit et al., 1980) can to some extent be used as indicators of caregiver QoL, but the interplay between patient status, caregiver QoL and burden is complex (Deeken et al., 2003).

In conclusion, the choice of outcome measure in economic evaluation in dementia is not an obvious one. As different outcome measures give different pieces of information, several outcome measures can be used.

12.6 RESOURCE UTILIZATION IN DEMENTIA

The costing process usually consists of two phases: first, resource utilization is expressed in terms of physical units (such as nursing home days), and second, the resource utilization figures are calculated into costs by the use of unit costs for each resource. RUD (Resource Utilization in Dementia) (Wimo et al., 1998b) is an example of a framework assessing the use of formal and informal resources, aiming at calculating costs from a societal perspective (Box 12.2). RUD has been used in several studies (Wimo *et al.*, 1999a; Wimo *et al.*, 2000; Wimo *et al.*, 2003a; Wimo *et al.*, 2003c). A comprehensive battery can be time-demanding and thus a short version, the RUD Lite (Wimo and Winblad, 2003b) was developed. It was possible to limit the number of variables in the RUD considerably without losing the societal perspective in the analysis (RUD Lite covers about 95 per cent of the costs resulting from the complete RUD – Wimo and Winblad, 2003b). One part of the RUD is the caregiver time subscale. Other instruments that assess caregiver time are the CATS

(Caregiver Activities Time Survey) (Clipp and Moore, 1995) and the CAS (Caregiver Activity Survey) (Davis *et al.*, 1997).

Since the organization of dementia care varies between countries, any resource use battery must be adapted to the specific situation in a country.

12.7 PHARMACO–ECONOMICAL STUDIES

Even if it would be advantageous to design studies purely for health economical purposes, pharmaco-economics will probably be part of comprehensive phase III/IV studies (Hill and McGettigan, 1998). It is, however, important to refine the methods used (Briggs and O'Brien, 2001). It has also been debated whether pharmaco-economic aspects are best included in phase III or phase IV studies (Schneider, 1998).

Several pharmaco-economical evaluations have been published, mainly on the cholinesterase inhibitors (one on memantine) with various approaches. The early tacrine studies focused on costs and they are also based on the same efficacy study (Knapp *et al.*, 1994). Even if treatment seems to be cost saving, the range is large in these studies, from about 1 to 17 per cent, indicating not only different methodological approaches but also problems. Few studies are empirical (Table 12.2) and most evaluations are based on models (Tables 12.3 and 12.4). In the donepezil models, Markov models have been used with QALYs or severity (avoided) as outcome, while survival analysis have been used in the rivastigmine models. In the galantamine studies, the AHEAD (assessment of health economics in Alzheimer's disease) concept is used (Caro *et al.*, 2001). In general, the results favour drug use, but sensitivity analyses show a range in the results, indicating uncertainty.

Drug trials are often criticized regarding representativeness. Schneider *et al.* (1997) showed that study populations in dementia drug trials only reflect about 7 per cent of a general dementia population. The progression rate of cognition is slower in placebo groups in most clinical studies than in

---

Box 12.2 *Components of a resource utilization battery*

Patient
- Accommodation/long-term care
- (Work status)
- Respite care
- Hospital care
- Outpatient clinic visits
- Social service
- Home nursing care
- Day care
- Drug use

Caregiver
- Informal care time (for patient)
- Work status
- (Respite care)
- Hospital care
- Outpatient clinic visits
- Social service
- Home nursing care
- Day care
- Drug use

Table 12.2 *Studies with empirical data. Costs are expressed as US$ 2003 (PPPs). Figures are rounded off.*

Drug	Treatment length (years)	Cost difference*	Cost difference (%) v controls	P	Comment	Ref
Donepezil	0.5	42	1.0	NS		Small *et al.*, 1998
Donepezil	1	4500	35.1	0.03	Long-term use	Hill *et al.*, 2002
		3800	29.9	NS	Short-term use	*ibid.*
Donepezil	1.9	−2.70	−25.4	?	Costs per day, direct medical mean costs	Fillit *et al.*, 1999
		−5.60	−46.8	?	Overall mean costs	*ibid.*
		2.30	63.7	0.02	Direct medical median costs	*ibid.*
		−1.60	−21.7	0.04	Overall median costs	*ibid.*
Donepezil	1	1200	4.2	NS	Total mean costs	Wimo *et al.*, 2003a
		−320	−1.8	NS	Total patient direct mean costs	*ibid.*
Memantine	0.5	1200	−13.3	0.01	Costs per month	Wimo *et al.*, 2003c

*A positive value indicates net savings with treatment

population-based studies. Another issue is whether study populations reflect the dementia care organization that the results are generalized to.

12.8 MILD COGNITIVE IMPAIRMENT

Health economical effects on mild cognitive impairment (MCI) can be divided into short-term and long-term effects (Wimo and Winblad, 2003a). In the short-term perspective, an intervention can perhaps result in a reduction of informal care in terms of IADL. Thus it is questionable whether the costs of a drug will be offset with a short-term viewpoint. In the long run, the question will be whether survival is affected and whether there will be any transitions of symptoms and resource use during the course of the dementia. To design studies to answer these questions is not easy. A synthetic approach with RCTs covering segments of the dementia course, modelling studies and open follow-up studies will probably be needed, resulting in some kind of 'best guess' judgement.

Table 12.3 *Cost analysis models. Costs are expressed as US$ 2003 (PPPs). Figures are rounded off.*

Drug	Model length (years)	Cost difference*	Cost difference (%) v comparator	Range in sensitivity analysis	Comment	Ref
Tacrine	4.4	2900	17.3	US$113–6595	Costs effects annualized by study's authors	Lubeck et al., 1994
Tacrine	5.3	11 500	7.5	US$698–26 687		Henke and Burchmore, 1997
Tacrine	9	2600	1.3	0.6–5.2%		Wimo et al., 1997a
Rivastigmine	2	2200**	NA	NA	Mild	Fenn and Gray, 1999
	0.5	18**	NA	NA		
Rivastigmine	2	4100**	NA	NA	All	Hauber et al., 2000b
	0.5	150**	NA	NA		

NA, not available
* A positive value indicates net savings with treatment with CHEIs
** The cost for rivastigmine is not included

Table 12.4 *Cost effectiveness (C/E) models. Costs are expressed as US$ 2003 (PPPs). Figures are rounded off.*

Drug	Model length (years)	Cost difference*	C/E or similar**	Range in sensitivity analysis (US$ 2003) (C/E)**	Comment	Source
Donepezil	5	−2500	10 000	1600–17 500 (all scenarios)	Mild; 10 mg	Stewart et al., 1998
Donepezil	5	880	<0	<0–8300 (all scenarios)	5 mg	O'Brien et al., 1999
Donepezil	5	410	<0	<0–3300	10 mg	Jonsson et al., 1999a
Donepezil	0.5	−610	185 000	<0–480 000 (all scenarios)	Mild AD at start	Neumann et al., 1999
	2	80	<0			ibid.
Donepezil	0.5	−1700	44 000	<0–44 000[†]	Mild AD at start	Ikeda et al., 2002
	2	250	<0			ibid.
Rivastigmine	0.5	−650	0.0337[†]	0.0067[§]	All stages	Hauber et al., 2000a
	2	410	0[†]	0[§]		ibid.
Galantamine	10	730	<0	<0–30 500	Mild–moderate	Getsios et al., 2001
Galantamine	10.5	1750	<0		Mild–moderate	Caro et al., 2002
Galantamine	10.5	3100	<0		All	Garfield et al., 2002
Galantamine	10	3800	<0	<0–14 300	24 mg	Migliaccio-Walle et al., 2003
Galantamine	10	−770	13 900	9300–27 900	16 mg	Ward et al., 2003
		−1000			24 mg	

* A positive value indicates net savings with treatment with CHEIs
** A positive value indicates a cost per gained QALY/avoided deterioration in severity; <0 cost savings and a positive outcome
[†] Included in presentation of main results
[‡] Threshold analysis: how many gained QALYs are needed to obtain cost effectiveness if Can$20 000/QALY is regarded as appropriate
[§] If Can$100 000/QALY
NA, not available

12.9 PHARMACO-ECONOMICS AND DRUG AUTHORITIES

New drugs go through several steps within drug authorities before entering the market. These steps are not necessarily handled within the same authorities. While the registration process in the European Union is being harmonized through EMEA (CPMP, 1997[1]), focusing on cognition, ADL and a global effect (Hill and McGettigan, 1998), decisions about pricing and reimbursement remain on the country level. Furthermore, there may be different forms of budget restrictions on various levels in the care organization.

In the USA, the specific guidelines for antidementia drugs presented by the FDA demands 'clinically meaningful effects' (Leber, 1997).

The drugs that are used in dementia are rather expensive and the fact that a drug is registered in a country does not mean that the drug will be available for all patients. The critical issue is the reimbursement decisions (Drummond, 2003). For example, in Sweden the cholinesterase inhibitors are reimbursed as other drugs. However, in Sweden a new authority has just been founded to handle questions about reimbursement on a national level. The drug authorities in Australia and Canada demand health economical evaluations as part of the reimbursement decision process (Hill and McGettigan, 1998). The Canadian Health Technology Assessment Guidelines for Pharmaco-economics (CCOHTA), focus on meta-analysis and epidemiological data and emphasize the use of cost benefit and cost utility analysis (CCOHTA, 1997).

12.10 INTERNATIONAL COMPARISONS

The way care is financed and organized as well as the relative supply of different forms of care, the general taxation level and the economical strength of countries are factors that make comparisons between countries difficult.

Comparing currencies also present problems. Usual currency exchange rates reflect trade between countries rather than purchase power. PPPs (purchase power parities) (OECD website), are probably better to use than exchange rates. Comparisons over time both within and between countries are also linked to uncertainty. Consumer price indexes are often used, but an index that reflects changes in the healthcare sector is better.

In multinational studies, the results should be aggregated in terms of resource use (and not in monetary terms) from every country. The cost calculations should then be performed in one currency, based on aggregated resource use. However, if there are great differences in care organization

between countries, aggregation of resource use results may also be problematic. For example, the concept of 'nursing home' can include a wide range of resources in terms of number of staff and their competence, physical environment, technical equipment, leading to different costs. There are also care concepts that are used just in one or only a few countries, such as DOMUS care in the UK (Beecham *et al.*, 1993), Group Living in Sweden (Wimo *et al.*, 1995)and Special Care Units (SCU) in the USA (Maas *et al.*, 1998). Home care may be dealt with by social services with poorly qualified staff, but also by specific teams focused on dementia. Even if a care organization can be roughly divided into levels (such as nursing home care – intermediate care alternatives – home care), such a simplistic division questions the validity of multinational intervention studies.

12.11 SEVERE DEMENTIA

Several years can pass in the stage of severe dementia (Winblad *et al.*, 1999). In a model of a Swedish cohort, the course of dementia with an estimated survival up to 9 years was simulated (Wimo *et al.*, 1998c). About 75 per cent of the total costs occurred in severe dementia, indicating that the total span for benefits during the total course in terms of cost reduction is only 25 per cent, if efficacy only is shown for mild to moderate dementia. The results indicate that severe dementia must be the focus for improved care and research. Many of the instruments we use today for outcome research show floor effects in severe dementia and they are not sufficiently sensitive to detect clinically relevant changes (Winblad *et al.*, 1999). Currently (March 2005) there is one drug, memantine (Reisberg *et al.*, 2003), approved for severe dementia, but studies on the cholinesterase inhibitors are underway.

12.12 CONCLUSION

The health economics of dementia is still in a premature state, even if the number of published studies is increasing. There is a great need for methodological improvement. There is also a great interest in the pharmaco-economics of dementia among the drug authorities in different countries and in the pharmaceutical companies who are engaged in antidementia drug research, illustrating that it is a hot topic.

REFERENCES

Allotey P, Reidpath D, Kouame A, Cummins R. (2003) The DALY, context and the determinants of the severity of disease: an exploratory comparison of paraplegia in Australia and Cameroon. *Society of Scientific Medicine* **57**: 949–958

Almberg B, Grafstrom M, Krichbaum K, Winblad B. (2000) The interplay of institution and family caregiving: relations between patient

---

[1]CPMP (Committee for Proprietary Medical Products) has changed its name to Committee for Medical Products for Human Use (CHMP). The EMEA acronym is unchanged, but the former European Agency for the Evaluation of Medical Products has now been replaced with the European Medicines Agency.

hassles, nursing home hassles and caregivers' burnout. *International Journal of Geriatric Psychiatry* 15: 931–939

Beecham J, Cambridge P, Hallam A, Knapp M. (1993) The cost of Domus care. *International Journal of Geriatric Psychiatry* 8: 827–831

Berg L. (1988) Clinical dementia rating (CDR). *Psychopharmacology Bulletin* 24: 637–639

Bergner M, Bobbitt RA, Carter WB, Gilson BS. (1981) The Sickness Impact Profile: development and final revision of a health status measure. *Medical Care* 19: 787–805

Birks JS and Harvey R. (2003) Donepezil for dementia due to Alzheimer's disease. (Cochrane Review). Oxford: Software Update, *Cochrane Library*, Issue 3

Blau TH. (1977) Quality of life, social indicators and criteria of change. *Professional Psychology* 8: 464–473

Bowling A. (1995) *Measuring Health. A review of quality of life measurement scales.* Milton Keynes, Philadelphia, Open University Press

Brane G, Gottfries CG, Winblad B. (2001) The Gottfries-Brane-Steen scale: validity, reliability and application in anti-dementia drug trials. *Dementia and Geriatric Cognitive Disorders* 12: 1–14

Briggs AH and O'Brien BJ. (2001) The death of cost-minimization analysis? *Health Economics* 10: 179–184

Brod M, Stewart AL, Sands L, Walton P. (1999) Conceptualization and measurement of quality of life in dementia: the dementia quality of life instrument (DQoL). *The Gerontologist* 39: 25–35

Buxton MJ, Drummond MF, Van Hout BA *et al.* (1997) Modelling in economic evaluation: an unavoidable fact of life. *Health Economics* 6: 217–227

Caro JJ, Getsios D, Migliaccio-Walle K, Raggio G, Ward A. (2001) Assessment of health economics in Alzheimer's disease (AHEAD) based on need for full-time care. *Neurology* 57: 964–971

Caro JJ, Salas M, Ward A, Getsios D, Mehnert A. (2002) Economic analysis of galantamine, a cholinesterase inhibitor, in the treatment of patients with mild to moderate Alzheimer's disease in the Netherlands. *Dementia and Geriatric Cognitive Disorders* 14: 84–89

Cavallo MC and Fattore G. (1997) The economic and social burden of Alzheimer disease on families in the Lombardy region of Italy. *Alzheimer Disease and Associated Disorders* 11: 184–190

CCOHTA. (1997) *Guidelines for economic evaluation of pharmaceuticals,* 2nd edition. Ottawa, The Canadian Coordinating Office for Health Technology Assessment

Clegg A, Bryant J, Nicholson T *et al.* (2002) Clinical and cost-effectiveness of donepezil, rivastigmine, and galantamine for Alzheimer's disease. A systematic review. *International Journal of Technological Assessment of Health Care* 18: 497–507

Clipp EC and Moore MJ. (1995) Caregiver time use: an outcome measure in clinical trial research on Alzheimer's disease. *Clinical Pharmacology and Therapeutics* 58: 228–236

Coucill W, Bryan S, Bentham P, Buckley A, Laight A. (2001) EQ-5D in patients with dementia: an investigation of inter-rater agreement. *Medical Care* 39: 760–771

CPMP. (1997) *Note for guidance on medical products in the treatment of Alzheimer's disease.* In: EMEA http://www.emea.eu.int/pdfs/human/ewp/055395en.pdf

Davis KL, Marin DB, Kane R *et al.* (1997) The Caregiver Activity Survey (CAS): development and validation of a new measure for caregivers of persons with Alzheimer's disease. *International Journal of Geriatric Psychiatry* 12: 978–988

Deeken JF, Taylor KL, Mangan P, Yabroff KR, Ingham JM. (2003) Care for the caregivers: a review of self-report instruments developed to measure the burden, needs, and quality of life of informal caregivers. *Journal of Pain and Symptom Management* 26: 922–953

Dolan P. (2000) A note on QALYs versus HYEs. Health states versus health profiles. *International Journal of Technological Assessment of Health Care* 16: 1220–1224

Drummond MF. (2003) The use of health economic information by reimbursement authorities. *Rheumatology (Oxford)* 42 (Suppl. 3): 60–63

Drummond MF, O'Brien B, Stoddart GL, Torrance GW. (1997) *Methods for the Economic Evaluation of Health Care Programmes.* Oxford, UK, Oxford University Press

Elstner K, Selai CE, Trimble MR, Robertson MM. (2001) Quality of Life (QoL) of patients with Gilles de la Tourette's syndrome. *Acta Psychiatrica Scandinavica* 103: 52–59

Ernst RL and Hay JW. (1994) The US economic and social costs of Alzheimer's disease revisited. *American Journal of Public Health* 84: 1261–1264

Ernst RL, Hay JW, Fenn C, Tinklenberg J, Yesavage JA. (1997) Cognitive function and the costs of Alzheimer disease. An exploratory study. *Archives of Neurology* 54: 687–693

Fenn P and Gray A. (1999) Estimating long-term cost savings from treatment of Alzheimer's disease. A modelling approach. *Pharmacoeconomics* 16: 165–174

Ferris SH and Mittelman MS. (1996) Behavioral treatment of Alzheimer's disease. *International Psychogeriatrics* 8: 87–90

Fillit H, Gutterman EM, Lewis B. (1999) Donepezil use in managed Medicare: effect on health care costs and utilization. *Clinical Therapeutics* 21: 2173–2185

Folstein MF, Folstein SE, McHugh PR. (1975) 'Mini-mental state'. A practical method for grading the cognitive state of patients for the clinician. *Journal of Psychiatric Research* 12: 189–198

Garfield FB, Getsios D, Caro JJ, Wimo A, Winblad B. (2002) Assessment of Health Economics in Alzheimer's Disease (AHEAD). Treatment with Galantamine in Sweden. *Pharmacoeconomics* 20: 629–637

Geldmacher DS, Provenzano G, McRae T, Mastey V, Ieni JR. (2003) Donepezil is associated with delayed nursing home placement in patients with Alzheimer's disease *Journal of American Geriatrics Society* 51: 937–944

Getsios D, Caro JJ, Caro G, Ishak K. (2001) Assessment of health economics in Alzheimer's disease (AHEAD): galantamine treatment in Canada. *Neurology* 57: 972–978

Gray A. (2002) Health economics. In: N Qizilbash, L Schneider, H Chui, P Tariot, J Brodaty, J Kaye, T Erkinjuntti (eds), *Evidence-Based Dementia Practice.* Oxford, Blackwell Publishing, pp. 844–854

Grutzendler J and Morris JC. (2001) Cholinesterase inhibitors for Alzheimer's disease. *Drugs* 61: 41–52

Hauber AB, Gnanasakthy A, Mauskopf JA. (2000a) Savings in the cost of caring for patients with Alzheimer's disease in Canada: an analysis of treatment with rivastigmine. *Clinical Therapeutics* 22: 439–451

Hauber AB, Gnanasakthy A, Snyder EH, Bala MV, Richter A, Mauskopf JA. (2000b) Potential savings in the cost of caring for Alzheimer's disease. Treatment with rivastigmine. *Pharmacoeconomics* 17: 351–360

Henke CJ and Burchmore MJ. (1997) The economic impact of the tacrine in the treatment of Alzheimer's disease. *Clinical Therapeutics* 19: 330–345

Hill S and McGettigan P. (1998) Drug authorities' policy on the assessment of drugs for dementia. In: A Wimo, G Karlsson, B Jönsson, B Winblad (eds), *The Health Economics of Dementia.* London, Wiley

Hill JW, Futterman R, Mastey V, Fillit H. (2002) The effect of donepezil therapy on health costs in a Medicare managed care plan. *Management Care Interface* 15: 63–70

Hux MJ, O'Brien BJ, Iskedjian M, Goeree R, Gagnon M, Gauthier S. (1998) Relation between severity of Alzheimer's disease and costs of caring. *Canadian Medical Association Journal* **159**: 457–465

Ikeda S, Yamada Y, Ikegami N. (2002) Economic evaluation of donepezil treatment for Alzheimer's disease in Japan. *Dementia and Geriatric Cognitive Disorders* **13**: 33–39

Jansson W, Almberg B, Grafstrom M, Winblad B. (1998) The Circle Model–support for relatives of people with dementia. *International Journal of Geriatric Psychiatry* **13**: 674–681

Johannesson M, Johansson PO, Jonsson B. (1992) Economic evaluation of drug therapy: a review of the contingent valuation method. *Pharmacoeconomics* **1**: 325–337

Johannesson M, Jonsson B, Karlsson G. (1996) Outcome measurement in economic evaluation. *Health Economics* **5**: 279–296

Jönsson L. (2003) *Economic evaluation of treatments for Alzheimer's disease*. Thesis. Stockholm: Karolinska Institutet

Jonsson L. (2003) Pharmacoeconomics of cholinesterase inhibitors in the treatment of Alzheimer's disease. *Pharmacoeconomics* **21**: 1025–1037

Jonsson L, Lindgren P, Wimo A, Jonsson B, Winblad B. (1999a) The cost-effectiveness of donepezil therapy in Swedish patients with Alzheimer's disease: a Markov model. *Clinical Therapeutics* **21**: 1230–1240

Jonsson L, Lindgren P, Wimo A, Jonsson B, Winblad B. (1999b) Costs of Mini-Mental State Examination-related cognitive impairment. *Pharmacoeconomics* **16**: 409–416

Jonsson B, Jonsson L, Wimo A. (2000) In: M May and N Sartorius (eds), *Dementia. WPA Series Evidence and Experience in Psychiatry*. London, John Wiley and Sons, pp. 335–363

Karlsson G, Jonsson B, Wimo A, Winblad B. (1998) Methodological issues in health economics of dementia. In: A Wimo, G Karlsson, B Jönsson, B Winblad (eds), *The Health Economics of Dementia*. London, Wiley, pp. 161–169

Kerner DN, Patterson TL, Grant I, Kaplan RM. (1998) Validity of the Quality of Well-Being Scale for patients with Alzheimer's disease. *Journal of Aging Health* **10**: 44–61

Knapp MJ, Knopman DS, Solomon PR, Pendlebury WW, Davis CS, Gracon SI. (1994) A 30-week randomized controlled trial of high-dose tacrine in patients with Alzheimer's disease. The Tacrine Study Group. *JAMA* **271**: 985–991

Knopman D, Schneider L, Davis K *et al.* (1996) Long-term tacrine (Cognex) treatment: effects on nursing home placement and mortality. Tacrine Study Group. *Neurology* **47**: 166–177

Koopmanschap MA. (1998) In: *The Health Economics of Dementia*. Wimo A, Karlsson G, Jonsson B, Winblad B (eds), London, John Wiley and Sons

Koopmanschap MA, Polder JJ, Meerding WJ, Bonneux L, van der Maas PJ. (1998) Costs of dementia in the Netherlands. In: A Wimo, G Karlsson, B Jönsson, B Winblad (eds), *The Health Economics of Dementia*. London, Wiley

Kronborg Andersen C, Sogaard J, Hansen E *et al.* (1999) The cost of dementia in Denmark: the Odense Study. *Dementia and Geriatric Cognitive Disorders* **10**: 295–304

Lamb HM and Goa KL. (2001) Rivastigmine. A pharmacoeconomic review of its use in Alzheimer's disease. *Pharmacoeconomics* **19**: 303–318

Langa KM, Chernew ME, Kabeto MU *et al* (2001) National estimates of the quantity and cost of informal caregiving for the elderly with dementia. *Journal of General Internal Medicine* **16**: 770–778

Leber P. (1997) Slowing the progression of Alzheimer disease: methodologic issues. *Alzheimer Disease and Associated Disorders* **11** (Suppl. 5): S10–21; discussion S37–39

Leung GM, Yeung RY, Chi I, Chu LW. (2003) The economics of Alzheimer disease. *Dementia and Geriatric Cognitive Disorders* **15**: 34–43

Lindgren B. (1981) *Costs of Illness in Sweden 1964–1975*. Lund, Liber

Logsdon RG, Gibbons LE, McCurry SM, Teri L. (2002) Assessing quality of life in older adults with cognitive impairment. *Psychosomatic Medicine* **64**: 510–519

Lovestone S. (2002) Can we afford to develop treatments for dementia? *Journal of Neurology, Neurosurgery, and Psychiatry* **72**: 685

Lubeck DP, Mazonson PD, Bowe T. (1994) Potential effect of tacrine on expenditures for Alzheimer's disease. *Medical Interface* **7**: 130–138

Lyseng-Williamson KA and Plosker GL. (2002) Galantamine: a pharmacoeconomic review of its use in Alzheimer's disease. *Pharmacoeconomics* **20**: 919–942

Lyseng-Williamson KA and Plosker GL. (2003) Spotlight on Galantamine in Alzheimer's Disease. *Disease Management and Health Outcomes* **11**: 125–128

Maas ML, Specht JP, Weiler K, Buckwalter KC, Turner B. (1998) Special care units for people with Alzheimer's disease. Only for the privileged few? *Journal of Gerontological Nursing* **24**: 28–37

Max W. (1996) The cost of Alzheimer's disease. Will drug treatment ease the burden? *Pharmacoeconomics* **9**: 5–10

Max W, Webber P, Fox P. (1995) Alzheimer's disease. The unpaid burden of caring. *Journal of Aging Health* **7**: 179–199

Migliaccio-Walle K, Getsios D, Caro JJ, Ishak KJ, O'Brien JA, Papadopoulos G. (2003) Economic evaluation of galantamine in the treatment of mild to moderate Alzheimer's disease in the United States. *Clinical Therapeutics* **25**: 1806–1825

Mohide EA, Torrance GW, Streiner DL, Pringle DM, Gilbert R. (1988) Measuring the wellbeing of family caregivers using the time trade-off technique. *Journal of Clinical Epidemiology* **41**: 475–482

Moore MJ, Zhu CW, Clipp EC. (2001) Informal costs of dementia care: estimates from the National Longitudinal Caregiver Study. *Journal of Gerontology, B Psychological Sciences and Social Sciences* **56**: S219–228

Neumann PJ, Hermann RC, Kuntz KM *et al.* (1999) Cost-effectiveness of donepezil in the treatment of mild or moderate Alzheimer's disease. *Neurology* **52**: 1138–1145

Neumann PJ, Sandberg EA, Araki SS, Kuntz KM, Feeny D, Weinstein MC. (2000) A comparison of HUI2 and HUI3 utility scores in Alzheimer's disease. *Medical Decision Making* **20**: 413–422

NICE. (2001) *Guidance on the Use of Donepezil, Rivastigmine and Galantamine for the Treatment of Alzheimer's Disease*. Technology Appraisal Guidance No.19. London, National Institute for Clinical Excellence, pp. 5–6

O'Brien BJ, Goeree R, Hux M *et al.* (1999) Economic evaluation of donepezil for the treatment of Alzheimer's disease in Canada. *Journal of American Geriatrics Society* **47**: 570–578

O'Shea E and O'Reilly S. (2000) The economic and social cost of dementia in Ireland. *International Journal of Geriatric Psychiatry* **15**: 208–218

OECD. PPP http://www.oecd.org/std/ppp/pps

OECD. (1996) *Caring for Frail Elderly People – Policies in Evolution*. Social Policy Studies No. 19. Paris, Organization for Economic Development

Olin J and Schneider L. (2003) Galantamine for Alzheimer's disease. Cochrane Review. Oxford, Software Update *Cochrane Library*, Issue 2

Ostbye T and Crosse E. (1994) Net economic costs of dementia in Canada. *Canadian Medical Association Journal* **151**: 1457–1464

Reisberg B, Ferris SH, de Leon MJ, Crook T. (1988) Global Deterioration Scale (GDS). *Psychopharmacological Bulletin* **24**: 661–663

Reisberg B, Doody R, Stoffler A, Schmitt F, Ferris S, Mobius HJ. (2003) Memantine in moderate-to-severe Alzheimer's disease. *New England Journal of Medicine* **348**: 1333–1341

Rice DP, Hodgson TA, Kopstein AN. (1985) The economic costs of illness: a replication and update. *Health Review* **7**: 61–80

Rice DP, Fox PJ, Max W *et al.* (1993) The economic burden of Alzheimer's disease care. *Health Affairs (Project Hope)* **12**: 164–176

Rosen WG, Mohs RC, Davis KL. (1984) A new rating scale for Alzheimer's disease, *American Journal of Psychiatry* **141**: 1356–1364

Salek SS, Walker MD, Bayer AJ. (1998) A review of quality of life in Alzheimer's disease. Part 2: Issues in assessing drug effects. *Pharmacoeconomics* **14**: 613–627

Sano M, Ernesto C, Thomas RG *et al.* (1997) A controlled trial of selegiline, alpha-tocopherol, or both as treatment for Alzheimer's disease. The Alzheimer's Disease Cooperative Study. *New England Journal of Medicine* **336**: 1216–1222

Schneider L. (1998) In: *Health Economics of Dementia*. Wimo A, Jonsson B, Karlsson G, Winblad B (eds), London, John Wiley and Sons. pp. 451–464

Schneider LS, Olin JT, Lyness SA, Chui HC. (1997) Eligibility of Alzheimer's disease clinic patients for clinical trials. *Journal of American Geriatrics Society* **45**: 923–928

Schulenberg J and Schulenberg I. (1998) Cost of treatment and cost of care for Alzheimer's disease in Germany. In: A Wimo, G Karlsson, B Jönsson, B Winblad (eds), *The Health Economics of Dementia*. London, Wiley

Schulz R and Beach SR. (1999) Caregiving as a risk factor for mortality: the Caregiver Health Effects Study. *JAMA* **282**: 2215–2219

Selai C, Vaughan A, Harvey RJ, Logsdon R. (2001) Using the QoL-AD in the UK, *International Journal of Geriatric Psychiatry* **16**: 537–538

Selai CE, Elstner K, Trimble MR. (2000) Quality of life pre and post epilepsy surgery. *Epilepsy Research* **38**: 67–74

Shukla VK, Otten N, Coyle D. (2000) *Drug treatments for Alzheimer's Disease III. a review of published pharmacoeconomic evaluations.* Report No. 11. Ottawa, Canadian Coordinating Office for Health Technology Assessment (CCOHTA), p. 37

Siegel JE, Torrance GW, Russell LB, Luce BR, Weinstein MC, Gold MR. (1997) Guidelines for pharmacoeconomic studies. Recommendations from the panel on cost effectiveness in health and medicine. Panel on Cost Effectiveness in Health and Medicine. *Pharmacoeconomics* **11**: 159–168

Small GW, Donohue JA, Brooks RL. (1998) An economic evaluation of donepezil in the treatment of Alzheimer's disease. *Clinical Therapeutics* **20**: 838–850

Smith KA and Shah A. (1995) The prevalence and costs of psychiatric disorders and learning disabilities. *British Journal of Psychiatry* **166**: 9–18

Sonnenberg FA and Leventhal EA. (1998) Modeling disease progression with Markov models. In: A Wimo, G Karlsson, B Jönsson, B Winblad (eds), *The Health Economics of Dementia*. London, Wiley, pp. 171–196

Spilker B. (1996) *Quality of Life and Pharmacoeconomics in Clinical Trials.* Philadelphia, Lippincott-Raven Publishers

Stewart A and Brod M. (1996) In: B Spilker (ed.), *Quality of Life and Pharmacoeconomics in Clinical Trials*. Philadelphia, Lippincott-Raven Publishers, pp. 819–830

Stewart A, Phillips R, Dempsey G. (1998) Pharmacotherapy for people with Alzheimer's disease: a Markov-cycle evaluation of five years' therapy using donepezil. *International Journal of Geriatric Psychiatry* **13**: 445–453

Stommel M, Collins CE, Given BA. (1994) The costs of family contributions to the care of persons with dementia. *The Gerontologist* **34**: 199–205

Torrance G. (1996) In: B Spilker (ed.), *Quality of Life and Pharmacoeconomics in Clinical Trials*. Philadelphia, Lippincott-Raven Publishers, pp. 1105–1121

Torrance GW. (1997) Preferences for health outcomes and cost-utility analysis. *American Journal of Management Care* **3** (Suppl.): S8–20

Torrance GW, Feeny DH, Furlong WJ, Barr RD, Zhang Y, Wang Q. (1996) Multiattribute utility function for a comprehensive health status classification system. Health Utilities Index Mark 2. *Medical Care* **34**: 702–722

Tsuchiya A, Dolan P, Shaw R. (2003) Measuring people's preferences regarding ageism in health: some methodological issues and some fresh evidence, *Society of Scientific Medicine* **57**: 687–696

Walker MD, Salek SS, Bayer AJ. (1998) A review of quality of life in Alzheimer's disease. Part 1: Issues in assessing disease impact. *Pharmacoeconomics* **14**: 499–530

Ward A, Caro JJ, Getsios D, Ishak K, O'Brien J, Bullock R. (2003) Assessment of health economics in Alzheimer's disease (AHEAD): treatment with galantamine in the UK. *International Journal of Geriatric Psychiatry* **18**: 740–747

Ware JE Jr and Sherbourne CD. (1992) The MOS 36-item short-form health survey (SF-36) I. Conceptual framework and item selection. *Medical Care* **30**: 473–483

Weinstein MC and Fineberg HV. (1980) *Clinical Decision Analysis.* Philadelphia, WB Saunders

Wimo A and Winblad B. (2002) Pharmacoeconomics of dementia: impact of cholinesterase inhibitors. In: S Gauthier S and J Cummings (eds), *Alzheimer's Disease and Related Disorders Annual 2002.* London, Martin Dunitz

Wimo A and Winblad B. (2003a) Pharmacoeconomics of mild cognitive impairment. *Acta Neurologica Scandinavica* **179** (Suppl.): 94–99

Wimo A and Winblad B. (2003b) Resource utilisation in dementia: RUD Lite. *Brain Aging* **3**: 48–59

Wimo A, Mattson B, Krakau I, Eriksson T, Nelvig A, Karlsson G. (1995) Cost-utility analysis of group living in dementia care. *International Journal of Technological Assessment of Health Care* **11**: 49–65

Wimo A, Karlsson G, Nordberg A, Winblad B. (1997a) Treatment of Alzheimer disease with tacrine: a cost-analysis model. *Alzheimer Disease and Associated Disorders* **11**: 191–200

Wimo A, Karlsson G, Sandman PO, Corder L, Winblad B. (1997b) Cost of illness due to dementia in Sweden. *International Journal of Geriatric Psychiatry* **12**: 857–861

Wimo A, Jonsson B, Karlsson G, Winblad BE. (1998a) *The Health Economics of Dementia.* London, John Wiley and Sons

Wimo A, Wetterholm AL, Mastey V, Winblad B. (1998b) Evaluation of the resource utilization and caregiver time in Anti-dementia drug trials – a quantitative battery. In: A Wimo, G Karlsson, B Jönsson, B Winblad (eds), *The Health Economics of Dementia*. London, Wiley, pp. 465–499

Wimo A, Witthaus E, Rother M, Winblad B. (1998c) Economic impact of introducing propentofylline for the treatment of dementia in Sweden. *Clinical Therapeutics* **20**: 552–566; discussion 550–551

Wimo A, Johansson L, von Strauss E, Nordberg G. (1999a) Formal and informal home care to Swedish demented patients, an application of RUD (Resource Utilization in Dementia) (abstract). *International Psychogeriatrics* **11** (Suppl. 1): 197

Wimo A, Winblad B, Grafstrom M. (1999b) The social consequences for families with Alzheimer's disease patients: potential impact of new drug treatment. *International Journal of Geriatric Psychiatry* **14**: 338–347

Wimo A, Nordberg G, Jansson W, Grafstrom M. (2000) Assessment of informal services to demented people with the RUD instrument. *International Journal of Geriatric Psychiatry* **15**: 969–971

Wimo A, von Strauss E, Nordberg G, Sassi F, Johansson L. (2002) Time spent on informal and formal care giving for persons with dementia in Sweden. *Health Policy* **61**: 255–268

Wimo A, Winblad B, Engedal K *et al.* (2003a) An economic evaluation of donepezil in mild to moderate Alzheimer's disease: results of a 1-year, double-blind, randomized trial. *Dementia and Geriatric Cognitive Disorders* **15**: 44–54

Wimo A, Winblad B, Stoffler A, Wirth Y, Mobius HJ. (2003b) Resource utilisation and cost analysis of memantine in patients with moderate to severe Alzheimer's disease. *Pharmacoeconomics* **21**: 327–40

Wimo A, Winblad B, Stöffler A, Wirth Y, Möbius HJ. (2003c) Resource utilization and cost analysis of memantine in patients with

moderate to severe Alzheimer's disease. *Pharmacoeconomics* **21**: 327–340

Winblad B, Hill S, Beermann B, Post SG, Wimo A. (1997) Issues in the economic evaluation of treatment for dementia. Position paper from the International Working Group on Harmonization of Dementia Drug Guidelines. *Alzheimer Disease and Associated Disorders* **11**: 39–45

Winblad B, Wimo A, Mobius HJ, Fox JM, Fratiglioni L. (1999) Severe dementia: a common condition entailing high costs at individual and societal levels. *International Journal of Geriatric Psychiatry* **14**: 911–914

Wolfson C, Oremus M, Shukla V *et al.* (2002) Donepezil and rivastigmine in the treatment of Alzheimer's disease: a best-evidence synthesis of the published data on their efficacy and cost-effectiveness. *Clinical Therapeutics* **24**: 862–886; discussion 837

Zarit SH, Reever KE, Bach-Peterson J. (1980) Relatives of the impaired elderly: correlates of feelings of burden. *The Gerontologist* **20**: 649–655

13

Cross-cultural issues in the assessment of cognitive impairment

AJIT SHAH, JAMES LINDESAY AND IAN O NNATU

Two types of cross-cultural studies will be discussed: cross-community studies comparing two or more ethnic groups in a single country, and cross-national studies comparing populations across two or more countries. We will focus on cross-community studies of ethnic groups within the United Kingdom (UK), using the Goldberg and Huxley (1991) model of pathways into care, and the significance of cultural factors. Cross-national studies will be examined with particular reference to methodology, aetiology and risk factors.

13.1 DEMOGRAPHY

13.1.1 International demographic changes

The size of the elderly population is increasing both in developed and developing countries, particularly the 'old old' (i.e. those >80 years) in developed countries (Ogunlesi, 1989; Zhang et al., 1990; Kalachie, 1991; Jorm and Henderson, 1993; Snowdon, 1993). It is estimated that 90 million people live outside their country of birth (Bohning and Oishi, 1995).

13.1.2 National changes in ethnic minority demography in the UK

The proportion of ethnic minority individuals >65 years in Britain has increased from 1 per cent in 1981 to 3 per cent in 1991 (OPCS, 1983, 1993); this figure is likely to increase when the figures from the 2001 census become available in the near future. This contrasts with 17 per cent of the indigenous population being over 65 years in 1991 (OPCS, 1993). In 1991, the composition of the ethnic elderly group was 41 per cent of 'Indian Subcontinent' origin, 34 per cent of 'Black Caribbean', 'Black African' and 'Black other' origin, 5 per cent of Chinese origin and 14 per cent from other ethnic groups (OPCS, 1993). Closer political and economic union with Europe may also lead to increased migration of elderly people between neighbouring states (e.g. English elderly retiring to Spain, France or Italy).

13.1.3 Implications of these demographic changes

The prevalence of dementia doubles every 5.1 years after the age of 60 (Jorm et al., 1987; Hofman et al., 1991). Thus, internationally, with the predicted increase in the elderly population (particularly of those >80 years), the absolute number of dementia cases will increase (Shah, 1992a, b; Jorm and Henderson, 1993; Ames and Flynn, 1994). There is, therefore, both a need and an opportunity to study the epidemiology, aetiology and risk factors, phenomenology, diagnosis, long-term outcome and prognosis of dementia cross-nationally and across different ethnic groups, to improve our understanding of dementia and enable adequate planning of services.

13.2 THE EPIDEMIOLOGY OF DEMENTIA AMONG ETHNIC GROUPS IN THE UK

There are several methodological difficulties related to epidemiological studies of dementia in different ethnic groups, notably the definitions of age and ethnicity, diagnostic issues, and lack of appropriately validated screening instruments.

13.2.1 Age

Epidemiological studies of dementia in developed countries usually focus on those aged 60–65 years and older. Some ethnic groups have a shorter life span, retire early and assume the social role of an elder at a younger age (Rajkumar *et al.*, 1997). Thus, an age cut-off in the range of 40–55 years has been used in some studies of ethnic groups in the UK (Barker, 1984; McCallum, 1990; Manthorpe and Hettiaratchy, 1993) and in developing countries (Yu *et al.*, 1989; Zhang *et al.*, 1990; Ganguli *et al.*, 1995; Vas *et al.*, 2001). Similarly, for indigenous Australians, old age has been officially defined as starting at age 50 years (Commonwealth Department of Health, Housing and Community Services, 1991). Use of younger age cut-offs makes comparison with studies of indigenous populations more difficult (Rait and Burns, 1997), but does allow for the generation of larger sample sizes. Using the same cut-off age will facilitate development of psychogeriatric services alongside those for the indigenous population, and avoid confusion and fragmentation of service delivery. However, study sample sizes will be smaller as ethnic minority populations are generally younger than their indigenous counterparts. Another issue is the difficulty in ascertaining the precise age of some ethnic elders (Chandra *et al.*, 1994; Rajkumar and Kumar, 1996; Rait *et al.*, 1997). This can be overcome to some extent by using an 'events calendar' (Rajkumar and Kumar, 1996).

13.2.2 Race, culture and ethnicity

Race, culture and ethnicity are often used interchangeably. Guidelines on the use of ethnic, racial and cultural definitions for research, audit and publication are emerging (Anonymous, 1996; Singh, 1997). Race is a phenomenological description based on physical characteristics (Bhopal, 1997). Culture describes features that individuals share, and which bind them together into a community. It is possible to be racially different but culturally similar. The definition and identification of ethnicity can pose difficulties (Lloyd, 1992; McKenzie and Crowcroft, 1996; Pringle and Rothera, 1996) because it incorporates some aspects of race and culture, and other related characteristics including language, religion, upbringing, nationality and ancestral place of origin (Rait and Burns, 1997). It may be a personal expression of identity influenced by life experience and place of habitation, and can change over time (Senior and Bhopal, 1984). Ethnic minority individuals have been defined as those with a cultural heritage distinct from the majority population (Manthorpe and Hettiaratchy, 1993). This definition may be appropriate in the UK where the indigenous white population forms the majority, but poses difficulties in countries like Australia where the indigenous population is a minority.

Using the above definitions, individuals of Indian subcontinent, African-Caribbean, African, Chinese, Irish, Jewish, South African and East European origin can be described as UK ethnic elders. Thus, ethnic elders comprise a heterogeneous group with unique individual and collective experiences (Barker, 1984; Manthorpe and Hettairatchy, 1993; Rait and Burns, 1997); they should not be amalgamated (Livingston and Sembhi, 2003), and consideration should be given to individual subgroups.

13.2.3 Other methodological issues

Epidemiological studies of dementia among ethnic elders in the UK are few in number. They are fraught with difficulties such as: ascertainment of age (Rait *et al.*, 1997); illiteracy (Lindesay *et al.*, 1997a, b); innumeracy; small sample sizes (Bhatnagar and Frank, 1997; Lindesay *et al.*, 1997b; Rait *et al.*, 1997); inappropriate sample frames (Richards *et al.*, 1996; Richards and Brayne, 1996; McCracken *et al.*, 1997); non-response (Bhatnagar and Frank, 1997; Lindesay *et al.*, 1997b; McCracken *et al.*, 1997) and refusal to participate (Bhatnagar and Frank, 1997); lack of valid tools to identify and quantify dementia (Lindesay, 1998; Shah, 1998); and lack of comparisons with the indigenous population (Bhatnagar and Frank, 1997).

Problems with sampling include: using an amalgamation of heterogeneous groups of ethnic elders (Bhatnagar and Frank, 1997; McCracken *et al.*, 1997; Livingston and Sembhi, 2003); an assumption that general practice patient lists are accurate and up to date (Bhatnagar and Frank, 1997; Lindesay *et al.*, 1997a, b; McCracken *et al.*, 1997); and the fact that many ethnic elders may be abroad for much of the time and only return to the UK when ill (Richards and Brayne, 1996; Bhatnagar and Frank, 1997).

In addition to using GP lists, sampling yield can be increased by means such as door knocking and snowballing, a technique whereby local community groups and ethnic elders themselves are asked to nominate other ethnic elders (Richards *et al.*, 1996; McCracken *et al.*, 1997; Rait *et al.*, 2000a, b).

13.2.4 Diagnostic issues

Psychiatric illnesses, including dementia, can be difficult to recognize among ethnic elders (George and Young, 1991). Cultural factors complicating diagnosis include: communication difficulties (George and Young, 1991; Shah, 1992c, 1997a, b; Livingston and Sembhi, 2003); taboo topics (Shah, 1992c); stigma attached to mental illness (Barker, 1984; Livingston *et al.*, 2002); bias and prejudice of clinicians (Solomon, 1992); institutional racism (Solomon, 1992); unfamiliarity with symptoms of mental illness by relatives (Manthorpe and Hettiaratchy, 1993); and illness being viewed as a function of old age. Another problem is the paucity of suitable screening and diagnostic instruments for dementia in this group (Shah, 1998). Cognitive tests standardized in one ethnic group may not be appropriate for another because they may be influenced by culture (Gurland *et al.*, 1992; Chandra *et al.*, 1994; Teresi *et al.*, 1995; Livingston and Sembhi, 2003; Prince *et al.*, 2003), education (Chandra *et al.*, 1994; Teresi *et al.*, 1995; Stewart *et al.*, 2003; Kim *et al.*, 2003a, b; Livingston and Sembhi, 2003; Prince *et al.*, 2003), language (McCracken *et al.*, 1997; Livingston and Sembhi, 2003; Prince *et al.*, 2003), literacy skills (Chandra *et al.*, 1994; Kabir and Herlitz, 2000; Livingston and Sembhi, 2003; Prince *et al.*, 2003), numeracy skills (Prince *et al.*, 2003), sensory impairments (Lindesay *et al.*, 1997b), unfamiliarity with test situations (Chandra *et al.*, 1994; Richards and Brayne, 1996) and anxiety (Lindesay, 1998).

Education can influence performance on cognitive tests like the Mini-Mental State Examination (MMSE) (Folstein *et al.*, 1975; Escobar *et al.*, 1986; Li *et al.*, 1989; Salmon *et al.*, 1989; Yu *et al.*, 1989; Phanthumchinda *et al.*, 1991; Tombaugh and McIntyre, 1992; Stewart *et al.*, 2003; Kim *et al.*, 2003a, b), and probably accounts for much of the difference in MMSE scores between immigrant groups and indigenous elders (Lindesay *et al.*, 1997b). The Chinese MMSE has developed different cut-off scores predicting dementia for different levels of education in respondents with good sensitivity and specificity (Katzman *et al.*, 1988; Zhang *et al.*, 1990; Sahadevan *et al.*, 2000); this has also been suggested in other ethnic groups (Murden *et al.*, 1991; Gurland *et al.*, 1992). An alternative approach that avoids using selective cut-off scores for two-stage population-based studies is to use operationally defined concepts of 'cognitively impaired' and 'cognitively declined' (Chandra *et al.*, 1998, 2001). For example 'cognitively impaired' has been defined as a score below the 10th percentile of the sample on a given cognitive test and is based on the reported 5 per cent average prevalence rate for dementia in Western countries. Illiterate subjects may be unable to complete tests that require reading, writing and drawing (Katzman *et al.*, 1988; Chandra *et al.*, 1994; Rajkumar and Kumar, 1996); illiteracy may also reduce access to information related to orientation in time and general knowledge (Lindesay, 1998). Innumerate subjects may be unable perform tests involving calculations (Chandra *et al.*, 1994; Livingston and Sembhi, 2003). A study of ethnic elders in Liverpool reported a higher prevalence of dementia in subjects unable to speak English (McCracken *et al.*, 1997); this may have been an artefact of their inability to speak English. Lack of education may also pose difficulties for the subject in understanding the nature of the test and therefore feeling that the questions are irrelevant and of little practical value (Chandra *et al.*, 1994; Richards and Brayne, 1996; Bhatnagar and Frank, 1997). Even if educational levels appear to be similar, there may be sociocultural inequality in access and quality (Bohnstedt *et al.*, 1994).

Tests identifying the discrepancy between age and date of birth (Bhatnagar and Frank, 1997; McCracken *et al.*, 1997) disadvantage ethnic elders born in remote villages with poor birth registration facilities, and those who have altered age and date of birth to facilitate migration and entry into institutions

(Rait *et al.*, 1997). Culture-specific questions (e.g. about royalty or politicians) also disadvantage ethnic elders (Bhatnagar and Frank, 1997; McCracken *et al.*, 1997), although these can be modified (e.g. dates of independence of the country of origin) (Chandra *et al.*, 1994; Rait *et al.*, 1997). Cultural concepts of orientation in time and place (Escobar *et al.*, 1986; Ganguli *et al.*, 1995; Lindesay *et al.*, 1997b) and preferential use of the Western or traditional calendar (Kua, 1992; Bhatnagar and Frank, 1997; Lindesay *et al.*, 1997b; Rait *et al.*, 1997) can also influence performance. Orientation items work well within the dominant culture but less well in some minority cultures (Rait *et al.*, 1997; Livingston and Sembhi, 2003); this was the case among Singaporean Chinese (Kua, 1992), but not in the Liverpool Chinese (McCracken *et al.*, 1997).

13.2.5 Developing new instruments for screening

There is a need to develop instruments that allow the subject to perform at their best without the influence of the extraneous factors listed above. Either new instruments can be developed, or existing instruments can be adapted and refined. Modifying existing instruments makes empirical and economic sense, and most research with well-developed techniques has adopted this strategy (Chandra *et al.*, 1994, 1998; Ganguli *et al.*, 1995; Hall *et al.*, 1993; Rait *et al.*, 1997).

Detailed knowledge of relevant cultural factors and their influence on ageing is required (Dein and Huline-Dickens, 1997). A Delphi panel of experts from the culture of interest or a more widespread consultation technique to examine each item for cultural relevance, translation, adaptation and modification has been used, with the aim of producing a culture-fair, education-free and analogous instrument (i.e. comparable meaning, difficulty, familiarity and salience) (Hall *et al.*, 1993; Chandra *et al.*, 1994, 1998; Graves *et al.*, 1994; Richards and Brayne, 1996; Richards, 1997). Both approaches can be combined (Rait *et al.*, 1997). The Delphi panel technique can use structured interviews, semistructured interviews, questions or vignettes (Rait *et al.*, 1997). The consultation approach involves professionals and/or lay members working closely, perhaps focusing on separate issues initially, and sharing them later (Rait *et al.*, 1997); this approach has been successfully used in developing a depression screening instrument for African-Caribbean elders in London (Abas, 1996).

Both translation and back-translation by separate groups of bilingual translators is necessary to ensure accuracy of translation (Brislin, 1970; Katzman *et al.*, 1988; Yu *et al.*, 1989; Chandra *et al.*, 1994; Lindesay *et al.*, 1997b). In addition, bilingual translators can ensure that the meaning and significance of the items are preserved as far as possible (Lindesay *et al.*, 1997b); this could be achieved by a Delphi panel when panel members originate from the same culture. Translation should endeavour to ensure content, semantic, technical, criterion and conceptual equivalence with the parent version of the scale for every item (Flaherty *et al.*, 1988; Rait *et al.*, 1997).

A sophisticated statistical technique employing item characteristic curves can be used to develop tests that are functionally equivalent (Gibbons *et al.*, 2002). Ideally, field pretesting is required to identify variations in dialect, logistic and conceptual problems, and practical difficulties (Li *et al.*, 1989; Yu *et al.*, 1989; Zhang *et al.*, 1990; Hall *et al.*, 1993; Chandra *et al.*, 1994, 1998; Ganguli *et al.*, 1995). Several rounds of field pretesting may be required (Chandra *et al.*, 1994; Ganguli *et al.*, 1995). This should, ideally, be followed by pilot testing to determine the distribution of scores (Chandra *et al.*, 1994; Ganguli *et al.*, 1996; Rait *et al.*, 2000a, b; Stewart *et al.*, 2001a, 2002) and their ability to discriminate between dementias of different severity (Chandra *et al.*, 1994; Lindesay *et al.*, 1997b).

Clear validation against a gold standard diagnosis of dementia is needed (Livingston and Sembhi, 2003). Ideally, this should be achieved by a standardized clinical interview (perhaps video or audio taped) with evaluation at two time points (Chandra *et al.*, 1994; Shah *et al.*, 1998) to confirm cognitive decline. Translated versions of the Geriatric Mental State Schedule (GMS) (Copeland *et al.*, 1976) have been used among older Asians, Chinese, Somali, African-Caribbean and British black people in Liverpool (Blakemore and Boneham, 1994; McCracken *et al.*, 1997), Indian subcontinent elders in Bradford (Bhatnagar and Frank, 1997), Chinese in Taiwan (Tsang *et al.*, 2002), and among respondents from India, China and southeast Asia, Africa, Latin America and the Caribbean (Prince *et al.*, 2003). An 'ad hoc' translated version of the Cambridge Cognitive Examination (CAMCOG) section of the Cambridge Mental Disorders of the Elderly Examination (CAMDEX) (Roth *et al.*, 1986) and the first part of the Schedules for Clinical Assessment in Neuropsychiatry (World Health Organization, 1992) have been used to gather systematic data to facilitate a clinical diagnosis of dementia in Gujarati elders (Lindesay *et al.*, 1997b; Shah *et al.*, 1998). Information from the CAMDEX interview and the Consortium to Establish a Registry for Alzheimer's Disease (CERAD) interview (Morris *et al.*, 1989) have been used by a panel of physicians to make consensus DSM-IIIR diagnosis of dementia among Cree Indians and English-speaking Canadians (Hall *et al.*, 1993). In most studies, the accuracy of the 'gold standard' instrument in diagnosing dementia has not been adequately examined; one useful method of validating such instruments is by serially following up dementia cases, whereupon true dementia cases are likely to demonstrate continuing decline in cognition (Shah *et al.*, 1998). The need for an assessment of functional impairment in the diagnosis of dementia in ICD-10 and DSM-IV can pose major problems in some cultures because of major conceptual difficulties in its definition and measurement across different cultures (Chandra *et al.*, 1994; Pollit, 1996; Richards and Brayne, 1996). Nevertheless, good interrater reliability between clinicians from six different countries in diagnosis of dementia using DSM-IIIR and ICD-10 criteria has been reported (Baldereschi *et al.*, 1994), suggesting that these diagnostic constructs can be used in cross-cultural research.

Important properties of instruments measuring features of dementia are listed in Box 13.1. Data on the sensitivity to

---

Box 13.1 *Important properties of instruments measuring features of dementia (Katzman et al., 1988; Chandra, 1994; Zaudig, 1996)*

- Patient characteristics
- User characteristics
- Type of instrument
- Setting for administration of instrument
- Source of data
- Output of instrument
- Psychometric properties
- Reliability (test-retest, interrater, intrarater and internal consistency)
- Validity (face, content, concurrent, predictive and incremental)
- Sensitivity to change
- Floor and ceiling effects
- Practical features
- Time frame of symptoms
- Training needs
- Duration of administration
- Availability of operational manual with glossary and definitions
- Qualification of users
- Costs

---

change are very important in incidence studies, because serial examination should be able to identify change in cognition as a measure of dementia (Chandra *et al.*, 1994). Ideally, most of these properties in the newly developed scale should be similar to or better than those of the parent version. In developing countries, either trained lay personnel or para-professionals are most likely to administer these instruments; even in developed countries, owing to limited research budgets, trained lay personnel may need to be used.

Versions of the MMSE have been developed in several languages, including Chinese (Serby *et al.*, 1987; Katzman *et al.*, 1988; Salmon *et al.*, 1989; Yu *et al.*, 1989; Xu *et al.*, 2003), Korean (Park and Kwon, 1990; Park *et al.*, 1991), Finnish (Salmon *et al.*, 1989), Italian (Rocca *et al.*, 1990), Yoruba (Hendrie, 1992), Spanish (Escobar *et al.*, 1986; Anzola-Perez *et al.*, 1996), Thai (Phanthumchida *et al.*, 1991), Cree (Hall *et al.*, 1993), Hindi (Ganguli *et al.*, 1995; Rait *et al.*, 2000a), Punjabi (Rait *et al.*, 2000a), Urdu (Rait *et al.*, 2000a), Bengali (Rait *et al.*, 2000a), Bangla (Kabir and Herlitz, 2000), Malyalum (Shaji *et al.*, 1996), Gujarati (Lindesay *et al.*, 1997b; Rait *et al.*, 2000a) and Sinhalese (de Silva and Gunatilake, 2002). However, comparisons between all these different versions are problematic as not all studies have followed a rigorous procedure for the development of screening instruments, and/or evaluated the psychometric and other properties adequately.

The abbreviated Mental Test Score (Quereshi and Hodkinson, 1974) has been developed in several south Asian languages for use among Gujaratis and Pakistanis and in

English for use among African Caribbeans in the UK (Rait et al., 1997; Rait et al., 2000a, b). A Korean version of the Alzheimer's Disease Assessment Scale (Rosen et al., 1984) has been developed (Youn et al., 2002). The MMSE, selected items from the CERAD neuropsychological test battery (Morris et al., 1989) and the CAMCOG component of the CAMDEX interview (Roth et al., 1986) have been evaluated in older African Caribbean people (Richards and Brayne, 1996; Richards et al., 2000). Orientation items of the MMSE, selected items of the CERAD battery and the clock drawing test have been further evaluated in elderly African Caribbeans and normative data are available (Stewart et al., 2001a). The 10-word list learning task from the CERAD battery has been shown to be successful in establishing a diagnosis of dementia in study populations from India, China and southeast Asia, Africa, Latin America and the Caribbean (Prince et al., 2003). The Alzheimer's Disease Risk Questionnaire (Breitner and Folstein, 1984), which obtains information on history of cognitive impairment among first-degree relatives, has been translated into Chinese and Spanish, and has been administered by bilingual workers (Silverman et al., 1992). The Informant Questionnaire on Cognitive Decline in the Elderly (IQCODE) (Jorm et al., 1991) has been developed for use in illiterate Chinese populations (Fuh et al., 1995). A dementia screening instrument, the Community Screening Interview for Dementia (CSI-D), with a cognitive test for the subject and an informant history, has been developed for use among Cree Indians in Canada (Hall et al., 1993; Hall et al., 2000), English-speaking Canadians (Hall et al., 1993; Hendrie et al., 1993; Hall et al., 2000) and Yoruba Nigerians in Ibadan (Hendrie et al., 1995a; Hall et al., 2000), African Americans in Indianapolis (Hall et al., 2000), Jamaicans (Hall et al., 2000) and in study populations in India, China and southeast Asia, Africa, Latin America and the Caribbean (Prince et al., 2003), with good psychometric and other properties. The Chula Mental Test, developed for elderly Thais by selecting and adapting items from several existing screening tests, has been found to reduce the influence of illiteracy on scores (Jitapunkul et al., 1996). A Spanish version (for use among Mexican Americans) (Royall et al., 2003) and a Brazilian version (Fuzikawa et al., 2003) of the clock drawing test have been evaluated; the Spanish version is reported to be education-free and acculturation-free.

A unique approach involving use of three instruments (the GMS, the CIS-D and the 10-word list-learning task from the CERAD battery appropriately translated into native languages) and an algorithm derived from these instruments has been shown to have high specificity and sensitivity in the diagnosis of dementia in culturally diverse populations from India, China and southeast Asia, Africa, Latin America and the Caribbean (Prince et al., 2003). Furthermore, this approach allows for educational bias.

Some commonsense rules should be followed when you are administering cognitive tests to ethnic elders. First, any sensory impairment should be corrected if possible; some ethnic groups, like the Gujaratis, have a higher prevalence of visual impairment (Lindesay et al., 1997b). Second, the nature,

purpose and duration of the test should be carefully explained and the instructions should be explicit and simple. This may need further facilitation by unscored trial runs on selected examples to ensure that the nature and purpose of the test is understood by the subject (Chandra et al., 1994, 1998). The latter may be particularly helpful in subjects who are not used to being examined in this way, or who are reluctant to share intellectual skills with a stranger (Richards and Brayne, 1996). Third, a calm, patient and reassuring approach by the assessor may help reduce anxiety and obtain the best possible performance. Finally, if possible, the individual should be assessed in their mother tongue (Shah, 1992c, 1999).

13.2.6 Prevalence studies of ethnic elders in the UK

Only a few prevalence studies have been carried out; there are no incidence studies. The literature suggests that the prevalence of dementia among ethnic elders of Indian subcontinent origin in the UK is either similar (Bhatnagar and Frank, 1997; Lindesay et al., 1997b; McCracken et al., 1997) or higher (McCracken et al., 1997) than among indigenous elders. A community study from Bradford, using the Hindi version of the GMS administered to Indian subcontinent elders, reported a dementia prevalence rate of 7 per cent (95 per cent CI 2.9–13.8 per cent) (Bhatnagar and Frank, 1997). However, using clinician's diagnosis, the prevalence was only 4 per cent (95 per cent CI 1.1–9.9 per cent), and there was poor agreement between the two diagnoses.

A two-stage community study from Leicester, using a Gujarati MMSE administered by trained personnel in Gujarati, a clinical interview and an ad hoc translated version of the CAMDEX and the SCAN interviews administered by a Gujarati-speaking psychiatrist, found prevalence rates of 0 per cent and 20 per cent (95 per cent CI 5.3–48.6 per cent) in the 65–74 and 75+ years age groups respectively (Lindesay et al., 1997b). This study included a comparison group of indigenous elders and the prevalence of dementia was higher in the Gujaratis, although this was not statistically significant. The stability of the diagnosis of dementia was confirmed at 27-month follow up by another Gujarati-speaking psychiatrist using similar diagnostic techniques (Shah et al., 1998).

A community study from Liverpool of African, Caribbean, Asian, Chinese and Middle Eastern elders used the GMS either in English or an ad hoc translation during interview (McCracken et al., 1997). The prevalence rates (95 per cent CI) of dementia in English-speaking individuals of black African, black Caribbean, black other, Chinese and Asian origin were 8 per cent (4–15), 8 per cent (4–15), 2 per cent (0.1–12), 5 per cent (1–26) and 9 per cent (2–41) respectively, similar to the 3 per cent (2–4) found in the indigenous population. Prevalence in the black African and Chinese who did not speak English was 27 per cent (10–50) and 21 per cent (11–33) respectively; these figures were higher than those for the indigenous population. The comparison group of indigenous elders was taken from another study that did not have the same complicated sampling frame. It is unclear whether the higher prevalence in the non-English speakers was real, or an artefact of communication or translation difficulties.

A community study in Islington used the shortened version of the Comprehensive Assessment and Referral Evaluation (Short-CARE) (Gurland *et al.*, 1984) in those born in the UK, Ireland, Cyprus, Africa and Caribbean and Europe (Livingston *et al.*, 2001). The prevalence of dementia in those born in the UK, Ireland, Cyprus, and Africa and the Caribbean was 10 per cent, 3.6 per cent, 11.3 per cent and 17 per cent respectively. Logistic regression analysis revealed that living in a residential home, age, being African or Caribbean and years of education were the only significant predictors of dementia. The Short-CARE interview was not translated and back-translated using any of the principles illustrated earlier and no information was provided about how the interview was administered to those who did not speak English.

A small pilot study of only 45 subjects reported a prevalence rate of 34 per cent for dementia in an African Caribbean group compared with 4 per cent in a white group (Richards *et al.*, 2000).

13.2.7 Other epidemiological issues

Most diagnostic systems emphasize the cognitive features of dementia (Fairburn and Hope, 1988), and non-cognitive features such as personality change, behaviour change, affective features, psychotic features and functional disability have been sparsely studied among ethnic groups (Jitapunkul *et al.*, 1996; Shah and Dighe-Deo, 1998). Data on the clinical presentation, natural history, risk factors, incidence rates, quality of life and carer stress are also sparse.

13.3 THE CONCEPT OF PATHWAYS TO CARE

In the UK, general practitioners (GPs) are traditionally the first port of call for patients requiring medical attention. Moreover, GPs act as gatekeepers for secondary services. Pathways into care encompass all stages from the first appearance of an illness in the community, patients consulting their GP, identification of the illness by the GP, management of the illness by the GP, referral by the GP to secondary care services, and the identification and management of the illness in secondary care (Goldberg and Huxley, 1991).

Ethnic elders and their carers in the UK, particularly from the African-Caribbean, Asian, Chinese and Vietnamese ethnic groups, are well aware of services provided by GPs and use them effectively (Bhalia and Blakemore, 1981; Barker, 1984; McCallum, 1990). Moreover, they have high general practice consultation rates (Donaldson, 1986; Balarajan *et al.*, 1989; Gillam *et al.*, 1989; Lindesay *et al.*, 1997a; Livingston *et al.*, 2002); up to 70 per cent have consulted their GP in the preceding month (Lindesay *et al.*, 1997a). However, there is a

---

Box 13.2 *Possible reasons for discrepancy in high general practice consultation rates but low service prevalence of ethnic elders in the UK*

- The prevalence of dementia may be low
- Dementia may be less severe
- Dementia may lack non-cognitive features that lead to clinical presentation
- Patient factors may influence primary care consultations
- Family factors may influence primary care consultations
- General practitioner factors may influence primary care consultations
- Secondary care services may not be ethnically sensitive

---

low prevalence of ethnic elders in contact with community or hospital mental health facilities (Blakemore and Boneham, 1994). This has more specifically been observed with dementia in psychogeriatric services (Lindesay *et al.*, 1997a; Rait and Burns, 1997; Jagger, 1998; Shah and Dighe-Deo, 1998). Several possible reasons for this discrepancy, as listed in Box 13.2, are systematically examined below.

13.3.1 The effect of patient and family factors on primary care consultations

The discrepancy between high GP consultation rates and low secondary psychogeriatric service use for ethnic elders may be influenced by factors related to patients and their families. Family members may not recognize symptoms of mental illness and dismiss dementia as a function of old age. Traditionally very few ethnic elders have reached old age and younger family members may be unfamiliar with symptoms of dementia (Manthorpe and Hettiaratchy, 1993; Rait and Burns, 1997). Moreover, both the DSM-IV and the ICD-10 diagnostic criteria for dementia require evidence of functional impairment, and this raises the possibility that different cultures may have different thresholds for diagnosis, depending upon the social roles and cognitive demands placed upon elderly people (Zhang *et al.*, 1990; Pollit, 1996). This may be enhanced if the patient is unable to communicate symptoms of mental illness to family members or the GP owing to lack of vocabulary or other language barriers (George and Young, 1991; Shah, 1992c, 1997a, b). Both family members and the patient may believe that nothing can be done; be unaware of existing services (Bhalia and Blakemore, 1981; Age Concern/Help the Aged Housing Trust (ACHAHT), 1984; Barker, 1984; McCallum, 1990; Lindesay *et al.*, 1997a); be unaware of the application procedure for these services (Lindesay *et al.*, 1997a); feel existing services are inadequate, inaccessible and culturally insensitive (Hopkins and Bahl, 1993; Lindesay *et al.*, 1997a); have had poor previous experience of services (Lindesay *et al.*, 1997a), and fear the stigma attached to mental illness (Barker, 1984; Manthorpe and Hettiaratchy, 1993; Livingston *et al.*, 2002).

The position of ethnic elders in some communities may be more advantageous than that of their white counterparts. In some cultures, notably Muslim, Sikh, Hindu and Jain, elderly people are well respected, and have a status and a role to give their life meaning and purpose. This applies to both men and women, and the latter can acquire a considerable degree of authority and independence with age. Family members may, therefore, feel obliged to look after the person with dementia at home. Thus, both the patient and family members may choose not to consult their GP. However, these hypotheses have not been systematically examined.

This gloomy situation may be changing in some areas. In two recent cross-sectional studies of UK psychogeriatric service users, ethnic elders received both health and social service resources at the same frequency as indigenous elders, despite having more individuals in the household and more children than indigenous elders (Redlinghuys and Shah, 1997; Odutoye and Shah, 1999). Similar findings were reported in a population-based community study for use of primary and secondary health services (excluding psychiatric services) and social services (Livingston et al., 2002). Thus, the traditional belief that ethnic elders do not access psychogeriatric and social services and are looked after by the extended family (Barker, 1984; Boneham, 1989; Manthorpe and Hettiaratchy, 1993) is changing, perhaps because younger family members lead a culturally different life style; work long hours and are busy (Barker, 1984); may have lived in the UK longer than their elders (Barker, 1984) and their elders may have migrated to join them contrary to their wishes (Silveira and Ebrahim, 1995); may experience family tensions (Boneham, 1989; Silveira and Ebrahim, 1995), and may experience financial hardship. Such factors may make it difficult for an extended family to provide support (Redelinghuys and Shah, 1997), thereby encouraging referral to services.

The clinical presentation of ethnic elders is influenced by their complex personal histories. Migration may have been enforced (e.g. from trauma and hardship) or elective (e.g. to join the family). First-generation migrants are less likely to assimilate into the host culture than subsequent generations, and may have greater problems with adjustment. This can lead to family conflicts and expose the individual to racist attitudes. The impact of these factors and that of the degree of acculturation on the clinical presentation of dementia is unclear.

13.3.2 The effect of GP factors on consultations

In the UK up to 70 per cent of Asians register with Asian GPs (Johnson et al., 1983). This, coupled with high GP registration and consultation rates among ethnic elders, should theoretically enable easier diagnosis and access to psychogeriatric and social services. The statutory offer of an annual physical and mental examination to all patients over the age of 75 (Secretaries of State for Health, Wales, Northern Ireland and Scotland, 1989), and the emphasis on the single assessment process and diagnostic protocols for dementia in primary care in the National Service Framework for Older People (Department of Health, 2001) should further facilitate this. However, it appears that relatively few ethnic elders receive this annual examination (Lindesay et al., 1997a). There are several reasons why dementia may not be identified during a routine GP consultation:

1. The prevalence of dementia among ethnic elders consulting their GPs may be low; some possible reasons for this were explored in the last section.
2. Even if the prevalence is similar or higher in ethnic elders consulting their GP than in the rest of community, then the severity of the dementia may be lower.
3. Non-cognitive features, which often lead to clinical presentations, may be less frequent or different to those in indigenous patients.
4. Data on clinical presentation, diagnostic features and natural history of dementia among ethnic elders are sparse, and GPs may lack the diagnostic skills to diagnose dementia in ethnic elders (Shah and Dighe-Deo, 1998).
5. Because ethnic elders with dementia are seen infrequently (Shah and Dighe-Deo, 1998), GPs lack experience of this condition in these groups; even psychiatrists experience this difficulty (Lindesay, 1998; Shah and Dighe-Deo, 1998; Shah, 1999). These difficulties may be further complicated by language and communication difficulties, the age and sex of the assessor, the context and setting of the assessment, attitude and expectations of both the patient and the family, and status of the patient in the family and the community (Lindesay, 1998). A careful informant history and assurance of confidentiality can help with this (Lindesay, 1998).
6. As discussed above there is a paucity of screening instruments with good psychometric and other properties. Diagnostic difficulties may lead to a lower rate of referral to secondary care services as shown in younger mentally ill primary care attenders of Indian subcontinent origin (Odell et al., 1997; Jacob et al., 1998).
7. The bias, prejudice and experience of clinicians (Solomon, 1992) can result in consultation difficulties. None of these hypotheses has been systematically studied.

Informant histories with ethnic elders can provide valuable information (Shah et al., 1998; Shah, 1999), but there are pitfalls. Well-intentioned family members may withhold valuable information if they feel it will present their family member in a 'bad light' (Shah, 1997a, b, 1999). Similarly, they may not volunteer any difficulties and problems for fear of being accused of failing in their duty of care.

Good communication between patients and professionals is paramount (Bhalia and Blakemore, 1981; ACHAHT, 1984; Jones and Gill, 1998; Shah, 1992c, 1999), as many ethnic elders do not speak English (Barker, 1984; Manthorpe and Hettiaratchy, 1993; Lindesay et al., 1997a). This has important consequences for the process of psychiatric assessment and for the communication of information about treatments and services. This problem can be minimized if staff members are able to speak the patient's language (Shah, 1992c, 1999). However, bilingual health workers are uncommon (Phelan and Parkman, 1995). Translation services, therefore, are usually required to communicate directly with patients (Shah, 1992, 1997a, b; Phelan and Parkman, 1995). Relatives, non-clinical staff, clinical staff and professional translators with and without special training in mental health can be used (Phelan and Parkman, 1995; Shah, 1997a, b). Translations can be done in person or via a three-way telephone conversation (Pointon, 1996; Jones and Gill, 1998). Ideally, professional translators should be used in person. The inherent difficulties and limitations in using translators in dementia (Shah, 1997a, b) and other mental disorders (Marcos, 1979; Kline et al., 1980; Shah, 1997a, b) are well described. For illiterate patients and carers, audiotapes, videos and diagrammatic representation with cartoons giving information on management and service related issues may be helpful (Lindesay et al., 1997a).

If dementia is identified it may or may not be treated. It may not be treated because the GP believes that nothing can be done, or considers that ethnically sensitive health and social services in the catchment area are inadequate, or has had poor response for previous referrals or be unaware of the procedure to access these services. If dementia in ethnic elders presenting to the GP is less severe and lacks troublesome non-cognitive features, the GP may consider that onward referral in unnecessary. The GP may feel that he or she can communicate better with the patient, particularly if they share the same ethnic background. Finally, the GP may wish to refer patients to secondary services, but the patient and/or family members may be reluctant. Reasons for this reluctance are similar to those discussed for patients or family not wanting to consult their GP in the first place.

13.3.3 Factors in secondary care that may influence diagnosis and management of dementia

There is a paucity of studies examining ethnic elders with dementia in psychogeriatric, geriatric and social services. Almost all the criticisms applied to primary care also apply to secondary care services. There are only two published studies of psychogeriatric service users (Redlinghuys and Shah, 1997; Odutoye and Shah, 1999), and both of these services may have been particularly accessible to elders of Indian subcontinent origin because of local service development factors.

13.4 THE CONCEPT OF MULTIPLE JEOPARDY

The difficulties faced by ethnic elders with dementia can be explained in terms of multiple jeopardy. The concept of double jeopardy owing to age- and race-related disadvantages was first developed in the USA (National Urban League, 1964) and later introduced to the UK (Dowd and Bengston, 1978). Sexism (Palmore and Manton, 1973) and social deprivation (Norman, 1985) have been added to develop a model of triple jeopardy. Boneham (1989) has developed a model of multiple disadvantages, which can be applied to all ethnic elders (Rait et al., 1996). Six factors contribute to this model of multiple jeopardy: ageism, racism, gender disparities, restricted access to health and welfare services, internal ethnic divisions and class struggle. These bring together all the issues discussed in earlier sections into a final common pathway, illustrating the difficulties that ethnic elders with dementia face in reaching secondary services. However, these models of disadvantage, whilst tantalizing, have been criticized and have not been systematically studied among ethnic elders with dementia.

13.5 THE DIFFERENTIAL PREVALENCE AND INCIDENCE OF THE DIFFERENT SUBTYPES OF DEMENTIA IN DIFFERENT CULTURAL AND NATIONAL GROUPS

Published studies of the prevalence of dementia in UK ethnic elders do not report on the relative prevalence of individual dementia subtypes. Anecdotally, it is believed that vascular dementia is more common than Alzheimer's disease (AD) among Indian subcontinent elders (Bhatnagar and Frank, 1997) and African Caribbeans (Richards et al., 2000; Stewart et al., 2001a; Livingston et al., 2001; Livingston and Sembhi, 2003) in the UK. Some risk factors for vascular dementia are more prevalent in these ethnic minority groups than in the indigenous population, such as diabetes in Asians (Mather and Keen, 1985; Samanta et al., 1987), and hypertension and cardiovascular disease in Asians and African Caribbeans (Balarajan, 1996; Ritch et al., 1996).

The prevalence rates of dementia in ethnic groups in other countries are also variable. A study of Chinese residents in USA nursing homes reported a prevalence rate of 95 per cent for dementia (Serby et al., 1987); the ratio of vascular dementia to AD was estimated as 4.4 to 1 (Serby et al., 1987), but there was no indigenous comparison group. Studies in the USA have reported a higher prevalence of dementia among African Americans (Still et al., 1990; Heyman et al., 1991; Perkins et al., 1997) and Hispanics (Perkins et al., 1997) than white Americans, although one study of severe dementia in African Americans did not find this (Schoenberg et al., 1985). The North Manhattan Ageing Study reported significantly higher prevalence and incidence rates of dementia in Latinos and African Americans compared with non-Latino white Americans (Gurland et al., 1995, 1999); however, these ethnic differences in prevalence and incidence disappeared after controlling for age and educational attainment. Also, there were no significant differences between the three groups for individual subtypes of dementia. Another study reported a higher prevalence of vascular dementia coupled with a higher prevalence of strokes and high blood pressure in African Americans (Heyman *et al.*, 1991; Perkins *et al.*, 1997).

In an American postmortem study of 144 cases of dementia, AD and dementia owing to Parkinson's disease were more common in white Americans, and alcohol-related and vascular dementias were more common in African Americans (de la Monte *et al.*, 1989). Another USA study, using an informant questionnaire (Alzheimer's Disease Risk Questionnaire) administered to non-demented elderly day centre attenders, reported a significantly increased risk of dementia in first-degree relatives of Jews and Italians compared with Chinese and Puerto Ricans (Silverman *et al.*, 1992). This raises the possibility of discrepant environmental exposure to risk factors, as the first two groups had migrated to the USA significantly earlier.

In one Canadian study, the prevalence of all dementias and AD was 4.2 per cent and 0.5 per cent respectively in Cree Indians, and 4.2 per cent and 3.5 per cent respectively in English-speaking Canadians (Hall *et al.*, 1993). An Israeli study of presenile dementia, using hospital discharge diagnosis as a proxy for incidence rates, reported age- and sex-adjusted incidence rates of presenile dementia of the Alzheimer's type to be higher in European and American Jews than those from Africa or Asia (Treves *et al.*, 1986), raising the possibility of both environmental and genetic risk factors. Pollit (1997), quoting Zann (1994), reported that the prevalence of dementia in Aborigines in Northern Queensland was 20 per cent, with alcohol-related dementia accounting for the majority of cases.

Some of the characteristics of prevalence studies of dementia from Asian and African countries are listed in Table 13.1. Although the rates are variable, the overall theme is one of low prevalence in these countries. The exceptions are studies from Shanghai (Zhang *et al.*, 1990), Korea (Park *et al.*, 1994), South Africa (Ben-Arie *et al.*, 1983) and Singapore (Lim *et al.*, 2003). The prevalence of AD in these countries is generally lower (Hasegawa *et al.*, 1986; Shibayama *et al.*, 1986; Li *et al.*, 1989, 1991) and that of vascular dementia generally higher (Hasegawa *et al.*, 1986; Shibayama *et al.*, 1986; Jorm *et al.*, 1987; Li *et al.*, 1989). Almost universally, the prevalence of dementia was reported to increase with age, and generally it was more common in women. Two incidence studies of AD in Japan showing an annual incidence of 1.1 per cent have been quoted in a review (Graves *et al.*, 1994). A meta-analysis of the world literature on incidence studies reported that the incidence of AD and vascular dementia exponentially increased with age (Jorm and Jolley, 1998); eastern countries had a lower incidence of AD and there was no difference in the incidence of vascular dementia between European and eastern countries.

The variable prevalence rates of dementia and its subtypes across different ethnic groups in a given country and across different countries may be due in part to methodological factors. These include differences in: the sensitivity of screening instruments and case-finding techniques (Jorm *et al.*, 1987; Amaducci *et al.*, 1991; Osuntokun *et al.*, 1992; Hall *et al.*,

1993; Prince *et al.*, 2003); diagnostic criteria (Jorm *et al.*, 1987; Amaducci *et al.*, 1991; Osuntokun *et al.*, 1992; Silverman *et al.*, 1992; Hall *et al.*, 1993); sampling frames and procedures (Jorm *et al.*, 1987; Amaducci *et al.*, 1991; Osuntokun *et al.*, 1992; Silverman *et al.*, 1992); screening personnel (Hall *et al.*, 1993) and interrater reliability (Osuntokun *et al.*, 1992); age and demographic characteristics of study populations (Li *et al.*, 1989; Yu *et al.*, 1989; Zhang *et al.*, 1990; Osuntokun *et al.*, 1992); educational attainment and literacy (Hall *et al.*, 1993; Prince *et al.*, 2003); and cultural factors. Some studies do not differentiate between different types of dementia (Kua, 1992).

13.5.1 Effect of life expectancy

Prevalence rates are influenced by several factors (Graves *et al.*, 1994; Suh and Shah, 2001). The overall incidence (and therefore overall prevalence) will be low in societies where life expectancy is short because fewer subjects will reach the age of risk. In general, socioeconomically less developed societies have shorter life expectancies than more developed societies. The selective survival of those not at risk of dementia may further compound such a trend. It is possible that early mortality selects for genetic and/or constitutional factors that protect against neurodegenerative disorders (Suh and Shah, 2001). Mortality and survival after the onset of dementia also influence prevalence rates. In regions where survival after the onset of dementia is short, the prevalence may be low even if the incidence is not (Suh and Shah, 2001). Consequently, lower prevalence in some countries may be due to reduced life expectancy, shorter survival from onset, or reduced age-specific incidence (White, 1992; Chandra *et al.*, 1994, 1998; Vas *et al.*, 2001). This difficulty can be reduced by using age-stratified samples to compare prevalence rates; however, the resulting sample size for older age groups is likely to be small in some developing countries. Another explanation for a low prevalence rate in an urban Indian area is selective migration, whereby people with dementia may return to their 'native' rural area (Vas *et al.*, 2001). An alternative approach is to compare incidence rates (Hendrie *et al.*, 1995a; Richards, 1997; Suh and Shah, 2001). However, incidence studies are time consuming, require large numbers of subjects and are expensive.

13.5.2 Genetic and environmental influences

If the differences in prevalence (or incidence) persist after these methodological problems are overcome, then cross-cultural and cross-national studies would allow investigation of underlying genetic and environmental risk factors and the interaction between them (Amaducci *et al.*, 1991; Osuntokun *et al.*, 1992; Silverman *et al.*, 1992; Brayne, 1993; Hall *et al.*, 1993; Chaturvedi and McKeigue, 1994). If the risk of dementia were solely due to genetic factors, then migrants would have the same incidence rate as in their country of origin (Graves *et al.*, 1994). Thus, comparison of the same ethnic group in different

Table 13.1   *Prevalence studies from African and Asian countries*

Country	Study	Sample size	Prevalence	Age	Stratified by age	Design	Gold standard
Nigeria	Osuntokun et al., 1992	326	Overall 0%	65+	?	Two-stage	DSM-IIIR dementia
Nigeria	Hendrie et al., 1995a	2494	Overall 2.29%; AD 1.41%	65+	Yes	Two-stage	DSM-IIIR and ICD-10 dementia
South Africa	Ben-Arie et al., 1983	139	Overall 8.6	65+	?	Mixed	?
India	Shaji et al., 1996	2067	Overall 3.39%; AD 41%; VaD 58%	60+	Yes	Two-stage	DSM-IIIR dementia
India (urban)	Rajkumar and Kumar, 1996	1300	Overall 2.7%	65+	Yes	Multi-stage	GMS and consensus by two psychiatrists
India	Rajkumar et al., 1997	750	Overall 3.5%; AD 42%; VaD 27%	60+	Yes	Two-stage	GMS and ICD-10 dementia
India	Chandra et al., 1998	5126	Overall 0.84%; AD 0.62%	55+	Yes	Two-stage	DSM-IV and NINCDS-ADRDA
India	Vas et al., 2001	2448	80.43%; 2.44%; AD 1.5%	40+	Yes	Three-stage	DSM-IV
Sri Lanka	de Silva et al., 2003	703	Overall 3.98%; AD 71%; VaD 14%	65+	Yes	Two-stage	DSM-IV and NINCDS-ADRDA
Israel (Arabs)	Bowirrat et al., 2001	821	20.5%	60+	Yes	One-stage	Unspecified
Singapore	Kua, 1991, 1992	612	Overall 2.3%	65+	Yes	One-stage	GMS-AGECAT
Singapore	Lim et al., 2003	234	Overall 7.7%	60+	No	One stage	ECAQ
Singapore	Lim et al., 2003		Overall 13.2%	60+	No	One-stage	IQCODE
Thailand	Phanthumchinda et al., 1992	500	Overall 1.8%; almost all AD	60+	Yes	Two-stage	DSM-IIIR dementia
Korea	Park et al., 1994	702	Overall 10.8%; AD 60%; VaD 12%; alcohol 8%	65+	Yes	Two-stage	DSM-IIIR dementia
Korea	Woo et al., 1998	1674	Overall 9.5%; AD 4.5%; VaD 2.5%	65+	Yes	Two-stage	NINCDS-ADRDA
Korea	Kim et al., 2003	1101	Overall 7.4%	65+	Yes	Three-stage	DSM-IIIR dementia
Hong Kong	Chiu et al., 1998	1034	Overall 6.1%; AD 65%; VaD 29%	70+	Yes	Two-stage	DSM-IV dementia
China	Li et al., 1989	1331	Overall 1.28%; AD 21%; VaD 57%	60+	Yes	Two-stage	DSM-III dementia
China	Zhang et al., 1990	5055	Overall 4.6% in 65+; AD 65%	55+	Yes	Two-stage	McKhann criteria
Taiwan	Liu et al., 1995	5297	Overall 2%	40+	Yes	Two-stage	DSM-IIIR dementia
Taiwan	Liu et al., 1994	455	Rates by age only	50+	Yes	One-stage	DSM-IIIR dementia
Taiwan	Liu et al., 1998	1736	Overall 2.5%; AD 80%; VaD 7%	65+	Yes	One-stage	DSM-IIIR dementia
Taiwan	Lin et al., 1998	2915	Overall 4%; AD 54%; VaD 23%	65+	Yes	Two-stage	ICD-10 Dementia; NINCDS-ARDRA and NINDS-AIREN
Taiwan	Liu et al., 1996	1016	Overall 4.4%; AD 49%; VaD 24%	65+	Yes	Two-stage	DSM-IIIR; NINCDS-ARDRA and NINDS-AIREN
Japan	Hasegawa et al., 1986	1507	Overall 4.8%; AD 24%; VaD 42%	65+	Yes	Two-stage	DSM-III dementia
Japan	Shibayama et al., 1986	3106	Overall 5.8%; AD 3%; VaD 2.8%	65+	Yes	Two-stage	DSM-III and ICD-9 dementia
Japan	Yamada et al., 1999	2222	Overall 7.2%; AD men 2%; women 3.8%; VaD men 2%; women 1.8%	60+	Yes	One-stage	DSM-IIIR dementia

communities, at different stages of economic development and differing environments, whilst maintaining genetic homogeneity, may allow identification of environmental risk factors (Graves *et al.*, 1994; Richards and Brayne, 1996). Environmental changes that accompany migration include dietary change, acculturation, occupational change, educational change and differences in water, air, pollution and climate, etc. (Graves *et al.*, 1994). The identification of genetic and environmental factors predisposing to dementia will allow better understanding of causal mechanisms, leading to improved treatments and, ultimately, preventative strategies (Graves *et al.*, 1994).

Cross-national and cross-cultural incidence and prevalence studies designed to overcome these methodological difficulties, using screening and diagnostic instruments that are culture-fair, education-free and analogous, with similar case-finding methods in age- and sex-stratified samples, are now emerging (White, 1992; Prince *et al.*, 2003). The 10/66 Dementia Research Group (2000a, b) of Alzheimer's Disease International has developed an algorithm using appropriately translated (into native languages) and validated (culture-fair and education-free) versions of the GMS, CIS-D and the 10-word list-learning test from the CERAD battery with high degree of sensitivity and specificity in the diagnosis of dementia in culturally diverse populations from India, China, southeast Asia, Latin America, Africa and the Caribbean (Prince *et al.*, 2003). Population-based prevalence studies using this algorithm in the same diverse populations and using similar methodology are currently underway. The findings of this large study will be of great interest because it will compare prevalence from many different and culturally diverse countries using the same culture-fair and education-free instruments and methodology.

13.5.2.1 ENVIRONMENT

Despite comparable rates of dementia in Japan and USA, prevalence of vascular dementia is highest in Japan, intermediate in Hawaii and lowest in the mainland USA and an opposite trend is observed for AD (Graves *et al.*, 1994). These rates are being systematically studied in a cross-national studies: the Ni-Hon-Sea study of Japanese in Japan, Hawaii and mainland US (Graves *et al.*, 1994, 1996), and the Honolulu-Asia Aging study of Japanese in Hawaii, Japan and Taiwan (White *et al.*, 1996). The prevalence of AD among Japanese Americans in Washington (Graves *et al.*, 1996) and Honolulu (White *et al.*, 1996) is closer to that of white Americans suggesting an environmental aetiology. A prospective cohort study of Japanese Americans has reported that those who lead a traditional Japanese life style had a slower decline in cognition over a 2-year period (Graves *et al.*, 1999), also suggesting the importance of environmental factors. However, a study of first-generation Japanese migrants from Miyagi prefecture in Japan to Brazil (Meguro *et al.*, 2001a) reported a similar prevalence of dementia, AD and vascular dementia to that in Miyagi prefecture in Japan (Ishii *et al.*, 1999) despite the migrants having a higher prevalence of

diabetes mellitus and cerebrovascular disease (Meguro *et al.*, 2001b). The authors concluded that the prevalence of dementia was not affected by the environment.

The Indo-USA cross-national study reported a prevalence of 0.84 per cent for all dementias among rural Indians near Delhi, a lower figure than in a community sample in Pennsylvania (Chandra *et al.*, 1998). An incidence study in the same geographical area reported one of the lowest incidences of AD in the world (Chandra *et al.*, 2001). A study of Singapore Chinese and Malays revealed a higher prevalence of dementia among Malays than the Chinese (Kua and Ko, 1995); this difference was largely accounted for by an increased prevalence of multi-infarct dementia among Malay women when compared with Malay men and Chinese women. A prevalence and incidence study comparing rates among Yoruba Nigerians in Ibadan and African Americans in Indianapolis has reported a lower prevalence and incidence for dementia and AD among the Nigerians (Hendrie *et al.*, 1995b, 2001).

13.5.2.2 GENETICS

An early pilot population-based prevalence study has reported a strong association between apolipoprotein E (ApoE) ε4 allele and AD in African Americans (Hendrie *et al.*, 1995a) suggesting that ApoE ε4 is a risk factor independent of ethnicity. However, this was not observed in Yoruba Nigerians in Ibadan (Osuntokun *et al.*, 1995), despite a high prevalence of ε4 allele in the community. This discrepancy was explained by differences in the expression of ApoE alleles or of ApoE receptors, interaction with unidentified modifier genes, or environmental factors interacting with genes. Furthermore, there was lower deposition of A4 β-amyloid in post-mortem brains of Nigerian subjects without dementia compared with a similar series in Melbourne, Australia (Osuntokun *et al.*, 1994). Both these factors may be important in explaining a lower prevalence and incidence of AD in Nigeria.

A strong association between ApoE ε4 homozygous status and AD has been observed among Caucasians (non-Hispanic white Americans), African Americans and Hispanics in America in population-based prevalence studies (Maestre *et al.*, 1995; Tang *et al.*, 1996; Sahota *et al.*, 1997); despite these associations, the relative risk of developing AD was the highest in Caucasians compared with African Americans and Hispanics suggesting a gene–environment interaction. However, when considering heterozygous ApoE ε4 status, this relationship was either weaker (Maestre *et al.*, 1995) or absent in African Americans (Tang *et al.*, 1996; Sahota *et al.*, 1997) in comparison with Caucasians and Hispanics.

A population-based incidence study, controlling for education, family history of AD and other risk factors such as hypertension, demonstrated a strong association between combined homozygous and heterozygous ApoE ε4 status and AD in whites, African Americans and Hispanics in America (Tang *et al.*, 1998); unfortunately, separate data on homozygous and heterozygous ApoE ε4 status were not available owing to a small number of individuals homozygous for ApoE ε4 in the three ethnic groups. Furthermore, in the presence of at least one ApoE ε4 allele, the cumulative risk of developing AD up to the age of 90 years was similar in each of the three ethnic groups. However, in the absence of the an ApoE ε4 allele, the cumulative risk of developing AD up to the age of 90 years was higher in both the African American and the Hispanic groups when compared with the white group (Tang et al., 1998). These observations taken together suggest that the effect of ApoE ε4 on AD is weaker and 'dose dependent' in African Americans compared with white Americans and to a lesser extent Hispanics. It is possible that the presence of other environmental factors or modifier genes may reduce the ApoE ε4-associated risk of developing AD in people of African origin (Sahota et al., 1997; Tang et al., 1998). These environmental factors or modifier genes may be able to alter the risk of one dose of ApoE ε4 more easily than two doses of ApoE ε4 (Maestre et al., 1995).

Another explanation for these findings is that there may be differential linkage disequilibrium between an unidentified AD susceptibility gene and ApoE ε4 alleles in different ethnic groups (Maestre et al., 1995). A further explanation is the differential survival of those with ApoE ε4 alleles, although this observation is not supported by reports that ApoE ε4 frequency in white subjects is unchanged with age (Maestre et al., 1995; Tang et al., 1996), and either unchanged (Tang et al., 1996) or increased (Maestre et al., 1995) with age in African American subjects. Also, the frequency of ApoE ε4 in white and African American AD patients is reported to decline (Maestre et al., 1995) or remain unchanged (Tang et al., 1996) with age. However, despite a decline in ApoE ε4 frequency in AD patients with age, other genetic or environmental factors may increase the risk of developing AD in African Americans and Hispanics in the absence of this allele (Tang et al., 1998), including ApoE allele, ε4 which has been reported in a population-based study to increase the risk of AD in African Americans compared with white Americans (Maestre et al., 1995). A population-based incidence study of Japanese American men reported a significant association between ApoE ε4 and AD (Havlik et al., 2000).

Chandra and Pandav (1998) have speculated that high serum levels of cholesterol may interact with ApoE ε4 alleles to produce AD based on evidence of the low serum cholesterol levels in rural Indians near Delhi and a low prevalence of AD (Chandra et al., 1998). However, their observations were not supported by the ApoE typing in the same population-based Indo-US prevalence study (Ganguli et al., 2000). The frequency of ApoE ε4 in the Indian sample was significantly lower than in the USA sample. However, the strength of association between ApoE ε4 and AD was similar in both samples. These findings taken together may be one explanation for one of the lowest prevalence rates for AD in the world to be reported in India (Chandra et al., 1998). The authors concluded that the different prevalence in the two samples cannot be explained by differential risk or modifier risk pertaining to ApoE polymorphism, and they speculated that there may be additional risk or protective factors, survival effects or contributory environmental factors.

In a convenience sample of Cherokee Indians in Texas the risk of developing AD declined with an increase in the genetic degree of Cherokee ancestry and this relationship was independent of ApoE ε4 status (Rosenberg et al., 1996); however, the protective effect of Cherokee ancestry declined with increasing age. These findings suggest a complex interaction between genetic and environmental factors and critical examination in population-based studies is needed.

13.5.3 Education

The role of educational attainment as a risk factor for dementia is controversial. However, examination of the role of education as an environmental factor across different ethnic groups may shed further light on the role of environmental factors or gene-environment interaction. In two USA studies of Latinos, African Americans and non-Latino white Americans, levels of education were strongly correlated with the prevalence of dementia (Gurland et al., 1995, 1999); however, the differences in prevalence rates across the three ethnic groups disappeared if age and education were controlled for (Gurland et al., 1999), suggesting education may be an important environmental risk factor independent of ethnicity. In a community study of African Caribbeans in London, hypertension and diabetes were specifically associated with cognitive impairment in those with low levels of education (Stewart et al., 2001b). In a South Korean study, a similar association was found between cognitive impairment and systolic blood pressure, previous diagnosis of diabetes and non-fasting glucose levels in subjects with no formal education (Stewart et al., 2003).

These collective findings may be explained by several hypothesis which could be rigorously tested in epidemiological studies:

- Subjects with lower levels of education may have less well-controlled hypertension or diabetes (Gurland et al., 1995, 1999; Stewart et al., 2001b, 2003).
- Cognitive test batteries may not be sufficiently sensitive to measure cognitive impairment accurately in those with high levels of education (Stewart et al., 2001b).
- Third, those with high levels of education may have developed sufficient cognitive reserve to be less vulnerable to the effects of hypertension and diabetes (Gurland et al., 1995, 1999; Stewart et al., 2001b, 2003).
- Cerebral damage owing to hypertension or diabetes may be more severe in those with lower levels of education (Stewart et al., 2003).

13.6 FUTURE DIRECTIONS

Most cross-cultural studies have concentrated on cognitive impairment. BPSDs have to date received little attention in cross-cultural settings and in developing countries (Shah and Mukherjee, 2000). Measures of BPSD that are culture-fair and analogous to those currently used in Western countries are emerging from developing countries (see Chapter 7b on measurement of non-cognitive symptoms of dementia). BPSD require close examination in cross-sectional and longitudinal studies of the prevalence and incidence of dementia in cross-cultural and cross-national settings; these studies should also be designed to examine genetic and environmental risk factors (and the interaction between them) for both cognitive impairment and BPSD. The 10/66 Dementia Research Group (2000a, b; Prince et al., 2003) from Alzheimer's Disease International is in a strong position to conduct such research. They have developed measurement instruments and a methodology that can be applied across cultures, and studies of prevalence and BPSD are in progress in India, southeast Asia, China, Africa, the Caribbean and south America.

Similarly, very few cross-cultural studies have examined neurochemical, neuroanatomical and neurohistological changes in post-mortem brains (Amaducci et al., 1992), and structural and functional neuroimaging techniques have not been used at all. These techniques should be applied in rigorous population-based cross-cultural studies of cognitive impairment and BPSD; this would be a further powerful means of exploring environmental and genetic risk factors, and the interaction between them. The clustering of less common dementias, such as Huntington's disease, prion dementias and Parkinson's dementia complex of Guam, in some cultural groups may shed light on the genetic and environmental aetiological factors (Graham et al., 1998). The development of these elaborate and sophisticated research programmes will require considerable development of specialist services for these groups in both developed and developing countries if they are to be feasible.

A theoretical model of the epidemiological transition in dementia has been developed using incidence and prevalence data from different countries (Suh and Shah, 2001). According to this model all societies sequentially move through four hierarchical stages:

1. low incidence–high mortality society;
2. high incidence–high mortality society;
3. high incidence–low mortality society; and
4. low incidence–low mortality society.

Several factors contribute to the prevalence of dementia:

- The overall incidence (and thus the prevalence) will be low in societies where life expectancy is low, as few individuals will reach the age of risk.
- Mortality and survival after the onset of dementia will also influence the prevalence rate. Thus, in regions where survival after the onset of dementia is short, the prevalence will be low even if the incidence is high.
- The incidence itself is very important because uneven geographical distribution of protective or risk factors of AD and vascular dementia will vary the incidence. In socioeconomically less developed societies, infectious diseases associated with poor socioeconomic factors will reduce life expectancy with fewer individuals reaching the age of risk for dementia. Such a society has been described as a low incidence–high mortality society. With improvement in basic medical care the average life expectancy will increase and reach the threshold age of risk for dementia. This will lead to a gradual transition from a low incidence–high mortality society to a high incidence–high mortality society. Furthermore, in socioeconomically more developed societies the mortality associated with dementia may decline because of greater availability of medical care and advances in medical care and technology. This will lead to a gradual transition to a high incidence–low mortality society.

- In socioeconomically well developed countries, efforts to improve the control of risk factors (such as those for vascular dementia) may reduce the incidence of dementia leading to a low incidence–low mortality society. The transition from a low incidence–high mortality society to a low incidence–low mortality society may unfold in several ways depending upon availability of medical services, advances in medical care and technology, public health policies and efforts undertaken to control risk factors for dementia in a given society.

A detailed discussion of all the evidence to support this hypothesis is beyond the scope of this chapter. However, cross-national and cross-cultural population-based prevalence and incidence studies, data on mortality and survival after the onset of dementia, and 'proxy' measures (such as infant mortality rates) of the quality of medical care can be used to rigorously examine this hypothesis.

REFERENCES

10/66 Dementia Research Group. (2000a) Dementia in developing countries. A preliminary consensus statement from the 10/66 Dementia Research Group. *International Journal of Geriatric Psychiatry* **15**: 14–20

10/66 Dementia Research Group. (2000b) Methodological issues in population-based research into dementia in developing countries. A position statement paper from the 10/66 Dementia Research Group. *International Journal of Geriatric Psychiatry* **15**: 21–31

Abas M. (1996) Depression and anxiety among older Caribbean people in the UK: screening, unmet need and the provision of appropriate services. *International Journal of Geriatric Psychiatry* **11**: 377–382

Age Concern/Help the Aged Housing Trust. (1984) *Housing for Ethnic Elders.* London, Age Concern

Amaducci L, Baldereschi M, Amato MP *et al.* (1991) The World Health Organization cross-national research program on age-associated dementias. *Aging* **3**: 89–96

Ames D and Flynn E. (1994) Dementia Services: an Australian view. In: A Burns and R Levy (eds), *Dementia.* London, Chapman Hall

Anonymous. (1996) Ethnicity, race, culture: guidelines for research, audit, and publication. *BMJ* **312**: 1094

Anzola-Perez E, Bangdiwala SI, De Llano GB *et al.* (1996) Towards community diagnosis of dementia: testing cognitive impairment in older persons in Argentina, Chile and Cuba. *International Journal of Geriatric Psychiatry* **11**: 429–438

Balarajan R. (1996) Ethnicity and variation in mortality from cardiovascular disease. *Health Trends* **28**: 45–51

Balarajan R, Yuen P, Raleigh VS. (1989) Ethnic differences in general practice consultation rates. *BMJ* **299**: 958–960

Baldereschi M, Amato MP, Nencini P *et al.* (1994) Cross-national interrater agreement on the clinical diagnostic criteria for dementia. *Neurology* **44**: 239–242

Barker J. (1984) *Research Perspectives on Ageing: Black and Asian Old People in Britain.* 1st edition. London, Age Concern Research Unit

Ben-Arie O, Swartz L, Teggin AF, Elk R. (1983) The coloured elderly in Cape Town – a psychosocial, psychiatric and medical community survey. Part II Prevalence of Psychiatric Disorders. *South African Medical Journal* **64**: 1056–1061

Bhalia A and Blakemore K. (1981) *Elders of the Minority Ethnic Groups.* Birmingham, AFFOR

Bhatnagar KS and Frank J. (1997) Psychiatric disorders in elderly from the Indian subcontinent living in Bradford. *International Journal of Geriatric Psychiatry* **12**: 907–912

Bhopal R. (1997) Is research into ethnicity and health racist, unsound or unimportant science? *BMJ* **314**: 1751–1756

Blakemore K and Boneham M. (1994) *Age, Race and Ethnicity: a Comparative Approach.* Buckingham, Open University Press

Bohning W and Oishi N. (1995) Is international migration spreading? *Migration Review* **29**: 3

Bohnstedt M, Fox PJ, Kohatsu ND. (1994) Correlates of Mini-mental Status Examination scores among elderly demented patients: the influence of race-ethnicity. *Journal of Clinical Epidemiology* **12**: 1381–1387

Boneham M. (1989) Ageing and ethnicity in Britain: the case of elderly Sikh women in a Midlands town. *New Community* **15**: 447–459

Bowirrat A, Treves TA, Friedland RP *et al.* (2001) Prevalence of Alzheimer's type dementia in an elderly Arab population. *European Journal of Neurology* **8**: 119–123

Brayne C. (1993) Research and Alzheimer's disease. An epidemiological perspective. *Psychological Medicine* **23**: 287–296

Breitner JCS and Folstein M. (1984) Familial Alzheimer's dementia: a prevalent disorder with specific clinical features. *American Journal of Psychiatry* **14**: 63–80

Brislin R. (1970) Back-translation for cross-cultural research. *Journal of Cross-Cultural Psychology* **1**: 185–216

Chandra V and Pandav R. (1998) Gene-environmental interaction in Alzheimer's disease: a potential role for cholesterol. *Neuroepidemiology* **17**: 225–232

Chandra V, Ganguli M, Ratcliff G *et al.* (1994) Studies of the epidemiology of dementia: comparison between developed and developing countries. *Aging, Clinical and Experimental Research* **6**: 307–321

Chandra V, Ganguli M, Pandav R, Johnston J, Belle S, DeKosky ST. (1998) Prevalence of Alzheimer's and other dementias in rural India: the Indo-US study. *Neurology* **51**: 1000–1008

Chandra V, Pandav R, Dodge HH *et al.* (2001) Incidence of Alzheimer's disease in a rural community in the Indo-US study. *Neurology* **57**: 985–989

Chaturvedi N and McKeigue PM. (1994) Methods for epidemiological surveys of ethnic minority groups. *Journal of Epidemiology and Community Health* **48**: 107–111

Chiu H, Lam LCW, Chi I *et al.* (1998) Prevalence of dementia in Chinese elderly. *Neurology* **50**: 1002–1009

Commonwealth Department of Health, Housing and Community Services. (1991) *Aged Care Reform Strategy Mid-Term Review 1990–1991. Report.* Canberra, Australian Government Publishing Service

Copeland JRM, Kelleher MJ, Kellett JM *et al.* (1976) A semi-structured interview for the assessment of diagnosis and mental state in the elderly. The Geriatric Mental State schedule. 1. Development and reliability. *Psychological Medicine* **6**: 439–449

de la Monte SM, Hutchins GM, Moore GW *et al.* (1989) Racial differences in the etiology of dementia and frequency of Alzheimer's lesions in the brain. *Journal of the National Medical Association* **81**: 644–652

de Silva HA, Gunatilake SB. (2002) Mini-Mental State Examination in Sinhalese: a sensitive test to screen for dementia in Sri Lanka. *International Journal of Geriatric Psychiatry* **7**: 134–139

de Silva HA, Gunatilake SB, Smith AD. (2003) Prevalence of dementia in a semi-urban population in Sri Lanka: report from a regional survey. *International Journal of Geriatric Psychiatry* **18**: 711–715

Dein S and Huline-Dickens S. (1997) Cultural aspects of ageing and psychopathology. *Ageing and Mental Health* **1**: 112–120

Department of Health. (2001) *National Service Framework for Older People.* London, Department of Health

Donaldson L J. (1986) Health and social status of elderly Asians. A community survey. *BMJ* **293**: 1079–1082

Dowd JJ and Bengston VL. (1978) Aging in minority populations: an examination of double jeopardy hypothesis. *Journal of Gerontology* **3**: 427–436

Escobar JI, Burnham A, Karno M *et al.* (1986) Use of the Mini-Mental State Examination (MMSE) in a community population of mixed ethnicity. *Journal of Nervous and Mental Diseases* **174**: 607–614

Fairburn CG and Hope A. (1988) changes in behaviour in dementia: a neglected area. *British Journal of Psychiatry* **152**: 406–407

Flaherty JA, Gaviria FM, Pathak D *et al.* (1988) Developing instruments for cross-cultural psychiatric research. *Journal of Nervous and Mental Diseases* **176**: 257–263

Folstein MF, Folstein SE, McHugh PR. (1975) 'Mini-mental State': a practical method for grading the cognitive state of patients for the clinician. *Journal of Psychiatric Research* **12**: 189–198

Fuh JL, Teng EL, Lin KN *et al.* (1995) The informant questionnaire on cognitive decline in the elderly (IQCODE) as a screening tool for dementia for a predominantly illiterate Chinese population. *Neurology* **45**: 92–96

Fuzikawa C, Lima-Costa MF, Uehoa E *et al.* (2003) A population-based study on the intra and inter-rater reliability of the clock drawing test in Brazil: the Bambui Health and Ageing Study. *International Journal of Geriatric Psychiatry* **18**: 450–456

Ganguli M, Ratcliff G, Chandra V *et al.* (1995) A Hindi version of the MMSE: development of a cognitive screening instrument for a largely illiterate rural population of India. *International Journal of Geriatric Psychiatry* **10**: 367–377

Ganguli M, Chandra V, Gilby JE *et al.* (1996) Cognitive test performance in a community-based nondemented elderly sample in rural India: the Indo-US cross-national dementia epidemiology study. *International Psychogeriatrics* **8**: 507–524

Ganguli M, Chandra V, Kamboh I *et al.* (2000) Apolipoprotein E polymorphism and Alzheimer's disease. *Archives of Neurology* **57**: 824–830

George J and Young J. (1991) The physician. In: AJ Squires (ed.), *Multicultural Health Care and Rehabilitation of Older People.* London, Edward Arnold

Gibbons LE, Van Belle G, Yang M *et al.* (2002) Cross-cultural comparison of the Mini-mental State Examination in United Kingdom and

United States participants with Alzheimer's disease. *International Journal of Geriatric Psychiatry* **17**: 723–728

Gillam S, Jarman B, White P *et al*. (1989) Ethnic differences in consultation rates in urban general practice. *BMJ* **299**: 953–958

Goldberg D and Huxley P. (1991) *Common Mental Disorders: A Biosocial Model*. London and New York, Tavistock and Routledge

Graham C, Howard R, Ha Y. (1998) Studies on dementia: Dementia and ethnicity. *International Psychogeriatrics* **10**: 183–191

Graves AB, Larson EB, White LR, Teng EL, Homma A. (1994) Opportunities and challenges in international collaborative epidemiological research of dementia and its subtypes. Studies between Japan and the US. *International Psychogeriatrics* **6**: 209–223

Graves AB, Larson EB, Edland SD *et al*. (1996) Prevalence of dementia in and its subtypes in the Japanese American population of King County, Washington State. *American Journal of Epidemiology* **144**: 760–771

Graves AB, Rajaram L, Bowen JD *et al*. (1999) Cognitive decline and Japanese culture in a cohort of older Japanese Americans in King county. *Journal of Gerontology Series B-Psychological Sciences and Social Sciences* **54**: S154–161

Gurland B, Golden Teresi JA *et al*. (1984) The Short-Care. An efficient instrument for the assessment for the assessment of depression and dementia. *Journal of Gerontology* **39**: 166–169

Gurland BJ, Wilder DE, Cross P *et al*. (1992) Screening scales for dementia: towards reconciliation of conflicting cross-cultural findings. *International Journal of Geriatric Psychiatry* **7**: 105–113

Gurland B, Wilder D, Cross P *et al*. (1995) Relative rates of dementia by multiple case definitions, over two prevalence periods in three sociocultural groups. *American Journal of Geriatric Psychiatry* **3**: 6–20

Gurland B, Wilder D, Lantigua R *et al*. (1999) Rates of dementia in three ethnoracial groups. *International Journal of Geriatric Psychiatry* **14**: 481–493

Hall KS, Hendrie HC, Brittain HM *et al*. (1993) The development of dementia screening interview in two distinct languages. *International Journal of Methods in Psychiatric Research* **3**: 1–28

Hall KS, Gao S, Emsley CL *et al*. (2000) Community screening interview for dementia (CIS D): performance in five disparate study sites. *International Journal of Geriatric Psychiatry* **15**: 521–531

Hasegawa K, Homma A, Imai Y. (1986) An epidemiological study of age-related dementia in the community. *International Journal of Geriatric Psychiatry* **1**: 45–55

Havlik RJ, Izmirlian G, Petrovitch H *et al*. (2000) ApoE ε4 predicts incident AD in Japanese American men: the Honolulu-Asia Aging Study. *Neurology* **54**: 1526–1529

Hendrie H. (1992) Indianapolis-Ibadan dementia project. In: JD Curb and AB Graves (eds), Multi-National Studies of Dementia. *The Gerontologist* **32** (Suppl. 2): 219

Hendrie H, Hall KS, Pillay N *et al*. (1993) Alzheimer's disease is rare in Cree. *International Psychogeriatrics* **5**: 5–15

Hendrie HC, Osuntokun BO, Hall KS *et al*. (1995a) Prevalence of Alzheimer's Disease and Dementia in two communities: Nigerian Africans and African Americans. *American Journal of Psychiatry* **152**: 1485–1492

Hendrie HC, Hall KS, Hui S *et al*. (1995b) Apolipoprotein E genotypes and Alzheimer's disease in a community study of elderly African Americans. *Annals of Neurology* **37**: 118–120

Hendrie HC, Ogunniyi A, Hall KS *et al*. (2001) Incidence of dementia and Alzheimer's disease in 2 communities: Yoruba residing in Ibadan, Nigeria, and African Americans residing in Indianapolis, Indiana. *Journal of the American Geriatrics Society* **285**: 739–747

Heyman A, Fillenbaum G, Prosnitz B. (1991) Estimated prevalence of dementia among elderly black and white community residents. *Archives of Neurology* **48**: 594–598

Hofman A, Rocca WA, Brayne C *et al*. (1991) The prevalence of dementia in Europe: a collaborative study of 1980–1990 findings. *International Journal of Epidemiology* **20**: 736–748

Hopkins A and Bahl V. (1993) *Access to Care for People from Black and Ethnic Minorities*. London, Royal College of Physicians

Ishii H, Meguro K, Ishizaki J *et al*. (1999) Prevalence of senile dementia in a rural community in Japan: the Tajiri project. *Archives of Gerontology and Geriatrics* **29**: 249–265

Jacob KS, Bhruga D, Lloyd KR *et al*. (1998) Common mental disorders, explanatory models and consultation behaviour among Indian women living in the UK. *Journal of the Royal Society of Medicine* **91**: 66–71

Jagger C. (1998) Asian elders. An under studied and growing population. *Old Age Psychiatrist* March (10): 8

Jitapunkul S, Lailert C, Worakul P *et al*. (1996) Chula Mental Test: a screening test for elderly people in less developed countries. *International Journal of Geriatric Psychiatry* **11**: 715–720

Johnson MRD, Cross M, Cardew S. (1983) Inner city residents, ethnic minorities and primary health care. *Postgraduate Medical Journal* **59**: 664–667

Jones D and Gill P. (1998) Breaking down language barriers. The NHS needs to provide accessible interpreting services for all. *BMJ* **316**: 1476

Jorm A and Henderson S. (1993) *The Problem of Dementia in Australia*, 3rd edition. Canberra, Australian Government Publishing Service

Jorm AF and Jolley D. (1998) The incidence of dementia: a meta-analysis. *Neurology* **51**: 728–733

Jorm AF, Korten AE, Henderson AS. (1987) The prevalence of dementia: a quantitative integration of the literature. *Acta Scandinavica Psychiatrica* **76**: 465–479

Jorm AF, Scott R, Cullen JS *et al*. (1991) Performance of Informant Questionnaire on Cognitive Decline in the Elderly (IQCODE) as a screening test for dementia. *Psychological Medicine* **21**: 785–790

Kabir ZH and Herlitz A. (2000) The Bangla adaptation of mini-mental state examination (BMASE): an instrument to assess cognitive function in illiterate and literate individuals. *International Journal of Geriatric Psychiatry* **15**: 441–440

Kalachie A. (1991) Ageing is a third world problem too. *International Journal of Geriatric Psychiatry* **6**: 617–618

Katzman R, Zhang M, Qu QY *et al*. (1988) A Chinese version of the Mini-mental State Examination: Impact of illiteracy in a Shanghai dementia survey. *Journal of Clinical Epidemiology* **41**: 971–978

Kim J, Jeong I, Chun JH *et al*. (2003a) The prevalence of dementia in a metropolitan city of South Korea. *International Journal of Geriatric Psychiatry* **18**: 617–622

Kim J, Stewart R, Prince M *et al*. (2003b) Diagnosing dementia in a developing nation: an evaluation of the GMS-AGECAT algorithm in an older Korean population. *International Journal of Geriatric Psychiatry* **18**: 331–336

Kline F, Acosta F, Austin W *et al*. (1980) The misunderstood Spanish speaking patient. *American Journal of Psychiatry* **137**: 1530–1533

Kua EH. (1991) The prevalence of dementia in elderly Chinese. *Acta Psychiatrica Scandinavica* **83**: 350–352

Kua EH. (1992) A community study of mental disorders in elderly Singaporean Chinese using the GMS-AGECAT package. *Australia and New Zealand Journal of Psychiatry* **25**: 502–506

Kua EH and Ko SM. (1995) Prevalence of dementia among elderly Chinese and Malay residents of Singapore. *International Psychogeriatics* **7**: 439–46

Li G, Shen YC, Chen CH et al. (1989) An epidemiological survey of age-related dementia in an Urban area of Beijing. Acta Psychiatrica Scandinavica 79: 557–563

Li G, Shen YC, Zhau YW et al. (1991) A three-year follow-up study of age-related dementia in an urban area of Beijing. Acta Psychiatrica Scandinavica 83: 99–104

Lim HJ, Lim JPP, Anthony P et al. (2003) Prevalence of cognitive impairment amongst Singapore's elderly Chinese: a community-based study using the ECAQ and the IQCODE. International Journal of Geriatric Psychiatry 18: 142–148

Lin RT, Lai CL, Tai CT et al. (1998) Prevalence and subtype of dementia in southern Taiwan: impact of age, sex, education and urbanisation. Journal of the Neurological Sciences 160: 67–75

Lindesay J. (1998) The diagnosis of mental illness in elderly people from ethnic minorities. Advances in Psychiatric Treatment 4: 219–226

Lindesay J, Jagger C, Hibbert MJ, Peet SM, Moledina F. (1997a) Knowledge, uptake and availability of health and social services among Asian Gujarati and white elders. Ethnicity and Health 2: 59–69

Lindesay J, Jagger C, Mlynik-Szmid et al. (1997b) The mini-mental state examination (MMSE) in an elderly immigrant Gujarati population in the United Kingdom. International Journal of Geriatric Psychiatry 12: 1155–1167

Liu HC, Chou P, Lin KN et al. (1994) Assessing cognitive abilities and dementia in a predominantly illiterate population of older individuals in Kinmen. Psychological Medicine 24: 763–770

Liu HC, Lin KN, Teng EL et al. (1995) Prevalence and subtypes of dementia in Taiwan: a community survey of 5297 individuals. Journal of the American Geriatrics Society 43: 144–149

Liu HC, Lin RT, Chen YF et al. (1996) Prevalence of dementia in an urban area in Taiwan. Journal of Formosa Medical Association 95: 762–768

Liu HC, Fuh JL, Wang SJ et al. (1998) Prevalence and subtypes of dementia in a rural Chinese population. Alzheimer Disease and Associated Disorders 12: 127–134

Livingston G and Sembhi S. (2003) Mental health of the ageing immigrant population. Advances in Psychiatric Treatment 9: 31–37

Livingston G, Leavey G, Kitchen G et al. (2001) Mental health of migrant elders – the Islington study. British Journal of Psychiatry 179: 361–366

Livingston G, Leavey G, Kitchen G et al. (2002) Accessibility of health and social services to immigrant elders: the Islington study. British Journal of Psychiatry 180: 369–374

Lloyd K. (1992) Ethnicity, primary care and non-psychotic disorders. International Review of Psychiatry 4: 257–226

McCallum JA. (1990) The Forgotten People: Carers in Three Minority Communities in Southwark. London, Kings Fund Centre

McCracken CFM, Boneham MA, Copeland JRM et al. (1997) Prevalence of dementia and depression among elderly people in black and ethnic groups. British Journal of Psychiatry 171: 269–273

McKenzie K and Crowcroft NS. (1996) Describing race, ethnicity and culture in medical research: describing the groups is better than trying to find a catch all name. BMJ 312: 1051

Maestre G, Ottman R, Stern Y et al. (1995) Apolipoprotein E and Alzheimer's disease: ethnic variation in genotypic risks. Annals of Neurology 37: 254–259

Manthorpe J and Hettiaratchy P. (1993) Ethnic minority elders in Britain. International Review of Psychiatry 5: 173–180

Marcos LR. (1979) Effects of interpreters on the evaluation of psychopathology in non-English speaking patients. American Journal of Psychiatry 136: 171–174

Mather H and Keen M. (1985) The Southall diabetes survey: prevalence of known diabetes in Asians and Europeans. BMJ 291: 1081–1084

Meguro K, Meguro M, Caramelli P et al. (2001a) Elderly Japanese emigrants to Brazil before world war II: II. Prevalence of dementia. International Journal of Geriatric Psychiatry 16: 775–779

Meguro M, Meguro K, Cramelli P et al. (2001b) Elderly Japanese emigrants to Brazil before World War II: I. Clinical profiles based on specific historical background. International Journal of Geriatric Psychiatry 16: 768–774

Morris J, Heyman A, Mohs R et al. (1989) The consortium to establish a registry for Alzheimer's disease (CERAD). Part 1. Clinical and neuropsychological assessment of Alzheimer's disease. Neurology 39: 1159–1165

Murden RA, McRae TD, Kaner S et al. (1991) Mini-mental state exam scores vary with education in blacks and whites. Journal of the American Geriatrics Society 39: 149–155

National Urban League. (1964) Double Jeopardy: the Older Negro in America Today. New York, NUL

Norman A. (1985) Triple Jeopardy: Growing Old in a Second Homeland. London, Centre for Policy on Ageing

Odell SM, Surtees PG, Wainwright NWJ et al. (1997) Determinants of general practitioner recognition of psychological problems in a multi-ethnic inner-city health district. British Journal of Psychiatry 171: 537–541

Odutoye K and Shah AK. (1999) The clinical and demographic characteristics of ethnic elders from the Indian subcontinent newly referred to a psychogeriatric service. International Journal of Geriatric Psychiatry 14: 446–453

Office of Population Censuses and Surveys. (1983) 1981: Census Country of Birth: Great Britain. London, HMSO

Office of Population Censuses and Surveys. (1993) 1991 Census: Ethnic Group and Country of Birth Great Britain. London, OPCS

Ogunlesi AO. (1989) Psychogeriatrics in Nigeria. Psychiatric Bulletin 13: 548–549

Osuntokun BO, Hendrie HC, Ogunniyi AO. (1992) Cross-cultural studies in Alzheimer's disease. Ethnicity and Diseases 2: 352–357

Osuntokun BO, Ogunniyi A, Akang EEU et al. (1994) A4-amyloid in the brains of non-demented Nigerians. Lancet 343: 56

Osuntokun BO, Sahota A, Ogunniyi AO et al. (1995) Lack of association between apolipoprotein E ε-4 allele and Alzheimer's disease in elderly Nigerians. Annals of Neurology 38: 463–465

Palmore E and Manton K. (1973) Ageism compared to racism and sexism. Journal of Gerontology 28: 363–369

Park JH and Kwon YC. (1990) Modification of the Mini-mental State Examination for use in the elderly in a non-western society. Part 1. Development of the Korean version of Mini-mental State Examination. International Journal of Geriatric Psychiatry 5: 381–387

Park JH, Park YN, Ko HJ. (1991) Modification of the Mini-Mental State Examination for use with the elderly in a non-western society. Part II: cut-off points and their diagnostic validities. International Journal of Geriatric Psychiatry 6: 875–882

Park J, Ko HJ, Park YN, Jung C. (1994) Dementia among the elderly in a rural Korean Community. British Journal of Psychiatry 164: 796–801

Perkins P, Annegers JF, Doody RS et al. (1997) Incidence and prevalence of dementia in a multiethnic cohort of municipal retirees. Neurology 49: 44–50

Phanthumchinda K, Jitapunkul S, Sitthi-Amorn C et al. (1991) Prevalence of dementia in an urban slum population in Thailand: validity of screening methods. International Journal of Geriatric Psychiatry 6: 639–646

Phelan M and Parkman S. (1995) Work with an interpreter. *BMJ* **311**: 555–557

Pointon T. (1996) Telephone interpreting service is available. *BMJ* **312**: 53

Pollit P. (1996) Dementia in old age: an anthropological perspective. *Psychological Medicine* **26**: 1061–1074

Pollit P. (1997) The problem of dementia in Australian Aboriginal and Torres Strait islander communities: an overview. *International Journal of Geriatric Psychiatry* **12**: 155–163

Prince M, Acosta D, Chiu H *et al.* (2003) Dementia diagnosis in developing countries: a cross-cultural validation study. *Lancet* **361**: 909–917

Pringle M and Rothera I. (1996) Practicality of recording patient ethnicity in general practice: descriptive intervention study and attitude survey. *BMJ* **312**: 1080–1082

Quereshi KN and Hodkinson HM. (1974) Evaluation of a ten-question mental test in institutionalised elderly. *Age and Ageing* **3**: 152–157

Rait G and Burns A. (1997) Appreciating background and culture: the south Asian elderly and mental health. *International Journal of Geriatric Psychiatry* **12**: 973–977

Rait G, Burns A, Chew C. (1996) Age, ethnicity and mental illness: a triple whammy. *BMJ* **313**: 1347

Rait G, Morley M, Lambat I, Burns A. (1997) Modification of brief cognitive assessments for use with elderly people from the South Asian sub-continent. *Ageing and Mental Health* **1**: 356–363

Rait G, Burns A, Baldwin R *et al.* (2000a) Validating screening instruments for cognitive impairment in older south Asians in the United Kingdom. *International Journal of Geriatric Psychiatry* **15**: 54–62

Rait G, Morley M, Burns A *et al.* (2000b) Screening for cognitive impairment in older African-Caribbeans. *Psychological Medicine* **30**: 957–963

Rajkumar S and Kumar S. (1996) Prevalence of dementia in the community: a rural urban comparison from Madras, India. *Australian Journal on Ageing* **15**: 9–13

Rajkumar S, Kumar S, Thara R. (1997) Prevalence of dementia in a rural setting: a report from India. *International Journal of Geriatric Psychiatry* **12**: 702–707

Redelinghuys J and Shah AK. (1997) The characteristics of ethnic elders from the Indian subcontinent using a geriatric psychiatry service in west London. *Ageing and Mental Health* **1**: 243–247

Richards M. (1997) Cross-cultural studies of dementia. In: C Holmes and R Howard (eds), *Advances in Community Care. Chromosomes to Community Care.* Petersfield, Wrightson Biomedical

Richards M and Brayne C. (1996) Cross-cultural research into cognitive impairment and dementia: some practical experiences. *International Journal of Geriatric Psychiatry* **11**: 383–387

Richards M, Brayne C, Forde C, Abas M, Levy R. (1996) Surveying African Caribbean elders in the community: implications for research on health and health service use. *International Journal of Geriatric Psychiatry* **11**: 41–45

Richards M, Brayne C, Dening T *et al.* (2000) Cognitive function in UK community dwelling African Caribbean and white elders: a pilot study. *International Journal of Geriatric Psychiatry* **15**: 621–630

Ritch AES, Ehtisham M, Guthrie S *et al.* (1996) Ethnic influence on health and dependency of elderly inner city residents. *Journal of the Royal College of Physicians London* **30**: 215–220

Rocca WA, Bonaiuto S, Lippi A *et al.* (1990) Prevalence of clinically diagnosed Alzheimer's disease and other dementing disorders. A door-to-door survey in Appigano, Macerata Province, Italy. *Neurology* **40**: 626–631

Rosen WG, Mohs RC, Davis KL. (1984) A new rating scale for Alzheimer's disease. *American Journal of Psychiatry* **141**: 1356–1364

Rosenberg RN, Richter RW, Risser RC *et al.* (1996) Genetic factors for the development of Alzheimer's disease in Cherokee Indians. *Archives of Neurology* **53**: 997–1000

Roth M, Tym E, Mountjoy CQ *et al.* (1986) CAMDEX: A standardised instrument for diagnosis of mental disorder in the elderly with special reference to the early detection of dementia. *British Journal of Psychiatry* **149**: 698–709

Royall DR, Espino DV, Polk MJ *et al.* (2003) Validation of a Spanish translation of the CLOX for use in Hispanic samples: the Hispanic EPESE Study. *International Journal of Geriatric Psychiatry* **18**: 135–141

Sahadevan S, Lim PPJ, Tan NJL, Chan SP. (2000) Diagnostic performance of the mental status tests in older Chinese: influence of education and age on cut-off values. *International Journal of Geriatric Psychiatry* **15**: 234–241

Sahota A, Yang M, Gao S *et al.* (1997) Apolipoprotein E-associated risk of Alzheimer's disease in the African American population is genotype dependent. *Annals of Neurology* **42**: 659–661

Salmon DP, Reikkinen PJ, Katzmman R *et al.* (1989) Cross-cultural studies of dementia- a comparison of the Mini-mental State Examination performance in Finland and China. *Archives of Neurology* **46**: 769–772

Samanta A, Burden AC, Fent B. (1987) Comparative prevalence of non-insulin-dependent diabetes mellitus in Asian and white Caucasians adults. *Diabetes Research and Clinical Practice* **4**: 1–6

Schoenberg BS, Anderson DW, Haerer AF. (1985) Severe dementia: prevalence and clinical features in a biracial US population. *Archives of Neurology* **42**: 740–743

Secretaries of State for Health, Wales, Northern Ireland and Scotland. (1989) *Working for Patients.* London, HMSO

Senior A and Bhopal R. (1994) Ethnicity as a variable in epidemiological research. *BMJ* **309**: 327–330

Serby M, Chou JC, Franssen EH. (1987) Dementia in an American Chinese nursing home population. *American Journal of Psychiatry* **144**: 811–881

Shah AK. (1992a) *The Prevalence and Burden of Psychiatric Disorders. A Report to the Department of Health.* London, Institute of Psychiatry

Shah AK. (1992b) The burden of psychiatric disorders in primary care. *International Review of Psychiatry* **4**: 243–20

Shah AK. (1992c) Difficulties in interviewing elderly people from an Asian ethnic group. *International Journal of Geriatric Psychiatry* **7**: 17

Shah AK. (1997a) Interviewing mentally ill ethnic minority elders with interpreters. *Australian Journal on Ageing* **16**: 220–222

Shah AK. (1997b) Straight talk. overcoming language barriers in diagnosis. *Geriatric Medicine* **27**: 45–4

Shah AK. (1998) The psychiatric needs of ethnic minority elders in the UK. *Age and Ageing* **27**: 267–26

Shah AK. (1999) Difficulties experienced by a Gujarati psychiatrist in interviewing elderly Gujaratis in Gujarati. *International Journal of Geriatric Psychiatry* **14**: 1072–1074

Shah AK and Dighe-Deo D. (1998) Elderly Gujaratis and psychogeriatrics in a London psychogeriatric service. *IPA Bulletin* **14**: 12–13

Shah AK and Mukherjee S. (2000) Cross-cultural issues in the measurement of behavioural and psychological signs and symptoms of dementia (BPSD). *Ageing and Mental Health* **4**: 244–252

Shah AK, Lindesay J, Jagger C. (1998) Is the diagnosis of dementia stable over time among elderly immigrant Gujaratis in the United Kingdom (Leicester). *International Journal of Geriatric Psychiatry* **13**: 440–444

Shaji S, Promodu K, Abraham T, Jacob RK, Verghese A. (1996) An epidemiological study of dementia in a rural community in Kerala, India. *British Journal of Psychiatry* **168**: 747–780

Shibayama H, Kashara Y, Kobyashi H et al. (1986) Prevalence of dementias in a Japanese elderly population. *Acta Psychiatrica Scandinavica* **74**: 144–151

Silveira E and Ebrahim S. (1995) Mental Health and health status of elderly Bengalis and Somalis in London. *Age and Ageing* **24**: 474–480

Silverman JM, Li G, Schear S et al. (1992) A cross-cultural family history study of primary progressive dementia in relatives of non-demented elderly Chinese, Italians, Jews and Puerto Ricans. *Acta Psychiatrica Scandinavica* **85**: 211–217

Singh SP. (1997) Ethnicity in psychiatric epidemiology: the need for precision. *British Journal of Psychiatry* **171**: 305–308

Snowdon J. (1993) How many bed days for an areas psychogeriatric patients? *Australia and New Zealand Journal of Psychiatry* **27**: 42–48

Solomon A. (1992) Clinical diagnosis among diverse populations: a multicultural perspective. Family in Society. *Journal of Contemporary Human Services* June: 371–377

Stewart R, Richards M, Brayne C et al. (2001a) Cognitive function in UK community-dwelling African Caribbean elders: normative data for a test battery. *International Journal of Geriatric Psychiatry* **16**: 518–527

Stewart R, Richards M, Brayne C et al. (2001b) Vascular risk and cognitive impairment in an older, British, African-Caribbean population. *Journal of the American Geriatrics Society* **49**: 263–269

Stewart R, Johnson J, Richards M, Brayne C, Mann A and Medical Research Council Cognitive Function and Ageing Study. (2002) The distribution of Mini-mental State Examination scores in an older UK African Caribbean population compared to MRC CFA study norms. *International Journal of Geriatric Psychiatry* **17**: 745–751

Stewart R, Kim J, Shin I et al. (2003) Education and the association between vascular risk factors and cognitive function: a cross-sectional study in older Koreans with cognitive impairment. *International Psychogeriatrics* **15**: 27–36

Still CN, Jackson KL, Brandes DA et al. (1990) Distribution of major dementias by race and sex in South Carolina. *Journal of South Carolina Medical Association* **86**: 453–456

Suh GH and Shah A. (2001) A review of the epidemiological transition in dementia – cross-national comparisons of the indices related to Alzheimer's disease and vascular dementia. *Acta Psychiatrica Scandinavica* **104**: 4–11

Tang MX, Maestre G, Tsai WY et al. (1996) Relative risk of Alzheimer's disease and age-at-onset distributions based on ApoE genotypes among elderly African Americans, Caucasians and Hispanics in New York City. *American Journal of Human Genetics* **58**: 574–584

Tang MX, Stern Y, Marder K et al. (1998) The ApoE ε4 allele and the risk of Alzheimer's disease among African Americans, whites and Hispanics. *Journal of the American Geriatrics Society* **279**: 751–755

Teresi JA, Golden RR, Cross P et al. (1995) Item bias in cognitive screening measures: comparisons of elderly white, Afro-American, Hispanic and high and low education subgroups. *Journal of Clinical Epidemiology* **4**: 473–483

Tombaugh TN and McIntyre NJ. (1992) The Mini-mental State Examination: a comprehensive review. *Journal of the American Geriatrics Society* **40**: 922–935

Treves T, Korczyn AD, Zilber N et al. (1986) Presenile dementia in Israel. *Archives of Neurology* **43**: 26–29

Tsang H, Chong M, Cheng TA. (2002) Development of the Chinese version of the Geriatric Mental State schedule. *International Psychogeriatrics* **14**: 219–226

Vas CJ, Pinto C, Panikker D et al. (2001) Prevalence of dementia in an urban Indian population. *International Psychogeriatrics* **13**: 439–450

White LR. (1992) Towards a program of cross-cultural research on the epidemiology of Alzheimer's disease. *Current Science* **63**: 456–469

White L, Petrovitch H, Ross GW et al. (1996) Prevalence of dementia in older Japanese-American men in Hawaii. *JAMA* **276**: 955–960

Woo JI, Lee JH, Yoo K et al. (1998) Prevalence estimation of dementia in a rural area of Korea. *Journal of the American Geriatrics Society* **46**: 983–987

World Health Organization. (1992) *SCAN: Schedules for Clinical Assessment in Neuropsychiatry.* Geneva, WHO

Xu G, Meyer JS, Huang Y et al. (2003) Adapting Mini-mental State Examination for dementia screening among illiterate or minimally educated elderly Chinese. *International Journal of Geriatric Psychiatry* **18**: 609–616

Yamada M, Sasaki H, Mimori Y et al. (1999) Prevalence and risks of dementia in the Japanese population: RERF's adult health study of Hiroshima subjects. *Journal of the American Geriatrics Society* **47**: 189–195

Youn JC, Lee DY, Kim KW et al. (2002) Development of the Korean version of Alzheimer's Disease Assessment Scale (ADAS-K). *International Journal of Geriatric Psychiatry* **17**: 797–803

Yu ESH, Liu WT, Levy P et al. (1989) Cognitive impairment among elderly adults in Shanghai, China. *Journal of Gerontology* **44**: S97–S106

Zann S. (1994) *Identification of support, education and training needs of rural/remote health care service providers involved in dementia care. Rural Health, Support, Education and Training (RHSET). Project Progress Report.* Queensland, Northern Regional Health Authority.

Zaudig M. (1996) Assessing behavioural symptoms of dementia of Alzheimer's type: categorical and quantitative approaches. *International Psychogeriatrics* **8** (Suppl. 2): 183–200

Zhang M, Katzman R, Salmon D et al. (1990) The prevalence of dementia and Alzheimer's disease in Shanghai, China: impact of age, gender, and education. *Annals of Neurology* **27**: 428–437

14

Helping staff and patients with dementia through better design

MARY MARSHALL

Nursing and care staff are the most precious resource in dementia care. Theirs is a challenging job, which requires them to be able to really focus on their relationship with the patient. They need to be able to relate at an emotional and practical level at the same time, all the time. They need to be able to keep patients stimulated whilst also keeping them safe. They need to be able to care for them, while also maintaining as much of the patients' independence as possible. They need to offer an environment that reinforces identity, while also offering group care. They also need dignity, privacy and choice in their work environment where they spend much of their lives.

We cannot expect nursing and care staff to value the individuals in their care if they do not feel valued. The buildings in which they are required to work can speak volumes about the extent to which their work is seen as valuable and important.

To enable nursing and care staff to give of their best requires buildings that are supportive. They need buildings, which, as far as possible, tell patients what is expected of them and how to find their way. They need buildings that make it easy to keep patients busy but also well supervised. They need it to be easy to modify buildings to reinforce identity.

This chapter will explain how buildings can be designed or modified to help nursing and care staff to provide the best possible care.

Unnecessary disability is a useful concept. A lot of buildings cause patients to be more disabled than they need to be and add to the burden of care for staff.

14.1 PROBLEMS FOR NURSING AND CARE STAFF CAUSED BY POOR DESIGN

If problems are clearly identified, design solutions are very obvious.

As far as staff are concerned there are many kinds of problems that make their lives difficult.

14.1.1 Front doors

Conspicuous front doors encourage patients to try to get out. Patients are constantly reminded that there is somewhere else to go by the constant traffic of people and trolleys in and out of the front door. Patients are mistaken for visitors and accompany people leaving. They also hang around the doors making everybody else feel bad about the fact that they can come and go, whereas the patients are trapped inside. We need to protect staff from the constant exposure to emotional pain that this causes (Samut, 2003).

14.1.2 Fire doors

Conspicuous fire doors, often at the end of corridors, keep everybody busy as patients depart through them and staff have to drop what they are doing to run after them. People with dementia often move towards light, so fire doors with windows in a dark corridor are very enticing.

14.1.3 Storage space

Lack of storage often means that bathrooms do not have the function that they should have because they are full of hoists, wheelchairs and zimmers. This is confusing for patients and infuriating for staff who need space to work. Patients need bathrooms to be places of calm and multisensory stimulation and instead they are full of rather frightening contraptions. Lack of storage can also mean that staff are unable to allow personal furniture in bedrooms because there is nowhere to put the furniture that belongs to the provider. Summerhouses and sheds, built to provide activities for men, are sometimes full of beds and chairs.

14.1.4 Dining rooms

Dining rooms that are too big are full of noise and distracting activity. Noise to people with dementia is as disabling as stairs are to people in wheelchairs (Hiatt, 1995). Given the levels of undernutrition in many establishments for older people (Walker and Higginson, 2000), every effort needs to be made to make dining a congenial experience where the patients can concentrate on eating without becoming stressed and agitated by other patients. Dining rooms need to be as small as possible (see Plate 2). Staff find it much easier to ensure that the atmosphere is calm and patients are getting individual attention if there are fewer than 10 people eating together at the one time. The lack of any sound-absorbing ceiling tiles, and other fabrics also makes it very hard for staff to ensure a quiet and calm atmosphere.

14.1.5 Household spaces

The lack of everyday household spaces and objects means that anxious old people, with no motivation to do anything or who spend the whole day running their hands across tabletops, have nowhere familiar to do what they have always done to pass the time. They simply exasperate staff and other residents. Given a kitchen they can happily spend hours keeping the surfaces clean or mopping the sink. Yet few units provide even the rudiments of a kitchen except for the occupational therapy activity kitchen and then it is behind closed doors and only available to certain patients at certain times. Washing poles and a line in the garden with an adjacent sink can keep some patients very happy (see Plate 3). An old car in the garden can be very good for older men to sit in or fidget in the engine.

14.1.6 Toilets

Out of the way or poorly identified toilets make it difficult for patients to find the toilet themselves. Levels of incontinence mean that staff spend much of their time taking people to the toilet and this can be very wearing and unrewarding. Many

staff can use this as an opportunity for individual interaction but motivation wears thin if you do little else. Yet a good part of the incontinence may be because patients cannot find the toilet. One nursing home reduced its use of incontinence pads by half when they painted the doorframe red and put a large sign on it with a picture and the words 'Toilet' (personal communication) (see Plate 4). Another home relocated their en-suite toilet doors to face the bed and again reduced incontinence (personal communication). Wilkinson *et al.* (1995) found the most effective sign was words and a picture.

14.1.7 Walking areas

Many places have little appropriate space for meaningful walking. Patients who walk a lot can be very wearing for staff and other patients. There can be many reasons for this. Allan (1994) lists the following possibilities:

- continuation of life style patterns
- occupation
- leisure
- response to stress
- neurological damage
- anxiety/stress/anger
- boredom
- need for toilet
- pain
- other physical/psychiatric illness
- loss of goal-directed behaviour
- faulty goal-directed behaviour
- need for exercise
- form of communication
- medication side effects.

Several of these are ameliorated by design. If a person needs exercise there ought to be healthy, positive ways that they can go on a walk, ideally through a garden so they can get fresh air and vitamin D. The design of the unit should take them on a journey that includes a pathway outside and back in again. Sadly too many buildings offer only corridors where patients go up and down, which is depressing for everybody. In other racetrack style units they go round and round, again making staff feel inadequate because it is demonstrably such a poor experience.

Faulty goal-directed behaviour could mean that the person could not find the toilet or their bedroom. Good basic design would mean that patients could see all the doors in their unit. If this is not possible, then good quality individual signage on bedroom doors can be very helpful. It is hard for staff to provide this if the basic name holders are not in place. Nothing looks worse than selotaped bits of paper or photographs. Fixed notice boards, picture frames or perspex holders make individualizing rooms very easy for staff. Better still is the glass-fronted cupboard by the door to hold much-loved objects and photographs.

Some people walk about because they are too hot or too cold. Staff need to be able to control the temperature of individual rooms so that people can have at least one place where the temperature suits them.

14.1.8 Observation

Poor design can make it very wearing for staff to keep an unobtrusive eye on all the patients. Many staff walk miles on each shift, at the expense of their backs and feet, in order to keep an eye on a population dispersed throughout a unit. It is much better for them to work on smaller units with everything watchable. This can be achieved with a more open plan. Clearly a completely open plan is impossible given fire safety regulations, but a great deal can be achieved if this is the starting point. Glazed walls on sitting/dining/kitchen rooms; kitchen areas with shuttering for when they are not in use; waist-high furniture acting as a room divider, alcoves rather than completely separate lounges; all help facilitate unobtrusive observation. It can be very hard for staff if the unit is full of little dogleg corridors and passages to fire doors. Patients can become invisible and cause great anxiety.

14.1.9 Garden access

Poor access to the garden can cause additional work for staff or can mean that patients rarely go out. Gardens need to be very accessible so that patients can go out without supervision. They also need to be safe, which means having a fence but concealing it behind planting so that it is not an invitation to climb over. Many gardens are only accessible through fire doors out of the way of the main body of the unit, thus depriving staff and residents of an important therapeutic resource. Gardens are an important place to benefit from vitamin D from sunlight, as well as a place for activities and normal exercise. Staff are only too well aware of the importance of exercise but some residents do not respond to organized groups.

14.1.10 Chairs

People with dementia sit in chairs for long periods. The chairs are sometimes lacking in support and cause pain or discomfort to the patients with dementia. This means that staff have to deal with patients who walk about to loosen up their limbs or lash out because they are stiff and sore. Staff often have to pack pillows around patients because the chairs offer no side support. More fit and active patients can fail to recognize their chair because they are all the same colour. Chairs have the potential to provide a positive touch experience; one which is seldom provided.

14.1.11 Staff facilities

Poor quality staff facilities can be very demoralizing. Nursing and care staff need places where they can laugh, cry, shower or put their feet up in private. These need to be of a decent quality so that they feel valued. Dignity, privacy and choice for staff means, in part, a space where they can get away to recharge their batteries. They also need offices, which are not near patient areas, so they can do their paperwork in peace. They need somewhere for training, counselling relatives and having meetings, space that is not invaded by patients.

14.1.12 Flooring

Flooring that is difficult to keep clean is a real source of exasperation to nursing and care staff as well as cleaning staff. Flooring is one of those issues where there is no right answer partly because the ideal flooring does not exist. The ideal would be a speckled carpet, which did not show every crumb and did not look as if it had crumbs on it. It would be a carpet because this feels safer to many people with dementia who are frightened of slipping. Carpets also provide a softer landing for people who do fall. Carpets are ideal because they soak up sound, they look domestic, do not reflect light and make the place look less clinical. But they are very difficult to keep stain- and smell-free. Some people are concerned that they can be a source of infection because they are so hard to wash. They rarely live up to the sales hype about being easy to wash. They often allow urine to penetrate and soak into the floor or concrete below. As a consequence staff prefer a hard floor surface that is easy to keep clean, and this is perfectly understandable. Ideally all floor covering would be the same colour because people with dementia cannot see the difference between a step and a change in floor colour.

14.1.13 Colour

Lack of differentiation between units means that patients often end up in the wrong place. Colour is often used with the intention of differentiating between units without a full understanding of the increasing impairments in colour differentiation that occur with age. Brawley (1997) has a good chapter on this. As we age we get less and less able to differentiate between pastel shades, initially, and this impairment starts at the blue end of the spectrum. Objects are much better than colour to orientate people with dementia. Strong colour contrast can be useful but it is best reserved for really crucial aspects such as toilet doors.

14.2 DESIGN THAT HELPS PATIENTS

Clearly staff are going to be most helped in their care activities if the patients are helped to function as well as they can, both because it means less work for staff and there is more job satisfaction. A therapeutic design for people with dementia will compensate for the following disabilities in every aspect:

- impaired memory
- impaired reasoning

- impaired learning
- high levels of stress
- increasing dependence on the senses.

In the same way that buildings can compensate for mobility problems and visual impairment, so they can compensate for these main disabilities of dementia and thereby help the person to remain as independent as possible. Some examples may illustrate how this thinking is applied.

14.2.1 Memory

If you have an impaired memory, it is helpful if you can see everywhere important that you need to go. You need to be able to see the toilet door and ideally the toilet itself; you need to be able to see the sitting or the dining room. Corridors are really difficult unless they are very short and very wide, because you cannot see the doors. For the same reason you need a lot of light, so that all available information is visible.

14.2.2 Learning

If you have impaired learning, you need lots of cues, so signage must include pictures and words. It also needs to be low enough for people who do not look upwards easily. If you find it difficult to learn where to go, you find it equally difficult to learn where you cannot go. Painting those doors that are not accessible the same colour as the walls, even to the extent of putting the handrail and skirting across them, can be helpful.

14.2.3 Reasoning

If you have impaired reasoning it is important that everything is understandable. The items that you are likely to use most often are those in the toilet: the tap, the flush handle and the paper holder. All need to be very easy to understand. A crosshead tap for example is much easier to understand than most lever taps especially the mixer versions (see Plate 5).

14.2.4 Stress

High levels of stress are much reduced by quiet, so acoustic tiles in the ceiling and lots of soft fabric surfaces can be very helpful, as can the availability of quiet sitting rooms and gardens.

14.2.5 Sensory abilities

Designing to take advantage of remaining sensory abilities for orientation is a real challenge. Impaired vision might mean using smell, touch or noise. Smell of disinfectant can lead people to a toilet and smell of food to a dining room, for example. The sense of smell can be very helpful in stimulating appetite, which is such a problem in people with dementia, so a kitchen or servery where toast can be made or bacon grilled can be very helpful – food generally arrives smell-free in trolleys. Impaired hearing means that everything possible needs to be done to make things visible.

14.3 SOME KEY DESIGN PRINCIPLES

There is not a great deal of research on design features. Day *et al.* (2000) provide an analysis of current research. Most of the literature is based on practice. It is tempting to give a checklist of design tips but this can never cover every aspect of a building, particularly when they have to be designed to help such a range of age groups and levels of disability. More helpful are principles against which actual buildings or proposed modifications can be judged. Many authors have presented design principles, starting with Uriel Cohen's book (Cohen and Weisman, 1991). There is a fair degree of international consensus (Judd *et al.*, 1997), which, if pulled together, gives a list of design points.

- Design should compensate for disability.
- Design should maximize independence.
- Design should enhance self-esteem and confidence.
- Design should demonstrate care for staff.
- Design should be orientating and understandable.
- Design should reinforce personal identity.
- Design should welcome relatives and the local community.
- Design should allow control of stimuli.

These principles are used as part of an audit tool to gauge the degree of 'dementia friendliness' of a building (Stewart and Page, 2000).

14.4 CONCLUSIONS

Buildings where people with dementia spend their days are also where nursing and care staff spend much of their lives. It is possible to design buildings to help nursing and care staff in their very complex and challenging work. It is also possible to design to help people with dementia to function at their best, which is clearly of assistance to staff. Perhaps the most important message of a building that takes staff needs properly into account is that the staff are valued and their work respected. This is a crucial message given the demands that are made of them.

REFERENCES

Allan K. (1994) *Wandering.* Stirling, Dementia Services Development Centre

Brawley EC. (1997) *Designing for Alzheimer's Disease.* New York, John Wiley and Sons

Cohen U and Weisman GD. (1991) *Holding on to Home: Designing environments for people with dementia.* Maryland, The Johns Hopkins University Press

Day K, Carreon D, Stump C. (2000) *The Therapeutic Design for Environments for People with Dementia.* Bristol, Policy Press

Hiatt LG. (1995) Understanding the physical environment. Pride Institute. *Journal of Long Term Care* **4**: 12–22

Judd S, Marshall M, Phippen P. (1997) *Design for Dementia.* London, Hawker Publications

Samut A. (2003) Developing an appropriate response to emotional pain. *Journal of Dementia Care* **11**(2)

Stewart S and Page A. (2000) Making design dementia friendly. *Conference Proceedings of the European Conference: Just Another Disability*, 1–2 October 1999, Glasgow

Walker J and Higginson C. (2000) The nutrition of elderly people and nutritional aspects of their care in long-term care settings. *Final audit report 1997–2000.* Glenrothes, CRAG

Wilkinson TJ, Henschke PJ, Handscombe K. (1995) How should toilets be labelled for people with dementia? *Australian Journal on Ageing* **13**:163–165

ADDITIONAL READING

There is a very expanding literature about design for dementia and increasing numbers of really sensitive buildings are being built. Some useful articles and books are listed below.

Benjamin LC and Spector J. (199) Environments for the dementing. *International Journal of Geriatric Psychiatry* **5**: 15–24

Bennett K. (1997) Cultural issues in designing for people with dementia. In: M Marshall (ed.), *State of the Art in Dementia Care.* London, Centre for Policy on Ageing

Calkins MP. (1988) *Design for Dementia Planning: Environments for the Elderly and the Confused.* Maryland, National Health Publishing

Cantley C and Wilson RC. (2002) *Put Yourself in my Place: Designing and Managing Care Homes for People with Dementia.* Bristol, Policy Press

Centre for Accessible Environments. (1998) *The Design of Residential Care and Nursing Homes for the Elderly.* London, Centre for Accessible Environments

Cohen U and Day K. (1991) *Contemporary Environments for People with Dementia.* Maryland, The Johns Hopkins University Press

Gitlin L, Liebman J, Winter L. (2003) Are environmental interventions effective in the management of Alzheimer's disease and related disorders? A synthesis of the evidence. *Alzheimer's Care Quarterly* **4**: 85–107

Kelly M. (1993) Designing for people with dementia. In: *The Context of the Building Standards.* Stirling, Dementia Services Development Centre

Peppard NR. (1991) *Special Needs Dementia Units: design, development and operations.* New York, Springer Publishing

Valins M. (1988) *Housing for Elderly People: a guide for architects and clients.* London, Architectural Press

15

The role of primary care in the management of dementia

BILL PETTIT

It is in a primary care setting that most of the care for those suffering from one of the dementia syndromes will be delivered. Changes in the demography of the population in association with changes in social and health policy mean that, in the United Kingdom (UK) at least, the burden of provision of health care will increasingly be that of the general practitioner or primary care physician. The population is ageing; by the middle of this century over one-quarter of the population will be aged over 60 years, with the over 85s being a significant proportion of those. The age-specific prevalence of dementia doubles every 5 years from 60 onwards and this presents a daunting prospect for those planning as well as those providing health and social care. Women are more at risk at all ages, and it has been speculated that this is due to an increased incidence of apolipoprotein E ε4 in women. Dementia is not just confined to the elderly, however, and there is a prevalence of 0.35/1000 in those aged 45–64 (Newens *et al.*, 1993).

Putting these numbers into a primary care context, the general practitioner with an average list size of 1800 people can expect to have perhaps 20 cases of dementia at any one time, although this will vary both by chance and the local age/sex distribution of the registered practice population. This is a similar order to those patients with other chronic diseases such as diabetes, past and present epilepsy and rheumatoid arthritis, almost all of whom will be known to the practice. With regard to the people with dementia, the general practitioner will know only of about 60 per cent of cases, and those at the more serious end of the disease spectrum. There is

great variation, however, and in one study (Illife *et al.*, 1991a) only about 8 per cent of those with severe cognitive impairment or depression were known to their general practitioner.

At present the role of the general practitioner with regard to dementia care will vary according to interest and perceived skills. General practitioners often do not seem to be active in the treatment of the dementias, probably owing to a form of therapeutic nihilism; feeling that there is nothing to be done.

Recent scientific developments, particularly with regard to the genetics, chemistry and treatment of Alzheimer's disease and vascular dementia have heightened the profile of the dementias. An increasing pressure from the public responding to the knowledge that there are drugs available that ameliorate some of the symptoms of some dementias will fuel this process. In the UK the National Service Frameworks for Older People has defined a care pathway for dementia and evidence-based best practice; by April 2004 all general practitioners should be using protocols agreed with their primary care organization (PCO) and local specialist services.

It is important that a person with dementia has their illness recognized by their general practitioner as soon as possible in the disease process. By early recognition it is possible to be proactive and plan a package of disease management to optimize the patient's quality of life, and perhaps modify the progress of the disease. The NMDA receptor antagonist memantine has a licence for use in moderate–severe Alzheimer's disease but the cholinesterase inhibitors donepezil, rivastigmine and galantamine are only licensed for use in mild–moderate cases. Dementia patients with this mild level of disease are just those cases of whom the general practitioner is not usually aware. At present the inception of a patient with dementia into primary care will usually be when a crisis occurs. This can happen when intercurrent illness produces a rapid deterioration in mental state or a carer is taken ill or dies, and a person with dementia becomes visible to the general practitioner for the first time. Patients with dementia often present to the Accident and Emergency department. In one study (Shaw et al., 1996), 24 per cent of those people over the age of 65 presenting to a casualty department after a fall were found to have cognitive impairment. This demonstrates the need for good liaison systems to be in place to alert primary care services to possible new dementia cases.

15.1 SCREENING FOR DEMENTIA

The general practitioner and the primary healthcare team will need to consider what strategies they wish to adopt in order to optimize dementia care by the early detection of the illness. There are no true screening tests to detect impending dementia in a presymptomatic latent phase at present, apart from those cases caused by relatively rare autosomal dominant gene defects. The ethical impact of such tests, if eventually developed, will be enormous, affecting many fundamental facets of life ranging from the ability to get employment to health and life insurance (Anonymous, 1996). For the foreseeable future, however, the general practitioner will have to rely upon early case finding coupled with a high index of clinical suspicion in order to detect cases of dementia. In UK general practice there was until recently a contractual framework in which registered patients aged 75 and over were offered an annual health assessment, including mental health. There is evidence, however, that this process is not very effective; it is also very demanding in resource terms. To 'screen' the average general practitioner's list of those over 75 years would take approximately 150 hours of face-to-face contact (Illife et al., 1991b). One study (Hallewell and Pettit, 1994) only found eight previously unknown cases of dementia and 16 previously identified cases in a screened population of 232 patients over the age of 75.

To date there is little evidence that cyclical population-based case finding produces much yield, particularly on a 12-monthly basis, owing to the relatively low incidence as opposed to the relatively high prevalence of the disease. It is becoming the norm for the use of computers in the clinical setting of the consultation in general practice. At a minimum this means that, for each encounter, a disease code and prescribing information is recorded in the computer databases. The end result of this is, over time, the generation of coded disease registers for a practice population. In the UK it is planned that such information will eventually be collected and shared on a PCO basis. In those practices where the disease register showed a lower than expected prevalence of dementia, then a stronger case for one cycle of case finding could be made. As the general practitioner will see up to 90 per cent of the practice population aged 75 and over in the setting of a consultation either at home or in the surgery in one year (Williams, 1984), case finding could be done on an opportunist basis; it could be said that this is good clinical practice. It is also quite feasible to seek out the 10 per cent not seen and administer rating scales to them. This does not have to be done by the general practitioner; community nurses of all disciplines can undertake this role, as could suitably trained lay people.

The type of practice population profile may well influence the approach taken to maximizing the number of dementia cases known. In socially deprived areas there tends to be a preponderance of patients from social classes III, IV and V. It is known that these groups use their general practitioner less than those from social classes I and II (Victor, 1991), despite having higher levels of morbidity for many diseases. In this sort of area, there is a stronger argument for active rather than opportunistic case finding, again for at least one cycle. As stated earlier, at present people with dementia often only become visible to primary care teams when the patient's support systems fail, perhaps owing to the death or illness of an elderly spouse. There is a need for primary care to be more proactive; the 'managed care' approach that some PCOs may adopt in the UK could be a vehicle for this. There will be many competitors for resources, however.

15.2 CASE FINDING

Although a question to a patient about their memory may be helpful, those patients presenting themselves with a complaint of memory loss are often found to be depressed rather than demented, even though depression and dementia coexist in up to 40 per cent of cases. Family and friends' comments about memory loss are much more significant, as are their comments about subtle problems with the instrumental activities of daily living (IADL). Deterioration in IADL, e.g. managing medication, using transport, handling finances and using the telephone, are significantly associated with cognitive impairment.

The general practitioner has a wide range of dementia-detecting or rating instruments that they can use as part of the consultation. There is reluctance for general practitioners to use these instruments, possibly as they feel the questions may be embarrassing. They are not alone in their reluctance: it has been reported that geriatricians have a similar attitude (Dunn and Lewis, 1993). This sense of embarrassment is misplaced; patients do not find the administration of the instruments intrusive (O'Connor et al., 1993; Hallewell and Pettit, 1994). The Abbreviated Mental Test Score (AMTS), clock face drawing and Mini-Mental State Examination (MMSE) are easy to use in a primary care setting, and take only a few minutes to administer. There are instruments such as the PHOTOs test (part of the CAMDEX and Rivermead behavioural memory test), that have been validated in a primary care setting (Hallewell and Pettit, 1994) and consist of seven photographs to be recognized and remembered. This test is even less intrusive, but will only detect cases and not measure severity. The MMSE offers severity rating, covers several domains and can be used serially, thus measuring rate of cognitive decline. It seems to be disliked by many general practitioners as it is thought to be a long instrument to administer. This is not so at all, and software versions are available for palm-top computers for the cost of a few pounds. At the moment simple instruments are being piloted as part of computer-aided decision-making software packages for use on primary care clinical computer systems. The patient's demographic information and past history, already held on the system, prompt the clinician to ask questions of the patient and enter the response into the computer, which will then score the responses and suggest if there is evidence of cognitive impairment. Until better instruments, perhaps with measures of ordinary and instrumental activities of daily living included in them, are developed, the MMSE may well be the instrument of choice. The main requirement is for the general practitioner to make the use of an instrument of their choice a regular part of routine clinical practice.

15.3 DIAGNOSIS

Having found a possible case of dementia, general practitioners can either refer to the specialist services at that point, or try to identify the type of dementia themselves. The natural history and clinical patterns of the dementia syndromes have been well described, particularly with regard to Alzheimer's disease (AD), which has a remarkably consistent natural history. The search continues for diagnostic markers of AD that do not require the neuropathological study of brain biopsy material, and so may be more accessible in a primary care setting. Blood tests such as analysis of the serum iron binding protein p97 (Kennard et al., 1996) showed early promise, but a truly sensitive and specific test has yet to be found. Magnetic resonance imaging of entorhinal cortex has been shown to be a potentially useful method of diagnosing early AD (Bobinski et al., 1999). This modality of investigation will not be in the primary care armamentarium for the foreseeable future!

Local shared care policy, where it exists, may influence the diagnostic input of the general practitioner. By taking a good history and carrying out a few investigations along with a physical examination, a general practitioner could make a diagnosis of dementia and probably the type of dementia syndrome in many cases. Most general practitioners would approach the diagnostic problem by excluding the reversible forms of dementia, and then trying to identify characteristic features of the remaining common dementia syndromes, those being AD, vascular dementia (VaD) and dementia with Lewy bodies (DLB). The other rarer causes of dementia such as neurosyphilis and Creutzfeldt–Jakob disease are very much in the specialist domain.

To aid diagnosis, a thorough history is essential – the more detailed the better. In the case of dementia this will need to be obtained from a relative or carer who knows the patient well, and has done so over a period of time. It is not sufficient to rely upon the patient alone for a history. The clinician will try to identify characteristic patterns of disease. In AD the indeterminate onset and insidious progress may be noted. Many areas of cognition are affected including memory, aphasia (loss of ability to understand the spoken or written word), apraxia (inability to perform familiar activities), agnosia (inability to recognize familiar objects) and disturbances in executive function (sequential organization, attention and planning). Functional disability results in deterioration in social and occupational activities. Early in AD, problems arise in the IADLs. As the disease progresses, the basic activities of daily living (ADL), including dressing, grooming and bathing, become restricted. In addition, behavioural changes are common and may include mood swings, wandering and agitation. In VaD a stepwise decline may be seen. There may be a history of transient ischaemic attacks or strokes. Other evidence of vascular disease history, such as angina, may be evident. It is important to remember that elements of VaD and AD may coexist. There is evidence to suggest that atherosclerosis is associated with both AD and VaD, and that there is an interaction between apolipoprotein E and atherosclerosis in the aetiology of AD (Hofman et al., 1997).

Visual hallucinations are more common in DLB, with up to 70 per cent of patients experiencing them, as is less severely impaired recent memory (Graham et al., 1997). DLB has a characteristic fluctuation in cognitive function, which may appear similar to a confusional state. Some 80 per cent of patients with DLB will demonstrate clouding of consciousness. It is very important that the general practitioner considers this diagnosis carefully, as patients with DLB are very sensitive to neuroleptic agents and administration of these agents may indeed prove fatal. The history itself should help distinguish the acute onset of a confusional state from the slow onset of any dementia syndrome. It is, of course, necessary to try to identify depression and delirium, and treat accordingly.

15.4 CLINICAL EXAMINATION

Examination will obviously include a dementia rating scale such as the MMSE. Evidence of disease in the cardiovascular system, such as ischaemic heart disease, hypertension and arterial bruits, would tend to support a hypothesis of VaD, although as previously stated, AD and VaD can coexist. A brief neurological examination may show evidence of extrapyramidal signs found in DLB. Evidence of cerebrovascular accident may be evident, such as focal neurological signs. A physical examination may reveal evidence of a reversible cause of dementia such as hypothyroidism or profound anaemia. It is stated that, overall, 5–10 per cent of dementias are reversible, but this is only true in about 1 per cent of dementia presenting in the elderly population. A younger patient presenting would increase clinical awareness of the possibility of a reversible dementia or one of the rarer dementia syndromes, and referral to a neurologist may be more appropriate than referral to old age psychiatry or memory clinic services.

15.5 INVESTIGATIONS

Laboratory tests will include glucose, full blood count, erythrocyte sedimentation rate, vitamin B_{12} and folate, thyroid function tests and biochemical profile. It has been traditional to undertake syphilis serology, but this is probably not cost-effective in primary care.

Neuroimaging is helpful in diagnosing a dementia, the cheapest option being a computed tomography (CT) brain scan without contrast. This will demonstrate structural changes in the brain typical of AD or VaD, and other abnormalities that may be a cause of cognitive decline such as tumours, haemorrhages and normal pressure hydrocephalus. Whether or not open access to CT imaging for general practitioners is practical is a matter for debate. The use of magnetic resonance imaging (MRI), functional MRI, single photon emission computed tomography (SPECT) and positron emission tomography (PET) are clearly not in the domain of primary care.

15.6 REFERRAL

Interestingly, almost three-quarters of UK general practitioners in one survey felt that a specialist opinion was not necessary to diagnose dementia (Grace, 1994). Now that drugs to ameliorate some of the symptoms of the dementias have a product licence or their equivalents are available for prescription, there has been a financial and clinical imperative in many areas to allow only initiation of prescribing by specialist clinicians. It is clearly essential that an accurate diagnosis of the type of dementia is needed to allow effective use of drugs. When considering specialist referral, the general practitioner will need to decide if he or she is going to refer and to whom. To aid this decision the practitioner needs to define and clarify purpose in referring: is it for diagnostic help, management help, prescription or a combination of these things?

The answers to these questions will make the type of referral clear. A neurologist may be appropriate for the younger or atypical case. The old age psychiatrist and their teams may be the most appropriate for cases where the patient is older and the diagnostic probabilities are more defined. If there is going to be a need for ongoing support, then the old age psychiatry teams will be the obvious choice; this is almost always the case. If the general practitioner is confident about the diagnosis, and the primary healthcare team is able to arrange appropriate support, then, arguably, no specialist referral is needed.

15.7 DRUG TREATMENT

It is probable that a patient with dementia will have other diseases also requiring treatment with drugs. It is important to review therapy to simplify the regimen as much as possible. The advice of the community pharmacist can be helpful regarding type of preparation and aids to compliance, such as 'dosette' boxes. Medication can be made up into blister packs with days and time of day clearly marked. Many people with dementia live on their own, and whilst it may be possible for someone to visit once daily to supervise medication, more frequent visits become problematic. If possible, once-a-day dosing with long-acting or modified-release agents should be arranged. There are several classes of drugs used in dementia, ranging from disease-modifying agents to those drugs used to modify behaviour. Donepezil, galantamine and rivastigmine have a UK product licence for the treatment of mild–moderate AD and memantine for moderate–severe AD. Prescribing guidelines such as those issued by the UK Standing Medical Advisory Committee (1998) and others (Lovestone *et al.*, 1997) exist for these agents. Initiation of this form of therapy is not, as yet, a primary care function, although continued prescription can be, as part of a shared care protocol. Other non-cholinergic agents are being developed and might be indicated in VaD as well as AD, but early results have been disappointing so far.

Aspirin therapy should be initiated in VaD to help prevent further ischaemic damage. Hypertension and atrial fibrillation should be treated vigorously. Other antiplatelet treatment, such as combined modified-release dipyridamole and aspirin may have a role if transient ischaemic attacks have been identified.

Wandering, agitation, aggression and insomnia are seen in dementia and can cause great distress to the carer. Aggression is often associated with delusions, and the general practitioner should try to identify the presence of this phenomenon. Non-drug interventions should be tried if at all possible, but there may be a need to prescribe medication at some stage. Small doses of a neuroleptic agent work well, but should be initiated carefully and the dose titrated to response. Patients with dementia are very susceptible to extrapyramidal side effects of these agents and, as has been previously stated, reactions can be fatal in those with DLB (Anonymous, 1994). In early 2004 it was reported that there was a two- to three-fold incidence of stroke in elderly patients with dementia treated with atypical antipsychotic agents. The Committee on the Safety of Medicines recommended that risperidone and olanzapine should not be used for the treatment of behavioural symptoms of dementia. Extrapyramidal side effects can be countered with agents such as orphenadrine, but these can cause confusion, delusions and hallucinations, so caution is required. Almost half of dementia patients may be depressed at some stage. Depression responds well to treatment in many cases; suitable agents are lofepramine, imipramine or a selective serotonin reuptake inhibitor (SSRI). The SSRIs have a better safety profile, and may be preferred if there are doubts about supervision or compliance.

15.8 FURTHER MANAGEMENT

There is no excuse for the continuing management of dementia in primary care to be one of crisis management. There has been a general interest in developing evidence-based guidelines for proactive management (Anonymous, 1995), especially in chronic disease management, and these well-described processes and principles for the management of chronic disease in primary care can be adapted for the dementia syndromes. Some excellent examples of evidence-based guidelines exist: *Interventions in the Management of Behavioural and Psychological Aspects of Dementia* produced by the Scottish Intercollegiate Guidelines Network in 1998, and the North of England evidence-based guidelines for the primary care management of dementia (Eccles *et al.*, 1998) are good examples. National guidelines are an excellent starting point, but need to be adapted and adopted locally in order to be 'owned' by a group of practitioners; anecdotal evidence suggests that 'top-down' guidelines tend to be ignored, whereas locally developed guidelines tend to be adhered to.

Dementia management should be anticipatory and there needs to be a system for regular review of the patient including some measure of disease progression and functional ability, with clearly defined triggers for carers to seek clinical help identified. There may be dedicated dementia care teams available or the primary care team may undertake the task itself. Computerized disease registers that can be associated with algorithms for care should make the task easier, but are not essential. The most important thing, as has been stated, is to develop a system for periodic review, including a definition of roles and responsibilities for the primary care team members. A package of care should include as much support for carers as possible; this has been shown to delay the admission of a patient with dementia to a nursing home (Mittleman *et al.*, 1996). In another study it was found that carers identified reliable, competent respite care, on a planned basis, as the single most important service to prevent premature long-term nursing home placement (Heagerty *et al.*, 1988).

A range of options for the care of the dementia patient in primary care exists, very much locally determined, however. This can vary from care at home by a spouse or other carer, with varying degrees of input from health professionals, to intensive home-based care from a community mental health team as an alternative to inpatient care (Stokes *et al.*, 1998). Other patients will attend day hospital or community facilities on a regular basis. The general practitioner should make sure that there is access to occupational therapy and the other non-drug therapies if felt appropriate. A holistic approach such as 'person-centred dementia care' (Thacker, 1998) is well suited to a nursing or residential home setting.

It should be remembered that a sudden deterioration in function may be due to a 'silent' intercurrent illness such as a chest infection, urinary tract infection or myocardial infarction and not part of the underlying dementia. Recognition of this is important as treatment of the intercurrent illness will restore cognitive function to its previous level.

15.9 CARERS AND THEIR SUPPORT

The vast majority of the burden of caring falls upon relatives, usually the spouse, of the patient. These carers are themselves often elderly and frail, and may also be ill. Research has confirmed that this is so, with only a minority of patients getting support from the statutory bodies (Luker and Perkins, 1987). The Alzheimer's Society found in a survey of UK health authorities (Anonymous, 1997) that there was inequality of service provision and access for people with dementia and, disturbingly, very little consultation with users and carers about how needs should be accessed and what services should be commissioned. It is to be hoped that changes in the structure of the UK National Health Service (NHS) in 1999, such as the formation of PCOs and the National Institute for Clinical Excellence (NICE), may go some way to mitigating this.

Along with the unremitting 24-hours-a-day, 365-days-a-year physical task of looking after a relative with dementia, there are other burdens that the carer will have to adapt to. Carers may have feelings of guilt or anger about they way they feel about the very different person they used to know, and may suffer from a form of grief reaction about the 'death' of an intellect when the body remains all too apparent. None of these things should be unexpected, and the primary care team should be able to anticipate problems and act in a proactive way.

One of the single most useful things that a general practitioner can do as soon as a diagnosis of dementia is made is to put relatives and carers (and also the patient, if appropriate) in contact with the local dementia self-help group. In the UK this would probably be the Alzheimer's Society or Alzheimer Scotland Action on Dementia. These organizations can provide a wealth of information and support, and are often able to provide literature and advice about topics such as sexuality, aggression, wandering and other emotive areas. Other voluntary groups such as Crossroads (the Association of Crossroads Care Attendant Schemes) in the UK can provide someone to sit with a person with dementia on a regular basis, allowing the caregiver time to him/herself. This can greatly improve the carer's quality of life.

15.10 LEGAL AND ETHICAL ISSUES

Dementia has an enormous impact on all aspects of life, and advice will be sought from the general practitioner about these. Sensitivity is needed when giving advice, particularly in the light of recent evidence (Meyers, 1997) that the majority (80 per cent) of carers feel that a person with AD should not be told the diagnosis. Interestingly, though, the carers themselves (70 per cent) felt they would want to know if they had the disease themselves. It is important that the person does know the diagnosis and prognosis in order to be able to put his/her affairs in order and consent to treatment whilst the intellectual capacity to do so remains. Relatives and carers do need to be given as much information as possible. Magazines, radio, television and the Internet have placed vast amounts of information about dementia in easily accessible form, but information overload is a risk and the quality of data variable, ranging from reputable science to dangerous quackery.

There are many major changes in the life of the person with dementia and his/her carers ahead and they need to be alerted to these to allow action to be taken. The doctor needs to be aware of legalities in order to alert the patient and carers, but it would be a foolish doctor or other member of the primary healthcare team who purported to give legal advice; this should be left to lawyers. Driving can be a cause of much concern, especially if the person and family rely on this form of transport. This is especially so in rural areas. The doctor may feel conflicts of interest when giving advice, not wanting to isolate the person with dementia and their dependants, but also not wanting to put the general public at risk. The patient should be advised to notify the vehicle's insurers of the nature of the illness. The British Medical Association suggests that any question from an insurance company regarding an opinion about whether a patient with dementia is fit to drive should not be answered by a family doctor in order to avoid risk of a charge of negligence in case of an accident. The person with dementia should be told to advise the competent authorities on the nature of the disability. The authorities will then gather such information as they require to make a decision about driving. A yearly licence may be issued, or the licence may be revoked. There is no doubt that people with mild cognitive impairment do drive, apparently safely. It is interesting to note, however, that in one study (Johansson et al., 1997) it was found that post-mortem evidence suggested a higher number of elderly drivers dying in a road traffic accident had evidence of Alzheimer's disease than age-matched controls. It would be advisable for the physician to contact the relevant professional organizations for expert advice, if needed. The general rule should be that, however uncomfortable a decision it may be, society's safety outweighs an individual's rights.

With regard to advice about making a will, the person with dementia will need to make a will while capable of understanding what a will is, what property there is to dispose of, and to whom. In order to satisfy these criteria, the family doctor is going to have to make absolutely sure that the person understands the nature of the illness, and its natural history, early on in the illness before cognitive impairment is fully established.

As the disease progresses, the need for Enduring Power of Attorney may be necessary. This gives another person (the attorney) the right to act for the patient (the donor). With ordinary Power of Attorney, this power becomes invalid if the donor becomes mentally incapable. Enduring Power of Attorney will allow the attorney to deal with the donor's affairs no matter what their mental state, as long as the donor had insight when appointing the attorney.

The general practitioner may also feel an ethical dilemma as he/she will often be caring for the dementia patient and the carer and family. Is facilitating the nursing home placement of a patient with dementia, perhaps against expressed wishes, in order to protect the mental and physical wellbeing of an exhausted carer the 'ethical' thing to do? Is it ethical to allow a crisis to develop by withholding support when a dementia patient is living alone and refusing help, in order to facilitate hospital admission and thus support the patient, perhaps by using statutory powers? There are no easy answers to any of these questions, but discussing the matter with colleagues and other members of the primary healthcare team sometimes make the solutions clearer.

15.11 PREVENTION

Until recently it would be unheard of for the subject of the prevention of dementia to be dealt with in a primary care context; indeed, very little about dementia per se was to be found in the primary care literature. There has been a sea of change, however. Much more is known about the pathogenesis of the dementia syndromes; although the evidence is not always based on robust randomized controlled trial work, there is mounting evidence that lifestyle modification and therapeutic interventions may be possible in the primary prevention of some of the dementia syndromes (Whalley, 1998). The general practitioner will need to be aware of this as an increasingly informed public may well require information from them. Recent published work regarding the adequate control of hypertension demonstrated in the elderly that, if hypertensive elderly people were treated for 5 years, 19 cases of dementia per 1000 of the population could be prevented (Forette et al., 1998) and these were cases of AD, rather than VaD, as may seem initially intuitive. Reducing vascular risk factors such as hypertension, obesity, hyperlipidaemia and smoking will reduce the risk of cerebrovascular accident and cognitive impairment.

There have been a number of robust trials, some (Forette et al., 1998) with the onset of dementia as an end point in its own right rather than transient ischaemic attacks and stroke used as proxy markers. The Study on Cognition and Progress in the Elderly (SCOPE) (Sever, 2002) looked at 5000 hypertensive patients aged between 70 and 89. At enrolment all subjects had a MMSE equal to or greater than 24. The subjects were randomized to placebo or angiotensin-converting enzyme (ACE) inhibitor plus other agents to control blood pressure. After 3.5 years there was a 24 per cent drop in stroke incidence in the treatment group and, although both arms showed a similar decline in MMSE, more sophisticated tests of cerebral function showed increased speed of cognition, increase in attention, improvement in episodic and working memory and better executive function in the treatment group compared with the controls. In the PROGRESS trial (PROGRESS Collaborative Group, 2001) over 6000 subjects with a history of transient ischaemic attack or stroke were enrolled. Importantly the inclusion criteria did not include hypertension, so normotensive subjects were included as well as hypertensive subjects. There was a reduction of cognitive decline of almost 20 per cent in the treatment group, which was more marked in the subgroup who did have another stroke. After 4 years the risk of dementia after a stroke was reduced by 34 per cent. The Antihypertensive and Lipid Lowering Treatment to prevent Heart Attack (ALLHAT) (ALLHAT Collaborative Research Group, 2002) introduced lipid lowering treatment as well as anti-hypertensive therapy with a favourable outcome in terms of cardiac and neurological events in the treatment groups. Other studies on statins have shown a reduction in AD in the treatment group (odds ratio 0.26) but only in subjects younger than 80. The available evidence suggests not only a reduction in VaD, which would be expected, but also AD, though the 'pure' form of either entity is probably rare and most cases sit on a continuum stretching between AD and VaD.

Diabetes is also associated with vascular problems and there is a relative risk for AD of 2.3 for men and between 1.4 and 2.0 for women who are diabetic. Good control of diabetes should help prevent both VaD and AD.

There was some evidence that the use of hormonal replacement therapy (HRT) may help prevent AD (Bonn, 1997); however, this is offset by the increased risk of breast cancer in users of HRT (Beral et al., 2003) and by the knowledge that HRT increases the relative risk of stroke by 1.41 after 5 years of use (Writing Group for the Woman's Health Initiative Investigators, 2002). More recent work has shown stroke itself is a risk factor for AD (hazards ratio for AD with a history of stroke 1.6) (Honig et al., 2003) so the role of HRT as protector against dementia is becoming clouded and may do more harm than good.

It has been suggested (Whalley, 1998) that a dementia prevention programme is possible. It should seek to lower the risk of dementia by reducing vascular risk factors, for example, by treating diabetes and hypertension, stopping tobacco use and normalizing lipids by drug therapy and diet. It is becoming increasingly likely that AD is a manifestation of insulin resistance (Rasgon and Jarvik, 2004) (Strachan M, 2003) and this theory gives a logical basis for the above approach. It has been suggested that a pill containing a statin, three blood pressure drugs (perhaps beta-blocker, ACE inhibitor and a thiazide all at half standard dose), low-dose aspirin and folic acid (to reduce serum homocysteine) be administered to persons over 55 years of age (Wald and Law, 2003). Using existing data, it is estimated that one-third of people so treated would gain an additional 11 years of life free from an ischaemic heart disease (IHD) event or stroke. It is true to say that there is considerable controversy about this proposal,

but the concept of IHD and stroke prevention is so similar to a dementia prevention programme that the two may really be the same thing. Only large-scale properly designed trials over some period of time are going to give the answers. The use of antioxidants and anti-inflammatory agents such as non-steroidal anti-inflammatory drugs (McGeer and McGeer, 1999) may have their place in the prevention of dementias by their actions as neuroprotectors.

Diet plays a role, especially in AD. Obesity itself is a risk factor for dementia independently of other comorbid factors with up to 74 per cent increased risk of dementia developing if the body mass index is greater than 30 (Whitmer et al., 2005). There is evidence (Grant, 1997) that a high fat and high calorie diet is associated with an increased prevalence of this disease, perhaps by adding to oxidative stress; conversely, fish consumption is associated with a reduced incidence. Vitamin C may protect against cognitive impairment in the elderly (Gale et al., 1996) as, indeed, does education (Ott et al., 1995). Modification of all these varied factors could potentially form part of a primary prevention package, but there is still a need for firmer, long-term prospective evidence before this can be recommended and such evidence may be hard to gather.

In primary care, especially in the UK, the same team will look after the same cohort of individuals over long periods of time. This means that they have the ability to note those people who are more at risk of developing a dementia syndrome, and there should be a raised index of clinical suspicion when dealing with these individuals. For example, in AD, about one-third of cases are familial. Risk factors for AD include previous Parkinson's disease (relative risk of 2.4), advanced parental age (relative risk 1.6) and head trauma (relative risk 1.8). Interestingly, a history of depression more than 10 years ago is said to carry a relative risk of 1.7 and more recent work (Green et al., 2003) in a large study shows a doubling of risk of AD in patients with a history of depression. We know that diabetes and hypertension are risk factors.

Primary care is now becoming highly computerized with many practices' 'paperless' and comprehensive disease databases being generated containing (when complete) most, if not all, of the information above. It has been suggested (Holt and Ohno-Machado, 2003) that there should be a nationwide adaptive prediction tool for coronary heart disease prevention. Adaptive predictive models are computer based and 'learn' to classify cases according to patterns. They include algorithms as well as more complex models such as neural networks. These systems are used in industry for pattern recognition and process control. Data collected under the new General Medical Services contract in the UK, along with pre-existing data, could populate an adaptive predictive tool and in essence stratify risk for each individual allowing targeted intervention for those highest at risk of coronary heart disease. By adding some of the dementia risk factors to this information, it would in theory allow the construction of a similar adaptive prediction tool for dementia prevention, especially as there is great overlap in the characteristics of the 'at CHD risk' and the 'at dementia risk' populations, again allowing for targeted intervention to 'prevent' dementia.

The prevalence of AD will quadruple by the year 2047 to 8.64 million cases in the USA unless effective preventive interventions can be developed. If the disease onset can be delayed by as little as 6 months then it is projected that in 50 years, 380 000 fewer people will be affected (Brookmeyer, 1998). This would have enormous resource implications.

15.12 THE FUTURE

The future of primary care is uncertain. There is a general trend for as much clinical and social care to be delivered to the patient as close to home as possible, hence firmly in the primary sector. There is also a trend for the introduction of managed care. The introduction of PCOs in the UK, with their similarities at trust level to US-style health maintenance organizations will accelerate this trend.

A main feature of health provision in primary and secondary care is the introduction of clinical governance. Clinical governance has been described as a system through which NHS organizations are accountable for continuously improving the quality of their services and safeguarding high standards of care by creating an environment in which excellence in clinical care will flourish (Scally and Donaldson, 1998). It involves standards, performance and quality review. It seems logical that patterns of care will be increasingly guideline-based and be capable of being audited both for process and outcome. The development of guidelines will no doubt be influenced by national guidelines, but need to be locally modified to be practical, as has been previously noted. Developing protocols and guidelines must not be taken lightly, and must be firmly evidence based. There can be apparent contradictions in the evidence, however. For example, with regard to the risks of smoking and dementia, one small study in the UK found the relative risk of AD in patients who smoked was 0.68 (Salib and Hillier, 1997), whereas a large population study in Rotterdam (Ott *et al.*, 1998) showed the relative risk to be 2.2. The difference may well be due to the presence or absence of the apolipoprotein E ε4 allele, but this example of apparent conflict in evidence demonstrates the need for expertise and care in developing a robust evidence base on which guidelines for care are based.

One of the outcomes of the introduction of care trusts has been a unification of clinical budgets with social care budgets. When this has truly happened, then the true cost of care (including clinical and social elements) is of prime importance. At the moment the fact that a modest outlay on anti-dementia drug costs might delay a patient entering very expensive residential or nursing care homes tends to be ignored, as different organizations are responsible for drug and social care budgets – the opportunity for overall cost saving is thus lost. With a unified or pooled budget this would not be the case. There is good evidence that the integration of medical and social care can result in reduced costs and reduced functional decline in the elderly (Bernabei *et al.*, 1998). A certainty is that patients of increasing levels of dependency will be cared for in the community in increasing numbers and this trend will continue (Stern *et al.*, 1993). Some general practitioners have found the increase in workload to date unmanageable (Williams *et al.*, 1992). The new General Medical Services contract introduced in the UK in April 2004 allows for enhanced services to be provided by some practices to special patient groups. This could be used as a mechanism for interested primary healthcare teams to develop a special interest in caring for people with dementia in a locality, including those registered with other practices.

REFERENCES

The ALLHAT Collaborative Research group. (2002) Major outcomes in high risk hypertensive patients randomized to angiotensin converting enzyme inhibitor or calcium channel blocker vs diuretic. *JAMA* **2888**: 2981–2997

Anonymous. (1994) Neuroleptic sensitivity in patients with dementia. *Current Problems in Pharmacovigilance* **20**: 6

Anonymous. (1995) *The Development and Implementation of Clinical Guidelines*. London, Royal College of General Practitioners

Anonymous. (1996) Apolipoprotein E genotyping in Alzheimer's disease (consensus statement). *Lancet* **347**: 1091–1095

Anonymous. (1997) *No Accounting for Health*. London, Alzheimer's Disease Society

Beral V and the Million Women Study Collaborators. (2003) Breast cancer and hormone-replacement therapy in the Million Woman Study. *Lancet* **362**: 419–427

Bernabei R, Landi F, Gambassi G *et al.* (1998) Randomised trial of impact of model of integrated care and case management for older people living in the community. *BMJ* **316**: 1348–1351

Bobinski M, de Leon M, Convit A *et al.* (1999) MRI of entorhinal cortex in mild Alzheimer's disease. *Lancet* **353**: 38–39

Bonn D. (1997) Oestrogen offers protection in Alzheimer's disease. *Lancet* **349**: 1889

Brookmeyer R. (1998) Projections of Alzheimer's disease in the United States and the public health implications of delaying disease onset. *American Journal of Public Health* **88**: 1337–1342

Dunn R and Lewis P. (1993) Compliance with standard assessment scales for elderly people among consultant geriatricians in Wessex. *BMJ* **307**: 606

Eccles M, Clarke J, Livingstone M *et al.* (1998) North of England evidence based guidelines development project: guidelines for the primary care management of dementia. *BMJ* **317**: 802–808

Forette F, Seux M-L, Staessen J *et al.* (1998) Prevention of dementia in randomised double-blind placebo-controlled systolic hypertension in Europe (Syst-Eur) trial. *Lancet* **352**: 1347–1351

Gale C, Martyn N, Cooper C. (1996) Cognitive impairment and mortality in a cohort of elderly people. *BMJ* **312**: 608–611

Grace J. (1994) Alzheimer's disease: your views. *Geriatric Medicine* **23**: 31–33

Graham C, Ballard G, Dass K. (1997) Variables which distinguish patients fulfilling clinical criteria for dementia with Lewy bodies from those with Alzheimer's disease. *International Journal of Geriatric Psychiatry* **12**: 314–318

Grant W. (1997) Dietary links to Alzheimer's disease. *Alzheimer's Disease Review* **2**: 42–55

Green R, Cupples LA, Kurz A *et al.* (2003) Depression as a Risk Factor for Alzheimer Disease. *Archives of Neurology* **60**: 753–759

Hallewell C and Pettit W. (1994) Liaison enhances primary care. *Care of the Elderly* **6**: 307–309

Heagerty MA, Dunn LM, Watson MA. (1988) Helping care-givers care. *Aging* **358**: 7–8

Hofman A, Ott A, Breteler M *et al.* (1997) Atherosclerosis, apolipoprotein E, and the prevalence of dementia and Alzheimer's disease on the Rotterdam Study. *Lancet* **349**: 151–154

Holt T and Ohno-Machado L. (2003) A nationwide adaptive prediction tool for coronary heart disease prevention. *British Journal of General Practice* **53**: 866–870

Honig LS, Tang MX, Albert S *et al.* (2003) Stroke and the risk of Alzheimer's disease. *Archives of Neurology* **60**: 1707–1712

Illife S, Haines A, Gallivan S *et al.* (1991a) Assessment of elderly people in general practice: social circumstances and mental state. *British Journal of General Practice* **41**: 9–12

Illife S, Haines A, Gallivan S *et al.* (1991b) Assessment of elderly people in general practice: functional abilities and medical problems. *British Journal of General Practice* **41**: 13–15

Johansson K, Bogdanovic N, Kalimo H *et al.* (1997) Alzheimer's disease and apolipoprotein E ε4 allele in older drivers who died in automobile accidents. *Lancet* **349**: 1143

Kennard M, Feldman H, Yamada T *et al.* (1996) Serum levels of the iron binding protein p97 are elevated in Alzheimer's disease. *Nature Medicine* **2**: 1230–1235

Lovestone S, Graham N, Howard R. (1997) Guidelines on drug treatments for Alzheimer's disease. *Lancet* **350**: 232–233

Luker K and Perkins E. (1987) The elderly at home, service needs and provision. *Journal of the Royal College of General Practitioners* **37**: 248–250

McGeer E and McGeer P. (1999) Brain inflammation in Alzheimer's disease: possible therapy with NSAIDs. *Progress in Neurology and Psychiatry* **3**: 25–28

Meyers BS. (1997) Telling patients they have Alzheimer's disease. *BMJ* **314**: 321–322

Mittleman MS, Ferris SH, Shulman E *et al.* (1996) A family intervention to delay nursing home placement of patients with Alzheimer's disease. A randomised controlled trial. *JAMA* **276**: 1725–1731

Newens AJ, Forster DP, Kay D *et al.* (1993) Clinically diagnosed presenile dementia of the Alzheimer's type in the Northern Health Region. *Psychological Medicine* **23**: 631–644

O'Connor D, Fertig A, Grande M *et al.* (1993) Dementia in general practice: the practical consequences of a more positive approach to diagnosis. *British Journal of General Practice* **43**: 185–188

Ott A, Breteler M, van Harskamp F *et al.* (1995) Prevalence of Alzheimer's disease and vascular dementia: association with education. The Rotterdam Study. *BMJ* **310**: 970–973

Ott A, Slooter A, Hofman A *et al.* (1998) Smoking and risk of dementia and Alzheimer's disease in a population-based cohort study: the Rotterdam Study. *Lancet* **351**: 1840–1843

PROGRESS Collaborative Group. (2001) Effects of a perindopril-based blood pressure lowering regimen amongst 6105 individual with previous stroke or transient ischaemia attack. *Lancet* **358**:1033–1041

Salib E and Hillier V. (1997) A case controlled study of smoking and Alzheimer's disease. *International Journal of Geriatric Psychiatry* **12**: 295–300

Scally G and Donaldson L. (1998) Clinical governance and the drive for quality improvement in the new NHS in England. *BMJ* **317**: 61–65

Sever P. (2002) The SCOPE Trial. *Journal of the Renin-Aldosterone System* **3**: 61–2

Shaw F, Richardson D, Bond J *et al.* (1996) Consequences and causes of falls in people with dementia. *Journal of Dementia Care* **4**: 28

Stern M: Jagger C, Clarke M *et al.* (1993) Residential care for the elderly: a decade of change. *BMJ* **306**: 827–830

Stokes G, Hope R, Khan M. (1998) 'The home team'. *Health Service Journal* **108**: 34–35

Strachan M. (2003) Insulin and cognitive function. *Lancet* **362**: 1253

Thacker S. (1998) Dementia – magic bullets versus holism. *Geriatric Medicine* **28**: 50–51

UK Standing Medical Advisory Committee. (1998) *The Use of Donepezil for Alzheimer's Disease*. London, NHS Executive

Victor C. (1991) *Health and Health Care in Later Life*. Milton Keynes, Open University Press

Wald NJ and Law MR. (2003) A strategy to reduce cardiovascular disease by more than 80 per cent. *BMJ* 2003; **326**: 1419–1423

Whalley LJ. (1998) Can dementia be prevented? *The Practitioner* **242**: 34–38

Whitmer R, Gunderson E, Barrett-Connor E *et al.* (2005) Obesity in middle age and future risk of dementia: a 27 year longitudinal population based study. *BMJ* doi 10.1136/bmj.38446.466z38.EO

Williams E. (1984) Characteristics of patients aged over 75 not seen during one year in general practice. *BMJ* **288**: 114–121

Williams E, Savage S, McDonald P, Groom L. (1992) Residents of private nursing homes and their care. *British Journal of General Practice* **42**: 477–481

Writing Group for the Woman's Health Initiative Investigators. (2002) Risks and benefits of estrogen plus progestin in healthy postmenopausal women. Principal results for the Woman's Heath Initiative Randomized controlled trial. *JAMA* **288**: 321–333

16

Multidisciplinary approaches in the management of dementia

16a

The role of nursing

PEGGY A SZWABO

Dementia presents with a progressive deterioration of cognitive abilities, increasing dependency on others for self-care and an emerging need for supervision. The role of nursing can be pivotal in that nurses work in a continuum of settings in which they provide care for the individual with dementia and their families. Nursing professionals have the benefit of face-to-face contact, be it in the clinic, home, or institution. The nurse may be the person who is most readily accessible and can coordinate the patient's care needs. Nurses are a valuable resource for understanding the difficulties of caring for the patient at home. Their role may be to observe changes in health status and to communicate these changes to the other members of the health team. It may be the nurse who talks most frequently to the family providing counselling and support. As a resource for assistance in day-to-day care, nurses can identify problems and give practical advice in caring for problems ranging from bathing to catastrophic reactions (Sloane et al., 1995).

The challenge of caring for patients with dementia is to become vigilant in identifying the range of symptoms of cognitive decline in the early stages to the more troubling behavioural symptoms of the later stages. Current research emphasizes the need for early identification. Backman and associates (2004) found that in preclinical dementia there is decline in cognitive functioning 3 years before diagnosis. These researchers observed that with increasing age and numbers of recent diseases there is a more rapid decline (Backman et al., 2003). Early identification of dementia is imperative. Individuals with mild symptoms may be eligible for cholinesterase inhibitors or inclusion in drug research trials that may delay the progression of the disease.

Though each setting in which the nurse provides care has specific issues, the care of patients with dementia falls into several components that are pertinent to all settings. These components are assessment with emphasis on self-care abilities and communication abilities; therapeutic interventions and symptom management; and support systems and resources. In addition, each stage of dementia presents unique challenges to nursing care. The overarching philosophy of care is to provide individualized care that enhances self-care abilities and encourages autonomy in the least restrictive setting for as long as possible. The patient with dementia requires a thorough and holistic evaluation including physical, psychiatric, psychosocial and environmental assessments. This chapter emphasizes assessment.

16.1 ASSESSMENT

Ongoing assessment is an essential part of the care of the patient with dementia. Geriatric prepared nurses have knowledge and understanding of age-related changes and common disease processes, as well as behavioural symptoms that can afflict the elderly patient. People with Alzheimer's disease (AD) have a full range of symptoms from those who have not yet come to medical attention, the mildly affected, to those with advanced symptoms (Albert et al., 1998). The progression of dementia symptoms jeopardizes the individual's ability to remain in an independent living situation.

All patients need to be evaluated for changes in cognition and functional abilities. The nurse's responsibility is to complete and continue a thorough nursing history to assess the stage of the disease, comorbid medical conditions, activities of daily living (ADL) and instrumental activities of daily living (IADLs), self-care abilities and competency to self-medicate. Various tools are available to document baseline abilities and change or decline (Katz et al., 1963, 1970; Lawton and Brody,

---

Box 16.1   *Mnemonic for dementia evaluation*

Drugs on board
Emotional disorders
Metabolic disorders
Ears, eyes – perception
Nutrition and normal pressure hydrocephalus
Infections
Arteriosclerosis and atherosclerosis
Sundowner's syndrome

1969). A review of systems is indicated owing to the high prevalence of comorbid medical conditions and susceptibility to delirium, particularly infections, inadequate nutrition and polypharmacy, being mindful of drug–drug interactions (Inouye, 1998). As noted previously, nurses should be suspicious of subtle declines in individuals not yet diagnosed but with the risk factors of increased age and numbers of recent medical conditions (Backman *et al.*, 2004).

Since dementia is to some degree a diagnosis of exclusion, specific reversible causes must be ruled out. Use of a mnemonic for evaluation of potentially treatable causes may be helpful (Box 16.1). Once the diagnosis is established, identification of the stage of disease development can be helpful in anticipating needs and to help the family plan for care.

Several authors have developed scales to stage dementia in general and AD in particular, such as the Global Deterioration Scale (GDS) (Reisberg *et al.*, 1982), the Clinical Dementia Rating scale (CDR) (Berg, 1988), the Blessed Memory-Information-Concentration Test (Blessed *et al.*, 1988), the Functional Assessment Staging (FAST) (Reisberg, 1988), and the Mini-Mental State Examination (MMSE) (Folstein *et al.*, 1975). In the outpatient setting, the 'SCOPED' assessment tool is a quick assessment of functional abilities (Dohrenwend *et al.*, 2003; Beck *et al.*, 1994). The questions revolve around the patient's safety, asking questions about **s**pending, **c**ooking, **o**perating automobiles, **p**ill taking, **e**veryday activities and **d**ecision-making.

All of these scales quantify the specific functional losses that occur with AD and in association with ageing. These scales plot symptoms from normal to severe and help clinicians track the course of the disease. This tracking helps identify where the individual is in the disease progression. Staging, used correctly, can assist the family in anticipating and preparing for problems rather than waiting until a crisis occurs, but if used inappropriately, can depersonalize the patient and limit options for therapeutic interventions (Cole *et al.*, 1998).

16.1.1 Mental health assessment

The nursing psychiatric assessment includes observation for depression, psychosis and behavioural change. The goal of the psychiatric assessment is to gather and integrate biological, psychological and socioeconomic data to provide comprehensive understanding of a person's psychosocial status.

Crucial information includes past ways of coping, identification of chronic and acute stressors, personality styles, family roles and dynamics, decision-making history, and past and family psychiatric history. Besides observing and documenting symptoms of depression and other psychiatric behaviours, nurses spend much time with the patient and can elicit pertinent information about the meaning and significance of behaviours and symptoms. An important hint in understanding the patient's current behaviour is to obtain information concerning who the patient was and behavioural styles prior to the onset of dementia. This information can give the clinician insight into and understanding of some of the behaviours exhibited by the patient. For example, a patient who worked nights may not have nocturnal wandering; a domineering personality may not respond to directives but needs to be 'in charge'.

16.1.2 Caregiver assessment

Holistic assessment of the patient with dementia includes evaluating how well the family or professional caregiver is handling the impact of the disease and the behaviours presented by the patient (see Chapters 4 and 11a). Caregiver burden is defined as the physical, emotional, social and financial challenge of providing care (George and Gwyther, 1986).

Caregivers have more stress symptoms, use more psychotropic medications and have less social activities. Depression and worsening behaviours in the person with dementia adversely affect the caregiver (Saad *et al.*, 1995). As part of the patient encounter, the caregiver's stress and issues with the person with dementia need to be assessed. The nurse can evaluate caregiver burden based upon the risk factors noted above and with one of the tools that measure caregiver burden such as the Zarit Burden Inventory (Zarit *et al.*, 1980) or the Screen for Caregiver Burden (Vitaliano *et al.*, 1991).

16.2 ENVIRONMENT AND SAFETY

Use of the milieu or environmental manipulation is a primary intervention for confused people. Important aspects of using the environment are for observation of behaviour, therapeutic interventions and to evaluate the efficacy of psychopharmacological options. The nurse in any setting is responsible for developing a therapeutic environment for the patient. Safety surveillance is emphasized, providing for the patient's needs and developing ways to tolerate their behaviours in a safe environment. Helping the family to remove safety hazards, toxins, inedibles, cords and throw rugs can ensure a more streamlined and safer habitat for the confused patient.

In a nursing facility (as well as the home), the environment should be streamlined to decrease confusion but stimulating enough to encourage the patient with dementia to be

Box 16.2 *Environmental strategies for dementia*

- Use of calendars, pictures and maps for visual and cognitive cueing
- Space for safe wandering, both inside and outside
- Use of wandering gardens (Hoover, 1995)
- Use of colour and signs to help with orientation and way-finding
- Use of light and small areas for conversation and quiet pursuits
- Decrease distracting, confusing noise levels
- Add appropriate music (Tabloski *et al.*, 1995)
- Comfortable home-like furniture
- Provision of activities that allow the patient success and interaction
- Use of electronic alarm systems and/or design to deter elopement, such as camouflaged doors, use of directional street signs, or dutch doors
- Assessment of area for fall prevention
- Good definition between walls and floors
- Availability of activities throughout the day and evening
- Access to portable foods and liquids for wanderers
- Physical activities to divert aggression

involved and interested. Teri and Wagner (1992) demonstrated that participation in pleasurable activities decreases depression in demented patients and lessens agitation. In designing the environment, several considerations need to be addressed. Box 16.2 refers to environmental considerations that benefit people with dementia and can provide a more therapeutic atmosphere for the confused.

The family trying to understand the disease may not consider changing the home environment as part of the treatment. The nurse can provide helpful, practical suggestions to assist the family to provide an optimal environment at home. Many family caregivers feel helpless and welcome practical advice that encourages their involvement in caring for their loved one.

16.3 COMMUNICATION

Language abilities deteriorate with dementia. Often the early symptoms include word-finding, receptive aphasia, derailing mid-sentence, confabulation (filling in missing gaps of information), tangentiality and circumstantiality. Many AD victims demonstrate remarkable conversational skills and social graces that fool the clinician. Family and caregivers need to be interviewed to validate patients' reports and abilities.

Techniques of communication require changes in approach and style. Conversation must be streamlined. Most sentences are too long and confused patients are not able to follow several thoughts or directions in one sentence. Slower paced conversation with fewer and more concrete words is indicated. Using as many of the senses as possible may imprint

the message more effectively – for example, using gentle touch to get a patient's attention; pointing to concrete objects like a water glass when asking to drink, or handing the glass with the request. Offering forced options, such as, 'Do you want an apple or an orange?' can help with decision making and foster autonomy. Repetitive questions can aggravate caregivers and upset patients. Sometimes ignoring or redirecting can help. Other patients need more reassurance and the nurse should attempt to divine the meaning behind the repetitious questions (Landreville *et al.*, 1998).

Asking the family about the patient's communication style or special language is necessary to continue to communicate and incorporate into treatment plans. Gathering this information can be instrumental in preventing frustration and agitated behaviours. Observation of the patient's non-verbal language and interpretation of its meaning can provide the nurse with insight into the patient as well as establishing more empathetic responses. Validation therapy proposed by Feil (1993) encourages interpretation of the patient's non-verbal behaviour as a way of validating feelings and emotions the patient can no longer express. Rocking behaviour can be interpreted as agitation or anxiety if vigorous but if it occurs in a gentle, relaxed fashion can be explained as comforting. In essence the nurse interprets to the patient his or her understanding that the behaviour may be expressing a positive or negative emotion, striving for a connection with the patient.

16.4 THERAPEUTIC INTERVENTION AND SYMPTOM MANAGEMENT

As dementia progresses, symptoms worsen and more troubling behaviours may present. These behaviours include agitation, aggression, wandering, sleep disorders, and inappropriate sexual behaviours.

Behavioural interventions designed for target symptoms can be instrumental in minimizing or defusing the escalation of those behaviours. They are the first line in handling milder behavioural and psychological symptoms of dementia (Cohen-Mansfield and Werner, 1995). The more aggressive or problematic behaviours may require a combination of pharmacological and non-pharmacological interventions (see Chapters 38 and 39). Patients with dementia require and benefit from more labour-intensive approaches, i.e. interventions and strategies that can be done by lay and professional caregivers and are easy to implement with widespread application to the home setting or the long-term care facility. As problematic behaviours arise, there is a need and opportunity for nursing intervention with the caregivers and the patient. Basic principles of behavioural intervention are summarized in Box 16.3. The rule of thumb of instituting behavioural approaches is based on the seven Rs – Reassess, Reconsider, Reassure, Rechannel, Redirect, Remove and Rethink (Kuhn, 1993).

16.4.1 Problematic behaviours

The nurse's role in managing agitation and aggressive behaviour is assessment of potential triggers and early intervention. Identification of individuals, situations and activities that provoke can prevent escalation and redirection to more appropriate activities. The nurse should evaluate how the patient is being approached. Is the approach calm and slow? Is the patient spoken to firmly and gently in advance so as not to startle and precipitate a spontaneous aggressive reaction? Is the use of touch helpful or counterproductive? Ryden and Feldt (1992) found that intrusive touching behaviours, which nurses and nursing assistants are likely to perform such as bathing and toileting, are likely to be perceived as threatening. Non-verbal behaviour and authoritarian postures can also set off aggressive responses. Use of redirection and reassurance can be the nurse's most valuable weapons. Assessing the reality of the situation and backing off to avoid escalation may be the most effective strategy. Helping the caregivers assess if the activity needs to be done now or if it can wait can prevent caregiver frustration and aggressive reactions. Assessing the patient's environment for too much stimulation and offering suggestions to provide quiet and less stimulating activities will help decrease outbursts. Prediction of possible behaviours and addressing the 'how to handle' before the behaviour occurs gives the family caregivers techniques to use and lessens their sense of helplessness. The potential for danger always needs to be addressed and treatment planning should include what to do and how to get help in whatever setting the patient is in.

Points to consider when assessing wandering and sleep disturbances include assessment of the environment for triggers that stimulate or induce the behaviour. Assessment of types of wandering helps define the appropriate intervention. Nurses need to ask the following questions. What was the patient like before dementia? Was the patient a high-energy person who never sat still and was always on the move? Is the current wandering a problem that requires intervention because of elopement concerns, striking out, a search for home and comfort or a risk to others? Is the confused patient upset because he/she knows where he/she is not? Or is the wandering purposeless, benign and tolerated in a safe environment (Butler and Barnett, 1991)?

Algase and colleagues (2003) have studied wandering and its meaning to the person with dementia. These researchers

found that by observing the pattern, duration and frequency, the nurse could differentiate between healthy and problematic wandering. By looking for the meaning of the wandering, the nurse is more apt to design an intervention that is more successful and relieving for people with dementia.

Related to wandering is the likelihood of becoming lost. The Alzheimer's Association of the United States predicts that 60 per cent of people with dementia will wander and become lost in their community (Rowe, 2003). This statistic highlights a potential public health problem. Nurses have the unique opportunity to educate families, law enforcement and the public of this potentially deadly behaviour. Educational information includes not leaving the person with dementia alone; securing the home environment to prevent inadvertent leaving; use of motion/tone detectors and alarms and security systems. Another resource is the Safe Return Programme of the Alzheimer's Association in the United States, which registers and photographs people with dementia and distributes vital information to local authorities if the need arises. Specific risk factors to be assessed are listed in Box 16.4 (Rowe, 2003).

Similarly for sleep disturbances, assessment of previous sleep patterns or occupational habits need to be incorporated into treatment plans. Assessment of environmental problems that interfere with sleep need to be addressed. Several studies (Hopkins *et al.*, 1992; Satlin *et al.*, 1992; Nelson, 1995) report that sleep patterns change with dementia, resulting in fewer hours of sleep and increased fragmented periods of sleep. Programming may need to be created to provide around-the-clock activities to provide for these changes. Nurses who provide 24-hour care have the opportunity to create innovative programming for patients on all three shifts from bedtime quiet time and snack activities to late-night groups and breakfast. It may be appropriate in future to provide institutional care more like a cruise ship with midnight buffets and recreation. Basic consideration includes avoidance or limited usage of caffeine, alcohol, or nicotine; evaluation of medication and avoiding night-time use of diuretics or stimulating medications; and establishing quiet, comforting, and regular bedtime rituals (Hopkins *et al.*, 1992; Rader and Tornquist, 1995; Rantz and McShane, 1995).

To treat sundowning, increased staffing, structured activities and environmental manipulation are indicated. Having one-on-one staffing or use of family and volunteers at shift change can decrease agitation, fear of abandonment and disorientation. Use of light and uncluttered rooms will decrease the patient's misinterpretation of the environment or illusions. Rescheduling of therapies from 3.00 to 5.00 pm can provide additional security and redirection (Rantz and McShane, 1995; Landreville et al., 1998).

New research on bright light therapy (BLT) indicates that morning BLT can delay evening agitation in patients with milder forms of dementia. BLT is less effective in more severe dementia because of more degeneration and deteriorating circadian activity rhythms. Bright light boxes for 2 hours of exposure 2500 lux every morning can be helpful in many patients with dementia (Ancoli-Israel et al., 2003).

Inappropriate sexual behaviours are troubling and difficult to deal with for both the nursing staff and the family. Medical conditions, such as urinary tract and vaginal infections, incontinence, chafing, rashes and other skin conditions can cause inappropriate sexual behaviours. Treating these conditions can prevent premature use of antipsychotics or other drugs used to lessen sexually inappropriate behaviour. Regular toileting schedules can lessen preoccupation with genitalia and voiding in inappropriate places. Choosing appropriate clothing that buttons from the back or jumpsuits can decrease embarrassing public scenes.

Information about the patient's past and present sexual functioning helps the nurse to provide opportunities for intimacy with spouse or partner, or at least to ensure privacy for masturbation or other intimacy needs. Assessment of loneliness and loss of companionship is a part of providing holistic care for the Alzheimer patient and family. In situations of inappropriate behaviours in public places, use of redirection and distraction is useful.

Education and information about sexuality and handling sexual behaviours is an important aspect of treatment for the staff, family and significant others, including ongoing in-services concerning acceptance, as well as their own reactions to sexual behaviours. There should be frank discussion of normal sexuality and self-assessment of individual practices that can encourage inappropriate behaviours or give the patient mixed messages. For example, some nursing staff are quite comfortable giving hugs and holding patients' hands whereas other staff would interpret a patient's hug as threatening and act accordingly. Staff need guidance and consistency in identifying intimacy needs versus inappropriate behaviours (Szwabo, 1998, 2003).

16.5   PSYCHOTHERAPEUTIC AND SUPPORTIVE THERAPIES

Alzheimer patients can remain physically active and may not exhibit frailty or disability until late stages of the disease. Their abilities to walk and wander about seeking stimulation challenge nurses to provide structured programming in the home or nursing facilities.

Use of the music therapy with groups and with individuals may soothe and calm. Music with the same beat as a normal heart rate of approximately 76 beats per minute has been found to calm agitation (Tabloski et al., 1995). Music can also stimulate memory and encourage participation in the present. A variety of 'touch' therapies and self-soothing techniques have been used widely for self-enhancement and to stimulate the senses as well as a tool for relaxing.

Small group work has proven successful with demented individuals. These groups range from leader-facilitated reminiscence therapy; current event discussion groups; object-oriented groups; supportive psychotherapy; breakfast groups that prepare food and encourage communication; task groups that develop successful 'jobs' and workplaces; and reduced stimuli activities. A variety of therapies – art, pet, exercise and spiritual – have a role in the treatment of patients with dementia.

The nurse can be the one professional who has the most contact with the person with dementia in multiple settings. This a unique opportunity and challenge to provide ongoing assessment, interventions, education and therapeutic options to patients, caregivers and the treatment team involved in caring for the Alzheimer family throughout the course of this disease. Keeping abreast of innovative and cutting edge research interventions are at the nurse's fingertips to share with families and other caregivers designing approaches to help people with dementia. Many successful therapies and interventions have found their way into recommended treatment strategies because nurses and the interdisciplinary team members continue to try to develop strategies to keep the demented patient as active, involved and independent as possible in the safest situation that can be provided.

REFERENCES

Albert S, Sano M, Bell K, Merchant C, Small S, Stern Y. (1998) Hourly care received by people with Alzheimer's disease: results from an urban community survey. The Gerontologist 38: 704–715

Algase D, Beel-Bates C, Beattie E. (2003) Wandering in long-term care. Annals of Long-Term Care 11: 33–39

Ancoli-Israel S, Martin J, Gehrman P et al. (2003) Effect of light in institutionalized patients with severe Alzheimer's disease. American Journal of Geriatric Psychiatry 11: 194–203

Backman L, Jones S, Small BJ, Aguero-Torres H, Fratiglione L. (2003) Role of cognitive decline in preclinical Alzheimer's disease: The role of comorbidity. Journal of Gerontology, Series B, Psychological Sciences and Social Sciences 588: 228–263

Backman L, Jones S, Small BJ, Aguero-Torres H, Fratiglione L. (2004) Role of cognitive decline in preclinical Alzheimer's disease: The role of comorbidity. Journal of Gerontology, Series B, Psychological Sciences and Social Sciences 588: 228–263

Beck J, Freeddan D, Warshaw G. (1994) Geriatric assessment: Focus on function. Patient Care (Feb): 12–37

Berg L. (1988) Clinical Dementia Rating (CDR). *Psychopharmacological Bulletin* **24**: 637–639

Blessed G, Tomlinson B, Roth M. (1988) Blessed-Roth Dementia Scale (DS). *Psychopharmacological Bulletin* **24**: 705–708

Butler J and Barnett C. (1991) Window of wandering. *Geriatric Nursing* **9**: 226–227

Cohen-Mansefield J and Werner P. (1995) Environmental influences on agitation: an integrative summary of an observation study. *American Journal of Alzheimer Care and Related Disease Research* **1**: 32–39

Cole MG, Primeau FJ, Elie LM. (1998) Delirium: prevention, treatment, and outcome studies. *Journal of Geriatric Psychiatry and Neurology* **11**: 126–137

Dohrenwend A, Kusz H, Eckleberry J, Stucky K. (2003) Evaluating cognitive impairment in the primary care setting. *Clinical Geriatrics* **11**: 21–29

Feil N. (1993) *The Validation Breakthrough.* Baltimore, Health Professions Press

Folstein M, Folstein S, McHugh P. (1975) Mini-mental state: a practical method for grading the cognitive state of patients for the clinician. *Journal of Psychiatric Research* **12**: 189–198

George L and Gwyther L. (1986) Caregiver well-being: a multidimensional examination of family caregivers of demented adults. *The Gerontologist* **26**: 253–259

Hoover R. (1995) Healing gardens and Alzheimer's disease. *American Journal of Alzheimer's Disease* **3**: 1–11

Hopkins R, Rindlisbacher P, Grant N. (1992) An investigation of the sundowning syndrome and ambient light. *American Journal of Alzheimer Care and Related Disease Research* **3**: 22–27

Inouye SK. (1998) Delirium in hospitalized older patients: recognition and risk factors. *Journal of Geriatric Psychiatry and Neurology* **11**: 118–125

Katz S, Ford A, Moskowitz R, Jackson B, Jaffe M. (1963) Studies of illness in the aged. The index of ADL: a standardized measure of physiological and psychosocial function. *JAMA* **185**: 94–98

Katz S, Downs T, Cash H, Grotz R. (1970) Progress in development of the index of ADL. *The Gerontologist* **10**: 20–30

Kuhn D. (1993) The 7 Rs of managing difficult behavior. *The Alzheimer's Disease Association of St Louis Newsletter* (August): 1

Landreville P, Bordes M, Dicaire L, Verreault R. (1998) Behavioral approaches for reducing agitation in residents of long-term-care facilities: critical review and suggestions for future research. *International Psychogeriatrics* **10**: 397–419

Lawton MP and Brody EM. (1969) Assessment of older people: self-maintaining and instrumental activities of daily living. *The Gerontologist* **9**: 179–186

Nelson J. (1995) The influence of environmental factors in incidents of disruptive behavior. *Journal of Gerontological Nursing* **5**: 19–24

Rader J and Tornquist E. (eds) (1995) *Individualized Dementia Care: Creative, Compassionate Approaches.* New York, Springer

Rantz M and McShane R. (1995) Nursing interventions for chronically confused nursing home residents. *Geriatric Nursing* **1**: 22–27

Reisberg B. (1988) Functional Assessment Staging (FAST). *Psychopharmacological Bulletin* **24**: 653–659

Reisberg B, Ferris S, de Leon M, Crook T. (1982) The Global Deterioration Scale (GDS): an instrument for the assessment of primary degenerative dementia (PDD). *American Journal of Psychiatry* **139**: 1136–1139

Rowe M. (2003) People with dementia who become lost. *American Journal of Nursing* **103**: 32–39

Ryden M and Feldt K. (1992) Goal-directed care: care for aggressive nursing home residents with dementia. *Journal of Gerontological Nursing* **37**: 35–41

Saad K, Hartman J, Ballard C *et al.* (1995) Coping by the carers of dementia sufferers. *Age and Ageing* **24**: 495–498

Satlin A, Volicer L, Ross V, Herz L, Campbell S. (1992) Bright light treatment of behavioral and sleep disturbances in patients with Alzheimer's disease. *American Journal of Psychiatry* **149**: 1028–1032

Sloane PD, Rader J, Barrick AL *et al.* (1995) Bathing persons with dementia. *The Gerontologist* **35**: 672–678

Szwabo P. (1998) Sexuality and Alzheimer's Disease. *Long-Term Links Newsletter* (Missouri Association of Long-Term Care Physicians and the Department of Community Medicine at the University of Missouri School of Medicine) Summer: 4–5

Szwabo P. (2003) Counseling Older Adults About Sexuality. *Clinics in Geriatric Medicine Clinics of North America* **19**: 595–604

Tabloski P, McKinnon-Howe L, Remington R. (1995) Effects of calming music on the level of agitation in cognitively impaired nursing home residents. *Journal of Alzheimer's Care and Related Disorders Research* **1**: 10–15

Teri L and Wagner A. (1992) Alzheimer's disease and depression. *Journal of Consulting Clinical Psychology* **3**: 379–391

Vitaliano P, Russo J, Yound H, Becker J, Maiuro R. (1991) The screen for caregiver burden. *The Gerontologist* **31**: 76–83

Zarit S, Reever K, Bach-Peterson J. (1980) Relatives of the impaired elderly: Correlates of feelings of burden. *The Gerontologist* **20**: 649–655

Social work and care management

DAVID CHALLIS, JANE HUGHES AND CAROLINE SUTCLIFFE

Social work, like any professional or occupational group, is inseparable from the organizational and legislative context in which it takes place since this defines the parameters of practice. Prior to the introduction of care management, descriptions of social work in services for adults, including older people, tended to focus on professional specific activities, to the neglect of outputs such as the function of linking the individual to networks of care. Moreover, social work with older people, including those with dementia, was typically short term (Hunter *et al.*, 1990). Assessments were often undertaken in a relatively narrow and service-oriented fashion (Social Services Inspectorate, 1987), followed by an allocation of service prior to closure. Continuing management of long-term problems for people living in the community was neglected. The advent of care management has required a useful redefinition of social work in relation to long-term care of older people. It can be most simply defined as a strategy for organizing and coordinating care services at the level of the individual client/patient. Care management therefore involves mobilizing and influencing various agencies and services to achieve clearly formulated goals, rather than each provider pursuing separate and perhaps diverse goals (Challis, 1993). It is helpfully understood in terms of six criteria: the performance of core tasks; effective coordination; explicit goals; a specific target population; a long-term care focus; and an impact on service development as well as individual cases. This is summarized in Box 16.5.

The Health Act 1999 has introduced new flexibilities that allow for pooled budgets, delegated commissioning and integration between services. Subsequently, the Health and Social Care Act 2001 was introduced to promote more integrated organizational structures for the delivery of health and social care through integrated care trusts to improve service delivery (Cm 4169, 1998; Cm 4818-I, 2000). More

---

Box 16.5 *Key characteristics of care management*

- **Core tasks**: case finding and screening; assessment; care planning; monitoring and review
- **Functions**: coordination and linkage of care services
- **Goals**: providing continuity and integrated care; increased opportunity for home-based care; make better use of resources; promote wellbeing of older person
- **Target population**: long-term care needs; multiple service requirements; risk of institutional placement
- **Differentiating features of long-term care**: intensity of involvement; breadth of services spanned; lengthy duration of involvement with older person
- **Multilevel response**: linking practice-level activities with broader resource and agency level activities

---

generally, with respect to the provision of health and social care for vulnerable older people, the National Service Framework for Older People (NSFOP) (Department of Health, 2001) has endorsed targets for the reform and development of particular services relevant to conditions more common amongst this group people, for example falls and stroke. Standard Seven of the NSFOP, which is specific to older people with mental health problems, advocates a multidisciplinary approach to a specialist mental health service, including social work input, with a core team member acting as a care coordinator for each older person referred for specialist care. These developments are important since research has demonstrated that the appropriate provision of services, such as day care, can have a positive impact upon the care of older people with dementia (Andrew *et al.*, 2000; Moriarty and Webb, 2000). Furthermore, respite care which can include day care, day or night sitting services in the older person's

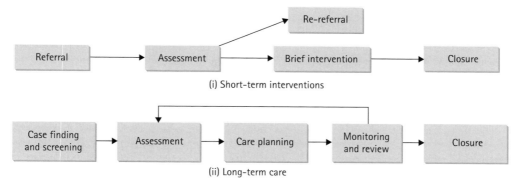

Figure 16.1   *A model of care (Challis et al., 1990).*

home, or relief care in a care home, has an important role in the context of community care (Levin and Moriarty, 1996).

16.6 CURRENT PATTERNS OF PRACTICE

Examination of existing services suggest there is considerable potential for development. A Department of Health inspection of services in the community for older people with dementia examined the core tasks of care management arrangements (Social Services Inspectorate, 1997a). In terms of assessment and care planning, formal links between health and social care were noted to be poor, although some evidence of good interprofessional collaborative working arrangements was observed. Furthermore, there was a lack of ongoing monitoring of people with dementia and their carers, and the monitoring and review of care plans were seen to be given insufficient priority. The report concluded that a more integrated approach to health and social care was required in order to meet the long-term care needs of people with dementia. More recently, concern has been expressed about the lack of specialist provision to support older people with mental health problems at home, and also regarding shortfalls in the long-term care sector for this group of people (Social Services Inspectorate, 2003).

The core tasks of long-term care embodied in care management, detailed in Figure 16.1, offer an approach suitable for the community-based care of vulnerable people with chronic conditions. Since older people with dementia typically have complex health and social care needs, it is important that agencies have in place procedures and protocols within care management arrangements that facilitate an appropriate response – a feature more likely to be associated with a differentiated approach to care management with procedures specific to those with complex needs. This is an approach in which a distinction is made between older people with complex needs often requiring a multiservice response and those with less complex needs, which are often met by a single service response provided by one agency. However, research has suggested that little progress was made in the development of a differentiated approach to care management immediately

Box 16.6   *Differentiated approach to care management*

- **Specialist assessment documents**: only 5 per cent for older people
- **Intensive care management for high-risk individuals requiring high levels of support**: rare and most not focused on older people

Source: Challis *et al.* (1999)

after the introduction of the community care reforms. Rather, care management services were, in the main, provided for the majority rather than for a selected group of older service users (Challis *et al.*, 1999; Weiner *et al.*, 2002). This is illustrated in Box 16.6. Nevertheless, a more differentiated approach to care management has been recommended by central government in order to assist social services departments in managing the volume of work and targeting resources on those in greatest need, such as people with dementia (Social Services Inspectorate, 1997a, b). It has identified three types of care management arrangements, each necessary to an integrated and comprehensive approach:

- a predominantly administrative type providing information and advice;
- a coordinating type that deals with a large volume of referrals needing either a single service or range of fairly straightforward services;
- an intensive type where there is a designated care manager who combines the planning and coordination of services with a more therapeutic, supportive role for a much smaller number of users with complex and changing needs.

The Single Assessment Process (SAP) (Department of Health, 2002) is consistent with the development of a differentiated approach to care management. At the outset, it was anticipated that comprehensive assessment would be the most appropriate for older people with dementia since it is specified as a prerequisite for residential and nursing home placements and intensive community support, where substantial packages of care at home are required. It will be undertaken by a range

Shorter-term care

> *Community mental health team for older people*
> doctors, nurses, psychologist,
> occupational therapists, social workers
> *Key workers*

+

Longer-term care

> *Case managers*
> Social workers with budget
> Service to patients with dementia
> *Care management*

Figure 16.2 *Lewisham Case Management Scheme: setting and roles (Challis et al., 1997).*

> **Box 16.7** *Practice interventions and strategies*
>
> - **Case finding and screening**: targeting of appropriate cases
> - **Assessment**
>   - structured approach
>   - severity of need assessed
> - **Implementing the care plan**
>   - goal defined
>   - strategies of intervention and resources identified
> - **Monitoring, review and case closure**
>   - achievement of goals reassessed
>   - problems reviewed
>   - outcome by domain of assessed need evaluated

of professionals or specialist teams, although geriatricians and old age psychiatrists are expected to take a prominent role in comprehensive assessment, particularly with regard to the development of approaches to assessment.

16.7 INTENSIVE CARE MANAGEMENT

The Lewisham Case Management Scheme offered a practical demonstration of care management designed to provide intensive community support to enable older people with dementia to live at home. It was one of a family of intensive care management studies designed to offer a community based alternative to institutional care (Challis and Davies, 1986; Challis et al., 1995, 2002a, b). Specifically, it was established in a multidisciplinary setting to develop a model of intensive care management for a target population of individuals with a diagnosis of dementia, identified as having unmet needs and likely to be at risk of entry to institutional care, despite input from statutory services (Challis et al., 1997, 2002a). The aim of the scheme was to provide effective integrated community-based long-term care that spanned the health and social service interface. The service was provided by social services case managers based in a community mental health team for older people. Most importantly, case managers were able to purchase care in response to identified need within defined parameters. This enabled the development of a specialist paid helper service that was available to those in the experimental group, receiving case management input. The service setting and roles are summarized in Figure 16.2. An evaluation of the scheme was undertaken using a quasi-experimental approach, where individuals in one community mental health team for older people received case management, the experimental group, and were compared with those in a similar community mental health setting without a case management service, the control group. A range of indicators were used covering aspects of needs, quality of

care, quality of life and wellbeing, encompassing the perspectives of the older person, carers (including family, friends and paid carers) and the assessing researcher.

Box 16.7 details the process of assessment and case management as it developed within the scheme. With regard to implementing the care plan, the goals of intervention in case management were identified by retrospective analysis of 80 care plans. These were analysed under seven categories: supportive, therapeutic, practical, preventive, social, destinational and organizational. The most frequently reported were supportive (68 per cent), therapeutic (66 per cent) and practical (56 per cent). Supportive goals were almost exclusively intended for the benefit of informal carers, the most frequently reported categories were to relieve carer burden, provide respite and assist carers. Therapeutic interventions were most often directed at devising strategies to reduce problem behaviours associated with the client's deteriorating state. Practical goals were directed towards the assistance of the client, with personal care, health care and domestic care being the most frequently mentioned. These demonstrate that the prime objective of case managers was to support, sustain and enhance the quality of life of the client in his/her own home, and thereby to assist the carers.

In the second year of the Lewisham Case Management Scheme its effects began to show in a lower rate of admission to care homes for older people with dementia in the experimental group, than under standard arrangements for those in the control group, also resulting in lower associated costs for residential care for the former. Hence the community tenure effect in this study appeared more muted than in other case management studies (Challis et al., 1995, 2002b). However, at 6 months, older people in the experimental group were more satisfied with their lifestyle at home, and there was evidence of a reduction in their needs specifically associated with activities of daily living. No differences were found between the groups in levels of depression, and there was no impact on levels of problem behaviours. With regard to the carers of the older people with dementia, there was a significant reduction in the amount of care input and distress at 12 months for carers in the experimental group.

It was, however, apparent that both experimental and control group clients were receiving support from a relatively resource-rich community-based old age psychiatry service, untypical of that to be found in most of the UK. Costs were higher for the group of older people receiving case management, in particular those accounted for by the social services department, since case manager visits and the paid helper service were not available to those receiving standard services. On the other hand, for carers of those in receipt of case management there was a positive gain, since financial and other costs were lower for this group compared with the carers of those receiving standard services. Moreover, when all costs to society were accounted for, including informal care, the weekly cost of supporting older people with dementia and their carers was not significantly higher for those receiving intensive case management, although the main component for statutory services was greater.

As demonstrated above, this specialist scheme was successful in providing care to older people with dementia to enable them to remain at home rather than be admitted to long-term care and provided effective support to their carers. This approach is consistent with other evidence relating to the provision of specialist care for this group of older people. Levin and colleagues (1994) noted factors that could make for improved care for people with dementia. These included a specialist integrated dementia care service, offering long-term care management to provide sufficiently intensive support, enabling a person to remain at home where appropriate and reflecting the wishes of cared for and the carer. This latter factor is particularly important since the centrality of support for carers remains a constant theme in policy and this service model is endorsed in the NSFOP (Cm 849, 1989; Cm 4169, 1998; Department of Health, 2001).

16.8 CONCLUSIONS

The change in the role, focus and setting for social workers and other professions in the UK working with people with dementia with the enactment of the community care legislation has been made more explicit in government guidance both at the inception of the community care reforms and subsequently (SSI/SWSG, 1991; Department of Health, 2001). A key theme in these has been the development of community-based multidisciplinary teams similar to those operating in mental health and learning disability services, as part of the move away from institution-based care. In order to fulfil the changed role accorded to UK social work, it is essential that arrangements are in place to facilitate the multidisciplinary assessment of people with dementia and particularly to ensure that specialist clinicians contribute to this process. A number of studies in the UK suggest potential gains from greater integration of secondary health care with the decisions made in the context of care management (Brocklehurst et al., 1978; Peet et al., 1994; Sharma et al., 1994; Challis et al., 2004). The experience of Australia, which has the community care reforms most analogous to those in the UK, gives credence to this type of arrangement (Challis et al., 1995; Howe and Kung, 2003).

It is anticipated that the effective care of people with dementia will benefit from the new service configurations, which pay less attention to traditional boundaries whether professional or organizational than hitherto. Within this, social work and care management have a distinct role in relation to the provision of long-term community-based care. The emergence of dementia-specific services as an outcome of the partnership initiatives may lead to further interprofessional role blurring which, if managed correctly, could be the basis of improved care for people with dementia and their carers. However, as distinct from similar developments in Ireland (Department of Health and Children, 2001), policy guidance in England requires that specialist dementia services develop within the more general framework for older age mental health services.

For social work there are two challenges consequent on these changes. First, the profession-specific contribution to the care of older people with dementia and their carers has changed to primarily that of responsibility for the care for people living at home and, by virtue of changes for the funding of long-term care, gate-keepers for admission to residential or nursing home care. There is now greater standardization in the process with recent guidance emphasizing the importance of assessment, care planning, monitoring and review. Second, and in antithesis to this clarity, the role of the social work profession in respect of the care of people with dementia has become less profession specific. Within multidisciplinary teams there are more opportunities for the sharing of tasks offering informal small-scale opportunities for service substitution. Research has found that the process of assessment of older people referred to a specialist mental health team for older people can be undertaken by any members of the professions within it (Lindesay et al., 1996), and more recently, increasing evidence of community nurses working within such teams for older people (Weiner et al., 2003). There is thus a tendency for there to be less specificity of role for staff as services become more community based. This leads unsurprisingly to a degree of insecurity among professional groups, because each derives their unique quality from a training and occupational function. Roles come to be negotiated rather than simply professionally defined within groups to a greater extent in community-based services and therefore may be seen as less clearly defined by individual professions. This process may well occur to a greater extent as the process of closer integration between health and social care develops.

REFERENCES

Andrew T, Moriarty J, Levin E, Webb S. (2000) Outcome of referral to social services departments for people with cognitive impairment. *International Journal of Geriatric Psychiatry* **15**: 406–414

Brocklehurst J, Carty M, Leeming J, Robinson J. (1978) Care of the elderly: medical screening of old people accepted for residential care. *Lancet* **2**: 141–142

Challis D. (1993) Alternatives to institutional care. In: R Levy, R Howard, A Burns (eds), *Treatment and Care in Old Age Psychiatry*. Petersfield, Wrightson

Challis D and Davies B. (1986) Case management. In: *Community Care*. Aldershot, Gower

Challis D, Chessum R, Chesterman J *et al.* (1990) *Case management in social and health care: The Gateshead community care scheme*. Canterbury, PSSRU

Challis D, Darton R, Johnson L, Stone M, Traske K. (1995) *Care Management and Health Care of Older People: the Darlington Community Care Project*. Aldershot, Arena

Challis D, von Abendorff R, Brown P, Chesterman J. (1997) Care management and dementia: an evaluation of the Lewisham Intensive Case Management Scheme. In: S Hunter (ed.), *Dementia: Challenges and New Directions*. London, Jessica Kingsley

Challis D, Darton R, Hughes J, Stewart K, Weiner K. (1999) Mapping and evaluation of care management arrangements for older people and those with mental health problems: An overview of care management arrangements. *Discussion Paper 1519/M009*. Personal Social Services Research Unit, University of Kent at Canterbury and University of Manchester [not publicly available]

Challis D, von Abendorff R, Brown P, Chesterman J, Hughes J. (2002a) Care management, dementia care and specialist mental health services: an evaluation. *International Journal of Geriatric Psychiatry* **17**: 315–325

Challis D, Chesterman J, Luckett R, Stewart K, Chessum R. (2002b) *Care Management in Social and Primary Health Care*. The Gateshead Community Care Scheme, Ashgate, Aldershot

Challis D, Clarkson P, Williamson J *et al.* (2004) The value of specialist clinical assessment of older people prior to entry to care homes. *Age and Ageing* **33**: 25–34

Cm 849. (1989) *Caring for People: Community Care in the Next Decade and Beyond*. London, HMSO

Cm 4169. (1998) *Modernising Social Services*. London, The Stationery Office

Cm 4818-I. (2000) *The NHS Plan: A Plan for Investment. A Plan for Reform*. London, The Stationery Office

Department of Health. (2001) *The National Service Framework for Older People*. London, Department of Health

Department of Health. (2002) The Single Assessment Process. Key implications, guidance for local implementation and annexes to the guidance. *Health Services Circular/Local Authority Circular* (HSC2002/001; LAC (2002)1). London, Department of Health

Department of Health and Children. (2001) *Quality and Fairness. A Health System for You*. Dublin, The Stationery Office

Howe A and Kung F. (2003) Does assessment make a difference for people with dementia? The effectiveness of the Aged Care Assessment Teams. *International Journal of Geriatric Psychiatry* **18**: 205–210

Hunter S, Brace S, Buckley G. (1990) The interdisciplinary assessment of older people at entry into long-term institutional care: lessons for the new community care arrangements. *Research Policy and Planning* **11**: 2–9

Levin E and Moriarty J. (1996) Evaluating respite services. In: R Bland (ed.), *Developing Services for Older People and Their Families*. London, Jessica Kingsley

Levin E, Moriarty J, Gorbach P. (1994) *Better for the Break*. London, HMSO

Lindesay J, Herzberg J, Collighan G, MacDonald A, Philpot M. (1996) Treatment decisions following assessment by multidisciplinary psychogeriatric teams. *Psychiatric Bulletin* **20**: 78–81

Moriarty J and Webb S. (2000) *Part of Their Lives: Community Care for Older People with Dementia*. Bristol, The Policy Press

Peet S, Castleden C, Potter J, Jagger C. (1994) The outcome of a medical examination for applicants to Leicestershire homes for older people. *Age and Ageing* **23**: 65–68

Sharma S, Aldous J, Robinson M. (1994) Assessing applicants for part 3 accommodation: is a formal clinical assessment worthwhile? *Public Health* **108**: 91–97

Social Services Inspectorate. (1987) *From Home Help to Home Care: An Analysis of Policy Resourcing and Service Management*. London, DHSS

Social Services Inspectorate. (1997a) *At Home with Dementia: Inspection of Services for Older People with Dementia in the Community*. London, Department of Health

Social Services Inspectorate. (1997b) *Better Management, Better Care*. Sixth Annual Report of the Chief Inspector Social Services Inspectorate 1996/97. London, HMSO

Social Services Inspectorate. (2003) *Modern Social Services: A Commitment to the Future*. Twelfth Annual Report of the Chief Inspector Social Services Inspectorate 2002/03. London, Department of Health

SSI/SWSG Social Services Inspectorate/Social Work Services Group. (1991) *Care Management and Assessment: Managers' Guide*. London, HMSO

Weiner K, Stewart K, Hughes J, Challis D, Darton R. (2002) Care management arrangements for older people in England: key areas of variation in a national study. *Ageing and Society* **22**: 419–439

Weiner K, Hughes J, Challis D, Pederson I. (2003) Integrating health and social care at the micro level: Health care professionals as care managers for older people. *Social Policy and Administration* **37**: 498–515

Occupational therapy

MICHAEL LOH

The clinical practice of occupational therapy (OT) involves the treatment of physical and psychiatric conditions through specific selected activities in order to help people reach their maximum level of function in all aspects of daily life (Hopkins and Smith, 1993). Fundamental to the philosophy of OT is the belief that purposeful activity is required to promote wellness and prevent disability (Rogers, 1994). It draws on a broad range of theoretical models, which is particularly useful in aged care where there is a significant interaction of biopsychosocial factors affecting the individual's functional status.

The OT process involves assessment, treatment planning, implementation and evaluation. Occupational therapists working in the field of dementia focus their approach on the maintenance of skills and the prevention of functional deterioration owing to the progressive nature of the disorder. The maintenance of a sense of self-worth is also a major consideration when working with people with dementia. Owing to the obvious debilitating symptoms of dementia, individuals can subsequently experience depression, anxiety, apathy and discouragement, which can have a detrimental effect on the dementing process (Pool, 1997). Therefore, in both areas of assessment and intervention, occupational therapy will encourage the individual's sense of wellbeing by allowing them some control over their personal life, and providing opportunities to achieve meaningful roles and to enjoy social interaction.

16.9 ASSESSMENT

16.9.1 Purpose of the occupational therapy assessment

Assessment is a major role of occupational therapy and is used to identify the impact of dementia on an individual's general daily functioning. Occupational therapists aim to assist older people to be as independent as possible, but first it is necessary to assess the individual's abilities, problems, wishes and interests (Pool, 1997). This information can then be used to plan and implement relevant therapeutic interventions.

OT assessments can provide specific information in the following areas:

- *activities of daily living (ADL)*: eating, dressing, grooming, bathing, toileting, medication management, home and money management, leisure, telephone use and transport;
- *cognitive function*: memory, judgement, problem solving, concentration;
- *perceptual and sensory function*: visual, auditory, proprioceptive sensation, stereognosis and praxis;
- *motor function*: balance, mobility and transfers, hand function, coordination;
- *communication skills*: verbal and non-verbal social skills, receptive and expressive dysphasia;
- *psychological state*: mood, anxiety and motivation.

Throughout the assessment process, therapists use both their physical and their psychiatric knowledge within the framework of the natural ageing process (Vincent, 1997). The information gathered from an OT assessment often overlaps, yet should also complement that gained from other professionals within the multidisciplinary team. However, the unique skills of the occupational therapist in dementia care usually lie in the area of ADL. That is, the therapist will assess the impact of a person's physical, cognitive, psychological and social disabilities on their day-to-day function (Atler and Michel, 1996).

In identifying an individual's functional ability in their living environment, the information may then be used in any of the following ways:

- assist in the formulation of a diagnosis;
- recommend support services to maintain the individual in their preferred living arrangement;
- recommend alternative accommodation options appropriate to the individual's level of functioning;
- advise on adaptive equipment to assist in maintaining independence;
- recommend leisure interests that can be maintained, adapted or introduced to promote quality of life and maintain self-esteem over the course of dementia;
- determine the individual's needs, and priorities for intervention, and to involve the person with dementia and family/carers in this process.

16.9.2 The process of the occupational therapy assessment

The progressive nature of dementia indicates that the process of assessing individuals is one that is ongoing and will change focus with the changing needs of the individual. In the early stages of dementia, the primary focus of assessment may be ADL and maintenance of individuals in their home environment. The later stages of dementia may call for the assessment of basic self-care tasks to determine the level and/or the type of residential care required. When an occupational therapist undertakes assessments of people with dementia, special considerations are required to ensure the assessment of performance is accurate. The use of simple language and repetition of instructions may be necessary to ensure that the person with dementia has sufficient time to process information and to respond to requests. The alleviation of the person's anxiety within the assessment situation is a consideration, particularly when the there is some degree of self-insight into deficits. Building a trusting and supportive relationship with individuals prior to the assessment process is important, as is providing positive feedback for the tasks that are done well, with less focus on problem areas.

Assessment may include one or all of the following techniques, and will be tailored to meet the needs of the individual and the overall purpose of the assessment.

16.10 INTERVIEW

The therapist will attempt to ascertain the individual's own perception of their skills and deficits. A person's ability to recognize difficulties in day-to-day functioning will be dependent on the level of dementia. It is therefore necessary to liaise with the family or a caregiver who may be able to provide a more accurate reflection of the person's current functional level. Family and caregivers can also provide

details of the life history, which can be used to promote communication and assist in the development of therapeutic relationships.

16.11 OBSERVATIONS

It is common for people with dementia to be poor historians and to embellish their current skill level. Observation of an individual's activity performance is used to enhance the information gained through the interview process. Observation of a person during activities can provide general information on many aspects of that person's functioning, such as cognition, motor, sensory and perceptual function, psychological state and skills in communication and ADL (Alexander, 1994).

The therapist may observe a person with dementia in a variety of different settings, both in groups and individually. In terms of the assessment of ADL, the specific activities assessed are selected according to their relevance to the individual's living situation, and where possible are carried out in a familiar environment. This aims are to reduce anxiety and limit the effects of the need to learn new skills and to orientate to new environments. Ideally, the assessment of a person's home management skills should occur in the home. The presence of unpaid bills, poor cleanliness of the house, and lack of evidence of fresh food may provide further evidence as to whether a person is managing daily tasks independently. Assessments over time provide a more accurate picture of a person's functioning than a single assessment, particularly when anxiety and performance deficits are observed.

16.12 STANDARDIZED TESTS

Assessment tools are often used by occupational therapists in conjunction with interviews and observation to gain a more specific picture of a person's performance in a particular area. Such tools can be used to determine a baseline functioning and can be used at a later date to monitor any change in performance that may have occurred.

There is a wide range of tools available for use with people who have dementia; however, many have not been designed specifically for this group. Commonly used ADL assessment tools suitable for use with dementia include the following:

- The Barthel Index (Mahoney and Barthel, 1965) is a simple index of independence to rate the self-care ability of individuals. It includes items on feeding, dressing, toileting and showering. Scores are determined by the amount of physical assistance a person requires to perform self-care tasks.
- Domestic and Community Skills Assessment (DACSA) (Collister and Alexander, 1991) may be used to assess an individual's knowledge of and practical skills in a variety of instrumental ADL (IADLs). It includes items such as

banking, bill-paying, shopping, meal preparation and house keeping. The assessment process involves both interview and observation of task performance.

- Assessment of Motor and Process Skills (AMPS) (Robinson and Fisher, 1996) measures a variety of motor and cognitive abilities during an individual's performance of IADLs. It involves the observation of an individual performing two or three tasks that are familiar and relevant to their living situation. They are then rated in the areas of motor skills and process (organizational adaptive) skills necessary for competent task performance.
- Assessment of Living Skills and Resources (Williams et al., 1991) is an IADL assessment tool that evaluates an individual's skill, and resources or support available for daily activities. The assessment determines the likelihood of an individual being able to carry out specific tasks given his/her current skill and resources in the home setting.

16.13 INTERVENTION

16.13.1 The use of activities

Performance in activities, which is the core of OT assessment, is also the major focus of intervention. OT treatment and techniques differ according to the individual and the stage of the disorder. Interventions aim to preserve a person's dignity and self-esteem while maximizing abilities and enabling improvement in quality of life. The occupational therapist achieves this through the medium of 'meaningful activities' that are selected also to be pleasurable, restore roles and enable friendship (Mace, 1987). A person with dementia has impaired learning ability, and so familiar and overlearnt activities tend to be most effective in treatment programmes (Zgola, 1987; Conroy, 1992; Vincent, 1997). However, individuals should also have the opportunity to be involved in a variety of both familiar and novel activities. Blair and Glen (1987) classified activities for people with dementia into four categories:

- *Activities designed to involve sensory stimulation.* The use of sensory activities is particularly useful when an individual's cognitive and communication abilities are severely impaired, and involvement in other activities is limited. Useful sensory activities include: visual (outings, photos, movies); tactile (massage, gardening, cooking, craft); auditory (appropriate and varied music, spending time outdoors); gustatory (different food experiences); and olfactory (flower collecting and arranging, cooking, aromatherapy).
- *Activities based on self-care and life skills.* Maintaining independence in daily living is a central activity for all people, and attention to these tasks helps to build self-esteem. These tasks can be structured and simplified to ensure that a person can still complete at least part of the activity. For example, verbal reminders can be used to

initiate bathing; or having essential ingredients and utensils on a kitchen table can assist a person to cook a simple meal.

- *Activities designed around realistic physical exercise.* Physical activity helps to maintain both physical and psychological wellbeing (Simpson, 1986). Physical exertion can also have beneficial effects on behaviour and sleep disturbances. Exercise programmes should be designed around enjoyable indoor and outdoor gross motor activities. These may include walking, bowling and dancing.
- *Activities designed to increase social interaction.* For many people with dementia, the use of group activities helps to promote social skills and verbal interaction. With the presence of impaired memory and concentration, small groups are more effective in facilitating communication. Activities useful for group settings include cooking, gardening, music and reminiscence. For example, reminiscence can be used as a social activity that encourages discussion as individuals recall past roles and interests.

16.13.2 Environment adaptations

The use of environmental modifications is an important non-pharmacological approach to the management of behavioural and psychological symptoms of dementia. Environmental modifications have been introduced in residential facilities, in hospitals as well as in home situations. Gitlin and colleagues' (2003) paper on the research in this area noted that, although 90 per cent of 63 studies reviewed reported positive findings, most studies were methodologically flawed, involved small samples, and were conducted in nursing homes. Environmental principles gleaned from these studies include:

- reducing environmental complexity by relaxing rules and expectations, and minimizing distractions;
- increasing orientation and awareness;
- creating a low stimulus, comfortable environment; and
- providing predictability, familiarity, and structure.

The environment can also be adapted for appropriate cuing. Objects can be placed in the environment to provide orientation; for example, laying out clothes cues a confused person to dress, or a night-light aids a person to locate the toilet. Objects can also be removed because of safety concerns; for instance, no longer hanging the car keys by the door eliminates a visual cue to drive (Gitlin and Corcoran, 1996).

Besides designing interventions to maximize a person's competency, the therapist also modifies the environment to facilitate the performance of daily activities. Changing immediate surroundings through home alterations, removal of objects, and simplification of tasks may reduce the external stressors that produce excess behavioural disturbances and disability in people with dementia (Gitlin and Corcoran, 1996).

Adding items to the environment can make the performance of activities easier. For example, the installation of a grab rail can assist a person to get in and out of the bath safely.

Environmental modifications should, where possible, be tailored to the requirements of the individual. They also need to be monitored on a regular basis to ensure that they are still assisting the current problem, or are replaced to address the individual's changing needs.

16.13.3 Working with families and carers

The family plays a crucial role in the care of the person dementia. An occupational therapist can assist in identifying the remaining strengths of the person with dementia. The therapist and the family can use this information to plan strategies jointly to maximize function and at the same time minimize the burden of care. Through education and support, carers are taught to support continued engagement of the person with dementia in meaningful activities (Baum and Edwards, 2003).

16.14 CONCLUSION

The specific role of occupational therapists in dementia care will be determined by the setting in which they work and the severity of the individual's dementia. Therapists may work as part of aged care assessment services, aged psychiatry community teams, day hospital or centres, acute inpatient units or long-term residential care facilities. It is therefore likely that therapists will be involved in the assessment and treatment of dementia anywhere from the very early to the late stages of the disorder. The general OT principles of practice will remain consistent across settings and disease stages, and will have an emphasis on maintenance of functional ability and attention to social and psychological needs to promote quality of life.

This chapter was originally written by Fiona Moffatt and Michael Loh and appeared as chapter 19c in the second edition of Dementia. It was updated by Michael Loh for this third edition.

REFERENCES

Alexander K. (1994) Occupational therapy. In: E Chiu and D Ames (eds), *Functional Psychiatric Disorders of the Elderly*. Cambridge, Cambridge University Press, pp. 522–543

Atler K and Michel GS. (1996) Maximizing abilities: occupational therapy's role in geriatric psychiatry. *Psychiatric Services* **47**: 933–935

Baum C and Edwards D. (2003) What persons with Alzheimer's disease can do: a tool for communication about everyday activities. *Alzheimer's Care Quarterly* **4**:108–118

Blair S and Glen A. (1987) Psychiatry in old age: occupational therapy and organic conditions. In: C Helm (ed.), *Occupational Therapy in the Elderly*. Edinburgh, Churchill Livingstone, pp. 87–114

Collister L and Alexander K. (1991) *The Occupational Therapy Domestic and Community Skills Assessment (DACSA) Research Edition*. Melbourne, Latrobe University

Conroy C. (1992) An evaluation of an occupational therapy service for persons with dementia. In: G Jones and B Miesen (eds), *Care-giving in Dementia: Research and Applications*. London and New York, Routledge, pp. 219–238

Gitlin L and Corcoran M. (1996) Managing dementia at home: the role of home environment modifications. *Topics in Geriatric Rehabilitation* **12**: 28–39

Gitlin L, Liebman J, Winter J. (2003) Are environmental interventions effective in the management of Alzheimer's disease and related disorders?: A synthesis of the evidence. *Alzheimer's Care Quarterly* **4**: 85–107

Hopkins A and Smith H. (1993) *Willard and Spackman's Occupational Therapy*, 8th edition. Philadelphia, JB Lippincott Co, p. 325

Mace N. (1987) Principles of activities for persons with dementia. *Physical and Occupational Therapy in Geriatrics* **5**: 13–27

Mahoney F and Barthel D. (1965) Functional evaluation: the Barthel Index. *Maryland State Medical Journal* **2**: 61–65

Pool J. (1997) Older people. In: J Creek (ed.), *Occupational Therapy and Mental Health*. New York, Churchill Livingstone, pp. 357–374

Robinson S and Fisher A. (1996) A study to examine the relationship of the assessment of motor and process skills (AMPS) to other tests of cognition and function. *British Journal of Occupational Therapy* **59**: 260–263

Rogers J. (1994) Statement: occupational therapy services for persons with Alzheimer's disease and other dementias. *American Journal of Occupational Therapy* **48**: 1029–1031

Simpson W. (1986) Exercise: prescriptions for the elderly. *Geriatrics* **41**:95–100

Vincent E. (1997) Occupational therapy for older persons. In: R Jacoby and C Oppenheimer (eds), *Psychiatry in the Elderly*. Oxford, Oxford University Press, pp. 357–374

Williams J, Drinka T, Greenberg J, Farrell-Holtan J, Euhardy R, Schram M. (1991) Development and testing of the Assessment of Living Skills and Resources (ASLAR) in elderly community-dwelling veterans. *The Gerontologist* **31**: 84–91

Zgola J. (1987) *Doing Things: A Guide to Programming Activities for Persons with Alzheimer's Disease and Related Disorders*. Baltimore and London, John Hopkins University Press, pp. 27–42

Speech and language therapy

BRONWYN MOORHOUSE

Communication is integral to successful living (Lubinski, 1991); however, its breakdown in dementia is well documented (e.g. Hopper and Bayles, 2001; Bourgeois, 2002). Eating and swallowing can also become problematic in this condition (Logemann, 2003). In 1991, Bourgeois reviewed dementia articles in the journals of the American Speech-Language-Hearing Association (ASHA). These articles focused strongly on how cognitive-linguistic profiles contributed to dementia diagnosis. Furthermore, in 1995 Clark observed that although ASHA advocated optimizing functional communication in older people, most clinicians still restricted themselves to assessment of Alzheimer's disease (AD). People with dementia, who can live for up to 20 years after diagnosis, also need help with communication to optimize quality of life (Bourgeois, 2002) and ease carer burden (Enderby, 2002). Hence, involvement of a speech and language therapist (SLT) in the diagnosis of dementia should be only the beginning of the clinical relationship. For a little over a decade, research exploring strategies to facilitate interactions in those with dementia has begun to emerge (e.g. Bourgeois, 1992; Baker, 2001; Spilkin and Bethlehem, 2003). It is appropriate that this chapter includes information about cognitive-linguistic difficulties observed in dementia and assessment tools used to examine these. In addition, it is imperative that it explores how SLTs can work with people who have dementia, significant others and care staff, in optimizing communication. Issues around the SLT's role in facilitating swallowing in dementia will also be explored.

16.15 SPEECH AND LANGUAGE CHANGES IN DEMENTIA

Reisberg et al. (1999) used the term retrogenesis to describe strong parallels between language acquisition and the loss of language in AD. Fried-Oken et al. (2000) noted that most research into communication difficulties in dementia relates to AD. Nonetheless, they concluded that many language changes seen in AD may also occur in other forms of dementia. As such, this section will refer primarily to language features of AD, according to stages of the Global Deterioration Scale (GDS) (Reisberg et al., 1982). Information regarding features of vascular dementia (VaD), dementia with Lewy bodies (DLB) and primary progressive aphasia (PPA) will then be outlined.

16.15.1 Alzheimer's disease

16.15.1.1 EARLY/MILD STAGE AD (GDS 3 AND 4)

Word-finding difficulties are commonly encountered early in AD (Bourgeois, 2002), affecting most recently acquired and least frequently used words (Haak, 2002). Conversation is therefore slightly empty with fewer ideas in the same amount of words (Bayles and Tomoeda, 1995). Communication is usually successful for brief interactions, but breaks down when lengthy (Haak, 2002). Comprehension of language sometimes remains intact (Bayles et al., 1992) or may decline for longer grammatically complex sentences (Clark, 1995), or material requiring inference (Fried-Oken et al., 2000) or abstraction (Haak, 2002). Failing memory and executive function impact on adherence to conversational rules around repetition, topic maintenance and turn-taking (Watson et al., 1999). There are often aborted phrases; however, talking may also be excessive (Bayles and Tomoeda, 1995). Oral reading and reading comprehension (Bayles et al., 1992) along with spelling and writing are often relatively preserved, but ability to generate written passages is reduced (Haak, 2002).

16.15.1.2 MIDDLE/MODERATE STAGE AD (GDS 5)

Intention to communicate and general message frameworks are still evident; however, utterances are depleted of content words (Haak, 2002), less concise and more repetitious with reference errors abounding (Bayles and Tomoeda, 1995). Content words are often replaced by indefinite labels (e.g. 'thing') consistent with pervasive lexical retrieval difficulty (Bourgeois, 2002). Sounds, syllables and whole phrases are repeated and the person often speaks excessively or withdraws (Clark, 1995). Automatic and social phrases are retained, but the person frequently forgets what he or she wishes to say (Haak, 2002). Paraphasias and confabulations begin to appear and discourse breakdown increases with poor propositional topic development, difficulty changing topic and maintaining discourse flow (Mentis et al.,1995; Fried-Oken et al., 2000). Expression and comprehension of complex grammar (e.g. embedded clauses or passives) is limited and abstract interpretation is lost, whilst comprehension of one (Haak, 2002) and sometimes two stage (Fried-Oken et al., 2000) commands is preserved. Reading aloud and mechanics of writing are relatively spared, but reading comprehension and writing are often limited to single words (Haak, 2002) and accuracy is markedly reduced (Bayles et al., 1992).

16.15.1.3 LATE/SEVERE STAGE AD (GDS 6 AND 7)

Initially use of automatic and social phrases may continue (Haak, 2002). Often utterances contain strings of non-words with occasional real words interspersed, but message form, simple grammar and intonation are basically present (Bayles and Tomoeda,1995). There is failure to adhere to speaker-listener conversational discourse roles (Clark, 1995). There may also be difficulty initiating speech, articulatory breakdowns and dysphagia (Clark, 1995). Eventually the person becomes completely non-verbal (Bourgeois, 2002), although conceptual knowledge may be preserved until very late (Fried-Oken et al., 2000). There is also failure to comprehend spoken or written language (Bayles and Tomoeda, 1995) and people rely increasingly on non-verbal cues and emotion to aid comprehension (Haak, 2002). Vocalizations may become disruptive – sometimes because of failure to access specific words describing basic needs and emotions, people, activities or objects wanted (Bourgeois, 2002). Resistance may reflect failure to understand verbal direction.

16.15.2 Vascular dementia

VaD occurs following multiple small infarcts occurring progressively over time (Hopper and Bayles, 2001) and can only be diagnosed where cardiovascular disease is documented (Tomoeda, 2001). Rather than the gradual language changes of AD, deterioration is usually stepwise with new deficits becoming evident suddenly after each new infarct (Hopper and Bayles, 2001; Tomoeda, 2001). As such, individual deficit profiles (depending on infarct locations) are often less uniform across different language areas than with AD (Hopper and Bayles, 2001). Nonetheless, Vuorinen, et al. (2000) found little difference, on average, in degree of language deficit across comprehension, naming and picture and object description tasks between individuals with mild to moderate AD versus VaD. Stevens et al. (1996) did find some heterogeneity in scoring between mild VaD and mild AD on a range of cognitive-linguistic tasks. Nonetheless, both groups were clearly differentiated from the 'worried well' on verbal fluency, naming, paragraph reading and immediate and delayed story recall. Powell et al. (1988) also reported greater motoric speech involvement in VaD (e.g. dysarthria and changes in intonation).

16.15.3 Dementia with Lewy bodies

DLB is possibly the second most common dementia after AD (Hopper and Bayles, 2001). To complicate diagnosis, many people with DLB also have AD lesions (McKeith et al., 1995). Most commonly reported characteristics are insidious in onset, beginning with forgetfulness, then word-finding and calculation difficulties and then other cognitive skills (McKeith et al., 1995). Fluctuating cognition (with periods of lucidity in early- to mid-stages), often mild extrapyramidal features (e.g. dysarthria and dysphagia) and a more rapid progression than AD are also observed (Tomoeda, 2001) – early on people with DLB often have more difficulty with visuospatial, problem solving and verbal fluency tasks (McKeith et al., 1995).

16.15.4 Primary progressive aphasia

In 1982, Mesulam described a syndrome of slowly progressive aphasia without generalized dementia. Gradually both number and severity of aphasic symptoms increase with sparing of non-language executive function for at least 2 years after onset (Weintraub et al., 1990). The most common problem is word-finding difficulty, followed by reduced comprehension with speech hesitancy, phonemic paraphasias, dysarthria, with slowed speech and stuttering also sometimes occurring (Westbury and Bub, 1997). Semantic dementia is a subtype of PPA where syntactic abilities are spared whilst naming, single word comprehension and reading are affected (Westbury and Bub, 1997). Phonology and comprehension of complex commands may also be intact in this condition (Stevens and Ripich, 1999). Progressive non-fluent aphasia (PNFA) is also another subtype of PPA (Thompson et al., 1997). Although it often also begins with word-finding difficulties, it progresses to reduced phrase length and complexity and then to telegraphic agrammatic output (Thompson *et al.*, 1997).

16.16 LANGUAGE ASSESSMENTS USED IN DEMENTIA

Individual profiles of cognitive-linguistic functioning ideally form part of a comprehensive memory clinic evaluation (including medical history and investigation, performance in activities of daily living and neuropsychological testing) (Ames *et al.*, 1992). Results of such assessment facilitate accurate diagnosis of presence and type of dementia for review upon repeated assessment(s). Appropriate cognitive-linguistic normative data help to distinguish those with early dementia from the 'worried well' (Bryan *et al.*, 2001). Such data also contribute towards differential diagnosis of depression, characterized by reduced concentration and slowed processing speed (Tomoeda, 2001) without primary verbal memory or language impairment (Stevens *et al.*, 1996). Accurate early dementia diagnosis is important in identifying any appropriate drug therapies and in providing informational counselling. Carers of those with AD are often more relaxed when they understand that language unravels sequentially (Haak, 2002). Furthermore, assessment allows for development of effective care plans (documenting impaired and spared abilities) and establishment of baselines for intervention effects or decline over time (Tomoeda, 2001). Other factors contributing to poor performance such as low hearing, vision or premorbid educational level (Tomoeda, 2001) as well as cultural biases (Lydall-Smith *et al.*,1996) should also be noted.

Recently, several tests assessing cognitive-linguistic function in dementia have emerged. Perhaps best known is the Arizona Battery for Communication Disorders of Dementia (ABCD) (Bayles and Tomoeda, 1993), which assesses performance in mild to moderate dementia across five constructs: linguistic comprehension, linguistic expression, verbal memory, visuospatial skills and mental status (orientation). It has norms from 86 people with probable AD (as described by McKhann *et al.*, 1984) and 86 normal elderly and takes 45–90 minutes to administer. Summary scores for each subtest indicate results in the high normal, low normal, mildly impaired or moderately impaired range. Results are averaged within constructs and a profile obtained to examine deficit pattern. The ABCD was developed in the USA, but norms have also been found to be appropriate with UK (Armstrong *et al.*, 1996) and Australian (Moorhouse *et al.*, 1999) samples.

Time taken to administer the ABCD in poorly resourced clinical settings may be excessive (Bryan *et al.*, 2001). Where only brief screening is possible, ABCD Story Retelling and Word Learning subtests are most sensitive to dementia (Tomoeda, 2001). Additionally, the Boston Naming Test has been found to detect early dementia (Stevens *et al.*, 1992). The Barnes Language Assessment (BLA) (Bryan *et al.*, 2001)

has also been developed to screen for dementia, assessing areas of expression, comprehension, reading and writing, memory and executive functions. It has items adapted from existing tests and includes a manual and set of test materials. It takes 40–60 minutes to administer and can be used with mild, moderate and, sometimes, severe dementia. Norms reported by Bryan *et al.* (2001) were preliminary.

Recent research into pragmatic or conversational abilities in dementia has used protocols rather than standardized assessments – for example, Watson, *et al.* (1999) who used Conversational Analysis (CA) to examine 'Trouble Indicating Behaviour' (TIB) and patterns and types of conversational repair trajectory. There are no dementia-specific protocols investigating function in this area. The only standardized dementia assessment touching on these abilities is the Functional Linguistic Communication Inventory (Bayles and Tomoeda, 1994). It assesses functional communication in moderate to severe AD. It takes 30 minutes to administer and includes items examining ability to greet, answer questions, reminisce and participate in conversations.

16.17 OPTIMIZING COMMUNICATION IN DEMENTIA

Interventions enhancing communicative success in AD will be grouped into three categories: direct, indirect (for caregivers) and environmental interventions (Clark, 1995). As some interventions overlap categories, they will be placed where they fit best. Although many findings cited below relate to intervention in AD, it may be helpful for the SLT to use or adapt this information for people with other dementia types – focusing on functional needs rather than diagnosis. Given relative sparing of executive function in PPA, additional strategies drawn from aphasia therapy may be used in optimizing communication. (For further ideas in this area see Graham *et al.* [1999]; Graham *et al.* [2001] and Rogers *et al.* [2000].)

16.17.1 Direct strategies

Direct interventions involve the SLT (or workers trained by the SLT) intervening face to face to modify communication in a person or group who have dementia. Some studies report on techniques devised by SLTs to target relearning or maintenance of ability to name specific word groups or learn key information in early to middle dementia. Spaced retrieval (SR) (involving rehearsal and recall at gradually increasing intervals) (Abrahams and Camp, 1993; Brush and Camp, 1998) or repeated exposure and questioning (by students) about related semantic properties (Arkin *et al.*, 2000) facilitated performance on specific tasks with some maintenance over several weeks (Abrahams and Camp, 1993). Potential functional communication improvements were not measured, however, Brush and Camp reported some functional use of learned information to achieve speech-language goals.

Some direct interventions devised by SLTs have targeted communicative processes that decline in early to middle AD. Arkin and Mahendra (2001) compared experimental (n = 7) and control (n = 4) groups over 20 weeks. All participants went to twice weekly exercise programmes. During one weekly exercise session students presented language and memory exercises, such as picture description, word association, simple discourse role plays and word category assignments. Controls experienced unstructured conversation with students. There were no significant differences between groups on the ABCD or on discourse meaningfulness; however, the experimental group had a significantly higher ratio of different nouns to total nouns at post test.

Clark and Witte (1991) advocated clinician training of those with early AD in the use of adaptive communication strategies to prolong effective communication – for example, learning when to use statements such as 'Please repeat exactly what you just said' or 'Say what you said more slowly', or 'Give me a little time. I'm having trouble finding the exact words'. or, 'I forgot what we were discussing'. Clark and Witte also suggested teaching facilitation strategies to assist self-cueing – for example, using circumlocution or a semantically related word. Furthermore, they suggested teaching a script strategy for simple storytelling (e.g. theme, characters, setting and events) to improve cohesion and topic maintenance. Clark and Witte recommended groups as ideal in early AD for practising these adaptive and facilitative strategies. In addition, they argued that sharing of useful conversational strategies and discussion of difficulties would help to reduce communicative stress. Clark (1988) (cited in Clark and Witte, 1991) used the above strategies with a group of eight people with mild to moderate AD. Carers reported maintained or increased functional communication, and scoring on aphasia test batteries was stable over six months.

Clark and Witte (1991) also advocated group programmes in later dementia with the clinician facilitating use of residual communication strengths by introducing tangible stimuli of interest to group members. Santo Pietro and Boczko (2001) used intact procedural memories to facilitate communication in groups for people in residential care with mild–moderate to moderate–severe AD. 'Breakfast Clubs' were run each working day for 12 weeks and involved members using greetings, discussing and choosing food for breakfast, helping one another prepare ingredients, setting the table, general conversation (e.g. 'The homes we grew up in'), cleaning up and then saying goodbye. Initially, speech–language clinicians and later trained facilitators provided visual and semantic cues, paired choices and trigger phrases to help members communicate choices and ingredients required. Participants reclaimed procedural memories for actions such as pouring, cutting, stirring and breaking eggs. Breakfast Club participants improved significantly with performance on the ABCD and had more self-initiated on-topic comments per session, more cross-conversation exchanges and increased initiation of procedural memories. Anecdotally, participants were observed laughing and singing together and had increased

involvement with activities of daily living and social pursuits, along with decreased agitation and wandering. Matched controls attending a conversation group, showed either no gains or slight declines over the same period.

Sonas aPc (activating potential for communication) is a multisensory packaged programme designed to activate communication and reduce social isolation in older people (mainly those with moderate to severe dementia – some non-verbal) (Threadgold, 2002). A group of eight older people meet once weekly with a trained facilitator – an SLT or other worker. Care staff have been trained in over 200 sites in Ireland and the UK (Connors 2001a). As participants arrive, a signature tune plays to trigger memories of previous meetings followed by sung individual greetings. There is then a sequence of gentle exercises with stimulation of the sense of smell, relaxing music during which taste and smell are stimulated, lively music for clapping, dance or percussion use, poetry reading (including opportunities for participant presentation), a singalong, sung individual leave-taking and final signature tune. Connors (2001b) evaluated the Sonas programme on 27 people with dementia over a 6-month period. They improved significantly with communication and cognition after 3 months. Initial gains were not maintained at 6 months; however, cross-programme difference scores approached significance for communication. Observation of videotaped sessions also indicated increased participation across the 6 months.

Fried-Oken et al. (2000) discussed the use Augmentative and Alternative Communication (AAC) to facilitate communication in late dementia. Although protocols guiding such work are still emerging, they suggested intervention over time would best meet individuals' complex and changing communication needs. They highlighted need for longitudinal studies to determine most appropriate use of intervention time (e.g. examining whether people benefit from learning to communicate with symbols and pictures when they can still read). They also asserted that cognitive-linguistic strengths and weaknesses would need to be carefully assessed to develop appropriate AAC input and/or output systems (e.g. instead of devising appropriate motoric access, determining if an alternative route could be found into the lexicon). They stressed the importance of also accommodating caregivers' needs, to increase chances of communication success.

In later dementia, SLTs can develop personal communication dictionaries to assist carers to interact with individuals with dementia – even with non-intentional communicators. Communication dictionaries were originally developed for early communicators (Siegel and Whetherby, 2000). Development of a communication dictionary requires careful observation and documentation of consistent non-verbal ways in which an individual behaves when wanting something. The SLT may involve carers in recording observations in specific categories – 'What Fred does' (e.g. takes your hand and pulls it towards his mouth), 'What it might mean' (e.g. 'I'm hungry or thirsty'), 'What you should do' (e.g. Give food or drink if appropriate or distract with another activity if not). A personal communication dictionary is useful in institutional settings where carers may not know the person. It should be easily accessible (e.g. a poster or notebook) for both reference and amendment. In addition, the dictionary may be helpful to familiar carers in structuring observations to best meet the person's needs.

16.17.2 Indirect strategies

Conversation is collaborative. Where one partner has AD, the other can use strategies to facilitate communication (Kessler et al., 2001). Enderby (2002) recommended SLTs' involvement in role play and group practice with carers to reinforce new techniques.

There are numerous documented strategies for optimizing comprehension in dementia. Generally, a person, when speaking to a partner with dementia, should to try to match language complexity to individual levels (Haak, 2002). In early dementia, using slightly slower speech with strategic pausing and reduced information is recommended (Bayles and Tomoeda, 1995; Bourgeois, 2002). As dementia progresses, it is best to converse about tangible things, simplify vocabulary, use non-verbal cues and restate when a message is not understood (Bayles and Tomoeda, 1995) or has been forgotten (Enderby, 2002). Before beginning, it may also be useful to orient the person to topic and then maintain and extend it (Kessler et al., 2001). In middle to late dementia, questions with alternatives (e.g. 'Do you want fish or chicken?'), short utterances and full names (rather than pronouns) are helpful (Haak, 2002). Demonstration to aid comprehension, avoidance of sarcasm and innuendo, use of native language and familiar wording (e.g. respectful title or maiden name) should also boost conversation. Where confusion is likely, carers should reintroduce themselves (Haak, 2002). Important topics should also be avoided where people are upset or tired (Enderby, 2002). In late dementia, sensory stimulation (e.g. tone of voice, smell, touch) can also be used to aid comprehension (Bourgeois, 2002) without patronizing or talking in front of the person as if they were absent (Haak, 2002).

There are fewer documented strategies for facilitation of expression in dementia. People with mild AD should be allowed to speak even when having word-finding difficulties (unless assistance is requested) and should be encouraged to use spared communicative abilities to reinforce self-worth (e.g. reading to a grandchild or writing letters to friends) (Haak, 2002). They may also benefit from encouragement to verbalize actions – for example, 'I'm going to have my dinner' (Haak, 2002). In keeping conversation flowing, Watson et al. (1999) found hypothesis formation more effective than requests for more information. Knowing the background of the person is also helpful in optimizing communication in institutional care settings (Enderby 2002; Haak, 2002). Greater response may be evoked if topics of interest are found. Sensitivity to use of words, gesture, tone of voice and context all help those with later dementia to feel comfortable making

communicative attempts (Enderby, 2002). Although people speak jargon or are mute, they may still have a message to communicate (Haak, 2002).

Despite the numerous strategies recommended regarding communication in dementia, there has been little work investigating frequency of use. Recently, Kessler et al. (2002) examined this question in five men with mild probable AD and their wives and a corpus of identified strategies. Videotaped 10-minute interactions indicated the strategies used by all wives – yes/no questions, facial expression, eye contact, allowing time to respond, showing as well as saying and cueing to topic. Further strategies were used by most, some or none. Overall, wives spontaneously used 60 per cent of identified strategies. This study provides a beginning in examining natural strategy use by carers. Watson et al. (1999) provided some insight into this complex question, observing that where a person has AD, interactants did not always repair misunderstandings, but rather preserved dignity of the speaker with AD. The following studies have all examined how education by SLTs might change carers interactions.

Bourgeois et al. (1997) trained seven home caregivers over 12 weeks to modify repetitive verbalizations in spouses with probable mild to moderate AD. In weekly 1-hour sessions, most troublesome verbalizations were identified and caregivers trained by the clinician to record behavioural baselines and to provide simple cue cards (e.g. with orientation information) in response. After baseline (2–7 weeks), the programme was implemented and spouses recorded additional data (4–10 weeks). Time series data indicated that four spouses recorded lower rates of repetitive verbalizations during intervention. Another recorded a low baseline, whilst the other two least consistently used the intervention. Follow-up data (recorded monthly rather than weekly) appeared quite similar to intervention. Seven control participants (whose caregivers recorded data without implementing strategies) showed increased repetitive verbalizations across phases.

Bourgeois (1992) explored introduction of personalized memory wallets to enhance communication in six people with mild to moderate AD. Using explanations of response definitions and role play, she trained carers in wallet use. Wallets contained individualized simple written information, drawings and photographs. Carers used the wallet daily across 4 or 5 days with participants to facilitate discussion about 'day', 'family' and 'yourself'. During this training and a maintenance period, participants made more novel on-topic statements and fewer ambiguous utterances. A further three participants also appeared to benefit from introduction of wallets even with minimal carer training. Most participants also used their wallets spontaneously to initiate conversations. Similarly, Baker (2001) reported on the use of life story books (LSBs) with people who had severe dementia and some retained language skills (verbal or non-verbal). SLTs compiled LSBs and trained relatives and staff (e.g. in pace of presentation and cueing). LSBs were initially monitored and changes made following feedback. After 6 months, reports from carer questionnaires indicated more focused and shared conversation, revived spousal involvement and changed staff attitudes towards the person. Staff also had greater understanding of the SLT's role and increased interest in future collaborations.

Spilkin and Bethlehem (2003) extended memory book use a little further. They collected two 10-minute baselines of interactions between a person with moderate to severe dementia and his daughter using a memory book. Initially, the daughter was given only a handout on basic strategies for book use. Spilkin and Bethlehem then used CA to analyse turn-taking, topic management and conversational repair. Results were used to identify breakdowns and the daughter was trained to use strategies (e.g. more close-ended and single-part questions, tolerating silences for longer, speaking about the pictures and elaborating) to modify interactions with her father. Immediately after training and 1 week later, they recorded two further 10-minute samples. After intervention, CA revealed the father used less minimal turns (e.g. 'mm'), more on-topic responses and he introduced and maintained more topics, whilst perseverating less. He was also more able to repair utterances and, overall, assumed a more active role, probably because his daughter provided more structure in conversation.

SLTs have a role in formal training of care staff to optimize communication in dementia. The FOCUSED programme emphasizes strategies based on an interactive discourse model – F – face to face, O – orient to conversation topic, C – continue the topic, U – unstick communication blocks, S – structure questions, E – exchange conversation and D – direct short sentences (Ripich and Wykle, 1996). Presented over several sessions, it involves role play, discussion and home assignments. In addition, Bryan and Maxim (1998) described communication training strategies used with care staff in the UK. Furthermore, Maxim *et al.* (2001) discussed factors that contribute towards SLTs successfully delivering workshops to care workers, and Pietro (2002) emphasized the importance of evaluating training outcomes on communicative behaviour in the real world.

16.18 ENVIRONMENTAL BARRIERS TO COMMUNICATION

As language devolves, the person with dementia relies increasingly on the environment as a dynamic contributor towards functioning (Clark, 1995). Given increasing problems with hearing and vision, it is critical that these problems be corrected optimally (with encouragement to wear aids) and that environments have limited background noise (e.g. using sound absorbing materials, turning televisions off) and good lighting (Enderby, 2002). In addition, good management of other medical conditions and drug regimens can affect communication positively (Clark, 1995). Although physical space is often quite limited and opportunities for solitude or intimacy rare, social interaction can also be minimal (Lubinski, 1991).

Use of space is important – for example, placing chairs and beds in proximity for comfortable interaction or using round tables at meal times (Morse and Intrieri, 1997). There are also sometimes attitudes that need to be challenged, such as ignoring those with severe communication problems (Lubinski, 1991), or inadequately trained staff speaking to residents only about physical care and failing to use effective communication techniques to reduce aggression (Pietro, 2002). If people have independent mobility, the environment needs to be set up (e.g. colour coding) so that they can find their way to spaces where they can interact (Lubinski, 1991). Unfortunately, when facilities are being designed or renovated, political will to prioritize communication-friendly environments can be lacking when features like cost, physical care and security are considered (Lubinski, 1991). Because more primitive senses of smell and taste may be relatively preserved in later dementia, stimulation of these senses via spice jars, scratch and sniff books, ethnic foods or texture of garden loam can also trigger conversation (Lubinski, 1991; Bourgeois, 1991). Recent studies have also suggested that having a pet or even a toy present can facilitate communication (e.g. Hopper *et al.*, 1998).

16.19 EATING IN DEMENTIA

In later dementia changes in swallow physiology and sensory loss often affect eating and swallowing (Logemann, 2003). Even in early AD, changes in duration of swallow phases have been noted (Priefer and Robbins, 1997). As such, SLTs have a role in optimizing swallowing and reducing the risk of aspiration pneumonia. Logemann observed that people can sometimes be taught strategies to upgrade food and drink consistencies that they can swallow safely, while others may be helped without learning, for example by changing consistencies to prevent aspiration, by triggering pharyngeal swallowing using certain intense tastes or bolus temperatures, or by positioning (Gillick and Mitchell, 2002). To reduce guesswork, it is important for SLTs to use an instrumental examination where pharyngeal dysphagia is suspected (Logemann, 2003). Nonetheless, people with advanced dementia cannot cooperate with such procedures (Gillick and Mitchell, 2002). Where people can no longer swallow safely, a percutaneous endoscopic gastrostomy (PEG) tube is sometimes inserted to administer liquid food directly into the stomach (Gillick and Mitchell, 2002). SLTs also have a role in recommending when this procedure may be considered. However, this decision is not just about swallowing status, but also PEG side effects (of diarrhoea and nausea in 10 per cent of people), likelihood of people pulling the tube out and findings that people with advanced dementia may well not benefit from PEG feeding in terms of survival or comfort (Gillick and Mitchell, 2002; Logemann, 2003). If there is no living will regarding medical intervention, guardians may have to make this difficult decision based on what people would choose for themselves (Gillick and Mitchell, 2002); however, in reality, PEG use can vary between countries or even doctors within the same hospital.

16.20 CONCLUSIONS

Communication, amongst other things, allows elderly people to vent anxieties, relieve loneliness, describe medical symptoms and stimulate cognition (Lubinski, 1991). As such, it seems obvious that SLTs should be increasingly involved in fostering communication in dementia. Nonetheless, in 2002 Bryan and Maxim observed that, in the previous 10 years, there had only been a very small rise in the numbers of SLTs specializing in dementia – despite the proportion of people over age 60 rising astronomically in coming decades. They advocated for SLTs becoming more committed to improving dementia services and gave four major reasons why this is timely – interest shown by the government, older people's increasing awareness of health issues, advances in understanding dementia and increasing evidence to support intervention. Exploring intervention has been a focus of this chapter. In addition to dementia assessment and dysphagia work, there is certainly evidence to support the SLT's role in working directly with those who have dementia, in educating carers and other professionals and in advocating for communication-friendly environments. Nonetheless, many studies reviewed have small sample sizes or generally lack methodological rigour. Future research should address issues such as: what constitutes success in these degenerative conditions and how, for whom and for how long communication interventions are effective in the real world. To address these issues effectively, single-case investigations require collection of lengthy baseline as well as intervention data, whilst group studies require strict selection criteria and well-matched control groups (see Lum, 2001). Given that future SLT resources are unlikely to be bountiful, research also needs to address where resources are best expended.

REFERENCES

Abrahams JP and Camp CJ. (1993) Maintenance and generalization of object naming training in anomia associated with degenerative dementia. *Clinical Gerontologist* **12**: 57–72

Ames D, Flicker L, Helme R. (1992) A memory clinic at a geriatric hospital: Rationale, routine and results from the first 100 patients. *Medical Journal of Australia* **156**: 618–622

Arkin S and Mahendra N. (2001) Discourse analysis of Alzheimer's patients before and after intervention: methodology and outcomes. *Aphasiology* **15**: 533–569

Arkin S, Rose C, Hopper T. (2000) Implicit and explicit learning gains in Alzheimer's patients: effects of naming and information retrieval training. *Aphasiology* **14**: 723–742

Armstrong L, Bayles K, Borthwick S, Tomoeda C. (1996) Use of the Arizona Battery for Communication Disorders of Dementia in the UK. *European Journal of Disorders of Communication* **31**: 171–180

Baker J. (2001) Life story books for the elderly mentally ill. *International Journal of Language and Communication Disorders* **36** (Suppl.): 185–187

Bayles KA and Tomoeda CK. (1993) *The Arizona Battery for Communication Disorders of Dementia*. Austin, Texas, Pro-Ed

Bayles KA and Tomoeda CK. (1994) *Functional Linguistic Communication Inventory*. Austin, Texas, Pro-Ed

Bayles KA and Tomoeda CK. (1995) *The ABCs of Dementia*. Phoenix, Arizona, Canyonlands Publishing, Inc

Bayles KA, Tomoeda CK, Trosset MW. (1992) Relation of linguistic communication abilities of Alzheimer's patients to stage of disease. *Brain and Language* **42**: 454–472

Bourgeois MS. (1991) Communication treatment for adults with dementia. *Journal of Speech and Hearing Research* **34**: 831–844

Bourgeois MS. (1992) Evaluating memory wallets in conversations with persons with dementia. *Journal of Speech and Hearing Research* **35**: 1344–1357

Bourgeois MS. (1997) Modifying repetitive verbalizations of community-dwelling patients with AD. *The Gerontologist* **37**: 30–39

Bourgeois MS. (2002) Where is my wife and when am I going home? The challenge of communicating with persons with dementia. *Alzheimer's Care Quarterly* **3**: 132–144

Brush JA and Camp CG. (1998) Using spaced retrieval as an intervention during speech-language therapy. *Clinical Gerontologist* **19**: 51–64

Bryan K and Maxim J. (1998) Enabling care staff to relate to older communication disabled people. *International Journal of Language and Communication Disorders*. **33** (Suppl.): 121–125

Bryan K and Maxim J. (2002.) Letter to the editor. *International Journal of Language and Communication Disorders*. **37**(2): 215–222

Bryan K, Binder J, Dann C *et al.* (2001) Development of a screening instrument for language in older people. *Ageing and Mental Health* **5**: 371–378

Clark LW. (1988) Enhancement of communication adequacy in early stage Alzheimer's disease patients. Unpublished research paper, New York, Hunter College of CUNY

Clark LW. (1995) Interventions for persons with Alzheimer's disease: Strategies for maintaining and enhancing communicative success. *Topics in Language Disorders* **15**: 47–65

Clark LW and Witte K. (1991) Nature and efficacy of communication management in Alzheimer's disease. In: R Lubinski (ed.), *Dementia and Communication*. Philadelphia, BC Decker

Connors TF. (2001a) *Sonas aPc for Family Carers of People with Dementia: a community study*. Dublin, Sonas aPc

Connors TF. (2001b) *Activating the Potential for Communication in People with Dementia in Residential Care*. Sonas Model Unit Project 2, Dublin, Sonas aPc

Enderby P. (2002) Promoting communication skills with people who have dementia. In: G Stokes and F Goudie (eds), *The Essential Dementia Care Handbook*. Bicester, Oxfordshire: Speechmark, pp. 102–108

Fried-Oken M, Rau MT, Oken BS. (2000) AAC and dementia. In: D Beukleman, K Yorkston and J Reichle (eds), *Augmentative and Alternative Communication for Adults with Acquired Neurological Disorders*. Baltimore, Paul H Brooks, pp. 375–405

Gillick MR and Mitchell SL. (2002) Facing eating difficulties in end stage dementia. *Alzheimer's Care Quarterly* **3**: 227–232

Graham K, Patterson K, Pratt K, Hodges J. (1999) Relearning and a case of subsequent forgetting of semantic category exemplars in a case of semantic dementia. *Neuropsychology* **13**: 359–380

Graham K, Patterson K, Pratt K, Hodges J. (2001) Can repeated exposure to 'forgotten' vocabulary help alleviate word-finding difficulties in semantic dementia? An illustrative study. *Neuropsychological Rehabilitation* **11**: 429–454

Haak NJ. (2002) Maintaining connections: understanding communication from the perspective of persons with dementia. *Alzheimer's Care Quarterly* **3**: 116–131

Hopper T and Bayles KA. (2001) Management of neurogenic communication disorders associated with dementia. In: R Chapey (ed.), *Language Intervention Strategies in Aphasia and Related Neurogenic Communication Disorders*, 4th edition. Philadelphia: Lippincott, Williams and Wilkins, 829–846

Hopper T, Bayles KA, Tomoeda CK. (1998) Using toys to facilitate communicative function in individuals with Alzheimer's disease. *Journal of Medical Speech Language Pathology* **6**: 73–80

Kessler T, Croot K, Togher L. (2001) Strategies to facilitate communication with a person with dementia of the Alzheimer type. *Proceedings of the 2001 Speech Pathology Australia National Conference*, Melbourne, 20–23 May, pp. 27–34

Kessler T, Croot K, Togher L. (2002) Recommended strategies for facilitating communication with people with dementia: Do spouses use them, do they know they use them, and how easy is it to know whether they help? *10th International Aphasia Rehabilitation Conference*, Brisbane, Australia 24–26 July, 2002

Logemann JA. (2003) Dysphagia and dementia. *ASHA Leader* **8**: pp. 1, 14

Lubinski R. (1991) Environmental considerations for elderly patients. In: R Lubinski (ed.), *Dementia and Communication*. Philadelphia, BC Decker Inc, pp. 257–273

Lum C. (2001) *Scientific Thinking in Speech and Language Therapy*. London, Lawrence Erlbaum

Lydall-Smith S, Moorhouse B, Gilchrist J. (1996) *Culturally Appropriate Dementia Assessment*. Canberra, Commonwealth of Australia

McKeith IG, Galasko GK, Wilcock GK, Byrne EJ. (1995) Lewy body dementia – diagnosis and treatment. *British Journal of Psychiatry* **167**: 709–17

McKhann G, Drachman D, Folstein M *et al.* (1984) Clinical diagnosis of Alzheimer's disease: report of the NINCDS-ADRDA work group under the auspices of Department of Health and Human Services task force on Alzheimer's disease. *Neurology* **34**: 939–944

Maxim J, Bryan K, Axlerod L, Jordan L, Bell L. (2001) Speech and language therapists as trainers: Enabling care staff working with older people. *International Journal of Language and Communication Disorders* **36** (Suppl.): 194–199

Mentis M, Briggs-Whittaker J, Gramigna GD. (1995) Discourse topic management in senile dementia of the Alzheimer type. *Journal of Speech and Hearing Research* **38**: 1054–1066

Mesulam MM. (1982) Slowly progressive aphasia without generalized dementia. *Annals of Neurology* **11**: 592–598

Moorhouse B, Douglas J, Pannacio J, Steel G. (1999) Use of the Arizona Battery for Communication Disorders of Dementia in an Australian context. *Asia Pacific Journal of Speech Language and Hearing* **4**: 93–107

Morse J and Intrieri R. (1997) 'Talk to me'. Patient communication in a long-term care facility. *Journal of Psychosocial Nursing* **35**: 34–43

Pietro MJS. (2002) Training nursing assistants to communicate effectively with people with Alzheimer's disease: A call for action. *Alzheimer's Care Quarterly* **3**: 157–164

Powell AL, Cummings JL, Hill MA, Benson DF. (1988) Speech and language alterations in multi-infarct dementia. *Neurology* **38**: 717–719

Priefer BA and Robbins J. (1997) Eating changes in mild-stage Alzheimer's disease: a pilot study. *Dysphagia* **12**: 212–221

Reisberg B, Ferris SH, De Leon MJ, Crook T. (1982) The global deterioration scale for assessment of primary degenerative dementia. *American Journal of Psychiatry* **139**: 1136–1139

Reisberg B, Franssen EH, Hasan SM *et al.* (1999) Retrogenesis: clinical, physiologic and pathologic mechanisms in brain ageing Alzheimer's and other dementing processes. *European Archives of Psychiatry and Clinical Neuroscience* **249**(S3): 111/28–111/36

Ripich DN and Wykle ML. (1996) *Alzheimer's Disease Communication Guide: the FOCUSED Program for Caregivers*. San Antonio, The Psychological Corporation

Rogers M, King J, Alarcon N. (2000) AAC and dementia. In: D Beukleman, K Yorkston and J Reichle (eds), *Augmentative and Alternative Communication for Adults with Acquired Neurological Disorders*. Baltimore, Paul H Brooks, pp. 305–337

Santo Pietro MJ and Boczko F. (2001) The breakfast club. *Alzheimer's Care Quarterly*. **2**: 56–60

Siegel E and Wetherby A. (2000) Nonsymbolic communication. In: M Snell and F Brown (eds), *Instruction of Students with Severe Disabilities*, 5th edition. Upper Saddle River, NJ, Prentice Hall, pp. 409–51

Spilkin ML and Bethlehem D. (2003) A conversational analysis approach to facilitating communication with memory books. *Advances in Speech-Language Pathology* **5**: 105–118

Stevens S and Ripich D. (1999) The role of the speech and language therapist. In: G Wilcock, R Bucks and K Rockwood (eds), *Diagnosis and Management of Dementia*. Oxford, Oxford University Press, pp. 137–57

Stevens S, Pitt B, Nicholl C *et al.* (1992) Language assessment in a memory clinic. *International Journal of Geriatric Psychiatry* **7**: 45–51

Stevens S, Harvey J, Kelly C *et al.* (1996) Characteristics of language performance in four groups of patients attending a memory clinic. *International Journal of Geriatric Psychiatry* **11**: 973–982

Thompson CK, Ballard KJ, Tait ME, Weintraub S, Mesulam M. (1997) Patterns of language decline in non-fluent primary progressive aphasia. *Aphasiology* **11**: 297–321

Threadgold M. (2002) Sonas aPc – a new lease of life for some. *Signpost Journal* **7**(2)

Tomoeda CK. (2001) Comprehensive assessment for dementia: A necessity for differential diagnosis and management. *Seminars in Speech and Language* **22**: 275–289

Vuorinen E, Laine M, Rinne J. (2000) Common pattern of language impairment in vascular dementia and in Alzheimer's disease. *Alzheimer Disease and Associated Disorders* **14**: 81–86

Watson CM, Chenery HJ, Carter MS. (1999) An analysis of trouble and repair in the natural conversations of people with dementia of the Alzheimer's type. *Aphasiology* **13**: 195–218

Weintraub S, Rubin N, Mesulam M-M. (1990) Primary progressive aphasia: Longitudinal course, neuropsychological profile, and language features. *Archives of Neurology* **47**: 1329–1335

Westbury C and Bub D. (1997) Primary progressive aphasia: a review of 112 cases. *Brain and Language* **60**: 381–406

Physiotherapy

IRENE SMITH LASSEN

Physiotherapy is based upon a comprehension of the human being as a dynamic whole with motor function as a part of an optimal psychosocial function. The body is the relation to the world (Merleau-Ponty, 1986) and it is seen as both a subject and an object. Through movements the human communicates knowledge and correlation to the environment, but movements are also a goal-directed solution of functional tasks and thereby a precondition of creating and maintaining a social life, an important topic when you are dealing with dementia.

The physiotherapist examines the body from an understanding of the mutual action between body and emotions, the body expressing and regulating emotions while being a biological and biochemical phenomenon, and evaluates the type and level of strain and resources in the patient. This information about the physical function contribute to diagnosis and therapy (Thornquist, 1992).

Elderly people with dementia often suffer from various somatic illnesses, neurological or musculoskeletal problems, that on the one hand may affect their motor function and state of mind, and on the other hand are reinforced by their mental and cognitive dysfunction.

Physiotherapy for demented people can take many forms with different foci depending on the severity of the illness and the purpose of the physiotherapeutic contribution.

In the early stage of dementia the object of physiotherapy is promoting awareness of the body and its possibly hidden resources working consciously with experiences of the body as a part of the whole identity. Later in the course the physiotherapy can be aiming at decreasing anxiety and depressive symptoms that may follow the progress of the disease.

Gradually, as the dementia develops and the patient's functions decline, the treatment focuses on activating the patient and establishing an environment that maintains and motivates movement and activities of daily living.

Owing to great variation in symptoms in patients with dementia, the physiotherapy must be directed to the individual's functional ability in order to stimulate and support the patient in making the most of their potential. This chapter will describe how physiotherapy is applied in the psychiatric field and how the discipline may contribute to the general management of dementia.

16.21 THE DEMENTED PATIENT

Dementia produces an appreciable decline in intellectual functioning and usually some interference with personal activities of daily living (World Health Organization [WHO], 1992). The decline affects different patients differently and must be managed individually depending on the patient's memory, thinking and reasoning capacity, emotional control, perception of stimulus and ability to orientate and learn, understand and communicate. However, all patients respond positively when treated with common courtesy, kindness and respect (Laerum, 2003).

Dementia patients are exposed to personality and behavioural changes and the progressive nature of the illness affects them psychologically. Their physical functions, however, are not debilitated necessarily concurrently with the other functions and here patients can use their remaining resources and gain a feeling of success, adding quality to their lives.

16.22 BODY AWARENESS THERAPY

Psychiatric physiotherapy has a short tradition, but in recent decades there has been an increasing acknowledgement of how the mind and the body influence each other, and the use of basic body awareness therapy (BAT) has been steadily growing in physiotherapy practice (Gyllensten, 2001).

BAT is the common name for a number of physiotherapeutic approaches using a holistic physiotherapy treatment (Roxendal, 1985). In the 1970s Gertrud Roxendal, physiotherapist and doctor of philosophy, established BAT in Scandinavian countries, integrating a number of techniques which inspired her. After meeting the French psychoanalyst and movement teacher Jacques Dropsy she recognized the value of his movement practice and theories and integrated his work in physiotherapy practice under the name of Basic BAT. In this branch of 'body awareness' the patient works with the basic functions of movements related to posture, coordination, free breathing and awareness (Roxendal, 1987). This work with the body constitutes the basis for the quality of movement in action, the expression of the self, interaction with others and involvement in activities in life (Dropsy, 1975, 1988; Roxendal, 1987). The treatment also inspired the creation of an assessment scale, the Body Awareness Scale (BAS), an instrument that measures the functions of grounding, posture, coordination, breathing and flow, that are the targets of Basic BAT practice.

Roxendal developed the theories of the body ego, an expression first used by Freud (1923), and she defined this as the bodily aspect of the inseparable unit body/mind that is the human being, or total identity (Roxendal and Wahlberg, 1995). She pointed out four cornerstones of important aspects in treatment:

- the encounter or interaction between the patient and the physiotherapist;
- the activation of the motivation of the patient;
- the conscious view of the human being; and
- the movement praxis of Basic BAT.

In this way Roxendal was a pioneer in establishing a broader view of factors active in physiotherapeutic treatment and the outcome of treatment (Gyllensten, 2001). Psychiatric physiotherapy has developed both theoretically and methodologically from Roxendal's work and is now practised outside Scandinavia.

16.23 CLINICAL PRAXIS OF BAT

In BAT one uses movements, breathing, massage and awareness to try to restore balance, flexibility and the unity of body and mind, working with the resources of the body as a whole. The therapist coordinator encourages the patient to move in better ways to attain postural control, balance, free breathing and coordination, using both body and words to guide the patient. The relation to the ground, vertical balance in the centre line, centring of movements and coordination from the solar plexus area, breathing, flow and awareness are seen as important aspects of the body ego trained in Basic BAT (Gyllensten, 2001). The movements in BAT are quite simple, fundamental and easy to learn, which makes them very suitable for demented patients, who often lack the ability to understand and perform more complicated exercises.

Basic BAT consists of movements of the body as a whole in lying, sitting, standing and walking positions. The work usually starts with stretching exercises on the floor or on a couch, and breathing exercises aimed at letting go of old compensations and control of the breathing and just letting it be. The patient progresses to the sitting or standing position in order to not get trapped in a regressive state. Here the work of becoming more aware and in contact with the antigravity muscles continues. The three basic coordinations starting in the trunk are practised:

- flexion-extension around the centre of movement in the solar plexus area;
- rotation around the vertical axis; and
- trunk rotation and counter rotation as seen in walking.

Mental presence and awareness are key words taught from the very first exercise – the person is stimulated by turning the attention both to doing and to what is experienced in the movements (Roxendal, 1987; Dropsy, 1988; Gyllensten, 2001).

Focusing on activating health promoting resources rather than on physical symptoms and limitations, BAT is a useful approach in the treatment of patients with dementia. The features of dementia include disturbances of cognitive functions and the sensorium as well as changes in physical functions (e.g. reduced trunk rotation); by initiating BAT at an early stage the basic elements of the body ego are stimulated and may help the patient to maintain functional skills and an experience of identity.

16.23.1 The role of the physiotherapist

The professional role of the physiotherapist is to guide and support the patient in the process of deepened awareness, and pictures and images can be used to facilitate the experience associated with the movement. Most of all, the physiotherapist is there to stimulate the search to become aware of dormant resources associated with vertical balance, freedom of breathing, movement and action. The therapist is able to support and give help only in accordance with their own level of awareness (Roxendal, 1987; Dropsy, 1988; Gyllensten, 2001).

16.24 MASSAGE, TOUCHING

The treatment is often supplemented by massage. The skin is the largest and most important sensory organ, and physical touch stimulates inner mental and physiological processes

(Mattson, 1998). Massage reduces muscle tension and rhythmical stroking of the skin has a medical effect in consequence of secreting oxytocin: reduced pain sensitivity, anxiety level, blood pressure and pulse indicating a calm wellbeing (Petterson *et al.*, 1996a, b).

The human being has a lifelong need for physical touch, and massage is an important form of communication. Touching is an intimate kind of contact that creates a connection between human beings (Montagu, 1986). Through the hands the therapist is in contact with respiration, emotionality, movements, tension and changes in tension in the patient. BAT incorporates special massage techniques that can activate both postural and autonomous reflexes (Mattson, 1998). Tactile stimulation of the skin evokes a more distinct sensation of the body and its centre, diverting attention from unpleasant thoughts and emotions and perhaps diminishing agitation and motor restlessness. Elderly demented patients are in physical contact with nursing staff when washing, dressing, feeding and having their personal hygiene attended to but, beyond that, massage can be given with the one purpose of yielding a positive bodily experience. Caregivers can profitably be instructed in therapeutic touching techniques to make nursing situations mutually pleasant.

16.25 INTERACTION

The importance of interaction between patient and physiotherapist is a central feature in clinical practice and studies have focused on the most important factors for successful treatment. Thornquist (1991) indicates the importance of the physiotherapist continuously using his or her body to communicate throughout the whole physiotherapy encounter. She argues that this communication is a central aspect of patient-centredness, and she also points to the problem of interpreting body language as an observer, since a gesture or a posture is dependent on the specific context (Thornquist, 1990). Self-experience and clinical experience develop knowledge in the cognitive, affective and psychomotor domains, and when working with demented people one has to deal with all these domains. According to Watzlawick *et al.* (1967) all behaviour in an interactional situation gives out messages and is thereby communication. Even nonsense, silence, withdrawal, immobility (postural silence) or any other form of denial is itself a communication. If the patient presents in this way, one should attempt to understand the underlying messages.

Establishing and maintaining contact focusing on the patient's resources are important aspects of the interaction and are vital for outcome (Gyllensten *et al.*, 1999, 2000). These might, however, be complicated in the treatment of demented patients if their motivation fluctuates. Clinical experience and reflecting on communication and the therapeutic process are important tools in interaction, as well as in forming an alliance.

The sooner in the dementia course the physiotherapy is implemented the easier it will be to develop an alliance with the patient, which can be maintained through subsequent years.

16.26 DEPRESSION AND ANXIETY

Changes in mood or emotion are prevalent in the spectrum of dementia (WHO, 1992). Having a depression is not just a matter of the mind but also affects the body. Patients with depression in comparison with non-depressed persons have more muscular tension, pain complaints, negative attitudes towards their own physical ability, restrained breathing and less freedom of movement (Jacobsen *et al.*, 2003). These symptoms are easily mixed up with and mistaken for symptoms owing to somatic illnesses and physical decline owing to ageing. However, they are the manifestation of depression in the body. In combination with depressive symptoms, a higher level of anxiety appears causing pain, provoking tension and unpleasant bodily symptoms. Clinical experience in physiotherapeutic treatment of depression and anxiety shows that patients benefit from BAT, which includes calming massage and relaxation techniques (e.g. stretching and releasing the body alternately). Treatment pays attention to normalizing the tension level and building up ego-forces, and the patient's focus on body management to be able to control the symptoms and use the body in a more harmonious way.

There are several studies showing that physical activity has a positive effect on the mental state, decreasing anxiety and depressive symptoms. Blumenthal *et al.* (1999) found that exercise training in older depressed patients accelerated the effect of medical treatment and follow up showed a significant decrease in depressive symptoms and a reduced number of relapses. The physical training must be individualized and supervised to include aerobic training and progressive resistance training (Veale *et al.*, 1992; Singh *et al.*, 1997; Lawler and Hopker, 2001).

16.27 PROMOTING MOBILITY

Physical ability deteriorates with increasing years and the physiological and pathological responses to ageing have a direct effect on movement and function. People with dementia may live a sedentary lifestyle and reach the limit of their physical ability simply in the performance of normal activities of daily living. Inactivity results in increasing dependency on the help of others. A number of age-induced changes that affect movement or function can be prevented, slowed down or even reversed by doing exercises (Trew, 1997).

Patients with dementia should be given opportunities for goal-directed movements in a plain and systematic way to maintain mobility and transfer skills (Oddy, 1998). Movement/mobility/transfer can be defined as movements that enable the patient to perform activities of daily living and to move around in their usual environment. These movements comprise standing up, walking inside/outside and on stairs, sitting down and getting in and out of bed.

The results of goal-directed physical training on impaired elderly people with dementia are significant improvements in the ability to walk and transfer, mobility and balance (Toulotte *et al.*, 2003). Earlier studies providing physiotherapy, including music and movement groups, body awareness and functional mobility training, also showed significant improvements in the mobility skills of elderly people with severe dementing illness (Pomeroy, 1993, 1994). An intervention study providing resistance exercise training proved that neuromuscular strength and function can be rehabilitated in elderly demented people (Thomas and Hageman, 2003).

From clinical experience weight resistance training is an effective, structured method to mobilize physical resources. Records should be kept to motivate patients showing progress and illustrating what they are capable of doing. Training and maintaining mobility skills may postpone the time when the demented patient needs personal care and social services.

16.28 COMMUNICATION

To initiate a movement or a transfer, the dementia patient needs to understand the purpose of the action. Using the voice and body in a certain way, the therapist can facilitate communication and get a successful result. Approaching the patient slowly from in front prevents them from being surprised or scared, and a friendly smile while keeping a distance can make them feel safe.

Verbal commands must be short, concise and simple, instructing the patient in positive phrases, e.g. 'Keep standing!' instead of 'Don't sit down!' because the patient may understand only some of the words (Laerum, 2003). In verbal explanation the words must accurately describe what is to be done. Demonstrating the movement using gestures, signs and touching may clarify to the patient how to move in the right way and in the right direction (Charman, 1997).

Throughout the session it is important to observe the facial expression and body language of the patient to receive an impression of how they respond to the treatment. Strategies for helping patients in daily activities are essential to promote mobility. Nursing staff and relatives are often without sufficient knowledge of techniques for activating the patient, but through instructions from a physiotherapist they can help arrange facilities creating a safe, stimulating environment drawing on the resources of the patient. Guidance and advice for the practical daily care of people with dementia are described in detail by Oddy (1998).

16.29 GROUP ACTIVITY

In some psychogeriatric wards and nursing homes movement groups are practised and have proven very useful to demented patients with similar mobility levels. The activity must be structured in an atmosphere that encourages spontaneous movements: adequate lightning, no interrupting background noises and no big empty spaces around the circle in which the patients are placed. Music can be used to give rhythm and an opportunity to join in the tunes. The patients may not remember the activity from one session to another and must be prepared and invited to participate.

Words and movements applied during the session must be recognizable for the patients, e.g. movements that are related to activities of daily living and that awaken memories. The elements include simple exercises stimulating muscle strength, mobility, balance, body awareness and spatial perception. Long instructions must be avoided in case patients are overstimulated with more information than is necessary. In order not to make patients uncomfortable or insecure, several repetitions are carried out for each exercise and the programme is repeated from one session to another comprising:

- *mobility training*: simple, soft movements related to activities of daily living functions performed at a moderate speed and with the sufficient time during and inbetween the exercises;
- *light aerobic training*: in order to increase the patient's circulation and staying power;
- *simple balance, stability and strength exercises*: such as weight transfer sideways sitting on chairs and pushing a medical ball around a circle;
- *body awareness and spatial exercises*: in which the physiotherapist designates the specific body part and direction for the movement;
- *non-verbal interaction between patients*: by rolling, throwing and kicking a ball or a balloon.

There are both medical and economical benefits of mobility groups. The social contact in the group is essential to prevent isolation and a passive life that usually follows reduced motor skills. The patients dare more in the group and, through visual stimulation, it is easier for them to revive the pleasure of movements. Staying in good physical shape may reduce the consumption of medicine and medical costs. In this way it is possible to avoid side effects and improve quality of life of patients.

16.30 SUMMARY

The demented population is a large and diverse group of patients who present various symptoms of the illness, different somatic symptoms and varying function levels. There is no recipe or formula for physiotherapy and the treatment must be based on individual ability, capacity and interest. A physiotherapeutic assessment contributes to a broader view of the patient in the multidisciplinary arena and, with the therapist's knowledge of the human body and the declining functions owing to ageing and dementia, attention can be focused on preventing the consequences and mobilizing existing physical possibilities. The patients benefit from the simplicity of basic BAT applied in individual treatment and exercise groups, activating physical resources and maintaining their motor skills. Positive sensations of the body can be evoked while the dementia causes loss of functions; promoting mobility and stimulating activities of daily living increases the patient's ability to cope with the dementia. The quality of life gained through physical training results in both personal and economic benefit.

REFERENCES

Blumenthal JA, Babyak MA, Moore KA et al. (1999) Effects of exercise training on older patients with major depression. *Archives of Internal Medicine* **159**: 2349–2356

Charman RA. (1997) Motor learning. In: M Trew and T Everett (eds), *Human Movement. An Introductory Text.* New York, Churchill Livingstone, pp. 87–104

Dropsy J. (1975) *Leva i sin Kropp (Living in your body).* Lund, Aldus

Dropsy J. (1988) *Den Harmoniske Krop (The harmonious body).* Copenhagen, Reitzels Forlag

Freud S. (1923) *The Ego and the Id.* (Standard edition of the complete psychological works of Sigmund Freud). London, Hogarth Press (republished 1961)

Gyllensten AL. (2001) *Basic Body Awareness Therapy: assessment, treatment and interaction.* Lund University, Sweden

Gyllensten AL, Gard G, Salford E, Ekdahl C. (1999) Interaction between patient and physiotherapist: a qualitative study reflecting the physiotherapist's perspective. *Physiotherapy Research International* **4**: 89–109

Gyllensten AL, Gard G, Hansson L, Ekdahl C. (2000) Interaction between patient and physiotherapist in psychiatric care – reflecting the physiotherapist's perspective. *Advances in Physiotherapy* **2**: 157–167

Jacobsen LN, Lassen IS, Friis P et al. (2003) Bodily symptoms in patients with severe depression (submitted).

Laerum M. (2003) Eldre med demens kan faa hjelp til optimal bevegelsesmulighet (Help can be given for optimal mobility of the aged with dementia). *Fysioterapeuten* **70**: 33–35

Lawler DA and Hopker SW. (2001) The effectiveness of exercise as an intervention in the management of depression: systematic review and meta-regression analysis of randomised controlled trials. *BMJ:* **322**: 763–767

Mattson M. (1998) *Body Awareness: applications in physiotherapy.* Umeaa University, Sweden

Merleau-Ponty M. (1986) *Phenomenology of Perception.* London, Routledge and Kegan

Montagu A. (1986) *Touching – the Human Significance of the Skin.* New York, Harper and Row

Oddy R. (1998) *Promoting Mobility for People with Dementia; a Problem-Solving Approach.* Age Concern, London

Petterson M, Alster P, Lundeberg T, Uvnäs-Moberg K. (1996a) Oxytocin causes a long-term decrease of blood pressure in female and male rats. *Psychology and Behaviour* **60**: 1311–1315

Petterson M, Alster P, Lundeberg T, Uvnäs-Moberg K. (1996b) Oxytocin increases nociceptive thresholds in a long-term perspective in female and male rats. *Neuroscience Letters* **212**: 87–90

Pomeroy VM. (1993) The effect of physiotherapy input on mobility skills of elderly people with severe dementing illness. *Clinical Rehabilitation* **7**: 163–170

Pomeroy VM. (1994) Immobility and severe dementia: when is physiotherapy treatment appropriate? *Clinical Rehabilitation* **8**: 226–232

Roxendal G. (1985) *Body Awareness Therapy and the Body Awareness Scale, Treatment and Evaluation in Psychiatric Physiotherapy.* Doctoral dissertation. Gothenburg, Department of Psychiatry, University of Gothenburg, Sweden

Roxendal G. (1987) *Ett Helhetsperspektiv – Sjukgymnastik i Framtiden (A Holistic Perspective – Physiotherapy in the Future.* Lund, Studentlitteratur

Roxendal G and Wahlberg C. (1995) *Behandling og Haandtering i Hverdagen – Haendernes Formidling (Everyday Treatment and Handling – Communicative Hands).* Copenhagen, Reitzels Forlag

Singh NA, Clements KM, Fiatarone MA. (1997) A randomized controlled trial of progressive resistance training in depressed elders. *Journals of Gerontology Series A: Biological Sciences and Medical Sciences* **52**: M27–M35

Thomas VS and Hageman PA. (2003) Can neuromuscular strength and function in people with dementia be rehabilitated using resistance exercise training? Results from a preliminary intervention study. *Journals of Gerontology Series A: Biological Sciences and Medical Sciences* **58**: M746–M751

Thornquist E. (1990) Communication: what happens during the first encounter between patient and physiotherapist. *Scandinavian Journal of Primary Health Care* **8**: 133–138

Thornquist E. (1991) Body communication is a continuous process. *Scandinavian Journal of Primary Health Care* **9**: 191–196

Thornquist E. (1992) *Fysioterapeutens funksjon og rolle innen psykisk helsevern (The function and roll of the physiotherapist in psychiatric health care).* University of Oslo, Norway

Toulotte C, Fabre C, Dangremont B, Lensel G, Thévenon A. (2003) Effects of physical training on the physical capacity of frail, demented patients with a history of falling: a randomised controlled trial. *Age and Ageing* **32**: 67–73

Trew M. (1997) The effects of age on human movement. In: M Trew and T Everett (eds), *Human Movement. An Introductory Text.* New York, Churchill Livingstone, pp. 119–128

Veale D, Le Fevre K, Pantelis C et al. (1992) Aerobic exercise in the adjunctive treatment of depression: a randomized controlled trial. *Journal of the Royal Society of Medicine* **85**: 541–544

Watzlawick P, Weakland JH, Jackson D. (1967) *Pragmatics of Human Communication. A Study of Interactional Patterns, Pathologies and Paradoxes.* New York, WW Norton

World Health Organization (1992) *The ICD-10 Classification of Mental Disorders and Behavioural Disorders. Clinical description and diagnostic guidelines.* Geneva, WHO

17

Sexuality and dementia

JAMES P WARNER

17.1 SEX AND NORMAL AGEING

Many publications about sexuality and sexual behaviour in older people begin with the same message, that it is time to dispel the stereotype that older people are asexual. Although many older people have an active sex life, this age group is more at risk of sexual dysfunction. Furthermore, age is a major risk factor for dementia and the impact a diagnosis of dementia has on sexual behaviour is complex and profound. This chapter outlines the sexual problems faced by individuals with dementia, and the effect that this has on partners and professional carers.

17.1.1 Sexual activity in older people

Although sexual activity appears to decline with advancing age (Schiavi et al., 1990; Kaiser, 1996), sexual activity does not stop, at least among many older individuals. One study of people attending a community centre in the USA (age range 42–82) found over two-thirds reported having a sexual partner (Wiley and Bortz, 1996). Over 90 per cent of this (self-selected) sample, including those over 70, desired sexual activity at least once a week, although less than half achieved this. Retrospective assessment of change in sexual activity over the previous 10 years in this study found no change in the pattern of preferred activity among women (kissing > intercourse > masturbation > oral sex), whereas men reported a decline in desire for intercourse over the same period (Wiley and Bortz, 1996). Bortz et al. (1999) surveyed 1202 community-dwelling men (mean age 74, range 58–94) attending luncheon clubs in California. Sixty-four per cent of men over 80 in this sample continued to masturbate, and 12 per cent reported intercourse at least weekly. Although the median frequency of intercourse fell from 3.6 episodes per month in men aged 55–59 to 1.3 per month in men aged 85–94, this is still a significant figure! Matthias et al. (1997) reported a large community survey of sexual activity and satisfaction based in the USA. They found that nearly 30 per cent of the sample (mean age 77, range 70–94) had experienced sexual activity in the past month; 69 per cent were reported to be 'satisfied' or 'very satisfied' with their sex life. In a small UK-based qualitative study of sexual satisfaction using purposive sampling, 13 of 21 participants over 70 rated their sex life as at least moderately important, with a few reporting that sex was more pleasurable or of increasing importance as they got older (Gott and Hinchliff, 2003). It appears sex does not even stop when people enter residential homes. In a study of residential home residents, again based in the USA, 62 per cent of men and 30 per cent of women had recently had intercourse (Bretschneider and McCoy, 1988).

17.1.2 Sexual dysfunction in older people

Older people are at risk of psychosexual dysfunction including loss of sex drive, erectile disorder and vaginal discomfort (Masters and Johnson, 1981). Loss of sex drive is commonly due to a mixture of psychogenic and organic factors, and may be related to a reduction in sex hormone levels in both sexes with age (Masters, 1986). Men are at risk of a number of age-related changes including: erectile disorder owing to organic causes including neuropathy and vasculopathy, and delayed ejaculation and longer refractory times (Masters, 1986; Carbone and Seftel, 2002). Older women may notice less effective vaginal secretion, reduced vaginal accommodation, fewer orgasmic contractions and vaginal irritation. Despite these difficulties in the mechanics of the sexual act, sexual activity remains important to many older people.

17.2 EFFECTS OF DEMENTIA ON SEXUALITY AND SEXUAL BEHAVIOUR

The onset of dementia may have a significant effect on the sex life of the individual and their partner, although the evidence base for changes in sexual behaviour in dementia is small. Wright (1991) undertook a controlled study of the impact of Alzheimer's disease (AD) on marital relationships. Eight of the 30 (27 per cent) couples of the dementia-affected group were sexually active, compared with 14 of the 17 (82 per cent) controls. In those individuals still sexually active, compared with controls sex took place more often in couples where one partner had dementia.

Derouesné et al. (1996) reported the findings of two surveys of married couples, where one individual had a diagnosis of possible or probable AD (Mini-Mental State scores 0–29). The first, a survey of 135 couples found that 80 per cent of spouses reported a change in the patient's sexual activity. This was not linked to degree of cognitive impairment or gender of the patient. The second study reported the results of a questionnaire about sexual relations before and after onset of AD. Indifference to sexual activity was common (63 per cent of respondents). Most respondents who reported a change in sexual activity noted a decrease, only four (8 per cent of respondents) reported an increase in sexual activity.

Although increased sexual demands were rare in this study of individuals with AD, this problem may be more common in other forms of dementia, especially frontal lobe dementias, which are often characterized by disinhibited behaviours. Furthermore, increased sexual demands may be underreported as they are particularly upsetting for carers, and very difficult to discuss with others.

In a survey of 40 partners of people with mild–moderate dementia, Ballard et al. (1997) found all nine (23 per cent) of the sample who continued to have sex were satisfied with their sexual relationship. Twelve (39 per cent) of the remaining sample who had ceased sexual activity were dissatisfied with this. There was a trend for continuance of sexual activity to be associated with better cognition scores.

17.2.1 Effects on the individual

Concerns over the diagnosis and prognosis, awareness of the stigma and likelihood of development of depression will all diminish sexual interest in an individual with dementia. There are few published studies on the impact of dementia on sexual function. Zeiss et al. (1990) in an uncontrolled survey of 55 men with AD, found that 53 per cent reported erectile

dysfunction. This was not related to age, degree of cognitive impairment or medication. The high rate of erectile disorder in partners of patients with dementia may be due to the additional stress placed on the relationship by the diagnosis (Litz et al., 1990). Dementia may also reduce libido and cause functional difficulties that adversely affect maintaining a sexual relationship (Jagus and Benbow, 2002). No published studies assess the prevalence of female sexual dysfunction in dementia.

17.2.2 Effect on the partnership

Changes in the balance of the relationship, especially a shift of role from partner to caregiver, may decrease sexual desire in the partner. Carers of individuals with dementia are also vulnerable to depression and anxiety as the carer burden increases. Apparent lack of interest, wandering, forgetting technique, incontinence and poor self-care also are likely to have an adverse effect on the sex life within a dyad. Despite this there is relatively little research in this area (Baikie, 2002). Although not all dementia-affected couples experience a change in sexual activity, an altered sexual relationship is a difficulty many people face after the onset of dementia within a dyad. The onset of dementia should not be assumed to herald cessation of an active sex life, and couples should be encouraged to think and act flexibly in order to adjust to the impact of the disorder (Davies et al., 1998).

Partners of individuals with dementia may confine themselves to celibacy at a time when the rewards of caring for the patient are becoming increasingly scarce. Some partners who retain their sex drive may seek sexual satisfaction elsewhere, through masturbation, visiting prostitutes or longer-term relationships outside the partnership. This may lead to guilt, especially if the patient is still living at home. This is a particularly difficult area to manage as partners are understandably reticent to talk about this. If they do, it is vital to have a nonjudgemental supportive approach. Partners will often blame themselves for the cessation of a sexual relationship. Counselling about the reasons for the patient's altered sex drive and an explanation that this is related to the dementia may help to reassure partners. It is important to stress to patients and carers that a lack of sexual activity should not preclude physical intimacy, and that physical intimacy, such as cuddling is unlikely to result in sexually inappropriate behaviour by the patient (Davies et al., 1992).

17.2.3 Sex in residential settings

Two principal issues should be considered when you are assessing the sexual behaviours of individuals in residential and nursing settings: (a) are the needs for appropriate sexual activity addressed and (b) are inappropriate activities identified and managed?

In an observational study of sexual behaviour in 40 men with dementia living in long-term care facilities, Zeiss et al.

(1996) found appropriate (defined as sitting close to someone, kissing or stroking face hands or arms) sexual behaviours were present in 20 per cent of the sample, compared with 35 per cent manifesting inappropriate or ambiguous behaviours. Mayers (1998) surveyed 33 professional caregivers working in medical facilities caring for people with dementia: 10 respondents reported observing consensual activity between patients. It is likely that, even if it is desired, sexual activity among couples will stop when one of them enters a residential setting. This may be due to a lack of facilities and privacy, perceived disapprobation of staff and professionals' concerns about defining what activities are 'consensual'.

17.2.4 Inappropriate sexual activity

Figures on the rates of inappropriate sexual activity among people with dementia consistently show that these behaviours are relatively uncommon, and rarely result in criminal proceedings. In one survey of 101 elderly sex offenders, only 1 per cent of the sample was diagnosed as having dementia (Fazel, 2002). Devanand et al. (1992) reported rates of sexual disinhibition of under 3 per cent in a survey of 106 individuals with AD. Burns et al. (1990) reported sexual disinhibition to be present in 7 per cent of a sample of 178 patients with AD in the UK with men and women affected equally. Inappropriate sexual behaviours (defined as sexually explicit comments, touching someone other than a partner on the breasts or genitals or exposing breasts or genitals in public) were recorded in 7 (18 per cent) of 40 subjects with dementia living in long-term care and were less common in patients with AD than other dementias (Zeiss et al., 1996). In a further study, Tsai et al. (1999) reported inappropriate sexual behaviour (overt sexual contact, self-exposure, hypersexuality or public masturbation) in 20 (15 per cent) of 133 individuals with dementia. No significant differences were noted with differing types of dementia. The largest study to date on individuals with dementia in care, involving 730 residents with dementia from 180 separate residential units, reported that inappropriate sexual behaviours were present in 5.3 per cent of the sample; far lower than other behavioural disturbances (Matsuoka-Hattori et al., 2003).

A large number of so-called inappropriate sexual behaviours have been reported. Mayers (1998) in her survey of professional caregivers for people with dementia found the most commonly reported sexualized behaviours observed over 1 year included touching breasts (85 per cent of respondents), buttocks (79 per cent) or genitals (73 per cent). Attempted intercourse by a patient was reported by 10 (30 per cent) respondents. Staff and other patients were both recipients of unwanted sexual activity in this survey. Interpretation of research into sexual problems is hampered by methodological limitations including sampling bias and the difficulty in coding the behaviour types. Despite this, it appears that oversexualized behaviours are not particularly common in individuals with dementia.

17.2.5 Summary

Given the extensive evidence of the frequency and importance of sex among older community-dwelling and care-home residents and the physiological impact of ageing on sexual function, assessment of the impact of the diagnosis on the sexual life of the individual with dementia, their spouse or partner and wider contacts becomes paramount. Ongoing reviews are necessary as dementia progresses, as difficulties may wax and wane as cognitive problems progress or with the advent of behavioural and psychological symptoms of dementia. Discussions about sexual difficulties should be initiated by clinicians, as people are often reluctant to volunteer to talk about their sex life. Older people may feel that sexual disorders are part of the ageing process, or that they are not a priority if they or their partner has dementia. If a sexual problem is suspected, then taking a history in a confident but sensitive manner can be very helpful.

17.3 ASSESSMENT

Most people faced with a sexual problem probably will discuss it first with their general practitioner, although many individuals are reticent about this and prefer an entrée in the guise of a physical complaint (d'Ardenne, 1988). Although there have been few studies about older people communicating their sexual problems, it is likely that they will be even more reluctant to discuss psychosexual difficulties. Therefore, it is often left to the clinician to elicit whether there are any sexual problems. Taking a psychosexual history is a delicate task that requires sensitivity and timing. With older couples, it may take more than one interview, and is probably best left altogether until a rapport has been established. Opinions differ about how to take a psychosexual history, particularly about whether to interview people separately or together. There are no hard and fast rules, and to a large extent, the method of history-taking depends on how advanced the dementia is. Where the dementia is mild to moderate, it probably is best to see the couple together and then see the informant alone. People respond to an open interviewing style, irrespective of their generation. Using euphemisms may lead to confusion and generate a sense of embarrassment among the interviewees.

17.3.1 Aims of taking a psychosexual history

There are several domains to a psychosexual history. First, an idea about how frequently a couple had sex before the onset of dementia and any pre-existing difficulties is useful. The next step is to elicit the presenting problem. This may be dysfunction of some sort (erectile difficulty, vaginismus), an increase or decrease in sexual drive (libido), sexual behaviour that the partner finds unwelcome or troublesome or infringes social/legal standards. The views of the individual with dementia and their partner about what outcomes are desired are also important.

17.3.2 Presenting problem

A comprehensive history may give useful clues as to whether the presenting problem has an organic or psychological basis. However, this organic/psychological dichotomy is often misleading, as many older individuals have a mix of aetiologies. Identify the presenting problem, its time scale, precipitating or alleviating factors and whether the problem is situation specific. For example, if a man presents with loss of erectile function, explore whether this is intermittent or sustained, and whether it occurs in all situations including masturbating alone, or only when having sex with a particular partner.

17.3.3 Current relationship

A detailed assessment of the current relationship (if any) is important. This includes quality of communication between the partners, the perceived strengths and weaknesses of the relationship, the impact the diagnosis of dementia has had on the relationship, and identifying issues of guilt or resentment. The nature of the sexual relationship and frequency of intercourse (if any) before the onset of the presenting problem should also be assessed.

17.3.4 Sexual development and past experiences

It is important to attempt a full assessment of the developmental history, whatever the age of the person. The scope may be limited by the dementia, but many patients may recall earlier details of their sexual development, and this part of the history often provides clues to the aetiology of the presenting problem. Attempt to seek information on age of puberty or menarche, first sexual experiences, length and quality of past relationships. It is important not to make assumptions about an individual's sexual orientation and it is possible to explore this sensitively by asking the first names of past partners. Asking about sexual abuse is another very sensitive task, but couching the question in terms of 'unwelcome sexual experiences' may help.

17.3.5 Assessment of risk

Altered sexual behaviour in the context of a dementia confers increased risk to the patient, carers and others. Although sexual disinhibition seems relatively rare, increased sexual appetite may occur as a result of frontal lobe damage, or increased demand for intercourse may result from forgetfulness of normal etiquette and conventions (Haddad and Benbow, 1993). Disinhibited sexual behaviour may result in conflict with others, and even in charges of assault. Rarely, a sexually disinhibited individual may commit rape (within or outside a marriage). Therefore an assessment of risk in cases of increased sexual arousal is mandatory, and treatment with antiandrogens or other sexual suppressants such as antipsychotic drugs

should be considered. Another area of risk for partners arises from delusions of infidelity. These may be intense and result in physical violence, so should be taken seriously.

17.3.6 Examination and investigations

All patients presenting with psychosexual difficulties should undergo a physical examination. Examination may reveal evidence of systemic disorders that are causing the sexual difficulties such as Parkinson's disease, diabetes or vascular disease. Assessment of the severity of dementia is useful in helping to plan treatment. Investigations for patients presenting with loss of sex drive or erectile dysfunction should include fasting glucose, prolactin, testosterone and sex hormone-binding globulin.

17.4 MANAGEMENT

17.4.1 Managing common sexual dysfunctions

Erectile disorder (ED) may be treated by behavioural and/or pharmacological approaches. Sensate focus (Masters and Johnson, 1966) is a graded programme of behavioural exercises that involves the couple engaging in mutual erotic exercise stopping short of intercourse. This change in focus of the sexual act away from intercourse may help reduce spectatoring (self-monitoring of erectile capacity) and performance anxiety. Applying this technique requires commitment and may be difficult for individuals with dementia.

Oral phosphodiesterase inhibitors such as sildenafil (Viagra) and vardenafil (Levitra) are an oral treatment for ED which is effective in most patients. Older age does not appear to be a contraindication *per se*, although these drugs should be avoided in patients with cardiovascular or hepatic disease, recent stroke and those on vasodilators (especially nitrates). Vaginal discomfort during intercourse is often related to atrophy and dryness of the vaginal mucosa, secondary to low oestrogen levels. Initially, these may respond to simple water-based lubricants or topical oestrogen creams.

17.4.2 Managing inappropriate behaviours

A variety of strategies to reduce unacceptable sexual behaviours has been suggested (Jensen, 1989; Howell and Watts, 1990). Most rely on behavioural modification, including removing reinforcement during the undesired behaviour and increasing reinforcement of appropriate alternative behaviours, allowing masturbation in private or using modified clothing that makes it difficult for the patient to undress. The utility of these approaches has not been established.

Drugs may help reduce the sexual response. Cyproterone acetate, medroxyprogesterone, conventional antipsychotics and beta-blockers all have an antilibidinal effect. Cyproterone acetate is a steroid analogue that is effective at reducing sexual drive and sexual responsiveness and has been advocated in treating older people with sex-offending behaviour (McAleer and Wrigley, 1998). It is a competitive antagonist of testosterone and reduces gonadotrophin release. Antipsychotics probably work by inducing hyperprolactinaemia, but may also increase confusion through their anticholinergic effects. The utility of these drugs in people with dementia is not established.

There are complex ethical considerations when antilibidinal drugs are used in patients unable to provide informed consent. However, the common law doctrine of necessity may be valid when capacity is lacking, especially where there is significant risk to the individual or others. Under these circumstances, clinicians should ensure they could justify that the sexual behaviour may result in significant risk to the patient or others, that they have attempted to discuss this with the patient, that they have discussed the proposed use of antilibidinal drugs in a multidisciplinary setting and documented the decision carefully. If the patient is unable to give informed consent, treatment with antipsychotic drugs rather than cyproterone, should probably be considered first.

17.4.3 Managing admission to nursing and residential homes

When an individual with dementia enters a residential facility, the sexual needs of that individual and their partner require assessment. This should include the provision of facilities for sexual expression and exploration of the needs of the partner who remains in the community (Kaplan, 1996). A survey of 300 health professionals about sexual expression of individuals with dementia in nursing homes showed a generally positive attitude (Holmes et al., 1997). Although interpretation was hampered by a low response rate (38 per cent), respondents were generally in favour of encouraging sexual expression among residents. Respondents appeared to favour masturbation rather than intercourse between residents. Training programmes for professional carers exist, focusing on exploring attitudes and information needs of carers, residents' rights and issues of capacity (Mayers and McBride, 1998; Heymanson, 2003). These workshops appear popular but their impact on managing sexuality in care settings has yet to be evaluated.

Some nursing and residential homes now provide married residents with double beds and shared facilities, although stricter rules exist for people developing new relationships and some have draconian rules prohibiting sex (in keeping with acute hospitals of all disciplines). This suppression of sexual activity probably stems from a number of reasons, including a belief among staff that older people are, or at least should be, asexual and that a diagnosis of dementia automatically invalidates the ability to consent to have sex. Neither is correct (Dickens, 1997). The former belief is strongly acculturated in the Western world and is difficult to shift. In an attempt to

obviate the problem about consent, Lichtenberg and Strzepek (1990) developed a structured assessment technique to aid decisions about patients' ability to consent to sexual relationships. This includes ascertaining the patient's awareness of the relationship, the ability to avoid exploitation and the awareness of potential risks. Although this instrument needs further evaluation, it provides a good framework for clinicians to make decisions about competency regarding sexual matters. In cases where consent to engage in sexual activity is established in both individuals, appropriate facilities (a double bed, privacy, time, condoms and water-based lubricants) should be provided by residential facilities for their residents.

There is sometimes a fine line between appropriate and inappropriate sexual behaviour, which is often dependent on the values of the staff and relatives of the individual concerned. However, some sexual behaviours are more clearly 'unacceptable'. These include masturbating or intercourse in public and sexual advances that are indiscriminate or clearly unreciprocated. In addition to the advice about controlling these behaviours it is helpful for staff on the unit to meet to discuss the issues. This not only allows a consistent approach from all staff members, but also allows individuals to vent their own anxieties. Explaining behaviours to other residents may help to reduce their anxiety.

17.5 GAY AND LESBIAN ISSUES

Specific problems faced by lesbian and gay couples include less understanding and tolerance by other family members and professional carers. If the dementia is HIV related, this may result in the patient and partner having to come to terms with being HIV positive, as well as the diagnosis of dementia. Gay partnerships may be discriminated against in terms of not being offered treatment for psychosexual disorders. In many countries, including the UK, gay partnerships still have no legal status and gay partners may not have the same pension and tenancy rights as heterosexual couples, leading to further worries for the partner.

17.6 SEXUAL ABUSE

Although much has been written about elder abuse, there is scant recognition of the potential of sexual abuse in older people with dementia. Estimates of the prevalence of all forms of elder abuse vary, but one study found rates of 16 per cent of a survey of 126 patients in a geriatric psychiatry service had experienced some abuse (Vida et al., 2002). There was a trend for individuals with dementia to experience more elder abuse. Sexual abuse was not classified in this study. In a statewide survey of elder abuse in Texas, of the 39 658 cases of abuse identified in individuals over 6592 (0.3 per cent) were cases of sexual abuse – nearly all of them women (Pavlik et al., 2001). This is likely to be a significant underestimate owing to lack of reporting and recognition. Benbow and Haddad (1993) highlighted the risk of sexual abuse of individuals with dementia, which is exacerbated by lack of definitions and awareness of the issue. Elder sexual abuse may occur at home or within residential or nursing homes, perpetuated by formal or informal carers or other residents. People with dementia may be physically frail and unable to resist sexual advances, and may not be able to report abuse when it occurs. Without a high index of suspicion, sexual abuse will be missed. Any suspicion of elder sexual abuse should be discussed within the multiprofessional team and the police, if appropriate.

17.7 CONCLUSIONS

Several issues about sexuality and dementia need to be considered. First, the impact on the individual with dementia in terms of altered sexual interest and comorbid psychosexual difficulties needs assessment. Second, inappropriate sexual behaviours, although uncommon, can result in misery for professional and family carers. Professionals of all disciplines need to be alert to these problems and offer support and help when necessary.

REFERENCES

Ballard CG, Solis M, Gahir M et al. (1997) Sexual relationships in married dementia sufferers. International Journal of Geriatric Psychiatry 12: 447–451

Baikie E. (2002) The impact of dementia on marital relationships. Sexual and Relationship Therapy 17: 289–299

Benbow SM and Haddad PM. (1993) Sexual abuse of the elderly mentally ill. Postgraduate Medical Journal 69: 803–807

Bortz WM, Wallace DH, Wiley D. (1999) Sexual function in 1,202 aging males: differentiating aspects. Journal of Gerontology 54: M237–M241

Bretschneider JG and McCoy NL. (1988) Sexual interest and behaviour in healthy 80–102-year-olds. Archives of Sexual Behaviour 17: 109–129

Burns A, Jacoby R, Levy R. (1990) Psychiatric phenomena in Alzheimer's disease. IV: Disorders of behaviour. British Journal of Psychiatry 157: 86–94

Carbone DJ and Seftel AD. (2002) Erectile dysfunction: diagnosis and treatment in older men. Geriatrics 57: 18–24

d'Ardenne P. (1988) Talking to patients about sex. The Practitioner 232: 810–812

Davies HD, Zeiss A, Tinklenberg JR. (1992) 'Til death do us part: intimacy and sexuality in the marriages of Alzheimer's patients. Journal of Psychosocial Nursing and Mental Health Services 30: 5–10

Davies HD, Zeiss AM, Shea EA, Tinklenberg JR. (1998) Sexuality and intimacy in Alzheimer's patients and their partners. Sexuality and Disability 16: 193–203

Derouesné C, Guigot J, Chermat V, Winchester N, Lacomblez L. (1996) Sexual behavioral changes in Alzheimer disease. Alzheimer Disease and Associated Disorders 10: 86–92

Devanand DP, Brockington CD, Moody BJ et al. (1992) Behavioral syndromes in Alzheimer's disease. International Psychogeriatrics 4 (Suppl. 2): 161–184

Dickens BM. (1997) Legal aspects of the dementias. Lancet 349: 948–950

Fazel S, Hope T, O'Donnell J, Jacoby R. (2002) Psychiatric, demographic and personality characteristics of elderly sex offenders. Psychological Medicine 32: 219–226

Gott M and Hinchliff S. (2003) How important is sex in later life? The views of older people. Social Science and Medicine 56: 1617–1628

Haddad PM and Benbow SM. (1993) Sexual problems associated with dementia: part 2. Aetiology, assessment and treatment. International Journal of Geriatric Psychiatry 8: 631–637

Heymanson C. (2003) Sexuality and intimacy in care homes. Journal of Dementia Care 11: 10–11

Holmes D, Reingold J, Teresi J. (1997) Sexual expression and dementia. Views of caregivers: a pilot study. International Journal of Geriatric Psychiatry 12: 695–701

Howell T and Watts DT. (1990) Behavioral complications of dementia: a clinical approach for the general internist. Journal of General Internal Medicine 5: 431–437

Jagus CE and Benbow SM. (2002) Sexuality in older men with mental health problems. Sexual and Relationship Therapy 17: 271–279

Jensen CF. (1989) Hypersexual agitation in Alzheimer's disease. Journal of the American Geriatrics Society 37: 917

Kaiser FE. (1996) Sexuality in the elderly. Urologic Clinics of North America 23: 99–109

Kaplan L. (1996) Sexual and institutional issues when one spouse resides in the community and the other lives in a nursing home. Sexuality and Disability 14: 281–293

Lichtenberg PA and Strzepek DM. (1990) Assessments of institutionalized dementia patients' competencies to participate in intimate relationships. The Gerontologist 30: 117–120

Litz BT, Zeiss AM, Davies HD. (1990) Sexual concerns of male spouses of female Alzheimer's disease patients. The Gerontologist 30: 113–116

McAleer A and Wrigley M. (1998) A study of sex offending in elderly people referred to a specialised psychiatry of old age service. Irish Journal of Psychological Medicine 15: 135–8

Masters WH. (1986) Sex and ageing – expectations and reality. Hospital Practice 21: 175–198

Masters WH and Johnson VE. (1966) Human Sexual Response. Boston, Little and Brown

Masters WH and Johnson VE. (1981) Sex and the aging process. Journal of the American Geriatrics Society 29: 385–390

Matsuoka-Hattori K, Miyamoto Y, Ito H, Kurita H. (2003) Relationship between behavioral disturbances and characteristics of patients in special units for dementia. Psychiatry and Clinical Neurosciences 57: 569–574

Matthias R, Lubben JE, Atchison KA, Schweitzer SO. (1997) Sexual activity and satisfaction among very old adults: results from a community-dwelling Medicare population survey. The Gerontologist 37: 6–14

Mayers KS. (1998) Sexuality and the demented patient. Sexuality and Disability 16: 219–225

Mayers KS and McBride D. (1998) Sexuality training for caretakers of geriatric residents in long-term care facilities. Sexuality and Disability 16: 227–36

Pavlik VN, Hyman DJ, Festa NA, Dyer CB. (2001) Quantifying the problem of abuse and neglect in adults – analysis of a statewide database. Journal of the American Geriatrics Society 49: 45–48

Schiavi RC, Schreiner-Engel P, Mandeli J, Schanzer H, Cohen E. (1990) Healthy aging and male sexual function. American Journal of Psychiatry 147: 766–771

Tsai S-J, Hwang J-P, Yang C-H, Liu K-M, Lirng J-F. (1999) Inappropriate sexual behaviours in dementia: a preliminary report. *Alzheimer Disease and Associated Disorders* **13**: 60–62

Vida S, Monks, RC, Des Rosiers P. (2002) Prevalence and correlates of elder abuse and neglect in a geriatric psychiatric service. *Canadian Journal of Psychiatry* **47**: 459–467

Wiley D and Bortz WM. (1996) Sexuality and ageing – usual and successful. *Journal of Gerontology* **51**: M142–M146

Wright LK. (1991) The impact of Alzheimer's disease on the marital relationship. *The Gerontologist* **31**: 224–37

Zeiss AM, Davies HD, Wood M, Tinklenberg JR. (1990) The incidence and correlates of erectile problems in patients with Alzheimer's disease. *Archives of Sexual Behaviour* **19**: 325–331

Zeiss AM, Davies HD, Tinklenberg JR. (1996) An observational study of sexual behavior in demented male patients. *Journals of Gerontology* **51**: M325–M329

18

Quality of life in dementia: conceptual and practical issues

BETTY S BLACK AND PETER V RABINS

Quality of life (QoL) is a state of being as determined by the evaluation of important aspects of an individual's life based on a set of values, goals, experiences and culture. While there is general agreement that QoL is a multidimensional concept, there is no consensus on how to define it or on what aspects of life should be considered when appraising one's QoL. For example, the World Health Organization's definition of QoL is 'the individual's perceptions of their position in life in the context of the culture and value system in which they live, and in relationship to their goals, expectations, standards and concerns' (WHO QoL Group, 1995). However, as Faden and German (1994) note, there are multiple valid and competing conceptions of the good life, that the meaning of QoL changes over the course of a lifetime and that adaptation to circumstances at the moment affect one's perception of QoL.

Health-related QoL (HRQoL) is a more narrow concept that focuses on aspects of life that are affected by a person's health conditions and treatment of those conditions (Kane, 2003). Though more specific than QoL, HRQoL is also a multidimensional concept that refers to one's social, psychological and physical wellbeing consonant with the individual's values and culture. This construct is broader than concepts such as mood and function and has attracted attention in recent years because its primary focus is on individuals' subjective global assessment of their situation as opposed to measures that assess standardized outcomes such as depression or activities of daily living. Although HRQoL is conceptualized as a broad construct, most researchers have concluded that it can be shown to be constructed of several domains, most commonly physical health, psychological wellbeing, function and social activity (Patrick and Erickson, 1993).

Lawton (1997) argued that QoL can and should be assessed both subjectively and objectively. He defined QoL as 'the multidimensional evaluation, by both intrapersonal and social-normative criteria, of the person-environment system of the individual' (Lawton, 1991; p. 6). He believed that there is a need for a frame of reference against which an individual's subjective assessment can be compared and that often there are consensual standards of quality (Lawton, 1997). Lawton suggested that subjective aspects of QoL (e.g. psychological wellbeing) and objective domains (e.g. physical safety) should be assessed in parallel to examine congruence and incongruence between the two approaches.

While HRQoL is conceptualized as a global construct and often examined using generic instruments such as the Quality of Wellbeing (QWB) scale (Kaplan and Bush, 1982) and the SF-36 (Ware and Sherbourne, 1992), many researchers have taken the approach of developing instruments specific to certain diseases because of the conclusion that the characteristics of those diseases have a significant impact on measurement of the construct. This approach can be particularly advocated in the case of dementia because the disease ultimately robs a person of the ability to express oneself owing to the progressive debilitating nature of most dementing illnesses and because of the unique value placed on thought and cognition, especially in the West.

QoL can contribute uniquely to the assessment of treatment interventions for persons with dementia. For example, agencies that approve pharmacological agents have chosen to emphasize cognitive improvement as a necessary attribute for drugs approved to treat cognitive disorders. However, these diseases also universally impair function and social capacity.

Therefore, it is plausible that effective treatments might improve the non-cognitive aspects of dementia more than the cognitive aspects. This suggests that QoL is potentially a unique approach for examining treatment outcomes. Brod and colleagues (1999) note that disease-specific instruments focus on domains most relevant to the disease and characteristics of the patients and their specificity increases the likelihood of capturing change over time.

18.1 GOALS OF QUALITY OF LIFE MEASUREMENT

In a general review of the concept of QoL and its measurement in dementia, Jennings (2000) delineates several broad issues. First he outlines the objections to the construct. These include the claim that it is so vague and so prone to misapplication that it is either useless or dangerous. Another objection is that it attempts to measure aspects of human existence that are ineffable and unmeasurable. Third, the construct can be seen as narrowing rather than expanding individual values since it claims to define a norm or a narrow view of QoL. Finally the term has within it some implication of judgement. Jennings concludes, however, that the value of the construct is that it can be used to improve aspects of life of the disenfranchised and that if we keep in mind the term's drawbacks they can be minimized.

Jennings concludes his analysis by suggesting that QoL has the great strength of setting positive goals and that this counteracts its negative application as a ranking and comparison of individuals or of the states of individuals. Ultimately, Jennings (2000) and Hughes (2003) conclude that the examination of QoL in persons with dementia emphasizes those with the disease and that this great strength counteracts the inherent drawbacks of the concept.

Measuring QoL can serve several important purposes. As Kerner and colleagues (1998) note, determining QoL increases our understanding of the impact that Alzheimer's disease (AD) and other dementias have on individuals over the course of their illness. Beyond specific aspects of the dementia syndrome, such as cognitive and functional impairments, QoL provides a more global indicator of how dementia influences wellbeing. Because dementia affects large numbers of people, has multiple causes and is non-linear in progression, Mack and Whitehouse (2001) suggest that QoL provides a common language for evaluating the effects of interventions. As new medications and other therapies become available, reliable measures of QoL are important for comparing pharmacological agents in terms of both benefits and side effects, for comparing non-pharmacological interventions with each other and for comparing pharmacological with non-pharmacological interventions (Rabins and Kasper, 1997). QoL is a key consideration in evaluating service programmes and in developing clinical guidelines (Brod et al., 1999). For those whose lives have been altered significantly by moving to long-term care facilities for healthcare reasons, Kane (2003) believes that we have a moral responsibility to understand and to improve QoL in nursing homes and other residential facilities. QoL also is a major consideration near the end of life when decision makers are often faced with choosing between more aggressive interventions or palliative approaches to care. Finally, we must also keep issues of QoL in mind not only when considering outcomes of treatment but also when allocating scarce resources at both the individual and societal levels (Whitehouse et al., 1997; Brod et al., 1999; Selai and Trimble, 1999).

18.2 THE CHALLENGES IN MEASURING QUALITY OF LIFE IN DEMENTIA

We have previously noted three challenges in assessing QoL in persons with dementia (Rabins and Kasper, 1997). The first is whether there are domains of QoL that are unique to dementia as opposed to other illnesses. Some of the hallmarks of dementia are that it impairs memory, it can affect attention, insight, judgement, problem solving, behaviour, personality, communication skills and it can lead to other non-cognitive symptoms (e.g. agitation, anxiety, depression, delusions, hallucinations) (Whitehouse et al., 1997). This constellation of possible features unique to dementia can markedly influence QoL. As Howard and Rockwood (1995) note, AD has many manifestations, not all of which are present in all patients. They emphasize the need to employ QoL measures that discriminate between patterns of symptoms across the course of the illness. The environment also has an influence on functioning and opportunities for social interaction which impacts HRQoL. Measures of QoL must be sensitive to the settings in which people with dementia reside, including at home in the community, in assisted living environments and in skilled nursing facilities.

A second issue relates to the subjective nature of the construct. Clearly, in the earlier stages of dementia when symptoms are mild to moderate and individuals can conceptualize the construct and express their opinions, the determination of self-rated QoL is most appropriate and informative. There is a growing interest in capturing the perspectives of those who have dementia, and there is a body of evidence that it is feasible to assess QoL directly from those with mild or moderate levels of severity (Logsdon and Teri, 1997; Brod et al., 1999; Logsdon et al., 1999; Selai et al., 2001a, b). However, since some individuals lose capacity to self-assess QoL, they must either be excluded from measurement or methods must be developed by which other individuals can rate the person's QoL. Reliance on others to determine an individual's QoL raises important concerns. Does another person have the right to make judgements about an individual's state of wellbeing from the rater's perspective? Concordance between patient and proxy responses are influenced by the nature of their relationship, time spent together, the degree of objectiveness of the questions and the patient's level of impairment (Brod et al., 1999). Albert and colleagues (1996) note that a proxy's rating of the frequency of an activity does not tell us if the person with dementia is engaging in the activity in a meaningful way or if the person is actually enjoying the activity. While many instruments used to measure QoL in dementia rely on proxies, proxy ratings have the drawback of filtering a subjective measure through the opinion of another person who may or may not share relevant values. This is a limitation that may be unavoidable, especially for those in the later stages of the illness. However, measures consisting of items that describe observable behaviours and expressions can help to minimize this limitation (Rabins and Kasper, 1997).

The third issue is establishing validity and reliability of instruments measuring QoL in a disorder in which some individuals are unable to conceptualize the construct. Establishing the validity of a measure (i.e. that it accurately measures what it purports to measure) is a challenge when there is no universally accepted definition of QoL and any definition is subject to an individual's interpretation and values (Rabins and Kasper, 1997). While criterion validity may not be possible, most developers seek to establish face validity and content validity by demonstrating the relevance and comprehensiveness of their instrument. Reliability of a measure can more readily be established than validity by demonstrating that its items have internal consistency, that it has good repeatability across administrations and that its use by multiple observers produces similar results. Another psychometric challenge for instruments measuring QoL in dementia is to demonstrate its responsiveness or sensitivity to change. This is a critical characteristic for its usefulness as an outcome measure.

In a thoughtful analysis, Hughes (2003) also identifies three somewhat overlapping problems assessing QoL in dementia. One is a determination of domains, second is the subjective-objective problem and third is how QoL should be assessed in the incapacitated person. Hughes suggests an ethical solution to these dilemmas. He identifies the construct of 'personhood' as the solution to these issues. In defining a person as a 'situated embodied agent' he suggests that both prior and current values and wishes of the person should be considered and that a person's social context of family, friends, neighbours and moral/spiritual values be incorporated.

18.3 METHODS AND INSTRUMENTS

Numerous approaches have been used to measure QoL in people with dementia. Differences relate to the general type of instrument used (i.e. generic versus disease-specific), the scope of the instrument (i.e. the domains of QoL examined) and the type of scores it produces and the method used for data collection. The approach selected by an investigator will depend on several factors. First, the purpose for measuring QoL may determine whether a generic or disease-specific instrument is most appropriate. While a disease-specific measure of QoL is most sensitive to the unique characteristics of dementia and its impact on people's lives, it cannot be used to compare the wellbeing of people with dementia with that of those with other types of illnesses. If QoL is being used as an outcome measure, it is important to consider whether the instrument's content will provide an appropriate measure of effectiveness of the therapy, intervention or programme being examined. Since most agree that QoL is multidimensional, investigators wanting to examine relationships between an intervention and particular aspects of QoL may prefer an instrument that provides subscale scores rather than one that provides only a single summary score. Instruments also vary in how items are scored. In many cases, the items of an instrument contribute equally to either a subscale score or the total score, while other measures have weighted scores based on the assumption that the issues reflected by different items vary in their contributions to the individual's QoL.

Characteristics of the study sample can influence the choice of methods and instruments. Some instruments have been designed to assess QoL of people across the course of their illness. These usually rely on proxy raters, such as family members or formal healthcare providers. Other instruments have been developed specifically for those with mild to moderate dementia who are likely to be able to self-assess their QoL or participate in the process along with an informant. Some measures have been designed to determine QoL in people with late-stage dementia, often relying on formal caregivers as proxy raters since so many of these individuals are cared for in nursing homes.

M. Powell Lawton, one of the most influential forces in how QoL is conceptualized and how instruments have been developed (Ready and Ott, 2003), has stated, 'I reject the idea that there can be one scale of QoL because "life" is composed of many facets' (Lawton, 1997, p. 91). Lawton argued that for clinical and research purposes it is important to know the separate content and salience values for each of the domains that compose QoL. Beyond the subjective measure of QoL involving self-report, he has described objective measures of QoL as those that deal with observable phenomena (Lawton, 1997). Lawton delineated two types of objective measures. First are attribute ratings, which are characteristics rated based on the rater's familiarity with or observation of the person's typical behaviour over a period of time. Instruments examining attributes (e.g. functional health, behavioural symptoms, social interaction and affect) are typically rated by a family member or a healthcare provider. The second type of objective measure is direct observation and coding of ongoing behaviour, which can include behaviours of the person with dementia, their displays of affect and interactions with care providers, or it can include aspects of the environment. Trained researchers typically complete observational measures.

18.4 MEASURES OF QUALITY OF LIFE IN DEMENTIA

The 12 instruments described below and summarized in Table 18.1 are examples of disease-specific measures for assessing QoL in people with dementia. This is not an exhaustive list,

Table 18.1 *Dementia-related measures of quality of life*

Instrument	Content/domains	Respondent	Patient population	Items
Activity and Affect Indicators of QoL	Positive affect Negative affect Activity	Proxy – formal and informal caregivers	Mild to severe	21
Alzheimer Disease Related Quality of Life (ADRQL)	Social Interaction Awareness of self Enjoyment of activities Feelings and mood Response to surroundings	Proxy – formal and informal caregivers	Mild to severe	47
Cognitively Impaired Life Quality Scale (CILQ)	Social interaction Basic physical care Appearance to others Nutrition/hydration Pain/comfort	Proxy – nursing caregivers	Severe	14
Cornell–Brown Scale for Quality of Life In Dementia (CBS)	Negative affectivity Physical complaints Positive affectivity Satisfaction	Clinician with patient's and caregiver's input	Mild to moderate	19
Dementia Care Mapping (DCM)	Well- or illbeing Personal detractions	Trained rater	Moderate to severe	24
Dementia QoL Instrument (DQoL)	Self-esteem Positive affect/humour Negative affect Feelings of belonging Sense of aesthetics	Patient	Mild to moderate	29
Pleasant Events Schedule-AD (PES-AD)	Passive–active Social–non-social	Proxy with patient's input	Mild	20
Progressive Deterioration Scale (PDS)	Extent patient can leave neighbourhood Ability to safely travel distances alone Confusion in familiar settings Use of familiar household implements Participation/enjoyment of leisure/cultural activities Extent patient does household chores Involvement in family finances, budgeting, etc. Interest in doing household tasks Travel on public transportation Self-care and routine tasks Social function/behaviour in social settings	Proxy	Mild to severe	27
Psychological Well-Being in Cognitively Impaired Persons (PWB-CIP)	Engagement behaviours Positive affect Negative affect	Proxy	Severe	16
Quality Of Life-AD (QoLAD)	Physical condition Mood Interpersonal relationships Ability to participate in meaningful activities Financial situation Overall assessment of self Life quality as a whole	Patient, proxy or both	Mild to moderate	13

(Continued)

Table 18.1   *(Continued)*

Instrument	Content/domains	Respondent	Patient population	Items
Quality of Life Assessment Schedule (QoLAS)	Physical Psychological Social/family Daily activities Cognitive	Patient and proxy	Mild to moderate	10
Quality of Life in Late Stage Dementia Scale (QUALID)	Activity Affect	Proxy	Severe	11

but it includes many of the instruments represented in the current literature on QoL in dementia. Investigators, including many who conduct clinical trials, have often chosen to use generic measures to examine QoL in people with dementia. For additional reviews of generic and disease-specific instruments, see Walker *et al.* (1998), Demers *et al.* (2000), Salek *et al.* (1998), Selai and Trimble (1999) and Ready and Ott (2003).

18.4.1 Activity and Affect Indicators of QoL

Albert and colleagues (1996, 1999) adapted two existing measures to assess QoL related to the domains of activity and affect in the previous 2 weeks as rated by caregivers. The 53-item Pleasant Events Schedule-AD (Teri and Logsdon, 1991; Logsdon and Teri, 1997) was reduced to 15 items, which are used to determine the frequency of, opportunity for and enjoyment of activities that take place either outside the home (5 items) or indoors (10 items). Affect is measured using Lawton's Affect Rating scale (Lawton, 1994, 1997), which consists of three positive affects (pleasure, interest, contentment) and three negative affects (anger, anxiety, depression). The frequency of each affect in the previous 2 weeks is determined based on a 5-point scale. A composite QoL indicator is then constructed by combining the affect and activity indicators.

The psychometric properties of this measure have been reported based on a sample of 130 outpatients diagnosed with AD. Test–retest reliability of the affect indicators ranged from correlations of 0.53 for pleasure to 0.92 for anger. Kappas were reported to be > 0.40 for 13 of the 15 activity items and > 0.60 for 12 of the 15 items, with low values for 'entertainment' (0.14) and 'radio/TV' (0.34) items. Reliability for the enjoyment of activities was reported to be excellent, with kappas > 0.70 for 14 items and a low value of 0.25 for the 'radio/TV' item. Validity was first assessed by comparing QoL ratings for patients who had family caregivers with those who had institutional caregivers. Data from the entire sample showed that QoL was rated significantly higher for patients with family caregivers than for those with institutional caregivers based on activities, but there were no differences in levels of positive or negative affect. For patients residing in nursing homes, family caregivers rated only the opportunity for activity as significantly higher than did the institutional

caregivers. Validity was also assessed based on the relationship of QoL ratings and cognitive status as measured by the modified Mini-Mental State Examination (MMSE) (Stern *et al.*, 1987). Lower cognitive status was significantly related to less opportunity, frequency and enjoyment of the 15 activities. Severity of dementia was significantly correlated with only one of the six affect items, with less frequent interest in the world among those with more advanced dementia. Data from both a clinic sample (n = 145), including few minority elders, and a population-based sample (n = 196), most of whom were either African American or Hispanic, showed that frequency of activity was significantly related to positive affect but not to negative affect in both samples and activity was significantly associated with three measures of disease severity in both samples (Albert *et al.*, 1999). The authors conclude that the affect measure, which is less clearly linked to observed behaviours, may be a less reliable indicator of QoL when reported by proxies.

18.4.2 Alzheimer Disease–Related Quality of Life (ADRQL)

Rabins and colleagues (1999) developed a proxy rated measure of QoL of people who have AD and other types of dementia across levels of severity. The content of the ADRQL was developed using an iterative process involving input from formal healthcare providers, informal care providers and a national panel of experts in the field of dementia research and treatment. The instrument contains 47 items with five domains (social interaction, awareness of self, enjoyment of activities, feelings and mood, response to surroundings) that describe primarily observable behaviours and actions. The ADRQL is administered using a structured interview format to either a formal or informal care provider who has extensive knowledge of the person with dementia in the previous 2 weeks. One assumption underlying the development of the ADRQL was that the included items and domains vary in their contribution to the concept of QoL. By developing preference weights for the items, these differences were incorporated into the measurement of health-related QoL. These preference weights were used to assign a scale value to each ADRQL item for scoring purposes. Scores ranging from 0 to 100 can be calculated for each domain and for an overall QoL score, with higher scores reflecting a higher QoL.

Psychometric properties of the ADRQL have been reported in the *User's Manual* (Black *et al.*, 2000) for the instrument. Internal consistency of the instrument has been examined based on data for residents in nursing homes and an assisted living facility. Both formal and informal caregivers were interviewed for a small sample (n = 17) of nursing home residents with AD. Cronbach's alphas were 0.77 using data from the formal caregivers and 0.84 based on the informal caregivers' data.

Gonzalez-Salvador and colleagues (2000) examined internal consistency of the ADRQL based on data for residents in an assisted living (AL) facility (n = 56) and in a skilled nursing facility (SNF) (n = 64). Their data resulted in Cronbach's alphas of 0.85 for data on the SNF residents, 0.91 for the AL residents and 0.89 for both groups combined. Their study also provided evidence of the instrument's validity. Based on data from the residents' formal caregivers (n = 120), the ADRQL was significantly correlated with MMSE (Folstein *et al.*, 1975) scores (r = 0.41; $P < 0.001$) and scores on the Severe Impairment Rating Scale (SIRS) (Rabins and Steele, 1996) (r = 0.44; $P < 0.001$), which is a cognitive measure for subjects with MMSE scores <6. Their data also showed that QoL was negatively associated with subscales of the Psychogeriatric Dependency Rating Scale (PGDRS) (Wilkinson and Graham-White, 1980) for orientation (r = −0.51; $P < 0.001$), behavioural disturbance (r = −0.37; $P < 0.001$) and physical dependency (r = −0.49; $P < 0.001$). Likewise, ADRQL scores were negatively correlated with the Cornell scale for Depression in Dementia (Alexopoulos *et al.*, 1988) (r = −0.42; $P < 0.001$), showing that fewer depressive symptoms were associated with a better QoL.

18.4.3 Cognitively Impaired Life Quality (CILQ) Scale

DeLetter and colleagues (1995) developed the CILQ scale to quantify differences in QoL of the severely cognitively impaired by nursing caregivers. Initially a 29-item version of the CILQ was developed based on focus groups with nursing staff members on rehabilitative, hospice and long-term care units. Factor analysis and clinical judgement were used to reduce the instrument to 14 items with five categories (social interactions, basic physical care, appearance to others, nutrition/hydration, comfort). Discriminate validity was established based on a sample of 12 cognitively impaired patients, who were categorized as either lower functioning or higher functioning. Scale scores based on ratings by 67 nursing caregivers were significantly different for the lower and higher functioning patients.

18.4.4 Cornell–Brown Scale (CBS) for Quality of Life in Dementia

Ready and colleagues (2002) developed the CBS by modifying the Cornell Scale for Depression (Alexopoulos *et al.*, 1988). The

CBS was developed based on the conceptualization that high QoL is indicated by the presence of positive affect, satisfactions, self-esteem and the relative absence of negative affect. This instrument is composed of 19 bipolar items in four categories (negative affectivity, physical complaints, positive affectivity and satisfaction) that yield a single QoL score. The CBS is completed by a clinician after the latter has conducted a joint semistructured interview with the patient and caregiver. Based on information obtained regarding the previous month, each item is rated on a 5-point scale from −2 to +2.

Psychometric data on the CBS are based on a sample of 50 patients from a hospital-based outpatient dementia clinic who were diagnosed as having either dementia or mild cognitive impairment (Ready *et al.*, 2002). The data for the entire sample showed good internal consistency based on a Cronbach alpha of 0.81 and very good interrater reliability as measured by intraclass correlation (r = 0.90). Validity data showed that the CBS was significantly correlated with a patients' self-rated mood using a visual analogue dysphoria scale (Spearman rho = 0.63). The data also showed a significant negative correlation (rho = −0.35) between CBS scores and Clinical Dementia Rating (Hughes *et al.*, 1982) scores but no significant relationship between CBS scores and MMSE scores. Reliability and validity findings were similar for the more mildly and more severely impaired halves of the sample.

18.4.5 Dementia Care Mapping (DCM)

Kitwood and Bredin (1994) devised the Dementia Care Mapping (DCM) method for evaluating the quality of care and wellbeing of people with dementia in residential care settings. The DCM methodology is based on the social–psychological theory of dementia care (Kitwood and Bredin, 1992), which holds that much of the decline among those with dementia is a consequence of social and environmental factors. DCM is a structured, observational method in which the wellbeing or illbeing (WIB) of patients is rated based on signs from the patient and the behaviour of staff towards the patient. Trained observers also record any personal detractors (PDs), which are any episodes that could lead to a reduction in self-esteem for the person with dementia (e.g. objectification, infantilization, disempowerment, etc.). Typically, five to ten patients are rated every 5 minutes over a 6-hour time period using 24 activity categories and indicators of social withdrawal. WIB values, which range from −5 (illbeing) to +5 (wellbeing), can be aggregated to determine an overall WIB score for the group and for each individual. Fossey and colleagues (2002) have shown that ratings for an abbreviated observation period during the hour 'before lunch' are significantly correlated with total scores for activities (r = 0.68; $P = 0.001$) and WIB (r = 0.50; $P = 0.02$) rated over the 6-hour assessment period.

The psychometric properties of the DCM method were evaluated by Fossey *et al.* (2002) using data from two cohorts of subjects (n = 123; n = 54). Internal consistency was established based on significant intercorrelations of the three main measures of the DCM method (activities, well/illbeing, social withdrawal), ranging from r = −0.27 to r = −0.63. In one cohort, however, the relationship between activities and social withdrawal (r = −0.16) was not statistically significant. Test–retest reliability was determined to be good for WIB scores (r = 0.55) and moderate for ratings of activities (r = 0.40) and social withdrawal (r = 0.43). Concurrent validity was determined based on data from a subset of 19 subjects from one cohort. The WIB score was strongly correlated (r = 0.73; $P < 0.0001$) with a pencil and paper generic measure of QoL, but the activities rating was not significantly associated with the generic QoL measure.

In a review of literature in which the DCM method was used, Beavis et al. (2002) found that interrater reliability was established in three of nine studies, with concordance ranging from 0.70 to 0.95. Criterion validity was established by Brooker et al. (1998) from data for a sample of 10 patients in which DCM scores were strongly correlated with levels of engagement (+0.81; $P = 0.01$). In their use of DCM for a large scale Quality Assurance Program, they demonstrated improvements in quality of care practice over a 3-year period based on changes in group WIB scores and declines in the numbers of PDs (Brooker et al., 1998). There is also limited evidence that DCM estimates of wellbeing correlate with other indicators of quality of care (e.g. pressure ulcer care, care planning and carer satisfaction) (Brooker et al., 1998; Beavis et al., 2002). Limitations of the DCM method as noted by Beavis and colleagues (2002) include sampling bias, small sample size, short evaluation periods, lack of consideration of the confounding variables commonly associated with dementia (e.g. psychiatric behavioural features, severity of impairment) and the required investments of time and nursing resources.

18.4.6 Dementia QoL Instrument (DQoL)

Brod and colleagues (1999) developed the DQoL, which was designed to be administered to people with dementia of mild to moderate severity. The DQoL is a 29-item instrument developed through an iterative process involving a literature review, focus groups, pilot testing and statistical examination of its psychometric properties. Screening questions are used to assess the individual's comprehension of the response format. The instrument consists of items rated on a 5-point visual scale that form five domain scales (self-esteem, positive affect/humour, negative affect, feelings of belonging, sense of aesthetics).

The psychometric properties of the DQoL were determined based on a sample of 99 people with mild to moderate dementia, 4 per cent of whom were unable to complete the instrument. Measures of internal consistency for the five scales ranged from 0.67 for feelings of belonging to 0.89 for negative affect. Two-week test–retest coefficients on a subsample of 18 subjects ranged from 0.64 for negative affect to 0.90 for positive affect/humour. There were no significant differences in scale reliabilities between those with mild

dementia and those with moderate dementia. Convergent validity was established by correlations of four DQoL scales with the Geriatric Depression Scale (GDS) (Yesavage et al., 1983) (self-esteem r = −0.48; positive affect/sense of humour r = −0.61; absence of negative affect r = −0.64; feelings of belonging r = −0.42). Those with lower GDS scores had significantly higher scores on the sense of belonging, absence of negative affect, positive affect and self-esteem scales than those with high GDS scores.

18.4.7 Pleasant Events Schedule–Alzheimer's Disease (PES-AD)

PES-AD is a checklist of events and activities for patients with AD that was derived from two earlier Pleasant Events Schedules, one for a general adult population (PES) and another version for older adults (PES-Elderly) (Logsdon and Teri, 1997). The 53-item PES-AD was developed by eliminating items from the PES-Elderly that were inappropriate for people with AD. This instrument has two domains (passive–active, social–non-social) and is designed for use with people who have mild dementia. Caregivers complete the PES-AD and involve the person with dementia as much as possible by asking questions and discussing each item with the patient. Items are rated according to their frequency and availability in the past month on a 3-point scale and are rated on whether the person enjoys the activity now and whether the activity was enjoyed in the past. A shorter 20-item version of the PES-AD (Short PES-AD) was devised by eliminating items difficult to rate, items not available to many people and items with item-to-total correlations below 0.35.

Logsdon and Teri (1997) provide psychometric properties of both the 53-item and 20-item PES-AD. Because the Short PES-AD is highly correlated with the PES-AD (r = 0.91 to r = 0.95), reliability and validity data will be presented here for only the Short PES-AD. Regarding the instrument's reliability, internal consistency was demonstrated by coefficient alphas ranging from 0.76 to 0.94 and split-half reliabilities ranged from 0.74 to 0.94 for the Short PES-AD. To assess the instrument's validity, correlations between the Short PES-AD and the MMSE and Hamilton Depression Rating Scale (HDRS) (Hamilton, 1960) were calculated. Both symptoms of depression and decreased cognitive function were associated with reduced frequency of enjoyable activity.

18.4.8 Progressive Deterioration Scale (PDS)

DeJong and colleagues (1989) developed the Progressive Deterioration Scale (PDS) to assess QoL in people with AD across levels of severity and to measure changes in QoL as the disease progresses. They used an iterative process of in-depth interviews with caregivers to determine how QoL was affected by the disease, preparation and testing of questionnaires to determine which factors would discriminate between levels of AD, based on the GDS (Reisberg, et al., 1982), and validation of the instrument. The final version of the PDS contains 27 items with 11 content areas that focus primarily on activities. The instrument is self-administered by the caregiver who scores each item using a bipolar visual analogue scale anchored with statements that describe the patient's characteristics. A composite score is calculated by averaging across the items, with higher scores reflecting a better QoL.

The reliability and validity of the PDS were reported by DeJong et al. (1989). Internal consistency of the PDS was established by Kuder–Richardson split-half reliability coefficients, which ranged from 0.92 to 0.95 for a sample of 151 subjects with AD. Test–retest reliability coefficients based on a sample of 123 subjects ranged from 0.775 for those with late stage AD to 0.889 for those with early AD, with an overall coefficient of 0.898. Preliminary versions of the PDS were shown to discriminate with 95 per cent accuracy between non-AD elders and AD patients, and to have 80 per cent overall accuracy in discriminating between four categories of subjects (controls, early AD, middle AD, late AD). For the final version of the PDS, construct validity was established based on significantly different mean scores across groups of patients (n = 151) categorized by the GDS as having early, middle and late stage AD.

Data on responsiveness to change were presented by Knopman and Gracon (1994). In a sample of 62 AD subjects in the placebo arm of a 12-week clinical trial, the mean change in PDS scores was −2.8 to +11.3. Their study showed large between-subject and within-subject variability, and they concluded that a reliable change score would be approximately four times larger than the mean change score. The review article by Salek et al. (1998) notes that the PDS has been used to measure QoL in some double-blind, placebo-controlled trials of tacrine that showed significant changes in PDS scores, but the significant results were not obtained for all treatment groups and only with certain doses of tacrine in each trial.

18.4.9 Psychological Wellbeing in Cognitively Impaired Persons (PWB–CIP)

PWB-CIP was developed by Burgener (Burgener and Twigg, 2002) to measure one aspect of QoL. Initially, the PWB-CIP was a 16-item observer-rated instrument that measures affective states and engagement behaviours. The instrument consisted of eight items reflecting positive affect and engaging behaviours and eight items that reflect negative affect and withdrawing behaviours. The internal consistency of the 16-item PWB-CIP was established based on a Cronbach alpha of 0.74 for the total scale. Validity of the instrument was supported by a moderate correlation of −0.59 with a measure of depression in the appropriate direction.

Longitudinal data from a sample of 96 outpatients with dementia (n = 73 at 18 months) were used to further refine the PWB-CIP and provide additional psychometric data (Burgener et al., 2002, in press). Based on factor analysis, five items were eliminated from the PWB-CIP, leaving 11 items

representing two factors (negative affect/interaction, positive affect/interaction). Item to total correlations ranged from 0.30 to 0.57 at baseline and 0.38 to 0.64 at 18 months. Internal consistency of the 11-item instrument was established based on Cronbach alphas of 0.79 at baseline and 0.82 at 18 months. The PWB-CIP was significantly associated (0.65 at baseline, 0.49 at 18 months) with a single item 'face' scale rated from sad to happy. Construct validity was also supported by significant correlations at baseline and at 18 months between the PWB-CIP and measures of personality, cognitive function, depression and productive behaviours, and at 18 months between the PWB-CIP and measures of interaction in the environment, including total social contacts and the PES-AD.

18.4.10 Quality of Life–AD (QoLAD)

Logsdon and colleagues (1999) developed the QoLAD to assess QoL as perceived by both the patient and the patient's caregiver. The content of the QoLAD was derived based on a review of relevant literature on QoL of older adults and other chronically ill populations and the input of patients, caregivers and experts in the fields of geriatrics and gerontology. This instrument consists of 13 items used to assess seven aspects of the patient's QoL (physical condition, mood, interpersonal relationships, participation in activities, financial situation, overall assessment of self, life quality as a whole). An interviewer administers the QoLAD to patients with mild to moderate severity of illness, and caregivers complete the measure in the form of a questionnaire. Each item is rated by the patient and by the caregiver on a 4-point scale, with 1 being 'poor' and 4 being 'excellent'. Total scores as rated by each range from 13 to 52. A weighted composite score is calculated by giving greater weight to the patient's rating than the caregiver's rating.

The psychometric properties of the QoLAD have been reported based on a sample of 77 community-dwelling AD patients and their caregivers (Logsdon et al., 1999). Measures of internal consistency included coefficient alphas of 0.88 and 0.87 for ratings by the patients and caregivers, respectively. Item-to-total correlations ranged from 0.41 to 0.67 for patient ratings and from 0.34 to 0.63 for the caregiver ratings. Ratings of items by the patients and by the caregivers were significantly correlated for 8 of the 13 items and for their total scores. Agreement was poorest on items related to ability to do chores and memory. Based on a subsample of 30 patient–caregiver pairs, 1-week test–retest reliability was established by intraclass correlation coefficients of 0.76 for patients and 0.92 for caregivers. Validity data showed that the patients' ratings on the QoLAD correlated significantly with the MMSE score, activities of daily living, measures of depression and the Pleasant Event Scale-AD. Higher scores on the QoLAD were associated with lower levels of depression, better day-to-day functioning and higher activity level. The caregivers' ratings on the QoLAD were not associated with the patient's MMSE or the patients' self-reported GDS measure. Measures of reliability and validity were examined separately for patients with lower cognitive status and those with higher cognitive status, and the authors concluded that moderate levels of cognitive impairment did not have a negative impact on either reliability or validity. However, QoLAD scores for those with mild cognitive impairment was significantly associated only with their GDS scores.

Logsdon *et al.* (2002) have also reported on the psychometric characteristics of the QoLAD based on a sample of 177 AD patient and caregiver pairs. The QoLAD was completed by 155 of the patients. Again, internal consistency for both patients (0.84) and caregivers (0.86) was good based on alpha coefficients. Agreement between patients and caregivers based on intraclass correlation coefficient was 0.28 and absolute agreement was 0.19. Validity was demonstrated by significantly higher QoL associated with less impairment in behavioural competence, better psychological status, less impaired physical function and a better interpersonal environment. QoLAD scores were examined across three levels of cognitive functioning. Patient rated scores were significantly different, with lower QoL reported among the lowest cognitive group, but there were no significant differences in caregiver-rated QoLAD scores across patients' cognitive functioning groups. The authors concluded that it was possible for individuals with mild to moderate dementia to reliably and validly rate their own QoL.

18.4.11 Quality of Life Assessment Schedule (QoLAS)

The QoLAS is an instrument derived from a technique called Quality of Life Assessment by Construct Analysis (QoLASCA) by Selai and colleagues (2001) for use with patients who have dementia. The QoLASCA method was a generic technique to assess QoL in patients with neurological disorders such as epilepsy. The QoLAS is an instrument tailored to individual patients and relies on both qualitative and quantitative approaches to measurement. This instrument is administered by interviewing the patient and the patient's caregiver regarding what is important for QoL and ways in which QoL is affected by one's current health condition. A total of 10 'constructs' are elicited, two each for five domains (physical, psychological, social/family, daily activities, cognitive functioning/wellbeing). The patient is asked to rate each construct on how much of a problem each item is on a scale of 0 to 5 from 'no problem' to 'it could not be worse.' The scores are totalled to give an overall QoLAS score out of 50.

The psychometric properties of the QoLAS were reported based on a sample of patient-caregiver dyads. Thirteen of the 37 patients, all of whom had MMSE scores less than 11, could not engage in the interview, and caregivers were not found for two other patients. In this sample of 22 dyads who were interviewed, the caregivers rated the patients as having a worse QoL than the patient had for each of the five domains. Correlations between patient and caregiver ratings for the five domains were higher for patients with mild dementia ($r = 0.29$ to $r = 0.79$) than for those with mild-to-moderate dementia ($r = -0.05$ to $r = 0.43$). Internal consistency was based on item-to-total correlations ranging from 0.59 to 0.86 for patient

ratings on the five domains and correlations for the caregiver ratings ranging from 0.64 to 0.81. Criterion validity was assessed based on ratings by both the patient and the caregiver. Patient ratings correlated with measures of affect, social life and activities, while caregiver ratings of the patients' QoL were associated with measures of mobility, activities of daily living and neuropsychiatric symptoms. Construct validity was established by demonstrating a significantly worse QoL among those with greater deterioration in daily activity skills.

18.4.12 Quality of Life in Late Stage Dementia Scale (QUALID)

Weiner and colleagues (2000) developed the QUALID for use in assessing QoL in persons with late-stage dementia residing in institutional settings. The items for this instrument were selected from the affect and activity measure devised by Albert *et al.* (1996). A group of clinicians experienced in assessing persons with AD selected the items by consensus to measure QoL in persons with late-stage dementia in long-term care facilities. The QUALID, which is administered as a structured interview, contains 11 items reflecting observable behaviours that are rated by frequency on a 5-point Likert scale by a nursing home technician who has at least 30 hours of exposure to the resident in the previous week. Scores range from 11 to 55, with lower scores reflecting a better QoL.

Reliability and validity of the QUALID have been reported based on a sample of 42 residents of a dementia special care unit (Weiner *et al.*, 2000). Internal consistency of the instrument, using data from 31 assessments, was established by a Cronbach's alpha of 0.77. Item-to-total correlations ranged from 0.17 to 0.70. Test–retest reliability based on a subsample of 19 residents was determined by intraclass correlation (ICC = 0.807; SEM = 0.080). Interrater reliability was established using data on 23 residents provided by two reporters interviewed by two recorders (ICC = 0.826; SEM = 0.07). To validate this instrument, QUALID scores were compared with those for measures of cognitive function, functional ability, depression and emotional/behavioural symptoms. The QUALID was not associated significantly with either the MMSE or the Physical Self-Maintenance Scale (Lawton and Brody, 1969) but was related to the GDS ($r = 0.36$; $P = 0.04$) and the Neuropsychological Inventory (Cummings *et al.*, 1994) ($r = 0.40$; $P = 0.01$).

18.5 CORRELATES OF QUALITY OF LIFE IN DEMENTIA

As researcher have developed disease-specific measures of QoL and attempted to establish their validity and as investigators have examined predictors of wellbeing for people with dementia, their findings reveal several fairly consistent correlates of QoL. First, studies often show that scores on QoL measures are associated with severity of illness (DeJong, 1989; Albert *et al.*, 1996, 1999, 2001; Gonzalez-Salvador *et al.*, 2000;

Ready *et al.*, 2002). Those with less cognitive and functional impairments are better able to engage in activities and their QoL is often reflected by less negative affect and more positive affect (Albert *et al.*, 1996, 1999; Logsdon and Teri, 1997). Having more impairments in activities of daily living (ADL) and greater physical dependency is associated with diminished QoL (Albert *et al.*, 1996; Logsdon *et al.*, 1999; Gonzalez-Salvador *et al.*, 2000; Ballard *et al.*, 2001; Logsdon *et al.*, 2002). However, some investigators have found no significant relationship between QoL and cognitive function as measured by the MMSE (Weiner *et al.*, 2000; Logsdon *et al.*, 2002; Ready *et al.*, 2002). These findings may be due to a limited range in the cognitive abilities of study participants. For example, Weiner and colleagues (2000) hypothesized that there would be no relationship between MMSE scores and the QUALID in their sample of nursing home residents with late-stage dementia.

QoL is also frequently associated with symptoms of depression among people with dementia (Logsdon and Teri, 1997; Brod *et al.*, 1999; Logsdon *et al.*, 1999; Gonzalez-Salvador *et al.*, 2000; Weiner *et al.*, 2000; Logsdon *et al.*, 2002; Burgener *et al.*, in press). Depression has a strong negative impact on QoL even when cognitive status is controlled for (Logsdon *et al.*, 2002). It is estimated that 15–30 per cent of people with AD experience clinically significant levels of depressive symptoms (Teri and Wagner, 1992). The strong relationships among dementia, depression and QoL highlight the importance of diagnosis and treatment, especially among residents of long-term care facilities where the risk of depression is high.

Some investigators have found significant relationships between the use of psychotropic medications and QoL among people with dementia. Albert and colleagues (1996) found that participants with low QoL in the Predictors Cohort were significantly more likely to use antipsychotic medications. In a sample of people with dementia living in either assisted living facilities or skilled nursing homes, residents taking anxiolytics had significantly lower scores on the ADRQL, while those on a cholinesterase inhibitor had higher QoL scores (Gonzalez-Salvador, 2000). Ballard *et al.* (2001) also found that people with dementia in residential facilities who used psychotropic medications had reduced QoL as assessed using DCM. Neuroleptic agents were most associated with wellbeing, social withdrawal and restriction of activities. It is important to note, however, that in cross-sectional studies it is not clear whether a medication diminishes QoL or whether a lower QoL is due to the psychiatric and behavioural problems being treated.

QoL instruments can be important tools for assessing quality of care. Several investigators have used the DCM method to examine residential care facilities with the goal of improving care practices (Williams and Rees, 1997; Younger and Martin, 2000; Innes and Surr, 2001; Kuhn *et al.*, 2002). For example, the Elderly Mentally Ill unit of a National Health Service trust in south Wales used DCM to assess quality of care in three types of facilities (continuing care/respite, assessment/day care and day centres) (Williams and Rees, 1997).

They determined that environmental/extraordinary circumstances (e.g. deaths, discharges, admissions) affect care by taking away qualified nurses, that staff to patient ratio is not as important as skill mix and role function and that a main theme was the need for more structure and continuity of care.

Younger and Martin (2000) reported findings from a DCM study conducted in two health districts of the UK that included six units (day units, assessment units, continuing care). They found more activity and less dependency in day units, but they determined that high dependency does not lead automatically to a lower quality of person-centred care. Innes and Surr (2001) used DCM to examine care practices in six residential and nursing homes in the UK. Overall, these facilities were meeting the physical care needs of residents but not the broader psychosocial care needs. The investigators found that activities requiring staff intervention generated higher wellbeing of residents and higher wellbeing was associated with fewer personal detractions.

In the USA, Kuhn and colleagues (2002) examined QoL in 10 assisted living facilities in a mid-western state using DCM. They found that residents in larger non-dementia specific sites fared better overall than those in small dementia-specific sites, with greater diversity of interactions and activities. These investigators also determined that these facilities were meeting basic care needs, but the psychological and social needs of residents were generally not given high priority. Woods (1999) suggests that the DCM method of assessing QoL and quality of care may be most valuable as part of the process of change, with feedback sensitively provided to staff and action plans developed to improve quality of care.

18.6 QoL AS AN OUTCOME MEASURE

Increasingly, efficacy studies are including QoL as an outcome measure of pharmacological and non-pharmacological interventions for people with dementia. In a review article, Howard and Rockwood (1995) identified 36 reports of anti-dementia drug trials for AD in which five mentioned and four measured QoL. They noted that only two of the QoL instruments used in those trials had been formally cross-validated in samples of patients with dementia, the PDS and the Italian QoL Scale (IQLS). A few years later, Salek and colleagues (1998) reviewed the use of QoL measures in assessing drug effects and identified six generic and three disease-specific measures used to assess QoL in clinical trials. They observed, however, that some studies referred to instruments such as the Physical Self-Maintenance Scale (PSMS) and the Instrumental Activities of Daily Living (IADL) scale as QoL measures, while other studies referred to these same instruments as measures of activities of daily living (ADL). This inconsistency illustrates an unresolved issue related to the multidimensionality of QoL, i.e. which constructs are aspects of QoL and which are correlates or determinants of QoL? Salek *et al.* (1998) espoused that an instrument classified as a

QoL measure must comprehensively assess all the components that constitute QoL. They concluded that efforts to develop and use QoL instruments for clinical trials had not yet produced a measure with satisfactory validity, reliability, sensitivity and feasibility.

In a review of outcome measures for drug trials, Demers and colleagues (2000) made a distinction between instruments used to measure function and those to assess QoL. They also noted the limited evidence of reliability and validity of the instruments they reviewed and the lack of data on responsiveness to change. In the absence of a 'gold standard' for measuring function and QoL in AD, they provide a stepwise set of guidelines to help investigators select and use the most appropriate scale for drug treatment trials. Their guidelines include:

- considering the objective of the scale and how it matches the goals of the study;
- making sure that the concept is clearly defined and has a sound theoretical base;
- considering the match between the population with whom the scale was developed and tested and the disability level of the study subjects;
- considering the instrument's test–retest reliability, especially if it is to be used repeatedly;
- considering the interrater reliability if multiple raters are involved;
- making sure that the unidimensionality of the scale has been established before relying on a summed score; and
- considering the expected magnitude of change with respect to the scale's responsiveness to change (Demers et al., 2000).

Woods (1999) reviewed the evidence from research studies of non-pharmacological interventions to increase independence and wellbeing in people with dementia. He noted that few of the studies he reviewed focused specifically on wellbeing. However, Woods included interventions designed to increase participation in activities among the studies that he categorized as promoting independence, such as those targeted at self-care, mobility, continence, orientation and environmental change, rather than with those promoting wellbeing. He suggested that often there is an implicit assumption that increased independence and increased interaction must be associated with a better QoL. The studies that he characterized as promoting wellbeing included interventions such as changes in the physical and social environment, reminiscence sessions, validation therapy, multisensory stimulation, dynamic psychotherapy and cognitive behaviour therapy. The outcomes of those studies included improved mood, improved life satisfaction and contentment or happiness rather than the more global concept of QoL.

To illustrate this, one non-pharmacological intervention that used QoL as a secondary outcome measure was conducted by Spector and colleagues (2003). They examined the efficacy of a cognitive stimulation therapy (CST) programme for people with dementia using a single-blind, multicentre randomized controlled trial that included participants from 18 residential homes and five day centres. They used strict inclusion criteria to identify suitable subjects (e.g. ability to communicate, no major physical illness or disability, MMSE between 10–24, etc.); 115 subjects participated in the intervention group and 86 were in the control group. Following the 14-session programme over 7 weeks, the intervention group had significant improvements on the MMSE, which was the primary outcome, and on the ADAS-cog (Rosen et al., 1984) and the QoLAD scale, which were two of the secondary outcome measures. They concluded that their results compare favourably with trials of drugs for dementia.

18.7 QUESTIONS AND ISSUES FOR THE FUTURE

We believe that the case has been made for the value of examining QoL as an important means of understanding the experience of people with dementia, evaluating and improving care practices and examining the efficacy of pharmacological and non-pharmacological therapies. However, the study of QoL in dementia is in the early stage of its development. Many questions and issues must be addressed in the future regarding how QoL is defined and measured in dementia and what the ethical and policy implications are of quantifying a fundamentally subjective, qualitative state of being for a group of vulnerable individuals.

While progress has been made over the past 15 years in the study of QoL and in the development of dementia-specific QoL instruments, there is no consensus on what domains comprise QoL in dementia. The selection of domains and items is sometimes guided by theory, sometimes seems arbitrary and often is based on judgements of professionals rather than the lay perspective (Bond, 1999). Among the instruments listed in Table 18.1, the most commonly included domains focus on mood or affect, involvement in activities and social interactions. However, as Whitehouse (2000) notes, there is less agreement on whether to incorporate functional status into QoL models or what beyond function should be included as components of QoL. Categories such as self-esteem, awareness of self, aesthetics or appearance to others are seen less often as components of QoL measures. Agreement is also lacking on whether spiritual wellbeing should be included as a component of QoL, especially for those in the early stages of dementia.

Equally important to achieving advancements in the study of QoL in dementia is the need to address the psychometric characteristics of our instruments. Salek and colleagues (1998) argue that future research should focus on using the available instruments cross-sectionally and longitudinally to identify their strengths and weaknesses rather than developing new instruments. They contend that such an effort would produce instruments that are sensitive to change and provide valid and reliable results. Most lacking for instruments currently in use are data on sensitivity to change, which is critical information for the selection of an appropriate outcome measure for practice and programme evaluation and treatment efficacy.

One of the limitations faced by measures that rely on proxies or on trained observers is that the QoL of the person with dementia is filtered by the experience, wellbeing and values of the rater. This is an unavoidable weakness when examining QoL of those in the latter stages of dementia when individuals lack the capacities needed to self-assess and/or communicate about their own QoL. However, research is needed to determine the most effective methods for enabling those with mild and moderate dementia to participate to the extent possible in the process of determining QoL. Whitehouse (2000) suggests that studies should examine how the varying patterns of neuropsychological disabilities affect patients' ability to engage in assessing their own QoL.

Currently, the primary outcome of interest for interventions directed towards dementia is improving or maintaining cognitive function or slowing its decline. When QoL is examined in either pharmacological or non-pharmacological trials, it is most often considered a secondary outcome, as the CST study by Spector et al. (2003) illustrates. Discussions are needed on whether QoL should be regarded as a primary outcome measure, especially for those in the advanced stages of dementia. QoL increasingly becomes an important factor when decisions are made near the end of life about the aggressiveness of care, the use of life-sustaining treatments or reliance on palliative care.

The assessment of QoL and its use in decision-making for people with dementia raise several ethical questions. Some may question the legitimacy of someone else making judgements about an individual's QoL. Faden and German (1994) contend that such judgements are made all the time in every arena of social policy and in private contexts. They suggest that the key moral questions turn on the legitimate uses of those judgements as justifications for consequential actions and policies. One controversy stems from '... whether, under what circumstances, and according to whose judgment diminished life quality is an appropriate indication for reduction or cessation of medical intervention' (Faden and German, 1994, p. 547). One concern is that the term QoL is sometimes used to refer to the moral worth or value of a person and that person's life (Jennings, 2000). Some may conclude that an assessment of QoL resulting in the lowest measure reflects a life not worth living. Such a conclusion is a misinterpretation of an instrument with a floor effect, not a reflection of the absence of quality (Rabins and Kasper, 1997). Jennings (2000) offers an alternative view of quality as marking 'the gap between actual circumstances and the possible circumstances of an intrinsically valuable life' (p. 169). He argues that QoL may tell us something about the experience of an individual but not the value of being human. As Selai and Trimble (1999) state, 'Given the important existential, moral and legal ramifications, the development of tools to assess QoL in patients with dementia must be scrupulously considered' (p. 103).

In a discussion of what counts as a 'good life' for people with dementia, Schermer (2003) concludes that differences in the philosophical theories about the good life manifest themselves in a number of controversies that may provide guidance for future research. First, he raises the issue of whether or not something can be good for people if they do not endorse it themselves. For example, how much value should be attached to the opinions of the person with dementia in order to determine what is good for them and which opinions should be relied on, those in the present or those that predate the dementia? Second is the controversy of whether or not things need to be experienced by a person in order to improve or diminish their wellbeing. For instance, is loss of decorum bad for an individual if the person does not experience it as such? Finally, there is the question of whether experiences should be rooted in reality. Can feelings such as happiness or belonging add to wellbeing if they are the product of some sort of illusion or delusion? Schermer suggests that research should focus more on the process of dementia and the effects of that process on patients' identities, self-conceptions, capacities, preferences and values. He also believes that a narrative perspective, in which life is conceived of as developing over time, including both the past and the present, can help in developing a more comprehensive account of what is a good life for the person with dementia.

REFERENCES

Albert SM, Del Castillo-Castaneda C, Sano M et al. (1996) Quality of life in patients with Alzheimer's disease as reported by patient proxies. *Journal of the American Geriatrics Society* **44**: 1342–1347

Albert SM, Castillo-Castanada C, Jacobs DM et al. (1999) Proxy-reported quality of life in Alzheimer's patients: comparison of clinical and population-based samples. *Journal of Mental Health and Aging* **5**: 49–58

Albert SM, Jacobs DM, Sano M, Marder K et al. (2001) Longitudinal study of quality of life in people with advanced Alzheimer's disease. *American Journal of Geriatric Psychiatry* **9**: 160–168

Alexopoulos GS, Abrams RC, Young RC, Shamoian CA. (1988) Cornell Scale for Depression in Dementia. *Biological Psychiatry* **23**: 271–284

Ballard C, O'Brien J, James I et al. (2001) Quality of life for people with dementia living in residential and nursing home care: the impact of performance on activities of daily living, behavioral and psychological symptoms, language skills and psychotropic drugs. *International Psychogeriatrics* **13**: 93–106

Beavis D, Simpson S, Graham I. (2002) A literature review of Dementia Care Mapping: Methodological considerations and efficacy. *Journal of Psychiatric and Mental Health Nursing* **9**: 725–736

Black BS, Rabins PV, Kasper JD. (2000) *Alzheimer Disease Related Quality of Life (ADRQL) User's Manual.* Baltimore, MD

Bond J. (1999) Quality of life for people with dementia: approaches to the challenge of measurement. *Ageing and Society* **19**: 561–579

Brod M, Stewart AL, Sands L, Walton P. (1999) Conceptualization and measurement of quality of life in dementia: The Dementia Quality of Life Instrument (DQoL). *The Gerontologist* **39**: 25–35

Brooker D, Foster N, Banner A, Payne M, Jackson L. (1998) The efficacy of Dementia Care Mapping as an audit tool: Report of a 3-year British NHS evaluation. *Aging and Mental Health* **2**: 60–70

Burgener S and Twigg P. (2002) Relationships among caregiver factors and quality of life in care recipients with irreversible dementia. *Alzheimer Disease and Associated Disorders* **16**: 88–102

Burgener SC, Twigg P, Popovich A. Measuring psychological well-being in cognitively impaired persons. *International Journal of Social Research and Practice* (in press)

Cummings JL, Mega M, Gray K et al. (1994) The Neuropsychiatric Inventory: An efficient tool for comprehensively assessing psychopathology in dementia. *Neurology* **44**: 2308–2314

DeJong R, Osterlund OW, Roy GW. (1989) Measurement of quality-of-life changes in patients with Alzheimer's disease. *Clinical Therapeutics* **11**: 545–554

DeLetter MC, Tully CL, Wilson JF, Rich E. (1995) Nursing staff perceptions of quality of life of cognitively impaired elders: instrumental development. *Journal of Applied Gerontology* **14**: 426–443

Demers L, Oremus M, Perrault A, Champoux N, Wolfson C. (2000) Review of outcome measurement instruments in Alzheimer's disease drug trials: psychometric properties of functional and quality of life scales. *Journal of Geriatric Psychiatry and Neurology* **13**: 170–180

Faden R and German PS. (1994) Quality of life: considerations in geriatrics. *Clinics in Geriatric Medicine* **10**: 541–551

Folstein MF, Folstein SE, McHugh PR. (1975) Mini-mental State: a practical method for grading the cognitive state of patients for the clinician. *Journal of Psychiatric Research* **2**: 189–198

Fossey J, Lee L, Ballard C. (2002) Dementia Care Mapping as a research tool for measuring quality of life in care settings: psychometric properties. *International Journal of Geriatric Psychiatry* **17**: 1064–1070

Gonzalez-Salvador T, Lyketsos CG, Baker A. (2000) Quality of life in dementia patients in long-term care. *International Journal of Geriatric Psychiatry* **15**: 181–189

Hamilton M. (1960) A rating scale for depression. *Journal of Neurology Neurosurgery, and Psychiatry* **23**: 56–62

Howard K and Rockwood K. (1995) Quality of life in Alzheimer's disease. *Dementia* **6**: 113–116

Hughes CP, Berg L, Danziger WL et al. (1982) A new clinical scale for the staging of dementia. *British Journal of Psychiatry* **140**: 566–572

Hughes JC. (2003) Quality of life in dementia: an ethical and philosophical perspective. *Expert Reviews in Pharmacoeconomics Outcomes Research* **3**: 525–534

Innes A and Surr C. (2001) Measuring the well-being of people with dementia living in formal care settings: The use of Dementia Care Mapping. *Aging and Mental Health*, **5**: 258–268

Jennings B. (2000) A life greater than the sum of its sensations: Ethics, dementia, and the quality of life. In: SM Albert and RG Logsdon (eds), *Assessing Quality of Life in Alzheimer's Disease*, New York, Springer Publishing Company

Kane RA. (2003) Definition, measurement, and correlates of quality of life in nursing homes: toward a reasonable practice, research and policy agenda. *The Gerontologist*, **43** (Special Issues II): 28–36

Kaplan RM and Bush JW. (1982) Health-related quality of life measurement for evaluation research and policy analysis. *Health Psychology* **1**: 61–80

Kerner DN, Patterson TL, Grant I, Kaplan RM. (1998) Validity of the Quality of Well-Being Scale for patients with Alzheimer's disease. *Journal of Aging and Health* **10**: 44–61

Kitwood T and Bredin K. (1992) A new approach to the evaluation of dementia care. *Journal of Advances in Health and Nursing Care* **1**: 41–60

Kitwood T and Bredin K. (1994) *Evaluating Dementia Care: The DCM Method*, 6th edition. University of Bradford, Bradford Dementia Research Group

Knopman D and Gracon S. (1994) Observations on the short-term 'natural history' of probable Alzheimer's disease in a controlled clinical trial. *Neurology* **44**: 260–265

Kuhn D, Kasayka RE, Lechner C. (2002) Behavioral observations and quality of life among persons with dementia in 10 assisted living facilities. *American Journal of Alzheimer's Disease and Other Dementias* **17**: 291–298

Lawton MP. (1991) A multidimensional view of quality of life. In: JE Birren, JE Lubben, JC Rowe, DE Deutchman (eds), *The Concept and Measurement of Quality of Life in the Frail Elderly.* New York, Academic Press, pp. 3–27

Lawton MP. (1994) Quality of life in Alzheimer's disease. *Alzheimer Disease and Associated Disorders* **8**: 138–150

Lawton MP. (1997) Assessing quality of life in Alzheimer disease research. *Alzheimer Disease and Associated Disorders* **11** (Suppl. 6): 91–99

Lawton MP and Brody E. (1969) Assessment of older people: self-maintaining and instrumental activities of daily living. *The Gerontologist* **9**: 179–186

Logsdon RG and Teri L. (1997) The Pleasant Events Schedule-AD: Psychometric properties and relationship to depression and cognition in Alzheimer's disease patients. *The Gerontologist*, **37**: 40–45

Logsdon RG, Gibbons LE, McCurry SM, Teri L. (1999) Quality of life in Alzheimer's disease: patient and caregiver reports. *Journal of Mental Health and Aging* **5**: 21–32

Logsdon RG, Gibbons LE, McCurry SM, Teri L. (2002) Assessing quality of life in older adults with cognitive impairment. *Psychosomatic Medicine* **64**: 510–519

Mack JL and Whitehouse PJ. (2001) Quality of life in dementia: state of the art report of the International Working Group for Harmonization of Dementia Drug Guidelines and the Alzheimer's Society Satellite Meeting. *Alzheimer Disease and Associated Disorders*, **15**: 69–71

Patrick DL and Erickson P. (1993) Concepts of health-related quality of life. In: *Health Status and Health Policy: Quality of Life in Health Care Evaluation and Resource Allocation.* New York, Oxford University Press

Rabins PV and Steele C. (1996) A scale to measure impairment in severe dementia and similar conditions. *American Journal of Geriatric Psychiatry* **4**: 247–251

Rabins PV and Kasper JD. (1997) Measuring quality of life in dementia: Conceptual and practical issues. *Alzheimer Disease and Associated Disorders* **11** (Suppl. 6): 100–104

Rabins PV, Kasper JD, Kleinman L, Black BS, Patrick DL. (1999) Concepts and methods in the development of the ADRQL: an instrument for assessing health-related quality of life in persons with Alzheimer's disease. *Journal of Mental Health and Aging* **5**: 33–48

Ready RE and Ott BR. (2003) Quality of life measures for dementia. *Health and Quality of Life Outcomes* **1**(11): 1–9

Ready RE, Ott BR, Grace J, Fernandez I. (2002) The Cornell-Brown Scale for Quality of Life in Dementia. *Alzheimer Disease and Associated Disorders* **16**: 109–115

Reisberg B, Ferris SH, de Leon MJ et al. (1982) The Global Deterioration Scale for assessment of primary degenerative dementia. *American Journal of Psychology* **139**: 1136–1139

Rosen WG, Mohs RC, Davis KL. (1984) A new rating scale for Alzheimer's disease. *American Journal of Psychiatry* **141**: 1356–1364

Salek SS, Walker MD, Bayer AJ. (1998) A review of quality of life in Alzheimer's disease. Part 2: Issues in assessing drug effects. *Pharmacoeconomics* **14**: 613–627

Schermer M. (2003) In search of 'the good life' for demented elderly. *Medicine, Health Care and Philosophy* **6**: 35–44

Selai C and Trimble MR. (1999) Assessing quality of life in dementia. *Aging and Mental Health* **3**: 101–111

Selai CE, Trimble MR, Rossor MN, Harvey RJ. (2001a) Assessing quality of life in dementia: Preliminary psychometric testing of the Quality of Life Assessment Schedule (QoLAS). *Neuropsychological Rehabilitation* **11**: 219–243

Selai C, Vaughan A, Harvey RJ, Logsdon R. (2001b) Using the QoL-AD in the UK. *International Journal of Geriatric Psychiatry* **16**: 537–542

Spector A, Thorgrimsen L, Woods B *et al.* (2003) Efficacy of an evidence-based cognitive stimulation therapy programme for people with dementia. *British Journal of Psychiatry* **183**: 248–254

Stern Y, Sano M, Paulson J *et al.* (1987) Modified Mini-Mental State Exam: Validity and reliability (abstract). *Neurology* **37** (Suppl. 1): 179

Teri L and Logsdon RG. (1991) Identifying pleasant activities for Alzheimer's disease patients: the Pleasant Events Schedule-AD. *The Gerontologist* **31**: 124–127

Teri L and Wagner A. (1992) Alzheimer's disease and depression. *Journal of Consulting and Clinical Psychology* **60**: 379–391

Walker MD, Salek SS, Bayer AJ. (1998) A review of quality of life in Alzheimer's Disease. Part 1: Issues in assessing disease impact. *Pharmacoeconomics* **14**: 499–530

Ware JE and Sherbourne DC. (1992) The MOS 36-item Short-Form Health Survey (SF-36) I. Conceptual framework and item selection. *Medical Care* **30**: 473–483

Weiner MF, Martin-Cook K, Svetlik DA, Saine K, Foster B, Fontaine CS. (2000) The Quality of Life in Late-Stage Dementia (QUALID) Scale. *Journal of the American Medical Directors Association* **1**: 114–116

Whitehouse PJ. (2000) Quality of life: Future directions. In: SM Albert and RG Logsdon (eds), *Assessing Quality of Life in Alzheimer's Disease*. New York, Springer Publishing Company

Whitehouse PJ, Orgogozo J, Becker RE *et al.* (1997) Quality-of-life assessment in dementia drug development: Position paper from the International Working Group on Harmonization of Dementia Drug Guidelines. *Alzheimer Disease and Associated Disorders* **11** (Suppl. 3): 56–60

Wilkinson IM and Graham-White J. (1980) Psychogeriatric Dependency Rating Scales (PGDRS): a method of assessment for use by nurses. *British Journal of Psychiatry* **137**: 558–565

Williams J and Rees J. (1997) The use of 'Dementia Care Mapping' as a method of evaluating care received by patients with dementia: an initiative to improve quality of life. *Journal of Advanced Nursing* **25**: 316–323

WHO QoL Group (1995) *WHO Quality of Life-100*. Geneva: World Health Organization Division of Mental Health

Woods B. (1999) Promoting well-being and independence for people with dementia. *International Journal of Geriatric Psychiatry* **14**: 97–109

Yesavage J, Brink T, Rose T. (1983) Development and validation of a geriatric depression screening scale: a preliminary report. *Journal of Psychiatry Research* **17**: 37–49

Younger D and Martin GW. (2000) Dementia Care Mapping: An approach to quality audit of services for people with dementia in two health districts. *Journal of Advanced Nursing* **32**: 1206–1212

19

Moral, ethical and legal aspects of dementia

19a

Ethical issues

STEPHEN J LOUW AND JULIAN C HUGHES

In the broad sweep of medical ethics, the issues affecting patients with dementia are sometimes amongst the most daunting for the clinician. They concern life and death and the very nature of personhood. Philosophical thought about the moral issues raised by clinical practice aims, at a meta-level, to show us the structure of our thoughts and decision-making processes; and, at a practical level, it aims to help us make up our minds. Thus, philosophy helps us to make practical decisions on a rational basis. We shall combine these two aims. First, we shall uncover the casuistic (case-by-case) basis to moral reasoning in clinical practice, using wandering as an example. Second, we shall discuss a characterization of personhood that stresses the importance of context and culture and shows the relevance of this way of thinking for issues (e.g. ethical issues around genetics) affecting families. Third, we shall show how virtue theory deepens our understanding of the several issues in connection with dementia that involve truth-telling. We believe it is virtue ethics that provides the most useful way to understand day-to-day ethical decision-making (see Chapter 19c).

In this chapter we cannot hope to mention all the ethical issues relating to dementia (for further discussion see Oppenheimer, 1999; Hughes, 2002). The literature is vast (Baldwin *et al.*, 2003). We hope, nevertheless, to indicate ways of thinking that might be broadly applicable.

19.1 MORAL REASONING AND CASUISTRY

It might be assumed that ethical reasoning is a linear, hierarchical process. So, in making ethical decisions we move from moral theories, such as consequentialism (which asserts that an action is right to the extent to which it promotes the best consequences) or deontology (which asserts that an action is right to the extent to which it reflects a correct moral rule or principle), to decisions regarding what to do in individual cases.

This approach had its origin in Hellenic times, when the successful method of Euclidian geometry was thought to be equally applicable to philosophy and ethics. Contrariwise, Aristotle (1925) suggested that we should argue from the details of an individual case towards the general principle, rather than the other way round. That is, induction, rather than deduction. Indeed, the rigorous demands of deductive thinking (e.g. that there should be an unbroken, logical chain of reasoning) are too susceptible to mistakes. As an alternative, casuistic reasoning is a practical, more familiar and reliable mode of ethical reasoning (Jonsen and Toulmin, 1988). It is not a new approach in ethics and it forms the basis of legal systems that incorporate case law.

In both the UK and the USA the establishment of and reference to *precedent cases* (case law) is fundamental to the progress of practical juristic reasoning. Judges immerse themselves in the details of a case, compare the facts of the present case with different precedents and decide the case accordingly. Rarely does a case undergo a formal deductive analysis based entirely on jurisprudential principles.

So, too, in clinical medicine many conditions are simply recognized and form the 'precedent cases' that help to establish the diagnosis of new cases. Occasionally general biological principles help to inform our clinical judgements by a sort of *nested deductivism*. For example, we know that anticholinergic medication can cause symptoms of delirium. So we can deduce that starting procyclidine might explain why this particular patient now has hallucinations. However, this deductive reasoning is *nested* in the broader recognition, which is more generally a process of induction, that the patient has a delirium.

In moral reasoning the process of casuistry similarly implies reference to a lexicon of generally accepted precedent cases. Developing such a lexicon of ethical cases itself requires a rigorous process, with cases being included from different perspectives. There must be *immersion in the particularities of the case* (the physical diagnoses, treatment options and prognosis in each instance, the wishes of the patient, the pros and cons of interventions, etc.), and into the *realities for a particular clinic* (what policies are in place, what is the norm of practice, what are the constraints on those norms, etc.); thereafter a process of *interpretation* should be very carefully conducted as to the moral relevance and meaning of theories being applied to the particular case in the light of previous cases. This process of *immersion* and *interpretation* typifies casuistry and, as will always be the case, can be undertaken well or badly (Murray, 1994).

Another important element of casuistry is that it accepts conclusions as being *presumptive* and emphasizes that they are revisable in the light of new experience; there is thus a resistance to dogma. This is also the case in Law, where a judge, having given a verdict, may give leave to appeal.

The justification of casuistic reasoning resides in the presumption that morality lies in the realm of practice, not of theory. Thus:

- arguments move from the particular to the general;
- ethical decisions are not presumed to be 'universal';
- the particularities of the case are given great weight, as are the circumstances of the clinical environment;
- the perspectives of different interested parties are important;
- moral theories and principles are informative, but not compelling, in the process of moral reasoning;
- whilst high value is necessarily placed on the precedent cases, these are in themselves open to revision.

19.1.1 An example of casuistic reasoning: wandering

There is increasing interest in using new technology to detect or prevent risky behaviour in dementia. Electronic tagging is seen as a way to prevent wandering, but it raises ethical issues (Hughes and Louw, 2002a). Approaching this problem using the principles of beneficence and non-maleficence would tend to lead to the conclusion that electronic tagging is a good thing, because it will reduce the risk of harm. Using the principle of autonomy, however, the libertarian will counter that tagging is an infringement of the person's freedom. Both sides start from ethical principles (Beauchamp and Childress, 1994), but they start from different principles, so there is a clash.

Casuistry would start from the details of the particular case: details about the protagonists, the available professional help, the psychological and social environment. The different perspectives of those involved would be considered as important. The principles of autonomy, beneficence and non-maleficence would not be ignored, but the particularities of the case would

be the main focus for discussion. A comparison with other cases might yield the conclusion, as so often in moderate to severe dementia, that it would be too unsafe to allow this person to wander. Casuistic reasoning, however, leaves open the possibility that there might be a case where the importance of getting out, where the person's deeply ingrained habits of walking a particular route, should not be restricted even if there were elements of risk. At the margin, in a case of very mild cognitive impairment, tagging would be an infringement of liberty. Making estimations about what to do at the margin – and (importantly) recognizing that there is a margin – is a feature of casuistic thought. Approaching decisions about tagging with openness (rather than with dogmatic principles) is appropriate and, we would argue, virtuous. By this means we accord individual people respect.

19.2 PRACTICE: PERSONS AND CONTEXT

We are suggesting, therefore, that just as in the ordinary course of our clinical development we rely on theoretical frameworks as well as practical experience, so too we should in ethical decision-making. The ethical lexicon we thus construct might be private or public, but to carry normative weight (i.e. to have the authority to direct the actions of others) it will have to be shareable in principle.

Thus, there is a background to which our lexicon must conform. Against this background, the lexicon must have some basic level of cogency and comprehensibility. The background will include our shared moral sentiments and reasoning, which will largely be inductive (but may include nested deductivism). However, the background to our decisions (clinical or ethical) will contain much more besides: it is multilayered and multifaceted. Indeed, it is the background of practice, the context in which clinical and ethical decisions must be made.

19.2.1 The situated-embodied-agent and cultural embedding

One way of putting this is to say that we are, as people, situated. We are situated as the bodily beings that we are, with our aims and intentions in a personal story, in a family and social context, in a particular culture and history (which includes a legal framework), in a space of moral and spiritual concerns (Hughes, 2001). Regarding the person against this multilayered background, as situated-embodied agents, is instructive when it comes to considering a whole raft of difficult clinical and ethical decisions (Hughes, 2002).

In keeping with the casuist approach, the clinician will need to be open to the background context. This might mean 'immersion' in (involving sensitivity to and respect for) a culture that could be quite different to his or her own. Some cultures involve views and taboos that have far-reaching clinical and ethical implications. The Chinese believe, for example, that it is bad luck to talk about death or serious, fatal diagnoses. The traditional Navajo American Indians believe that thought and language shape reality and influence events; thus, positive language may have a healing effect and negative language may be harmful (Braun *et al.*, 2000).

The point, however, is not just about cultural politeness. Looking at different cultures also challenges our own predominant view that self-rule (autonomy) is paramount. Consider, for example, the African notion of *ubuntu*, which encapsulates the idea that an individual can exist only in the context of relationships. Similarly, while the Navajo American Indians include autonomy as part of their belief system, this is necessarily in the context of the principle of cooperation or consensus. There is a blurring of the boundaries between the individual and his or her community. Consequently the emphasis shifts from individual autonomy towards communal justice or fairness. In relation to a patient who is developing dementia, the family circle and the community traditionally draw in closer and sustain the individual's identity, by continued respect for his or her personality and traditional roles as an elder.

Cultures might learn from one another. For instance, in these 'non-Western' cultures it is assumed that the community will share the cause of an individual's distress. Hence, issues relating to confidentiality require to be seen from the family and community perspective. But this should be no different in 'Western' societies (Hughes and Louw, 2002b). Indeed, there are several strands of ethical thought that stress the extent to which the person cannot be regarded as a detached atom, but must be seen as embedded in a multi-layered context.

Feminine ethics, for instance, move away from the (masculine) emphasis on rights and autonomy to consider the intrinsic importance of our caring interrelationships (Noddings, 1984). Similarly, narrative ethics suggests that we will understand a person by understanding his or her story. It is in the context of narrative, therefore, that judgements about right and wrong for people must be made. However, our stories interconnect: we do not make them up alone (Jones, 1999).

19.2.2 Interrelationships: from genetics to families

The pace of genetic research in dementia means that ethical issues in this area become ever more pressing (Farmer and McGuffin, 1999). One of the main complexities here highlights the problem of our embeddedness. We each have a unique genetic make-up. Yet genetics link us to the rest of the human species (as well as to the animal kingdom and the living world generally). In particular, knowing about an individual's genetics might give us sensitive information about the person's family. The issue is to do with privacy in a world that interconnects. The interconnections are ultimately, in this case, to those who have to pay higher premiums on their health insurance because of the burden placed on insurers by high-risk individuals and families.

The genetics of dementia has not yet afforded us the ethical experience that would allow the construction of the sort of lexicon to which we have referred above. This is not, however, a problem for casuistry. It simply means we have to look at other cases to make our comparisons (e.g. Huntington's disease). Moreover, it stresses that casuistry provides a process, but not the basis, for our ethical decisions. At root our suggestion is that we should follow the example of the virtuous clinician (see Chapter 19c). How would he or she approach an individual asking for information that might affect the whole family? It would surely be by carefully, empathically negotiating that the person should consider the impact of any decision on others. More broadly, how would the virtuous clinician deal generally with confidential information? This would surely be by maintaining confidence whilst recognizing the limits of this duty with respect to those others who are intimately involved.

Cultural comparisons, as we have seen, demonstrate different perspectives. The ethicist-clinician, in developing the skills of understanding and reasoning, must be aware of the subtle nature and implications of these different perspectives. However, as the issues relating to genetics demonstrate, the different perspectives are not just cross-cultural. The perspective of family carers has long been largely overlooked in the professional literature relating to ethics (Hughes *et al.*, 2002a). The ethical issues for family carers are, however, different from those facing professionals precisely because they arise in a personal context and reflect long-term relationships (Hughes *et al.*, 2002b).

If, however, we should take the views of family carers seriously, how much more seriously should we take the views of people with dementia themselves? The tendency to ignore their perspectives undoubtedly reflects the supposition that they are, in one sense or another, incompetent. There is evidence, however, that even in the moderate to severe stages of the disease people with dementia continue to convey meaning (Sabat and Harré, 1994). Hence, there has been increasing interest in and concern to express the views of people with dementia (Bond and Corner, 2001). It seems important that ethical research should take the same path of involving people with dementia, typically through qualitative research, backed up by rigorous philosophical thought and analysis (Hughes, 2003).

19.3   TOWARDS THE VIRTUES

So, recognizing ourselves as situated-embodied agents means that we see people, including people with dementia, as interconnecting and interrelating in a context. The shared nature of this context is the background against which our interpretive judgements concerning the goodness or badness of particular actions are made. It is the context in which we must immerse ourselves, in keeping with the casuistic approach, in order to understand the particularities of the case. It is the context against which our interpretations, with reference to our lexicon of ordinary and salient cases, must be made.

All of this involves a building up of experience through practice. It should be the epitome of what Aristotle termed *phronesis*, or practical wisdom. This is the virtue that allows us to make practical judgements about what is good or bad for human beings. It cannot be taken for granted that we shall all acquire this type of wisdom. Some of us will be temperamentally better at it than others, but it is inescapable that we shall have to make decisions and we shall naturally wish to make good decisions, by which we mean decisions that will be good for us generally. To quote Aristotle (1925: pp 138–9):

> ... since moral virtue is a state of character concerned with choice, and choice is deliberate desire, therefore both the reasoning must be true and the desire right, if the choice is to be good, and the latter must pursue just what the former asserts.

What the virtues, including *phronesis*, require is some sense of what we should be as human beings. Well, whatever this might entail, it is likely to be arrived at by a careful application of the casuistic process against the background of our shared, interconnecting, interrelationships and experience.

19.3.1 Deepening analysis: the virtue of fidelity in dementia

Many of the ethical issues that arise in connection with dementia are to do with truthfulness. Here are examples:

- Should Mrs A be told that she has Alzheimer's disease?
- Should Mr B's son be told that his father has dementia?
- Should Ms C, who has mild cognitive impairment, be told that this might progress to dementia?
- Should Mrs D, with a moderately severe dementia, be told that correspondence is being copied to her daughter, the social worker and the local Alzheimer's Society?
- Should Mr E's medication be hidden in his drinks?
- Should Mrs F's husband tell her he is taking her for respite care, or should he pretend it is just a drive in the country?
- Should Miss G's nephew and niece agree to an admission to long-term care, having promised they would keep her at home?

When such ethical issues are discussed in the literature, appeal is usually made to the principles of medical ethics, or to consequentialist or deontological considerations. Despite the concern that telling the diagnosis might cause depression (and so be maleficent), being truthful is a way of respecting the person's autonomy (Pinner and Bouman, 2002). Covert drug administration may be the best way of relieving a person's agitation and of satisfying the duty of care but is, nevertheless, a breach of trust (Treloar *et al.*, 2001). Interestingly, in a study that consulted people with dementia, although the discussion still centred on conflicting principles (autonomy versus paternalistic beneficence and non-maleficence), 'veracity' was recognized as the underlying 'difficult virtue' (Marzanski, 2000).

Virtue theory offers a deeper analysis of the need to be truthful (May, 1994). First, virtues underlie the principles we have mentioned above. Arguments about telling the truth may reveal a concern for the person's *welfare*. Maybe the truth will have good consequences or bad consequences. Either way, the underlying virtue is that of benevolence. Alternatively, it might be argued that the person has a *right* to know the truth (whatever the consequences) and an appeal can be made to the virtues of honesty and respect. Respect for the person's autonomy is also supported by the virtue of candour. However, there is a deeper link between telling the truth and the virtue of fidelity. As May (1994) suggests:

> The virtues with which the professional dispenses the truth may condition the very reality he or she offers the patient ... The professional relationship, though less comprehensive and intimate than marriage, is similarly promissory and fiduciary ... The moral question for the professional becomes not simply a question of telling truths, but of *being true to his promises*. Conversely, the total situation for the patient includes not only his disease but also whether others ditch him or stand by him in extremity ... The fidelity of the professional *per se* will not eliminate the disease ... but it can affect mightily the context in which the trouble runs its course.

Writing from the perspective of professionals, we should not overlook how this sort of analysis also helps to explain the profound sense of guilt family carers feel when, for instance, they have to place the person with dementia in a residential or nursing home. The intimacy of family or similar relationships makes it all the more difficult to break faith: guilt then becomes a manifestation of not being true.

19.4 SUMMING UP: HERMENEUTICS AND VIRTUES

The care of people with dementia requires great understanding. This may in part be instinctive, but it is also certainly acquired and can be improved by careful, critical reflection. Hermeneutic philosophers talk of a pre-understanding, the common background perhaps, that allows meanings to be interpreted. They seek out the common ground in different positions as a way of understanding shared and disputed values. This desire to find a way forward, by attention to what all parties are conveying (through words and actions), requires that a practical solution should be found. Hence, hermeneutics also involves *phronesis*:

> ... this type of wisdom includes a certain attitude, a certain condition, obtained by practice. Virtues are based on education and training; they are acquired in the process of acting and living. Virtues grow from experience. Only those who have had to deal with numerous ethical questions ... may possess practical wisdom. Understanding dementia is in the end a practical matter, a matter of being experienced (Widdershoven and Widdershoven-Heerding, 2003).

In this chapter we have sketched an ethical meta-landscape and pointed towards the practical usefulness of theories that stress the importance of experience, that recognize our interrelationships and encourage careful and empathic negotiation. We have suggested how our decisions in ethical and clinical matters require the building up, case by case, of a lexicon against which our judgements can be made. However, the judgements that inform the lexicon are embedded in a background of interrelationships and interconnections, where people are situated in multilayered contexts of shared and disputed valued. Openness to the corrective that this background might impose is itself a sign of the sort of virtue that allows us to negotiate the moral landscape in a practical way.

REFERENCES

Aristotle. (1925) *The Nichomachean Ethics* (translated by D Ross). Oxford, Oxford University Press

Baldwin C, Hughes J, Hope T, *et al.* (2003) Ethics and dementia: mapping the literature by bibliometric analysis. *International Journal of Geriatric Psychiatry* **18**: 41–54

Beauchamp T and Childress J. (1994) *Principles of Biomedical Ethics*, 4th edition. New York, Oxford University Press

Bond J and Corner L. (2001) Researching dementia: are there unique methodological challenges for health services research? *Ageing and Society* **21**: 95–116

Braun KL, Pietsch JH, Blanchette PL. (eds) (2000) *Cultural Issues in End of Life Decision Making*. London, Sage

Farmer A and McGuffin P. (1999) Ethics and psychiatric genetics. In: S Bloch, P Chodoff, SA Green (eds), *Psychiatric Ethics*, 3rd edition. Oxford, Oxford University Press, pp. 479–493

Hughes JC. (2001) Views of the person with dementia. *Journal of Medical Ethics* **27**: 86–91

Hughes JC. (2002) Ethics and the psychiatry of old age. In: R Jacoby and C Oppenheimer (eds), *Psychiatry in the Elderly*, 3rd edition. Oxford, Oxford University Press, pp. 863–895

Hughes JC. (2003) Ethics research in dementia: the way forward? In: EM Welsh (ed.), *Focus on Alzheimer's Disease Research*. Hauppauge (NY), Nova Science Publishers, pp. 245–266

Hughes JC and Louw SJ. (2002a) Electronic tagging of people with dementia who wander. *BMJ* **325**: 847–848

Hughes JC and Louw SJ. (2002b) Confidentiality and cognitive impairment: professional and philosophical ethics. *Age and Ageing* **31**: 147–150

Hughes JC, Hope T, Savulescu J, Ziebland S. (2002a) Carers, ethics and dementia: a survey and review of the literature. *International Journal of Geriatric Psychiatry* **17**: 35–40

Hughes JC, Hope T, Reader S, Rice D. (2002b) Dementia and ethics: a pilot study of the views of informal carers. *Journal of the Royal Society of Medicine* **95**: 242–246

Jones AH. (1999) Narrative based medicine: narrative in medical ethics. *BMJ* **318**: 253–256

Jonsen AR and Toulmin S. (1988) *The Abuse of Casuistry: a History of Moral Reasoning*. Berkeley, University of California Press

Marzanski M. (2000) Would you like to know what is wrong with you? On telling the truth to patients with dementia. *Journal of Medical Ethics* **26**: 108–113

May WF. (1994) The virtues in a professional setting. In: KWM Fulford, GR Gillett, JM Soskice (eds), *Medicine and Moral Reasoning*. Cambridge, Cambridge University Press, pp. 75–91

Murray TH. (1994) Medical ethics, moral philosophy and moral tradition. In: KWM Fulford, GR Gillett, JM Soskice (eds), *Medicine and Moral Reasoning*. Cambridge, Cambridge University Press, pp. 91–105

Noddings N. (1984) *Caring: a Feminine Approach to Ethics and Moral Education*. Berkeley, University of California Press

Oppenheimer C. (1999) Ethics in old age psychiatry. In: S Bloch, P Chodoff, SA Green (eds), *Psychiatric Ethics*, 3rd edition. Oxford, Oxford University Press, pp. 317–343

Pinner G and Bouman WP. (2002) To tell or not to tell: on disclosing the diagnosis of dementia. *International Psychogeriatrics* **14**: 127–137

Sabat SR and Harré R. (1994) The Alzheimer's disease sufferer as a semiotic subject. *Philosophy, Psychiatry, and Psychology* **1**: 145–160

Treloar A, Philpot M, Beats B. (2001) Concealing medication in patients' food. *Lancet* **357**: 62–64

Widdershoven GAM and Widdershoven-Heerding I. (2003) Understanding dementia: a hermeneutic perspective. In: KWM Fulford, K Morris, JZ Sadler, G Stanghellini (eds), *Nature and Narrative: an Introduction to the New Philosophy of Psychiatry*. Oxford, Oxford University Press, pp. 103–111

19b

Legal issues

BERNARD M DICKENS

19.5 CAPACITY

Underlying most legal issues raised by patients' dementia is the question of capacity. Comprehensive legal criteria of capacity are elusive. Specific determinations are often governed more by processes of assessment than by tests that produce uniformly replicable conclusions. Courts pay attention to persons' classifications for instance as moderately or severely demented, and to the cognitive deficits associated with each status. Judicial proceedings achieve legally compelling assessments of individuals' capacities for particular functions, but are frequently prohibitively costly and inaccessible. Physicians' assessments, particularly but not only by psychiatrists, are usually convincing, especially when confirmed by a second, independent opinion. Clinical psychologists' assessments of patients' cognitive capacities are often valuable. However, for testamentary capacity, a lawyer's finding that a client can give adequate instructions, answer standard questions about property and family composition, and make reasonable choices, is usually sufficient to show capacity to make an effective will.

A tendency until recent times, that occasionally persists, was to consider a finding of capacity or incapacity as 'global', or all or nothing. A finding made for one purpose, whatever it was and by whomsoever made, governed all other purposes. Now, however, capacity is considered specific to separate functions, so that a patient who is competent for one purpose, such as to consent to medical care, may not be competent for another, such as making contracts or other financial arrangements.

Competent persons can make decisions on the basis of their wishes, even when these are against their best interests as physicians and others assess them. Patients do not lose the right to be governed by their wishes simply because they become incapable of expressing them, or of confirming them. Incapable persons should therefore be treated according to their wishes as shown when competent, unless they indicate otherwise when treatment is imminent or they would be seriously endangered. It is not legally justifiable to discount people's wishes just because others, such as their family members, can make better decisions for them.

19.5.1 Medical care capacity

The law sets a fairly low threshold of capacity to consent to medical care recommended by a patient's physician. Patients must be able to understand what the care entails, its alternatives, the risks of each and consequences of forgoing all care. Some legal systems and enacted laws set capacity to refuse consent at the same level as capacity to accept it, on the principle that a person with contractual capacity may accept or reject a contract. A more refined approach where services are available without direct charge to patients, is that higher competency is required to refuse indicated medical care, because that choice may expose individuals to higher risks of harm (see Chapter 19c). Physicians may appear manipulative if they accept competence of patients who accept their recommendations and question that of patients who decline, but since courts respect clinicians' disinterested professional judgment, this is analytically sound.

When patients are incompetent to consent to medical care, others may decide on their behalf. If patients' wishes made when competent are known, they may be legally binding (above). If their wishes are unknown, or would be seriously harmful, care decisions may be made by guardians appointed according to locally prevailing laws. Where these are uncertain, closest family members may decide, such as patients' spouses, children or parents. It is a misnomer to describe this as 'substituted consent'; the patient is treated non-consensually, on the *de jure* or a *de facto* guardian's authorization. A limit may be that *de facto* guardians have no power to authorize payments for care from the patients' assets, where payment is required.

19.5.2 Medical research capacity

When research is not intended for their personal benefit, patients' capacity to consent requires higher levels of competency. The risks and non-beneficial purpose of treatment must be clearly comprehended. Guardians' powers are limited to therapy, and they cannot authorize invasive research on incompetent patients. They may approve medical record inspections and, for instance, monitoring of patients' therapy as control subjects, however, if confidentiality is protected, and allow the drawing of a few extra drops of blood for research when venepuncture is lawfully undertaken for therapeutic, diagnostic or monitoring purposes.

19.5.3 Contractual capacity

It is commonly supposed that cognitively impaired adults lack contractual capacity, in the same way as legal minors. In many circumstances this is true, because the law recognizes, and aims to protect impaired persons against, their vulnerability to exploitation and undue influence. The contractual principle *caveat emptor*, let the purchaser beware, relies on purchasers possessing ordinary capacity to exercise common prudence, and not be misled by delusions, confusion or defective perception. When cognitively impaired persons lack the ability to be wary or cautious on their own behalf, the law may afford them the protection of contractual incapacity.

However, the law does not discriminate against demented persons by precluding them from acting on their own behalf to acquire items, supplies and services they need for their sustenance, protection and comfort. Accordingly, they enjoy contractual capacity to make binding agreements for the food, shelter, clothing, medical care and other goods and services that will maintain them in a manner appropriate to their accustomed circumstances, known in law as 'necessaries'. Impaired purchasers are protected against exploitation in bargaining for necessaries by the courts requiring that they pay not necessarily the contractually agreed price, but only as much as is merited (*quantum meruit*) for a necessary supplied. In case of dispute, the courts will determine the payment due, on the basis of parties' equal bargaining power. When payments are so determined or are set, for instance, as standard rates that parties cannot vary by bargaining, such as for public services like domestic heating or electricity, impaired persons are liable, and legally able, to pay for them from their assets.

A demented person can avoid a contract for non-necessaries if the contractual partner is aware of the disability, and if the disabled person did not take any advantage under the contract. The partner cannot avoid the contract, however, and is entitled to only a *quantum meruit* payment if the disabled person leaves the contract binding.

19.5.4 Testamentary capacity

In many countries, laws on distribution of estates without wills are patterned on distribution with wills, reducing disadvantages of testamentary incapacity. Nevertheless, legal property transactions, including by will, usually require relatively high levels of capacity. Testators must have a reasonable awareness of their assets and how they can be determined, of their family structures and moral obligations, and of liabilities their estates may have to settle. Lawyers uncertain of clients' capacity cannot proceed without reliable, independent assurance. Witnesses to wills observe only that they were signed without coercion, not testators' mental capacity.

A legal concern is the influence of cognitive and affective disorders on testamentary capacity, and their interaction. Provided that prospective testators know how to determine their general assets, although not necessarily their current market value, and key participants in family structures, they have capacity. This is so even if they hold particularly strong and even irrational sentiments about individuals and institutions, whether positive or negative. Capacity should be questioned, however, when evidence arises that an individual's attitude may be based on a demented or serious delusion. It is a matter of professional judgement, of physicians, lawyers and, for instance, accountants, how far to go in probing the convictions that have conditioned what appears an irrational attitude toward a close family member who is a potential beneficiary, or a person or institution named by an intending testator. A legal duty of care may exist to protect a patient or client against the undue influence of those deliberately seeking testamentary advantages. No duty exists to protect potential beneficiaries against irrational exclusion from benefits, although they may contest testators' capacity after provisions of wills become known.

Wills are 'ambulatory', meaning that they are to be understood in the context of the testator's circumstances as at the time of death, or earlier loss of capacity to vary the will, for instance by an added codicil. A common practice is to propose residual provisions to accommodate accidental oversights. For instance, when monetary gifts are made to named grandchildren, any who may have been inadvertently overlooked, and any not anticipated to be born when the will is drafted, may be included by language such as 'and the same to other offspring of my children's unions'.

Wills can usually be revoked more easily than they are made. Testators may tear or deface them or throw them away, without witnesses or requirements of clear capacity. Capacity to repudiate a will is less exacting than capacity to make one, involving only rejection of what was previously arranged.

19.5.5 Matrimonial capacity

Historically, marriages united families, and family property, rather than just individuals. Today, however, matrimonial capacity requires only the affectionate intention to spend one's life faithfully with another. Incapacity to rear future children is not necessarily a barrier, particularly when partners are beyond childbearing age, such as in second marriages. Because marriage introduces new family and moral obligations, its legal effect in many countries is automatically to revoke existing wills. A dysfunction of this law is that when elderly couples have capacity to enter second marriages, agreeing that both will leave their property not to each other but to their own children of earlier marriages, their existing wills are revoked but they may lack capacity to make new wills giving effect to their agreement. On death with no will, the survivor of them will usually inherit the other's estate, contrary to their intentions. This may be overcome only by complex legal property arrangements, for which again their competence may be suspect, unless they have only modest means and obvious intentions.

19.5.6 Child care capacity

Even mild dementia, in contrast to mild mental retardation, may disqualify individuals from eligibility to adopt children, since courts usually apply relatively high standards of suitability for placement of babies and young children. This is not a barrier, however, to capacity to marry a partner with a dependent child. A more common issue is suitability of patients as caregivers to their grandchildren. The legal approach is less to assess potential caregivers than to consider the best interests of each child. A decision balances its competing interests in physical and, for instance, nutritional protection against the value of maintenance of familiar relationships. Decisive factors are patients' degrees of cognitive impairment and children's ages and degrees of dependency. Mildly or moderately demented patients may be more suitable for short-term placements of children, such as when a single parent is confined to give birth to another child.

19.6 ADVANCE MEDICAL DIRECTIVES

Laws increasingly permit, and encourage, competent people to anticipate times to come when they are no longer competent, and to take the earlier opportunity to arrange how they then want to be treated. Advance directives have been called 'living wills' and often focus on terminal care. As more is learned, however, of genetic predictors of future dementia, and, for instance, AIDS-related dementia, directives will come to focus more on future life than on future death. The value of advance directives is that they can address future residential and healthcare arrangements, medical treatment related and unrelated to advance of dementia, and for instance, acceptance and limits of involvement in research. When people make advance directives while they are undoubtedly competent, the directives are of legal significance whether or not they conform to legally-set formulae. Mildly or moderately demented patients may also create credible directives

concerning matters within their cognitive grasp. Even at advanced stages of dementia, however, spoken directives can be given that effectively deny consent to interventions that cause distress or discomfort. Further, no advance directive can be enforced so as to apply invasive treatment that the patient resists at the time of attempted administration, except perhaps to avoid premature death.

19.7 INVOLUNTARY DETENTION AND CHOICE OF RESIDENCE

Perhaps the most difficult area of legal policy concerning persons with more advanced dementia is their involuntary detention in psychiatric facilities. Beyond determination of correct policy, difficulty arises from the law itself when legislation permits but does not compel such persons' involuntary detention, and when involuntary detention not authorized by legislation may be held excusable on grounds of necessity to protect demented persons against their risk of suffering serious bodily harm.

There is an historical record of severe legal oppression of demented people, related to a conviction that those with cognitive impairments are unpredictable, and therefore dangerous. There is also a more benign record of belief that they merit care, and that needs may be met that they cannot themselves supply, in the safety of suitable residential care. Their detention was therefore justified on grounds both of protecting the public, and of protecting them against those who would abuse and exploit them, and against themselves. The issue of correct policy remains unresolved, and legislation often reacts to publicized tragedies, such as demented people living at home who die from starvation or cold, or people involuntarily detained for years who, on release, prove capable of living safe and fulfilling lives.

The recent, liberal trend has been towards deinstitutionalization. Human rights principles support demented persons' rights to live where and how they wish, unless they can be proven, by legal process, to be significantly dangerous to others, or to risk suffering serious impairment. Danger to others may take the form of physical violence, but may also include non-violent sexual molestation of others, perhaps owing to disinhibition of instinctive behaviour. Danger to self may take the form of failing to eat or to keep warm, with risk of malnutrition or hypothermia, forgetting to watch cooking food, with risk of causing fires, or lapses in personal hygiene that risk infections. Involuntary long-term detention in psychiatric facilities is increasingly legally based only on dangerousness, to others or self. It is legally justified only on proof that no less invasive alternative is available. Short-term detention may be excusable, but only until an episode of dangerousness to self or others has ended. Less invasive for those dangerous to themselves are regular home visits to ensure nutrition and adequacy of heat and, for instance, fitting automatic time switches to turn off cooking appliances.

There is concern, however, associated with reduced budgets for public health and social welfare services, that so-called community care of the mentally impaired is liable to become community neglect. So-called open door policies applied by psychiatric institutions, by which mental health patients may freely enter institutions that offer care, as voluntary or informal patients, and may freely leave when they wish, operate in fact as revolving door facilities through which impaired patients circulate. Demented people do not always achieve the dignity, comfort or protection in the community intended by deinstitutionalization, but often live wretched, abbreviated lives of chaos, neglect, dependency, and sometimes, as an ironic alternative to psychiatric detention, imprisonment.

Although, in many countries, demented patients may be involuntarily detained only on grounds of their dangerousness, family members such as patients' children may achieve the same effect by removing them from their residences of choice, the patients' homes, and taking them into their own care or delivering them to care facilities. By legal action taken on their behalf, patients may insist on remaining in, or being reinstated in, their own homes. However, such action is often hard to initiate through public guardians, and private action may be barred by patients' incapacity to act by themselves or to contract for legal services. Family members may legally defend removal of demented patients from their own homes by showing that, even though they are not dangerous owing to violence or risk of severe self-injury, they cannot live securely without constant care and supervision.

19.8 CRIMINAL LIABILITY

Serious crimes consist not simply in doing prohibited acts, but in doing them with a prohibited intention or state of mind, i.e. like much else in law, the issue turns on capacity. When demented persons lack capacity to form the mental element that makes an act criminal, they may be found not guilty by reason of mental disorder, which in some jurisdictions is called insanity. In some countries, this 'not guilty' verdict has no penal consequences, but the facts may trigger a hearing under mental health legislation to see if the person meets dangerousness criteria and, like any other non-criminal but dangerous person, is liable to involuntary detention in a psychiatric facility.

In many countries, those found not guilty by reason of mental disorder are liable to detention in secure psychiatric facilities, from which they will not be released until considered to be no threat to the public. They are often detained for longer than they would have been imprisoned had they been found mentally capable and guilty. The justification is that they receive necessary treatment in detention, although demented patients may not be amenable to treatment. Under some legal procedures, a criminal court cannot hear a prosecutor's evidence of a defendant's mental disability until the prosecutor has shown that the likely trial outcome, if there is no such disability, would be a guilty verdict. This is to reduce the risk of detaining an innocent person in a secure psychiatric facility on grounds of mental disability. However, a defendant who wishes to plead not guilty on grounds of mental disorder may do so earlier.

A special problem in facilities where demented patients reside, both involuntarily and voluntarily, comes from sexual behaviour. Molestation of staff members may not be violent, but is conduct against which they are entitled to legal protection. Sexual behaviour with other residents may be consensual, but those with whom such behaviour is initiated may lack legal capacity to consent. Legal models of capacity may be based on adolescents, whose consent to or initiation of consensual sexual behaviour may be legally ineffective, leaving their partners convictable. Further, facility staff may involve police, for fear of their own legal liability for negligence in protection of residents, particularly when a participant in such behaviour has a spouse, or has children who complain of the parent's sexual abuse. Staff members' or police officers' disapproval of or discomfort with demented patients' expressed sexuality may underlie their reactions of invoking criminal law.

A particular problem in criminal proceedings arises when a defendant of borderline competence charged with a serious crime insists on pleading guilty. The problem is aggravated in those jurisdictions, such as in the USA and Caribbean, where the death sentence is retained, and a defendant refuses to appeal against its imposition. The problem involves not only defence counsel, who may be court-appointed, but also prosecuting counsel who, as officers of the court, often acting in a quasi-judicial capacity, cannot knowingly be party to a risk of injustice. Prosecuting authorities may accordingly engage psychiatrists to conduct inquiries into criminal defendants' fitness to plead and fitness to stand trial, and to help them to decide on launching any appeal proceedings.

FURTHER READING

British Medical Association. (1995) *Advance Statements About Medical Treatment*. London, BMA

Burns FR. (2003) The elderly and undue influence *inter vivos*. *Legal Studies* 23: 251–283

Grubb A. (ed.) (2004) *Principles of Medical Law*, 2nd edition. Oxford, Oxford University Press (especially Ch. 4)

Law Commission. (1995) *Mental incapacity*. (Law Com. No.231). London, HMSO

Lord Chancellor's Department. (1997) *Who Decides? Making decisions on behalf of mentally incapacitated adults*. (Cm 3803). London, HMSO

Perlin ML. (1997) *Mental Disability Law: Civil And Criminal*. Charlottesville, Virginia, Michie

Picard EI and Robertson G. (1996) *Legal Liability of Doctors and Hospitals in Canada*, 3rd edition. Scarborough, Ontario: Carswell (especially Ch. 2)

Silberfeld M and Fish A. (1994) *When the Mind Fails: a Guide to Dealing With Incompetency*. Toronto, University of Toronto Press

Skene L. (1998) *Law and Medical Practice: Rights, Duties, Claims and Defences*. Sydney, Butterworths (especially Ch. 5)

Wendler D and Prasad K. (2001) Core safeguards for clinical research with adults who are unable to consent. *Annals of Internal Medicine* 135: 514–523

End-of-life decisions

JULIAN C HUGHES AND STEPHEN J LOUW

The end of life, speaking literally, is awful. Our attitude towards death will colour our attitude towards life. Being light-hearted about death is a perfectly reasonable attitude, but death is also a matter of profound seriousness, partly because of the shape it gives to our lives. Whether or not we believe in an after-life, death is a matter of great awe.

In this chapter, which is concerned with end-of-life issues, we shall focus on virtue ethics. In a sense, what virtue ethics does – to good purpose – is to change the questions that arise. In the remainder of this introduction we shall flesh out some of our earlier discussion of *virtue ethics* (see Chapter 19a). Our aim is not to provide a full account of virtue ethics (see Hursthouse, 1999), but simply to indicate its usefulness.

Virtue ethics suggest that an action is right inasmuch as it is the act that a virtuous person (one who has the virtues and uses them) would perform, where a virtue is understood as a disposition required for people to flourish or live well. Thus, virtue ethics does not just tell us about what human beings are like, nor does it simply give us rules or principles to follow. Rather, the virtues gesture at that which we should *become* as human beings. They point us in the direction of what it is to do well humanly. The virtues tell us how to act.

People will question how we can *know* what is virtuous? One easy answer is that we should ask a virtuous person. As Hursthouse (1999) comments:

> This is far from being a trivial point, for it gives a straightforward explanation of an important aspect of our moral life, namely the fact that we do not always act as 'autonomous', utterly self-determining agents, but quite often seek moral guidance from people we think are morally better than ourselves (p. 35).

Doctors might note how this mirrors clinical experience: we talk to senior colleagues about difficult clinical decisions.

Hursthouse has a second response to the question about knowing what is virtuous. She points out that, even if we know that we are not fully virtuous, it does not follow that we know *nothing* of the virtues. Our knowledge of the virtues is part of the background context in which our practical decisions are embedded (see Chapter 19a). We know about honesty, truthfulness, prudence etc. Moreover, in the clinical arena, when we want expert advice, we do not choose just anyone. We can pick out clinical expertise judiciously.

Furthermore, it does not seem too unreasonable to notice that such difficult clinical cases often involve a value judgement, or something akin to an ethical dimension. If it were simply a factual question about the next step in therapy, any colleague might do. Where, however, the question is about the real value of pursuing treatment for this individual, we need someone who is streetwise, who shows practical wisdom. So we can recognize virtuous people even as we are aware of our own deficiencies.

Virtue ethicists are sensitive to the accusation that they concentrate more on the agent than on the act. As we have already seen, this is not the case. What is *done* is virtuous or vicious, and right or wrong accordingly. Nevertheless, the dispositions of the agent seem far from irrelevant to the goodness or badness of the act. Our final point in this introduction is that this, too, is a reason for doctors to take the virtues seriously.

> What people often complain about is not whatever decision the doctors made, but the manner in which they delivered it or acted on it ... A dose of virtue ethics might make [doctors] concentrate more on how they should respond, rather than resting content with the thought that they have made the right decision (Hursthouse, 1999, p. 48).

In the remainder of this chapter we shall start by discussing the philosophical issues raised by advance directives in dementia and show the difference that virtue ethics makes. The same approach will then be used to discuss, first, artificial nutrition and hydration and the ethical distinction between ordinary and extraordinary means; second, withdrawing and withholding treatment and the principle of futility. We shall also discuss the palliative care approach to dementia and the case against resuscitation.

We shall, however, pass over the topics of assisted suicide and euthanasia (but see Keown, 1995). Virtue theory makes us take seriously what is important in our lives, what makes a life worth living, what makes it good or bad. In this way it has more in keeping with the palliative care approach than with an attitude that aims at death. The question in virtue ethics is: What do we become by aiming at the death of the person with dementia? And the related question is: What do we become if we aim to keep the life of the person with dementia as good as it can be on its natural trajectory towards death? These are difficult questions, which we cannot do justice to, but it is worth recalling that Aristotle said, in relation to courage, that the exercise of the virtues is not always pleasant.

19.9 ADVANCE DIRECTIVES AND PRACTICAL WISDOM

Advance directives are underpinned by the ethical principle of autonomy. The aim is to extend the patient's autonomy into the future, even in the face of incompetence. There is growing recognition that the liberal idea of autonomy does not take account of the importance of personal relationships and mutual dependency (Agich, 2003). Advance directives raise other philosophical concerns too. These have now been rehearsed many times. We shall give a summary account:

- One way to think of personal identity is to regard it as tied to consciousness and, in particular, to memory (Locke, 1690).
- Personal identity becomes a matter of psychological continuity and connectedness (Parfit, 1984).
- In dementia, memory loss means that there is not sufficient psychological continuity or connectedness to say that personal identity has been maintained.
- So the person with dementia cannot be regarded as the same person as the previous person who did not have dementia.
- But then, if they are different persons, the advance directive made earlier by the non-demented person cannot now be applicable to the demented person (Hope, 1995).

It has even been argued that the demented individual will eventually not satisfy the requirements for personhood and cannot then be called a person at all (Buchanan, 1988). This line of thought is disrupted by the broader notion of the person as a situated embodied agent, which importantly allows that the person's memories are significant, but shows that being a person is to be embedded in a social structure, involving

family and friends, legal advisers, spiritual leaders and advocates (Hughes, 2001). It follows that the individual's personhood may, in a moral and philosophical sense, continue to be expressed through established social connections. In which case, we remain persons even when we have dementia; thus, our advance directives retain their validity.

Another valuable perspective, which squares with the situated-embodied agent view, is to be found in narrative ethics.

> From a narrative perspective, a person's identity is formed in stories, which both express and create the unity of a person's life. As stories, advance directives presuppose the unity of the patient's life, and try to contribute to that unity, not by making the different phases identical, but by trying to create a meaningful whole which covers all of them (Widdershoven and Berghmans, 2001).

The idea of taking the person's life as a whole has been used by Dworkin (1993) to develop his notion of 'critical interests', which are those interests that help to shape a person's life. These are contrasted with 'experiential interests', which are the interests we have in current experiences. Critical interests are deemed more central to our lives and, therefore, 'precedent autonomy', as expressed by an advance directive, should rule the day when the person is deemed 'incompetent'. The opposing view has been put by Dresser (1995). She argues that it is an affront to disregard the needs and wishes of the person *now*. To this debate Jaworska (1999) has added that the person with dementia is still a 'valuer', so should still be taken seriously. This chimes with the suggestion that advance directives should be accompanied by a 'values history', to help determine with greater confidence the true wishes of the person who now lacks capacity.

So, at a philosophical level, advance directives in dementia raise questions about personal identity and, in the Dworkin–Dresser debate, raise the issue as to whether the wishes of the 'then-self' or the 'now-self' should take precedence.

These questions and issues, however, seem less important from the perspective of virtue ethics. Confronted by this individual with severe dementia, whose current wishes are difficult to ascertain, but whose advance directive states that he or she would not wish to receive life-sustaining treatment in the event of dementia, what would the virtuous clinician do? Well, any doctor of 'good sense' would, if practicable, talk to as many people involved as possible. It would certainly do no harm to talk with the person with dementia. This might not be easy, but it is wrong to position the person with dementia as 'incompetent' when this might not be the case. From the perspective of the individual with dementia, good communication and empathic understanding will enhance his or her standing as a person (Sabat, 2001).

There are three points to make:

- 'Good sense' is another translation of Aristotle's notion of *phronesis* (see Chapter 19a). It is good sense to talk with people. Weighing up their views in the particular circumstances of the case, against a background of experience and moral judgements, requires practical wisdom.

- What we are describing is exactly the process commended (e.g. in recent draft UK legislation) as necessary to determine a person's best interests, which is what we should be doing when the person lacks capacity to make a decision (Hughes, 2000).
- The virtuous doctor will wish to do what is best for the patient. This is not because the principle of beneficence dictates that we must do such and such, it is because taking people seriously is the mark of someone who has the virtues of charity, justice and *phronesis*.

The issue is not, then, about whether or not this is a person, nor is it about which self to take seriously (the then-self or the now-self), it is about a right attitude in the face of a tragic and difficult situation. It is about what we do in these particular circumstances; but it is also about how we do it. Paying attention to the person, with all that this entails, is the first step. Practical wisdom is required to determine what decisions will be best in these particular circumstances. This will depend on some concept of what is humanly best. These decisions must be made with the right attitude of concern towards the patient, which is a mark of charity. Finally, the weighing up implied in the adjudication of what is best for this particular person will reflect the virtues of fairness and friendship.

Hence, virtue ethics changes the subject. We move from rarefied debates about whether or not the individual is a person, to a more straightforward discussion about how we respond to, how we help, this fellow human being now in this dreadful predicament. And suddenly it seems outlandish to ignore his current state in favour of something he might have said in the past; yet churlish to ignore what he so clearly wrote previously. However difficult it might seem, we have to weigh things up in the light of the concrete circumstances that now obtain. The advance directive, therefore, sits in a context and serves a useful purpose, but only insofar as it contributes to the good and allows human flourishing, albeit flourishing circumscribed by worldly realities.

19.10 WITHHOLDING AND WITHDRAWING LIFE-SUPPORTIVE TREATMENT

The question whether it is in the patient's best interests to withhold or withdraw life-prolonging treatment arises in a variety of contexts for the person with dementia. The woman with a moderate dementia falls and fractures her hip, but there are postoperative complications. At what stage are supportive therapies withdrawn? The man with severe dementia develops a chest infection that does not clear with a variety of antibiotics. Should intravenous antibiotics be withheld? (Should oral antibiotics ever have been commenced?)

19.10.1 Ordinary and extraordinary means

One way of approaching the general issue of withholding or withdrawing life-prolonging therapy is to consider whether there is proportionality between the complexity of the intervention and the apparent benefit that the patient might derive. The distinction between 'ordinary' and 'extraordinary means' allows that 'ordinary means' can differ from person to person and may be 'extraordinary' in other circumstances.

Clearly this moral approach is essentially casuistic: whether something is ordinary or extraordinary must be assessed on a case-by-case basis. It also involves virtues: it is a matter of practical wisdom that such and such a treatment would be disproportionate in terms of the benefits it might bring. Let us presume that the decision involves whether or not to treat the infection of the person with dementia. It is a difficult decision precisely because it involves both factual and evaluative judgements. The virtue of *practical* wisdom suggests precisely that the wisdom is rooted in the doing: it is the experience of clinical practice, supported by a relevant evidence base, that will count. Hence, a study that showed aggressive treatment of infections did not affect the underlying disease and, in fact, was associated with an acceleration in the severity of the disease (Hurley *et al.*, 1996) would be very relevant to the decision.

19.10.2 Palliative care in severe dementia

This brings to mind the suggestion that, in considering end-of-life ethical issues in dementia, we have much to learn from hospices (Volicer and Hurley, 1998). Palliative care involves:

- an affirmation of life, but one in which dying is regarded as a normal process, so that death should neither be hastened nor postponed;
- providing relief from distressing symptoms;
- integrating the psychological, social and spiritual aspects of care;
- offering support to dying people so that they might live as actively as possible until death;
- offering support to families coping with the person's illness and their bereavement (World Health Organization, 1990).

These principles can equally well be applied to people with dementia as they are to people with cancer. Indeed, there are grounds for arguing that palliative care in dementia can be regarded in the same light as person-centred care, since both are motivated by a concern for the person, where what it is to be a person is understood broadly (Hughes *et al.*, 2004). It will at some stage be the case that people with dementia require terminal care. Our suggestion is that seeing end-stage dementia in this light demonstrates an appropriate attitude – one in keeping with notions of what it is to live well humanly – to the final stages of a terminal disease. Such an attitude is hardly likely to be oblivious to quality of life and certainly would not involve a commitment to a lingering death (Post and Whitehouse, 1998).

In this regard, Coetzee *et al.* (2003) considered the attitudes of carers and old age psychiatrists towards the treatment of potentially fatal events in end-stage dementia. Clinicians appeared to be less keen on active treatment; but the carers set greater store by 'patient-centred' issues, such as dying with dignity. One of the interesting things here is the possibility that the disagreement between clinicians and carers might disappear in the face of a uniting concern for some humanly important values to do with what can, in the circumstances, constitute a good life. The virtues required, then, are to do with understanding and discernment. The professional virtues of respect and humility towards the families of people with severe dementia may allow the right sort of mutual understanding and, in a way, also suggest respect for the person with dementia. This is not to say that we must simply do whatever the family wishes. Taking their concerns seriously, however, and showing how we share them and how we shall attend to them is a matter of practical wisdom, charity and compassion.

One defining characteristic of hospice care is that cardiopulmonary resuscitation is normally excluded as an option in terminal conditions. Such treatment would be disproportionate in terms of its likely effects on someone with metastatic cancer. The same sort of reasoning (strangely) is not applied to dementia. Practical wisdom would caution against the wholesale adoption of policies that make the resuscitation of people with dementia in the event of cardiopulmonary arrest the norm. Not only might there be harm to the patients (e.g. rib fractures), transgressing the principle of non-maleficence, but also attempts to resuscitate people with severe dementia could be regarded as obscene.

To make this charge is to point towards an incompatibility between the motivation behind such attempts at resuscitation and the thought that death at some point is both natural and can rightly be regarded as a relief. This latter thought says more about how to live well as a human being than the former motivation, which is more concerned with the avoidance of litigation. As such, it is the balanced acceptance of death that is likely to be the stance taken by the virtuous person.

19.10.3 Futility

There has been an increasing trend to think of these issues in terms of futility. At first sight this approach appears deceptively devoid of complex conflicts of values – an intervention is adjudged futile on entirely empirical grounds (e.g. Awoke *et al.*, 1992). Nevertheless, the objective criteria for what may or may not count as 'futile' do not take into account the full details of the individual case, bringing to bear the perspectives of all those involved.

Once again, virtue theory changes things. Resuscitation in severe dementia is wrong, not simply because it is estimated to be futile, but because it suggests an inappropriate attitude towards the human condition when faced by the inevitability

of death. To have the appropriate attitude is to have some notion of what it is to live fully and well, even in circumscribed circumstances. It is also to demonstrate the virtue of courage in the face of a terminal state.

19.11 ARTIFICIAL NUTRITION AND HYDRATION

Recent evidence points to the likelihood that percutaneous endoscopic gastrostomy (PEG) or nasogastric tube (NGT) feeding does not materially affect survival in severely demented patients (e.g. Finucane *et al.*, 1999). These procedures carry a significant morbidity and even the risk of death. Hence, the moral case for using these 'extraordinary' means of support becomes less persuasive (e.g. Gillick, 2000).

The uneasy feeling, however, is that by not using these treatments the patient is effectively being deliberately dehydrated or starved to death. Some would claim, indeed, that this is not a matter of medical treatment; it is a matter of basic human care that people should receive food and drink. It would be a failure in charity, on this view, not to pursue treatment by NGT or PEG. Again, we would need to immerse ourselves in the details of a case in order to make a decision, based on our interpretation in the light of the underlying moral principles. But these should reflect a variety of virtues. So an alternative view would be that it shows a lack of charity not to take seriously the risks and a failure of empathy not to seek some other way of attending to the person with dementia.

It might then be better to accept that giving food and drink constitutes basic human care, whilst at the same time accepting that NGTs and PEGs are a disproportionate response. Hence, feeding could still take place using thickened foods and the correct posture, in the knowledge that the person's life might be shortened if aspiration were to occur. The intimate contact of careful feeding continues, therefore, as a matter of charity and practical wisdom. This will achieve for the person the best quality of life within the confines of the difficult situation. The risk that is taken, which is serious, nevertheless can still be viewed as a matter of honouring the person's ability to interact and interconnect humanly.

The artificial means of treatment provide a technical solution but one that lacks meaningful content, which comes from the embedded nature of food and drink in our lives. Recognition of this broader picture is a matter of practical wisdom, for it keeps in view the overall purpose of our lives in a practical sort of way. We are made to interrelate (think of feminine ethics) and interconnect (think of narrative ethics) through our giving and taking of food and drink. But PEG tubes and NGT feeding do not inherently involve interrelationship or interconnectivity. In other cases, where they will restore the person's ability to interrelate and interconnect, they would seem to be the right choice, but not in severe dementia. To see this is to show virtue, by showing a grasp of the real purposes that make our lives good.

19.12 CONCLUSION

The end of life comes in dementia in a variety of ways. What is required is often a practical matter. We have contended that clinical practice at the end of life in dementia will be enhanced by attention to what might constitute living (and dying) humanly well.

REFERENCES

Agich GJ. (2003) *Dependence and Autonomy in Old Age: An Ethical Framework For Long-Term Care.* Cambridge, Cambridge University Press

Awoke S, Mouton CP, Parrott M. (1992) Outcomes of skilled cardiopulmonary resuscitation in a long-term-care facility: futile therapy? *Journal of the American Geriatrics Society* **40**: 593–595

Buchanan A. (1988) Advance directives and the personal identity problem. *Philosophy and Public Affairs* 17: 277–302

Coetzee RH, Leask SJ, Jones RG. (2003) The attitudes of carers and old age psychiatrists towards the treatment of potentially fatal events in end-stage dementia. *International Journal of Geriatric Psychiatry* **18**: 169–173

Dresser R. (1995) Dworkin on dementia: elegant theory, questionable policy. *Hastings Center Report* **25**: 32–38

Dworkin R. (1993) *Life's Dominion. An Argument About Abortion and Euthanasia.* London, Harper Collins

Finucane TE, Christmas C, Travis K. (1999) Tube feeding in patients with advanced dementia. *JAMA* **282**: 1365–1370

Gillick MR. (2000) Rethinking the role of tube feeding in patients with advanced dementia. *New England Journal of Medicine* **342**: 206–210

Hope T. (1995) Personal identity and psychiatric illness. In: AP Griffiths (ed.), *Philosophy, Psychology and Psychiatry.* Cambridge, Cambridge University Press, pp. 131–143

Hughes JC. (2000) Ethics and the anti-dementia drugs. *International Journal of Geriatric Psychiatry* **15**: 538–543

Hughes JC. (2001) Views of the person with dementia. *Journal of Medical Ethics* 27: 86–91

Hughes J, Hedley K, Harris D. (2004) Palliative care in severe dementia: philosophy and practice. *Nursing and Residential Care* **6**: 27–30

Hurley AC, Volicer BJ, Volicer L. (1996) Effect of fever-management strategy on the progression of dementia of the Alzheimer type. *Alzheimer Disease and Associated Disorders* **10**: 5–10

Hursthouse R. (1999) *On Virtue Ethics.* Oxford, Oxford University Press

Jaworska A. (1999) Respecting the margins of agency: Alzheimer's patients and the capacity to value. *Philosophy and Public Affairs* **28**: 105–138

Keown J. (ed.) (1995) *Euthanasia Examined: Ethical, Clinical and Legal Perspectives.* Cambridge, Cambridge University Press

Locke J. (1690) *An Essay Concerning Human Understanding.* AD Woozley, ed., (1964) Glasgow, William Collins/Fount Paperbacks

Parfit D. (1984) *Reasons and Persons.* Oxford, Oxford University Press

Post SG and Whitehouse PJ. (1998) The moral basis for limiting treatment: hospice care and advanced progressive dementia. In: L Volicer and A Hurley (eds), *Hospice Care for Patients with Advanced Progressive Dementia.* New York, Springer, pp. 117–131

Sabat SR. (2001) *The Experience of Alzheimer's Disease: Life Through a Tangled Veil.* Oxford, Blackwell

Volicer L and Hurley A. (eds) (1998) *Hospice Care for Patients with Advanced Progressive Dementia.* New York, Springer

Widdershoven G and Berghmans R. (2001) Advance directives in psychiatric care: a narrative approach. *Journal of Medical Ethics* 27: 92–97

World Health Organization. (1990) *Technical Report Series 804.* Geneva, World Health Organization

19d

Driving

DESMOND O'NEILL

At the core of the syndrome of dementia is the loss of social or occupational function. In the early days of specialist medicine and psychiatry of old age, assessment of function centred on activities of daily living, concentrating on a relatively basic set of skills. An increase in the sophistication of the disciplines, as well as the need to probe relatively high-level loss of function in early dementia has led to an increased attention to instrumental activities of daily living, such as managing financial affairs. Driving is an instrumental activity that has attracted particular attention because of a false perception of hazard to other people as well as increasing numbers who drive at all ages (Wang and Carr, 2004). The United States Transportation Research Board, the Organization for Economic Cooperation and Development and the European Conference of Ministers for Transport have all prepared reports on ageing and transport within the last 3 years (CEMT, 2001; OECD, 2001; US Department of Transportation, 2003). It is a definite health issue: drivers in Finland, the UK, Ireland and the US report health as primary cause of driving cessation, usually without a formal consultation to ensure maximal remediation (Persson, 1993; Rabbitt *et al.*, 1996; Hakamies-Blomqvist and Wahlstrom, 1998; O'Neill *et al.*, 2000). It is a fascinating topic and, while the knowledge base is still relatively slender, the issues involved have major practical, ethical and societal implications for patients, their family carers and healthcare professionals. There are widely differing agendas on the part of those involved: the patient, the carers, the physician, the statutory licensing authority and the insurance companies, both motoring and health.

As dementia is a largely (but not exclusively) age-related disease, it is of note that the developed world is experiencing an exponential rise in the proportion of older drivers among the driving population. In the USA only 5.9 per cent of drivers were over 60 in 1940: this had increased to 7.4 per cent by 1952 and to 11.4 per cent by 1960 (McFarland *et al.*, 1964). Elderly drivers should comprise 28 per cent of the driving population in the USA by the year, 2000 and 39 per cent by 2050 (Malfetti, 1985). Over a third of those aged over 80 in 1990 drove at least once a year in Ontario, Canada (Chipman *et al.*, 1998). In the UK there has been an increase of 600 per cent in the number of women drivers over the age of 65 between 1965 and 1985 (Department of Transport, 1991). Although most will drive personal automobiles, this is not exclusively the case. On the one hand, licensing regulations for drivers of public service vehicles and heavy transport vehicles is nearly always more restricted and uses a more algorithmic approach than for drivers of personal automobiles. On the other hand, those who develop dementia at a younger age are more likely to be driving heavy goods or public service vehicles, and the abolition of mandatory retirement age in the USA has resulted in school bus drivers being able to continue into their mid-80s, and there has been litigation concerning this group.

19.13 WHAT PUBLIC HEALTH ISSUES ARISE WITH OLDER DRIVERS?

One of the most important, and underrecognized, public health hazards arising from dementia is the consequences of loss of mobility for those with dementia who stop driving (Taylor and Tripodes, 2001). One of the other key questions about the ageing of the driving population is whether they add significantly to hazard on the roads. This question is in itself symptomatic of an ageist approach to older driver issues: it is likely that the predominant problem is that older people give up driving without sufficient remediation (White and O'Neill, 2000). The crash rate for older drivers for a given period of time is considerably lower than that for the driving population as a whole (Gebers et al., 1993). Many safety experts defend older drivers as a relatively safe group (Evans, 1988) and in some road tests healthy older drivers perform better than younger controls (Gebers et al., 1993). The increased crash rate per miles driven noted in elderly populations in comparison to middle-aged controls is not only academic while older people continue to drive a lower mileage: it also is a product of driving a low mileage, which is in itself intrinsically risky. If younger and older people who drive a low mileage are compared, this apparent increase disappears (Hakamies-Blomqvist et al., 2002).

Low mileage exposes them to more dangers per mile than high-mileage drivers as they encounter disproportionately more intersections, congestion, confusing visual environments, signs and signals (Janke, 1991), yet older drivers cope at least as well with this.

Crashes involving the elderly are also more likely to be fatal, by a factor of 3.5 in two-car accidents (Klamm, 1985), reflecting the increased frailty and reduced reserve of older adults, while raising suspicions that automobile design may not be tailored for maximum safety of this group (Schieber, 1994; Li et al., 2003). Opposing these trends is the fact that the accident rates for young adults often arise from behaviour that leads to high-risk situations; accident rates in older drivers occur despite a trend to avoid high-risk situations (Planek et al., 1968) and the lowest proportion of crashes while under the influence of alcohol (National Center for Statistics and Analysis, 1995).

Janke (1994) has suggested a reasonable interpretation of these apparently contradictory findings. A group's average crash rate per year may be considered as an indicator of the degree of risk posed to society by that group, whereas average accident rate per mile indicates the degree of risk posed to individual drivers in the group when they drive, as well as to their passengers. The increased risk to individual drivers is most likely due to age-related illnesses, particularly neurodegenerative and vascular diseases (O'Neill, 1992; Johansson et al., 1997).

19.14 IS DRIVING WITH DEMENTIA A PUBLIC HEALTH HAZARD?

The precise contribution of the dementias to overall crash hazard is uncertain. Although Johansson suggested a major role for dementia as cause of crashes among older drivers on neuropathological grounds (Johansson et al., 1997), subsequent interview with families did not reveal significant problems with memory or activities of daily living (Lundberg et al.,

1999). The Stockholm group also showed that older drivers who had a high level of traffic violations had a high prevalence of cognitive deficits (Lundberg et al., 1998). Retrospective studies of dementia and driving from specialist dementia clinics tend to show a high risk (Friedland et al., 1988; Lucas-Blaustein et al., 1988; O'Neill, 1993b), whereas those which are prospective and look at the early stages of dementia show a less pronounced pattern of risk. In the first 2 years of dementia the risk approximates that of the general population (Drachman and Swearer, 1993; Carr et al., 2000). The most carefully controlled study yet of crashes and dementia showed no increase in crash rates for drivers with dementia (Trobe et al., 1996). Likely causes for this counter-intuitive finding include a lower annual mileage and restriction of driving by the patient, family and physicians.

Extrapolating from special populations may skew predictions of risk. For example, epilepsy, for which there are relatively clear-cut guidelines in most countries, would seem to pose a clear threat to driving ability as viewed from a clinic setting. Recent population-based studies seem to suggest that the increased risk is relatively low (Hansotia and Broste, 1991; Drazkowski et al., 2003). In a population renewing their licences in North Carolina, the lowest decile had a relative crash risk of 1.5 in the 3 years previous to the cognitive testing (Stutts et al., 1998), A somewhat reassuring finding from this cohort is that those with the poorest scores for visual and cognitive function also drove less and avoided high-risk situations (Stutts, 1998). A reasonable conclusion from these studies is that dementia among drivers is not yet a public health problem. Although increasing numbers of older drivers may change this situation, it is also possible that 'Smeed's law' will operate, whereby increasing numbers of drivers among a defined population are associated with a drop in fatality rates per car (Smeed, 1968).

19.15 IS THERE A ROLE FOR SCREENING OLDER POPULATIONS OF DRIVERS?

Despite the lack of convincing evidence for an older driver 'problem', ageist policies in many jurisdictions has led to screening programmes for older drivers. In the absence of reliable and sensitive assessment tools, this approach is flawed, as illustrated by data from Scandinavia (Hakamies-Blomqvist et al., 1996). In Finland there is regular age-related medical certification of fitness to drive, whereas Sweden has no routine medical involvement in licence renewal. There is no reduction in the number of older people dying in car crashes in Finland but an increase in the number of those dying as pedestrians and cyclists, possibly in part by unnecessarily removing drivers from their cars. A more minimalist and less medical approach using very simple measures, such as a vision test and a written skill examination, may be more helpful (Levy et al., 1995); unfortunately this approach is also associated with a reduction in the number of older drivers, a possible negative health impact (Levy, 1995). Another approach is opportunistic health screening, perhaps of those older drivers with traffic violations (Johansson *et al.*, 1996). It remains to be seen whether these and other screening policies reduce mobility among older people, a practical and civil rights issue of great importance. Another problem is the uncertainty about the outcome of screening, as there is currently a limited repertoire.

19.16 PHYSICIANS AND DRIVING ASSESSMENT

Another problem is the relative ignorance of physicians about the effects of illness on driving. Some of this relates to the predominantly negative tone of much of the medical regulations for driving (White and O'Neill, 2000), and it is likely that doctors are insufficiently aware of healthcare interventions that have been shown to improve driving comfort and safety: examples exist for arthritis, stroke and cataract (van Zomeren *et al.*, 1987; Jones *et al.*, 1991; Monestam and Wachtmeister, 1997). Doctors are unaware of the driving habits of their patients when prescribing drugs that may affect driving (Cartwright, 1990) and also have a patchy knowledge of medical regulations for driving (Strickberger *et al.*, 1991; O'Neill *et al.*, 1994). As the regulations are rarely based on evidence-based criteria and are negatively presented, this 'failure' by doctors to acquaint themselves with the regulations may in fact reflect a healthy cynicism about the current official medical fitness criteria. There may also be an element of ageism by which doctors may assume that older patients do not drive: a review of dementia from the UK seemed to take this attitude (Almeida and Fottrell, 1991), whereas US reviewers have been aware of the high number of older drivers for over a decade (Winograd and Jarvik, 1986).

Drivers may not only be unaware, but also may wilfully ignore medical advice and regulations. In many countries they continue to drive despite failing to comply with regulations for diabetes, visual disease and automatic implantable cardioverter defibrillators (Frier *et al.*, 1980; Eadington and Frier, 1988; McConnell *et al.*, 1991; Finch *et al.*, 1993). It must be stated that there is no evidence that this under reporting results in any increased crash risk!

We have little information on advice given to drivers with dementia by family physicians or physicians at specialist clinics for the evaluation of dementia. This would be of interest because of the wide range of answers given for patients with life-threatening arrhythmias (Strickberger *et al.*, 1991). In any event, a major shift of emphasis is required by healthcare professionals to consider driving ability in the functional assessment of older people.

The procedures for intervention after the opportunistic detection of illnesses relevant to driving also vary widely. In the UK the doctor's duty is to inform the patient that he/she must contact the Driver and Vehicle Licensing Authority (DVLA); direct contact by the doctor with the DVLA is only allowed if there is evidence of continued driving that constitutes a hazard to others, and if persuasion through other family members and carers has been unsuccessful. This contrasts with the position in several states in the US and provinces in Canada where the doctor is bound by law to report patients with certain illnesses to the licensing authorities. The disparity between these practices is confusing, but cross-national comparisons may prove a boon to researchers who wish to establish the most appropriate methods for screening and reporting of age-related diseases.

19.17 ASSESSMENT PROCEDURES

The placing of driving issues in an appropriate therapeutic context is the most important task. Rather than focusing on the difficult case of patients who present late with impaired driving ability and insight, we need to recognize that the assessment of dementia provides the potential for a range of interventions, one of the most important of which is the establishment of a framework for advance planning in a progressive disease. Just as this is commonly recognized for such practical matters as enduring power of attorney in many jurisdictions, so too we need to start a process that encompasses an assessment, a commitment to maximizing mobility and also an awareness-raising process for the patient and carers that the progression of the disease will inevitably result in a loss of driving capacity. This latter component has been termed a Ulysses contract, after the hero made his crew tie him to the mast on the condition that they did not heed his entreaties to be released when seduced by the song of the sirens (Howe, 2000). Developing this process incorporates some new stances in dementia care, in particular of the diagnosis disclosure in at least general terms – the patient who drives needs to be told that he/she has a memory problem that is likely to progress and hamper driving abilities. In general, carers are fearful of diagnosis disclosure but older people seem to want to be told if they have this illness. There is also evidence such a process may facilitate driver cessation, by enhancing a therapeutic dimension to disease diagnosis and advance planning (Bahro *et al.*, 1995). It forms the basis of a useful patient and carer brochure from the Hartford Foundation which is also available online (Hartford Foundation, 2000). This type of approach also seems to have worked with older, visually-impaired drivers (Owsley *et al.*, 2003). The most useful model of assessment is that of an assessment cascade (Figure 19.1).

Not all levels will be required by all patients: a patient with a homonymous hemianopia is barred from driving throughout the European Union, and referral to the social worker to plan alternative transportation is appropriate. Equally, a mild cognitive defect may only require a review by the physician and occupational therapist. The overall interdisciplinary assessment should attempt to provide solutions to both maintaining activities and exploring transport needs. The on-road test may be helpful as it may demonstrate deficits to

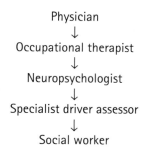

Physician
↓
Occupational therapist
↓
Neuropsychologist
↓
Specialist driver assessor
↓
Social worker

Figure 19.1   *Assessment cascade.*

a patient or carer who is ambiguous about the patient stopping driving. At a therapeutic level, members of the team may be able to help the patients come to terms with the losses associated with stopping driving. The occupational therapist may be able to maximize activities and function and help focus on preserved areas of achievement, whereas the social worker can advise on alternative methods of transport.

The assessment of fitness to drive should only take place after a thorough evaluation of the underlying medical condition(s). The evaluation of dementia, both clinically and investigative, is well covered in other chapters but dementing illnesses may coexist with other conditions that affect driving ease and ability. Important components of the history and examination of theoretical relevance to the driving task are medication and alcohol use (Doege and Engelburg, 1986), perception, cognitive status and psychomotor ability. Perception is probably more important than vision. Cognition may be usefully measured by the physician using one of the many brief mental status schedules (O'Neill, 1993a), and the elements of general clinical assessment of older drivers for medical fitness to drive are now described on both sides of the Atlantic (Carr, 1993; O'Neill, 1993a, b). Although the Mini-Mental State Examination (MMSE; Folstein and Folstein, 1975) correlates with driving performance (Odenheimer et al., 1994; Fitten et al., 1995; Fox et al., 1997), it is not sufficiently sensitive or specific to be used as a determinant of driving ability (Lundberg et al., 1997).

The basic thrust of the assessment is to catalogue and remedy all pathologies that may be relevant to driving: vision, cognitive function, neurological and musculoskeletal disorders, as well as conditions that may give rise to transient loss of consciousness such as diabetes and syncope. In any one illness there may be multiple facets that affect driving: in Parkinson's disease, this includes motor, cognitive and affective aspects. Each component needs to be maximally remedied before a final decision is made. A collateral history of driving behaviour is very important, although one small study has shown a poor correlation between carer rating of driver behaviour and on-road testing (Hunt et al., 1993).

Medications should be minimized; although the data are preliminary, long-acting benzodiazepines (Hemmelgarn et al., 1997), tricyclic antidepressants (Ray et al., 1993) and neuroleptics should be targeted.

19.18 FURTHER ASSESSMENT

In cases of very mild cognitive impairment or very severe cognitive impairment, the judgement may be relatively easy and require little by way of supplementary testing. For those falling in between, the precise nature of the further evaluation is not yet standardized, just as the neuropsychological evaluation of dementia is not yet standardized; and just as not all chest pains arise from pulmonary emboli, clinicians need to have access to appropriate specialist expertise and technology to exclude it in such cases. So too, old age psychiatrists may need to invoke the assistance of a driving specialist centre, the components of which are medical, occupational therapy, sometimes neuropsychology, and specialist driving assessors. A first effort may be made with a suitably trained occupational therapist (Ranney and Hunt, 1997): this profession is notable for upskilling in driving assessment in Australia, Canada and the USA.

The choice of tests will be relatively arbitrary and, as in any memory clinic where geriatricians or psychiatrists of old age will familiarize themselves with the battery of tests carried out by the occupational therapist or psychologist in the local area, it is likely that good communication between professionals and familiarity with the chosen tests is as important as the precise tests chosen.

While a number of screening and evaluation test batteries have been proposed, it makes more sense to choose some core areas of interest, and to allow some room for clinical judgements on areas such as patient judgement and impulsiveness. The task is rendered more complex by the sophistication of models of driving, which do not conform easily to traditional cognitive test batteries. At least five main types of model have been explored: psychometric, motivational, hierarchical controls, information processing and error theory (O'Neill, 1996). At a minimum, a test battery should contain a general measure of overall cognitive function, a dementia grading and include tests of attention, particularly visual attention, information processing and perception. Some matching to dementia type will be appropriate: perception in visual dementia, attention in subcortical dementias, judgement in frontotemporal dementia.

Neuropsychology test in themselves show a relatively modest correlation with driving skills in dementia and are unlikely to ever completely replace on-road driving tests (Reger et al., 2004). The British Psychological Society has stated that at present no single test or test battery can be recommended as clearly predictive of fitness to drive (British Psychological Society Multidisciplinary Working Party on Acquired Neuropsychological Deficits and Fitness to Drive, 1999). Specific tests that show correlation with driving ability in more than one study include the MMSE (above), the Trail Making Test (Maag, 1976; Janke and Eberhard, 1998; Mazer et al., 1998; Stutts et al., 1998), and a range of tests of visual attention (Klavora et al., 1995; Marottoli et al., 1998; Owsley et al., 1998; Trobe, 1998; Duchek et al., 2003), including the 'Useful Field of View', a composite measure of preattentive processing, incorporating speed of visual information processing, ability to ignore distractors (selective attention) and ability to divide attention (Owsley *et al.*, 1991). A range of other tests have been assessed in single studies (an interesting one is traffic sign recognition; Carr *et al.*, 1998) and a comprehensive review is available from the US National Highway Traffic Safety Administration (Staplin *et al.*, 1999). In conjunction with the clinical assessment and collateral history, these tests will help to decide which patients require on-road testing, as well as those who are likely to be dangerous to test!

A more promising approach may be by way of using a hierarchical/behavioural model. This divides the driving task in strategic, tactical and operational levels. The assessment tool examines questions of driving behaviour at strategic and tactical levels. In a preliminary study using this instrument, drivers who select driving tasks below their capacities and compensate by adapting their driving style cause fewer accidents than those who do not apply these strategies (de Raedt and Ponjaert-Kristoffersen, 2000).

Simulator testing is in its infancy: although sophisticated simulator techniques are sensitive (and safe!) (Rizzo *et al.*, 1997), the cost and complexity of an adequate simulator render the technique experimental rather than practical.

19.19 ON-ROAD TESTING

If this assessment is inconclusive, an on-road assessment is advisable. In the UK, such assessments are available from the Forum group of driver assessment centres. In the US, the Association of Driver Rehabilitation Specialists (ADED, www.aded.net) can provide the list of suitably qualified driving assessors. It is important to emphasize to the patient that this test is not the driving test used for learner drivers. Rather, this is an assessment to gain insight into both the capabilities and difficulties of the driver. A good relationship with a specialist driving assessor is an important part of the assessment process. The assessor will require a full clinical report, and may choose to use one of the recently developed scoring systems for on-road testing of patients with dementia. These include the Washington University Road Test (Hunt *et al.*, 1997) or the Alberta Road Test (Dobbs *et al.*, 1998). The latter is of interest as the authors have classified the errors made by drivers with dementia into categories of increasing significance, providing a basis for future studies.

19.20 DECISION-MAKING AND INTERVENTIONS

If the assessment points to safe driving practice, the decision to continue driving entails several components. These are:

- duration before review
- possible restriction
- driving accompanied

- licensing authority reporting relationship
- insurance reporting responsibility.

As dementia is a progressive illness, it is prudent to make any declaration of fitness to drive subject to regular review: a recent study suggests that a review period of 6 months is probably reasonable (Duchek *et al.*, 2003), or sooner if any deterioration is reported by the carer. Following evidence that the crash rate is reduced if the driver is accompanied (Bédard *et al.*, 1996), it could be considered sensible to restrict driving to exclusively when there is someone else in the car, using the co-pilot syndrome (Shua-Haim and Gross, 1996). There is also preliminary evidence from the state of Utah that those drivers with restricted driving licences have lower crash rates (Vernon *et al.*, 2002): patients should be advised to avoid traffic congestion as well as driving at night and in bad weather. The patient and carers should be advised to acquaint themselves with local driver licensing authority requirements as well as the policy of their motor insurance company. All the above should be clearly recorded in the medical notes. Except for jurisdictions where there is mandatory reporting of drivers with dementia (e.g. California and some Canadian provinces), there is no obligation on the doctor to break medical confidentiality in these cases.

19.21 WHEN DRIVING IS NO LONGER POSSIBLE

If the assessment supports driving cessation, patients and carers should be advised of this, and a social worker consulted to help maximize transportation options. Giving up driving can have a considerable effect on lifestyle. Driving is probably both a right and a privilege; however, 42 per cent of the elderly think that driving is a right as opposed to 27 per cent who think that it is a privilege (AA Foundation for Road Safety Research, 1988). However, normal elderly drivers accept that their physician's advice would be very influential in deciding to give up driving (AA Foundation for Road Safety Research, 1988) and many patients with dementia will respond to advice from families or physicians (Adler and Kuskowski, 2003).

For the probable minority who are still resistant to persuasion, removal of a driving licence represents a potential breach of civil rights (Reuben *et al.*, 1988). The way we deal with driving reflects how we help the patient to deal with the reality of the deficits caused by dementia. A more positive approach has been suggested whereby the issue of driving is treated as a part of a therapeutic programme. A case was described whereby the patient's feelings and fears about giving up driving were explored with him (Bahro *et al.*, 1995). The intervention was designed with the patient as collaborator rather than patient and by dealing with the events at an emotional rather than at an intellectual level. The patient was able to grieve about the disease and in particular about the loss of his car. This in turn enabled him to redirect his attention to other meaningful activities that did not involve driving. Although this approach may be hampered by the deficits of dementia, it reflects a more widespread trend towards sharing the diagnosis of dementia with the patient.

If this positive approach is not successful, confidentiality may have to be broken for a small minority of cases. Most professional associations for physicians accept that the principle of confidentiality is covered to a degree by a 'common good' principle of protecting third parties when direct advice to the patient is ignored (General Medical Council, 1985; Retchin and Anapolle, 1993). Removal of the driving licence is not likely to have much effect on these patients, and the vehicle may need to be disabled (Donnelly and Karlinsky, 1990) and all local repair services warned not to respond to calls from the patient!

In the event of a decision to advise cessation of driving, advice from a medical social worker helpful in planning strategies for using alternative modes of travel. This may be difficult in a rural setting: one estimate of community transport exclusively for older people in the USA was $US5.14 for a one-way trip in 1983 (Rosenbloom, 1993) and the political system has not woken up to the need for adequate paratransit, i.e. tailored, affordable and reliable assisted transport acceptable to older adults with physical and/or mental disability (Freund, 1991). Tailored transport (paratransit) is expensive, but may have benefits in reducing institutionalization and in improving quality of life. Psychiatrists of old age and geriatricians have an advocacy role to ensure that public policy on transportation is developed to take account of the deficiencies of transit and paratransit systems.

19.22 THE FUTURE

Several developments may attenuate the problems of the older driver with dementia. At a population level, preventive strategies for dementia may lessen the burden of cognitive disability, and strictures on the prescribing of agents such as long-acting benzodiazepines may have a positive impact on reducing crash susceptibility. Improvements in highway design, signage and Intelligent Transportation Systems may make travel safer for all.

For the individual, we still do not know whether anticholinesterase-inhibitor therapy can help driving skills in early Alzheimer's disease. There is also a suggestion that cognitive training with useful field of view can help driving skills in non-demented older adults (Ball and Owsley, 1994); this form of cognitive rehabilitation may be useful. Finally, older drivers can benefit from environmental and technological cueing (Dingus *et al.*, 1997); developments in this form of technology may also benefit drivers with cognitive impairment.

REFERENCES

AA Foundation for Road Safety Research. (1988) *Motoring and the Older Driver.* Basingstoke, AA Foundation for Road Safety Research

Adler G and Kuskowski M. (2003) Driving cessation in older men with dementia. *Alzheimer Disease and Associated Disorders* **17**: 68–71

Almeida J and Fottrell E. (1991) Management of the dementias. *Reviews in Clinical Gerontology* **1**: 267–282

Bahro M, Silber E, Box P, Sunderland T. (1995) Giving up driving in Alzheimer's disease – an integrative therapeutic approach. *International Journal of Geriatric Psychiatry* **10**: 871–874

Ball K and Owsley C. (1994) Predicting vehicle crashes in the elderly: who is at risk? In: K Johansson and C Lundberg (eds), *Aging and Driving.* Stockholm, Karolinska Institutet, pp. 1–2

Bédard M, Molloy M, Lever J. (1996) Should demented patients drive alone? *Journal of the American Geriatrics Society* **44**: S9

British Psychological Society Multi-Disciplinary Working Party on Acquired Neuropsychological Deficits and Fitness to Drive. (1999) *Fitness to Drive and Cognition.* Leicester, British Psychological Society

Carr DB. (1993) Assessing older drivers for physical and cognitive impairment. *Geriatrics* **48**: 46–48, 51

Carr DB, LaBarge E, Dunnigan K, Storandt M. (1998) Differentiating drivers with dementia of the Alzheimer type from healthy older persons with a Traffic Sign Naming test. *Journal of Gerontology: Biological Sciences and Medical Sciences* **53**: M135–139

Carr DB, Duchek J, Morris JC. (2000) Characteristics of motor vehicle crashes of drivers with dementia of the Alzheimer type [see comments]. *Journal of American Geriatrics Society* **48**: 18–22

Cartwright A. (1990) Medicine taking by people aged 65 or more. *British Medical Bulletin* **46**: 63–76

CEMT. (2001) Report on transport and ageing of the population. Paris, CEMT

Chipman ML, Payne J, McDonough P. (1998) To drive or not to drive: the influence of social factors on the decisions of elderly drivers. *Accident Analysis and Prevention* **30**: 299–304

Department of Transport. (1991) *The Older Driver: Measures for Reducing the Number of Casualties among Older People on our Roads.* London, Department of Transport

de Raedt R and Ponjaert-Kristoffersen I. (2000) Can strategic and tactical compensation reduce crash risk in older drivers? *Age and Ageing* **29**: 517–521

Dingus TA, Hulse MC, Mollenhauer MA, Fleischman RN, McGehee DV, Manakkal N. (1997) Effects of age, system experience, and navigation technique on driving with an advanced traveler information system. *Human Factors* **39**: 177–199

Dobbs AR, Heller RB, Schopflocher D. (1998) A comparative approach to identify unsafe older drivers. *Accident Analysis and Prevention* **30**: 363–370

Doege TC and Engelburg AL. (eds) (1986) *Medical Conditions affecting Older Drivers.* Chicago, American Medical Association

Donnelly RE and Karlinsky H. (1990) The impact of Alzheimer's disease on driving ability: a review. *Journal of Geriatric Psychiatry and Neurology* **3**: 67–72

Drachman DA and Swearer JM. (1993) Driving and Alzheimer's disease: the risk of crashes. *Neurology* **43**: 2448–2456 [published erratum appears in *Neurology* 1994; **44**: 4]

Drazkowski JF, Fisher RS, Sirven JI *et al.* (2003) Seizure-related motor vehicle crashes in Arizona before and after reducing the driving restriction from 12 to 3 months. *Mayo Clinic Proceedings* **78**: 819–825

Duchek JM, Carr DB, Hunt L *et al.* (2003) Longitudinal driving performance in early-stage dementia of the Alzheimer type. *Journal of American Geriatrics Society* **51**: 1342–1347

Eadington DW and Frier BM. (1988) Type 1 diabetes and driving experience: an eight-year cohort study. *Diabetic Medicine* **6**: 137–141

Evans L. (1988) Older driver involvement in fatal and severe traffic crashes. *Journal of Gerontology* **43**: S186–S193

Finch NJ, Leman RB, Kratz JM, Gillette PC. (1993) Driving safety among patients with automatic implantable cardioverter defibrillators. *JAMA* **270**: 1587–1588

Fitten LJ, Perryman KM, Wilkinson CJ et al. (1995) Alzheimer and vascular dementias and driving. A prospective road and laboratory study [see comments]. *JAMA* **273**: 1360–1365

Folstein ME and Folstein SE. (1975) Mini-Mental State. A practical method for grading the cognitive state of patients for the clinician. *Journal of Psychiatric Research* **12**: 189–195

Fox GK, Bowden SC, Bashford GM, Smith DS. (1997) Alzheimer's disease and driving: prediction and assessment of driving performance. *Journal of the American Geriatrics Society* **45**: 949–953

Freund K. (1991) The politics of older driver legislation. *The Gerontologist* **31** (special issue II): 162

Friedland RP, Koss E, Kumar A et al. (1988) Motor vehicle crashes in dementia of the Alzheimer type [see comments]. *Annals of Neurology* **24**: 782–786

Frier BM, Matthews DM, Steel JM, Duncan LJ. (1980) Driving and insulin-dependent diabetes. *Lancet* **1**: 1232–1234

Gebers MA, Romanowicz PA, McKenzie DM. (1993) *Teen and Senior Drivers.* Sacramento, California Department of Motor Vehicles

General Medical Council. (1985) *Professional Conduct and Discipline: Fitness to Practice.* London, General Medical Council

Hakamies-Blomqvist L and Wahlstrom B. (1998) Why do older drivers give up driving? *Accident Analysis and Prevention* **30**: 305–312

Hakamies-Blomqvist L, Johansson K, Lundberg C. (1996) Medical screening of older drivers as a traffic safety measure – a comparative Finnish-Swedish Evaluation study. *Journal of the American Geriatrics Society* **44**: 650–653

Hakamies-Blomqvist L, Ukkonen T, O'Neill D. (2002) Driver ageing does not cause higher accident rates per mile. *Transportation Research Part F, Traffic Psychology and Behaviour* **5**: 271–274

Hansotia P and Broste SK. (1991) The effect of epilepsy or diabetes mellitus on the risk of automobile accidents [see comments]. *New England Journal of Medicine* **324**: 22–26

Hartford Foundation. (2000) *At the Crossroads: a Guide to Alzheimer's Disease, Dementia and Driving.* Hartford, CT, Hartford Foundation

Hemmelgarn B, Suissa S, Huang A, Boivin JF, Pinard G. (1997) Benzodiazepine use and the risk of motor vehicle crash in the elderly [see comments]. *JAMA* **278**: 27–31

Howe E. (2000) Improving treatments for patients who are elderly and have dementia. *Journal of Clinical Ethics* **11**: 291–303

Hunt L, Morris JC, Edwards D, Wilson BS. (1993) Driving performance in persons with mild senile dementia of the Alzheimer type. *Journal of the American Geriatrics Society* **41**: 747–752

Hunt LA, Murphy CF, Carr D, Duchek JM, Buckles V, Morris JC. (1997) Reliability of the Washington University Road Test. A performance-based assessment for drivers with dementia of the Alzheimer type. *Archives of Neurology* **54**: 707–712

Janke MK. (1991) Accidents, mileage, and the exaggeration of risk. *Accident Analysis and Prevention* **23**: 183–188

Janke MK. (1994) *Age-related Disabilities that may impair Driving and their Assessment.* Sacramento, California Department of Motor Vehicles

Janke MK and Eberhard JW. (1998) Assessing medically impaired older drivers in a licensing agency setting. *Accident Analysis and Prevention* **30**: 347–361

Johansson K, Bronge L, Lundberg C, Persson A, Seideman M, Viitanen M. (1996) Can a physician recognize an older driver with increased crash risk potential? *Journal of the American Geriatrics Society* **44**: 1198–1204

Johansson K, Bogdanovic N, Kalimo H, Winblad B, Viitanen M. (1997) Alzheimer's disease and apolipoprotein E ε4 allele in older drivers who died in automobile accidents. *Lancet* **349**: 1143–1144

Jones JG, McCann J, Lassere MN. (1991) Driving and arthritis. *British Journal of Rheumatology* **30**: 361–364

Klamm ER. (1985) Auto insurance: needs and problems of drivers 55 and over. In: JL Malfetti (ed.), *Drivers 55+: Needs and Problems of Older Drivers: Survey Results and Recommendations.* Falls Church, VA, AAA Foundation for Road Safety, pp. 87–95

Klavora P, Gaskovski P, Martin K et al. (1995) The effects of Dynavision rehabilitation on behind-the-wheel driving ability and selected psychomotor abilities of persons after stroke. *American Journal of Occupational Therapy* **49**: 534–542

Levy DT. (1995) The relationship of age and state license renewal policies to driving licensure rates. *Accident Analysis and Prevention* **27**: 461–467

Levy DT, Vernick JS, Howard KA. (1995) Relationship between driver's license renewal policies and fatal crashes involving drivers 70 years or older [see comments]. *JAMA* **274**: 1026–1030

Li G, Braver ER, Chen LH. (2003) Fragility versus excessive crash involvement as determinants of high death rates per vehicle-mile of travel among older drivers. *Accident Analysis and Prevention* **35**: 227–235

Lucas-Blaustein MJ, Filipp L, Dungan C, Tune L. (1988) Driving in patients with dementia. *Journal of the American Geriatrics Society* **36**: 1087–1091

Lundberg C, Johansson K, Ball K et al. (1997) Dementia and driving – an attempt at consensus. *Alzheimer Disease and Associated Disorders* **11**: 28–37

Lundberg C, Hakamies-Blomqvist L, Almkvist O, Johansson K. (1998) Impairments of some cognitive functions are common in crash-involved older drivers. *Accident Analysis and Prevention* **30**: 371–377

Lundberg C, Johansson K, Bogdanovic N, Kalimo H, Winblad B, Viitanen M. (1999) Follow-up of Alzheimer's disease and apolipoprotein E ε4 allele in older drivers who died in automobile accidents. In: D O'Neill (ed.) *The Older Driver, Health and Mobility.* Dublin, ARHC Press

Maag F. (1976) [Practical driving tests – experiences and resulting problems]. *Beitrage zur Gerichtlichen Medizin* **34**: 111–115

Malfetti JL. (ed.) (1985) *Drivers 55 plus: Needs and Problems of Older Drivers: Survey Results and Recommendations.* Washington, DC, AAA Foundation for Road Safety

Marottoli RA, Richardson ED, Stowe MH et al. (1998) Development of a test battery to identify older drivers at risk for self-reported adverse driving events [see comments]. *Journal of the American Geriatrics Society* **46**: 562–568

Mazer BL, Korner-Bitensky NA, Sofer S. (1998) Predicting ability to drive after stroke. *Archives of Physical Medicine and Rehabilitation* **79**: 743–750

McConnell RA, Spall AD, Hirst LH, Williams G. (1991) A survey of the visual acuity of Brisbane drivers. *Medical Journal of Australia* **155**: 107–111

McFarland RA, Tune GS, Welford AT. (1964) On the driving of automobiles by older people. *Journal of Gerontology* **19**: 190–197

Monestam E and Wachtmeister L. (1997) Impact of cataract surgery on car driving: a population based study in Sweden. *British Journal of Ophthalmology* **81**: 16–22

National Center for Statistics and Analysis: National Highway Traffic Safety Administration. (1995) *Traffic Safety Facts 1994: Older*

Population. Washington, DC, National Highway Traffic Safety Administration

O'Neill D. (1992) Physicians, elderly drivers and dementia. *Lancet* **339**: 41–43

O'Neill D. (1993a) Brain stethoscopes: the use and abuse of brief mental status schedules. *Postgraduate Medical Journal* **69**: 599–601

O'Neill D. (1993b) Illness and elderly drivers. *Journal of the Irish College of Physicians and Surgeons* **22**: 14–16

O'Neill D. (1996) The older driver. *Reviews in Clinical Gerontology* **6**: 295–302

O'Neill D, Neubauer K, Boyle M, Gerrard J, Surmon D, Wilcock GK. (1992) Dementia and driving. *Journal of the Royal Society of Medicine* **85**: 199–202

O'Neill D, Crosby T, Shaw A, Haigh R, Hendra TJ. (1994) Physician awareness of driving regulations for older drivers. *Lancet* **344**: 1366–1367

O'Neill D, Bruce I, Kirby M, Lawlor B. (2000) Older drivers, driving practices and health issues. *Clinical Gerontology* **10**: 181–191

Odenheimer GL, Beaudet M, Jette AM, Albert MS, Grande L, Minaker KL. (1994) Performance-based driving evaluation of the elderly driver: safety, reliability, and validity. *Journal of Gerontology* **49**: M153–M159

OECD. (2001) *Ageing and Transport: Mobility Needs and Safety Issues.* Paris, OECD

Owsley C, Ball K, McGwin G Jr et al. (1998) Visual processing impairment and risk of motor vehicle crash among older adults. *JAMA* **279**: 1083–1088

Owsley C, Ball K, Sloane ME, Roenker DL, Bruni JR. (1991) Visual/cognitive correlates of vehicle accidents in older drivers. *Psychology and Aging* **6**: 403–415

Owsley C, Stalvey BT, Phillips JM. (2003) The efficacy of an educational intervention in promoting self-regulation among high-risk older drivers. *Accident Analysis and Prevention* **35**: 393–400

Persson D. (1993) The elderly driver: deciding when to stop. *The Gerontologist* **33**: 88–91

Planek TW, Condon ME, Fowler RC. (1968) *An Investigation into Problems and Opinions of Older Drivers.* Chicago, National Safety Council

Rabbitt P, Carmichael A, Jones S, Holland C. (1996) *When and Why Older Drivers give up Driving.* Basingstoke, AA Foundation for Road Safety Research

Ranney TA and Hunt LA. (1997) Researchers and occupational therapists can help each other to better understand what makes a good driver: two perspectives. *Work* **8**: 293–297

Ray WA, Thapa PB, Shorr RI. (1993) Medications and the older driver. *Clinics in Geriatric Medicine* **9**: 413–438

Reger M, Welsh RK, Watson GS, Cholerton B, Baker LD, Craft SA. (2004) The relationship between neuropsychological functioning and driving ability in dementia: a meta-analysis. *Neuropsychology* **18**: 85–93

Retchin SM and Anapolle J. (1993) An overview of the older driver. *Clinics in Geriatric Medicine* **9**: 279–296

Reuben DB, Silliman RA, Traines M. (1988) The aging driver. Medicine, policy, and ethics. *Journal of the American Geriatrics Society* **36**: 1135–1142

Rizzo M, Reinach M, McGehee D, Dawson J. (1997) Simulated car crashes and crash predictors in drivers with Alzheimer disease. *Archives of Neurology* **54**: 545–551

Rosenbloom S. (1993) *Will Older Persons lose Mobility?* Washington, DC, American Association of Retired Persons

Schieber F. (1994) High-priority research and development needs for maintaining the safety and mobility of older drivers. *Experimental Aging Research* **20**: 35–43

Shua-Haim JR and Gross JS. (1996) The co-pilot driver syndrome [see comments]. *Journal of the American Geriatrics Society* **44**: 815–817

Smeed R. (1968) Variations in the patterns of accident rates in different countries and their causes. *Traffic Engineering and Control* **10**: 364–371

Staplin L, Lococo KH, Stewart J, Decina LE. (1999) *Safe Mobility for Older People Notebook.* DOT HS 808 853. Washington, DC, National Highway Traffic Safety Administration

Strickberger SA, Cantillon C, Friedman PL. (1991) When should patients with lethal ventricular tachyarrhythmias resume driving? *Annals of Internal Medicine* **115**: 560–563

Stutts JC. (1998) Do older drivers with visual and cognitive impairments drive less? *Journal of the American Geriatrics Society* **46**: 854–861

Stutts JC, Stewart JR, Martell C. (1998) Cognitive test performance and crash risk in an older driver population. *Accident Analysis and Prevention* **30**: 337–346

Taylor BD and Tripodes S. (2001) The effects of driving cessation on the elderly with dementia and their caregivers. *Accident Analysis and Prevention* **33**: 519–528

Trobe JD. (1998) Test of divided visual attention predicts automobile crashes among older adults. *Archives of Ophthalmology* **116**: 665

Trobe JD, Waller PF, Cook-Flannagan CA, Teshima SM, Bieliauskas LA. (1996) Crashes and violations among drivers with Alzheimer disease. *Archives of Neurology* **53**: 411–416

US Department of Transportation. (2003) *Safe mobility for a maturing society: challenges and opportunities.* Washington, DC, US Department of Transportation

van Zomeren AH, Brouwer WH, Minderhoud JM. (1987) Acquired brain damage and driving: a review. *Archives of Physical Medicine and Rehabilitation* **68**: 697–705

Vernon DD, Diller EM, Cook LJ, Reading JC, Suruda AJ, Dean JM. (2002) Evaluating the crash and citation rates of Utah drivers licensed with medical conditions, 1992–1996. *Accident Analysis and Prevention* **34**: 237–246

Wang CC and Carr DB. (2004) Older driver safety: a report from the older drivers project. *Journal of American Geriatrics Society* **52**: 143–149

White S and O'Neill D. (1988) Health and relicensing policies for older drivers in the European union. *Gerontology* **46**: 146–152

Duchek JM, Hunt L, Ball K, Buckles V, Morris JC. (1998) Attention and driving performance in Alzheimer's disease. *Journal of Gerontology: Psychological Sciences and Social Sciences* **53**: 130–141

White S and O'Neill D. (2000) Health and relicensing policies for older drivers in the European Union. *Gerontology* **46**: 146–152

Winograd CH and Jarvik LF. (1986) Physician management of the demented patient. *Journal of the American Geriatrics Society* **34**: 295–308

20

Services to people with dementia: a worldwide view

Africa

OLUSEGUN BAIYEWU AND ADESOLA O OGUNNIYI

Africa is a multiracial, multicultural society, inhabited predominantly by people of the Arabian stock in the north, while in west, east and southern Africa Negroid people predominate. There is, however, a substantial number of white settlers in southern Africa. The population of people aged 65 years and over in Nigeria is about 3 per cent (National Population Census, 1994). The figures for most countries in sub-Saharan Africa are similar. In 1997 life expectancy at birth in most African countries ranged between 38 and 59 years except for South Africa, Mauritius, Egypt, Morocco, Libya and Algeria where the figure was over 65 years. Life expectancy will increase to between 51 and 70 years in these countries by the year 2025 (World Health Organization [WHO], 1998). Many elderly in Africa are impoverished with little education and low occupational pursuit.

Epidemiological data on dementia are available from few countries in Africa; notably Nigeria, South Africa, Egypt and Ethiopia. The first report available was by Ben-Aire et al. (1986) who reported a prevalence of 8.6 per cent for dementia among the coloured older persons in South Africa. The Ibadan–Indianapolis study, a comparative study involving elderly African Americans in Indianapolis and elderly Nigerians in Ibadan, reported a dementia prevalence rate 4.8 per cent for community residents of Indianapolis, compared with 2.29 per cent for residents of Ibadan (Hendrie et al., 1995). In the incidence study the figures were 3.24 per cent and 1.35 per cent for Indianapolis and Ibadan respectively (Hendrie et al., 2001). The rates in Ibadan were much lower than the rates from Western societies.

Farrag et al. (1998) reported a dementia prevalence rate of 4.5 per cent, among community dwellers in Egypt, a rate which is close to the reports from Western societies. In a small study of two nursing homes in Lagos, Nigeria, 48 per cent of destitute occupants had dementia (Baiyewu et al., 1997). It would therefore appear that dementia is commoner

in nursing homes even in Africa as found in Western societies. Behavioural symptoms of dementia have been reported in Nigerians (Hendrie et al., 1995; Baiyewu et al., 2003). Generally, the reports point to the fact that caregivers see both dementia and behavioural disorders as symptoms of ageing, so little effort is made to seek orthodox medical treatment. However, there are incontrovertible evidences that behavioural symptoms are distressful (Baiyewu et al., 2003).

20.1 CARE ARRANGEMENTS

Very few facilities are available for caring for demented persons in Africa, in fact most African countries have no policies on ageing. Services available vary from country to country depending on resources. In this chapter, Nigeria and South Africa will be used as representative countries for the continent.

In Nigeria, the family provides care for the demented elderly, with little or no public assistance. Baiyewu et al. (2003) observed that caregivers are mostly daughters of the elderly. In a community survey in Ibadan, Nigeria 15 per cent of the elderly lived alone, while 62 per cent lived in multigenerational living arrangements (Ogunniyi et al., 2001), which reinforces the role of family care. Despite the belief that dementia is part of ageing, substantial amounts of money are spent by family members seeking alternative care for dementia in the form of sacrifices with herbalists and prayers and fasting in syncretic churches (Uwakwe, 2001). Medical treatment for the elderly in Nigeria is provided through the network of primary, secondary and tertiary care facilities (Akanji et al., 2002). There are psychiatric units in teaching hospitals, there are also specialist psychiatric hospitals spread all over the country. These hospitals provide treatment for all forms of mental disorders including dementia. There are about

10 nursing homes dotted all over southern Nigeria, most of which are run by churches and voluntary agencies for destitute elderly. In all they hold less than 1000 beds; this is obviously not in agreement with the recommendation of WHO that advises adequate nursing home beds for those who need them (Wertheimer, 1997).

In 2001 a geriatric psychiatry clinic was set up in the University College Hospital, Ibadan; at the same time there are emerging programmes on psycho-education for caregivers of demented individuals, pilot studies based in the community in the eastern part of Nigeria (Uwakwe, 2001). Assessment of services like these are necessary in order to determine their relevance, acceptability and effectiveness.

In South Africa there appear to be more structured programmes. There are six outpatient psychiatric facilities for the elderly and two psychogeriatric inpatient units as well as a number of nursing homes (Baiyewu and Potocnick, in press).

20.2 CONCLUSION

There is a need for more psychogeriatric assessment centres in many African countries. Establishment of such centres by both government agencies and non-governmental organizations will give elderly persons with dementia access to required help and caregivers will be assisted to look after demented individuals in the community for as long as possible.

REFERENCES

Akanji BO, Ogunniyi A, Baiyewu O. (2002) Health care for older persons, a country profile: Nigeria. *Journal of American Geriatrics Society* **50**: 1289–1292

Baiyewu O, Adeyemi JD, Ogunniyi AO. (1997) Psychiatric disorders in Nigerian nursing home residents. *International Journal of Geriatric Psychiatry* **12**: 1146–1150

Baiyewu O, Smith-Gamble V, Akinbiyi A *et al.* (2003) Behavioral and caregivers reaction of dementia as measured by Neuropsychiatry Inventory in Nigerian community residents. *International Psychogeriatrics* **15**: 399–409

Baiyewu O and Potocnick F. (2005) Psychogeriatric services: current trends in Nigeria and South Africa. In: B Draper, P Melding, H Brodaty (eds), *Psychogeriatric Services Delivery: an International Perspective.* Oxford, Oxford University Press (in press)

Ben-Aire O, Swartz L, Teggin AF, Elk R. (1986) The coloured elderly in Cape Town – a psychological, psychiatric medical survey. *South African Medical Journal* **64**: 1506–1561

Farrag AKF, Farwiz HM, Kheds EH, Mahfouz RM, Omran SM. (1998) Prevalence of Alzheimer's disease and other dementing disorders: Assiut-Upper Egypt Study. *Dementia and Geriatric Cognitive Disorders* **9**: 323–328

Hendrie HC, Osuntokun BO, Hall KS *et al.* (1995) Prevalence of Alzheimer's Disease and Dementia in two Communities: Nigerian Africans and African Americans. *American Journal of Psychiatry* **152**: 1485–1492

Hendrie HC, Baiyewu O, Eldermire D, Prince C. (1996) Behavioural disorders in dementia: cross-cultural perspectives: Caribbean, Native American, Yoruba. *International Psychogeriatrics* **8**: 483–486

Hendrie HC, Ogunniyi AO, Hall HS *et al.* (2001). The incidence of dementia in two communities, Yoruba, residing in Ibadan, Nigeria, and African Americans in Indianapolis, USA. *JAMA* **285**: 739–747

National Population Commission of Nigeria. (1994) *Census 1991 – National Summary.* Nigeria, National Population Commission

Ogunniyi AO, Baiyewu O, Gureje O *et al.* (2001) Morbidity pattern of elderly Nigerian residents of Idikan Ibadan. *West African Journal of Medicine* **20**: 227–231

Uwakwe R. (2001) The financial (material consequences of dementia in a developing country: Nigeria. *Alzheimer Disease and Associated Disorders* **15**: 56–57

Wertheimer J. (1977) Psychiatry of the elderly: A consensus statement. *International Journal of Geriatric Psychiatry* **12**: 432–435

World Health Organization. (1998) *The World Health Report – Life in the 21st Century: A vision for all.* Geneva, WHO

Australia

DINA LOGIUDICE, ELEANOR FLYNN AND DAVID AMES

Australia is the oldest continent in geological terms and has been inhabited by modern humans for much longer than North America or northern Europe (Flannery, 1995), but until relatively recently its population was rather young because of high immigration rates. The country is now experiencing very rapid growth in its aged population with a consequent steep rise in the number of people with dementia (Access Economics, 2003).

Most of Australia's 20 million inhabitants live in cities (60 per cent of the population lives in the five state capitals of Sydney, Melbourne, Brisbane, Perth and Adelaide). The country is a federation of six states and two territories. The state governments are responsible for hospital care, but the national government provides the states with much of their revenue and administers the universal health insurance scheme, Medicare. The economy is heavily reliant upon exports of agricultural and mining products and has been in relative decline compared to other developed countries since the late 1950s. Per capita foreign debt levels are among the highest in the world (Australian Institute of Health and Welfare, 2003). In March 2005 one Australian Dollar (A$) was worth $US0.78, £0.41 and €0.60.

20.3 DEMOGRAPHY

There are three distinct groups of older people: the Anglo-Celtic majority, the descendants of the original indigenous Australians, and post-war migrants from Europe. One quarter of Australians aged above 60 years are migrants and 25 per cent of them come from a non-English speaking background. Aboriginals and Torres Strait Islanders account for barely 1 per cent of the elderly (Access Economics, 2003).

The number of people with diagnosed dementia in Australia in 2002 was estimated to be 162 300 or 0.8 per cent of the country's total population (Access Economics, 2003). This represents an increase from 0.6 per cent in 1993, but this rise will be dwarfed over the half century to 2051, during which time the number of people with diagnosed dementia is projected to increase to 581 300, while the country's total population rises by only 36 per cent. This rate of anticipated increase is one of the highest for any OECD country (Henderson and Jorm, 1998). The numbers would be much higher if individuals with undiagnosed mild to moderate dementia were included.

20.4 HEALTH AND WELFARE SERVICES

The Australian health and welfare system is pluralistic and complex. Services are provided by national, state and local governments and various private organizations. Medicare, a universal health insurance system financed through taxation and a compulsory income levy, reimburses part or all of the costs incurred by patients for primary medical care, diagnostic and ambulatory specialist medical care. The Pharmaceutical Benefits Scheme (PBS) pays most of the cost of approved drugs for ambulatory patients. The national government also subsidises the cost of residential aged care for eligible people. The total expenditure on health and residential care for the year 1996–97 was $A43 billion, which represented 8.5 per cent of Gross Domestic Product. For 1993–94 the average health cost per person over 65 was $A4919 and $A1301 for persons under 65 (Australian Institute of Health and Welfare, 2003).

Dementia costs in 2002 were estimated at $A6.6 billion of which $A5.6 billion were 'real' and $A1billion 'transfer' costs.

The costs include residential care ($A2.9 billion p.a. in 2002), indirect carer costs ($A1.7 billion p.a. in 2002) and A$592 million of tax foregone, carer payments of A$324 million and additional welfare payments of A$52 million. These costs are expected to double by 2010 (Access Economics, 2003). The hospital sums were determined from principal diagnoses alone and would therefore be a gross underestimate as there is no indication of hidden costs. Many individuals with dementia who enter hospitals for other conditions stay there longer than those who are free of cognitive impairment (Ames and Tuckwell, 1994). By comparison, $A831 million was spent on hypertension, $A894 on ischaemic heart disease and $A630 million on cerebrovascular disease in the same year.

In the Australian health system patients see their general practitioner (GP) for initial consultations. Most GPs work in group practices and bill their older and pensioner patients only for the amount that they will be reimbursed by Medicare. Patients' visits to specialists are reimbursed by Medicare only if the patient has been referred by a GP and many specialists charge fees that exceed the Medicare reimbursement. Patients choose their own GP, may visit more than one GP, and often do, which can lead to imperfect hospital discharge planning.

The six state and two territory governments provide free hospital care, primarily to inpatients but also for some ambulatory care visits. The increasing number of people requiring hospital care and constraints on hospital funding have led to significant delays for admission for 'non-urgent' treatment (e.g. joint replacements). Funding for public hospitals comes from the national government by way of grants to the states from funds raised by income tax. Private health insurance covers hospital and some non-hospital care, but premiums have risen faster than inflation in recent years. Until the end of the last century and introduction of a subsidy scheme financed by the national government, there had been a marked decrease in the number of people in private health insurance, though the fall was least in those on the old age pension. This trend has reversed and over one-third of Australians have private health insurance now. Extra health and welfare benefits are provided for war veterans, most of whom are elderly.

Community services, such as home care and delivered meals, used to be provided by local government, with funding from both state and national governments. Although the funding sources remain unchanged, these days the services are often delivered by private or not-for-profit organizations, which have tendered to provide them.

The disparate nature of the funding and service provision means that organizations providing services for older people are often required to contract with several levels of government and various programmes of the same government to obtain funds. Trials of pooling funding and coordinating care are underway, but the impediments to change are enormous and include the Australian Medical Association, who see this as the 'thin edge of the managed care wedge' (Messenger, 1999).

20.5 ASSESSMENT OF PEOPLE WITH DEMENTIA

20.5.1 General practitioners (GPs)

Reviews show that most GPs have difficulties diagnosing and managing dementia, and that assessment protocols could prove useful (Brodaty et al., 1994), especially those that indicate when to use cognitive instruments; this need is being addressed (Brodaty et al., 1998, 2002). The GP is often the first point of contact for a patient or carer seeking help, yet there is a perceived need for increased coordination between the GP and local services, and better understanding by the GP of the possibilities of 'shared care' for those affected by dementia (Pond et al., 1994; Shah and Harris, 1997). The assessment and management of a person with dementia and their carer is time consuming; however, the reimbursement structure has been adjusted to pay GPs for time spent meeting families or contacting other services.

20.5.2 Aged persons' psychiatry services

The state governments provide psychiatric services. Services for the old in the state of Victoria comprise a regional network of community aged psychiatry assessment and treatment teams (APATTs), linked to specialist aged psychiatry inpatient units with 15–30 beds in modern hospitals, co-located with aged care and adult psychiatry services. The teams are multidisciplinary and cover the entire state. Patients are assessed in their usual abode at the request of a GP, another health worker, family member or other carer. The APATTs provide a continuing care and support service to help patients to remain at home or to return there after discharge from an acute ward.

Limitations on these services relate to a relative lack of psychiatrists willing to undertake salaried public practice and to modest funding for other staff, which limits the community services to office hours, but service provision has expanded in recent years. Old age psychiatry services in other states are variable, but less well developed than in Victoria. The best of the rest are in New South Wales and South Australia.

20.5.3 Geriatric services and Aged Care Assessment Services (ACASs)

The ACASs were set up in 1984 and cover all of Australia (Howe, 1997). They may be co-located with regional geriatric hospital services or with specialist mental health services for the aged, or other health or welfare services. ACASs are funded by the national government to ensure that all people referred to residential care actually need it. Referrals are taken from patients, carers and health workers, including GPs and hospitals. Those referred are assessed at home or in hospital. The teams are multidisciplinary. Occupational therapists, physiotherapists, community nurses and geriatricians often see patients whose needs can be met at home with supports, which the ACAS will arrange. Other allied health staff (e.g. pharmacists and dietitians) are attached to some teams. ACASs provide assessment but do not offer continuing care. The majority of people assessed by an ACAS have evidence of dementia or other cognitive impairment (LoGiudice et al., 1995).

20.5.4 Memory clinics

In 1998 the Victorian government, acting on the report of a Ministerial Task Force (Ministerial Task Force on Dementia Services in Victoria, 1997) established 14 regional Cognitive, Dementia and Memory Services (CDAMSs) across the state to provide multidisciplinary assessment of people with dementia, and their carers. CDAMSs aim to provide integrated services throughout the 'pathway of dementia' at all levels of the healthcare system. A number of clinical indicators are used to evaluate the services. They include: prompt response to and assessment of referrals, adequate counselling of carers and the development of links with GPs and other care services. Patients have the option of being assessed at home.

Specialized memory clinics operate in major cities outside Victoria but have no distinct pattern or specific government funding, each being the brainchild of a particular specialist. Some are privately operated. Attendance by people with dementia at a memory clinic, which provides education, counselling and referral to services, seems to improve the quality of life of family carers (LoGiudice et al., 1999).

20.5.5 Private specialists

Many patients with dementia see psychiatrists, neurologists or general physicians for initial assessment. There are no complete data on these referrals but younger and wealthier dementia patients are more likely to be referred to a private specialist. The patient may then be referred on to an assessment service for further assistance.

20.6 CARE AND TREATMENT OF PEOPLE WITH DEMENTIA

20.6.1 Community and non-residential services

Family and other informal carers provide most care to those with dementia. They experience high levels of stress (Brodaty and Hadzi-Pavlovic, 1990) and the carer's own GP is often unaware that they are looking after an older person (Payda et al., 1999). A range of community options is provided to help people with dementia to continue living in the community, especially straight after discharge from a hospital. Many of these services are provided by brokerage from a case manager and are part of broader schemes to replace residential care with community care.

20.6.2 Alzheimer's Australia

An Alzheimer's Disease and Related Disorders Society was set up in 1985. It has undergone two changes of name and is now known as Alzheimer's Australia. Branches operate in each state and territory. Its goals include national dementia policy development, sharing of resources and expertise, and liaison with Alzheimer's Disease International. State branches provide education and counselling for those with dementia, their families, other carers and paid care workers. Alzheimer's Australia provides a national telephone advisory service ('Dementia Helpline').

20.6.3 Residential care

Residential care is provided by a variety of organizations including state governments, private operators and charitable organizations. People with dementia are heavy users of residential care. The national government subsidises and regulates residential care facilities. Two levels of care are provided. Low care facilities (previously called hostels) provide meals and assistance with activities of daily living including the administration of medication. High level care facilities (formerly called nursing homes) offer 24-hour nursing care and the majority of residents in these facilities have dementia (Henderson and Jorm, 1998). Some patients in low level care can have additional help funded to enable them to remain where they are instead of moving to high level care ('Ageing in Place').

20.6.4 Access to drug treatments for dementia

Since February 2001 it has been possible for patients to have most of the cost of treatment with a cholinesterase inhibitor paid for by the PBS if they have been assessed by a physician or psychiatrist who has certified that they have Alzheimer's disease of mild to moderate severity and that they meet other cognitive score-based criteria. The complexity of, and frequent changes to, these rules, and a relative lack of specialists interested in dementia probably cause cholinesterase inhibitors to be underprescribed and commenced at a later stage of the illness than would be ideal. Memantine is available but unsubsidized so few patients take it. Many patients with behavioural and psychological symptoms of dementia receive drug treatments. The prescription of subsidized novel antipsychotics via the PBS as limited to individuals whose doctors would state that they have a diagnosis of schizophrenia, until 2005 when low-dose risperidone was approved for subsidy when prescribed to patients with behavioural disturbance in the context of dementia.

20.7 RESEARCH AND REVIEWS OF SERVICES

20.7.1 Research

Australian researchers have made major contributions to knowledge about dementia, especially in epidemiology, neuropathology, new drug evaluation and carer support (Ames, 1997) and despite modest government research funding, this effort continues.

20.7.2 Reviews

There have been multiple reviews of existing services and of pilot schemes to provide new or integrated services for patients and carers. The national government released a National Action Plan for Dementia Care (NAPDC) in 1992, a mid-term report of the Plan in 1996 (Howe, 1997) and two national mental health plans in 1992 and 1998. An evaluation of the NAPDC indicated a need for further integration and development of demonstration programmes, resources and education strategies. Populations who were highlighted as requiring special attention included Aboriginal and Torres Strait islanders, immigrants of non-English-speaking background, and younger people with dementia. The desirability of managing dementia in the acute healthcare and primary care settings was emphasized. A Ministerial Working Party Report to the Victorian government led to the funding of regionalized CDAMS (Ministerial Task Force on Dementia Services in Victoria, 1997) and a recent review supported the ongoing role and funding of these clinics (Department of Human Services, 2003).

20.8 EDUCATION AND TRAINING

Australian medical education has undergone great change since 1990. Of the 10 established and three new medical schools, five offer graduate-only programmes and all are implementing new curricula. Nearly all of these curricula are integrated, combining basic science with clinical teaching and use problem-based learning. These curricula are too new for their outcomes to be judged. There are five professors of old age psychiatry and most medical schools have an old age psychiatrist at senior lecturer level or above. Departments of geriatric medicine are well developed and are usually led by a professor.

All nursing education is university based. There are chairs of gerontic and psychiatric nursing with postgraduate training available in these and other fields. Allied health training is via an undergraduate degree with additional postgraduate study for some disciplines such as psychologists.

The medical colleges all expect their fellows to undertake continuing medical education and for some, such as the Royal Australian College of General Practice, there is a financial incentive to do so. Academics provide some courses for GPs on the basics of assessment and management of dementia. Since cholinesterase inhibitors started to be reimbursed through the PBS some pharmaceutical companies have paid for GPs to receive education about aspects of dementia.

20.9 THE FUTURE

Changes in education for health professionals, both at undergraduate and continuing medical education level, provide opportunities for educators to develop and implement modules that teach the basics of dementia assessment and care to a majority of health professionals in Australia.

There is hope that the steady improvements in services for people with dementia that have occurred since the mid-1980s will continue. All levels of government acknowledge the rapid ageing of Australia's population and that this phenomenon will be associated with a huge rise in the number of people affected by dementia (Howe, 1997). The costs of providing services to a rapidly growing elderly population in the context of relative economic decline may constrain further improvements and even the maintenance of services in the end, but this has not happened yet.

REFERENCES

Access Economics. (2003) *The Dementia Epidemic: Economic Impact and Positive Solutions for Australia.* Canberra, Alzheimer's Australia

Ames D. (1997) Geriatric psychiatry in Australia. *International Journal of Geriatric Psychiatry* **12**: 143–144

Ames D and Tuckwell V. (1994) Psychiatric disorders among elderly patients in a general hospital. *Medical Journal of Australia* **160**: 671–674

Australian Institute of Health and Welfare. (2003) *Australia's Health: the Sixth Biennial Publication of the Australian Institute of Health and Welfare.* Canberra, Australian Institute of Health and Welfare.

Brodaty H and Hadzi-Pavlovic D. (1990) Psychosocial effects on caregivers of living with persons with dementia. *Australian and New Zealand Journal of Psychiatry* **24**: 351–361

Brodaty H, Howarth GC, Mant A, Kurrle S. (1994). General practice and dementia. A national survey of Australian GPs. *Medical Journal of Australia* **160**: 10–14

Brodaty H, Clarke J, Ganguli M *et al.* (1998) Screening for cognitive impairment in general practice: toward a consensus. *Alzheimer Disease and Associated Disorders* **12**: 1–13

Brodaty H, Pond D, Kemp NM *et al.* (2002) The GPCOG: a new screening test for dementia designed for General Practice. *Journal of the American Geriatrics Society* **50**: 530–534

Department of Human Services Victoria. (2003) *Review of the Cognitive Dementia and Memory Service Clinics.* Melbourne, Lincoln Gerontology Centre

Flannery T. (1995) *The Future Eaters: an Ecological History of the Australian Lands and People.* New York, George Braziller

Henderson AS and Jorm AF. (1998) *Dementia in Australia*, 4th edition. Canberra, Australian Government Publishing Service

Howe A. (1997) From states of confusion to a National Action Plan for Dementia Care: the development of policies for dementia care in Australia. *International Journal of Geriatric Psychiatry* **12**: 165–171

LoGiudice D, Waltrowicz W, McKenzie S, Ames D, Flicker L. (1995). Dementia in patients and carers referred to an Aged Care Assessment Team, and stress in their carers. *Australian Journal of Public Health* **19**: 275–280

LoGiudice D, Waltrowicz W, Brown K, Burrows C, Ames D, Flicker L. (1999) Do memory clinics improve the quality of life of carers? A randomised trial. *International Journal of Geriatric Psychiatry* **14**: 626–632

Messenger A. (1999) Who will control care? *Australian Medicine* **11**: 15

Ministerial Task Force on Dementia Services in Victoria. (1997) *Dementia Care in Victoria. Melbourne: Aged, Community and Mental Health Division.* Victoria, Victorian Government Department of Human Services

Payda C, Draper B, Luscombe G, Ehrlich F, Maharaj J. (1999) Stress in carers of the elderly. *Australian Family Physician* **28**: 233–237

Pond CD, Mant A, Kehoe L, Hewitt H, Brodaty H. (1994) General practitioner diagnosis of depression and dementia in the elderly: can academic detailing make a difference? *Family Practice* **11**: 141–147

Shah S and Harris M. (1997) A survey of general practitioners' confidence in their management of elderly patients. *Australian Family Physician* **26** (Suppl. 1): S12–S17

China

YU XIN

20.10 AGEING IN CHINA

The proportion and absolute number of elderly people in the total population of China has increased in recent years as the rate of ageing has accelerated. Chinese life expectancy reached 70 years in 1993. In 2000, elderly people comprised 10.2 per cent of the population, 129 million elderly (Lu Zhishan, 1994) (Table 20.1). In Shanghai, the largest city in China, people over 60 form 18.2 per cent of the city's 14 million population.

China became an elderly nation by the end of last century, but professional and social infrastructures have not been organized to meet the challenge of ageing. The 1 per cent sampling survey showed that the average family size in 1995 was 3.7, a 0.3 reduction compared to the 1990 national population survey (Chinese National Statistical Bureau, 1995). Thus in China, the traditionally valued extended family in which three or even four generations live together has weakened. Although the one child per family policy (which was first initiated in the 1980s) has been implemented mainly in urban areas, rural families are getting smaller in the same way. There are several reasons for this change.

- People have the freedom to choose where they live since housing has become a commodity. Young people prefer to move out from old dormitories which were allocated by the government to new apartments, leaving their elderly parents at home.
- People have more freedom of migration. Because of the disparity of economic development and a continuous decrease of arable land in the countryside, labourers tend to move from western and central parts of China to the east and coastal areas. More importantly, living and working in cities is no longer a crime for country boys and girls but the right of a citizen. Thus villages are more and more forgotten places full of elderly people and children.
- In the final quarter of last century, many unpredicted changes occurred in China. For the first time in thousands of years, the authority of the elderly is being questioned, especially when they are living on limited pensions while their children are enjoying the fruits of the market economy. 'Reverence to elderly' is repeatedly emphasized in the media, not because the Chinese are still proud of it but because it is felt that this virtue is threatened by social reform.

Table 20.1 *Prediction of the ageing population in China*

	1985	1990	1995	2000	2025	2050
Total population in China (millions)	1049.00	1143.33	1197.00	1270.00	1498.00	1547.00
Aged population (millions)	86.00	98.21	116.00	129.00	264.00	331.00
Aged/total population(%)	8.2	8.6	9.7	10.2	17.6	21.4

20.11 EPIDEMIOLOGY OF DEMENTIA IN CHINA

Dementia used to be an unusual condition even for psychiatrists. Not only were the elderly a small portion of the total population two decades ago, but people with dementia were rarely seen in clinical practice.

In 1986 the first epidemiological study of age-related dementia on a population aged 60 and over in China was conducted in an urban area of Beijing (Li Ge *et al.*, 1989). In this study, 1090 elderly people were screened using the Mini-Mental State Examination (MMSE), the suspected cases were interviewed by psychiatrists, DSM-III was adopted for diagnostic criteria, and Dementia Differential Diagnostic Schedule (DDDS) for differential diagnosis. Fourteen cases of moderate and severe dementia were identified, with a prevalence rate of 1.3 (≥60) and 1.9 per cent (≥65), respectively.

Table 20.2 lists important epidemiological studies on dementia in the past 10 years. Lai Shixiong and colleagues (2000) did a survey in a group of people older than 75 and showed that the prevalence rate of dementia especially Alzheimer's disease (AD) was much higher in this age group. Zhang Mingyuan and his colleagues (1990) indicated that loss of spouse and lower economic status were more common in dementia patients.

A nationwide survey on the epidemiology of dementia included 42 890 people aged 55 and over in six rural and six urban areas of China (Twelve Areas Epidemiological Investigation on Mental Disorders Coordinating Group, 1986). Although the final paper has not yet appeared some reports have been published and some of the results are listed in Table 20.2. The survey suggests that AD is the major type of dementia in old age and more prevalent in men. Vascular dementia seems more common in rural areas.

20.12 CAREGIVERS AND CARE-SETTINGS FOR PEOPLE WITH DEMENTIA

20.12.1 Where are the aged living?

Most of the Chinese elderly age at home. A survey by the ministry of social welfare demonstrated that 11 per cent of the elderly intended to live in nursing homes, i.e. 14 million people felt difficulty in living alone. However, there are only 1.04 million beds in a total of 51 000 residential institutions for the elderly. Furthermore, among these 1.04 million beds, the occupancy rate is only 70 per cent.

What makes these residential institutions unpopular with elderly people? First, these institutions are usually located in the countryside, far away from families, necessary facilities, and medical services. Second, these institutions are under-resourced, understaffed, and poorly equipped. They have no qualifications to take care of elderly people with medical conditions, much less of dementia.

20.12.2 Psychiatric services for people with dementia

With the astonishing recent changes in society and public health, Chinese psychiatrists also face a great challenge never

Table 20.2 *Prevalence rates* of dementias in China*

Author	Location	Population	Diagnostic Criteria	Results
Zhang Mingyuan *et al.* (1990)	Shanghai, urban area	5055 (≥55)	DSM-III-R	>55:2.57%; >65:4.61%
Chen Changhui *et al.* (1992)	Beijing, urban community	5172 (≥65)	DSM-III	1.03%
Gao Zhixu *et al.* (1993)	Shanghai, both rural and urban areas 3779 rural/urban:	2560/1219	DSM-III-R	4.21%
Tang Muni *et al.* (1999)	Si Chuan, rural areas	5987	DSM-III-R NINCDS-ADRDA	1.74%
Lai Shixiong *et al.* (2000)	Guangzhou, urban area	3825 (≥75)	DSM-III-R, NINCDS-ADRDA	8.90%
Qu Qiumin *et al.* (2000)	Xian, both rural and urban areas	4850 (≥55)	DSM-IV, NINCDS-ADRDA	3.53%
Zhou Bin *et al.* (2001)	Shanghai, both rural and urban areas	17018 (≥55)	DSM-IV, NINCDS-ADRDA	2.03%
Zhang Zhenxin *et al.* (2001)	Beijing, both rural and urban areas	5743 (≥55)	DSM-IV, NINCDS-ADRDA	4.2%
Tang Zhe *et al.* (2002)	Beijing, both rural and urban areas	2788 (≥60)	DSM-III-R, NINCDS-ADRDA	5.1%

* Except for two prevalence rate studies on vascular dementia (VaD) conducted in Beijing in the early 1990s, all studies indicate that the prevalence rate of VaD is lower than that of AD seen before. In 1997 there were 485 psychiatric hospitals in China, which could offer 107 362 beds; 13 912 doctors were working in psychiatric hospitals. Unfortunately, facilities for elderly patients are very limited. Accurate figures are not available, but it is estimated that fewer than 10 per cent of beds in each psychiatric hospital serve the elderly. Qualified geriatric psychiatrists are even fewer, proportionally.

20.12.3 Living in communities

Two studies in Beijing and Shanghai indicated that demented people were mainly looked after by their families at home (96.3 per cent vs 87.3 per cent) (Li Yongtong *et al.*, 1990; He Yanling *et al.*, 1995). Wu Wenyuan *et al.* (1995) evaluated the total burden of dementia caregivers compared with normal controls. The study suggested that dementia caregivers had more care burden, especially when the caregivers were female, and those with dementia were male. He Yanling *et al.* (1995) also indicated that dementia caregivers had more depressive and somatic symptoms than normal controls. Taking care of people with dementia is distressing work. The work is harder if the family is living in a community in which few resources are available.

20.13 KEY FACTORS IN SERVICE DELIVERY FOR PEOPLE WITH DEMENTIA

20.13.1 Government

The government plays a leading role in each aspect of social activities in China. Medical services are regarded as one part of the social welfare system. The government plans to build up the tertiary medical service delivery system in which the focus is on community health care. However, in China, there was no such thing as a community until a decade ago. The Chinese used to live in government dormitories assigned by work units (known in Chinese as *danwei*). A professor's next door neighbour could be a cleaner who worked in the same unit. Only when housing became merchandise and free mobility was allowed, could people live together according to their income, taste, and other social characteristics. The modern community is just developing in China. 'The Dormitory form' community was closely linked to where people worked, thus administration and supervision were easy and simple. The old primary care service was based on this system. With the collapse of old communities and rise of new ones, the primary healthcare system needs to be reformed. The pathway from community-based care to tertiary care is not well structured. The deficiency was completely exposed during the outbreak of the severe acute respiratory syndrome (SARS): the primary healthcare system did not work as a doorkeeper to keep suspected cases in communities, thus more and more people rushed into tertiary hospitals and got infected or infected others. The government has been aware

of the importance of community health care, but feels perplexed when putting it into practice. No referral system between primary, secondary and tertiary health care is established yet. Primary healthcare workers are usually poorly trained. Medical insurance companies are not willing to cover primary health care since they are not confident in the quality of service provided. The government encourages neighbourhood committees to set up nearby residential institutions for local elderly people, but medical services, administrative arrangements and personnel resources are not ready for these institutions to admit people with dementia.

20.13.2 Non-governmental organizations (NGOs)

Many NGOs, both academic and non-academic, can help in building up care systems for people with dementia. The Chinese Society of Psychiatry is drafting treatment guidelines for dementia in the elderly. The Chinese Society of Neurology conducted a nationwide survey on the prevalence of dementia in the elderly in four areas in China. Alzheimer's Disease of China has organized public education campaigns on World Alzheimer's Disease Day for three years. The Chinese Federation for the disabled and handicapped has helped to establish nursing homes for poorly functioning elderly people.

20.14 FUTURE PROSPECTS

When Japan became an elderly nation in 1970, its GDP per capita was $US1689. China transformed to an elderly nation with a GDP per capita of less than $US800 in the year 2000. Moreover, the government has no accumulated monies for the current generation of elderly since their working years were in the period of the 'planned economy', when there were no such things as insurance, or savings for pensions. Institutional care for people with dementia is completely unaffordable for most families. An optional solution for providing a decent service for dementia patients is to develop home care. In order to keep people with dementia at home as long as possible, the following considerations should be taken into account:

- The community should be empowered for self-administration in order to make the welfare of its members its first priority.
- Facilities and resources in the community can be available for families who are taking care of people with dementia at home.
- Primary health care should be qualified to provide necessary services for those with dementia.
- Tertiary, secondary, and primary healthcare systems should be organically integrated so that people with dementia can be shifted freely if needed.
- Social welfare agencies, and medical insurance organizations should adopt more flexible policies

to cover part of the expenses of caring for people with dementia at home and to compensate family caregivers.

- Finally, nursing homes, which are specific to dementia care, should be established. Some of the 5 million people with dementia will always need decent places for the final phase of their lives.

20.15 CONCLUSIONS

China is becoming an ageing society with surprising speed, while dementia becomes a challenge as prominent as it is in Western countries. Social and economic development is at a relatively low level that cannot meet the needs of people with dementia in any existing models. A unique service delivery system for dementia care should be developed which takes account of Chinese realities.

REFERENCES

Chen Changhui, Shen Yucun, Li Shuran *et al.* (1992) The investigation on prevalence rate of elderly dementia in urbane area of Beijing. *Chinese Mental Health Journal* **6**: 49–52

Chinese National Statistical Bureau. (1995) *Statistical Report on 1995 1% Sampling Survey of China.* Beijing, CNSB

Gao Zhixu, Liu Fugen, Fang Yongsheng *et al.* (1993) A study of morbidity rate of senile dementia among aged in urban and rural areas. *Journal of Neurology and Psychiatry of China* **26**: 209–211

He Yanling, Zhang Mingyuan, Qiu Jianyin *et al.* (1995) The mental health status of dementia caregivers. *Chinese Journal of Clinical Psychology* **3**: 200–204

Lai Shixiong, Wen Zehuai, Liang Weixiong *et al.* (2000) Prevalence of dementia in an urban population aged 75 and over in Guangzhou. *Chinese Journal of Geriatrics* **19**: 450–455

Li Ge, Shen Yucun, Chen Changhui *et al.* (1989) An epidemiological survey of age-related dementia in an urbane area of Beijing. *Acta Psychiatrica Scandinavica* **79**: 557–563

Li Yongtong, Chen Changhui, Luo Hechun *et al.* (1990) The psychological well-being of caregivers of elderly dementia. *Chinese Mental Health Journal* **4**: 1–5

Lu Zhishan. (1994) Current status of elderly and its development tendency in China. *Chinese Journal of Geriatrics* **14**: 194–198

Qu Qiumin, Qiao Jin, Yang Jianbo *et al.* (2001) Study of the prevalence of senile dementia among elderly people in Xian, China. *Chinese Journal of Geriatrics* **20**: 283–286

Tang Muni, Guo Yangbo, Xiang Mengze, Huang Mingsheng. (1999) Epidemiology of senile dementia and Alzheimer's disease in rural area. *Chinese Journal of Psychological Medicine* **9**: 20–22

Tang Zhe, Meng Shen, Dong Huiqing *et al.* (2002) Prevalence of dementia in rural and urban parts of Beijing. *Journal of Geriatrics of China* **22**: 244–246

Twelve Areas Epidemiological Investigation on Mental Disorders Coordinating Group. (1986) The summary of prevalence rates of various mental disorders from 12 areas epidemiological investigation. *Chinese Journal of Neurology and Psychiatry* **19**: 80–82

Wu Wenyuan, Zhang Mingyuan, He Yanling *et al.* (1995) A study on well-being and related factors of caregivers of dementia patients. *Chinese Mental Health Journal* **9**: 49–52

Zhang Mingyuan, Rober Katzman, William Liu *et al.* (1990) Prevalence study on dementia and Alzheimer's disease. *Chinese Journal of Medicine* **70**: 424–428

Zhang Zhenxin, Wei Jing, Hong Xia *et al.* (2001) Prevalence of dementia and major subtypes in urban and rural communities of Beijing. *Chinese Journal of Neurology* **34**: 199–203

Zhou Bin, Hong Zhen, Huang Maosheng *et al.* (2001) Prevalence of dementia in Shanghai urban and rural area. *Chinese Journal of Epidemiology* **22**: 368–371

The Former Soviet Union

ROBIN JACOBY

In the previous edition of this book, Poznyak and Solodkaya (2000) described very clearly the services available, or rather the lack of them, for older people living in the former USSR. In summary, they depicted countries with large populations in which overall life expectancy was decreasing, especially for males, but the proportion of older people was increasing. Rates of mental illness were high; levels of service provision were low; the focus of care was essentially institutional; and professional training was only just beginning to develop. What, therefore, has changed since then?

20.16 DEMOGRAPHY AND EPIDEMIOLOGY

United Nations data and projections continue to demonstrate a marked divide between declining overall populations in former Soviet countries and a growth in the proportion of those aged 65 and over. This is shown in Table 20.3 using the same countries as in Poznyak's and Solodkaya's table (2000, p. 349). The divide is greatest in the two most populous countries, Russia and Ukraine, which contain about 190 million people. Put crudely, but accurately, Russians and Ukrainians eat diets high in saturated fats, smoke tobacco excessively, and have high rates of alcoholism, tuberculosis (TB) and HIV/AIDS. Together with poorer standards of public health provision than were offered by the USSR, these facts conspire to reduce survival in adults of working age, especially males. As in Western countries, although for different reasons, there are fewer economically active persons to provide resources for more old people.

Poznyak and Solodkaya (2000) indicated that ICD-10 was beginning to make an impact in former Soviet countries. There is no doubt that this is increasingly true, helped by dissemination of relevant literature in Russian (Cooper, 2000; Goldberg, 2000). However, given the geographical vastness of the USSR, modern epidemiological literature is extremely sparse. In a survey of 1109 people of 60 and over in part of the Moscow area, Gavrilova and Kalyn (2002) found that 36.6 per cent suffered from some form of disorder definable by ICD-10. Furthermore, when they compared the results of one study conducted 10 years before with another 10 years after the collapse of the USSR, they found an increase in mental disorders that they attributed to the stress caused by the immense social disruption and poverty of the immediate post-Soviet period.

20.17 OLD AGE PSYCHIATRY SERVICES

The basic structure of services, insofar as they exist, has not changed since Poznyak and Solodkaya (2000) described them in the last edition. There are very few psychiatrists whose practice is only with older patients. The focus remains institutional. At primary care level there are polyclinics in which psychiatrists sometimes work. Mostly, however, polyclinics are staffed by primary care physicians (PCPs), so-called *terapyevty* (терапевты). Boundary disputes between PCPs and psychiatrists are common, with psychiatrists claiming that only they are qualified to treat mental disorders. Given that there are not nearly enough psychiatrists and secondary resources in rich Western countries to treat all patients with mental disorders, and that the majority have to be treated in primary care, it is clearly nonsensical for psychiatrists in former Soviet countries to claim such restrictive practices. In some places, however, encouraged by Western non-governmental organizations (NGOs) who provide teaching and written material in Russian, PCPs are being taught to diagnose and treat suitable cases of depression and other disorders.

Specialist psychiatric resources include:

- outpatient clinics at so-called dispensaries (диспансеры);

Table 20.3 *Population data and projections from four former Soviet Republics (Source: United Nations Population Division)*

Country	Year	Total population (millions)	Age 65+ (%)
Belarus	2000	10 034	13.7
	2005	9 809	14.9
	2010	9 612	14.4
	2020	9 208	16.3
Kazakhstan	2000	15 640	6.9
	2005	15 354	8.6
	2010	15 130	8.4
	2020	15 422	10.1
Russia	2000	145 612	12.5
	2005	141 553	14.1
	2010	137 501	13.3
	2020	129 018	16.7
Ukraine	2000	49 688	13.8
	2005	47 782	15.9
	2010	46 038	15.9
	2020	42 605	17.5

- inpatient wards at large mental hospitals;
- and beds in institutions for the chronic mentally ill (*internaty*/интернаты).

Both hospitals and *internaty* do have some wards specifically for older patients, but many of the latter are treated in standard general adult psychiatry wards, not unusually containing around 70 patients, with two or three nurses per shift. Whether housed on specialist old age psychiatry or general adult wards, older patients have to put up with facilities that would be considered scandalous in richer Western countries (see Plates 6 and 7), reflecting not only the low status of the mentally ill, but also the lack of resources that the authorities wish or feel able to put into psychiatric services.

Many old persons with mental disorders, including dementia, live at home, some, but not all, known to psychiatric services. Apartments are small and often house three generations of one family. The younger adults have to work hard, frequently doing two or three jobs to maintain a reasonable standard of living. If a grandparent suffers from dementia, enormous strain is placed on the shoulders of younger members. Since it is known how bad the alternative to home care is, efforts are made to keep elderly relatives at home beyond a stage that would be considered tenable in Western countries. On the other hand, families are forced frequently to institutionalize a demented relative simply in order to maintain a reasonable income.

In most former Soviet countries the Ministry of Social Protection provides some home-care services, but with untrained staff who are generally reluctant to be involved with mentally ill clients, the latter being regarded as problems

for the health services. Thus, community services are poorly coordinated between healthcare and social welfare, exacerbated by an unwillingness for the two relevant ministries to collaborate.

20.18 FUTURE DEVELOPMENTS

Although it is difficult to avoid the conclusion that too little has been done to improve services for the elderly mentally ill in former Soviet countries and that a huge injection of resources is needed to bring them up to acceptable levels, it would be wrong assume that the future is entirely bleak. There is no shortage of manpower and no lack of enthusiasm in younger professionals to see change. Resistance to change comes from the old Soviet *nomenklatura* (establishment) who remain in positions of power but are not, of course, immortal. Western NGOs, such as the Geneva Initiative on Psychiatry*, raise money to print material in Russian (e.g. Jacoby and Oppenheimer, 2003), and organize courses in old age psychiatry given by Russian-speaking Western psychiatrists. The demand for the written material and the courses outstrips the ability to provide them. A great deal of time and money are required to repair the harm done by Soviet power to all aspects of life in the countries it dominated for 70 years, but the peoples of these countries want change and are certainly intelligent and resourceful enough to achieve it.

REFERENCES

Cooper J. (2000) *Karmannoe Rukovodstvo k MKB-10: klassifikatsiya psikhicheskikh i povedencheskikh rasstroistv.* Kiev, Sphera (Russian translation of *Pocket Guide to the ICD-10 Classification of Mental and Behavioural Disorders, 1998.* Edinburgh, Churchill Livingstone)

Gavrilova SI and Kalyn Ya B. (2002) Social and environmental factors and mental health in the elderly. *Vestnik Rossiiskoi Akademii Nauk* **9**: 15–20 (in Russian with summary in English)

Goldberg D. (ed.) (2000) *Posobie Po Prakticheskoi Psikhiatrii Kliniki Modsli.* Kiev, Sphera (Russian translation of *The Maudsley Handbook of Practical Psychiatry,* 3rd edition. Oxford, Oxford University Press, 1998)

Jacoby R and Oppenheimer C. (ed.) (2003) *Psikhiatria Posdnego Vozrasta.* Kiev, Sphera (Russian translation of *Psychiatry in the Elderly,* 2nd edition. Oxford, Oxford University Press, 1997)

Poznyak V and Solodkaya T. (2000) Services for dementia in the developing world: a view from the new independent states of the former Soviet Union. In: J O'Brien, D Ames, A Burns (eds), *Dementia,* 2nd edition. London, Arnold, pp. 349–352

*GIP grew from a group of activists opposed to Soviet political abuse of psychiatry into the largest NGO currently helping to reform psychiatric services and adherence to human rights in the former USSR. For a more detailed account of its work visit its website at www.geneva-initiative.org

20e

France

BRUNO VELLAS, B BOS, BENOIT LAVALLART AND L GREGOIRE

Alzheimer's disease (AD) is a common disease in France, with more than 700 000 patients and approximately 140 000 new cases each year. Owing to the burden related to this disease many initiatives has been realized in the past few years to care those patients.

20.19 ALZHEIMER'S DISEASE CLINICAL AND RESEARCH CENTRES

The French government developed recently an Alzheimer Plan. Part of this plan was the accreditation of 16 CMRRs (Centres Memoire de Recherche et de Resources – Memory Research and Resource Centres). These centres of excellence comprise clinics, research and education in the field of AD at the top levels. They are formed from Neurology, Psychiatry or Geriatric departments.

The four CMRRs from the South of France (Bordeaux [Pr Dartigues], Toulouse [Pr Vellas], Montpellier [Pr Touchon], Nice [Pr Robert]) decided to create the F-CMRR-SF (Federation of the Alzheimer's Centres from the South of France). The advantage of this federation is to associate four CMRR from different specialities (neurology, psychiatry, geriatric and public health). Medical directors have a weekly telephone conference.

A national federation of the CMRR is in process. Some projects of the F-CMRR-SF and the national federation are:

- a common computerized patient medical chart;
- common educational projects;
- jointly research projects.

20.20 LOCAL MEMORY CENTRES

Moreover, approximately 200 local memory centres (CMPs, Centres Memoire de Proximité) have been identified. To be selected each centre must have a multidisciplinary team including neurologist, geriatrician, psychiatrist and neuropsychologist.

Some other initiatives are also being developed such as a standardized neuropsychological and geriatric assessment for each of these memory centres, as well as a standardized form to follow the patients.

The PHRC (Programme Hospitalier de Recherche Clinique), financed by the French ministry of health, decided to fund some large collaborative programmes. One is the ReAl.Fr project (Reseau Français sur la Maladie d'Alzheimer). The aim of this project is to follow for 4 years a cohort of 700 elderly patients with AD living at home, with a monthly assessment follow up (Principal Investigator: Pr Vellas).

One other programme aims to develop and validate a 'Care Plan Project' for the AD patients, with a standardized follow up every 6 months; 1200 AD patients over France will be part of this programme, involving 80 CMPs, half in the control group and half in the care plan intervention group.

There is also one other PHRC again financed by the French Ministry of Health – Focus on MCI Patients (Principal Investigator: Pr Dubois).

20.21 INPATIENT UNITS

The first acute care unit for AD patients was created over 10 years ago in the Toulouse Alzheimer's Centre, Toulouse

University Hospital. Since that date, acute care units for AD patients have been created in several university hospitals in France. These acute care units, usually part of a department of internal medicine and geriatrics, are able to receive patients with AD 24 hours a day, all year round. Usually 30 per cent of the patients come for difficult diagnosis, 40 per cent for complications related to the disease, mostly behaviour disorders, and 30 per cent for associated disease like pneumonia, weight loss or anorexia. These units play a major role in the care of the patients, linking together with home care and nursing home care. They work also closely with the emergency department of hospitals.

20.22 DAY HOSPITALS

We have two kinds of day hospital in France: those related to CMRR or CMP are involved in the diagnosis and patient follow up; and respite day care for AD patients. These respite day care centres are mostly in the community.

20.23 NURSING HOMES

They are approximately 10 000 nursing homes in France, around 30 per cent of which have special care units for severely demented patients. The criteria for special care are:

- to receive demented patients;
- to have a special care plan for dementia;
- to have special environmental design;
- to keep the family involved;
- to have a special training programme.

Every 2 years a national congress on SCU is organized, with more than 1000 participants attending.

20.24 HOME CARE

Home care for AD patients is largely developed in France, with special funding to care for the elderly with loss of autonomy, giving them money to receive help to perform basic activities of daily living at home. Nurses and physicians are likely to visit their elderly patients at home. More than 25 per cent of AD patients from the REAL-FR study are living at home alone with help.

20.25 FAMILY ASSOCIATION

Family associations like France Alzheimer are very much involved and active in France at the both national and regional levels. There are also many other initiatives presently being developed in France in the field of AD care, including aspects of ethics. However, there is more to be done in France: as in many other countries, only 50 per cent of AD patients are diagnosed, 30 per cent are undertreated, and still fewer have a really long-term and well-evaluated healthcare plan programme.

FURTHER READING

Vellas B and Fitten J (eds) (2004), *Alzheimer's Disease: Research and Practice*, Vol. 9. Paris, *L'Année Gérontologique*. (2004), Vol. 18. Paris

Germany

SIEGFRIED WEYERER AND MARTINA SCHÄUFELE

20.26 LONG-TERM CARE INSURANCE AND MEDICAL TREATMENT OF INDIVIDUALS WITH DEMENTIA

Among the population in Germany who are over the age of 65 years, about 1 million individuals suffer from moderately severe to severe dementia (Bickel, 2001). About 40 per cent of them are institutionalized in residential and nursing homes, while 60 per cent live in private households and are generally cared for by family members.

In Germany statutory health insurance generally covers the costs of medical services. However, the provision of long-term care for elderly patients suffering from chronic disorders such as dementia places an enormous emotional and financial burden on both patients and their families. To alleviate this situation, legislation establishing a system of statutory long-term care insurance came into effect on 1 January 1995, with automatic coverage for people who are covered by statutory health insurance. The system of statutory long-term care insurance offers financial aid ranging from 205 € (Euros) to 1688 € per month depending on the nature and extent of the demand for basic nursing care and household help. However, the need for general care and supervision of persons with mental disorders (which accounts for a major portion of the costs for care of those with dementia) is not taken into consideration when long-term care insurance benefits are assessed. In order to better meet their needs, since 2002 those in need of care who are residing in private households and who can justifiably claim for substantial general care and supervision can claim additional financial aid up to a total of 460 € per year. However, no current figures are available as to the number of claims filed or the sum of benefits paid on behalf of dementia patients.

Over 90 per cent of the adult population visit a primary care physician at least once a year. The percentage among the elderly is even higher and their annual consultation rate is well above average. Most patients with dementia first consult a primary care physician, many of whom are not well enough informed about or trained to deal with gerontopsychiatric disorders. They rarely refer patients with dementia to mental healthcare institutions. Results of various studies show that the use of psychiatric institutions and services drops sharply from roughly 25 per cent by the 65–74-year-olds in need of care to less than 10 per cent by those over the age of 75 years (Bickel, 2003). This seems due in part to a sense of nihilism with regard to dementia patients. This attitude is also reflected by the relatively low number of prescriptions for antidementia drugs. From 1992 to 2000 the number of prescribed daily doses of antidementia drugs in Germany dropped by 60 per cent, from 516 million to 215 million. This indicates a marked and increasing undersupply of the affected population with these medications. Two regional studies showed that on average only 10 per cent of Alzheimer patients are treated with acetylcholine esterase inhibitors (Demling and Kornhuber, 2002).

Over the past 20 years, more than 70 memory clinics have been established. These outpatient services specialize in the early recognition of cognitive problems, the diagnosis of dementia, pharmacological treatment and clinical trials, the development of non-pharmacological treatment strategies, the support and counselling of patients and their relatives and the support and advanced training of primary care physicians and psychiatrists (Kurz et al., 2003). Memory clinics are usually integrated into university hospitals and are heavily committed to research. Their services are generally not covered by statutory health insurance. Owing to the limited number of memory clinics and the particularities of their funding, they are not a standard component of the system of ambulatory dementia care (Stoppe, 2002).

Facilities and services that play an important role in the care of dementia patients in Germany will now be discussed.

20.27 CARE FOR COMMUNITY-DWELLING PATIENTS

20.27.1 In-home services

In-home services provide mainly medical treatment measures (dressing of wounds, administration of injections, etc.), basic nursing care (personal hygiene, etc.), and – to a lesser extent – household help for patients living at home. Upon the introduction of long-term care insurance, which prioritizes ambulatory care over inpatient care, it was expected that there would be a regular rush by claimants on such ambulatory care providers. Indeed, their number has increased markedly since then: from roughly 3000 in 1993 to 12 596 licensed services in October 2000. Nonetheless, only about 27 per cent of those eligible for benefits of long-term care insurance and who reside in private households file claims for the care or household help available from the ambulatory services (Bundesministerium für Familie, Senioren, Frauen und Jugend, 2002). Claims solely for financial benefits were filed on behalf of 73 per cent of eligible patients, meaning that their care will be provided exclusively by private caregivers, usually family members. At present, no estimate of the current demand by dementia patients for in-home services is available. Results of an earlier study indicate that approximately 1 out of 10 dementia patients living at home in the southern Germany city of Mannheim made use of an ambulatory care service (Schäufele et al., 1995). The study also revealed that the services in themselves cannot provide the necessary complete support. In particular, weekend service, in-home supervision, or activating care, all of which are essential in dementia care, are available on a limited basis, if at all. Moreover, the costs for these services are not covered by the long-term care insurance but must be borne by the patients themselves.

20.27.2 Geriatric day and night care

Semi-inpatient services constitute the link between in-home and institutional long-term care. They are an important component of the system of geriatric care, providing elderly individuals in need of aid with qualified assistance on workdays from the morning throughout the afternoon (day care) or from the evening throughout the night (night care).

The first geriatric day care centres in Germany were established in 1973 with the aim of preventing or at least prolonging the often unwanted and expensive referral to a nursing home. Despite the strong increase in the number of day care centres within the past 25 years, they remain less important than institutional long-term care. A study carried out in 17 centres providing geriatric day care revealed that slightly more than half (58.6 per cent) of their clients suffered from dementia (Weyerer and Schäufele, 1999). Dementia patients who regularly wander off or who exhibit a high potential for aggression cannot be cared for in geriatric day care centres (Kurz et al., 2003).

Disorders of circadian rhythm particularly complicate the in-home care of dementia patients. For this reason, night care has been available in Germany for a number of years. Approximately 1400 night-care beds were created; however, at 13 per cent the demand lags far behind the supply (Schneekloth and Müller, 2000).

20.28 CARE FOR RESIDENTS OF OLD-AGE HOMES

The type of care provided by old-age homes has changed greatly in Germany over the last 20 years: the original focus on residential care has since given way to nursing care. In 1999 the number of old-age homes in Germany totalled 8859, most of them nursing homes, with altogether 645 456 beds (Bundesministerium für Familie, Senioren, Frauen und Jugend, 2002). In Germany, as in most other industrialized nations, nursing-care facilities are key providers of dementia care. Cost estimates for dementia indicate that long-term institutional care in nursing homes accounts for 50–75 per cent of the total direct costs (Bickel, 2001).

A move into institutional care is all the more probable in cases of advanced dementia. Recent results indicate that up to 80 per cent of the affected population will enter a nursing home during the course of dementia, remaining there until their death, because in-home care can no longer be guaranteed. Residential nursing-care facilities in Germany were unprepared for the shift in the numbers of demented patients, who now constitute the majority of residents: currently approximately 60 per cent (Weyerer et al., 2001). The work load and stress upon nursing staff have increased accordingly. This development is a major challenge to the principle of integrated care. Lately political efforts have been made to improve the institutional care of dementia patients. Special types of augmented care, such as partially integrated approaches (special day care for dementia patients) or segregated approaches (for example, special care units) have been introduced, accompanied by architectural and conceptual changes and advanced training for the nursing staff.

The forerunner of this development in Germany was the city of Hamburg, which in 1991 made 750 beds available in 30 nursing-care facilities as part of the so-called 'Hamburg Model'. These beds were designated specifically for the special institutional care of dementia patients. The Hamburg Model encompasses both domus units, in which solely dementia patients are cared for, as well as integrated units. In the latter, dementia patients reside on the same ward as those without dementia, but are cared for separately, either all day or for a few hours every day. Like the domus unit arrangement, segregated daytime care also includes group play, music, physical activities and certain therapy measures oriented to the capabilities and deficits of the residents. The care beds in the Hamburg Model are more expensive than those in traditional nursing homes since the staff is larger and better qualified. Admission to the Hamburg Model is governed by specific requirements: the presence of a medically diagnosed advanced dementia in conjunction with marked behaviour disturbances and the capacity to participate in group activities (patients cannot be bed-ridden). A recent study carried out in traditional nursing homes in Mannheim revealed that one out of six nursing-home residents with dementia fulfils these criteria.

As an alternative to hospital-like care in nursing homes, sheltered households for dementia patients have been established by various social welfare institutions in recent years that feature a normal daily routine and a family-like environment. The success and effects of this type of living arrangement are not yet known.

No official figures are available on the number of facilities in Germany that offer special dementia care programmes. However, they are still outweighed by the number of traditional nursing homes. Partially integrated care (i.e. segregated daytime care) seems to be the most popular specialized concept, offered by approximately 10–15 per cent of the German nursing homes.

20.29 SUMMARY AND CONCLUSIONS

Dementia patients are the most frequent users of long-term care facilities. However, several studies have shown that many care-providers, as well as physicians, hospitals, and nursing homes are inadequately prepared and lack adequate training. Training opportunities and quality of service are in dire need of improvement. Dementia care is still strongly characterized by the dichotomy between the in-home care provided by family members, augmented by ambulatory care services, and the residential care provided by nursing homes. Contrary to expectation, ambulatory care services or semi-inpatient services such as day or night care have been used less frequently than was originally anticipated (Bundesministerium für Familie, Senioren, Frauen und Jugend, 2002). This is most likely due to the fact that the supply and the operation of these services do not sufficiently match the needs of the dementia patients and their families.

Moreover, statutory long-term care insurance does not cover the costs generated by the specific needs of the severely mentally ill elderly: supervision, instruction, activation, occupational therapy. Although it is a step in the right direction, the recently passed Act Supplementing Domiciliary Care

Services (Pflegeleistungs-Ergänzungsgesetz) fails to meet the needs of demented patients and their caregivers.

The number of dementia patients in Germany is expected to double within the next 40 years, while at the same time the number of family caregivers will continue to decrease, giving rise to an enormous demand for professional geriatric care (Bickel, 2001). Nursing homes will see the number of dementia patients among their residents soar to at least 75 per cent. In view of these demographic data, the development of specialized types of institutional care for dementia patients, which began later in Germany than in other countries, is an urgent matter.

REFERENCES

Bickel H. (2001) Demenzen im höheren Lebensalter: Schätzungen des Vorkommens und de Versorgungskosten. *Zeitschrift fur Gerontologie und Geriatrie* **34**: 108–115

Bickel H. (2003) Epidemiologie psychischer Störungen im Alter. In: H Förstl (ed.), *Lehrbuch der Gerontopsychiatrie und -psychotherapie.* Stuttgart, New York, Georg Thieme, pp. 11–26

Bundesministerium für Familie, Senioren, Frauen und Jugend (ed.). (2002) *Vierter Bericht zur Lage der älteren Generation in der Bundesrepublik Deutschland. Risiken, Lebensqualität und Versorgung Hochaltriger, unter besonderer Berücksichtigung demenzieller Erkrankungen.* Eigendruck, Berlin

Demling J and Kornhuber J. (2002) Stand der Pharmakotherapie. In: JF Hallauer and A Kurz (eds), *Weissbuch Demenz.* Stuttgart, New York, Georg Thieme, pp. 85–86

Kurz A, Jansen S, Tenge B. (2003) Gerontopsychiatrische Versorgungsstrukturen. In: H Förstl (ed.), *Lehrbuch der Gerontopsychiatrie und-psychotherapie.* Stuttgart, New York, Georg Thieme, pp. 11–26

Schäufele M, Lindenbach I, Cooper B. (1995) Die Inanspruchnahme von Sozialstationen vor und nach Inkrafttreten des Leistungstatbestandes Schwerpflegebedürftigkeit – eine Studie in Mannheim. *Gesundh-Wes* **57**: 55–62

Schneekloth U and Müller U (eds). (2000) *Wirkungen der Pflegeversicherung. Forschungsprojekt im Auftrag des Bundesministeriums für Gesundheit, durchgeführt von I + G Gesundheitsforschung, München, und Infratest Burke Sozialforschung, München. Schriftenreihe des Bundesministeriums für Gesundheit Bd 127.* Baden-Baden, Nomos

Stoppe G. (2002) Gedächtnissprechstunden/Memory-Kliniken. In: JF Hallauer and A Kurz (eds), *Weissbuch Demenz.* Stuttgart, New York, Georg Thieme, pp. 85–86

Weyerer S and Schäufele M. (1999) Epidemiologie körperlicher und psychischer Beeinträchtigungen im Alter. In: A Zimber and S Weyerer (eds), *Arbeitsbelastung in der Altenpflege.* Göttingen, Bern, Toronto, Seattle, Hogrefe, pp. 3–23

Weyerer S, Schäufele M, Hönig T. (2001) Demenzkranke in der stationären Versorgung: Aktuelle Situation. In: Bundesministerium für Familie, Senioren, Frauen und Jugend (eds): *Qualität in der stationären Versorgung Demenzerkrankter.* Stuttgart, W Kohlhammer, pp. 9–18

20g

Hong Kong

HELEN CHIU

Hong Kong is situated on the South China coast. It returned to Chinese sovereignty in 1997 and is now a Special Administrative Region of China with a high degree of autonomy under the policy of 'one country two systems'. As Hong Kong was a British colony for over 100 years, it is more westernized than the rest of China, and the development of dementia services is also different. The current population is 6.8 million and the percentage of population aged 65 or above is 11 per cent. Service development for dementia care has only started in the last few years under the pressure of a rapidly ageing population. Long-term care of people with dementia is a great problem because of the breakdown of traditional family care in Hong Kong in recent years. This may be related to growing westernization and attrition of filial respect, combined with a decreasing trend of extended families.

20.30 PREVALENCE OF DEMENTIA

A local study involving 1034 older people has found that the prevalence of dementia was 4 per cent for people aged 65 or above (Chiu *et al.*, 1998). Alzheimer's disease and vascular dementia accounted for 65 per cent and 29 per cent of cases respectively; 45 per cent of the subjects with dementia were living in residential homes, which is a high figure compared with the rest of China and Taiwan.

20.31 MEDICAL SERVICES

Most medical services for dementia are provided by psychogeriatric teams whereas geriatricians treat many elderly with vascular dementia, as well as those with physical problems. At present, there are seven multidisciplinary psychogeriatric teams serving different catchment areas in Hong Kong. These teams provide services to patients with dementia and functional psychiatric illness, including inpatient, outpatient, consultation and limited day hospital services. These teams also run an outreach programme to assess and treat elderly people living in subvented old-age and care-and-attention homes. Five memory clinics have been set up for early diagnosis of and intervention for dementia.

Protocols for assessment and clinical management of dementia have been developed by the Psychogeriatric Working Group, which consists of leaders of all the psychogeriatric teams. Guidelines for use of cholinesterase inhibitors are very similar to the NICE guidelines in the UK. However, the drug budget in the public health sector is very tight, and there are financial constraints on prescription of these drugs even if patients fulfil the criteria to receive antidementia drugs. Traditional Chinese medicine is rarely used for dementia. Besides medication, input from other members of the multidisciplinary team, including nurses, occupational therapists, physiotherapists, social workers and clinical psychologists, is an important part of management.

20.32 COMMUNITY SUPPORT SERVICES

Elderly health centres run by the Department of Health offer health education and screening for a number of disorders including dementia. In addition, general practitioners play an important role in screening for patients with dementia. Financial support to the elderly is available in the form of old-age allowance and disability allowance.

Community support services include home help, home-delivered meals (meals-on-wheels) and day care centres for the elderly. The Alzheimer's Association was established in Hong Kong in 1995. In 1998, the Hong Kong Psychogeriatric Association was founded and one of its targets has been to promote public awareness and facilitate training as well as research on dementia.

Residential services for the elderly are provided by care-and-attention homes and nursing homes. Care-and-attention homes provide accommodation, general personal care and limited nursing care. Nursing homes serve those who require a higher level of nursing care. In general, the subvented facilities are of better quality than the private ones but some of them do not like to accept patients with dementia and behavioural problems. Many of these elderly are thus admitted to privately run care-and-attention homes, some of which are not up to standard, and physical restraints are frequently used.

20.33 LEGAL ISSUES

A major gap in dementia care concerns legal provision. The Mental Health (Amendment) Ordinance 1997 set up a Guardianship Board to appoint guardians to make decisions on behalf of people who are mentally incapacitated. In addition, enduring power of attorney is now available, but it does not cover healthcare issues. Development on the issue of advance directives remains very slow.

20.34 SPECIAL DEMENTIA SERVICES

Extra funding to subvented care-and-attention homes to look after the elderly with dementia was given in the form of dementia care supplement. In 1999, the government funded a pilot project to set up several dementia residential units and dementia day care centres. However, because of lack of funding, these special dementia services were not supported after 4 years.

A major advance in dementia care recently is the establishment of a specially designed dementia centre, the Jockey Club Centre for Positive Ageing in 2000. This centre is funded by the Hong Kong Jockey Club with the objective to promote dementia care in Hong Kong. The service arm comprises of day care and respite residential service. The training and public education arm provides training to professionals,

front-line workers and informal carers, as well as education to the public. In addition, there is a resource centre and a website (www.jccpahk.com). The research arm conducts studies on dementia care as well as opinion surveys on human rights issues in dementia care, including physical restraints, advance directives, etc.

20.35 RESEARCH

The Department of Psychiatry at the Chinese University of Hong Kong has a dementia research unit, which is linked with the Jockey Club Centre for Positive Ageing. Studies conducted in the last few years include development of neuropsychological tests for use in the Chinese elderly, epidemiological surveys on dementia, genetic investigations of Alzheimer's disease and vascular dementia, neurobiological correlates of behavioural and psychological symptoms in dementia, as well as studies on dementia care.

20.36 THE FUTURE

Hong Kong has made significant progress in the development of dementia care over the last 5 years. For instance, the Jockey Club Centre for Positive Ageing is evolving into a centre of excellence in the region of South-east Asia. However, there is still no clear or consistent policy on dementia care by the government. In addition, after the outbreak of the severe acute respiratory syndrome (SARS), a lot of funding and resources in the health sector will be channelled to the prevention and control of infectious diseases. The economic downturn in the recent few years, as well as the shift of priority in health care after SARS outbreak (Chiu et al., 2003) are two major challenges in the further development of dementia care in Hong Kong.

REFERENCES

Chiu HFK, Lam LCW, Chi I et al. (1998) Prevalence of dementia in Chinese elderly in Hong Kong. Neurology 50: 1002–1009

Chiu HFK, Lam LCW, Li SW, Chiu E. (2003) SARS and psychogeriatrics – perspective and lessons from Hong Kong. International Journal of Geriatric Psychiatry 18: 871–873

India

KALYANASUNDARAM S AND MATHEW VARGHESE

Projections indicate that by the year 2020, there will be 470 million people aged 65 and older in developing countries, more than double the number in developed countries. Three countries projected to have the largest number of old people in the year 2025 are China, India and Indonesia (Siegel and Hoover, 1982). India's elderly population, which was 57 million in 1990, is expected to cross 100 million in 2013. From a mere 5.1 per cent of the population in 1901, the elderly will become 21 per cent of the population by the year 2050. The elderly constituted 7.7 per cent of the total population in the India census 2001, and this figure is expected to rise to 11 per cent by the year 2020. With the country's population exceeding a billion, India ranks second in the entire world in the number of 'aged' citizens.

20.37 AGEING SCENARIO IN INDIA

As most elderly people live at home, family members shoulder caregiving responsibilities. The existing healthcare facilities are not geared to meet these challenges posed. In India life expectancy has gone up from 20 years in the beginning of the twentieth century to 62 years today. The erstwhile joint family, the natural support system, has crumbled. The fast-changing pace of life has added to the woes of the older person: 30 per cent of older persons live below the poverty line, and another 33 per cent just marginally over it; 80 per cent live in rural areas; 73 per cent are illiterate, and can only be engaged in physical labour; 55 per cent of women over 60 are widows, many of them with no support whatsoever. There are nearly 200 000 centenarians in India.

20.38 CARE ARRANGEMENTS

Old age was never seen as a social problem in ancient India. Respect towards elders and the concept of obligation towards parents (*pitra rina*) forms part of the cultural value system (Venkoba Rao, 1993). In contemporary Indian society, however, the position and status of the elderly and the care and protection that they have traditionally enjoyed have been undermined by several factors. Urbanization, migration, the break-up of the joint family system, growing individualism, the change in the role of women from being full-time caregivers, and increased dependency status of the elderly are some of the prominent factors.

20.39 ISSUES CONCERNING PEOPLE WITH DEMENTIA

Studies by the 10/66 Dementia Research Network in Goa and Chennai examined the impact of care giving for elders (Dias *et al.*, 2004). Carers of people with dementia spent significantly longer time providing care than did carers and co-residents of depressed persons and controls. The highest proportion of time was spent in communicating, supervising, and helping with eating and toileting. Levels of carer strain were notably higher among carers of people with dementia. They were 16 times more likely to have a common mental disorder than other carers. Economic strain was indicated by high proportion of caregivers of people with dementia who had given up work to provide care, coupled with the increased likelihood that the family had to meet relatively high healthcare costs.

20.40 SERVICES IN INDIA

20.40.1 Hospital-based services

Most of the hospitals in India see persons with old age problems. However, most physicians do not recognize dementia as a medical problem. Also, other than the routine coverage in the psychiatry training curriculum, there are no specific training courses in geriatric (or old age) psychiatry. At present only a handful of hospitals offer special outpatient psychiatric services for the old age population.

20.40.2 Non-governmental agencies

There are two well-known non-governmental agencies, which have been operating in India in the care of the elderly. These are the Alzheimer's and Related Disorders Society of India (ARDSI) and Helpage India.

20.40.2.1 THE ALZHEIMER'S AND RELATED DISORDERS SOCIETY OF INDIA (ARDSI) (WWW.ALZHEIMERINDIA.ORG)

ARDSI was founded in June 1992. At present ARDSI has 14 Chapters in various cities across the country, with another 9 Chapters proposed. The Registered Office is in Cochin, Kerala. ARDSI also offers a range of community-based services such as:

- community care
- domiciliary care
- day care
- community geriatric nursing training
- dementia care fund
- memory clinic
- research.

Their website is WWW.ALZHEIMERINDIA.ORG

20.40.2.2 HELPAGE INDIA (WWW.HELPAGEINDIA.ORG)

HelpAge India is a national level voluntary organization that was formed in 1978. It has 37 offices all over India with its headquarters in New Delhi. It aims to foster the welfare of the aged in India especially the needy aged. It also helps to raise funds and increase social awareness about the problems of the elderly. HelpAge India has implemented 3084 projects and made a difference to the lives of over 7 million persons. Its programmes focus on improved access to health and eye care facilities, community-based services, livelihood support,

and training. In addition, the organization also supports welfare programmes like old-age homes, day care centres and the Adopt-A-Grandparent scheme.

20.41 DISCUSSION

Mental disorders in the elderly in India are a major public health issue for four major reasons:

- Because of increased population of elders, the number of people with mental disorders is rising rapidly.
- There is very poor awareness about these disorders.
- Traditional family and social support systems for elders are rapidly changing.
- There are virtually no health services geared for the special needs of elders in India.

Caregiver strain has not been acknowledged; instead, a near mythical strength is attributed to the abilities of families to cope. This distracts from the need for a rational debate regarding the future balance between informal family support and formal care services, and hinders evidence-based policymaking. Prioritizing home-based support for elderly persons with serious mental disorders and their carers should be given serious consideration. Removing stigma may require integrating the subject of mental disorders of elders into community and general health programmes. Collaboration is required with non-governmental organizations (such as the Alzheimer's and Related Disorders Society of India) that are pioneering programmes to empower the elderly and support families. Working with the existing manpower and health and social service infrastructure is likely to be more successful in meeting the mental health needs of elders in India than developing specialized psychogeriatric services throughout the country.

REFERENCES

Dias A, Samuel R, Patel V, Prince M, Parameshwaram R, Krishnamoorthy ES. (2004) The impact associated with caring for a person with dementia: a report from a 10/66 Dementia Research Group's Indian Network. *International Journal of Geriatric Psychiatry* **19**: 182–184

Siegel JS and Hoover SL. (1982) Demographic aspects of the health of the elderly to the year 2000 and beyond. *World Health Statistical Quarterly* **35**: 132–202

Venkoba Rao A. (1993) Psychiatry of old age in India. *International Review of Psychiatry* **5**: 165–170

Italy

ANGELO BIANCHETTI AND MARCO TRABUCCHI

Dementias, and Alzheimer's disease (AD) in particular, affect an increasing number of people in the developed countries and also in less developed regions of the world (Wimo *et al.*, 2003). Worldwide there lacks a homogeneous approach to neurodegenerative disorders, and various health services follow different lines of development, not always supported by scientific evidence (Bianchetti and Trabucchi, 2003).

Italy has only a short history in this field. The regional organization of its health system causes variability both in the number and in the quality of interventions for people affected by dementia (Dello Buono *et al.*, 1999).

In Italy interest in dementia started in the early 1980s mostly from the commitment of Luigi Amaducci. In the early 1990s Trabucchi, Bianchetti and Zanetti started the first National Research and Clinical Center for AD and related disorders (IRRCS San Giovanni di Dio Fatebenefratelli) in Brescia (Lussignoli *et al.*, 1998). In 1997 the Italian Association of Psychogeriatrics was founded, involving neurologists, psychiatrists and geriatricians.

In this short review the most important steps of the Italian organization of care for demented patients are summarized.

AD is the most common dementing disorder. Once considered rare AD is now recognized as a major cause of death and a growing public health challenge (Bianchetti and Trabucchi, 2001). On the basis of a multicentre longitudinal survey carried out in Italy (Italian Longitudinal Study on Ageing – ILSA), started in 1992/1993, it has been estimated that approximately 6.4 per cent of the population over 64 years of age is afflicted by dementia (2.5 per cent for AD and 1.4 per cent for vascular dementia), with a higher prevalence in women (7.2 per cent) than in men (5.3 per cent) (ILSA, 2002). The prevalence of dementia increases with age, both for AD and vascular dementia (VaD) (Figure 20.1). The incidence rates are 12.47 per 1000 person-years and 6.55 for AD (Di Carlo *et al.*, 2002). On

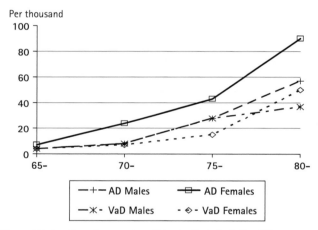

Per thousand

Figure 20.1 *Prevalence rates of dementia in Italy for different age groups (based on ILSA study).*

these bases about 150 000 new cases of dementia per year are expected. The ILSA study demonstrated that dementia is a major causes of mortality and disability in individuals aged 65 to 84 years; the 2-year mortality risk ratio (MRR) was 3.61 for the demented elderly, higher than for neoplasm (MRR = 2.01), heart failure (MRR = 1.87), and diabetes (MRR = 1.62) (Baldereschi *et al.*, 1999).

20.42 HEALTH SERVICES FOR DEMENTIA PATIENTS IN ITALY

Despite progress in the development of new treatment strategies for AD, many patients and caregivers receive inadequate care (Bianchetti and Trabucchi, 2001). Health service organizations do not satisfy the complex needs of demented patients. In

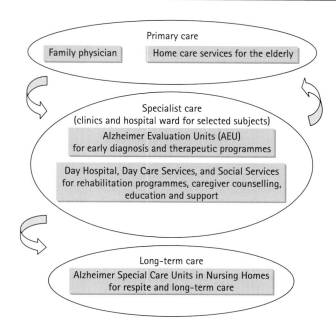

Figure 20.2 *Comprehensive care network for demented patients.*

recent years different health services were designed to diagnose dementia more accurately and to improve the care of patients (Bianchetti and Trabucchi, 2003). The aims of these services (diagnostic evaluation, treatment/referral, case management, research, training and continuing education, rehabilitation programmes, special care programmes), their target subjects (outpatients, inpatients, nursing home residents), organization and costs are substantially different, but still not thoroughly studied (Dello Buono *et al.*, 1999; Doody *et al.*, 2001).

In 1994 the regional government of Lombardy (northern Italy, 8.5 million inhabitants) started a comprehensive care network of services called 'Piano Alzheimer', aimed at the care of patients in different dementia phases (Trabucchi *et al.*, 1995). The care network delineated by Piano Alzheimer is summarized in Figure 20.2. On the basis of the results of a pilot study, 20-bed Special Care Units (SCUs) in 70 nursing homes (corresponding to 4.5 per cent of the total nursing home beds in the Region) were opened and dedicated to demented patients with high levels of behavioural disturbance (Bianchetti *et al.*, 1997; Frisoni *et al.*, 2000).

To assess the efficacy of SCU in comparison to traditional nursing home models of care, a study (SCUD project) has been performed (Frisoni *et al.*, 1998). Ambulating patients with moderate to severe dementia and severe behavioural disturbances on the modified Neuropsychiatric Inventory were enrolled in 18 SCUs and 25 traditional nursing homes. Patients were assessed at baseline and after 6 months. Baseline behavioural disturbances significantly improved at follow up in both groups (38 and 41 per cent change, respectively), with no increase in the percentage of patients taking neuroleptic and non-neuroleptic drugs (ranging from 46 to 56 per cent for both groups at baseline and follow up). Indicators of adverse effects of psychotropic medications (cognitive performance and falls) remained unchanged. In the case group the reduction of

behavioural disturbances was achieved with lower use of physical restraints: 10 per cent of cases and 32 per cent of controls ($P = 0.02$) at follow up respectively (Frisoni *et al.*, 1999).

The mean daily cost for patients in the SCUs is approximately 100 €. In Italy, 50 per cent of nursing home costs are paid for by the National Health System, which contributes a further 11 per cent of the cost of patients in SCUs. The cost/effectiveness analysis demonstrated that, with a cost increase of only 11 per cent, a considerable improvement in quality of life may be attained, with a reduction in physical and pharmacological restraints (Trabucchi, 1999). The role of SCUs in the care of demented patients is widely debated, and the importance of the quality of life as outcomes of these type of services has been emphasized recently (Albert, 2004).

The Piano Alzheimer also planned a number of day centres specifically devoted to demented subjects. They follow patients during day time (from 8 am to 6 pm), 6 or 7 days a week, and work in collaboration with family doctors in providing disease evolution, performing non-pharmacological interventions and a general surveillance of therapy. However, their costs are very high (about 70 € a day) almost completely charged to the families; for this reason day centres have not developed successfully.

Piano Alzheimer of the Lombardy region also provides an acute hospital ward offering medical care to the demented elderly, with the aim of studying specific guidelines for all hospitals of the region that have a high prevalence of patients affected by dementia (about 50 per cent of over 65 admitted to acute medical wards have a Mini-Mental State Examination (MMSE) score <24).

Others Italian Regions (i.e. Emilia, Tuscany, Marche, Liguria) organized specific projects for demented patients, on the assumption that their care needs a devoted organization, with employees (physicians, nurses, social workers) expressly devoted and skilled. Most of these projects are based on geriatric services. The projects include a number of Alzheimer Centres for coordination, research, education, and second or third level diagnosis (the allocation and the number of these centres differs between regions), SCUs in nursing homes, and a great effort for the education of personnel. In all projects the role of the primary physician is central, but it is well known that family doctors often do not comply with the psychological and time-consuming involvement needed by the care of persons affected by dementia. Caregivers and patients' families are considered not only targets of treatment, but also partners in care. In general, great differences are observable in the different regions in the dissemination of services, emphasis on home care in comparison with residential care, economic interventions in favour of persons affected by dementia and their families.

The most recent and important step in service organization in Italy has been the implementation of 'Progetto Cronos', born with the aim to standardize prescriptions of cholinesterase inhibitors (AchE-I) and to assess their effects on defined outcomes (cognition, functional status, behaviour) in non-selected subjects (Bianchetti *et al.*, 2003). This national project

Table 20.4 *Clinical characteristics at baseline of 1362 patients enrolled in Piano Alzheimer in the Cremona area*

	Total (n = 1362)	Females (n = 1007)	Males (n = 355)
Age	77.4 ± 6.9 [48–95]	78.0 ± 6.77	5.9 ± 7.4
Sex (% female)	73.9		
Education (years)	5.4 ± 2.7 [0–21]	5.2 ± 2.4	6.1 ± 3.4
Disease duration (months)	26.9 ± 15.7 [5–96]	26.6 ± 15.2	27.6 ± 17.0
Co-occurrent chronic diseases	[0–4]		
None (%)	41.0	40.9	41.4
1 or more (%)	59.0	59.2	58.6
MMSE score	19.2 ± 3.9 [10–26]	18.9 ± 3.8	19.9 ± 3.9
ADL (preserved)	4.8 ± 1.5 [0–6]	4.8 ± 1.6	5.1 ± 1.4
IADL (preserved)	3.8 ± 2.6 [0–8]	3.6 ± 2.5	4.3 ± 2.8
Previous use of ChE-I (%)	38.6	37.8	41.1
AChE-I drugs prescribed			
Donepezil (%)	67.0	67.7	64.8
Rivastigmine (%)	23.9	23.6	24.8
Galantamine (%)	9.1	8.6	10.4

started in October 2000 and involved about 500 Alzheimer Evaluation Units (AEUs), embracing all health districts. Besides helping to adopt a definite attitude towards the reimbursement of AchE-I, the project aimed to build up a nationwide network of centres with a homogeneous level of diagnostic and therapeutic competence. It has been a great effort with good results, since it stimulated the *ex novo* organization of centres, with standardized protocols and a database collected by the Ministry of Health. At the end of the project (March 2003) about 40 000 mild to moderate AD patients had been recruited. This pattern of prescription is lower than expected, revealing insufficient attention to the early detection of the disease. Data collected from AEUs of a northern Italian area (Cremona) on 1362 AD patients in the mild-moderate stage of the disease are presented in Table 20.4. Mean MMSE values in patients starting treatment were 19.2 ± 3.9, 19.8 ± 4.5 after 3 months ($P < 0.05$, t-test for paired samples), and 18.9 ± 4.9 after 9 months (not significant by t-test for paired samples versus baseline). Data replicate in the real world those obtained in controlled clinical trials. This fact further confirms that non-selected AD patients with a mild to moderate cognitive decline seldom enrolled in randomized controlled trials may benefit from AchE-I treatment. The specific role of drugs compared with the positive effect exerted by the care given at AEUs remains to be clarified. In the near future the AEUs system will be in charge of data monitoring regarding the efficacy and the risk ratio of atypical antipsychotic drugs in dementia. The availability of data on thousands of patients will be of great value for the definition of guidelines regarding the prescription of these drugs for behavioural and psychological symptoms of dementia.

In all Italian regions one of the main unresolved problems is the education of professionals at various levels. Historically, universities demonstrated only moderate interest in chronic diseases of the elderly, neglecting teaching both during undergraduate and postgraduate curricula. Today, education-information in the field of dementias is almost completely in the hands of the pharmaceutical industry, with the risk that

---

Box 20.1 *Characteristics of AD caregivers in Italy: results of a national survey**

- 73.8% of principal caregivers were females (72.1% in mild AD, 81.2% in severe AD)
- 69.1% were <60 years old (71.1% in mild AD, 63.1% in severe AD)
- 49.6% were children, 34.1% spouse
- 65.0% lived with the patient (59.1% in mild AD, 75.5% in severe AD)
- 58.6% of caregivers received help from other family members (73.6% in mild AD, 50.9% in severe AD), and 37.3% from paid personnel (21.6% in mild AD, 40.0% in severe AD)
- 26.3% of caregivers reported a direct impact on working activity (17.5% stopped working activity)
- 60.4% reported a worsening of quality of life
- 33.6% used drugs after the beginning of caregiver activity (72.2% psychotropic drugs; 15.7% somatic drugs and 12.1% unconventional drugs)

* Adapted from CENSIS, 1999

---

the quality and quantity of messages are modulated by the needs of the drug market.

20.43 BURDEN OF CARE ASSOCIATED WITH ALZHEIMER'S DISEASE

The care of a demented patient induces high levels of psychological, physical and economic burden on individuals, their caregivers, families and society as a whole. Caregivers play a key role in the management of dementia and are the main social buffer against the early institutionalization of patients (Prince, 2004).

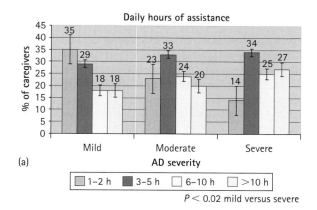

(a)

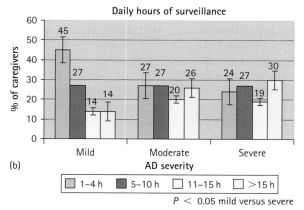

(b)

Figure 20.3 *Caregivers' time spent for the assistance (a) and surveillance (b) of AD patients in Italy: results of a national survey. (Adapted from CENSIS, 1999.)*

In 1999 the Geriatric Research Group collaborated with the Italian Association for Alzheimer Disease (AIMA) and the Centre for Social Studies (CENSIS) in the conduct of a national survey on 802 AD principal caregivers equally distributed between Italian Regions (CENSIS, 1999). The AD patients were females in 68.1 per cent of cases, and 80.0 per cent were aged 65 years or older. The characteristics of caregivers are summarized in Box 20.1. The data confirm that caregivers experienced a substantial burden in the assistance and surveillance of patients (Figure 20.3).

The use of supportive and educational programmes has been regarded as the most reliable way to reduce distress and decrease the risk of institutional placement of demented patients (Schulz *et al.*, 2004). In Italy many interventions were conducted using different strategies, the elements of which can be categorized into three broad aspects: psychological, educational, and social. It has been possible to demonstrate that caregiver interventions (psychological and educational programme) significantly reduce burden in carers and improves their quality of life (Zanetti *et al.*, 1998).

In the field of caregiving, in Italy a new phenomenon has occurred in the last 5 years, i.e. the presence of a large number of paid caregivers, mostly coming from Eastern European countries (Poland, Moldavia, Ukraine), who demonstrate a high level of humane attitudes, and have good ability both to

learn the Italian language and to perform basic home care. These persons, mostly females (80 per cent), with a mean age of about 50 years, plan a stay in Italy to collect sufficient money for specific purposes (building a house in their original country, funding a university degree for their children, etc.). Their mean wage is about 800 € per month plus housing and food. In the area of Brescia (1 million inhabitants) the number of these workers has been estimated at 10 000–12 000.

20.44 THE COSTS OF ALZHEIMER'S DISEASE IN ITALY

Recent funding changes in many developed countries have left AD patients and their families responsible for many costs that were previously reimbursed, such as those for medication, hospitalization or nursing care. Indeed, it has been estimated that a major component of the total cost of the care of an AD patient falls upon the family caregiver who is caring for the patient at home.

In Italy economic pressures stimulated a large debate on the need for a new tax specifically devoted to the support of the chronically ill elderly. Although no decisions have so far been taken by the Parliament, a yearly amount of about 10 million € is considered necessary to maintain the present level of care in the northern part of the country and to build even a rudimentary network in the southern regions.

One study conducted in Italy calculated that the family's expenditure for the non-medical care of the patient at home was $US8218 annually (about 9000 €) (Cavallo and Fattore, 1997).

The Geriatric Research group conducted a cost-of-illness study (CoDem – Cost of Dementia), designed to give a profile of the total economic costs of AD in Italy, based upon measurement of the direct and indirect costs associated with the care of community-dwelling AD patients (Trabucchi *et al.*, 1996). As a result of the onset of dementia, 35.4 per cent of patients were forced to stop work, while 20.4 per cent of caregivers either reduced their working hours or stopped work altogether. Thirty-five per cent of all caregivers made some modifications to their house to make it more suitable for the patient (mean cost $US7900). Total mean weekly costs for a patient's care were estimated to be $US585, including paid providers (housekeeping, cooking, transportation, medication and drug administration) and an estimate of the indirect costs associated with family caregiving. The estimated cost of direct and indirect home care increases with disease severity (from $US852 to $US1062 per annum, as calculated using the cost replacement method) (Bianchetti *et al.*, 1998).

In the CoDem study, the principal predictor of the weekly costs for home care (direct and indirect) was the number of instrumental archives of daily living functions (IADLs) lost, with an increase in weekly costs of $US72 per function (Bianchetti *et al.*, 1998). Total annual nursing home costs increased from $US1200 to $US4000 from mild (1) to severe

(3) dementia ratio with the Clinical Dementia Rating (CDR) scale, and the ability to perform IADLs was the single best predictor of nursing home placement (Trabucchi, 1999).

20.45 CONCLUSION

The management of AD is multimodal, guided by the stage of illness and focused on the specific symptoms of the patient. While no current therapy can reverse the progressive cognitive and functional decline of AD, several pharmacological and psychosocial techniques have been proven to be effective to control behavioural symptoms, to slow cognitive and functional decline and to improve the quality of life of patients and caregivers (Cummings, 2004). They have special needs; programmes, environments and care approaches must reflect this uniqueness, and the organization of health services must make the different possible effective interventions available. Whatever the cost–benefit outcome of a particular treatment option, it is the responsibility of physicians to determine the optimal quality of care for their patients. However, physicians also have a responsibility to ensure that scarce resources are not squandered. To do so outcomes must be shown such as those involving drug treatment, rehabilitation procedures or the organization of services.

In the near future Italy will be challenged by historical events: an economic crisis as in many other developed countries, ageing of the population with an increased number of chronic patients owing also to their prolonged survival, and uncontrolled immigration from Africa and Eastern Europe where the outcomes are unpredictable. Only strong political control of this scenario will allow us to assist the most frail citizens, such as demented subjects in an appropriate way in future.

REFERENCES

Albert SM. (2004) The Special Care Unit as a quality-of-life intervention for people with dementia. *Journal of the American Geriatrics Society* **52**: 1214

Baldereschi M, Di Carlo A, Maggi S *et al.* (1999) Dementia is a major predictor of death among the Italian elderly. ILSA Working Group. Italian Longitudinal Study on Aging. *Neurology* **52**: 709–713

Bianchetti A and Trabucchi M. (2001) Clinical aspects of Alzheimer's disease. *Ageing* **13**: 221–230

Bianchetti A and Trabucchi M. (2003) Health services and economic perspectives in Alzheimer's Disease. *Italian Journal Psychiatry and Behavioural Science* **13**: 19–27

Bianchetti A, Benvenuti P, Ghisla KM, Frisoni GB, Trabucchi M. (1997) An Italian model of Dementia Special Care Unit: results of a pilot study. *Alzheimer Disease and Associated Disorders* **11**: 53–56

Bianchetti A, Frisoni GB, Ghisla KM, Trabucchi M. (1998) Clinical predictors of the indirect costs of Alzheimer's disease. *Archives of Neurology* **55**: 130–131

Bianchetti A, Padovani A, Trabucchi M. (2003) Outcomes of Alzheimer's disease treatment: the Italian CRONOS project. *International Journal of Geriatric Psychiatry* **18**: 87–88

Cavallo MC and Fattore G. (1997) The economic and social burden of Alzheimer's disease on families in the Lombardy region of Italy. *Alzheimer Disease and Associated Disorders* **11**: 184–190

CENSIS. (1999) *La Mente Rubata. Bisogni e Costi Sociali della Malatti di Alzheimer.* Milano, Italy, Franco Angeli Ed

Cummings JL. (2004) Alzheimer's Disease. *New England Journal of Medicine* **351**: 56–67

Dello Buono M, Busato R, Mazzetto M *et al.* (1999) Community care for patients with Alzheimer's disease and non-demented elderly people: use and satisfaction with services and unmet needs in family caregivers. *International Journal of Geriatric Psychiatry* **14**: 915–924

Di Carlo A, Baldereschi M, Amaducci L *et al.* (2002) Incidence of dementia, Alzheimer's disease and vascular dementia in Italy. The ILSA Study. *Journal of the American Geriatrics Society* **50**: 41–48

Doody RS, Stevens JC, Beck C *et al.* (2001) Practice parameter: management of dementia (an evidence-based review). Report of the Quality Standards Subcommittee of the American Academy of Neurology. *Neurology* **56**: 1154–1166

Frisoni GB, Gozzetti A, Bignamini V *et al.* (1998) Special care units for dementia in nursing homes: a controlled study of effectiveness. *Archives of Gerontology and Geriatrics* (Suppl. 6): 215–224

Frisoni GB, Bianchetti A, Pignatti F, Gozzetti A, Trabucchi M. (1999) Holoperidol and Alzheimer's disease. *American Journal of Psychiatry* **156**: 2019–2020

Frisoni GB, Aleotti F, Bianchetti A, Trabucchi M. (2000) Special care for dementia in Europe In: *Special Care Units, Research and Practice in Alzheimer's Disease* Vol. 4, pp. 114–121

ILSA [The Italian Longitudinal Study on Ageing Working Group]. (1997) Prevalence of chronic diseases in older Italians: comparing self-reported and clinical diagnoses. *International Journal of Epidemiology* **26**: 995–1002

Lussignoli G, Frisoni GB, Bianchetti A, Trabucchi M. (1998) Measurement of outcomes in Alzheimer's Disease. In: B Vellas, J Fitten, G Frisoni (eds), *Research and Practice in Alzheimer's Disease.* Pan's, Serdi Publisher, pp. 437–446

Prince M for the 10/66 Dementia Research Group. (2004) Care arrangements for people with dementia in developing countries. *International Journal of Geriatric Psychiatry* **19**: 170–177

Schulz R and Martire LM. (2004) Family caregiving of persons with dementia: Prevalence health effects and support strategies. *American Journal Geriatric Psychiatry* **12**: 240–249

Trabucchi M. (1999) An economic perspective on Alzheimer's Disease. *Journal of Geriatric Psychiatry and Neurology* **12**: 29–38

Trabucchi M, Bianchetti A, Zanetti O. (1995) An Italian network for the care of demented patients. *The Gerontologist* **35**(S1): 90

Trabucchi M, Ghisla KM, Bianchetti A. (1996) CODEM: a longitudinal study on Alzheimer disease costs. In: E Giacobini and R Becker (eds), *Alzheimer Disease: Therapeutic Stragies.* Boston, Birkhäuser, pp. 561–565

Wimo A, Winblad B, Aguero-Torres H, von Strauss E. (2003) The Magnitude of Dementia Occurrence in the World. *Alzheimer Disease and Associated Disorders* **17**: 63–67

Zanetti O, Metitieri T, Bianchetti A, Trabucchi M. (1998) Effectiveness of an educational programme for demented persons' relatives. *Archives of Gerontology and Geriatrics* (Suppl. 6): 531–538

Japan

MASAHIRO SHIGETA AND AKIRA HOMMA

The circumstances that surround the elderly drastically changed in 2000. One reason was the public Long-Term Care Insurance (LTCI) programme which started in 1 April 2000 (Maeda, 2003; Shimizu, 2003). Many Japanese people think that daughters and their sons' wives should take care of their aged parents. Even women who work feel a strong sense of responsibility to take care of their own and their husband's aged parents. However, social care for the elderly has started after the implementation of LTCI and it is likely that many people will change their attitude towards care with this new programme in the future. It will become easier to use various services for the elderly and the burden on relatives will be reduced. Another dramatic change has been the review of the Adult Guardianship System (Maeda, 2003). Previously adult guardianship in Japan had several drawbacks, because its simplicity and strictness (Arai, 1999). When a person was judged as incompetent by a psychiatrist, the Japanese legal term of incompetent was a significant discriminator – for example, this is documented in the census registration (family register). Moreover, a relative nominated as a guardian might not always do things in the best interest of the demented older person. For instance, a child nominated as a guardian for the child's mother or father might have used his or her property only for child's advantage. However, the most important drawback was that there was no legal system for a person to nominate a guardian voluntarily while the person was still mentally intact. A new Japanese Guardianship System was legislated for in order to solve these problems.

20.46 THE NEW PUBLIC LONG–TERM CARE INSURANCE (LTCI) PROGRAMME

The LTCI system covers Japanese citizens aged 40 and over. There are two types of insuree: Type I insuree and Type II insuree. Type I insurees are aged 65 or over and in need of long-term institutional or domiciliary services. Type II insurees are aged between 40 and 65, have age-related diseases such as Alzheimer's disease and stroke, and are in need of institutional or domiciliary services because of the disease. When the insuree wants to use the services of the LTCI (see Box 20.2), he or she should apply to the insurer, which is the local government where he/she lives, for the assessment of needs for care and services. A designated care service agency can act as proxy for the insuree. Once the assessment committee of the local government determines that the applicant is in need of the services, the cost of services used after the date of application is covered by the Insurance. As the application is

---

Box 20.2 *Services to be covered by Long-term Care Insurance*

Community care services
- Home care service (including domiciliary services)
- Visiting bathing service
- Visiting nurse service
- Visiting rehabilitation service
- Use of the services in a rehabilitation centre
- Physician's or dentist's call on
- Use of the services in a day care centre
- Short-term stay service
- Group home service for the demented
- Care services at the retirement home
- Rental service or purchase of technical aids
- Costs for improvement of housing

Institutional care service
- Care service in a nursing home
- Care service in a healthcare facilities for the elderly
- Care services in a long-term care geriatric hospital

approved, a care plan is made either by the insuree or by a licensed care-manager, although the insurer pays for a care plan made by a care manager. The care plan is made in accordance with the approved degree of care needs and there are six degrees of care needs. The care plan made by the insuree or a licensed care-manager is then presented to the insurer. The insurer pays the cost of services to the designated home care service agency according to these care plans presented prior to the start of services. In the case of community services, the insuree is required to pay the cost of meals and 10 per cent of the total cost of services.

20.47 THE NEW ADULT GUARDIANSHIP SYSTEM

The new Adult Guardianship system consists of the Guardianship, Curatorship and Help system. Previously, when someone was declared by the Family Court to be incompetent in the management of the property, he or she lost all legal capacity and a guardian was mandated to take over all the legal authority to make decisions on their behalf. Under the new Adult Guardianship system, even an incompetent person may keep the capacity to decide acts related to daily living for themselves.

Previously when someone was declared as quasi-incompetent, he or she partially lost all legal capacity. Under the new Curatorship System, he or she loses only the capacity for specified acts written in the Civil Code. The newly legislated Help System is for those who suffer from intellectual deterioration such as dementia as well as mental disability, and thereby lack a sufficient level of mental ability as a normal adult, but the level of incompetence is less than that of quasi-incompetence. For these persons, the Family Court may nominate a Helper in accordance with the application of a client, a spouse, a close relative or a public prosecutor, with the informed consent of the client. The Court may nominate more than one person including a legal person. A Guardian, a Curator or a Helper is obliged to give as much attention as possible so that the client can receive appropriate health and medical care, live in a decent dwelling, use a welfare institution and have adequate rehabilitation, although the Helper is only responsible for the management of the client's property and for the arrangements of and care service needed.

The most important innovation in the Adult Guardianship system is that anyone can nominate a guardian for oneself voluntarily while still mentally intact. 'The Law for Voluntary Nomination of Adult Guardian' was enacted by the Diet along with the revision of the Civil Code. Voluntary nomination is made in the form of a notarial deed and registered according to the 'Adult Guardianship Registration Act'. However, despite these improvements one serious drawback remains. Consent to medical examination and treatment can be done by neither Guardian nor Curator. A system that clarifies who legally consents regarding medical decisions for an incompetent subject needs to be developed.

REFERENCES

Arai M. (1999) *Adult Guardianship System in Aged Society*, revised edition (in Japanese). Tokyo, Yuhikaku

Maeda D. (2003) Social security, health care, and social services for the elderly in Japan. In: *Aging in Japan, 2003*. Tokyo, Japan Aging Research Center

Shimizu Y. (2003) Development of public long-term care insurance and future direction of elderly care. In *Aging in Japan 2003*. Tokyo, Japan Aging Research Center

Mexico

DAVID RESNIKOFF AND ALONSO RIESTRA

Latin America is a vast and heterogeneous region, approximately 10 times the size of Europe. It can be divided into four regions: North America, Central America, South America and the Caribbean. Languages spoken in Latin America are predominantly Spanish and Portuguese. Almost 512 million people live in Latin American countries, including Mexico, Central America, the Latin Caribbean and the Latin population of the USA (Encyclopaedia Britannica, 2003).

20.48 MEXICAN POPULATION

Mexico comprises 31 states and a federal district, which is the national seat of government (Alba, 1982). The 2000 census showed that 7.1 per cent of the population speak one of 68 indigenous languages (INEGI, 2000). In the case of the elderly it is often their only language. These languages are unrelated to each other and are widespread across the country.

Mexico is undergoing a demographic transition that will be complete by the year 2050. During this transition, changes in life expectancy, fecundity rate and migration will impact on the demographic structure resulting in progressive ageing of the population. Ageing is one of the most important risk factors for dementia. In industrialized countries it has been estimated that the prevalence of dementia of about 3 per cent for the 60–65-year-old population doubles every 5 years to reach about 50 per cent for the population older than 80 years. In Mexico from the year 2000 to 2050 the life expectancy of 74 years will increase up to 81.3 years (men 79, women 83.6). The probability of dying in the first year of life will decrease from 23/1000 to 5/1000 in the same time period. The fecundity rate will also fall from 2.11 children/woman in 2000 to 1.85 children/woman in 2050 and there is also an expected rise in the age of marriage and the age at the time of first childbirth. All these changes, including also migration factors, will result in an increase of the Mexican population from 100.6 million to 129 million inhabitants by the year 2050. In this same period the median age of the population will increase from 26.6 years to 42.7 years and the percentage of people of 60+ years old will also increase from 6.8 per cent to 28 per cent. On the other hand the economically productive population (15–59.8-year-olds) will remain relatively constant from 59.8 per cent in 2000 to 62.2 per cent in 2030 and 55.3 per cent in 2050 (INEGI, 2000). According to the analysed data in Mexico there were 6.8 million people 60 years old or older in 2000 and there will be 36 million people of this age group in 2050. The estimated number of people with dementia is likely to increase from approximately 980 000 people to 6.7 million in the same period; in other words in 2050 there will be as many demented people as adults older than 59 years are today. This numbers may be conservative considering that the estimated prevalence of dementia is taken from industrialized countries. Lower level of education, decreased access to health services and other factors that accompany poverty in the elderly might make these estimates larger in Mexico.

The health of the Mexican population is well below the minimum World Health Organization's (WHO) standards and more than 30 per cent of the population is malnourished (Campos Ortega, 1992); 10.6 million Mexicans are marginated from the rest of the population (CONAPO, 2003). The enormous population increase has been caused partly by a drop in the mortality rate, owing to both massive vaccination programmes and acute treatment for dehydration related to gastrointestinal infections, and partly by a very high birth rate. Although standards of health are gradually improving, central government has found it almost impossible to offer adequate health education and other social services (SSA, 1992).

Official unemployment figures are around 7.5 per cent (INEGI, 2000) but 40 per cent of the population work outside the formal employment sector in occupations such as windscreen washers at traffic lights and illegal street vendors. Since the 1994 economic crisis, there has also been a large increase in a well organized and still growing delinquency industry (gang robberies, automobile theft, kidnapping and drug trafficking). The majority of the population live between a state of survival and tremendous poverty. The extreme poor constitute 15 per cent of the population, 47 per cent live under the minimum level of decent living, and 36 per cent have no access to good medical services (SSA, 2000).

The majority of health-related problems have their origin in poverty, ignorance, malnutrition and a deficient healthcare infrastructure; in the 2000 general census it was estimated that 9.5 per cent of the population >15 years could not read and write (INEGI, 2000). In Mexico City this is aggravated by land, water and air pollution. Bearing in mind the pressure on public spending, government spending on programmes for the elderly have had a low priority. However, the elderly are high consumers of health resources. Up to 30 per cent of the beds in the public sector were occupied by the old in 1992 (Ruiz and Salvador, 1994) – an increasing tendency that places insurmountable pressure on the healthcare system. Recent figures show that in recent years the elderly occupancy of beds in the public sector has increased by 12 per cent in the last 8 years (SSA, 2000).

20.49 GENERAL STRUCTURE OF HEALTHCARE SERVICES

The Mexican healthcare system is a complicated network of different institutions, which offer service in all areas of care. Government-provided health care is organized into three levels as follows:

- *Primary care.* These services aim to solve 70–85 per cent of health problems. Their main objectives are the promotion of health, prevention of disease and detection of initial treatable or chronic conditions. They mainly constitute unsophisticated and low-budget health clinics, attended by family and general practitioners. Since the collapse of the Mexican economy in 1995, the government is redirecting resources to this level of care.
- *Secondary level.* The purpose of this level is to solve between 10 and 15 per cent of healthcare demands. It constitutes an organized network of hospitals and outpatient clinics with low-level trained doctors in different specialties. This level of care has been crippled owing to the budget deficits of overspending governments.
- *Tertiary care.* At this level, highly specialized centres treat the 3–5 per cent of the problems previously unresolved. Scientific investigation, research and education are major objectives (Resnikoff *et al.*, 1991).

The type of population served and supporting finance also define Mexico's healthcare institutions. Various groups of workers are catered for by occupational health schemes including those who work for the nationalized petroleum industry, and civil servants. There is a private sector, which accounts for 12 per cent of the medical facilities in the country and caters for 17 per cent of the population (SSA, 2003).

20.50 PSYCHIATRY

Historically, Mexico was a pioneer, ahead of other American countries in providing care for those who, during colonial times, were malnourished and wandered the streets. In 1566 the first psychiatric hospital of the Americas was founded in Mexico City. In the recent past, dependent mainly on charitable donations, these sorts of institutions have decayed and many have disappeared (Campillo and De la Fuente, 1976). In 1910 President Díaz inaugurated the building of a new national general asylum called 'La Castañeda'. During the next few decades several private institutions for the care of the mentally ill were built, and along with La Castañeda contributed to the development of psychiatry as a medical specialty. Between 1950 and 1960 the Health Ministry (Secretaría de Salubridad y Asistencia; SSA) established a network of 11 psychiatric institutions to substitute for the failing general asylum. Unfortunately, appropriate technical and economic resources were not made available for their maintenance and, over a period of several years of poverty and neglect, they suffered severe deterioration. Other institutions to emerge from the Mexico City Council (DDF) and hospitals belonging to the workers unions (IMSS) have suffered the same fate. Only two hospitals in the public sector have been able to overcome some of these problems and they have played an important role in the teaching of psychiatry (De la Fuente, 1982). In one of these institutions, the Fray Bernardino Hospital in Mexico City, the country's first psychogeriatric unit was created 4 years ago with 20 short-term beds for the assessment and initial treatment of psychiatric disorders (including dementia) in the elderly.

In 1991 the SSA mental health services comprised 17 hospital units with a total of 5200 beds and 24 mental health clinics. Other public and private institutions provide 3300 more beds. Of the total number of psychiatric beds, 57 per cent are in SSA hospitals, 24 per cent are in other government hospitals and 19 per cent are run privately (Resnikoff *et al.*, 1991); 60 per cent of the psychiatric beds (1 for every 5453 inhabitants) are located in the Mexico City area, while in central and south-eastern regions the figure is 1 bed for every 55 315 and 44 115 inhabitants respectively (Pucheu, 1984).

Unfortunately, recent data are unavailable; however, many public institutions catering for the mentally ill have disappeared owing to the economical pressures on the governmental budget.

Personnel specializing in the field of mental health (doctors, psychologists, nurses, occupational therapists and social workers) are scarce and badly distributed. The WHO recommends a minimum of five psychiatrists for every 100 000 inhabitants. In Mexico we calculate 3.1 psychiatrists for every 100 000. Recent figures from the national psychiatric Council state that there are 2800 trained psychiatrists, but only 200 are certified. In 1985 there were 1108 practising psychiatrists in Mexico; 85 practised child psychiatry and 170 were psychoanalysts. The rest were a mixed bag of general psychiatrists. Of these 7 per cent dedicated the whole of their time working in public institutions, 23 per cent solely to private practice and 63 per cent combined both activities. Only 10 per cent of all psychiatrists have carried out any documented scientific investigation and 20 per cent participate in teaching activities (De la Fuente *et al.*, 1988). With regard to other workers in the mental health field, the deficit is even more acute. Notwithstanding an intensive programme of training, there are only 126 social workers in the field of mental health and 35 nurses with formal training in the management of psychiatric patients.

20.51 PSYCHOGERIATRICS AND GERIATRICS

In Mexico as a whole there are only eight trained psychogeriatricians and a handful of psychiatrists and neurologists committed to treating the aged. In other words less than 1 per cent of trained psychiatrist dedicate their practice to old age. In Mexico City there is the aforementioned psychogeriatric inpatient unit at the Fray Bernardino Hospital, with 20 beds, and three informal units at private hospitals amounting to a total of 550 beds for a population of 20 million. Teaching of psychogeriatrics is poor and limited to three main programmes, and there has not been an improvement in this area in the last 5 years:

- Diploma in Psychogeriatrics – training in mental health of the aged for mental health workers;
- psychogeriatrics as a subject for general psychiatrists in training in two city hospitals comprising 10 sessions of 2 hours each and no practical placement;
- a 2-year course in psychogeriatrics run by the national university, that also falls down on clinical training and experience.

In the central state of Jalisco there is a small psychogeriatric unit run privately by one of the few trained psychogeriatricians, which involves some teaching of trainees.

Most of the specific knowledge acquired by psychiatrists in the treatment of the elderly therefore comes from experience gathered during general psychiatric training – there is little formal training. Very recently the Ministry of Health has acknowledged the lack of resources for old age psychiatry and for the first time there is to be serious planning concerning the future of mental health caring for the elderly.

The field of geriatric medicine is better organized with a long-standing tradition in teaching and training. The 400 geriatricians distributed throughout the main cities have traditionally covered the shortfall in services for the elderly mentally ill.

20.52 SERVICES FOR DEMENTIA

It is clear that services for dementia are scarce in Mexico, and are mainly located at the tertiary level of the healthcare system, which caters for the unresolved problems or those who have slipped through the previous levels of care. Only a minority of patients with dementia are seen and treated by health professionals. At this level, diagnosis and outpatient care are priorities, with most patients being cared for at home or in unregulated nursing homes. There are eight specialized centres in Mexico City for assessment, diagnosis and follow up of patients with dementia. Each centre works individually with few guidelines for diagnosis and treatment strategies. Five of these centres are part of the IMSS system and three are private centres; four are within geriatric areas of general hospitals and one belongs to a neurological institute. In the private sector three memory clinics cater for patients with dementia. All centres lack both medical and nursing care at community level and there is little input from social services. Respite care and crisis intervention services are virtually non-existent. The rest of the country has no specialized care except for simple small units for assessment of patients in the private sector.

In real terms private family doctors treat patients diagnosed with dementia at home or in private nursing homes by professionals with little training or understanding of the problem.

20.53 DEMENTIA AND THE COMMUNITY

There are two national non-profit organizations for patients with dementia and their families. the Asociación Médica de Alzheimer y enfermedades similares (AMAES) was founded by relatives of patients with dementia in 1988, affiliated to Alzheimer's Disease International (ADI) and hosted the ADI international conference in 1989. The objectives of AMAES are:

- family counselling and support;
- promotion of and assistance of support groups around the country (20 exist);
- education of the public;
- training for primary and secondary carers;
- promotion of clinical and epidemiological investigation;
- leadership in public policy (AMAES, 1988).

Fondo de Apoyo para la Enfermedad de Alzheimer (FAEA) was initially part of AMAES. Subsequently it has concentrated on the specific objective of creating respite through day care centres around the country. At present it manages two day care centres for patients with dementia capable of handling 20 patients each. One is located in Mexico City and the other in the city of Queretaro. The centres are privately administered and non-profit making (FAEA, 1992).

20.53.1 The Mexican national plan for dementias

The demographic explosion has many implications both for today and the future, creating a huge demand on education, employment and health services, especially for the under-privileged and particularly for our ageing population.

The Mexican family has survived as a powerful and conservative institution, and it is very important for political stability. Traditions and moral and religious values are passed on through the family. The extended family gives a supportive structure to the young and to the old. Nevertheless, a number of factors have greatly affected the familial structure in recent years. These include:

* demographic changes;
* migration to urban areas;
* illegal migration to the USA;
* westernization;
* diminished religious influence.

Taking all these factors into account, and with the recent changes in the political structure, with a new ruling party after 70 years without any political change, the scenario is changing towards a more humane and politically sound system that will take into account the needs and future demands of Mexican society.

In the year 2001, the Ministry of Health started to develop a National Plan of Health. Within its core, the mental health of the citizens was contemplated and it became clear that as a national priority the health of the elderly, and particularly the need to develop public policy related to the dementing illnesses, was urgently needed.

A National Advisory team that could promote a plan for tackling this problem was created. I (first author) was asked to develop the team structure and within 6 months produced with my six-member team a National Plan for Alzheimer Disease and Related Disorders that could be working within the next year.

This is not the time or place to state our plan; however, let me put forward the four main objectives that we are trying to achieve.

20.53.1.1 SERVICE DELIVERY

This refers to all the measures needed to promote quality and presence in our services, especially at primary care level promoting integral management of patients with intellectual decline and for their families.

We need to create services for each community for prevention, early diagnosis, treatment, rehabilitation and respite, basically at primary care level with support of secondary units for more precise diagnosis and cases with special needs. At the same time, there is an urgent need to promote social services to assist the families in need, with help and feedback from non-governmental agencies like Alzheimer support groups and associations.

20.53.1.2 HEALTH EDUCATION

Health education within the programme includes all aspects related to the improvement of health preventative measures when applicable to the dementing illnesses. They include means to tackle poverty, social inequality and education. In the specific area of education *per se* the following are clear objectives of the plan:

* to promote changes in the curriculum in the educational programmes, which would include dementias in the Medical Faculties and postgraduate training programmes in Medicine, plus programme changes in the psychology, nursing and social workers training programmes;
* to promote the development of a Diploma in Intellectual Decline and Dementias as a formal 2-year course for medical and paramedical personnel;
* to provide behavioural and psychological signs and symptoms of dementia (BPSD) training packages for nurses, primary care physicians and families;
* to initiate public awareness programmes.

For the educational programmes we are attempting to use novel educational systems via the internet and educational packages to promote service delivery in remote areas of Mexico.

20.53.1.3 RESEARCH

Our programme is aware that without formal research no public policy can be established. With very limited resources in our country, we must find the means to optimize the economic resources and establish guidelines for those specific areas urgently needed to support policy changes in the area of the dementing disorders.

20.53.1.4 LEGISLATION

To be able to consolidate the National Plan for Dementias, we should take into consideration the changes needed to promote both patients' and health providers' rights.

We are aware that the plan we have produced has to have short- and long-term objectives and we know that results will not be seen for some years. One major problem is clouding the whole success of this enterprise: lack of resources and bureaucracy can limit success.

20.54 THE INTERNATIONAL PSYCHOGERIATRIC ASSOCIATION'S (IPA) LATIN AMERICAN INITIATIVE

The elderly population of Latin America is projected to increase dramatically over the next 20 years (Liviv-Bacci, 1995), and with this in mind the IPA has launched an initiative to promote the development of psychogeriatric services in this area (Resnikoff, 1997). Of a worldwide IPA membership of 1112 in 1998 only 6.11 per cent were Latin American professionals even though the total population of Latin America is greater than that of Europe and the USA combined.

Latin American countries are beginning to recognize the impact of an ageing population on their cultures and societies. This in turn will dramatically affect policy-making and general health service delivery in countries where old age has traditionally been the responsibility of extended family networks. Owing to rapid changes in the economy of the region and resultant social restructuring, traditional family values and support systems are collapsing and extended families are often no longer capable of caring for elderly relatives, leading to a demand for social intervention policies.

The IPA'S Latin American Initiative has three primary concerns:

- *Policy*. The IPA is concerned with giving assistance to healthcare professionals in the area of education of policy-makers, with the aim of a healthy approach to an ageing population. The IPA has active members who have tackled similar problems in their respective countries and who are willing to share their experiences with Latin American countries.
- *Education*. Education in geriatric and psychogeriatrics is still underdeveloped in this part of the world. The IPA will advise and assist on general principles of developing educational programmes.
- *Communication*. The flow of information in and out of Latin American countries, between them and with other nations is developing at a very slow rate. The IPA intends to promote a better system of information sharing (Resnikoff, 1997).

REFERENCES

Alba F. (1982) *The Population of Mexico: Trends, Issues and Policies.* Mexico, Transaction Press

AMAES. (1988) *Establecimiento legal de la Asociación Mexicana de Alzheimer (Bylaws).* Mexico, AMAES

Campillo C and De la Fuente R. (1976) La psiquiatría en México: una perspectiva histórica. *Mexico DF, Gaceta Médica de México* 11: 3

Campos Ortega S. (1992) Análisis demográfico de la morbilidad en México. Mexico DF, El Colegio de México

CONAPO (Consejo Nacional de Población). (2003) *Statistical Analysis of the Mexican Population.* Mexico, CONAPO

De la Fuente R. (1982) Acerca de la Salud Mental en México. *Salud Mental* 5: 22–31

De la Fuente R, Diaz Martinez A, Fouillouz C. (1988) La formación de psiquiatras en la República Mexicana. *Salud Mental* 11: 3–7

Encyclopaedia Britannica. CD-Rom, 2003

FAEA. (1992) *Establecimiento legal del Fondo de Apoyo para la enfermedad de Alzheimer. (Bylaws).* Mexico, FAEA

INEGI (Instituto Nacional de Estadística, Geografía e información). (2000) *Análisis de la Población y Proyecciones.* Mexico, INEGI

Liviv-Bacci R. (1995) Notas sobre la transición demográfica en Europa y America Latina. *Memorias de la IV Conferencia Latinoamericana de Población.* México, INEGI 1, pp. 13–28

Pucheu C. (1984) *Panorama actual de la psiquiatría y la Salud mental en México. Cuadernos de Salud mental 7.* Mexico, UNAM Publishers

Resnikoff D. (1997) *Latin-American Initiative. Report to the International Psychogeriatric Board of Directors.* Jerusalem

Resnikoff R, Pustilnik S, Resnikoff D. (1991) Mexico: struggling for a better future. In: L Appleby and R Araya (eds), *Mental Health in the Global Village.* London, Royal College of Psychiatrists

Ruiz L and Salvador A. (1994) *El cambio estructural de la Salud Pública en México, 29.* Mexico, SSA

SSA (Secretaría de Salud). (1992) *Encuesta Nacional de Salud.* Mexico, SSA

SSA (Secretaría de Salud). (2000) *Encuesta Nacional de Salud.* Mexico, SSA

SSA (Secretaría de Salud). (2003) *Encuesta Nacional de Salud.* Mexico, SSA

Netherlands

THEA J HEEREN

In the Netherlands the development of specific services for people with dementia started in the 1950s with the setting up of Psychogeriatric Nursing Homes. There were both quantitative and qualitative reasons: the shortage of beds in the general psychiatric hospitals and the feeling that people suffering from dementia needed specialized care (Robben, 2002).

In the 50 years that followed, the number of beds for people with dementia in nursing homes has grown to 30 813 in 2003. The nursing homes take care of patients with severe dementia for whom care at home or other residential care facilities is no longer possible. However, only 18 per cent of people with dementia reside in a nursing home (Health Council, 2002) and therefore services have been established to meet the needs of those living on their own with mild or moderate dementia. The estimated growth of the number of elderly with dementia underlines the necessity of adequate services. Whereas in the year 2000 it was estimated that 1 in 93 people in the Netherlands was demented, this figure will be 1 in 81 in 2010, 1 in 71 in 2020 and 1 in 44 in 2050 (Health Council, 2002)

In this chapter an overview of services available in the Netherlands will be given. At the moment not all services exist in every healthcare region; the Dutch Government has asked the Netherlands Institute for Care and Welfare to develop a National Dementia Care Programme giving guidelines with regard to services that should minimally be available in each healthcare region.

20.55 DIAGNOSIS AND TREATMENT

20.55.1 General practitioners

In the Netherlands the general practitioner (GP) diagnoses the majority of people with dementia. The main reasons for referral to a specialist service are (The Dutch College of General Practitioners [NHG], 1998):

- dementia with an indication for neuroimaging (suspicion of tumour, infarcts etc.)
- rapid progressive dementia
- young age (<65)
- uncharacteristic features or course, and doubt about diagnosis
- non-cognitive symptoms that need specialist treatment
- indication for treatment with cholinesterase-inhibitors.

20.55.2 Memory clinics; multidisciplinary dementia team

Specialist services for diagnosis and treatment of dementia have in common that they work with a multidisciplinary team consisting of medical specialists, (neuro)psychologists and specialized nurses. Regional differences exist in the location of the service and the medical department from which it originates. Memory clinics usually are part of the general (or university) hospital, organized either by the department of neurology, geriatrics or psychiatry. Multidisciplinary dementia teams generally are based in community mental healthcare centres or in the general psychiatric hospital. The memory clinics usually focus more on a disease-related diagnostic work-up, whereas the mental healthcare-based teams lay more emphasis on needs assessment, case management and treatment of non-cognitive and behavioural disturbances.

20.56 CARE

20.56.1 Ambulatory

The GP can ask for support from home care (for both nursing and household tasks). When more support is needed, day care, usually in either a residential home or a nursing home, can be obtained, including transportation to and from the day care facility. Also night care and care during a holiday by the caregiver can be arranged. Support for the family caregiver is available through meetings with other caregivers organized by either the regional community mental healthcare centres or by the Dutch Alzheimer Foundation. Forms of integrated support (in which both patient and relative participate) are 'the Alzheimer cafe' (available in more than 50 cities in the Netherlands) (Miesen, 2002) and support programmes where healthcare professionals attend to both the needs of the patients and their caregivers (called 'meeting centres') (Droes, 2000).

20.56.2 Residential

When it is no longer feasible to take care of a patient with dementia in the home, the GP and/or the family will request long-term care. As mentioned before, long-term care is organized in psychogeriatric nursing homes, where a specialized Nursing Physician is responsible for the care of the patients. A recent development is the establishment of small-scale housing for people with dementia. Small-scale housing consists of separate units and of small units within a larger context (nursing home, residential care home or other type of residential care) where 8–12 persons live together. Small-scale units give a better overview, which is important for patients with dementia, allowing them to retain some degree of control over their environment. Furthermore, if a limited number of permanent carers are linked to small groups of patients, this has the benefit of promoting the individualization of care. The small-scale approach also offers the opportunity of forming groups of people who are better suited to one another in terms of background, interests or disease stage. The main problem at the moment, however, is a shortage of places both in large and small scale nursing homes.

20.57 COOPERATION AND COORDINATION

The basic principle of the current policy in the Netherlands is 'tailored care': care on the basis of a sound personal needs assessment. Dementia patients often require various types of care, treatment and counselling, delivered either simultaneously or in sequence. Many informal and professional carers, as well as various organizations, are involved in this. Integration and coherence are needed for a good quality of care. The above mentioned National Dementia Care Programme will have to provide a framework for coordination of the care delivered by many different organizations, institutions and disciplines, including GPs. High expectations are placed upon the concept of case management, in order to promote the cohesion of care.

REFERENCES

Robben PBM. (2002) *Kwartet voor ouderen*. Houten, Bohn Stafleu Van Loghum

Droes RM, Breebaart E, Ettema TP, van Tilburg W, Mellenbergh GJ. (2000) Effect of integrated family support versus day care only on behavior and mood of patients with dementia. *International Psychogeriatrics* **12**: 99–115

Dutch College of General Practitioners (NHG). (1998) *Practice Guideline Dementia*. (http://nhg.artsennet.nl)

Health Council of the Netherlands. (2002) *Dementia*. The Hague, Health Council of the Netherlands, publication no. 2002/04E. (http://gr.nl)

Miesen B. (2002) *Het Alzheimer Café. Vragen, antwoorden, gevoelens en ervaringen van mensen die te maken hebben met dementie*. Lifetime, Kosmos/Z and K Uitgevers Bv

New Zealand

PAMELA S MELDING

*E ngā iwi, e ngā reo, e ngā karangatanga maha o ngā hau e whā –
tenei te mihi atu ki a koutou kātoa. Tēnā koutou, tēnā koutou,
tēnā koutou kātoa.* [To all people, all voices, all the many relations from the four winds, greetings to you all] (Māori Greeting)

20.58 EPIDEMIOLOGY

New Zealand is an independent bicultural nation of 4 million
people living in a group of South Pacific Islands covering an
area of 268 000 square kilometres, slightly greater than the
United Kingdom. Much of New Zealand is rural and the
majority of the population is concentrated in the cities of
Auckland, Hamilton, and Wellington in the North,
Christchurch, and Dunedin in the South. One-third of New
Zealanders live in the Auckland region alone. Currently, about
11 per cent of the population is over 65 years but in common
with the worldwide trend of population ageing this figure is
expected to rise to over 18 per cent by 2030. In New Zealand,
about 3500 people die annually of various forms of dementia.
The only survey on dementia to date (Campbell *et al.*, 1983)
estimated 7.7 per cent of people over 65 years had dementia.
In present day terms this suggests about 30 000–35 000 older
New Zealanders have dementia and require services and care.

20.59 ASSESSMENT FOR DEMENTIA

For the majority of people with dementia, access to services is
through geriatric or geriatric psychiatry teams via primary
care. Most base hospitals have geriatric services, but geriatric
psychiatry services are confined to the more populated centres.
While both specialties accept patients with dementia, the
geriatric psychiatry teams assess and manage patients with
the more difficult or complex behavioural, psychological
symptoms of dementia (BPSD), patients for whom the diagnosis is indeterminate, need neuropsychiatric evaluation, or
their dementia is complicated by a pre-existing psychiatric
disorder. About 25–50 per cent of a geriatric psychiatry
team's workload is with cognitively impaired or demented
older people. Most of these demented patients have complications of BPSD, delirium or comorbid depression (Melding
and Osman, 2000). In most major centres, geriatric and geriatric psychiatry teams work closely together either as conjoined or co-located services with cross-referral systems.

Geriatric and geriatric psychiatry services use a commu-
nity/outreach-based model of assessment and treatment.
Multidisciplinary community teams are the norm for geriatric
psychiatry and are becoming more common in geriatrics
also. One or more members of a geriatric or geriatric psychiatry multidisciplinary team will usually assess a patient with
possible dementia in their place of residence and if necessary,
cross-refer for further assessment or admit to inpatient
assessment treatment and rehabilitation (ATR) services (the
term ATR is used for both disciplines). Home assessment is
preferred as this gives the opportunity to assess the home situation and family burden of care. Day clinic services are in
short supply with one-third of geriatric and over one-half of
geriatric psychiatry services lacking such facilities. Only a few
larger geriatric psychiatry services can offer a memory clinic.
In the hinterland of the major cities and towns are many
small rural towns and a higher proportion of older people
live in these outlying areas (20 per cent as opposed to urban
15 per cent). Service delivery and provision of facilities for
people with dementia in these areas are limited and provision is often by outreach clinics to these areas (national range
2–6 clinics per service) from the base hospital.

20.60 CARE FOR PEOPLE WITH DEMENTIA

20.60.1 Care in the home

The majority of people with early stages of dementia and less significant functional impairment (70–80 per cent) usually are cared for in their own homes, by family caregivers (National Health Committee, ADARDS, 1997; Richards 2001). Current health policy advocates 'ageing in place' (Howden-Chapman *et al.*, 1999) as the preferred option. Certainly, the majority of patients prefer to continue in their own homes for as long as possible and this option is cheaper than providing government-subsidized residential care. To enable this policy, New Zealand has a system of Need Assessment Service Coordinators (NASC), attached to all older people's services, who design packages of home support for patients with early dementia (meals on wheels, home assistance, district nursing, etc.) When applicable, they arrange placement in a rest home or private hospital. A patient can be admitted to a rest home, state funded, for up to 28 days annually for respite. The care may be taken flexibly, a day, a week or *en bloc* to allow the hardworking family caregivers a break or perhaps a holiday. At the present time, the total number and range of services available through NASC varies throughout the country, but the recent adoption of the *Best Practice, Evidenced Based Guideline: Assessment Process for Older People* (New Zealand Guidelines Group, 2003) and the proposed use of a common assessment tool should, in the next few years, make access to home care services more equitable, nationwide.

As dementia progresses, patients will often need more specialist or greater levels of care than NASC can provide in the home environment. The most common reasons for relatives to relinquish care to institutions are: mental confusion, particularly where agitated or disruptive behaviour occurs, or frequent nocturnal disturbance, together with urinary incontinence (Richmond *et al.*, 1995).

20.60.2 Hospital care

Traditionally, older people with advanced dementia were cared for in geriatric wards in public hospitals. In the 1960s and 1970s, government policy of that time provided means-tested subsidies for patients requiring rest home or private hospital care, who were occupying public hospital beds. This policy encouraged mushrooming development of rest homes and private hospitals by the 'not for profit religious and welfare' sector and 'for profit' private operators. Over the next 25 years, the policy had the effect of devolving geriatric patients from public hospital wards to the private sector. Currently, very few long-stay beds exist within the public hospital system, and the few that remain are only on the West Coast and Northland, large rural areas with few facilities other than the base hospital. At the present time, contracted to the Ministry of Health (subsidised beds) are 21 411 rest home plus 9509 private hospital beds (Ministry of Health, 2002). These establishments are graded into levels of care with the highest levels being for those most disabled. Eighty per cent of residents are over 75 years (MOH, 2002), of whom well over half have dementia (NZ Department of Statistics) as their main disability. In addition, there are 2315 specific beds for people with behavioural disturbance and dementia, taking about 7–8 per cent of patients with dementia who need care that is more specialized. These special dementia units attract a higher subsidy and patient entry to them is only through the geriatric psychiatry teams, who also provide consultation and liaison services to these units and indeed to the residential sector.

20.60.3 Non-Governmental Organizations (NGOs)

NGOs provide many services for people with dementia. A major contributor of services is the Alzheimer Association, which has branches in most areas of the country. The local Alzheimer societies provide help and support to family members and particularly to those caring for relatives at home. They often provide short educational courses for caregivers on managing a demented relative at home and their field workers provide caregiver support. Age Concern is another major NGO that provides advocacy and support services. Age Concern also plays a key role in health promotion (Age Concern, 1999), organizing 'elder abuse' local teams and providing welfare guardianship services for people without kin. Quite a few rest homes also provide day care services as well as respite care for people with dementia, services not usually available in the public sector.

20.61 MĀORI ISSUES

The constitutional basis, legislature and ethos of New Zealand is the country's founding document, *The Treaty of Waitangi*, which in 1840 protected the 'rights' of the *tangata whenua* (lit. 'The people of the land'), the indigenous Māori, while granting sovereignty of the Islands to the British Crown. Today, 15 per cent of New Zealand's population is Māori. The Treaty is a living document and an important current 'right' to be protected is health. Another is the special status of Māori elders amongst their communities. *Kaumāmuā* (male elder) status is associated with the cultural practices of older age, wisdom, experience and knowledge of the culture, and they are the traditional leaders of the Māori people.

Despite improvements over the last few decades, there are still marked disparities between Māori health and life expectancy when compared with the European population of New Zealand. Māori have been prone to vascular disease, stroke, renal disease, cancer, respiratory disease and diabetes, which result in untimely deaths, early onset ageing and premature dementia, particularly cerebrovascular dementia.

Ill health commences approximately 5 years earlier than in other New Zealanders and life expectancy of Māori males is 10 years less and for females 8 years less than for New Zealanders as a whole (NZ Department of Statistics). Debate is ongoing as to whether the legal definition of 'elderly' for Māori on which eligibility for national superannuation is determined should be a lower age than for other New Zealanders (Māaka, 1993). Māori ill health, poor life expectancy and the diminishing number of kaumātua as a result are major health priorities for New Zealand.

Ability to provide assessment, treatment and placement options for older Māori with dementia that are also culturally appropriate is a major challenge for all services. Many teams have limited access to cultural advisors and there is a major shortage of Māori professional staff within the teams. Māori concepts of health are more holistic than those espoused by their European treaty partners. For Māori, and particularly older Māori, health has a framework of taha tinana (physical health), taha hinengaro (emotional and psychological), taha whānau (health family), and taha wairua (spiritual health) (Durie, 1998). This latter dimension involves concepts of inter-connectedness with their papatūānuku (lit. 'Mother Earth', i.e. traditional lands and landscape). Older Māori are much more likely to be living close to their ancestral Maraes (traditional meeting places) in provincial or rural areas that often lack geriatric services. Traditionally, Māori culture is rooted in the whānau (extended family) in contrast to the Western ethos of personal autonomy; their individualism is subsumed within the whānau so that, for Māori, all matters relating to a patient's health need discussing with the family. The whānau and not the individual make the key decisions.

Not only are Māori prone to dementia at an earlier age, but services for Māori older people and elders are lacking in traditional Māori areas, and attempts at residential placement of patients with dementia far away from the whānau contradicts the Māori framework of health and cause more distress. In common with most other ethnic groups, the older Māori population is increasing and these issues are increasing in significance for a New Zealand health service delivery.

The New Zealand Government has recently begun to take considerable interest in older people's health. The ageing of the population, the 'baby boom' generation reaching retirement in the next 10 or 20 years, and the increases in cost of disability support for older people have pressed the urgent need for a national Strategy for the Health of Older People (Minister for Disability Issues, 2002). The guiding principles are person- (and their family) centred care, personal choice in options for care, together with provision of a range of inpatient, community geriatric and geriatric psychiatry services, residential assessment, treatment and rehabilitation, and residential care to be available for patients in each District Health Area, nationwide. Other requirements include administrative processes that enable integrated services, are needs based, are responsive and flexible to changing patient needs, are based on best practice, supported by research and, of course, affordable to the individual and state. It remains to be seen if the individual District Health Boards can achieve this utopian vision by the due date of 2010.

New Zealand has one of the highest rates of subsidized institutionalization for older people in the world with over 6 per cent of total public health expenditure and 25 per cent of all health expenditure for the over-65s funding residential care subsidies for older people, the majority of whom have dementia. To control burgeoning expenditure, residential services have to contract with the Ministry of Health through their local District Health Authorities, who require measurable quality criteria, including provisions for training of staff, staffing levels, medication practices and restraint minimization, all of which are subject to auditing and monitoring of facilities.

A particularly thorny issue is lack of provision of medications for the treatment of dementia. The anticholinesterase inhibitor drugs are licensed for use and therefore available but not subsidized, as the funding body believes that there is insufficient evidence of their efficacy to make them freely available. Therefore, patients have to pay the full cost of these drugs. This is seen by older persons' advocacy groups as inequitable and unfair, as many elderly patients are not able to afford them. For clinicians, inability to provide these drugs at reasonable cost for those who might benefit is extremely frustrating.

Whilst there will always be challenges to overcome, one strength of dementia care in New Zealand are that there is good cooperation between geriatrics and geriatric psychiatry. There is a clear national strategy and the policy direction is towards conjoined services nationwide by 2010 to ensure the 'continuum of care'. The strength is that there is a well-developed residential sector when patients need higher levels of care and generally, the residential, community, advocacy organizations and public arms of care are happy to work with each other for the betterment of the patients. There is political will to improve dementia care for elderly people and there is clinical will to develop the flexible community support programmes desired by patients and their families.

REFERENCES

Age Concern. (1999) Ageing is Living. An educational and training resource to prepare for positive ageing. Wellington, Age Concern

Campbell AJ, McCosh LM, Reinken J, Allen BC. (1983) Dementia in old age and the need for services. Age and Ageing 12: 11–16

Durie M. (1998) Whaiora, Maori Health Development. Auckland, Oxford University Press

Howden-Chapman P, Signal L, Crane J. (1999) Housing and Health in older people: ageing in place. Social Policy Journal of New Zealand 13: 14–30

Māaka R. (1993) Te Ao o te Pakeketanga: The world of the aged. In: P Koopman-Boyden (ed.), New Zealand's Ageing Society: The Implications. Wellington, Daphne Brasell, pp. 213–254

Melding PS and Osman N. (2000) The view from the bottom of the cliff. Old age psychiatry services in the patients and the resources. New Zealand Medical Journal 113:439–442

Minister of Disability Issues. (2002) *The Health of Older People Strategy. Health Sector Action to 2010 to support Positive Ageing.* Wellington, Ministry of Health

Ministry of Health. (2002) *Health of Older People in New Zealand. A Statistical Reference.* Wellington, Ministry of Health

Minister for Senior Citizens. (2001) *The New Zealand Positive Ageing Strategy.* Wellington: Ministry of Health

National Health Committee, ADARDS. (1997) *Guidelines for the support and management of people with dementia.* Wellington, Ministry of Health

New Zealand Guidelines Group. (2003) *Best Practice Evidenced Based Guideline, Assessment Processes for Older People.* Wellington, Ministry of Health

Richards J. (2001) Dementia: The privilege of caring. *New Zealand Family Physician* **28**: 19–21

Richmond D, Baskett J, Bonita R, Melding P. (1995) *Care of Older People in New Zealand.* Wellington, New Zealand Government Press

Nordic countries

KIRSTEN ABELSKOV

'Services are based on local culture, politics, skills and education of the staff who provide the service.' This was one of the main conclusions of a symposium on Service Delivery at the 11th IPA (International Psychogeriatric Association) Chicago Congress 2003 (IPA, www.IPA-online.org).

20.62 LOCAL CULTURE AND DEMOGRAPHIC DATA

The Nordic countries Iceland, Finland, Sweden, Norway and Denmark to some extent have a common Scandinavian model of the service delivered to older people. The Scandinavian model means that nearly all education, hospital treatment, social support and services to the elderly are free and paid through taxation. In Finland 25 per cent of the social costs are paid privately. The social expenditure in the Nordic countries ranges from 5.0–11.3 per cent of Gross Domestic Product. (GDP, Nordic Council of Ministers, 2003) (Table 20.5). It is striking that Denmark has the lowest life expectancy for men (74.6 years) and women (79.2 years) and has the highest expenses per elderly, while Iceland has the lowest expenses and the highest life expectancy for both men (78.5 years) and women (82.1 years). However, this might in part reflect differences in statistical estimates between the countries.

The burden of the elderly differs between countries. The demographic data in Table 20.6 shows that the percentage of the population who are over 65 varies from 11.6 (Iceland) to 17.2 (Sweden). In some counties in Sweden, more than 35 per cent of the population is over 65 (www.nordregio.se/population). Norway has the highest rate of nursing home facilities, Finland has the lowest. It is difficult to compare the resources for the elderly in the five countries as different admission criteria are used for nursing home places, sheltered nursing facilities and special apartments etc. Only Norway and Denmark have special statistics (*Statistical Yearbook*, 2003).

In Denmark, no new nursing homes have been established for the last 15 years and 15000 nursing home places have been replaced with two-room flats, which may be unsuitable for people with dementia.

All Nordic countries have psychogeriatric services, but not in all counties within those countries.

The Municipals are responsible for the services for older people, and as nursing home places are reduced, home service in the Municipals has increased. In the middle of the 1980s a saying became popular among the local authorities: 'Stay as long as possible in your own home'. Nursing home places were reduced and a new development began in a communal nursing system.

All countries have day facilities and different ways of providing help in the patients' own homes. Personal care, meals on wheels, administration of medication in special boxes daily and weekly, cleaning help and help in the garden are some of the possibilities. There are also day care centres.

Table 20.5 *Social expenditure in the Nordic countries*

Social expenditure	Iceland	Finland	Sweden	Norway	Denmark
Per cent of GDP	5.5	8.1	11.3	7.4	10.9
Euro (millions, 2001)	412.8	10 156.7	23 885.1	11 108	15 578.5

Table 20.6   *Demographic and old age care place data of Nordic countries*

	Iceland	Finland	Sweden	Norway	Denmark
Population (in millions)	0.29	5.19	8.90	4.55	5.38
(1) and (2)		0.3			0.1
65+ population per 1000	33.8	787.3	1532.1	673.5	798.4
Institutions or Serving Houses (2001)	3073	54 881	127 124	72 219	63 037
Nursing Home Places				36 000	26 037
Protected dwellings				8000	3926
Receiving home help (2001)	6334	84 210	121 741	94 882	173 370

1 Aaland Islands (Finland)
2 Faroe Islands and Greenland (Denmark)

Table 20.7   *Acts that govern the following situations*

	Social service	Public health	Patients rights	Old age housing	Legal guardianship	Psychiatry
Denmark	+	+	+	+	+	+
Norway	+	+	+		+	+
Finland	+	+	+		+	+
Sweden	+	+	+	+		+
Iceland	+	+	+	+	+	

Most of the Nordic countries provide reduced fares for transportation on buses and trains, and one municipal has provided a free holiday tour to southern Europe.

Sweden has, from late in the 1970s established 'housing and living' facilities, a house for 6–8 people with dementia and full-time staff, who try to make the day as natural as possible instead of an ordinary nursing home placement. This has become more fashionable in recent years in the Nordic countries.

In 2002, the municipal staff in Denmark had risen to 129 930, and the number of people over 65 receiving help from the community nursing system stood at 324 661. Forty-one per cent of 65+-year-old Danish people get help in their own home, some of these for 24 hours (*Statistical Yearbook*, 2003).

20.63 LAWS

The laws in Finland point out that the client must be treated so that the dignity of the elderly is preserved and that his or her convictions and privacy are respected (Vaarama *et al.*, 2001). The Danish laws, especially the Social Services Act (www.sm.dk/english/Legislation/Act) emphasize patients' integrity and autonomy. The conflict between autonomy and helplessness may lead to loss of dignity, care desertion and, in the extreme situation, senile squalor. After the first Social Services Act (2000), this conflict has left nursing staff with an ethical dilemma – tension between respect for the elderly person's autonomy and need of care.

The second Social Service Act (2003) has reduced some of the negative effects, but it still highlights the autonomy of the patient and care is still perceived, in some way, as paternalistic.

All the Nordic countries have laws concerning mental health and social service, all have a policy of patients' rights and most have legal guardianship regulations (Table 20.7).

20.64 EDUCATION

The staff in the municipal home nursing system are 'Health and Social' helpers with 14 months of basic training, 'Health and Social' assistants with 3 years (www.sosu.dk – English version not available) in basic training and nurses have 3 1/2 years training. (www.sygeplejerskeuddannelsen.dk – English version available).

20.65 CONCLUSION

Services for the care of older people in the Nordic Countries is, in most cases, functioning well, but legislation does not cover but complicates the lives of 5–10 per cent of the most disabled demented elderly.

REFERENCES

Nordic Statistical Yearbook (2003) Copenhagen, Nordic Council of Ministers

Statistical Yearbook (Statisk årbog) Denmark 2003

Vaarama M, Luomahaara J, Peiponen A, Voutilainen P. (2001) *The Whole Municipality Working Together With Old People. Perspectives on development of elderly people's independent living care and services.* Helsinki, National Research and Development Centre for Welfare and Health (STAKES)

Romania

NICOLETA TĂTARU

In Romania, around 12 per cent of the population are over the age of 65 years. The increased prevalence of mental health problems in the elderly requires different approaches to the development of the old age psychiatry.

20.66 WHAT DO WE EXPECT FROM OLD AGE PSYCHIATRY?

The most developed countries have policies, programmes and facilities to address mental health problems associated with the ageing of their populations. Because developing countries lack such specific organization, the World Health Organization promotes such developments and has collaborated with the World Psychiatric Association and other European and international psychiatry associations to elaborate on consensus statements and technical documents. These assist the development of the care for old people with mental disorders. (World Health Organization, 1996, 1997, 1998, 2002).

20.67 OLD AGE PSYCHIATRY IN ROMANIA

Old age psychiatry is recognized as a specialty in only a few countries. It requires a grounding in general psychiatry, general medicine and gerontology. In Romania, old age psychiatry has been a recognized subspecialty of psychiatry since 2001. There is a training postgraduate course organized in Bucharest leading to a diploma in psychogeriatrics for psychiatrists, geriatricians and medical residents (World Health Organization, 1998; Camus *et al.*, 2003).

20.68 MENTAL HEALTH SERVICES FOR THE ELDERLY IN ROMANIA

In the last few years, in most countries the psychiatric services have been more and more orientated towards the community (Jolley and Arie, 1992; Arie, 1994; Wattis, 1994; Philpot and Banerjee, 1996; Wertheimer, 1997). The special needs of older people were not always recognized and respected by generic services (Wattis, 1994). Any new mental health service strategy must take the following into consideration: integration of mental health care, creation of services adequate to specific needs of patients, continuity of care by cooperation among various services providers, multidisciplinary team work, community involvement and geographic catchment areas (Cooper, 1997; Tăturu, 1997).

Stigma remains an obstacle in ensuring access to good care for the elderly. Stigma against the elderly mentally ill leads to the development of negative attitudes, including the attitudes of professionals and services, and consequent poor quality treatment and care, and inadequate funding at both national and local levels (World Health Organization, 2002). In most developing countries, including Romania, no national programme for care of the elderly exists or has been financed.

Only recently have we started to add community healthcare services to the traditional system of hospital care. The Mental Health Law appeared in Romania in August 2002. In Chapter 4 of the law the forms of specific mental health services existing in Romania are listed, along with the care standards for people with mental disorders (Mental Health Law, 2002).

20.68.1 Inpatient services

The elderly with acute or chronic mental disorders are treated in:

- *psychiatric hospitals* for acute mental disorders – in most districts
- *long-stay accommodation/continuing hospital care*
- *geropsychiatric wards in psychiatric hospitals* (Nucet only; in Iaşi the department is only for dementia patients)
- *psychiatric wards in general hospitals* (in areas where psychiatric hospitals do not exist)
- *Liaison Psychiatry Department* in University General Hospital Bucharest
- *psychiatric department in geriatric hospitals.*

In developed countries some mentally ill people are treated in general hospitals in consultation-liaison psychiatry departments as a new way of integrating care for patients with physical and psychiatric comorbidity (Lipsitt, 2003). In Romania and other developing countries, traditionally the mentally ill were treated for financial reasons in general or geriatric hospitals as there were insufficient psychiatric hospitals.

Older people with dementia and no behavioural disorders or significant physical disabilities are also admitted to *nursing homes* and other *social service long-stay* units organized by the state, non-governmental organizations (NGOs) or churches.

20.68.2 Outpatient units

- *Outpatient or community assessment units – day care centres* (Bucharest, Brasov, Cluj, Iaşi, Oradea, Sibiu, Timişoara)
- *Primary care/Residential care*
- *Hostel respite care* (Oradea)
- *Community mental health centre for older people.* Organized in Oradea in 1996 by the Foundation 'Worrying about Grandparents'. The centre is a link between the patients and their families, general practitioners and hospitals for acutely or chronically mentally ill people (Tătaru, 1997; Tătaru *et al.*, 2002; Tătaru, 2003)
- *Memory Centre Bucharest.* Opened in 2000 within the 'Professor Doctor Alexandru Obregia' University Hospital in Bucharest by the Rumanian Alzheimer Society. The Memory Centre is a modern ambulatory facility for diagnosis and intervention (Tătaru *et al.*, 2002; Tătaru, 2003)
- *Community and social support services* (organized by NGOs and churches in almost all districts)
- *Clubs for elderly.*

In Romania the above services operate only in few districts and there is still a severe lack of resources.

Day programmes contribute to reducing stigma and discrimination by reducing isolation and furthering the ability to face to daily life. (Tătaru *et al.*, 2002; De Mendonca Lima *et al.*, 2002; Tătaru, 2003).

20.68.3 Residential care

In 2003 a programme was started for residential care and follow up for patients of all ages. The elderly with mental disorders including dementia are also cared for by this programme (Health Department, 2003).

Medical treatment and also the domiciliary services, including meals-on-wheels, home helps and mobile laundry help handicapped elderly to remain at home. The latter are now only provided by NGOs and churches.

There is also some financial support from the Labour and Social Protection departments as compensation for families or caregivers of the chronically ill with handicap (including those with dementia), who are treated at home.

In Romania there is no intermediate stage between home care support and the nursing home, which provides sheltered accommodation for elderly people, or those with less severe dementia and behavioural disorders (Lovestone and Gauthier, 2001).

Most Romanians with dementia who have a family are treated at home. It is difficult for families to place them in a long-stay unit, not only because of attitudes, shame and feelings of guilt, but also because patients who have families or relatives are not admitted to state nursing homes.

Patients with dementia who have behavioural disturbances, psychotic symptoms or agitation require admission to a psychiatric hospital for acute or chronic illness, both those who live in nursing homes and the ones who live in their own homes.

Cooperation between social and medical services is difficult, because they are separately organized. The role of NGOs and of churches in the system of community care for the elderly is increasing in Romania, but is still very limited.

The extension of outreach services of nursing homes and residential homes in conjunction with day care centres, day hospitals and residential care could be a valuable alternative to the high degree of institutionalization of Romanian elderly people with or without mental disorders (Tudose, 2001; Tătaru *et al.*, 2002, 2003).

General practitioners and community nurses are also involved in the care of the elderly and it would be opportune for them to participate in domiciliary visits by psychiatrists (Jolley and Arie, 1992; Wattis, 1994). To this end we have initiated an educational programme that includes courses for family doctors who are involved in the primary care of dementia. The objectives of the training are to promote development at every level for all those concerned and indicate the groups to whom education should be offered, what to teach them and which teaching methods to use (World Health Organization, 1998; Cazmus *et al.*, 2003).

One of the key theoretical issues for the future development of community services is likely to be the distinction between care and treatment. Psychogeriatric services will need to retain a proportion of their long-stay beds for rehabilitation and treatment of elderly people with functional illnesses and demented people with behavioural problems (Wattis, 1994).

20.69 CONCLUSIONS

Today in Romania, in the care of mentally ill people we are trying to reorientate the mental health services from old-fashioned psychiatric hospitals towards community care services. We started by reducing the number of beds, but without ensuring care programmes and community services for these patients. A great number of long-stay psychiatric wards were transferred to the social services. The elderly with chronic mental disorders as well as those with dementia are looked after both in psychiatric long-stay hospitals and in social services facilities whose staff are inadequately trained to care for these patients. However, most dementia patients are still in the care of their families, if they have one. It is a pity, but we do not have either a clear picture of all services for elderly care or local epidemiological studies in this field.

In spite of the professionals' endeavours specializing in teaching and educational programmes, there are only a few psychogeriatric services and even fewer special care services for dementia patients. The national programme for elderly care is only a project that, for the time being, lacks financial support.

REFERENCES

Arie T. (1994) The development in Britain. In: JRM Copeland, MT Abou-Saleh, DG Blazer (eds), *Principles and Practice of Geriatric Psychiatry*. Chichester, John Wiley, pp. 6–10

Camus V, Katona C, De Mendonca Lima CA. (2003) Teaching and training in old age psychiatry: a general survey of the World Psychiatric Association member societies. *International Journal of Geriatric Psychiatry* **18**: 694–699

Cooper B. (1997) Principles of service provision in old age psychiatry. In: R Jacoby and C Oppenheimer (eds), *Psychiatry in the Elderly*, 2nd edition. Oxford, Oxford University Press, pp. 357–375

De Mendonca Lima CA, Kuhne N, Bertolote JM. (2002). Day hospitals in old age psychiatry: past goals and future challenges, *IPA European and Mediterranean Regional Meeting*, 7–20 April, Rome

Health Department /318. (2003) *Standards for Residence Care.* Monitorul Oficial al Romaniei, XV, Nr 255

Jolley D and Arie T. (1992) Developments in psychogeriatric services. In: T Arie (ed.), *Recent Advances in Psychogeriatrics*, 2nd edition. London, Churchill Livingstone, pp. 117–135

Lipsitt DR. (2003) Psychiatry and the general hospital in an age of uncertainty. *World Psychiatry* **2**: 87–92

Lovestone S and Gauthier S. (2001) *Management of Dementia.* London, Martin Dunitz, pp. 109–119

Mental Health Law. (2002) Monitorul Oficial al Romaniei, XIV, Nr 589

Philpot M and Banerjee S. (1996) *Mental Health Services for older people In London, London's Mental Health.* London, King's Foundation, pp. 46–64

Tătaru N. (1997) Project for the development of an ambulatory and semi-ambulatory centre for the third age. *Dementia and Geriatric Cognitive Disorders* **8**: 128–131

Tătaru N. (2003) Mental health services for the elderly in central and eastern European countries. *IPA Regional European Meeting*, April, Geneva

Tătaru N, Dicker A, Tudose C. (2002). The Old Age Psychiatry in Eastern European Countries. *The 30th Symposium of the European Association of Geriatric Psychiatry*, 14–16 November 2002, Padova, Italy

Tudose C. (2001) *Dementele, o Provocare Pentru Medicul de Familie.* Bucharest, Infomedica pp. 98–103.

Wattis JP. (1994) The pattern of psychogeriatric services. In: JRM Copeland, Abou-Saleh, DG Blazer (eds), *Principles and Practice of Geriatric Psychiatry.* Chichester, John Wiley, pp. 779–883

Wertheimer J. (1997) Psychogeriatric organisation in the medico-social network: the experience of the canton of Sand, Switzerland. *Dementia and Cognitive Disorders* **8**: 143–145

World Health Organization Division on Mental Health and Prevention of Substance Abuse (1996) *Psychiatry of the Elderly – a Consensus Statement.* Geneva, WHO

World Health Organization Division on Mental Health and Prevention of Substance Abuse, and World Psychiatric Association (1997) *Program on Mental Health, Organization of Care in Psychiatry of the Elderly: a Technical Consensus Statement.* Geneva, WHO

World Health Organization Department of Mental Health and World Psychiatric Association (1998) *Education in Psychiatry of the Elderly: a Technical Consensus Statement.* Geneva, WHO

World Health Organization Division on Mental Health and Prevention of Substance Abuse and World Psychiatric Association (2002) *Management of Mental and Brain Disorders Reducing Stigma and Discrimination against Older People with Mental Disorders: a Technical Consensus Statement.* Geneva, WHO

Latin America and the Caribbean

JOÃO CARLOS BARBOSA MACHADO

20.70 AGEING IN LATIN AMERICA AND THE CARIBBEAN

Population ageing usually has been associated with the more industrialized countries of Europe and North America, where a fifth or more of the entire population typically is aged 60 or over. What is less known is the fact that population ageing has occurred and is occurring in less industrialized countries and is growing much more rapidly than the ageing population in more-developed nations. Uruguay, for example, currently has a higher percentage of older (60+) population than does Canada and the USA. Outside of Europe and North America, the Caribbean is the 'oldest' region of the world, with 10 per cent of its aggregate population aged 60 years and over.

According to the Pan American Health Association (PAHO), Latin America and the Caribbean region can be divided in four subregions for the socioeconomic profiles of older persons: Andean Countries; Central America with the Spanish-speaking Caribbean and Haiti; English-speaking Caribbean and Netherlands Antilles, and Southern Cone and Mexico, which together have two-thirds of the total older population in Latin America and the Caribbean. Brazil and Mexico alone have 50 per cent of all older people in the region.

During the first quarter of the new century, the ageing population of Latin America and the Caribbean will grow by more than 138 per cent, increasing from 42 million in 2000 to 100 million by 2025, according to a report on *The State of Ageing and Health in Latin America and the Caribbean* (PAHO and the Merck Institute of Aging and Health, 2004) (Figure 20.4).

By 2025, in every country of the region at least 10 per cent of all those aged 60 or older today will then be aged 80 or older. In Argentina, Brazil, Chile and Uruguay this proportion will be even higher. The region's oldest old percentage is projected to grow significantly during the coming decades, more than

doubling between 1990 and 2020. Brazil will likely see more than a tripling of its oldest old during this period, from 1.9 million to 7.1 million. After 2020, the growth of the oldest old will further accelerate as the large baby-boom cohorts born after World War II begin to reach age 75 (CEPAL, 2002).

Latin American and the Caribbean have a heterogeneous ethnic and racial origin population with different socio-economic and cultural profiles. It is estimated that 60 per cent of the region's older population are women. The majority of older people have only a primary level of education. With the exception of Argentina and Cuba, the illiteracy rate among the elderly is above 10 per cent all over Latin America and the Caribbean, being over 20 per cent in most of the countries, including Brazil, Colombia and Mexico (PAHO and the Merck Institute of Aging and Health, 2004). Around two-thirds of this population lives in urban areas and there are

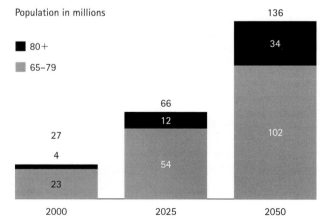

Figure 20.4 *Projection of the population aged 65 or older, Latin America, 2000, 2025 and 2050. (CEPAL 2002, reprinted with permission)*

51 cities with more than 1 million inhabitants. Some cities, such as Buenos Aires, Lima, Mexico City, Rio de Janeiro and São Paulo, are among the 30 largest cities in the world (United Nations, 2003).

In contrast to industrialized societies which have witnessed a steady increase in overall standards of living, in Latin America and the Caribbean access to sources of income by the elderly is usually far below what is required to secure self-sufficiency. The difference persists between the most and the least equitable societies in terms of the distribution of income. Forty per cent of men 60 years and older are still working while only 8 per cent of women have any paid employment. A higher proportion of women than men do not live with a spouse or partner, but with a child or another relative, with a decline in traditional family support.

Government efforts and resources have been insufficient to guarantee adequate healthcare and social support systems and the policy-makers do not prioritize ageing issues. Not surprisingly therefore information and research programmes are lacking and the issues of long-term care, institutionalization and pension reform have not yet been addressed.

The ageing process of the population has coincided with an increase in chronic and degenerative diseases and disabilities. As a result of these demographic changes there also have been changes in the pattern of diseases at the regional level. Two mortality patterns currently coexist: one typical of poor societal living conditions (infectious and parasitic communicable diseases) and the other of more developed societies (chronic and degenerative non-communicable diseases) are combined with high mortality from accidents and violence. The resulting 'epidemiological polarization' magnifies the persistence of significant health gaps between different social groups and geographical areas within countries (PAHO, 1997, 2002).

20.71 EPIDEMIOLOGY: DEMENTIA PREVALENCE

Despite the scarcity of available epidemiological data it is reasonable to consider the dementias as a major public health problem in Latin America and the Caribbean, although it is not recognized as such at either governmental or community levels (Arizaga et al., 1999).

A MEDLINE-based search to assess the epidemiology of dementia in Latin America and the Caribbean by Caramelli (2003) found a total of 16 studies of which only seven were population-based studies carried out in Brazil (The Catanduva Study) (Herrera et al., 2002), Colombia (The Aratoca Study) (Rosselli et al., 2000; Pradilla et al., 2002), Cuba (The La Habana Study) (Llibre et al., 1999) and Uruguay (The Villa del Cerro Study) (Ketzoian et al., 1997). In addition there are two other ongoing studies being conducted in Mexico (C Zunica, personal communication) and Venezuela (The Maracaibo Aging Study) (Maestre et al., 2002).

Methodology for dementia screening, as well as criteria and tools used for dementia diagnosis varied widely in the different studies. In Uruguay, Ketzoian et al. (1997) estimate a prevalence of 4.03/1000 when the entire population of Villa del Cerro is considered. Herrera et al. (2002) found a prevalence of dementia of 7.1 per cent among 1156 randomly selected subjects (25 per cent of the total elderly population) aged more than 65 years in Catanduva, Brazil. Llibre et al. (1999) found a prevalence of dementia of 8.2 per cent among subjects aged more than 60 years in Havana, Cuba. Pradilla et al. (2002) estimate a prevalence of dementia of 10.5/1000 subjects (all ages) in a rural area in Aratoca, Colombia. The differential diagnosis of dementia subtypes is not available in all studies, but when it is described, Alzheimer's disease (AD) or degenerative dementia is the leading cause, ranging from 47.4 per cent to 62.5 per cent of all dementia cases. Mixed dementia or AD with cerebrovascular disease is the second most common diagnosis in three out of five studies and vascular dementia is the second leading cause in the remaining two population studies.

20.72 ORGANIZATION OF SERVICES FOR PEOPLE WITH DEMENTIA

Although overall improvements in dementia care can be seen in this region, improvements are not uniform for all countries or for all social groups within a single country (Mangone et al., 2000). However, some similarities are still present. Patients and their families have misconceptions about normal ageing and dementia. Resignation and lack of expectations are very common.

In a study conducted in 24 centres in developing countries including Latin America and the Caribbean, 706 persons with dementia and their caregivers were interviewed. It was found that older people are indivisible from their younger family members. Most caregivers were women, living with the person with dementia in extended family households. Nonetheless, despite the traditional apparatus of family care, levels of caregiver strain were at least as high as in the developed world. Many had to curtail employment in order to provide care and also faced the additional expense of paid carers and health services. Families from the poorest countries were particularly likely to have used expensive private medical services, and to be spending more than 10 per cent of the per capita GNP on health care. It is suggested that the high levels of family strain feed into the cycle of disadvantage and thus should be a concern for policy-makers (The 10/66 Dementia Research Group, 2004).

An overview of the healthcare system in the region shows that it is a mixed public-private system in both insurance and provision, with most elderly persons being forced into the public system (Marin and Wallace, 2002). The dominance of the public system in the care of the elderly has the potential to improve the organization and delivery of needed services, but up to now health care for older persons has not been a top priority compared to broader macrosystem issues.

Specialized services for the elderly are fairly scarce across Latin America and the Caribbean. Most are based in big cities at large teaching hospitals with few psychogeriatric hospital wards, day hospitals, dementia reference centres and memory clinics or day centres. In recent years there has been a rising awareness by the health and social services acknowledging the lack of resources available for the elderly and the need for a change.

In Brazil, after the approval of the National Policy Act for the Health of the Aged by the Ministry of Health in 1999, 13 reference centres out of 78 planned are now open for the care of demented patients and their families. These centres offer free distribution of cholinesterase inhibitors and atypical antipsychotics under rigid medical control. In 2003, the Elderly Act was approved by the national parliament with the intention to ensure social, health, citizenship and human rights for the Brazilian elderly population.

In Mexico, the Ministry of Health began the development of a National Plan for Alzheimer's Disease and Related Disorders, now considered a national priority with the following components: service delivery, health education, research and legislation (Resnikoff, 2001).

The healthcare services usually are divided into primary, secondary and tertiary care. In most primary care settings, the professionals have inadequate working conditions combined with time constraints. General practitioners (GPs) often consider memory problems as part of the normal ageing process. Most professionals have scarce knowledge of dementia recognition and management with poor understanding and training in the use of diagnostic tools (Sarasola et al., 2003). To illustrate this fact a study was conducted in Brazil (Bertolucci and Ferretti, 2002), which surveyed 1500 medical practitioners with regard to time of graduation, specialty, study habits, work setting and basic questions about dementia. Lack of knowledge was noticed in 942 doctors from different specialties who participated in the survey, especially among those who had graduated 7 years and over, as well as GPs. Not surprisingly, patients are not adequately investigated and, as a result, if they are referred to the reference centres, it is often late in the course of their dementias.

Specialists are concentrated in big cities working mainly on their own in private practice. At the universities, services are not prepared to see the number of patients in need and in general there are few properly trained specialists in dementia care. Specialist doctors are usually geriatricians, neurologists or psychiatrists and a multidisciplinary team is rarely available (Machado, 2003).

Most countries in the region have the availability of diagnostic studies, genetic testing, neuroimaging (cranial computed tomography, magnetic resonance imaging and single-photon emission tomography) as well as neuropsychological testing, although they are available mainly in reference centres, which are considered expensive and not always readily accessible to the population (Mangone and Arizaga, 1999).

Support groups for patients and their carers have sprung up in the region over the past 10 years. Alzheimer's Disease International (ADI) as well as private groups offer a range of activities for the aged, and support family members and

carers; these are appreciated, but are of insufficient number to cover the needs of the population, little publicized and difficult to access.

20.73 EDUCATION, TRAINING AND RESEARCH

Despite the growing interest of the professionals in the field there are a small number of specialists. Most countries (if not all of them) lack a national framework for postgraduate education in dementia. There is no unique specialty or society for the care of demented patients. In most countries national geriatric, psychiatric and neurological societies usually have special interest groups on dementia. By valuing the importance of an interdisciplinary approach to dementia and other neuropsychiatric disorders in old age, Argentina, Brazil and Chile have successfully founded interdisciplinary associations of geriatric neuropsychiatry, although the medical councils do not recognize geriatric neuropsychiatry as a medical subspecialty (Machado, 2003; Sarasola et al., 2003).

In the years to come, the development of public health strategies to cope with dementia will be very challenging for Latin America and the Caribbean. Therefore, efforts should be made for a permanent collaboration among academics, clinicians, national medical societies, governmental and national/international non-governmental organizations. Initiatives in that direction will be crucial for raising awareness of the dementias, which should influence political action, policy-making and general heath service delivery in the region.

With this purpose, Latin American members of the International Psychogeriatric Association (IPA) have established an interest group named the Latin American Initiative (IPA LAI) (Resnikoff, 1997). Of the worldwide IPA membership in 2004 only 5 per cent were Latin American professionals, even though the total population of Latin America is greater than that of Europe and the USA combined.

IPA LAI aims to help in the development and implementation of educational programmes in Latin America as well as to support collaborative multinational epidemiological studies. The IPA LAI Educational Program Group is directed to primary care physicians and the healthcare team working in primary care (Machado, 2001).

The programme includes the design of educational strategies to allow the transfer of new knowledge to the daily practice of professionals dealing with dementia, as well as to provide direct training to healthcare professionals giving them the necessary tools to train the caregivers. Moreover, aims are:

- to assess the impact of sociodemographic variables on dementia diagnosis such as education and illiteracy;
- to develop or adapt assessments for sociodemographic factors relevant to the diagnosis;
- to adapt screening and diagnostic instruments that are reliable, practical, easy to implement and interpret; and

- to develop diagnostic decision trees for expensive diagnostic studies in dementia considering the local financial situation and other health priorities.

Another example of a partnership reported to have been very effective in helping to direct and support advocacy was between The 10/66 Dementia Research Group with ADI and its national Alzheimer's Associations (Prince *et al.*, 2004).

20.74 CONCLUSIONS

The care of persons with dementia has shown considerable and steady improvement in Latin America and the Caribbean. In spite of this progress, governmental funds are not enough to provide all the needs, societal awareness is low, socio-economic problems are great and the number of specialists in the public and private sector is very low.

According to Gutierrez-Robledo (2002), the fast epidemiological transition faced by Latin America countries has created an enormous opportunity to develop systems that differ from those in more developed countries by capitalizing on the lack of infrastructure to produce more home-based rather than institution-based long-term care systems. Since dementia treatment is a dynamic process, it should be approached through programmes that range from health promotion strategies to the establishment of support networks for long-term care in the community. These programmes should be part of a public policy that involves all sectors of society to provide adequate care for patients with or without family support, family members and carers. Involvement of the elderly in the planning of their own futures will be also of paramount importance.

Considering the important cultural and historical links present between Latin American and the Caribbean countries, a joint effort to determine and share common solutions for the significant challenges in providing better care and in promoting a higher quality of life for dementia patients in the region should be mandatory.

REFERENCES

Arizaga RL, Mangone CA, Allegri RF, Ollari JA. (1999) Vascular dementia: the Latin American perspective. *Alzheimer Disease and Associated Disorders* 13 (Suppl. 3): S201–S205

Bertolucci PHF and Ferretti CEL. (2002) Knowledge of dementia among doctors in Brazil. *Neurobiology of Aging* 23 (Suppl. 1): S168

Caramelli P. (2003) The current and future rapid growth of older people in Latin America: implications in Psychogeriatrics. *International Psychogeriatrics* 15 (Suppl. 2): 7

CEPAL (Comisión Económica para América Latina y el Caribe). (2002) América Latina y Caribe: estimaciones y proyecciones de población, 1950–2050, *Boletín demográfico* 69 (LC/G.2152-P), Santiago de Chile, Centro Latinoamericano y Caribeño de Demografía (CELADE) División de Población de la CEPAL, enero.

Gutierrez-Robledo LM. (2002) Looking at the future of geriatric care in developing countries. *Journal of Gerontology, A: Biological Sciences and Medical Sciences* 57: M162–M167

Herrera Jr E, Caramelli P, Silveira ASB, Nitrini R. (2002) Epidemiologic survey of dementia in a community-dwelling Brazilian population. *Alzheimer Disease and Associated Disorders* 16: 103–108

Ketzoian C, Rega I, Caseres R et al. (1997) Estudio de la prevalencia de las principales enfermedades neurologicas en una población del Uruguay. *La Prensa Medica Uruguaya* 17: 9–26

Llibre JJ, Guerra MA, Perez-Cruz H et al. (1999) Dementia syndrome and risk factors in adults older than 60 years old residing in Habana. *Revista Neurológica Argentina* 29: 908–911

Machado JCB. (2001) *Latin-American Initiative*. Report to the IPA Board of Directors. Nice, IPA

Machado JCB. (2003) Evolving strategies for the integration of the related specialties devoted to the field of clinical neurosciences and aging: a view from geriatric medicine. *International Psychogeriatrics* 15 (Suppl. 2): 66

Maestre GE, Pino-Ramirez G, Molero AE et al. (2002) The Maracaibo Aging Study: population and methodological issues. *Neuroepidemiology* 21: 194–201

Mangone C and Arizaga R. (1999) Dementia in Argentina and otter Latin-American countries: an overview. *Neuroepidemiology* 18: 231–235

Mangone CA, Arizaga RL, Allegri RF, Ollari JA. (2000) La demencia en Latinoamérica. *Revista Neurológica Argentina* 25: 108–112

Marin PP and Wallace SP. (2002) Health care for the elderly in Chile: a country in transition. *Aging Clinical and Experimental Research* 14: 271–278

PAHO. (2002) *Health in the Americas, Pan American Health*. Washington, DC, PAHO

PAHO/WHO, National Institute on Aging and US Bureau of the Census. (1997) *Aging in the Americas into the XXI century*. PAHO, Washington, DC

PAHO and the Merck Institute of Aging and Health. (2004) *Report on The State of Aging and Health in Latin America and the Caribbean*. Washington, DC, PAHO

Pradilla G, Ardila A, Vesga Angarita BE, Leon-Sarmiento FE. (2002) Grupo de estúdio GENECO. Study of neurological diseases prevalence in Aratoca, a rural area of eastern Colombia. *Revista Médica de Chile* 130: 191–199

Prince M, Graham N, Brodaty H et al. (2004) Alzheimer Disease International's 10/66 Dementia Research Group – one model for action research in developing countries. *International Journal of Geriatric Psychiatry* 19: 178–181

Resnikoff D. (1997) *Latin-American Initiative*. Report to the IPA Board of Directors. IPA, Jerusalem

Resnikoff D. (2001) Programa de acción para la atención del deterioro intelectual y las demencias. Boletín especial de Alzheimer: http://www.ssa.gob.mx/unidades/conadic

Rosselli D, Ardila A, Pradilla G et al. (2000) The Mini-Mental State Examination as a selected diagnostic test for dementia: a Colombian population study. GENECO. *Revista Neurológica Argentina* 30: 428–432

Sarasola D, Tragano FE, Allegri RF. (2003) The Geriatric Neuropsychiatry in Argentina. *International Psychogeriatrics* 15 (Suppl. 2): 134

The 10/66 Dementia Research Group. (2004) Care arrangements for people with dementia in developing countries. *International Journal of Geriatric Psychiatry* 19: 170–177

United Nations. (2003) World Population Prospects: The 2003 Revision Population Database. New York, United Nations Population Division of the Department of Economic and Social Affairs (http://esa.un.org/unup)

Spain

RAIMUNDO MATEOS, MANUEL MARTÍN-CARRASCO AND MANUEL SÁNCHEZ-PÉREZ

20.75 SOCIOPOLITICAL FRAMEWORK

20.75.1 Unity versus diversity among autonomies

It is not possible to understand the organization of the Spanish health system services without knowing the key points of the sociopolitical context. Spain is a highly aged state of around 43 million inhabitants (17 per cent are more than 65 years old, and this percentage reaches up to 25 per cent in some provinces). A crucible of languages and cultures, it is politically organized into 17 autonomous governments, very different in their extension, number of inhabitants, degree of urban development, economic growth and cultural heritage. Although the general principles are guaranteed by some national laws, for instance, the Health General Law (Ley General de Sanidad, 1986) or the Gerontology National Plan (Ministerio de Asuntos Sociales, 1992), each autonomous government is concerned with the development of some specific laws, standards of performance and budgetary endowments. Therefore, there are remarkable territorial differences in practice.

20.75.2 Service systems

In this context, dementia care is mainly exercised by the three main public systems (Health System, Social Services and so called 'Welfare-Health Service') complemented by a private system of irregular implementation.

The National Health System guarantees the right to complete, free health care for almost all the population. It is complemented by the Social Service System, which manages retirement pensions and all kinds of social welfare (for illness, unemployment, poverty, etc.). In the last few decades, the capabilities of both systems (and their economic expenses) have increased in an exponential way, with serious coordination failures between both. This is especially noticeable when diligence is needed for groups with many health and welfare needs (a situation for which dementia patients and their families are a typical example).

With the purpose of palliating the aforementioned deficiency, the Catalonian autonomous government started a decade ago the programme 'Vida als Anys', addressed to chronic patients (80 per cent were elderly). This integrated model of resources, which was accompanied by a specific budget, has succeeded in showing its judicious points and has become a referential point for other autonomies (e.g. Galicia).

Finally, with regard to the private sector of Health and/or Social Services, two facts must be pointed out:

- it has an unequal representation in the different autonomies of the state;
- given the wide basis of public health and social services, it aspires to 'sell' its product to the public system rather than 'competing' with it.

20.75.3 Public opinion

The mass media quickly showed great interest on the subject. The degree of social alert has increased remarkably during over the last years. The Spanish situation will be outlined by considering the assets and the liabilities of Spanish systems of care for dementia patients and their carers.

20.76 THE ASSETS OF HEALTH AND SOCIAL RESOURCES

There is some epidemiological information available, regarding the magnitude of the problem (Lobo *et al.*, 1992; López-Pousa *et al.*, 1995) and the relationship between cognitive impairment and other pathologies (Mateos *et al.*, 1997, 2000).

The family is still the main source of social support in Spain. Consistently, the diminution of its members, the increasing involvement of women in the professional world and a decrease of the birth rate has turned the situation into an untenable one. Some devices to measure carer burden and needs have recently started to be introduced into clinical (Martín-Carrasco *et al.*, 1996) and epidemiological (Mateos *et al.*, 1998; Ybarzábal *et al.*, 2002) studies.

Public health coordination was successfully achieved some time ago in some provinces such as Alava, by reason of its unusual administrative autonomy, its high socioeconomic level and prevailing urban organization, as well as its small territory.

At some health centres there are psychogeriatric teams with full-time interdisciplinary staff, a community philosophy and team work (Martín-Carrasco *et al.*, 1991; Mateos *et al.*, 1994; Martín-Carrasco and Artaso, 1996; Sánchez-Pérez, 1997, 2002; Sánchez-Pérez *et al.*, 1997).

Social centres include modern residences/nursing homes with a community projection (SEGG, 1995) and home help respite care (SEGG, 1997).

Carers' self-help movements rely on two big state associations and an increasing number of regional offices.

Several universities give postgraduate courses on gerontology and the autonomous University of Barcelona still offers, in its sixth edition, the unique postgraduate Diploma and Master of Psychogeriatrics held in Spain (Sánchez-Pérez, 2003).

The autonomous governments of first Cataluña and then Galicia, Cantabria and Asturias, have created advisory commissions for psychogeriatrics. Their task is to set up the philosophy and to reach an agreement on protocols for performance and coordination of resources needed for dementia care, including modalities of treatment for those disorders (Servei Català de la Salut, 1988a, b; Comisión Asesora en materia de Psicoxeriatria, 1999).

We are witnessing an increase in the number of psychiatrists interested in taking care of dementia patients and carers as a result of the improvement of the young psychiatrists' training not only in dementia, but in geriatric psychiatry in general. This is due to a conjunction of interests and opportunities. On the one hand, those professionals working within the limited welfare points are enthusiastic and available for teaching and training residents. On the other hand, some scientific societies, like the Sociedad Española de Gerontopsiquiatría y Psicogeriatría

(SEGP), have played a stimulating role by means of congresses and monographic courses.

20.77 LIABILITIES OF HEALTH AND SOCIAL RESOURCES

The coordination between the different departments is still deficient, not only between Health and Social Services, but also within both areas:

- between primary and specialized health care;
- between the three specialties mostly involved – psychiatry, neurology and geriatrics; and
- between basic and specialized social services.

The success of the first Alzheimer conference, under the leadership of neurology, created the hope that the rest of the involved medical specialties (psychiatry and geriatrics, as well as primary health care) would join forces with other professional sectors and patients' informal carers. After the fourth conference, the feeling is that such an effective and supportive coordination in daily welfare activities will take much longer than relatives and many professionals had imagined and still hope for.

There is a lack of basic resources including places in nursing homes, day hospitals and home care, and there are few specialized services with specific programmes for dementia care. If residential facilities for elderly people develop too quickly, a disconcerting diversity is created, in such a way that besides centres equipped with modern technologies and medical staff *in situ*, suitable for housing dementia patients, there persists the out-of-date asylum model where philanthropic organizations assume care for patients without enough professional support. The current regulations in this sector need to be improved.

There is an increasing debate over the proliferation of clinics exclusively focused on the diagnosis of dementia and that are not always equipped with interdisciplinary teams. This model contrasts the principle of welfare continuity emphasized by the World Health Organization (WHO) and the World Psychiatric Association (WHO, 1997).

Geriatric and psychogeriatric teaching is not yet consolidated in the undergraduate courses of the medical faculties in most of the universities of the country. Many professionals lack awareness and training, especially within primary health care and community social services (Mateos, 2000).

The plight of carers has still not been recognized by society. We lack legal regulation to lighten their economic burden and to help them continue their job.

20.78 CONCLUSION

At present the balance is negative (Mateos, 2003). The Spanish House of Commons decided in 1997 to urge the Government to develop a National Plan on Alzheimer's disease. It seems that the National Health Ministry wants to revitalize this unfinished project, which should outline concrete actions to improve the deficiencies discussed above. It is a way for hope, not only for carers but also for those professionals entrusted with the task of delivering and improving dementia care in Spain.

REFERENCES

Comisión Asesora en materia de Psicoxeriatria. (1999) *Plan Galego de atención ó enfermo de Alzheimer e outras demencias.* Santiago de Compostela: Xunta de Galicia

Ley General de Sanidad (14/1986 de 25 de Abril). BOE España 29/4/1986

Lobo A, Dewey M, Copeland J, Día JL, Saz P. (1992) The prevalence of dementia among elderly people living in Zaragoza and Liverpool. *Psychological Medicine* **22**: 239–243

López-Pousa S, Vilalta J, Linas J. (1995) Epidemiología de las demencias en España. *Revista de Gerontologia* **5** (Suppl.): 28–33

Martín-Carrasco M and Artaso B. (1996) Economic evaluation of the psychogeriatric day-care center: methodological aspects. *Revista Espanola de Geriatria y Gerontologia* **31**: 29–36

Martín-Carrasco M, Abad R, Nadal S. (1991) Instituciones intermedias en el tratamiento de las demencias y otros trastornos psiquiátricos en la vejez: El Centro de Día Psicogeriátrico. *Revista Espanola de Geriatria y Gerontologia* **26** (Suppl. 2): 39–45

Martín-Carrasco M, Salvadó I, Nadal S *et al.* (1996) Adaptación para nuestro medio de la Escala de Sobrecarga del Cuidador (Caregiver Burden Interview) de Zarit. *Revista de Gerontologia* **6**: 338–346

Mateos R. (2000) Formación específica en Psicogeriatría: necesidads y situación actual. *Informaciones Psiquiátricas* **162**: 335–340

Mateos R. (2003) The organization of psychogeriatric services in Spain. In: Abstracts of the XI Congress of the International Psychogeriatric Association (IPA), Chicago, August. *International Psychogeriatrics* **15** (Suppl. 2): 77

Mateos R, Camba MT, Gomez R, Landeira P. (1994) La Unidad de Psicogeriatría del Area de Salud. Un dispositivo asistencial novedoso en la red de Salud Mental de Galicia. In: *Saúde Mental e Sociedade. Proceedings of II Congreso da Asociación Galega de Saúde Mental,* Santiago de Compostela, pp. 259–275

Mateos R, Garcia MC, Camba MT *et al.* (1997) Epidemiological, clinical and treatment implications of the demential syndromes in Galicia (Spain). *Cadernos do IPUB (Brasil)* **10**: 133–55

Mateos R, Ybarzábal M, García MJ *et al.* (1998) Dificultades, estrategias de afrontamiento y satisfacción de los cuidadores de pacientes psicogeriátricos. Estudio piloto de validación del CADI, CAMI, CASI. *Proceedings of VIII Reunión de la Sociedad Española de Gerontopsiquiatría y Psicogeriatría,* Cádiz. September

Mateos R, Droux A, Páramo M *et al.* (2000) The Galicia Study of Mental Health of the Elderly II: The use of the Galician DIS. *International Journal of Methods in Psychiatric Research* **9**: 174–182

Ministerio de Asuntos Sociales. (1992) *Plan Gerontológico.* Madrid, Ministerio de Asuntos Sociales

Sánchez-Pérez M. (1997) El modelo de atención sociosanitario en la atención a los problemas de salud mental del anciano. *III Jornada de Actualización en Psicogeriatría.* Martorell (Barcelona), April

Sánchez-Pérez M. (2002) Asistencia sociosanitaria en Salud Mental: evaluación de una experiencia. Informaciones Psiquiátricas. In: *Proceedings of VI Jornadas de Actualización en Psicogeriatría,* Martorell, May 2001, no. 167, pp. 95–103

Sánchez-Pérez M. (2003) Training in Geriatric Psychiatry in Spain. *International Psychogeriatrics* **15** (Suppl. 2): 77

Sánchez-Pérez M, Rodríguez JP, Nin J. (1997) Asistencia en una Unidad Psicogeriátrica Sociosanitaria. *Proceedings of VII Reunión de la Sociedad Española de Gerontopsiquiatría y Psicogeriatría.* Salamanca, September

Servei Català de la Salut. (1988a) *The Working Groups of the Psychogeriatric-Advisory Council: Cognitive and Behavioural Disorders in Social Health Care* (bilingual document). Pla de Salut, Quadern no. 10. Barcelona, Bayer

Servei Català de la Salut. (1988b) *Consell Assessor Sobre el Tractament Farmacològic de la Malaltia d'Alzheimer.* Informe no 1/1998, Barcelona

SEGG (Sociedad Española de Geriatría y Gerontología). (1995) In: Rodríguez P. (ed.), *Residencias para Personas Mayores. Manual de Orientación.* Madrid, SG Editores

SEGG (Sociedad Española de Geriatría y Gerontología). (1997) In: Rodríguez P and Valdivieso C. (eds), *El Servicio de Ayuda a Domicilio. Programación del Servicio. Manual de Formación para Auxiliares.* Madrid, Fundación Caja Madrid and SEGG

World Health Organization. (1997) Organization of Care in Psychiatry of the Elderly: a technical consensus statement. (Doc.: WHO/MSA/MNH/MND/97.3). Geneva, World Health Organization

Ybarzábal M, Mateos R, García-Álvarez MJ, Amboage MT, Fraguela I. (2002) Validación de la versión española del CANE. Escala de Evaluación de Necesidades para Ancianos de Camberwell. *Revista de Psicogeriatría* **2**: 38–44

Britain

MARTIN BROWN, COLIN GODBER AND DAVID G WILKINSON

Since the last edition of this book a number of major events have influenced the practice of old age psychiatry in Britain. Five years ago we were optimistic about the impending Royal Commission report on long-term care, yet disappointingly the Government did not fully accept their recommendations, which has led to divisiveness between the different countries within Britain. The National Health Service had been organized for a while through acute trusts, which were mostly concerned with running the general hospitals, and community trusts providing the rest of the services, which contained most of the psychogeriatric services. Community trusts have now been abandoned in favour of primary care trusts (PCTs) who purchase care from the acute and mental health trusts. In some cases the old age services have been incorporated into the new mental health trusts, whereas elsewhere they are provided directly by PCTs. Other changes include the publication of a *National Service Framework for Older People* (Department of Health, 2001) and the appointment of an older persons' 'tsar'. Whilst these initiatives are welcome they have largely focused on physical health issues and have not been accompanied by extra readily visible monies, and the impact of their development appears at best neutral.

On a more positive note the last 5 years have seen a huge expansion in the use of cholinesterase inhibitors in the management of mild to moderate Alzheimer's disease endorsed by the recommendations of the National Institute for Clinical Excellence (NICE, 2001). The emergence of these drugs has led to differing patterns of referral from primary care with a tendency for patients to be seen and diagnosed at a much earlier stage of their illness than would have been the case 10 years ago. However, there are still up to four-fold differences in uptake between different strategic health authorities within the UK (T Gosden and C Baker, personal communication).

20.79 THE CLIENTELE

20.79.1 People with dementia

The prevalence of dementia in the UK has increased by at least 50 per cent in the last 30 years and is estimated to increase by the same proportion between 1991 and 2021; by this time over 900 000 people are likely to be affected (Challis *et al.*, 2002).

A small proportion of those with dementia have illnesses starting before the age of 65 (early onset dementia). These patients usually present first to adult psychiatric services or neurologists, but, whereas the latter may have a particular role with initial diagnosis and assessment, the overall management often falls to old age psychiatry services who tend to exhibit a more holistic approach. The development of memory clinics has increased the role of old age psychiatry in the initial diagnosis and treatment of these early onset cases. However, only a minority of districts have services specifically geared to their support in the community or indeed their longer-term care.

20.79.2 Informal carers

The bulk of care in the UK is provided by informal carers and it has been estimated that the replacement cost of the care provided by friends and family for chronic disorders such as dementia exceeds £20 billion. There is a great recognition of the need to provide services that not only help patients but also support and offer respite to their carers. Most services offer carers support groups, both educational and supportive, sitting services and respite care. Voluntary services like MIND and the Alzheimer's Society work with carers to provide continuing support including helplines and advocacy. Most carers wish to keep the patient at home but features such as aggression, agitation, insomnia and incontinence make this difficult and are correlated with the need for residential care. One study has shown that whilst only 10 per cent of carers wished their relatives could be taken into residential care, this was shown to be the only intervention that had a positive impact on the mental health of carers.

20.80 ORGANIZATION OF SERVICES IN BRITAIN

20.80.1 Health care

The bulk of health care in Britain is provided by the National Health Service (NHS) funded through taxation and predominantly free at the point of delivery. The NHS has struggled to keep up with the pressures of technological and demographic change and has only managed by the encouragement of growth in private health insurance and a narrowing of the definition of health care. The latter has been achieved by moving much of the responsibility of care for chronic disability and illness, such as dementia, onto social services, people with dementia and their families.

General practice remains the cornerstone of the NHS and manages the vast majority of mental disorder without referral to secondary care. However, the last 40 years have seen the emergence of Geriatric Medicine and Old Age Psychiatry as specialties. Although geriatric medicine has become increasingly engrossed in the acute hospital care of older people, old age psychiatry has focused much more on community-based assessment, treatment and support of carers. This, together with an active approach to the treatment of functional illness and close work with primary and social care has made it an attractive branch of psychiatry expanding 15-fold since the mid 1970s. Whilst the specialty continues to grow, some areas of the country fail to attract or retain consultants. Psychiatry has failed to attract more than 4 per cent of the medical graduates who are necessary to fuel consultant expansion. Most services in Britain manage the mental health needs of all the population over 65, i.e. depression, alcohol misuse, paranoid states, as well as dementia, though a few old age psychiatrists will work with dementia alone. Treatments for depression have improved greatly in the last 10 years and this, combined with the emergence of cholinesterase inhibitors, the continuing closure of hospital-based long-stay beds and demographic changes, have all led to a higher proportion of community-based referrals relating to dementia care.

20.80.2 Housing, social and voluntary services

A major problem in coordinating care for people with chronic disability in Britain has been the lack of co-terminosity, different management and funding arrangements between health and social services and again between the latter and local authority environmental services, e.g. housing, transport and leisure. Initiatives to ensure closer working between health and social services have been slow to materialize for the over 65s and have lagged behind a closer working between the same agencies dealing with mental illness in younger people, a process accelerated by the *National Service Framework* (NSF) for mental illness (which specifically excluded any coverage of mental disorder in those over the age of 65). In many areas old age psychiatrists now work more closely with geriatricians than with their colleagues practising general adult psychiatry.

The last decade has seen a continued expansion in the care, both in the community and within institutional settings, provided by the commercial sector. However, the voluntary sector provides a significant proportion of day care and specialized domiciliary support. Organizations such as Age Concern, the Alzheimer's Society and MIND continue to play key roles as pressure groups, as sponsors of research and pilot developments, and as instigators of a wide range of information, self-help and relative support groups.

20.80.3 Financial support

Care provided by the NHS is free and people with at least moderate disability are eligible for non-means-tested allowances, e.g. attendance allowance, subject to independent medical assessment. These grants are designed to allow the individual to purchase care to cater for the disability but the attendance allowance would, for example, purchase about 10 per cent of the weekly cost of nursing home care.

The Royal Commission on Long-Term Care of the Elderly (1999) recommended that all personal care should be provided free regardless of assets, and that residents of homes should be responsible only for the hotel charges. The Government in England rejected this recommendation as too costly and instead introduced free nursing care. In reality most care provided in nursing homes was again deemed to be personal care with the Government restricting the NHS contribution to the funding of care provided by registered nurses alone. This free nursing care is assessed as falling into one of three bands attracting payments of between £40 and £135, each a fraction of the total care costs. The Scottish Parliament, however, accepted the recommendations of the Royal Commission. These different practices have helped fuel a lively debate about long-term care and have attracted considerable media attention.

20.81 COMMUNITY SUPPORT

20.81.1 Primary health care

Nearly all patients with dementia live in the community and hence the bulk of their medical care comes from GPs. Although their skills and confidence in diagnosis and management appear to be improving, there are still wide variations as a result of inconsistencies in training with little exposure to old age psychiatry at undergraduate or GP training level. In primary care many district nurses have been seconded as care managers, which has improved liaison between health and social services, as has the development of older persons' healthcare coordinators. These initiatives have probably brought some cases of dementia, where carers are under considerable stress, to secondary care at an earlier stage than otherwise would have been the case. These initiatives have had more impact on dementia care than GPs' contractual needs to screen all patients over 75 annually or through specific inputs of health visitors who are predominantly involved with families and young children.

20.81.2 Domiciliary support and day care

For the demented person living with a resident carer, social care aims to provide support in the form of domestic tasks, shopping, aspects of personal care and respite to allow the carer to go out. For the demented person living alone, such care is targeted at aspects of personal and domestic care, in which skills have been lost, e.g. maintenance of adequate diet and compliance with medication. The limiting factor to the successful introduction of home-based care will often be the degree of insight of the patient. Unwillingness to accept help will lead to increased risks through self-neglect and wandering. Here the community psychiatric nurse (CPN) visiting the home and developing a rapport with the patient is crucial and, where paranoid symptoms exist, the judicious use of an antipsychotic may be vital.

Day centres, as opposed to day hospitals, are run by social services departments or voluntary agencies and may form an important part of a package of care that allows a demented person to continue living at home. They cater for a wide range of clients with varying degrees of confusion and physical disabilities, with some day centres setting up separate days for those patients with more advanced dementia often associated with mild behavioural problems such as wandering.

Day care has been shown to form part of the package of support in up to two-thirds of patients with dementia. Studies have emphasized the positive effects on both the carers and those with the dementia themselves, particularly for the latter at the relatively early stages of the illness.

20.82 SPECIALIST SERVICES

In the UK with its ageing population, people with dementia are seen in all areas of medicine but the specialist management and assessment per se is largely the province of old age psychiatry. Very few neurologists provide dementia services, with most only being involved in the diagnosis of younger and atypical cases. Geriatricians have always managed dementia in the physically frail, and as they become more proactive in the

management of risk in stroke patients, running clinics for falls and 'funny turns', they are much more likely to be involved in the diagnosis and management of vascular dementia.

20.82.1 Assessment

Although most dementia referrals are still assessed in the home setting by an old age psychiatrist, increasingly this is delegated to one of the members of the multidisciplinary community mental health team. The aim of any assessment is to establish a diagnosis, identify any treatable disorders, ascertain the suitability of current living environment, and make some estimation of care requirements and future prognosis.

Some centres have always used day hospitals to undertake these initial assessments rather than home visits, and the trend to outpatient assessment is increasing with the advent of symptomatic treatments and the consequent development of memory clinics. Patients tend to be seen much earlier in the disease process and outpatient attendance is quite appropriate.

Old age psychiatry services have tended to devote most of their energies to developing community assessment and treatment programmes with a great emphasis on caregiver support, though increasingly attention is turning to the multitude of patients admitted to general hospitals with physical illness complicated by dementia. A few experiments with joint psychiatric and geriatric assessment units aimed at treating both physical and behavioural problems have not been widely adopted. Most services now favour 'inreach' or liaison services to the general hospital wards often employing specialist nurses to great effect.

20.82.2 Treatment

The rapid expansion of memory assessment clinics, prompted by the enthusiasm following the licensing of the first cholinesterase inhibitor in 1997, has not been uniform across the UK. This has not only been based on lack of resources, although no additional funding was made available to provider trusts who would bear the costs of prescriptions and monitoring, but also on the traditional conservatism of the UK medical establishment who felt the evidence of efficacy was not sufficiently robust.

Some impetus to prescribe these treatments was given by the NICE guidelines although these have also provided hurdles. Their guidance suggested that treatment with one of the three licensed cholinesterase inhibitors should be made available to patients with mild to moderate Alzheimer's disease with Mini-Mental State Examination (MMSE) scores above 12, provided that the diagnosis had been made in secondary care and that treatment was monitored regularly by the specialist team or as part of a shared care protocol with primary care (NICE, 2001).

This advice has neither been justified scientifically nor implemented fully owing to the debate about whether the budgetary responsibility should fall to primary or secondary care. Although it was a laudable attempt to promote the rational use of these drugs, it has effectively removed the management of uncomplicated cognitive impairment from primary care where it must belong. The guidance has paradoxically complicated management and escalated costs, with the need to develop numerous specialist clinics to monitor the treatment, and has effectively deskilled GPs who now feel unable to take responsibility for what is quintessentially a primary care problem. Despite the introduction of the NSF for older persons, with its attempt to root out age discrimination, the NICE guidance has introduced a hurdle to the NHS treatment with a licensed drug for a common, disabling and distressing illness in older people unparalleled in any other age group. Its attempt to resolve the marked variations in availability across the country, up to four-fold differences in use, for which the term 'post code prescribing' was coined, has been unsuccessful. Prescription levels have increased overall but the geographical inequities remain. One benefit from the resultant infrastructure is that more patients with early Alzheimer's and younger onset cases are being assessed and the systems are now established to enable the utilization of new treatments as they evolve. It is interesting to note that the use of these treatments is much higher in Northern Ireland, which has combined health and social service boards and may reflect an understanding that the use of these drugs could provide savings in long-term care costs.

20.82.3 Community support

The increasing emphasis on community-based support has led most services towards a model based on community mental health teams (Coles *et al.*, 1991). These multidisciplinary teams usually comprising psychiatrist, CPN, social worker and occupational therapist, take a generic approach to the allocation of assessments at a team meeting, although the person designated as the key worker or care manager can call on the specialist advice of other team members as required. For most services the CPN is the team member most involved with continuing care and carer support for dementia patients. They often take on the role of liaising with primary care, social services and private community care and residential providers as well as accessing secondary care in the form of assessment or respite admissions. They often run carers' groups both as support and education and are usually able to respond quickly to avoid crises. Some services have now developed 24-hour services to allow continuity of care. Increasingly charities are involved in providing community support in terms of helplines, sitting services and advocacy programmes, which add considerably to the quality of the support provided by statutory services.

20.82.4 Day hospital and respite care

While day hospitals have a definite role in the initial assessment of dementia patients, continued attendance has often been criticized as being synonymous with day centre supportive care, providing social and diversional activities for the patient and respite for the carers. However, they provide skilled ongoing support for the increasing numbers of cases of dementia living in the community with high dependency needs and behavioural disturbance, who can be very disruptive in a day care facility, and they appear to identify and meet the needs of such patients (Rosenvinge, 1994; Howard, 1995; Ashaye *et al.*, 2003). Many patients had been offered planned regular respite admissions in hospital as part of a care package to enable carers to continue looking after their relative at home. However, there is increasing pressure on beds and respite is now limited to those patients whose continuing care needs cannot be met in residential settings. The lack of frequent regular respite has had the effect of increasing the number of patients requiring full-time care as carers give up, and many of these now ironically occupy the same short-term beds as a result of the lack of public funding of nursing home care beds.

20.83 INSTITUTIONAL CARE

20.83.1 Historical perspective

The advent of specialist services such as geriatrics and old age psychiatry shifted the emphasis from long-stay care towards acute care and rehabilitation. In old age psychiatry many long-stay wards were closed to support investments in community care and day hospitals. At that time there were very few nursing homes, and local authorities, then the major providers of residential care, were directing funding to sheltered housing and domiciliary support. The 1980s saw the private sector take on an increasing proportion of the provision of residential and nursing home care, with the financial costs picked up by Social Services, patients and their families with the heavy means testing mentioned earlier. Perverse incentives applied by the Thatcher government led to a massive increase in institutional care and starvation of community developments of the previous decade. It was also used as an opportunity for the NHS to withdraw heavily from its role in continuing care.

20.83.2 NHS and Community Care Act, 1990

Following criticism by the Audit Commission and new models such as the Kent Community Care Scheme, this important legislation (DHSS, 1990) attempted to redress the imbalance of the 1980s. It gave Social Services the responsibility for assessing need and commissioning appropriate care, with the emphasis on supporting people in their own homes where possible. Unfortunately inadequate funding and continued cost shifting by the NHS handicapped the efforts of Social Services' domiciliary provision and was slow to take off; the growth of 'warehousing' in residential care continued well into the 1990s. The low tariffs offered by Social Services have often resulted in poor quality and inadequate training by the private providers, a situation in which the continuing care of those with dementia tends to suffer most. This with a fall-off of capacity owing to unprofitability in the institutional sector has resulted in increasing resort to hospital admission when social care breaks down and then blocking of beds through delays in the care packages and placements necessary for discharge. The rising tide of blocked beds has caused much consternation to the Government as it contributes to problems in achieving targets on waiting times for elective procedures, such that from 2004 Social Services are being fined for 'bed blocking' that occurs in acute beds. At present such arrangements will not apply to delayed discharges from dementia assessment beds as they are not considered as acute.

20.83.3 Settings for long-term care

Changes described earlier in this section have led to an increasing proportion of people in residential homes suffering from dementia. Those residential care homes specializing in dementia care are often termed Elderly Mentally Infirm (EMI) homes. Most of these homes have responded well to the challenge of managing behavioural problems and fears of overreliance on sedative medication are not borne out by recent research (Lindesay *et al.*, 2003). At least 50 per cent of residents of non-EMI homes nevertheless have dementia. Research suggests that in these homes the recognition and skills in the management of dementia, even by registered general nurses, is often poor (Macdonald and Carpenter, 2003).

Those with the most difficult behaviour may need to receive ongoing care in an Old Age Psychiatry Unit or in an EMI nursing home environment. Since 1996 health and social services have had to produce jointly agreed criteria for those people entitled to receive free NHS continuing care (Department of Health, 1995). This process has accelerated a rapid decline in the number of NHS continuing care beds, though there is widespread variability in the existence of such beds from one health authority to another (Audit Commission, 2000). These often operate as medium stay units for patients with disturbed behaviour, often in the middle stages of their illness.

20.84 OPPORTUNITIES FOR THE FUTURE

A new millennium has continued to bring a frenetic pace of change to health services but, while the health service as a whole has started to receive real extra investment, little of this as yet has found itself directed towards dementia care. Fortunately old age psychiatry continues to expand as a specialty and appears an increasingly attractive career option for doctors choosing to work in mental health. The expansion in use of cholinesterase inhibitors and other drugs for dementia has changed the practice of old age psychiatry and exciting opportunities exist for further developments in this sphere. These factors, having coincided with increasingly responsible coverage of dementia issues in many areas of the national press, promise to make the next few years challenging but rewarding for all those who work in this important area.

REFERENCES

Ashaye OA, Livingston G, Orrell MW. (2003) Does standardised needs assessment improve the outcome of psychiatric day hospital care for older people? A randomised controlled trial. *Ageing and Mental Health* 7: 195–199

Audit Commission. (2000) *Forget me not – Mental health services for older people*. London, Audit Commission

Challis D, von Abendorff R, Brown P, Chesterman J, Hughes J. (2002) Care management, dementia care and specialist mental health services: an evaluation. *International Journal of Geriatric Psychiatry* 17: 315–325

Coles RG, von Abendorff R, Herzberg JL. (1991) The impact of a new community mental health team on an inner city psychogeriatric service. *International Journal of Geriatric Psychiatry* 6: 31–39

Department of Health. (1995) NHS *Responsibilities for Meeting Continuing Health Care Needs*. HSG(95)8, LAC(95)5. London, DoH

Department of Health. (2001) *National Service Framework for Older People*. London, HMSO

DHSS. (1990) National Health Service and Community Care Act. London: HMSO

Howard R. (1995) The place of day hospitals in old age psychiatry. *Current Opinion in Psychiatry* 8: 240–241

Lindesay J, Matthews R, Jagger C. (2003) Factors associated with antipsychotic drug use in residential care: changes between 1990 and 1997. *International Journal of Geriatric Psychiatry* 18: 511–519

Macdonald AJD and Carpenter GI. (2003) Recognition of dementia in non-EMI nursing home residents in SE England. *International Journal of Geriatric Psychiatry* 18: 105–108

National Institute for Clinical Excellence. (2001) *Guidance on the use of Donepezil, Rivastigmine and Galantamine for the Treatment of Alzheimer's Disease*. Technology Appraisal Guidance No 19. London, NICE

Rosenvinge HP. (1994) The role of the psychogeriatric day hospital. *Psychiatric Bulletin* 18: 733–736

Royal Commission on Long-term Care of the Elderly. (1999) *With Respect to Old age: Long-term Care – Rights and Responsibilities*. London, HMSO

20s

North America

ROBIN J CASTEN AND BARRY W ROVNER

Dementia is the most common psychiatric disorder of late life. It is characterized by progressive cognitive impairment, behavioural disturbances, and functional decline. Given the range and progression of symptoms over time, healthcare services for demented patients are varied and dynamic in order to respond to patients' changing needs.

An important goal of care is to optimize the time the patient is able to reside in the community while simultaneously minimizing the burden to caregivers and families (American Psychiatric Association, 1997). This is important as caregiver burden can have serious consequences for both the family and the patient. The substantial demands on time and energy, coupled with the reality that a family member will not get better, often lead to depression and/or ill health for care-givers. In extreme cases, this can lead to elder abuse and/or neglect. The following discussion describes various types of services, the population for which they are most appropriate, and the characteristics of ideal clinical programmes.

Regardless of type of service, quality clinical programmes share some common characteristics, the most important of which is the recognition that the management of dementia should address both physical and mental health. As other authors in this book indicate, there is a high rate of psychiatric symptoms among demented patients but many do not receive mental health services. Barriers include:

- a shortage of geriatric mental health professionals;
- a lack of training identifying and treating behavioural problems; and
- a lack of adequate reimbursement rates for mental health services.

A second characteristic of quality programmes is the use of non-pharmacological approaches to manage behavioural problems when possible, and to recognize the need for pharma-cological treatments when appropriate. Both are preferable to restraints, which are not only inhumane but do little to encourage positive social interactions and feelings of wellbeing.

Another characteristic of exemplary programmes is that their physical settings are conducive to the needs of demented people both with and without sensory impairments. Some people with dementia have a tendency to wander; environments in nursing homes, for example, that promote safety (e.g. secure boundaries), while at the same time allow patients freedom of mobility, are optimal. Further, colour coded rooms and hallways may help disorientated patients find their way, and furniture and fixtures in contrasting colours may help them navigate safely.

A final attribute of optimal clinical programmes is the involvement of the family in care planning. Families are an invaluable source of data for the physician as they can provide detailed information about patients' histories and responses to previous interventions. Conversely, information should flow the other way as well; physicians can educate families about the disorder's progressive nature so that they can adequately plan for future care and have reasonable expectancies.

20.85 CARE FOR COMMUNITY–DWELLING PATIENTS

Services for patients living in the community can serve as a bridge between independence and institutionalization. They can give caregivers peace of mind with respect to the care and safety of their demented relatives, while allowing them the freedom to attend to other aspects of their lives. Further, in many instances, patients are able to continue living in their homes, affording them the comfort of being in familiar surroundings. There are two types of services for community-dwelling patients: in-home services and adult day care (see Zarit *et al.*, 1999 for a review).

20.85.1   In-home services

In-home care is a general term referring to a multitude of services (e.g. housekeeping, companionship) that are provided in the home. Their overall goal is to provide assistance with tasks of daily living or respite care so caregivers can have some relief from care duties. Specific services can consist of home-delivered meals, nursing care, homemaker services, occupational therapy, transportation services and companionship.

There are several problems with in-home services. First, they are underused by minorities, low-income people, those without families, and people living in rural areas (Advisory panel on Alzheimer's Disease, 1996). Ironically, these individuals are often those who have the greatest need for assistance. Accessibility is a major barrier to care since services are simply not available in areas where these individuals are likely to reside (e.g. poverty stricken areas and rural areas). Services are most likely to be solicited by family members since dementia often renders people incapable of seeking care. Thus socially isolated people are not likely to be recipients of in-home services. Clearly, outreach programmes that target demented people who are socially and/or geographically isolated are needed. One such programme, Gatekeepers, relies on referrals from unconventional sources (e.g. utility companies, postal workers) to identify older people living alone who may be in need of services (Florio *et al.*, 1996).

Another problem with in-home services is the employment of unskilled personnel. When an agency is being selected to provide in-home care, it is essential that licensing requirements, intensity and type of training, and background checks be specified. In-home care is also problematic because it can be quite costly. Finally, because it often has poor linkages to other services, appropriate referrals are unlikely to be made. In fact, there is no evidence that in-home services delay or prevent nursing home placement (Cohen, 1991).

In sum, in-home services can provide a useful service for both patients and their families. However, it is important that families thoroughly investigate the qualifications of staff, and do not rely on in-home care as the sole source of information and care. In-home services are probably best viewed as an adjunct to more comprehensive care.

20.85.2   Adult day care

Adult day care is an attractive option for older people who are able to live in the community yet are not capable of functioning

independently. There are two general models of care: medical and social. Medical programmes provide rehabilitation and other medical care, while social programmes focus on social functioning and recreation. In general, day care provides a structured and safe environment where patients receive cognitive and social stimulation. Patients may receive psychological counselling (either individually or in a group) to help them adjust to the dementia, and to provide emotional support. Many centres allow families to arrange for ancillary services such as transportation, personal care, respite care and rehabilitation therapy.

Quality day care programmes employ adequately trained staff with a staff/patient ratio of 1:7. At least some staff members should be qualified to dispense and manage medication. Nursing services should also be available, and there should be special protocols for incontinent patients. The activities should be planned and overseen by an experienced activities coordinator. The activity schedule should include both individual and group level activities. Since some patients, especially those who are depressed, may have little motivation to participate in activities, staff should strongly encourage patient involvement. At least one meal is provided daily at day care centres, so special diets should be available, and staff should be on hand to assist with eating.

For the most part, research evaluating the effects of day care has noted positive outcomes for both patients and their caregivers (see Gaugler and Zarit, 2002 for a thorough review). With respect to patients, while overall day care does not appear to lead to improved functional outcomes, it does have positive effects on subjective well being. Day care can also benefit caregivers. Zarit *et al.* (1998) compared caregivers of patients who used adult day care to caregivers whose family members did not. Caregivers whose family members were enrolled in day care for at least 3 months for at least 2 days per week reported less stress, less depression, and lower feelings of overload compared to control caregivers. It is important to note that the positive effects for caregivers are only apparent when services are used frequently and consistently.

The biggest problem with adult day care is a shortage of services. There are currently 4000 programmes available, but approximately 10 000 are needed. Lack of transportation is another obstacle to care. Finally, adult day care is not funded by Medicare, and all costs are absorbed by the patient or families. Daily costs can range from $US50 to $US180.

20.86   CARE FOR NON-COMMUNITY-DWELLING ADULTS

For demented adults with severe cognitive impairment, or co-morbid physical or psychiatric disease, residing in the community may not be feasible. For these patients there are three types of care: adult foster care homes, assisted living, and nursing homes.

20.86.1 Adult foster care homes

Adult foster care homes are state-regulated, small sites that provide supervised housing for demented adults. There are currently 60 000 such homes available. Care at the homes is family oriented, and patients have the opportunity to interact with other people. The major problem with foster care is that most homes are not licensed and personnel are not highly trained, creating a situation where abuse and/or inadequate care can flourish. Further, there is a lack of federal guidelines regulating such homes (Advisory Panel on Alzheimer's Disease, 1996).

20.86.2 Assisted living

Assisted living is any residential programme that is not licensed as a nursing home, yet is equipped to respond to needs for assistance (e.g. tasks of daily living). Patients usually reside in congregate apartment-like settings where they live alone or with a spouse, and they are able to bring their own furnishings. Meals may or may not be eaten in a dining hall-like setting. A great deal of autonomy is available, and only needed services are purchased (e.g. meal preparation, house-keeping, transportation). This can be an ideal arrangement for patients who desire a certain degree of privacy and are capable of some independence. Further, as the dementia progresses, additional services are available so that changing needs for assistance are met.

20.86.3 Nursing homes

Severely demented adults usually reside in nursing homes. In 1995, there were 1.8 million nursing home beds in the United States, and half of all patients were demented. Fifty per cent of the demented residents are over age 85, and 75 per cent are female. Many are incontinent. Greater than one-third have psychiatric symptoms, and over half exhibit behavioural problems.

The major problem with nursing homes is that they are modelled after standard medical hospitals, and are thus unlikely to provide adequate psychiatric care (Rovner et al., 1996). Consequently, dementia and other psychiatric disorders (e.g. depression, delirium) are often undiagnosed. Staff are usually not knowledgeable about dementia and how to manage its associated behavioural problems. According to a report issued by the Office of Technology Assessment (1992), these issues are manifested in a lack of continuity of care, no provision of space to wander, inappropriate levels and type of stimulation, and the encouragement of patient dependency on staff. Nursing home patients are also likely to be over-medicated with psychoactive drugs, which can have profound side effects (Avorn et al., 1992).

A recent trend in nursing home care is the implementation of Special Care Units (SCUs), which are self-contained units housed within nursing homes. While there are no agreed-upon criteria as to what constitutes an SCU, care is usually specialized and individualized to meet the needs of demented patients. Patients' strengths are identified and elicited, reversible medical and psychiatric disorders are treated, and behavioural disorders are viewed as a product of patient/nurse/environment interactions rather than the disease (Rovner, 1994; Rovner et al., 1996). Patients are usually free to wander and there are fewer patients per staff member than is typically found in a nursing home.

Research regarding the benefits of SCUs are mixed, in part because of a lack of uniformity concerning what constitutes an SCU. Among the more favourable findings were that SCU patients were less likely to experience functional decline after 1 year compared to a control group comprising demented nursing home residents (Rovner et al., 1990). Further, SCU patients were more inclined to participate in activities, and less prone to have behaviour problems, be restrained or receive antipsychotics (Rovner et al., 1996; Bellelli et al., 1998). SCU patients are also less likely to have falls (Rovner et al., 1990). Other research found less favourable results. For example, Phillips et al. (1997) found that SCU placement did not lead to slower functional decline.

It should be noted that it is impossible to apply rigorous clinical trial methodology to the study of SCUs (i.e. residents cannot be randomized to an SCU versus a non-SCU), and this could account for discrepant findings. In addition, there is a lack of standardization concerning what constitutes an SCU, and this too could account for conflicting results. In theory, SCUs should possess the following characteristics:

- assessment and diagnosis;
- staff specialization and education;
- minimal restraint use;
- flexible care routines; and
- specialized environmental design.

In an attempt to determine the extent to which SCUs actually possess these ideal characteristics, Chappell and Reid (2000) examined 510 institutionalized Canadian residents. The sample represented 77 care facilities, and 51 per cent of the sample were residing in an SCU. Results indicated that SUCs were no more likely than traditional units to possess these characteristics. In a similar study of long-term care facilities in Arkansas, very few SCUs met all of the requirements for an SCU as mandated by state legislature (Gerdner and Beck, 2001). In theory, SCUs appear to be a viable alternative to nursing home care for the severely demented patient. However, placement should be done with the caveat that many SCUs do not meet the requirements of an exemplary unit.

20.87 SERVICES FOR BOTH COMMUNITY AND NON–COMMUNITY-DWELLING PATIENTS

Three types of services, case management, inpatient geriatric psychiatry units and dementia clinics, are used by patients presenting with a range of cognitive decline.

20.87.1 Case management

Case management attempts to aid clients and families negotiate the fragmented and institutionally based United States long-term care system. The basic components of case management include identifying the target population, screening assessment, care planning, linkage to services, monitoring, advocacy and reassessment. While case management for long-term care became popular in the 1970s to provide chronically ill elderly with adequate access to appropriate and reasonably priced community-based services, its focus has shifted. More recently it has evolved into a gatekeeping mechanism for containing healthcare expenses. Several studies have demonstrated that case management services for the elderly can be cost effective (Eggert and Brodows, 1984). The services can be provided by public agencies, but more recently, private for-profit firms have proliferated.

Various legislative proposals addressing the long-term care system for the elderly have been introduced. For example, the Elder-Care, Long-term Care Assistance Act of 1988 provides assistance for a full range of home care and adult day care services, and expands benefits for nursing home care. While there is considerable variation as to the type of organization that should be providing case management, some common themes emerge. Among them is that case management should be provided for persons who are limited in two to three activities of daily living (ADL) and or need substantial supervision due to mental/cognitive problems. It appears that the evolving case management system will play an increasing important role in the long-term care of individuals with dementia in the future.

20.87.2 Inpatient geriatric psychiatry units

Demented patients often experience comorbid psychiatric illnesses and symptoms. Mental health problems among demented people include agitation (55 per cent), depressive symptoms (42 per cent), hallucinations/delusions (33 per cent), sleep disorder (26 per cent), and weight loss or anorexia (22 per cent). These disorders frequently necessitate admission to an inpatient geriatric psychiatry unit (Rabins and Nicholson, 1991). The primary goals of hospitalization are:

- the assessment and provision of safety;
- treatment of psychiatric symptoms that may be contributing to excess disability; and
- the monitoring of such treatment.

Demented patients may exhibit suicidal and/or violent thoughts or behaviours. A psychiatric unit provides a safe environment where patients can express their thoughts and feelings, while at the same time reducing the risk of harm to self or others. Electroconvulsive therapy (ECT) is occasionally used to treat depression in demented patients. The invasive nature of this procedure requires that it be performed on an inpatient basis. Further, prescribing of several antidepressants

needs to be closely monitored, and this is best accomplished when the patient is an inpatient. Finally, psychiatric illness can worsen or exacerbate existing dementia, so a thorough neurological assessment is often warranted to identify and treat any comorbid psychiatric conditions. For example, among older people, depression can be manifested as a mild dementia, and depression treatment may improve cognitive function. Some easily treatable or manageable diseases (e.g. thyroid disease, syphilis) may cause symptoms of dementia, and a complete diagnostic evaluation can identify these conditions. In fact, a recent study found that 34 per cent of inpatients had a previously unknown illness at admission (Perry et al., 1995). In sum, a geriatric psychiatry unit provides an opportunity for close monitoring and assessment so that psychiatrists and other professionals trained in geriatrics can determine the most appropriate treatment needs.

Few studies have examined the impact of inpatient units for dementia. One recent study examined 15 patients admitted to an inpatient unit for an average of 2 weeks to treat agitation and disruptive behaviours. Results showed that most of the patients exhibited less agitation at discharge (Wiener et al., 2001).

20.87.3 Dementia clinics

Accurate clinical diagnosis of all individuals with suspected dementia is essential given the multiplicity of medical and psychiatric conditions that may mimic dementing syndromes.

Dementia clinics have existed more or less in the United States for about 10–15 years and provide a multidisciplinary assessment of the patient and family. Clinics of this nature can both facilitate entry to the dementia care system and be a resource for optimal long-term management. It appears, however, that they select for patients whose cognitive deficits are complicated by emotional or behavioural problems and whose conditions are of significant duration. Coyne and associates (1990) found that the average age of clients coming to their clinic was 73.16, and that symptoms of cognitive impairment had been displayed for 4.2 years. It appears that less than 10 per cent of referrals are living in health-related facilities at the time of evaluation (Larson et al., 1984; Coyne et al., 1990), with the overwhelming majority living at home or with relatives. Not surprisingly given this data, family members prove to be the most common source of referral (Larson et al., 1984; Coyne et al., 1990).

The majority of patients receive a standard examination battery. Components include patient history, past medical history, complete physical and neurological examination, comprehensive blood work (including measurements of blood counts, electrolytes, thyroid function, blood urea nitrogen, creatinine, B_{12}, folic acid, sedimentation rate, and serological test for syphilis and urinalysis). Additionally, electrocardiography, electroencephalography and neuroimaging studies are routinely done in the United States. Psychometric tests, including the Mini-Mental State Exam (MMSE), and the

Boston Naming Test are frequently used. Additional neuropsychological testing as well as lumbar puncture are performed when clinically indicated. While the National Institute of Aging task force recommends this extensive and expensive evaluative process, a number of investigators have advocated a selective approach to diagnostic testing. Larson and colleagues (1986) found that a careful history and physical exam accompanied by complete blood cell count, chemistry battery and a thyroid function test are effective in diagnosing treatable illness causing cognitive impairment. Larson and associates (1986) likewise found that most patients could be diagnosed with careful bedside evaluations and a few screening tests.

Dementia evaluation centres are of diagnostic value, providing relatives, and where appropriate patients, with clear comprehensive information about diagnosis and prognosis. More often, however, working with families to plan appropriate short-term and long-term management of the demented individual proves to be the clinic's primary responsibility.

REFERENCES

Advisory Panel on Alzheimer's Disease. (1996) *Alzheimer's Disease and Related Dementias: Acute and Long-Term Care Services.* US Government Printing Office, Washington DC

American Psychiatric Association. (1997) Practice Guidelines for the treatment of patients with Alzheimer's disease and other dementias of late life. *American Journal of Psychiatry* **154**: 1–39

Avorn J, Soumerai S, Everitt D *et al.* (1992) A randomized trial of a program to reduce the use of psychoactive drugs in nursing homes. *New England Journal of Medicine* **327**: 168–173

Bellelli G, Frisoni GB, Bianchetti A *et al.* (1998) Special care units for demented populations: A multicenter study. *The Gerontologist* **38**: 456–462

Chappell NL and Reid RC. (2000) Dimensions of care for dementia sufferers in long-term care institutions: Are they related to outcomes? *Journal of Gerontology: Social Sciences* **55B**: S234–S240

Cohen C. (1991) Integrated community services. In: J Sadavoy, L Lazarud, L Jarvik (eds), *Comprehensive Review of Geriatric Psychiatry.* Washington DC, American Psychiatric Press, pp. 613–634

Coyne A, Meade H, Petrone M. (1990) The diagnosis of dementia: demographic characteristics. *The Gerontologist* **30**: 339–344

Eggert G and Brodows B. (1984) Five years of ACCESS: What have we learned. In: R Zawadski (ed.), *Community-Based Systems of Long-Term Care.* New York, Haworth Press, pp. 27–48

Florio ER, Rockwood TH, Hendryx MS, Jensen JE, Raschko R, Dyck DG. (1996) A model gatekeeper program to find the at-risk elderly. *Journal of Case Management* **5**: 106–114

Gaugler JE and Zarit SH. (2001) The effectiveness of adult day services for disabled older people. *Journal of Aging and Social Policy* **12**: 23–47

Gerdner LA and Beck CK. (2001) Statewide survey to compare services provided for residents with dementia in special care units and non-special care units. *American Journal of Alzheimer's Disease and Other Dementias* **5**: 289–295

Larson E, Reifler B, Featherstone H, English D. (1984) Dementia in elderly outpatients: A prospective study. *Annuals of Internal Medicine* **100**: 417–423

Larson E, Reifler B, Sumi S. (1986) Diagnostic tests in the evaluation of dementia. *Archives of Internal Medicine* **146**: 1917–1922

Perry DW, Milner E, Kirshman VHR. (1995) Physical morbidity in a group of patients referred to a psychogeriatric unit: A 6-month prospective study. *International Journal of Geriatric Psychiatry* **10**: 151–154

Phillips CD, Sloane PD, Hawes C *et al.* (1997) Effects of residence in Alzheimer's Disease Special Care Units on functional outcomes. *JAMA* **278**: 1340–1344

Rabins P and Nicholson M. (1991) Acute psychiatric hospitalization of patents with irreversible dementia. *International Journal of Geriatric Psychiatry* **6**: 209–211

Rovner BW. (1994) What is therapeutic about special care units?: The role of psychosocial rehabilitation. *Alzheimer Disease and Associated Disorders* **8**: S355–S359

Rovner BW, Lucas-Blaustein J, Folstein MF, Smith SW. (1990) Stability over one year in patients admitted to a nursing home dementia unit. *International Journal of Geriatric Psychiatry* **5**: 77–82

Rovner BW, Steele CD, Shmuely Y, Folstein MF. (1996) A randomised trial of dementia care in nursing homes. *Journal of the American Geriatrics Society* **44**: 7–13

US Congress, Office of Technology Assessment. (1992) *Special Care Units for People with Alzheimer's Disease and Other Dementias: Consumer Education, Research Regulatory, and Reimbursement Issues.* Washington, DC, US Government Printing Office.

Wiener PK, Kiosses DN, Klimstra S, Murphy C, Alexopoulos G. (2001) A short-term inpatient program for agitated demented nursing home residents. *International Journal of Geriatric Psychiatry* **16**: 866–872

Zarit SH, Stephens MAP, Townsend A, Greene R. (1998) Stress reduction for family caregivers: Effects of adult day care use. *Journal of Gerontology Social Science* **53B**: S6–S77

Zarit SH, Gaugler JE, Jarrot SE. (1999) Useful services for families: Research findings and directions. *International Journal of Geriatric Psychiatry* **14**: 165–181

21

Services for younger people with dementia

ROBERT C BALDWIN AND MICHELLE MURRAY

According to the Alzheimer's Society (AS) in the United Kingdom (UK), there are approximately 18 500 younger people with dementia (Alzheimer's Society, 2001). For the purpose of this chapter 'young' is defined as less than 65 years of age. The needs of these individuals do not readily fit into existing health and social care systems. As numbers are small, their needs tend to be invisible to planners. Even those who receive care find the services fragmented. Unmet need has led to a 'declaration of rights' for younger people with dementia from one of the pioneering services in Merseyside, UK. This is reproduced in Box 21.1. Although quite old, it has formed the basis for several innovative services and is the basis for the principles of service development to be outlined (Alzheimer's Society, 2001).

21.1 EPIDEMIOLOGY

Table 21.1 illustrates the findings from two epidemiological studies of young-onset Alzheimer's disease (AD) in the UK, one in Scotland (McGonigal *et al.*, 1993) and the other in the North of England (Newens *et al.*, 1993). The latter authors calculated a point-prevalence of 34.6 per 100 000 for AD in the age band 45–64. They also estimated a further 11.7 per 100 000 for vascular dementia (VaD) and 7.0 per 100 000 for other forms of dementia. The latter included alcohol-related dementia, traumatic brain damage, frontotemporal dementia, Creutzfeld–Jakob disease, multisystem failure, cerebral tumour

and normal pressure hydrocephalus. There are other causes not included or not found in these studies:

- Huntington's disease, a genetic disorder with a peak incidence of symptoms between the ages of 30–45, has important diagnostic implications as predictive testing is possible and protocols for this are available (Cetnarskyj and Porteous, 1999). AIDS-related dementia poses special demands for multi-agency working (Murray, 2003).
- Prion disease is a recent highly publicized cause of early-onset dementia (although very uncommon).
- Dementia in Down's syndrome will become more common as patients with learning disability age (Neary and Snowden, 2003). It is estimated that 13 per cent of people with a learning disability develop dementia, rising to 22 per cent in those aged 65 years (Cooper, 1999).
- Alcohol-related dementia remains a controversial entity although undeniably excess alcohol consumption causes multiple handicaps, including cognitive impairment (Crowe, 1999).

It is important to have accurate estimates of non-AD causes of dementia when planning new services. In a study, which did not focus on AD alone (Harvey, 1998), the latter accounted for less than 50 per cent of all cases of young-onset dementia. Of importance, frontotemporal dementia was the third most common form of dementia, after VaD, with a similar prevalence to alcohol-related dementia.

In summary, taking into account all causes of dementia, in an area serviced by an average primary care trust in England

Box 21.1 *Declaration of rights for younger people with dementia**

- *Full informed medical assessment.* General practitioners should have the relevant skills to recognize the symptoms of dementia in all age groups and be aware of the need to refer on to appropriate consultants
- *Recognition of the need for specialist services.* Identification of consultants with special responsibilities for this group of people who will make a diagnosis where possible and from whom caregivers are entitled to ongoing medical supervision
- *After diagnosis* people with dementia and their caregivers should have access to the following services organized on at least a subregional basis:
  - *specialist day care services* organized in a flexible way so that caregivers can continue to work. The aim should be for appropriate stimulation with an emphasis on constructive occupational therapy for those who are able to benefit from it and, for those who cannot, diversional activities. Within the service should be properly funded resource centres providing comprehensive and accurate information and counselling, and support for caregivers with a drop-in facility
  - *appropriate residential care* when required – not elderly persons' homes or acute psychiatric establishments
  - *implementation of care management* so that services are assessed at the time of need, enabling a progressive build-up of care as the person's health deteriorates
- *Access to welfare benefits.* Easy access to welfare benefits currently available plus some benefits:
  - *a specialist caregiver's benefit*
  - *a benefit equivalent to Disability Living Allowance* (mobility component) payable to people with dementia irrespective of age
  - *universal acceptance of Alzheimer's as a 'terminal' illness irrespective of age*
  - *money* to provide care for the person in the community on the scale now available to pay for residential care
- *Retrospective reinstatement of rights and benefits* for people who have had to terminate their employment either voluntarily or through dismissal and who have later been diagnosed as having dementia and who have consequently been discriminated against. Employers should be directed to recognize dementia as a reason for early retirement so that pension rights and other benefits are not affected
- *Appropriate training and information* to be made available at all levels for public and professionals alike, including general practitioners

*This declaration was originally prepared for and on behalf of people with dementia under pensionable age in the Mersey Regional Health Authority (February, 1991)

Table 21.1 *Estimated age and prevalence of young onset Alzheimer's disease in two studies from the UK*

Age range	Prevalence per 100 000	
	Scotland[1]	Northern Region[2]
40–44	1.4	0
45–49	8.1	2.4
50–54	27.6	11.8
55–59	39.7	35.6
60–64	37.8	87.3

[1] McGonigal *et al.* (1993)
[2] Newens *et al.* (1993)

(about 100–150 000 individuals), there will be between 75–100 patients with young-onset (age of onset under 65 years) dementia. In the UK specialist mental health trusts serve populations upward of 1 million, with correspondingly larger predicted numbers. The main diagnoses in young-onset dementia are AD, VaD, frontotemporal dementia and alcohol-related dementia.

21.2 THE NEED FOR A SERVICE

The epidemiological data above demonstrate that the number of younger people with dementia is miniscule in proportion to the 500 000 or so people in all with dementia in the UK, the majority of whom are elderly. Why then should effort be expended developing specialist services? There are three main reasons.

- The diagnosis of young-onset dementia is complex and specialized.
- The needs of people with dementia in younger adult life are largely unmet and differ from older persons with dementia.
- National policy is important. In England and Wales the *National Service Framework for Older People* (Department of Health, 2001) proposes that Old Age Psychiatry take a strategic lead for this patient group, a position supported by the Royal College of Psychiatrists (Royal College of Psychiatrists, 2001).

21.2.1 Diagnosis and assessment

The causes of early-onset senile dementia include diagnoses that psychiatrists rarely encounter, such as prion diseases and multisystem failure. The spectrum of diagnoses of dementia in younger people differs from that in old age. For example, frontotemporal dementia, which often presents with behavioural problems, may account for 20 per cent of young-onset dementias but is rare in later life (Neary *et al.*, 1988). Diagnosing dementia in younger people is complex and requires a team with specialist skills, including neurological, neuroimaging and neuropsychological evaluation. Access to genetic counselling for conditions such as Huntington's disease, familial Alzheimer's disease (which usually has an onset in mid-life) and frontotemporal dementia are essential. Varma *et al.* (2002) showed that in three dementias occurring in relatively younger patients (Alzheimer's disease, VaD and frontotemporal dementia) diagnostic accuracy using a combination of magnetic resonance imaging (MRI) and single photon emission computed tomography (SPECT) was very high. This is different from late-onset dementias where mixed pathology and medical co-morbidity make diagnostic precision harder.

A major complaint by caregivers is the inordinate time to diagnosis, over 3 years in one study (Luscombe *et al.*, 1998). In research conducted in the 1990s, which compared the diagnostic practices of two teaching hospital departments, one in neurology and the other geriatric psychiatry, it was found that the neurology department, which specialized in the diagnosis of presenile dementia, conducted a much more comprehensive medical assessment than did the old age psychiatry department. Those referred to the neurology service were more than twice as likely to receive detailed neuropsychological testing. The rates for neuroimaging were likewise double those of the geriatric psychiatry service (Allen and Baldwin, 1995). In the study of Luscombe *et al.* (1998), better diagnostic accuracy was achieved by neurologists when compared to that by psychiatrists. The contemporary picture remains far from ideal, with evidence that neurologists are still more complete diagnosticians while old age psychiatrists are better at involving support services, organizing follow up and prescribing antidementia treatment (Cordery *et al.*, 2002). Perhaps the optimum model is for a neurologist and a psychiatrist to work together. There are examples of this in practice (Allen and Baldwin, 1995; Ferran *et al.*, 1996).

The audit of Allen and Baldwin (1995) took place when neuroimaging was hardly available to psychiatrists. Improvements in old age psychiatry services, better training of old age psychiatrists and markedly improved access to brain imaging by psychiatrists means that some psychiatric services are perfectly competent to make a diagnosis of dementia in younger people. Also, the arrival of the antidementia drugs (currently donepezil, rivastigmine, galantamine and memantime) has been an impetus to old age psychiatrists to improve diagnostic accuracy. In a given geographical locality clinicians from the specialties of neurology and psychiatry should develop their own protocols to enable a competent assessment of a younger person presenting with dementia. These should include how to access a range of diagnostic services, including genetic counselling and must be able to offer advice about fitness to drive a motor vehicle.

Another major area of development since the previous edition of this book is the Memory Clinic (Lindesay *et al.*, 2002). Although these have arisen largely in response to the growing demand for cholinesterase inhibitors they are often sufficiently well resourced to undertake the specialist assessment of a range of cognitive disorders including dementia of younger adulthood (Lindesay *et al.*, 2002). They have the added advantage of reducing the stigma attached to the terms dementia and psychiatry.

Lastly, a common diagnostic error is to overlook an affective disorder in a younger person with memory problems (Nott and Fleminger, 1975; Ferran *et al.*, 1996). This should not be forgotten.

21.2.2 The needs of young people with dementia and their caregivers

In England a person with young-onset Alzheimer's disease may receive outpatient care from a neurologist, a social worker from the social services adult mental health team, psychiatric nursing support from the provider adult mental health team, day care and respite care from the social services elderly team and continuing (long-term) care from an old age psychiatrist. A similar person in his or her 70s will receive a 'package' of care delivered by an old age psychiatry team, with one person named as the care coordinator with responsibility for coordinating services under the Care Programme Approach (Department of Health, 1999). This inconsistency in management underpins the need for a specialist service.

A common myth is that younger people with dementia die quickly thus obviating the need for elaborate 'packages' of community care. In a study by Newens *et al.* (1995), of 109 subjects, the median survival time from onset to death was over 9 years; 57 per cent were still living at home 5 years from the date of survey, which contradicts this view. Moreover, of those who remained at home 20 per cent required some assistance in each of six areas of activity of daily living.

There have been a few surveys specifically of need of patients with young-onset dementia and of their caregivers. Baldwin (1994) in a survey of 44 patients, the majority in the community, found higher morbidity from non-cognitive symptoms (aggression, wandering, delusions and hallucinations) than from cognitive impairment, as assessed by the Clifton Assessment Procedures for the Elderly (CAPE) (Pattie and Gilleard, 1979). Other studies have confirmed this (Sperlinger and Furst, 1994; Delany and Rosenvinge, 1995; Harvey, 1998), the importance being that non-cognitive symptoms have a direct impact on increasing perceived burden in caregivers (Harvey, 1998; Ballard *et al.*, 2001). Stress among caregivers is very high (Baldwin, 1994; Delany and Rosenvinge, 1995; Luscombe *et al.*, 1998). Harvey (1998) found that anxiety and depression were the most typical symptoms of stress and that females were most affected. The type of dementia did not appear to influence the degree of stress.

Financial hardship is very common and often not recognized (Harvey, 1998). In surveys that have asked about employment status (Baldwin, 1994; Sperlinger and Furst, 1994; Delany and Rosenvinge, 1995), nearly all those with dementia were unemployed. In the survey of Sperlinger and Furst (1994), three-quarters had to give up their jobs because of their dementia. Lastly, younger people with dementia tend to be relatively physically fit, unlike patients accessing old age psychiatry services.

21.3 THE ECONOMIC BURDEN

Harvey (1998) conducted an economic analysis of the costs of young-onset dementia. The average community costs were £1560 per patient, whereas for those who were in residential or nursing home care it was £20 924. The costs overall were higher per patient than have been estimated for older people with dementia and this effect was accounted for by the younger patients using more residential or nursing home care. While one cannot read too much into these findings, the implication is that better community care may reduce or delay the need for institutionalization, thereby lowering overall costs.

21.4 PRINCIPLES OF SERVICE DEVELOPMENT

Drawing upon the studies summarized above, when caregivers are asked what they would like, better coordination of services, welfare and benefits advice, day care and respite, including respite in the home are regularly requested. In reality these needs are not met. Baldwin (1994), Delany and Rosenvinge (1995), Newens *et al.* (1995) and Cordery *et al.* (2002) found that the most common support offered was a visit from a community psychiatric nurse (CPN), but only for fewer than half of those surveyed. In these studies availability of and contact with social workers was minimal.

The epidemiological data summarized in Table 21.1 illustrate an important point of relevance in service planning. The majority of people with young-onset Alzheimer's disease are in the age range of 50–64 years. Harvey (1998) has calculated that there are only 2500 individuals with AD in the UK under the age of 50. This poses difficulties for a service that is attempting to meet the needs of such a wide age range. The offspring of the youngest are likely to be teenagers whereas the older patients are likely to have offspring who themselves are approaching middle age.

In the UK the Faculty of Old Age Psychiatry of the Royal College of Psychiatrists has proposed guidelines for planning services for younger people with dementia (Box 21.2). These place a responsibility on purchasers of social care and health to develop specific contracts for the care of younger people with dementia and their caregivers in areas covering upward of half a million. It is important that neurological and psychiatric services collaborate and that relevant caregiver organizations are consulted. One way to start a service is to identify a lead psychiatrist, a community psychiatric nurse and a named person to provide a link with social services. In England the *National Service Framework for Older People* specifies that old age psychiatric services should take the lead (Department of Health, 2001). However, this will require additional funds.

Large numbers of beds in institutions was not a priority for caregivers in the surveys cited earlier. However, Harvey (1998) has calculated that there is a need for 10 residential or

---

> **Box 21.2** *Summary of recommendations from the Royal College of Psychiatrists**
>
> - Purchasing agencies should have specific contractual arrangements for a specialized service for younger people with dementia, and a named consultant with special responsibility and sessions over and above that available for older patients with dementia.
> - In each area there should be one named consultant, often an old age psychiatrist, responsible for the service, drawing from a population base of 500 000.
> - Close collaboration with neurology and neuropsychiatry for accurate diagnosis is needed.
> - For a population of 500 000 a specialist multidisciplinary team is justified. For smaller populations a named community health nurse is needed, while each local authority should have a named social worker.
> - Relevant caregiver and voluntary organizations should be involved in planning.
> - Initial service development should focus on diagnostic and community services. Specialist services should only be developed where traditional services are deficient.
> - A comprehensive service comprises the above plus day and respite care and long-stay care, with provision separate to that for older people with dementia.
>
> *The Royal College of Psychiatrists, 2001

nursing home places per 100 000 population at risk; enough for a small unit, or for a contracting arrangement between a number of purchasers and a provider with specialist expertise.

The needs of younger people with dementia are best met by a small multidisciplinary team comprising input from a consultant psychiatrist, mental health nurse or nurses, an occupational therapist, psychologist and social worker, with additional services as required by speech and language therapist, podiatrist, physiotherapist, etc. The team should ideally have its own community support workers. Such a team can offer outreach in to the home, day care and access to respite resources, ideally in a special facility and will serve a population of approximately half a million. The roles and tasks of the specialist multidisciplinary team have recently been described by Baldwin and Murray (2003).

21.5 GENERIC VERSUS SPECIALIST SERVICES

The Royal College of Psychiatrists cautions against overdevelopment of specialist services. Wherever possible it is best to make full use of existing age-appropriate services, such as home helps, welfare and benefits advice, etc. The principle should be to optimize cooperation and collaboration across existing statutory and other services. The latter include not only social services and the voluntary sector but also child support agencies, child and adolescent psychiatric services and family therapy services (Garrod, 2003; Murray, 2003).

Box 21.3 *Preliminary data for planning a service*

- Estimate local prevalence
- Estimate diagnostic heterogeneity (e.g. alcoholic and vascular dementia)
- Identify lead consultant
- Identify lead nurse
- Identify local relevant resources (e.g. welfare and benefits advice)

Box 21.4 *Practical issues in planning a service for younger people with dementia*

- Single point of access
- Clear arrangement and protocols about who makes the diagnosis
- Right of access to all existing relevant services
- Care coordination by a key worker
- Access to a reasonable range of specific services
- Clear protocols for respite care
- Clear protocols for emergency psychiatric admission

21.6 PLANNING SERVICES

In the last edition of this book we recommended that each locality conduct a survey to estimate prevalence and need. The advent of good quality epidemiological data means that accurate estimates can be made without doing this (Box 21.3). In the UK the Alzheimer's Society offers web-based information about need in specific localities (Alzheimer's Society, 2001; www.alzheimerers.org.uk). However, diagnoses can vary from area to area; for example in Baldwin's (1994) study there were more cases of VaD and alcohol-related dementia than there were of AD. This is probably because the location was a deprived inner city area. Likewise, local resources, some of which may be relevant to those with young-onset dementia, can vary enormously. If it is thought necessary to garner more detailed estimates of need, this can be crudely ascertained by conducting a survey of local specialists in the fields of psychiatry, neurology, medicine, trauma, rehabilitation and neurosurgery. Local social service offices can also be approached. The neuroimaging department may also have a register with information about diagnoses as well as age. Some specialist organizations such as the Huntington's society and Headway (a head injury charity in the UK) may also be of help. Lastly, it is relatively easy and cheap in the UK to conduct a postal survey of general practitioners.

Box 21.4 summarizes some of the practical issues which must be addressed before setting up a new service. A single point of access must be organized. Agreement must be reached about how a diagnosis is to be made and by whom, with protocols for respite care and acute admission on psychiatric grounds. Given that the patients are quite fit physically, an old age psychiatric ward may not be the best place to admit a disturbed younger person with dementia and there should be an agreed protocol addressing where such patients should be admitted and under whose care.

21.7 CARE FOR CAREGIVERS

Luscombe *et al.* (1998) conducted a survey of 102 caregivers of patients with young-onset dementia. They describe the plight of the typical caregiver as: 'an harassed person, beset by psychological problems, financial worries, loss of employment and family conflicts'. Those most distressed were young females caring for male patients and children caring for a parent.

CANDID (Counselling and Diagnosis in Dementia) (Harvey *et al.*, 1998) has been established at the National Hospital for Neurology and Neurosurgery, London. The aims of CANDID are to increase accessibility to advice, diagnosis and counselling for the person with a young-onset dementia, their caregivers and other health professionals. CANDID also offers information and education to increase the general awareness of the needs of the younger person with dementia for nurses, doctors, social workers and others working within this specialized area. The service is available on the Internet (http://dementia.ion.ucl.ac.uk/DRG_Website/Candid/welcome_to_the_candid_home_page.htm). Another site offering specialist advice and support is the Pick's Disease Support Group (http://www.pdsg.org.uk/).

21.8 EXAMPLE OF A LOCAL SERVICE

Manchester offers a needs-led service which has been provided through the collaboration of health and social services (Baldwin and Murray, 2003). The service works closely with both the local and regional branch of the Alzheimer's Society. It is multidisciplinary with a whole-time specialist nurse, 0.6 whole-time equivalent occupational therapist, half-time social worker and sessional input from a psychologist and speech and language therapist. There is a team manager. The service has a single point of access, but referrals are closely monitored by the lead consultant and specialist nurse, to ensure a thorough diagnosis has been made. It does not offer a diagnostic service.

The Manchester service has expanded to develop day care and outreach care, which often incorporate social activities and special interests. It also offers basic personal care and support. A caregivers' support group and campaigning group help to promote the needs of this group of people and ensure that young-onset dementia is very much on the local agenda. Views of users and caregivers are systematically collected and inform service development (Shlosberg *et al.*, 2003).

A specialist nurse is able to provide support and advice and is able to direct and link people to other appropriate services, for example care management, welfare rights information and advice. He/she can act as care coordinator for a proportion of the clients.

21.9 OTHER INITIATIVES

From 1998 to 2000 there was a national young-onset dementia initiative in the United kingdom (http://www.alzheimers. org.uk/Younger_People_with_Dementia/index.htm). It was aimed at caregivers, professionals and local branches of the Alzheimer's Society requiring support or advice about service development.

Regional forums have been developed to raise the profile at regional level, provide support for users and caregivers, to encourage service development and to learn from the practice and experience of others. They exist largely as partnerships between statutory services and providers, the independent and voluntary sectors, and usually meet quarterly. For a disorder like younger-onset dementia they provide an invaluable source of support and networking. They may also guide local service commissioners. The above website provides a link to regional forums, the numbers of which are increasing. For example in the north west of England there were two specialist services for younger people in the mid-1990s but by 2002 this had grown to 10.

The Clive Project (http://www.thecliveproject.demon. co.uk/) in Oxfordshire, England, has formed a group in collaboration with MHA Care Group (formerly Methodist Homes, an independent sector provider), to develop suitable accommodation for younger people with dementia. MHA hopes to offer the following three options: short breaks, independent supported living and enhanced support. These should offer the person and their family flexible choices and continuity of care and support. Appropriate accommodation is not currently available in most areas of the UK. Where caregiver preferences have been sought, the following have emerged as relevant: small-scale domestic-type houses accommodating around four to six people, which are close to a welcoming and accepting community and accessible to local leisure facilities and social activities. The accommodation should be as 'normal' as possible, with care tailored to the individual and able to promote independence appropriate to the person's abilities. Appropriate accommodation for younger people with dementia may be the next step in the evolution of specialist services.

21.10 SUMMARY

Dementia services have arisen largely to address the needs of older people. The prevalence and needs of younger people with dementia is now much better understood. Services for these people, some of which should be specialized, can be organized around a population base of around half a million. At a minimum there should be clear local protocols for diagnosis and assessment and a named consultant and specialist nurse to take the lead in service development in partnership with other relevant bodies, such as social service departments and the local Alzheimer's Society.

REFERENCES

Allen H and Baldwin B. (1995) The referral, investigation and diagnosis of presenile dementia: two services compared. *International Journal of Geriatric Psychiatry* **10**: 185–190

Alzheimer's Society. (2001) *Younger People with Dementia: A Guide to Service Development and Provision.* London, Alzheimer's Society

Baldwin RC. (1994) Acquired cognitive impairment in the presenium. *Psychiatric Bulletin* **18**: 463–465

Baldwin R and Murray M. (2003) *Younger People with Dementia: A Multidisciplinary Approach.* London, Martin Duntiz

Ballard C, O'Brien J, James I, Swann A. (2001) *Dementia: Management of Behavioural and Psychological Symptoms.* Oxford, Oxford University Press

Cetnarskyj R and Porteous M. (1999) Huntington's disease. In: S Cox and J Keady (eds), *Younger People with Dementia: Planning, Practice and Development.* London, Jessica Kingsley, pp. 107–120

Cooper S-A. (1999) Learning disabilities and dementia. In: S Cox and J Keady (eds), *Younger People with Dementia: Planning, Practice and Development.* London, Jessica Kingsley, pp. 121–134

Cordery R, Harvey R, Frost C, Rossor M. (2002) National survey to assess current practices in the diagnosis and management of young people with dementia. *International Journal of Geriatric Psychiatry* **17**: 124–127

Crowe S. (1999) Alcohol-related brain impairment. In: S Cox and J Keady (eds), *Younger People with Dementia: Planning, Practice and Development.* London, Jessica Kingsley, pp. 135–150

Delany N and Rosenvinge H. (1995) Presenile dementia: sufferers, carers, and services *International Journal of Geriatric Psychiatry* **10**: 597–601

Department of Health. (1999) *Effective Care Co-ordination in Mental Health Services: Modernizing the Care Programme Approach.* London, DoH

Department of Health. (2001) *National Service Framework for Older People.* London, DoH

Ferran J, Wilson KCM, Doran M *et al.* (1996) The early onset dementias: a study of clinical characteristics and service use. *International Journal of Geriatric Psychiatry* **11**: 863–869

Garrod K. (2003) Support for families. In: R Baldwin and M Murray (eds), *Younger People with Dementia: A Multidisciplinary Approach.* London, Martin Dunitz, pp. 155–162

Harvey RJ. (1998) *Young-onset dementia: Epidemiology, Clinical Symptoms, Family Burden and Outcome.* London, NHS Executive, Imperial College

Harvey RJ, Roques PK, Fox NC, Rossor MN. (1998) CANDID – counselling and diagnosis in dementia: a national telemedicine service supporting the care of younger patients with dementia. *International Journal of Geriatric Psychiatry* **13**: 381–388

Lindesay J, Marudkar M, van Diepen E, Wilcock G. (2002) The second Leicester survey of memory clinics in the British Isles. *International Journal of Geriatric Psychiatry* **17**: 41–47

Luscombe GA, Brodaty H, Freeth S. (1998) Younger people with dementia: diagnostic issues, effects on carers and use of services *International Journal of Geriatric Psychiatry* **13**: 323–330

McGonigal G, Thomas B, McQuade C, Starr JM, MacLennen WJ, Whalley LJ. (1993) Epidemiology of Alzheimer's presenile dementia in Scotland, 1974–88. *BMJ* **306**: 680–683

Murray M. (2003) Multiagency working. In: R Baldwin and M Murray (eds), *Younger People with Dementia: A Multidisciplinary Approach.* London, Martin Dunitz, pp. 173–178

Neary D and Snowden J. (2003) Causes of dementia in younger people. In: R Baldwin and M Murray (eds), *Younger People with Dementia: A Multidisciplinary Approach.* London, Martin Dunitz, pp. 7–41

Neary D, Snowden JS, Northen B. (1988) Dementia of frontal lobe type. *Journal of Neurology, Neurosurgery, and Psychiatry* **51**: 353–361

Newens AJ, Forster D, Kay D, Kirkup W, Bates D, Edwardson J. (1993) Clinically diagnosed presenile dementia of the Alzheimer type in the Northern Health Region. *Psychological Medicine* **23**: 631–644

Newens AJ, Forster DP, Kay D. (1995) Dependency and community care in presenile Alzheimer's disease. *British Journal of Psychiatry* **166**: 777–782

Nott PN and Fleminger JJ. (1975) Presenile dementia: the difficulties of early diagnosis. *Acta Psychiatrica Scandinavica* **51**: 210–217

Pattie AH and Gilleard CJ. (1979) *Manual of the Clifton Assessment Procedures for the Elderly (CAPE).* Sevenoaks, Hodder and Stoughton

Royal College of Psychiatrists. (2001) *Services for Younger People with Alzheimer's Disease and Other Dementias.* Council Report CR77. London, Royal College of Psychiatrists

Shlosberg E, Browne C, Knight A. (2003) In: R Baldwin and M Murray (eds), *Younger People with Dementia: A Multidisciplinary Approach.* London, Martin Dunitz, pp. 179–192

Sperlinger D and Furst M. (1994) The service experiences of people with presenile dementia: a study of carers in one London Borough. *International Journal of Geriatric Psychiatry* **9**: 47–50.

Varma AR, Adams W, Lloyd JJ *et al.* (2002) Diagnostic patterns of regional atrophy on MRI and regional cerebral blood flow change on SPECT in young onset patients with Alzheimer's disease, frontotemporal dementia and vascular dementia. *Acta Neurologica Scandinavica* **105**: 261–269

22

Alzheimer (disease and related disorders) Associations and Societies: supporting family carers

HENRY BRODATY, ALISA GREEN, NORI GRAHAM AND LEE-FAY LOW

National Alzheimer Disease Associations and Societies have become a powerful force throughout the world, advocating on behalf of people with dementia and their carers. The growth in these voluntary organizations has been brought by the quantum leap of public awareness about Alzheimer's disease (AD) and related dementias, particularly in developed countries. This rise in public awareness has occurred as a result of a number of converging factors.

First was the relabelling of senility and senile dementia following the landmark clinicopathological study of Blessed *et al.* (1968). Suddenly, what had previously been accepted as normal ageing was dignified as a disease, albeit one with a somewhat unusual name. Prior to 1968, AD had been regarded as a relatively rare dementia in younger people.

Second, the demographics of the developed world changed. Average life expectancy in developed countries now extends beyond 75 years for men and 80 years for women. The percentage of older people is the highest ever recorded, with the proportion of those over 65 years in some countries such as Sweden and the United Kingdom exceeding 15% of their population. There were estimated to be 25 million people with dementia worldwide in 2000. This number is projected to increase to 63 million in 2030 (with 41 million in less developed regions) and to 114 million in 2050 (41 million in less developed regions) (Wimo *et al.*, 2003). As age is the major risk factor for dementia, affecting 6% of those 65 or older and 20% of those aged 80 years or more, the greying of the world's population has resulted in a marked rise in the number of people with dementia.

With so many people affected by dementia, the number of people caring for them is even greater. It is therefore a common experience for many in the developed world to know of someone suffering from dementia. It is now people's

expectation to live a long and healthy life as so many physical diseases have been eliminated. AD is one of the few diseases one is likely to develop in old age.

A third factor has been increasing public awareness, as demonstrated in the press and media. This is partially the result of publicized cases, such as those of Rita Hayworth, Ronald Reagan and Charlton Heston in the USA, Iris Murdoch in Great Britain and Hazel Hawke, the ex-wife of a former prime minister, in Australia. Sensational media stories abound, be they medical 'breakthroughs' (e.g. discovery of genes that cause AD, the role of aluminium, the suggestion that red wine protects against AD, and trial of an AD vaccine) or heartbreaking tragedies. This has fuelled the public's fascination with, and fear of, AD.

A fourth factor is the upsurge of research activities on so many fronts: molecular biology, epidemiology, genetic studies, the search for more accurate diagnoses and assessment, and the search for better treatments for both cognitive and non-cognitive symptoms. Effective prevention and treatment may be on the horizon, but meanwhile there are many millions of people affected by dementia, and for every person with dementia there is at least one, and often several, carers under stress. It is therefore important to highlight social research on the impact of AD on carers, and to identify practical ways to reduce the stress and burden of caring.

Certain factors can reduce stress, such as adequate home help to assist with the practical hard work, giving carers the opportunity to go out and have some time for themselves (Levin *et al.*, 1989). The importance of recognition of the disease by the general practitioner and other primary care workers, the need for referral to a specialist for diagnosis, and ongoing follow up and advice have also been stressed. Most of these will be required for the rest of the life of the person with dementia.

A fifth factor is the breakdown of traditional family structures with the changing roles of women and adult children, and the diminution of the sense of moral obligation to care for the older members of the family. This is putting great pressure on health and social care systems, and governments are being forced to consider how to provide a system to meet the needs of dementia and their carers. In the developed world it is beginning to be recognized, if not acted upon, that there is a limit to what families can tolerate or can be expected to tolerate.

The problem of caring for someone with dementia at home has led carers to seek each other out, to talk together and support one another. This has resulted in the growth of Alzheimer Associations all over the world. In the larger developed countries – USA, UK, Canada, Australia – these Associations have been able to exert a powerful voice about carers' needs.

22.1 SELF-HELP GROUPS

The late twentieth century witnessed the rise of consumer organizations and the self-help group (SHG) movement. SHGs are now available for almost every chronic condition, and should be part of the armamentarium of every clinician.

SHGs may be formed by groups of people who feel themselves to be powerless or stigmatized. They may see themselves as different from the general community or disadvantaged, e.g. 'Alcoholics' Anonymous', or may seek political advantage such as 'Grey Power' or they may consider that their condition is being ignored, as was the case for people with dementia and their families. SHGs may be composed of people who share a similar status or condition, such as the 'Nursing Mothers' Association'. Some SHGs are formed by people connected in some way to a group for whom they are advocating or for whom they have a specific concern, be they friends, for example the 'Association of Relatives and Friends of the Mentally Ill', or professionals dedicated to the same cause.

Many SHGs are linked to medical conditions: 'Arthritis Foundation', 'Autism Association', 'Colostomy and Ileostomy Society', 'Epilepsy Association', 'National Heart Foundation', and the 'Schizophrenia Fellowship'.

The advantages of SHGs, such as the Alzheimer Association, are several:

- support
  - emotional
  - practical
- education for professionals
- universalization – a sense of belonging, a feeling of no longer being alone
- identity – a sense of purpose
- political power – lobbying
- influence and advocacy
- public awareness.

Potential disadvantages are that:

- the SHGs can become a substitute culture;
- charismatic leaders can subvert the primary goals for their own personal objectives;
- governments can abandon provision of care to non-government organizations;
- rival SHGs may squabble for members or influence and internal divisions can beset any organization.

Support groups are distinct from group psychotherapy in that participants in support groups are not viewed as 'patients', but rather as 'normal' people who, as result of their caring role, are at an increased risk of becoming overburdened and developing psychological and physical problems (Cuijpers *et al.*, 1996).

Support groups can be led either by professional support group leaders, or by peer group leaders. In professionally led groups, the leader has professional qualifications and/or training, and the group tends to be more formally structured. By contrast the facilitator of a peer-led group usually is, or has been, a carer himself or herself. Peer-led groups tend to be less structured, and use more of a self-help approach by focusing on sharing common problems and information gained from participants' personal experiences (Toseland *et al.*, 1989). Other methods of support link carers by computer and telephone networks (Gallienne *et al.*, 1993; Smyth and Harris, 1993) and are particularly useful for reaching isolated carers such as those living in rural and remote areas. There are also support groups for people with dementia themselves, particularly in the early stage of the disease (Yale, 1995) including an internet-based virtual support group run by 'Dementia Advocacy Support Network International' (www.dasninternational.com).

22.1.1 Alzheimer SHGs

At a local level, support groups primarily for family carers, meet regularly and frequently, usually monthly. Support groups tend to be led by a health professional, such as a social worker, often in combination with a carer. Some support groups are led by carers alone, and some by professionals alone. Meeting may be structured (see above) so that there is a formal speaker, viewing of a videotape or discussion of a set topic, followed by general discussion; or unstructured in order to allow for more interaction between attendees. Practical arrangements for people with dementia during the support group vary. Some support groups only allow family carers to attend, others allow people with dementia to come too, or provide a separate room for patients' activities. Carers' groups are sometimes held adjacent to day centres. Interested health professionals, students and observers sometimes attend too, although only with the prior permission of the group.

Anecdotal evidence suggests that some carers attend SHGs regularly over many months, even years. Others come for one or two meetings, perhaps feeling that they have achieved all they need, or may feel that support groups are not suitable for them. Other carers may never come because they have no need, have enough support from their own networks of friends and family, have obtained the support that they need from one-to-one counselling, or, most often, have never been told of the existence of such groups (Thomson *et al.*, 1997).

Telephone and internet education and online support networks are becoming more common and used by caregivers (Harvey *et al.*, 1998; White and Dorman, 2000; Glueckauf and Loomis, 2003). Caregivers express particular interest in using telephone support lines (Colantanio *et al.*, 2001).

22.1.2 The efficacy of support groups

Participation in support groups may have a positive impact on the wellbeing of carers. Support group participation, in cross-sectional studies, has been found to be associated with lower levels of objective and subjective burden; the more frequent and the longer the periods of support group participation, the less the subjective burden (Gonyea, 1990). Carers who attend support groups have also been found to have higher levels of morale than carers who do not attend support groups (Gonyea, 1990). Additionally, support group attendees have been found to experience a significant increase in feelings of self-efficacy (Lovett and Gallagher, 1988; Gallagher *et al.*, 1989), and improvements in their psychological functioning.

In the only randomized trial we could locate, the Cleveland Alzheimer's Managed Care Demonstration evaluated the effects of integrating 'Alzheimer Association' care consultation with a not-for-profit managed healthcare organization. Care consultation is a telephone-based information, support and referral service with follow up supplied by professional staff. Care consultation decreased use of some services and caregiver depression but did not alter satisfaction with healthcare services or strain (Bass *et al.*, 2003).

Comparatively, professionally led groups appear to produce greater improvement in carers' psychological functioning, whereas peer-led groups have been found to increase informal support networks and the extent to which carers feel able to handle the caregiving role more (Toseland *et al.*, 1989). Finally, most importantly, carers themselves tend to value support groups, and often report them to be informative, useful and meaningful (Clark and Rakowski, 1983; Gallagher, 1985; Kahan *et al.*, 1985; Mohide *et al.*, 1990; Jansson *et al.*, 1998).

The findings to date regarding the efficacy of support groups are, however, equivocal, since some studies have not found support groups to result in statistically significant gains. In their review of eight studies that examined the effects of support groups, Cuijpers *et al.* (1996) found that only three demonstrated a significant reduction in carers' depression and stress and an improvement in their wellbeing. In one study, while carers who attended support groups were found to have significantly better help-seeking coping efforts compared to carers who did not attend support groups, there

was no significant difference found between the two groups of carers in terms of their wellbeing (Gage and Kinney, 1995). A study published since this review reported that the level of carer distress decreased and quality of life improved (Fung and Chien, 2002).

There is also evidence to suggest that support groups may be more beneficial for some carers than for others. For instance, SHGs have been found to be more effective for carers whose social network lacks contact with others who have similar caring experiences and for caregivers in more stressful situations (Pillemer and Suitor, 1996, 2002). Additionally, Cuijpers *et al.* (1996) found that support groups were more effective for carers who were dissatisfied about their role as a carer or who had a paid job, where the person with dementia was more apathetic and/or lived in a nursing home, and where participation in the support groups incurred a small cost ($5–$20).

In spite of the benefits of support group attendance that have been reported, many carers do not attend support groups, either by choice or because of barriers. Cuijpers *et al.* (1996) reported that there were three main reasons that affected carers' decision to attend support groups – for information, for help with dealing with problems, or for help dealing with their feelings of severe burden. Molinari *et al.* (1994) reported that the reason given by 80 per cent of carers who did not attend support groups was that they had not received advice encouraging them to attend a support group. Analysis of data from 608 dementia caregivers found that enabling variables such as knowledge of services, cost and access, explained more variation in service use than predisposing and need variables such as demographics, patient behaviour and caregiver burden (Toseland *et al.*, 2002). Communication problems between caregivers and general practitioners (GPs) may impede timely referrals for appropriate information and support (Bruce and Paterson, 2000; Bruce *et al.*, 2002). These findings suggest that it is incumbent upon relevant health professionals to provide information about local support groups to carers as part of their management plan.

22.1.3 The impact of cultural factors

In Western countries such as the USA and Australia, ethnic minorities often underuse community services such as support groups (Henderson *et al.*, 1993). Researchers have started to examine the factors that prevent ethnic minorities from participating in support groups, and to look at the extent to which the traditional structure of support groups can be modified to meet the needs of ethnic minority populations (Henderson, 1992: Henderson *et al.*, 1993). For instance, Henderson and colleagues (1993) attempted to set up more culturally sensitive support groups, when they noted that despite widespread advertising and promotion, attendees at local AD support groups were exclusively white. After surveying African American and Hispanic communities on issues of late life, health and wellbeing, and dementia, they started up several African American and Hispanic support groups, and demonstrated that ethnic minority groups responded to AD support groups when they were implemented in a manner that was consistent with the cultural values of their community. In particular, Henderson (Henderson, 1992; Henderson *et al.*, 1993) recommended that in order for support groups to reach ethnic minority populations successfully, it is important:

- to get acquainted with ethnic communities;
- to recruit and train ethnic support group leaders;
- to find a culturally neutral site for the group to meet; and
- to let the participants determine the form of the group.

22.1.4 Special support groups

Young people with dementia, people with unusual forms of dementia and people who are very prominent in their community and their families often find traditional support groups do not suit them. Attempts have been made to meet their needs by setting up special groups for them, e.g. for younger people with dementia, for people with frontotemporal dementia (such as Pick's disease) (Armstrong, 2003; Diehl *et al.*, 2003). There is increasing emphasis on providing support groups for people with early dementia themselves while they retain insight (Chung, 2001; Coaten, 2002).

22.2 NATIONAL ALZHEIMER ASSOCIATIONS

The overarching aim of all Alzheimer Associations is to improve the quality of life for people with dementia and for their carers. (The term 'Alzheimer Association' is used generically hereafter to include the more correctly named 'Alzheimer Disease and Related Disorders Association', as well as similarly named organizations such as the 'Alzheimer Disease Society'; see www.alz.co.uk and follow the links to find Alzheimer Association in your country. They are also listed in the appendix on page 805.) Alzheimer Associations have a number of important aims.

22.2.1 Information

One of the most important aims is the provision of information. It is well recognized that information brings power. It is fundamental that people with dementia, their carers, professionals, members of the general public and government should have easy access to accurate information. National offices of Alzheimer Associations throughout the world meet an ever-increasing number of enquiries about the disease itself, about financial and legal matters, and about nursing homes. They provide a shoulder to cry on, and information on up-to-date research findings, and where to get help and how to manage particularly difficult problems. For these enquiries to be dealt with in an efficient manner, it is necessary to have an office, staffed by one or more people, paid or unpaid, and a telephone line. A regular newsletter sent out to all members is invaluable. In addition good publications and fact sheets written in response to the most frequent enquiries (written by knowledgeable professionals) are all essential. It is helpful to start building up a library of books, videos and papers to meet the demand. A new national society can take articles from existing publications elsewhere, as there are many topics that come up again and again. The Internet has revolutionized the availability and speed with which information is available to all those who need it.

22.2.2 Membership

Caring for someone with dementia can be a very isolating experience and the knowledge that there are others around who understand the problems and who can be contacted can be very reassuring. In the UK, for example, the membership of the 'Alzheimer's Society' is now over 20 000. This has been achieved by having a single national body to which all members from all over the country belong. The national office ensures that members know where to find a local branch or group so that they can take part in local activities. Having a large membership gives the Association more power and clout and is impressive to politicians and professionals.

22.2.3 Training

Alzheimer Associations often play an important role in the training and education of family members as well as care workers in residential nursing homes, day care and domiciliary services. The situation is similar all over the world. Care workers often have no background in this sort of work and have been given little if any information about the care recipient's illness or behavioural problems, or any sort of guidance as to how to do their work. Better training and information for family and professional carers are key to ensuring better care for people with dementia. Training and counselling programmes conducted by or in conjunction with Alzheimer Associations may reduce carer distress and delay nursing home admission (Mittelman *et al.*, 1996; Brodaty *et al.*, 1997; see Chapter 11a). In Australia, the Commonwealth Government has funded 'Alzheimer's Australia' to conduct the 'Living with Memory Loss Program', anecdotally a highly successful parallel 7-week course for people with early dementia and for their partners. A pilot of this programme demonstrated a decrease in distress in the person with dementia (Brodaty and Low, 2004).

A partnership between the New Jersey police department and their local Alzheimer Association educated police on wandering reduction in AD, increased enrolment of people with AD in a national registration programme, and increased police sponsored AD community outreach programmes (Lachenmayr *et al.*, 2000).

22.2.4 Services

There are several types of services that are used by carers: home care, day care, in-home (sitting) and residential respite care, and permanent care, although each carer may have a different requirement. Finding the right solution reduces the stress on carers and makes institutionalized care less likely (Mittelman *et al.*, 1996). The 'Alzheimer's Connection Demonstration Program' in the USA was an attempt to link families with needed services and resources using case management (Cox and Albisu, 2001). Individual carers' needs cannot always be met because resources either do not exist or are very patchy. Adequate provision of services for carers is a major problem in most (or all) countries around the world. This problem presents differently in every country and sometimes is the main reason that dementia has reached the top of many political agendas, as care is often needed well beyond the capacity of the family to provide or the government's willingness to pay.

The challenge to all governments in all countries is how to provide cost-effective resources for carers of people with dementia and their families, as well as improving the quality of training of professional carers. Worldwide there is immense pressure by governments on the private and voluntary sectors to deliver these services. Whichever sector provides these services, a national association has an extremely important part to play in defining how to deliver and monitor services with reasonable standards of care and at economic cost.

22.2.5 Research

Whilst well established and wealthy societies such as the US and UK are able to fund research, most Alzheimer Associations are not. Associations can and do act as an advocacy group to pressure other funding bodies and government to provide more money for dementia research and to ensure that such funding is available for investigation of the best way to help people with dementia and their families as well as for basic sciences and drug studies.

Alzheimer Associations can help researchers in various ways. They can provide access to people with dementia and their families. They can advise researchers on their projects, giving the carer perspective, which is immensely valuable. Researchers can help Alzheimer Associations by advising, contributing to newsletters and giving talks. Most Alzheimer Associations have found it important to have a strong supportive medical and scientific committee to provide advice to the Association.

It is important that the relationship between carers and interested professionals is worked out in a sensitive way. Ultimately, support for persons with dementia and their carers must remain the main focus of all Alzheimer Associations.

22.2.6 Public awareness

Good publications, training materials and courses are a fundamental way of increasing public awareness and respect amongst professionals and politicians. As public awareness grows, and more people become involved and interested, so gradually there is more coverage in radio, television and the press. Time spent lobbying politicians and other professionals is time well spent. Links established with other associations, with politicians and with professionals foster recognition of AD and the other dementias as a priority area of concern, underscored by their increasing prevalence in the community. Alzheimer Associations are in a powerful position to prioritize their concerns on behalf of the family, and these may well vary from country to country.

22.2.7 Fund raising

Inevitably funds have to be raised to pursue the aims of the Association. Government grants are important, not only for the actual amounts of money but also because of the recognition such money offers. In many countries governments give no money. Many countries find that the major amount of funding come from individuals, trusts, industry and legacies. Some countries find having a membership and members paying a fee in exchange for receiving a newsletter and other information is helpful; many members give a donation as well as their membership fee. It must, however, be remembered that, although having sufficient funds is important, equally important is how to use the money as efficiently as possible, with careful budgeting along prepared activity lines. Every Alzheimer Association needs people with financial experience to help guide it, and a fusion of personal, business and professional experience is of primary importance to achieve these aims.

Building a strong national Alzheimer Association is difficult and can be a long process. It is essential that from the start the Association decide on its aims. It will need a good team of staff and volunteers and some good information and training materials. It will also need to put into place parliamentary lobbying. In order to carry this out it is necessary to have an efficient office with up-to-date computerization and a fundraising strategy in order to raise the money to pursue these aims.

22.3 ALZHEIMER DISEASE INTERNATIONAL

The first Alzheimer Disease Association was founded in 1978 in Canada. In 1984 'Alzheimer's Disease International' (ADI), the World Federation of Alzheimer's Disease and Related Disorders Associations and Societies, was formed at a special meeting in Washington. There are now 66 countries with National Associations which are members of ADI and the number is growing every year (see Figure 22.1).

All National Associations face a serious array of tasks which are going to become more important as the years go by. ADI draws on international expertise to support its member societies and encourage new countries to form National Associations.

In the office of ADI, which was originally based in Chicago but is now in London, there are four paid staff who

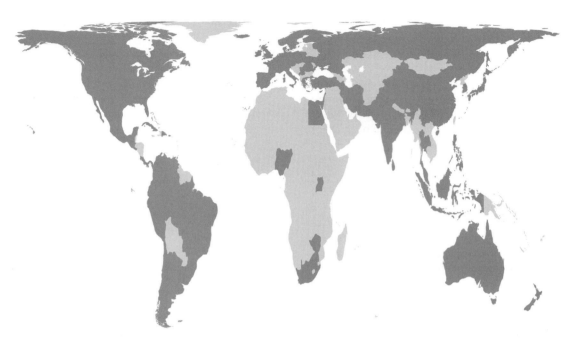

Figure 22.1   *Map of the world with those countries belonging to ADI shown in dark grey. (Source: Alzheimer's disease International, Member Countries map 2004–2005. Reprinted by kind permission of Alzheimer's Disease International.)*

are responsible for the administration of the organization. The organizational structure includes an elected Executive Committee and Board and a general Council that meets annually. The organization is run on a tight budget with money from membership fees and donations.

Criteria for ADI membership are that:

- The member must act as the national carer based organization and produce evidence that it is the representative body of families of people with AD and related disorders in that country.
- The organization needs to have national credibility and to have reached organizational maturity with a Board of Directors with adequate representation of family members.
- The Association needs to be able to pay the reasonably modest dues to participate in ADI.
- It should provide services for family carers, e.g. helpline, support groups, public information and education programmes.

The primary aim of ADI is to assist Alzheimer Associations who have already become members and to encourage the formation of Associations in countries where they do not exist. In order to pursue this primary aim, ADI has developed the 'Alzheimer University Course', with the assistance of the Open University in the UK. Since 1998 ADI has conducted an annual 3-day course for members of new and emerging Alzheimer Associations, consisting of workshops aimed at assisting and strengthening new organizations. Alzheimer University Courses on focused issues are also run for more established associations.

ADI disseminates information and acts as a resource point for enquiries and requests for help around the world. A regular newsletter is published which many countries translate for their own purposes. It produces several basic publications including help for carers, how to set up and run an Alzheimer Association, how to influence public policy, and how to set up a support/self help group.

It has also produced a number of important fact sheets dealing with issues of international importance such as demography, prevalence and genetics and drug treatment. All the publications are available on the webpage and can be downloaded from there (www.alz.co.uk). Publications are translated into Spanish. Communication between countries and people has been made greatly easier by email (adi@alz.co.uk). A list of national Alzheimer Association websites providing information on AD and other dementias in different languages is also available from the webpage.

ADI is officially affiliated with the World Health Organization and is closely linked with many international associations with similar interests, such as the International Psychogeriatric Association, World Psychiatric Association, and the World Federation of Neurology. The pharmaceutical industry increasingly looks to ADI for advice about dementia and consumer needs.

Every year ADI hosts an international conference focused on carers and carer issues, which provides a unique opportunity for carers and professionals of all disciplines from many countries to come together and learn from one another.

ADI encourages research and there is a large medical and scientific panel with representatives from many countries around the world. This panel acts as an advisory board and its members act as ambassadors for ADI when people travel to countries to attend meetings; they also give help with articles and talks at conferences.

ADI's major research commitment is the 10/66 Dementia Research group (http://www.alz.co.uk/1066) that brings together a collaboration of researchers from developed and developing countries. 10/66 refers to the less than one-tenth of all population-based research into dementia that is directed towards the two-thirds or more of people with dementia who live in developing countries. 10/66 was formed to redress this imbalance, encouraging active research collaboration between centres in different developing countries and between developed and developing countries. Since its establishment in 1998, 10/66 has published the results of pilot investigations in 26 centres from 16 developing countries. These studies aimed to establish a culture-fair method for diagnosing dementia in older populations characterized by very low levels of education (Prince *et al.*, 2003), and to describe the care arrangements for people with dementia in the developing world (Prince, 2004). The 10/66 group has also highlighted the lack of awareness and understanding of the nature of the dementia syndrome, and the unresponsiveness of healthcare services as currently constituted (Shaji *et al.*, 2002a, Patel and Prince, 2002). The group has developed and described services for people with dementia in developing countries using local health workers, who can be can be trained to identify cases of dementia with reasonable accuracy (Shaji *et al.*, 2002b).

Stimulating national and international political and public awareness is an important objective of ADI. This is partly being achieved by more countries developing Alzheimer Associations and all of the Associations becoming stronger. However AD is a global problem. World Alzheimer's Day is 21 September and was launched in September 1994 when ADI celebrated its tenth anniversary. ADI supplies its members with a world bulletin with a special focus each year. It produces badges, posters, and ideas for activities which countries can organize themselves according to their different cultures and languages.

22.4 CONCLUSION

Very few governments, even of Western countries are fully aware of the significance of the problem of AD and related disorders and their impact on families. Even if they are aware, the social and economic implications are not fully recognized. Every country, whatever its level of economic development, has a duty to put the dementias and their consequences high on its political agenda. It also represents responsible planning and will be cost effective to work in conjunction with Alzheimer Associations to meet the current and future needs now. The challenge for ADI and all National Associations is to find ways of influencing governments worldwide to take seriously the impact of AD and related disorders on the individual and family, while simultaneously providing support, information and other services to people with dementia and their families.

REFERENCES

Armstrong M. (2003) The needs of people with young-onset dementia and their carers. *Professional Nurse* **18**: 681–684

Bass DM, Clark PA, Looman WJ *et al.* (2003) The Cleveland Alzheimer's managed care demonstration: outcomes after 12 months of implementation. *The Gerontologist* **43**: 73–85

Blessed G, Tomlinson BE, Roth M. (1968) The association between quantitative measures of dementia and of senile change in the cerebral grey matter of elderly subjects. *British Journal of Psychiatry* **114**: 797–811

Brodaty H and Low L-F. (2004) 'Making Memories' a quasi-experimental pilot evaluation of a new program for people with dementia and their caregivers. *Australasian Journal of Ageing* **23**: 1441–1446

Brodaty H, Gresham M, Luscombe G. (1997) The Prince Henry Hospital Dementia Caregivers' Training Programme. *International Journal of Geriatric Psychiatry* **12**: 183–192

Bruce DG and Paterson A. (2000) Barriers to community support for the dementia carer: a qualitative study. *International Journal of Geriatric Psychiatry* **15**: 451–457

Bruce DG, Paley GA, Underwood PJ *et al.* (2002) Communication problems between dementia carers and general practitioners: effect on access to community support services. *Medical Journal of Australia* **177**: 186–188

Clark NM and Rakowski W. (1983) Family caregivers of older adults: Improving helping skills. *The Gerontologist* **23**: 637–642

Chung JC. (2001) Empowering individuals with early dementia and their carers: an exploratory study in the Chinese context. *American Journal of Alzheimer's Disease and Other Dementias* **16**: 85–88

Coaten R. (2002) A support group for people with early stage dementia. *Dementia: The International Journal of Social Research and Practice* **1**: 383–392

Colantonio A, Kositsky AJ, Cohen C, Vernich L. (2001) What support do caregivers of elderly want? Results from the Canadian study of health and aging. *Canadian Journal of Public Health* **92**: 376–379

Cox C and Albisu K. (2001) The Alzheimer's Connection Demonstration Program: instituting a national case management program. *American Journal of Alzheimer's Disease* **16**: 279–284

Cuijpers P, Hosman CMH, Munnichs JMA. (1996) Change mechanisms of support groups for caregivers of dementia patients. *International Psychogeriatrics* **8**: 575–587

Diehl J, Mayer TF, Hans D, Alexander F. (2003) A support group for caregivers of patients with frontotemporal dementia. *Dementia* **2**: 151–161

Fung W-Y and Chien W-T. (2002) The effectiveness of a mutual support group for family caregivers of a relative with dementia. *Archives of Psychiatric Nursing* **XVI**: 134–144

Gage MJ and Kinney JM. (1995) They aren't for everyone: the impact of support group participation on caregiver's well-being. *Clinical Gerontologist* **16(2)**: 21–34

Gallagher DE. (1985) Intervention strategies to assist caregivers of frail elders: Current research a future research directions. *Annual Review of Gerontology and Geriatrics* **5**: 249–282

Gallagher D, Lovett S, Zeiss A. (1989) Interventions with caregivers of frail elderly persons. In: M Ory and K Bond (eds), *Aging and*

Health Care: Social Science and Policy Perspectives. London, Routledge Press

Gallienne RL, Moore SM, Brennan PF. (1993) Alzheimer's caregivers: psychosocial support versus computer networks. *Journal of Gerontological Nursing* **19(12)**: 15–22

Glueckauf RL and Loomis JS. (2003) Alzheimer's caregiver support online: lessons learned, initial findings and future directions, *Neurorehabilitation* **18**: 135–146

Gonyea JG. (1990) Alzheimer's disease support group participation and caregiver well-being. *Clinical Gerontologist* **10**(2): 17–34

Harvey RJ, Roques PK, Fox NC, Rossor MN. (1998) CANDID – counselling and diagnosis in dementia: a national telemedicine service supporting the care of younger patients with dementia. *International Journal of Geriatric Psychiatry* **13**: 381–388

Henderson JN. (1992) The power of support: Alzheimer's disease support groups for minority families. *Aging* **363–364**: 24–28

Henderson JN, Gutierrez-Mayka M, Garcia J, Boyd S. (1993) A model for Alzheimer's disease support group development in African-American and Hispanic populations. *The Gerontologist* **33**: 409–414

Jansson W, Almbergy B, Grafstrom M, Winblad B. (1998) The circle model – support for relatives of people with dementia. *International Journal of Geriatric Psychiatry* **13**: 674–681

Kahan J, Kemp B, Staples FR, Brummel-Smith K. (1985) Decreasing the burden in families caring for a relative with a dementing illness: A controlled study. *Journal of the American Geriatrics Society* **33**: 664–670

Lachenmayr S, Goldman KD, Brand FS. (2000) Safe return: a community-based initiative between police officers and the Alzheimer's Association to increase the safety of people with Alzheimer's disease. *Health Promotion Practice* **1**: 268–278

Levin E, Sinclair I, Gorbach P *et al.* (1989) *Family Services and Confusion in Old Age*. Avebury, Aldershot

Lovett S and Gallagher D. (1988) Psychoeducational interventions for family caregivers: Preliminary efficacy data. *Behavior Therapy* **19**: 321–330

Mittelman MS, Ferris SH, Shulman E *et al.* (1996) A family intervention to delay nursing home placement of patients with Alzheimer's disease. A randomized controlled trial. *JAMA* **276**: 1725–1731

Mohide EA, Pringle DM, Streiner DL *et al.* (1990) A randomised trial of family caregiver support in the home management of dementia. *Journal of the American Geriatrics Society* **38**: 446–454

Molinari V, Nelson N, Shekelle S, Crothers MK. (1994) Family support groups of the Alzheimer's association: an analysis of attendees and non-attendees. *Journal of Applied Gerontology* **13**: 86–98

Patel V and Prince M. (2001) Ageing and mental health in a developing country: who cares? Qualitative studies from Goa, India. *Psychological Medicine* **31**: 29–38

Pillemer K and Suitor JJ. (1996) 'It takes one to help one': effects of similar others on the well-being of caregivers. *Journal of Gerontology* **51B**: S250–S257

Pillemer K and Suitor JJ. (2002) Peer support for Alzheimer's caregivers: It is enough to make a difference? *Research in Aging* **24**: 171–192

Prince M. (2004) 10/66 Dementia Research Group. Care arrangements for people with dementia in developing countries. *International Journal of Geriatric Psychiatry* **19**: 170–177

Prince M, Acosta D, Chiu H *et al.* (2003) Dementia diagnosis in developing countries: a cross-cultural validation study. *Lancet* **361**: 909–917

Shaji KS, Smitha K, Praveen Lal K, Prince M. (2002a) Caregivers of patients with Alzheimer's disease: a qualitative study from the Indian 10/66 Dementia Research Network. *International Journal of Geriatric Psychiatry* **18**: 1–6

Shaji KS, Arun Kishore NR, Lal KP, Prince M. (2002b) Revealing a hidden problem. An evaluation of a community dementia case-finding program from the Indian 10/66 dementia research network. *International Journal of Geriatric Psychiatry* **17**: 222–225

Smyth KA and Harris PB. (1993) Using telecomputing to provide information and support to caregivers of persons with dementia. *The Gerontologist* **33**: 123–127

Thomson C, Fine M, Brodaty H. (1997) *Carers support needs project: Dementia carers and the non-use of community services: report on the literature review*. (Commissioned by the Ageing and Disability Department, University of New South Wales). Sydney, Social Policy Research Centre

Toseland RW, Rossiter CM, Labrecque MS. (1989) The effectiveness of peer-led and professionally led groups to support family caregivers. *The Gerontologist* **29**: 465–471

Toseland RW, McCallion P, Gerber T, Banks S. (2002) Predictors of health and human services use by persons with dementia and their family caregivers. *Social Science and Medicine* **55**: 1255–1266

White MH and Dorman SM. (2000) Online support for caregivers. Analysis of an Internet Alzheimer mailgroup. *Computers in Nursing* **18**: 168–176

Wimo A, Winblad B, Aguero-Torres H, von Strauss E. (2003) The magnitude of dementia occurrence in the world. *Alzheimer Disease and Associated Disorders* **17**: 63–67

Yale R. (1995) *Developing Support Groups for Individuals with Early Stage Alzheimer's Disease*. Baltimore, Health Professions Press

Mild cognitive impairment

A historical perspective

KAREN RITCHIE AND SYLVAINE ARTERO

23.1 COGNITIVE IMPAIRMENT AS A FEATURE OF NORMAL AGEING

Alterations in cognitive functioning in the absence of dementia have long been considered a normal aspect of ageing-related brain changes. Affecting principally episodic verbal memory, such changes are generally distinguished from neuro-degenerative disorders by their far slower progression, their lesser impact on ability to perform activities of daily living, and the relative sparing of linguistic and visuospatial functions. Increased interest in the nature and long-term prognosis of ageing-related modifications in cognitive performance have now led us to question to what extent they may be considered 'normal'. The past 50 years have seen numerous attempts to define these subclinical alterations in cognitive functioning and to establish their aetiology with greater precision than the general notion of 'ageing brain changes' to which they have formerly been attributed.

One of the earliest attempts to characterize subclinical cognitive disorder was Kral's notion of benign senescent forgetfulness (BSF) (Kral, 1962) which referred to patient complaints of a persistent difficulty in recalling detail, commonly with accompanying depressive symptoms. While Kral initially considered such complaints to characterize a depressive state, which he referred to as depressive pseudodementia, long-term follow up of some of these patients showed that a significant proportion went on to develop vascular dementia. BSF was diagnosed by Kral by an open psychiatric interview and no formal algorithm was proposed. Formal diagnostic criteria for non-dementia cognitive impairment were first proposed by Crook *et al.* in 1986 for the National Institute of Mental Health. Referring to 'age-associated memory impairment' (AAMI); they defined these changes as subjective complaints of memory loss in older (aged > 50) people verified by a decrement of at least one standard deviation on a formal memory test in comparison with means established for young adults. Blackford and La Rue (1989) later suggested suitable tests of non-verbal and verbal secondary memory tests, proposing that AAMI be defined as performance at least one standard deviation below the mean for young adults on one or more of these tests. They also differentiate AAMI from the more severe state of 'late-life forgetfulness' (LLF), defined as performance between one and two standard deviations below the mean on at least 50 per cent of a battery of at least four tests.

Levy *et al.* (1994) argued that there is little reason *a priori* that cognitive decline in normal old age should be confined to memory functions exclusively, and in collaboration with the International Psychogeriatric Association and the World Health Organization proposed an alternative concept of ageing-associated cognitive decline (AACD). The criteria for AACD not only admit to the possibility of a wider range of cognitive functions being affected (attention, memory, learning, thinking, language, visuospatial function), but also stipulate that the deficit should be defined in reference to norms for older and not young adults to avoid confounding of decline with age and cohort effects. This refinement takes into account the observations of researchers such as Schaie and Willis (1991) who have demonstrated that much of the difference in cognitive performance observed between young and elderly cohorts is attributable to generation differences (notably in education and health care) rather than to ageing-related brain changes. Studies comparing the performance of AACD and AAMI criteria have concluded that they do not identify the same individuals within general population studies, AACD targeting a more severe state of impairment within a larger AAMI group (Richards *et al.*, 1999).

Recognition by the major international classifications of disease of subclinical cognitive deterioration linked to the normal ageing process began with the appearance in DSM-IV (1994) of the concept of age related cognitive decline (ARCD). Like AACD it refers to an objective decline in cognitive functioning owing to the physiological process of ageing; however, no operational criteria or cognitive testing procedures were specified. It is rather loosely defined as a complaint of difficulties in recalling names, appointments or in problem-solving, which cannot be related to a specific mental problem or a neurological disorder. Subsequent attempts to operationalize ARCD using data from two general population studies in France and the USA have concluded that the concept has little value either in predicting clinical outcomes or in identifying comparable populations for research purposes (N Quizilbash, personal communication).

23.2 DISEASE MODELS OF SUBCLINICAL COGNITIVE IMPAIRMENT

Early conceptualizations of subclinical cognitive deficit have in common the theoretical assumption that such changes are distinct from dementia and other pathologies, being the consequence of inevitable ageing-related cerebral changes such as cortical atrophy, which may be considered a normal feature of the ageing process. As parallel research into the causes of dementia and cerebrovascular disease has now led to a clearer understanding of their aetiology, it has also been shown that many of the physiological abnormalities seen in these disorders are also present to a lesser extent in subjects identified as AAMI and AACD. Consequently elderly persons with subclinical cognitive deficits have become the subject of neurological as well as psychogeriatric research, the underlying question being whether cognitive deficits of this type may be due to underlying brain pathology, which might be potentially treatable. Alternative concepts have subsequently appeared in the literature linking cognitive disorder to various forms of underlying pathology. For example, the 10th revision of the *International Classification of Diseases* (1993) described 'mild cognitive disorder' (MCD) which refers to disorders of memory, learning and concentration, often accompanied by mental fatigue, which must be demonstrated by formal neuropsychological testing and attributable to cerebral disease or damage, or systemic physical disease known to cause dysfunction. MCD is secondary to physical illness or impairment, excluding dementia, amnesic syndrome, concussion, or postencephalitic syndrome. The concept of MCD, which was principally developed to describe the cognitive consequences of autoimmune deficiency syndrome but then expanded to include other disorders in which cognitive change is secondary to another disease process, is applicable to all ages, not just the elderly. Attempts to apply MCD criteria to population studies of elderly persons suggest it to be of limited value in this context, casting doubt on its validity as a

nosological entity (Christensen *et al.*, 1995) for this age group. DSM-IV (American Psychiatric Association, 1994) has proposed a similar entity, mild neurocognitive disorder (MNCD), which encompasses not only memory and learning difficulties but also perceptual-motor, linguistic and central executive functions. While the concepts proposed by the two international classifications, MCD and MNCD, do not provide sufficient working guidelines for application in a research context, they do provide formal recognition of subclinical cognitive disorder as a pathological state requiring treatment, and as a source of handicap, and are thus likely to be important within a legal context.

A similar concept of cognitive change secondary to multiple underlying disease processes, but in this case referring to elderly populations, is that of CIND (cognitive impairment no dementia). The concept was developed within the context of the Canadian Study of Health and Aging and is defined by reference to neuropsychological testing and clinical examination (Graham *et al.*, 1997). Persons with CIND, like MCD and MNCD, are considered to have cognitive impairment attributable to an underlying physical disorder, but may also have a 'circumscribed memory impairment', which is a modified form of AAMI. CIND encompasses a wider range of underlying pathologies than MCD and MNCD, including disorders such as delirium, substance abuse and psychiatric illness, which are excluded from the ICD and DSM categories.

23.3 MILD COGNITIVE IMPAIRMENT – SUBCLINICAL COGNITIVE CHANGE AS PRODROMAL DEMENTIA

MCD, MNCD and CIND are constructs that have been developed principally for research purposes and consider cognitive disorder in the elderly to be heterogeneous, not necessarily progressive, with treatment being determined by the nature of the underlying primary systemic disease. On the other hand many clinical observations of the long-term outcome of cognitive complaints, particularly those presenting to memory clinics and neurology departments, led to the general conclusion by many neurologists that subclinical cognitive disorder in the elderly is in fact principally, if not exclusively, early-stage dementia. Thus whereas dementia was considered by many in the early 1990s to be an extension of a 'normal' process of progressive ageing-related cognitive deterioration, by the end of the decade subclinical cognitive deficit began to be perceived as an extension of a pathological process. Numerous studies have referred vaguely to mild cognitive disorders in relation to dementia and in 1997 Petersen and colleagues (Petersen *et al.*, 1997) proposed diagnostic criteria for the concept of mild cognitive impairment (MCI), initially defined as complaints of defective memory and demonstration of abnormal memory functioning for age, with normal general cognitive functioning and conserved ability to perform activities of daily living. MCI was considered to be a prodrome of Alzheimer's disease (AD). MCI criteria proved difficult to apply as it referred to poor cognitive functioning as assessed at one point in time, thus precluding appreciation of decline over time, and difficult to differentiate from cohort effects, low IQ and education. A later definition refined the initial concept by referring to memory impairment beyond that expected for both age and education level (Petersen et al., 1999). An alternative approach has been to define it in terms of early-stage dementia. For example Krasuki et al. (1998) refer to cognitive impairment with a score of 20 or more on the MMSE, and Zaudig (1992) defines MCI as a score of more than 22 on MMSE or 34–47 on the SIDAM dementia scale. Others have referred to criteria based on Clinical Dementia Rating Scale or Global Deterioration Scale scores (Flicker et al., 1991; Kluger et al., 1997). The concept of MCI subsequently became the focus of considerable interest as it opened up the possibility of widescale treatment of a subclinical state by the new cholinergic therapies developed for dementia.

23.4 OPERATIONALIZING MILD COGNITIVE IMPAIRMENT CRITERIA

Subsequent studies using MCI criteria have encountered numerous difficulties. These have been principally due to the lack of a working definition based on designated cognitive tests and other clinical measures. The result has been that population prevalence, the clinical features of subjects identified with MCI, and their clinical outcomes, vary widely between studies and even within studies where there has been longitudinal follow up. A consensus conference held in Chicago in 1999 confronted the many difficulties facing the MCI concept (Petersen et al., 2001), notably its two underlying assumptions that it should be confined exclusively to isolated memory impairment and whether it constitutes a prodrome of AD, or alternatively a more clinically heterogeneous group at increased risk of dementia owing to any cause. While there is some limited evidence that a purely amnesic syndrome may exist (Richards et al., 1999), these appear to represent only a very small proportion (6 per cent) of elderly persons with cognitive deficit when the full range of cognitive functions are examined. Higher rates of 'circumscribed memory deficit' (31.7 per cent of CIND cases) are observed within the Canadian Longitudinal Study (Graham et al., 1997), but only subjects with a score below a cut-off on the MMSE are examined, and the test battery itself consists predominantly of memory tasks. Memory tests also involve cognitive capacities other than memory, notably attentional and linguistic capacities, so that it is difficult in the absence of a detailed neuropsychological examination to conclude that an individual has an isolated amnesic impairment. Many of the studies that observe principally memory deficits in MCI have used almost exclusively memory tests in their diagnostic examination.

The Chicago consensus group concluded that subjects with MCI have a condition different from normal ageing and are likely to progress to AD at an accelerated rate; however, they may also progress to another form of dementia or improve. This group thus proposed subtypes of MCI according to type of cognitive deficit and clinical outcome distinguishing MCI Amnestic (MCI with pronounced memory impairment progressing to AD), MCI Multiple Domain (slight impairment across several cognitive domains leading to AD, vascular dementia or stabilizing in the case of normal brain ageing changes), and MCI Single Non-Memory Domain (significant impairment in a cognitive domain other than memory leading to AD or another form of dementia). It has subsequently been suggested that MCI be further subdivided according to the suspected aetiology of the cognitive impairment, in keeping with international classifications of dementing disorders: for example MCI-AD, MCI-LBD, MCI-FTD and so on.

23.5 THE FUTURE OF MILD COGNITIVE IMPAIRMENT

A number of concepts now exist to describe subclinical cognitive disorder in the elderly. Application of these concepts in general population studies gives quite different prevalence rates both between concepts and even between studies using the same concept (Table 23.1).

Clearly such deficits have multiple causes. A longitudinal study of a general population sample with subclinical cognitive deficits has demonstrated multiple patterns of cognitive change with variable clinical outcomes including dementia, depression, cardiovascular and respiratory disorders (Ritchie et al., 1996). However, it is the identification of those cases likely to evolve towards dementia that have been given priority, especially given the development of treatments that may delay dementia onset. The potential treatment window for dementia is large, with twin studies indicating that insidious changes in cognitive performance may occur up to 20 years before disease onset (La Rue and Jarvik, 1987). For this reason at a conceptual level, MCI has been the principal focus of interest as longitudinal studies confirm the high risk rates of MCI for dementia, with conversion estimates ranging from 10 to 15 per cent per year (Petersen et al., 1997), 40 per cent over 2 years (Johnson et al., 1998), 20 per cent over 3 years (Wolf et al., 1998), 30 per cent over 3 years (Black, 1999), 53 per cent over 3 years (McKelvey et al., 1999), to 100 per cent over 4.5 years (Krasuki et al., 1998). Population studies show, however, lower dementia conversion rates (2–8 per cent per annum; Tierney et al., 1996; Johanssen and Zarit, 1997; Kluger et al., 1999; Hogan and Ebly, 2000; Artero et al., 2001; Morris et al., 2001) than those observed in clinical studies (12–31 per cent; Flicker et al., 1991; Bowen et al., 1997; Devanand et al., 1997; Huang et al., 2000) as they include a wider range of cognitive impairments, which are probably also less severe than those presenting in clinical settings. These studies suggest that alternative cognitive criteria (notably those for ARCD) in conjunction with subtle measures of loss of ability to perform activities of everyday living

Table 23.1   *Characteristics and estimated prevalence rates (where available) of nosological entities designating cognitive impairment in elderly persons without dementia*

Concept	Reference	Criteria	Population prevalence (%)
BSF	Kral (1962)	Memory complaints, forgetting details. Depression	–
AAMI	Crook *et al.* (1968)	Memory impairment with decrement on formal cognitive test compared to young adults	7–38
LLF	Blackford and LaRue (1989)	AAMI with greater decrement on 50% of a test battery	–
AACD	Levy *et al.* (1994)	Impairment on any formal cognitive test compared to peers	21–27
ARCD	DSM IV (APA, 1994)	Objective decline in cognitive functioning due to old age	8
MCD	ICD-10 (WHO, 1993)	Disorders of memory learning and concentration demonstrated by testing. Due to disease	4
MNCD	DSM IV (APA, 1994)	Difficulties in memory, learning, perceptual-motor, linguistic and central executive functioning. Due to disease	–
CIND	Graham *et al.* (1997)	Circumscribed memory impairment and low MMSE score due to disease or age	30–80
MCI	Petersen *et al.* (1997)	Complaints of defective memory, demonstrated by deficit on cognitive tests with normal general intellectual functioning compared to peers. Due to dementia	3–15

and anatomical changes on cerebral imaging (volume loss in hippocampal and entorhinal cortex) may ultimately provide better dementia prediction (Tierney *et al.*, 1996; Touchon and Ritchie, 1999; Artero *et al.*, 2001, 2003; Ritchie *et al.*, 2001; Visser *et al.*, 2002; Palmer *et al.*, 2003).

While the recognition of MCI as a potentially pathological entity marks an early step towards the recognition of non-dementia cognitive disorder as an important clinical problem with a potential treatment, it does not now meet the necessary validation criteria for a formal nosological entity (Ritchie *et al.*, 2001). The feasibility of widescale treatment will very much depend on the development of more precise diagnostic criteria. Premature application of MCI criteria for the identification of subjects for clinical trials is likely to lead to either the inclusion of high numbers of non-cases (yielding high failure rates and subsequent discreditation of a treatment that may have been successful on sample subgroups) or alternatively by restriction to subjects in reality already manifesting early dementia, in which case potential preventive/delaying effects will be minimized. The future of MCI development will depend very much on close collaboration between specialist clinical units refining clinical criteria and epidemiologists monitoring screening efficiency within the general population where MCI will principally be detected.

REFERENCES

Artero S, Touchon J, Ritchie K. (2001) Disability and mild cognitive impairment: a longitudinal population-based study. *International Journal of Geriatric Psychiatry* **16**: 1092–1097

Artero S, Tierney MC, Touchon J, Ritchie K. (2003) Prediction of transition from cognitive impairment to senile dementia: a prospective longitudinal study. *Acta Psychiatrica Scandinavica* **107**: 390–393

Black SE. (1999) Can SPECT predict the future for mild cognitive impairment? *Canadian Journal of Neurological Sciences* **26**: 4–6

Blackford RC and La Rue A. (1989) Criteria for diagnosing age associated memory impairment: proposed improvements from the field. *Developmental Neuropsychology* **5**: 295–306

Bowen J, Teri L, Kukull W, McCormick W, McCurry SM, Larson EB. (1997) Progression to dementia in patients with isolated memory loss. *Lancet* **349**: 763–765

Christensen H, Henderson AS, Jorm AF, MacKinnon AJ, Scott R, Korten AE. (1995) ICD-10 mild cognitive disorder: epidemiological evidence on its validity. *Psychological Medicine* **25**: 105–120

Crook T, Bartus RT, Ferris SH, Whitehouse P, Cohen GD, Gershon S. (1986) Age associated memory impairment: proposed diagnostic criteria and measures of clinical change – Report of a National Institute of Mental Health Work Group. *Developmental Neuropsychology* **2**: 261–276

Devanand DP, Folz M, Gorlyn M, Moeller JR, Stern Y. (1997) Questionable dementia: clinical course and predictors of outcome. *Journal of American Geriatrics Society* **45**: 321–328

Flicker C, Ferris FH, Reisberg B. (1991) Mild cognitive impairment in the elderly: predictors of dementia. *Neurology* **41**: 1006–1009

Graham JE, Rockwood K, Beattie EL *et al.* (1997) Prevalence and severity of cognitive impairment with and without dementia in an elderly population. *Lancet* **349**: 1793–1796

Hogan DB and Ebly EM. (2000) Predicting who will develop dementia in a cohort of Canadian seniors. *Canadian Journal of Neurological Sciences* **27**: 18–24

Huang C, Wahlund LO, Dierks T, Julin P, Winblad B, Jelic V. (2000) Discrimination of Alzheimer's disease and mild cognitive impairment by equivalent EEG sources: a cross-sectional and longitudinal study. *Clinical Neurophysiology* **111**: 1961–1967

Johanssen B and Zarit SH. (1997) Early cognitive markers of the incidence of dementia and mortality: a longitudinal population-based study of the oldest old. *International Journal of Geriatric Psychiatry* **12**: 53–59

Johnson KA, Jones K, Holman BL. (1998) Preclinical prediction of Alzheimer's disease using SPECT. *Neurology* **50**: 1563–1572

Kluger A, Gianutsos JG, Golomb J, Ferris SH, Reisberg B. (1997) Motor/psychomotor dysfunction in normal aging, mild cognitive decline, and early Alzheimer's disease: diagnostic and differential diagnostic features. *International Psychogeriatrics* **9**: 307–316

Kluger A, Ferris SH, Golomb J, Mittelman MS, Reisberg B. (1999) Neuropsychological prediction of decline to dementia in nondemented elderly. *Journal of Geriatric Psychiatry and Neurology* **12**: 168–179

Kral VA. (1962) Senescent forgetfulness: benign and malignant. *Canadian Medical Association Journal* **86**: 257–260

Krasuki JS, Alexander GE, Horwitz B *et al.* (1998) Volumes of medial temporal lobe structures in patients with Alzheimer's disease and mild cognitive impairment (and in healthy controls). *Biological Psychiatry* **43**: 60–68

La Rue A and Jarvik LF. (1987) Cognitive function and prediction of dementia in old age. *International Journal of Aging and Human Development* **25**: 79–89

Levy R on behalf of the Aging-Associated Cognitive Decline Working Party. (1994). Aging-associated cognitive decline. *International Psychogeriatrics* **6**: 63–68

McKelvey R, Bergman H, Stern J. (1999) Lack of prognostic significance of SPECT abnormalities in elderly subjects with mild memory loss. *Canadian Journal of Neurological Sciences* **26**: 23–28

Morris JC, Storandt M, Miller JP *et al.* (2001) Mild cognitive impairment represents early-stage Alzheimer disease. *Archives of Neurology* **58**: 397–405

Palmer K, Fratiglioni L, Winblad B. (2003) What is Mild Cognitive Impairment? Variations in definitions and evolution of nondemented persons with cognitive impairment. *Acta Neurologica Scandinavica* **179**: 14–20

Petersen RC, Smith GE, Waring SC, Ivnik RJ, Kokmen E, Tangelos EG. (1997) Aging, memory and mild cognitive impairment. *International Psychogeriatrics* **9**: 65–69

Petersen RC, Smith GE, Waring SC, Ivnik RJ, Tangalos EG, Kokmen E. (1999) Mild cognitive impairment: clinical characterization and outcome. *Archives of Neurology* **56**: 303–308

Petersen R, Doody R, Kurz A *et al.* (2001) Current concepts in mild cognitive impairment. *Archives of Neurology* **58**: 1985–1992

Richards M, Touchon J, Ledésert B, Ritchie K. (1999) Cognitive decline in ageing: are AAMI and AACD distinct entities? *International Journal of Geriatric Psychiatry* **14**: 534–540

Ritchie K, Leibovici D, Ledésert B, Touchon J. (1996) A typology of subclinical senescent cognitive disorder. *British Journal of Psychiatry* **168**: 470–476

Ritchie K, Artero S, Touchon J. (2001) Classification criteria for mild cognitive impairment: a population-based validation study. *Neurology* **56**: 37–42

Schaie KW and Willis SL. (1991) Adult personality and psychomotor performance: cross-sectional and longitudinal analyses. *Journal of Gerontology* **46**: 275–284

Tierney MC, Szalai JP, Snow WG, Fisher RH, Nores A, Nadon G. (1996) Prediction of probable Alzheimer's disease in memory-impaired patients: a prospective longitudinal study. *Neurology* **46**: 661–665

Touchon J and Ritchie K. (1999) Prodromal cognitive disorder in Alzheimer's disease. *International Journal of Geriatric Psychiatry* **14**: 556–563

Visser PJ, Verhey FR, Hofman PA, Scheltens P, Jolles J. (2002) Medial temporal atrophy predicts Alzheimer's disease in patients with minor cognitive impairment. *Journal of Neurology, Neurosurgery, and Psychiatry* **72**: 491–497

Wolf H, Grunwald M, Ecke GM *et al.* (1998) The prognosis of mild cognitive impairment in the elderly. *Journal of Neural Transmission* **54**: 31–50

World Health Organization. (1993) *The ICD-10 Classification of Mental and Behavioural Disorders. Diagnostic Criteria for Research.* Geneva, World Health Organization

Zaudig M. (1992) A new systematic method of measurement and diagnosis of 'Mild Cognitive Impairment' and dementia according to ICD-10 and DSM-III-R criteria. *International Psychogeriatrics* **4**: 203–219

24

Clinical characterization

SELAM NEGASH, YONAS ENDALE GEDA AND RONALD C PETERSEN

In recent years, increasing attention is being paid to the transitional state between normal ageing and early Alzheimer's disease (AD). As research on ageing and dementia moves toward prevention, and as baby-boomers advance into the age at which they are at risk for AD, it has become important to characterize individuals who are at the earliest stage of a cognitive impairment, and to distinguish them from those experiencing normal ageing. Mild cognitive impairment (MCI) is a term used to describe this transitional zone between normal ageing and very early AD. Mild cognitive impairment represents a condition where individuals show memory impairment greater than expected for their age, but otherwise are functioning well and do not meet the commonly accepted criteria for dementia (Petersen et al., 1999).

Inherent in the definition of MCI and in its differentiation from normal ageing is the question of 'What is normal?'. While there are well-established diagnostic and research criteria for dementia, the picture has been less clear with regards to what constitutes normal ageing. In discussing normal ageing, it is useful to differentiate between what is being referred to as 'successful ageing' and typical normal ageing. Successful ageing represents a state of health that allows individuals to function effectively and successfully as they age (Kaye et al., 1994). In this setting, there is likely very little cognitive decline over one's life span, and cognitive function can be preserved well into the 10th decade or beyond. However, this definition of normal pertains to a very small segment of the population. What characterizes many of the elderly is normal typical ageing, where individuals encounter comorbidities, such as hypertension, coronary artery disease and sensory abnormalities, as part of ageing. In this discussion, the latter definition of normal is used.

Historically, attempts at characterizing cognitive changes at the normal tail-end of the continuum have produced several terms such as, benign senescent forgetfulness (Kral, 1962),

age-associated memory impairment (AAMI) (Crook et al., 1986), and ageing-associated cognitive decline (AACD) (Levy, 1994). These terms are generally meant to reflect the extremes of normal ageing, rather than to describe a precursor of pathologic ageing. Mild cognitive impairment, on the other hand, is recognized as a pathological condition, rather than manifestation of normal ageing, and it has recently received a great deal of attention as a clinically useful entity.

24.1 CLINICAL ASPECTS

Most clinicians recognize patients in their clinical practice who have some cognitive impairment, but are not sufficiently debilitated as to warrant the diagnosis of dementia or AD. These intermediate groups of patients are common in everyday practice, and their characterization is becoming increasingly important. While the diagnosis of probable AD, and its correspondence to definite AD, is well defined, the picture has been less clear concerning this group of patients who are in the boundary between normal ageing and very early AD. As the theoretical model in Figure 24.1 depicts, the current challenge is to move to the left on the function curve to allow clinicians to make the diagnosis of a cognitive impairment prior to reaching the threshold for clinically probable AD. This region on the curve has recently been characterized as 'MCI'. During this phase, individuals experience subtle cognitive deficits, usually forgetfulness, but otherwise have largely intact cognition and activities of daily living.

24.1.1 Criteria

At present, there is no consensus in the field on a single set of criteria for MCI. A great deal of research is moving forward

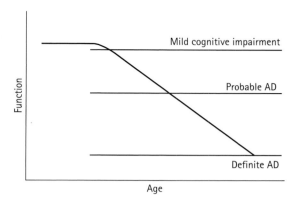

Figure 24.1 *Hypothetical characterization of function by age. As function declines, subjects go through a transitional stage of mild cognitive impairment prior to reaching the threshold for the diagnosis of clinically probable Alzheimer's disease (AD). (With permission from Petersen, 2000.)*

Box 24.1   *Criteria for amnestic mild cognitive impairment (a-MCI)*

- Memory complaint usually corroborated by an informant
- Objective memory impairment for age
- Essentially preserved general cognitive function
- Largely intact functional activities
- Not demented

---

to characterize certain features of the construct and additional work will likely continue. The most typical and well-studied scenario of MCI pertains to individuals who have impairment in a single domain of memory, and recently, this form of MCI has been termed amnestic MCI (a-MCI) (Petersen, 2003). The criteria for a-MCI are outlined in Box 24.1. It is important to note that these are clinical criteria, and that while neuropsychological testing can be very helpful, the ultimate diagnosis is a clinical judgement. The operationalization of these criteria has generated considerable research, and is currently being examined by a number of investigators worldwide. In general, these criteria are satisfied as follows.

The first criterion concerns the subjective memory complaint, which preferably is corroborated by an informant who knows the subject well. Several studies have indicated that a cognitive impairment substantiated by an informant is more likely to be reliable (Morris *et al.*, 1991; Tierney *et al.*, 1996), as subject's memory complaints are of variable reliability (Ritchie *et al.*, 1996; Smith *et al.*, 1996). As such, this criterion is 'soft' and may be a challenge to implement, but without prior cognitive function testing, it is critical for the purpose of excluding individuals with life-long static cognitive deficits (Graham *et al.*, 1997).

A second criterion concerns an objective memory impairment for age. This criterion can be fulfilled by use of neuropsychological testing, where tasks commonly used for this purpose include the Auditory Verbal Learning Test, the

Wechsler Memory Scale-Revised, Logical Memory II, or Visual Reproductions II (Rey, 1964; Wechsler, 1987). It is important to note here, however, that no particular test or cut-off score is specified for this criterion; rather, this was left to the judgement of the clinician in the appropriate clinical context. In the literature, the cut-off score of 1.5 standard deviations (SD) below age norms has been suggested by some investigators. In the original description of the MCI cohort followed at the Mayo Clinic, subjects with MCI scored approximately 1.5 SD below age- and education-matched controls on measures of learning and delayed recall, and their performance was more similar to patients with AD than to normal controls. However, this level of performance was not used as a cut-off score. Rather, these persons have a mean memory impairment of 1.5 SD; as such, there is a range of performance around the mean, where nearly half of the group had performance score somewhat less than 1.5 SD below the mean. Thus, it is important that this criterion is interpreted in conjunction with the first criterion. The memory complaint is meant to represent a change in function for the person. The clinician may be challenged by persons who are of either high intellect (whose performance is now in the statistically 'normal' range, but this level of performance represents a change for that person), or by persons with low education level (whose lower cognitive performance may not represent a change from baseline). The preferable approach to this challenge is to allow the clinician to use judgement in combining all of these criteria. As such, a precise history from the patient and an informant coupled with neuropsychological testing can be invaluable.

Third, general cognitive function is essentially normal. Subjects with MCI usually show mild impairments in non-memory cognitive domains such as language, attention and visuospatial skills; however, these impairments are not of sufficient magnitude to compromise functional abilities, or to warrant a diagnosis of dementia. It should be noted here again that performance in these domains should be judged relative to age-appropriate standards, but no specific instruments or cut-off scores are predetermined. Ultimately, the judgement of the clinician is required in making these determinations.

The fourth criterion pertains to largely intact activities of daily living (ADL). Subjects with MCI might show slower performance in complex ADL, but they are still able to complete them without difficulty and their slight impairments are of insufficient magnitude to constitute dementia. This criterion, however, can also be a challenge to implement especially in older adults. That is, the criterion requires that the slight functional impairments observed be due to a decline in cognitive function, which can be difficult to delineate in older subjects who may have several medical comorbidities and physical limitations. This once again underscores the necessity of assimilation of all of the data available in making the clinical judgement.

Finally, the last criterion is that subjects are not demented. This criterion hinges on the degree of functional impairment and is also made on the basis of the clinician's best judgement.

Many of these subjects will have a slight degree of general cognitive impairment, but it will not be of sufficient magnitude to meet the standard *Diagnostic and Statistical Manual of Mental Disorders IV* (American Psychiatric Association, 1994) criteria for dementia.

In general, subjects with MCI appear more normal than not. As such, the difficult distinction is between normal ageing and MCI rather than between MCI and AD. In the older subjects, a degree of memory impairment is frequently associated with ageing and consequently, the demarcation between normal ageing and early MCI can be a challenge. Nevertheless, the concept is a reasonable one, and several multicentre studies have now documented that these criteria can be implemented on a reliable basis across institutions (Grundman *et al.*, 2004).

24.1.2 Clinical subtypes

Although most research has focused on a-MCI, as the field of MCI has advanced, it has become apparent that other clinical subtypes exist as well (Petersen *et al.*, 1999; Petersen, 2003). More recently, the concept of MCI has been expanded to include at least three more subtypes.

- *Multiple domain amnestic MCI* pertains to individuals who, in addition to memory deficit, also have impairments in at least one other cognitive domain such as language, executive function or visuospatial skills.
- *Multiple domain non-amnestic MCI*, on the other hand, pertains to individuals who have impairments in multiple cognitive domains, but not including memory.
- *Single domain non-amnestic MCI*, which is the least common subtype, pertains to individuals with impairment in a single non-memory domain such as language, executive function or visuospatial skills. Other cognitive domains, including memory, are essentially normal.

Individuals in the non-amnestic subtypes are likely to have a different outcome from those with memory impairment. It is also imperative that individuals in all of these subtypes of MCI have minimal impairments in functional activities that do not represent a significant change in function from a prior level, and they also do not meet the criteria for dementia.

In addition to the clinical subtypes, there can also be multiple aetiologies or causes for each subtype, as depicted in Figure 24.2. Therefore, if one selected the single domain a-MCI subtype of a presumed degenerative aetiology, this would likely represent a prodromal form of AD. However, one could also add the subtype of the multiple domain a-MCI since this subtype has a high likelihood of progressing to AD as well (Petersen *et al.*, 2004). In contrast, the other subtypes emphasizing impairments in non-memory domains such as executive function and visuospatial skills, may have a higher likelihood of progressing to a non-AD dementia, such as dementia with Lewy bodies (Boeve *et al.*, 2004). Therefore, the combination

Clinical classification		Aetiology: Degenerative	Vascular	Psychiatric	Trauma
Amnestic MCI	Single domain	AD		Depr	
	Multiple domain	AD	VaD	Depr	
Non-amnestic MCI	Single domain	FTD			
	Multiple domain	DLB	VaD		

Figure 24.2 *Classification of clinical subtypes of mild cognitive impairment (MCI) with presumed aetiology. (Modified from Petersen and Morris, 2003.)*

of clinical subtypes and putative aetiologies can be useful in predicting the ultimate type of dementia to which these diseases will evolve.

24.1.3 Proposed diagnostic scheme

One logical question that can arise from the above, then, is based on these criteria and classifications: How does one generate a diagnosis of MCI in a new patient? Figure 24.3 depicts the scheme proposed to help guide this diagnostic process, and ultimately, this scheme will lead to the classification outlined in Figure 24.2. The diagnostic process usually begins with a person, or an informant who knows the person well, expressing some complaint about the person's cognitive function. For example, the person may note forgetfulness for names, or that they are misplacing objects, such as car keys. When presented with these complaints, the clinician's first task is to make a judgement as to normal cognition or suspected dementia based on the person's history and a mental status exam. For example, a score of 18/30 on the Mini-Mental State Examination along with clear signs of impairments in functional activities may suggest dementia, while a score of 28/30 on this exam added to no signs of impairment in complex ADL may suggest that the person, despite subjective complaints, is likely normal. The clinician at this point should also entertain other explanations, such as depression, for this complaint. In cases, however, where the clinician is uncertain as to the precise cognitive status of the person, the diagnosis of MCI may be entertained, and here, the flow chart depicted in Figure 24.3 can be useful (Petersen, 2004).

Once the diagnosis of MCI is entertained, the next step for the clinician is to assess the decline in cognitive function to determine whether it constitutes a diagnosis of very mild dementia. This can be accomplished through a careful history from the patient and preferably a collateral source. If the clinician determines that the decline in cognition does not constitute a significant impairment in functional activities as to warrant the diagnosis of a very mild dementia, then the

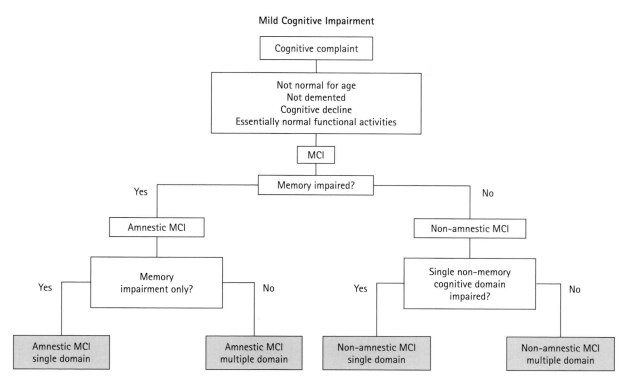

Figure 24.3 *Flow chart of decision process for making diagnosis of subtypes of mild cognitive impairment. (With permission from Petersen, 2004.)*

diagnosis of MCI is further assumed, and the next step is to identify the clinical subtype. Here, the clinician should first ask, 'Is memory impaired?' and assess memory more carefully. Although there are no generally accepted instruments for this purpose, neuropsychological tests involving word list learning or paragraph recall can be useful. If memory is determined to be impaired for age, the clinician can assume that this is an a-MCI. If, on the other hand, memory is found to be relatively spared, but the person has impairment in other non-memory cognitive domains, such as language, executive function, or visuospatial skills, this constitutes a non-amnestic subtype of MCI.

Once this determination has been made, the next step for the clinician is to ask, 'Are other cognitive domains also impaired?' This can also addressed using neuropsychological testing or other relatively brief office instruments. If these assessments reveal, for example, that a person with an a-MCI has impairment only in the memory domain, but that other cognitive domains are relatively intact, this constitutes the diagnosis of single domain a-MCI. If, on the other hand, other cognitive domains are also found to be compromised in addition to memory, this constitutes the diagnosis of multiple domain a-MCI. Likewise, if a person with non-amnestic MCI is found to have impairments only in a single non-memory domain, such as language, executive function or visuospatial skills, this constitutes the diagnosis of single domain non-amnestic MCI. However, if multiple non-memory domains are found to be mildly impaired, the diagnosis of multiple domain non-amnestic MCI is warranted.

Although this type of classification of MCI may appear cumbersome, it may be important if one is to gain more insights into the various subtypes of cognitive impairments. It can also have practical utility in so far as the medical treatments for the prodromal forms of dementia are specific to the presumed underlying aetiology of the developing dementing disorder, and are different depending on the presumed outcome of the subtype of MCI.

24.1.4 Outcome

As interest in MCI increases, several studies using the construct are being conducted around the world in a variety of research settings. As indicated above, most of the literature to date pertains to individuals with memory impairment, and it is useful to review these studies to determine the outcome of these individuals. At the Mayo Alzheimer's Disease Research Center/ Alzheimer's Disease Patient Registry, a group of approximately 220 individuals with a mean age of 79 years has been followed for 3–6 years using the original Mayo criteria, which focused on amnestic MCI (Petersen *et al.*, 1999). The subjects in these studies have progressed to dementia at a rate of approximately 12 per cent per year, which is in contrast to the normal elderly cohort that developed dementia at the rate of 1–2 per cent per year (Petersen *et al.*, 2003). Further, over the course of 6 years, up to 80 per cent of them will have converted to dementia, suggesting that this group represents a population at risk. In addition, as is shown in Figure 24.4, when individual measures such as mental status are examined,

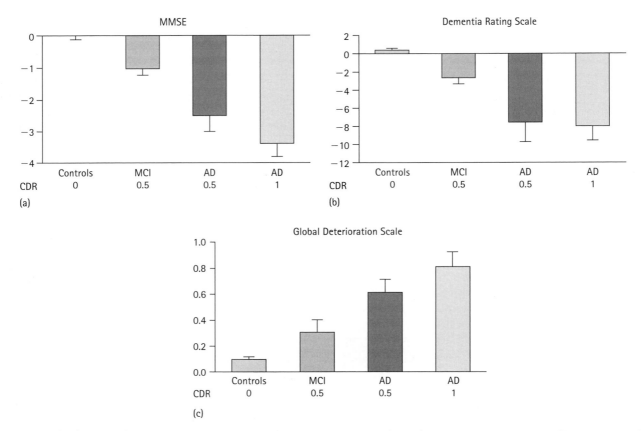

Figure 24.4 (a–c)   *Annual rates of change on the Mini-Mental State Examination (MMSE), Dementia Rating Scale and Global Deterioration Scale. (With permission from Petersen* et al., *1999.)*

subjects with MCI tend to fall midway between normal elderly controls and patients with very mild AD, and their progression rate also indicates a similar pattern.

In evaluating the measures that could predict a more rapid progression to dementia, Mayo investigators have also shown apolipoprotein E (ApoE) ε4 allele carrier status to be one of the most prominent variables (Petersen *et al.*, 1995). Performance on a cued memory task and several neuroimaging measures such as volumetric measurements of the hippocampus were also found to be useful predictors (Petersen *et al.*, 1991; Jack *et al.*, 1999).

Similarly, Tierney and colleagues in Toronto followed a group of 123 patients who had been identified by primary care physicians as having memory impairments. Over the course of two years, they found that 29 of these individuals had developed AD (Tierney *et al.*, 1996). Further, in evaluating predictors for the progression, they found delayed recall and an index of mental control to be better indicators, with ApoE ε4 carrier status being a reliable predictor only when combined with memory tests.

Investigators from the Alzheimer's Disease Patient Registry in Seattle followed a cohort of patients with an isolated memory impairment for 5 years and found that 10 of 21 subjects developed dementia over this time period, with the mean duration to dementia of 3.8 years (Bowen *et al.*, 1997). In this

study, no individual memory test was found to be better indicator than any other.

Investigators from New York University identified a group of individuals with a Global Deterioration Scale (GDS) of 3 whom they characterized as representing mildly impaired subjects and followed them for two years (Flicker *et al.*, 1991). They found that 23 of 32 subjects progressed to dementia over this time frame.

Daly and colleagues from Harvard recruited their subjects from media advertisements and identified a cohort of individuals who were mildly impaired but not demented (Daly *et al.*, 2000). These investigators modified the Clinical Dementia Rating to make it more sensitive in detecting individuals with subtle memory impairment and a CDR of 0.5. Of the 123 individuals characterized in this fashion, 23 progressed to AD over 2 years at the rate of 6 per cent per year. This rate is lower than seen in other studies and may reflect the combination of recruitment strategy and use of the CDR as the instrument of evaluation and progression.

In an epidemiological study from France, Ritchie and colleagues evaluated a cohort of 833 subjects they had followed longitudinally (Ritchie *et al.*, 2001). These investigators retrospectively applied neuropsychologically based criteria to create a group of MCI subjects and compared their outcome to a group meeting criteria for AACD. They found that the MCI criteria when applied retrospectively through the use of neuro-psychological instruments were unstable, and that AACD subjects actually demonstrated a higher conversion rate. The instability in this study, however, may have arisen from the literal, neuropsychologically based interpretation of the MCI criteria, rather than the clinical application of the criteria used in other studies.

In the PAQUID study from several south-western regions of France, Larrieu and colleagues followed a population-based sample of 1265 subjects who were at risk of developing cognitive impairment by virtue of age (Larrieu *et al.*, 2002). They found that overall MCI was a good predictor of AD but that the concept was unstable over time. They also found that over 2–3 years, 40 per cent of the sample had reverted to normal, which is quite unusual relative to other studies. It is possible that some of the instability may have been related to their use of the Benton visual retention test as their only memory measure.

Investigators from Rush Alzheimer's Disease Center studied individuals from the Religious Order Study, a research project constituting a volunteer cohort of nuns and priests who are being followed longitudinally (Bennett *et al.*, 2002). They identified a group of 211 nuns and priests with multiple domain MCI including memory, and followed them for a mean of 4.5 years. Their findings showed that persons with MCI developed AD at a rate 3.1 times higher than those who did not meet criteria for MCI.

In the first population-based study to yield prevalence data on MCI subtypes, investigators from the Cardiovascular Health Study assessed prevalence rates from the sample they had applied the criteria for a-MCI and multiple domain MCI (Lopez *et al.*, 2003). They found that the overall MCI prevalence in the Pittsburgh site was 22 per cent, with a-MCI accounting for 6 per cent and multiple domain MCI representing 16 per cent.

The Canadian Study of Health and Ageing used subjects with cognitive impairment, no dementia (CIND) to investigate the relative contributions of each of the features of the criteria for a-MCI. They felt that subjective complaint and impairment in ADL might not be necessary for the definition of MCI. Nonetheless, most people with MCI, regardless of the definition, were found to progress to dementia, usually AD (Fisk and Rockwood, 2003).

Using the Kungsholmen Project, investigators from Stockholm evaluated the outcome of subjects with CIND defined by Mini-Mental State Exam scores (Palmer *et al.*, 2002). They found that the risk of developing dementia in these subjects was associated with the level of severity of CIND, and that those who improved from CIND did not show increased risk of subsequently progressing to dementia.

Dawe and colleagues reviewed the concept of MCI a decade ago and concluded that there was a wide discrepancy in the rates of progression, which ranged from 1–25 per cent (Dawe and Philpot, 1992). These investigators put forth several factors that could account for the variability, including the source of subjects, specific criteria used and methods for implementing

them, and length of follow up. Interestingly, all these factors continue to be relevant today.

More recently, Luis and colleagues at Mount Sinai Medical Center in Miami reported a review of MCI with recommendations for future research (Luis *et al.*, 2003). These included additional research to develop appropriate and sensitive neuropsychological and functional measures, reliable methods to assess progression, and epidemiologically oriented instruments that are sensitive to multiple cultures.

In summary, as is apparent from the literature, considerable variability exists in the characterization of subjects with MCI. This variability is more likely due to lack of consistent criteria and to variable neuropsychological instruments employed to measure progression. As such, these findings emphasize the need for more consistent criteria and instruments that can allow comparability of studies across various subject populations and settings. Nevertheless, it is also apparent from these studies that the concept of MCI, regardless of the definition, is a valid construct and as such, merits further study (Petersen *et al.*, 2001a).

24.2 NEUROIMAGING

Recently, neuroimaging has become an important tool in the diagnosis of MCI and subsequent prediction of its progression. Several neuroimaging studies have indicated that magnetic resonance (MR)-based measurements of hippocampus can differentiate MCI from normal ageing and AD, and predict the rate progression to AD. Jack and colleagues have shown that hippocampal volumes of subjects with MCI falls midway between normal controls and patients with mild AD (Jack *et al.*, 1997). More recently, Jack and colleagues also demonstrated the usefulness of MRI volume measurements in assessing progression to AD by showing that hippocampal volumes in MCI subjects were predictive of conversion to AD, even after controlling for age, oestrogen use, neuropsychological test performance, ApoE status, history of ischaemic heart disease and hypertension (Jack *et al.*, 1999). Kaye and colleagues have demonstrated the predictive ability of hippocampal volume measurements by showing that subjects who progressed to develop dementia had smaller hippocampal volumes at the time of presentation compared with those individuals who did not progress to dementia (Kaye *et al.*, 1997).

Further, based on the theoretical rationale that AD pathology first appears in the transentorhinal cortex, several studies have recently focused their attention on the entorhinal cortex. While some of these studies found the entorhinal cortex to be a better discriminatory measure of early cognitive impairment than hippocampus (Bobinski *et al.*, 1999; Killiany *et al.*, 2000; Du *et al.*, 2004), others have found both structures to be equally useful in differentiating MCI from normal ageing and very mild AD (Xu *et al.*, 2000). Although it is quite likely that the disease initiates in the entorhinal cortex, measurement of hippocampus may be preferable because MRI depiction of the borders of the entorhinal cortex can be obscured by technical difficulties in imaging this area.

More recently, magnetic resonance spectroscopy (MRS) studies performed to assess MCI have proven useful. Kantarci and colleagues used myoinositol/creatine ratios and *N*-acetylaspartate/creatine ratios to compare MCI subjects to normal controls and to patients with very mild AD (Kantarci *et al.*, 2000). These investigators found increased myoinositol/creatine ratio in MCI subjects relative to normal controls, and in AD patients relative to those with MCI. In contrast, the *N*-acetylaspartate/creatine ratio did not decline until the subjects had reached the stage of AD. Even though this area requires further investigation, the data suggest that myoinositol/creatine ratio, which likely reflects glial activity, may be more useful earlier in the disease than *N*-acetylaspartate/creatine ratio, which may reflect neuronal integrity.

Thus, the existing literature indicates that the field of neuroimaging is well situated to provide a powerful tool for evaluation of MCI. Larger studies with prospective follow up would be needed to establish the reliability of these techniques in routine use.

24.3 NEUROPATHOLOGY

Despite the increased focus on MCI, the neuropathological basis of this condition is unknown. This is mainly because subjects with MCI are unlikely to die of the disease; as such, neuropathological confirmation of the condition is relatively uncommon. Nonetheless, the few data that are available have shed important light on the neuropathological substrates of MCI. A recent report from the Nun Study examined the neuropathological characteristics of individuals whose cognitive function ranged from normal to mild cognitive impairments to dementia (Riley *et al.*, 2002). The findings indicated that the development of Alzheimer's neurofibrillary pathology was one of the neuropathological substrates of mild cognitive impairments.

DeKosky and colleagues (2002) evaluated choline acetyltransferase activity in the hippocampus and frontal cortex using subjects enrolled in the Religious Order Study. Using a classification of MCI that allowed for multiple cognitive domains to be impaired, they found that 44 per cent of their sample of MCI had low likelihood of AD pathology while another 44 per cent showed intermediate likelihood of AD pathology according to NIA-Reagan criteria. Further, a study from Washington University focusing on subjects with very mild AD (CDR 0.5) has shown that 84 per cent of these subjects had neuropathological features of AD upon autopsy. Finally, a study from the Mayo Clinic identified 15 subjects who died while their clinical classification was a-MCI and found that all of the subjects had some form of medial temporal lobe pathology accounting for their memory impairment (Petersen, 2002).

Thus, the findings from these neuropathological studies suggest that MCI patients do not have fully expressed features

Table 24.1 *Clinical trials in MCI*

Sponsor	Duration	End point	Treatments
ADCS*	3 years	AD	Vitamin E Donepezil
Merck	2–3 years	AD	Rofecoxib
Novartis	3 years	AD	Rivastigmine
Janssen	2 years	Symptoms	Galantamine
Pfizer	6 months	Symptoms	Donepezil
UCB	1 year	Symptoms	Piracetam

* Alzheimer's Disease Cooperative Study supported by National Institute on Aging, Pfizer Inc., Eisai Inc. and Roche Vitamins.

of AD. As such, they are an important group to identify for possible intervention.

24.4 CLINICAL TRIALS

As the focus of AD research moves toward prevention, numerous clinical trials on MCI are being undertaken. A recent report from the Memory Impairment Study, which conducts multicentre trials on MCI, indicates that the operational criteria for MCI are successful in distinguishing MCI from normal ageing and AD (Grundman *et al.*, 2004). Thus, AD prevention trials involving MCI patients appear to be promising in detecting, intervening in and delaying the disease while it is still in a transitional clinical stage. As outlined in Table 24.1 the therapeutic agents currently being tested are cholinesterase inhibitors, antioxidants, anti-inflammatories, nootropics and glutamate receptor modulators. In their recent review, Geda and Petersen (2001) indicate that several clinical trials are undertaken by ADCS (Alzheimer's Disease Cooperative Study) and a number of pharmaceutical research groups. These clinical trials are similar in their design, hence the authors discussed the ADCS study as a prototype of these trials. About 70 institutions in North America participating in this study funded by National Institute on Aging, Pfizer Inc., Eisai Inc. and Roche Vitamins. It is a randomized, double-blind, placebo-controlled trial involving three arms with 240 subjects per arm. The objective is to assess the safety and efficacy of vitamin E (2000 IU/day) and donepezil (10 mg/day), and is powered to bring about a 33 per cent reduction of the conversion of MCI to AD over the 3-year period of the study. Over the course of the study donepezil reduced the risk of progressing to AD for the first 18 months of the trial. Vitamin E had no therapeutic effect. The secondary cognitive measures supported the overall group progression rates. No unexpected adverse events were observed. This was the first therapeutic trial to demonstrate an ability to delay the clinical diagnosis of AD.

24.5 CONCLUSION

MCI is becoming an increasingly popular clinical entity. The American Academy of Neurology has recently reviewed the literature on this topic and made recommendation that, while the precise outcome of these subjects is uncertain, MCI is a useful clinical concept worthy of attention and further investigation (Grundman *et al.*, 2004). As clinicians draw their attention to the earliest presentation of a cognitive impairment, this could translate into earlier and possibly more effective treatment options.

REFERENCES

American Psychiatric Association. (1994) *Diagnostic and Statistical Manual of Mental Disorders*, 4th edition. Washington DC, American Psychiatric Association

Bennett DA, Wilson RS, Schneider JA. (2002) Natural history of mild cognitive impairment in older persons. *Neurology* **59**: 198–205

Bobinski M, de Leon MJ, Convit A. (1999) MRI of entorhinal cortex in mild Alzheimer's disease. *Lancet* **353**: 38–40

Boeve BF, Ferman TJ, Smith GE *et al.* (2004) Mild Cognitive Impairment preceding dementia with Lewy Bodies. *Neurology* **62** (Suppl. 5): A86

Bowen J, Teri L, Kukull W, McCormick W, McCurry SM, Larson EB. (1997) Progression to dementia in patients with isolated memory loss. *Lancet* **349**: 763–765

Crook T, Bartus RT, Ferris SH, Whitehouse P, Cohen GD, Gershon S. (1986) Age-associated memory impairment: Proposed diagnostic criteria and measures of clinical change – Report of a National Institute of Mental Health Work Group. *Developmental Neuropsychology* **2**: 261–267

Daly E, Zaitchik D, Copeland M, Schmahmann J, Gunther J, Albert M. (2000) Predicting conversion to Alzheimer disease using standardized clinical information. *Archives of Neurology* **57**: 675–680

Dawe BPA and Philpot M. (1992) Concepts of mild memory impairment in the elderly and their relationship to dementia–a review. *International Journal of Geriatric Psychiatry* **7**: 473–479

DeKosky ST, Ikonomovic M, Styren S *et al.* (2002) Upregulation of choline acetyltransferase activity in hippocampus and frontal cortex of elderly subjects with mild cognitive impairment. *Annals of Neurology* **51**: 145–155

Du AT, Schuff N, Kramer JH *et al.* (2004) Higher atrophy rate of entorhinal cortex than hippocampus in AD. *Neurology* **62**: 422–427

Fisk JDMH and Rockwood K. (2003) Variations in case definition affect prevalence but not outcomes of mild cognitive impairment. *Neurology* **61**: 1179–1184

Flicker C, Ferris SH, Reisberg B. (1991) Mild cognitive impairment in the elderly: predictors of dementia. *Neurology* **41**: 1006–1009

Geda YE and Petersen RC. (2001) Clinical trials in mild cognitive impairment. In: S Gauthier and J Cummings (eds), *Alzheimer's Disease and Related Disorders*. London, Martin Dunitz

Graham JE, Rockwood K, Beattie BL *et al.* (1997) Prevalence and severity of cognitive impairment with and without dementia in an elderly population. *Lancet* **349**: 1793–1796

Grundman M, Petersen RC, Ferris SH *et al.* (2004) Mild cognitive impairment can be distinguished from Alzheimer disease and normal aging for clinical trials. *Archives of Neurology* **61**: 59–66

Jack CR Jr, Petersen RC, Xu Y-C *et al.* (1997) Medial temporal atrophy on MRI in normal aging and very mild Alzheimer's disease. *Neurology* **49**: 786–794

Jack CR Jr, Petersen RC, Xu Y-C *et al.* (1999) Prediction of AD with MRI-based hippocampal volume in mild cognitive impairment. *Neurology* **52**: 1397–1403

Kantarci K, Jack CR, Xu YV *et al.* (2000) Regional metabolic patterns in mild cognitive impairment and Alzheimer's disease: a 1H MRS study. *Neurology* **55**: 210–217

Kaye JA, Oken BS, Howieson DB, Howieson J, Holm LA, Dennison K. (1994) Neurologic evaluation of the optimally healthy oldest old. *Archives of Neurology* **51**: 1205–1211

Kaye JA, Swihart T, Howieson D *et al.* (1997) Volume loss of the hippocampus and temporal lobe in healthy elderly persons destined to develop dementia. *Neurology* **48**: 1297–1304

Killiany RJ, Gomez-Isla T, Moss M *et al.* (2000) Use of structural magnetic resonance imaging to predict who will get Alzheimer's disease. *Annals of Neurology* **47**: 430–439

Kral VA. (1962) Senescent forgetfulness: benign and malignant. *Canadian Medical Association Journal* **86**: 257–260

Larrieu S, Letenneur L, Orgogozo JM *et al.* (2002) Incidence and outcome of mild cognitive impairment in a population-based prospective cohort. *Neurology* **59**: 1594–1599

Levy R. (1994) Aging-associated cognitive decline. *International Psychogeriatrics* **6**: 63–68

Lopez OL JW, DeKosky ST, Becker JT *et al.* (2003) Prevalence and classification of mild cognitive impairment in the cardiovascular health study cognition study. *Archives of Neurology* **60**: 1394–1399

Luis CA LD, Acevedo A, Barker WW, Duara R. (2003) Mild cognitive impairment: Directions for future research. *Neurology* **61**: 438–444

Morris JC, McKeel DW, Storandt M *et al.* (1991) Very mild Alzheimer's disease: informant based clinical, psychometric, and pathologic distinction from normal aging. *Neurology* **41**: 469–478

Palmer K, Wang HX, Backman L, Winblad B, Fratiglioni L. (2002) Differential evolution of cognitive impairment in nondemented older persons: results from the Kungsholmen Project. *American Journal of Psychiatry* **159**: 436–442

Petersen RC. (2000) Aging, mild cognitive impairment, and Alzheimer's disease. *Neurologic Clinics* **18**: 789–805

Petersen RC. (2002) Mild cognitive impairment. *Neurobiology of Aging* **23**: S145

Petersen RC. (2003) Conceptual overview. In: Petersen RC (ed.), *Mild Cognitive Impairment: Aging to Alzheimer's Disease*. New York, Oxford University Press, pp. 1–14

Petersen RC. (2004) Mild cognitive impairment as a diagnostic entity. *Journal of Internal Medicine* **256**: 183–194

Petersen RC and Morris JC. (2003) Clinical features. In: Petersen RC (ed.), *Mild Cognitive Impairment: Aging to Alzheimer's Disease*. New York, Oxford University Press, pp. 15–40

Petersen RC, Smith GE, Ivnik RJ, Kokmen E, Tangalos EG. (1991) The free and cued selective reminding test: clinical utility with demented populations. *Journal of Clinical and Experimental Neuropsychology* **13**: 65

Petersen RC, Smith GE, Ivnik RJ *et al.* (1995) Apolipoprotein E status as a predictor of the development of Alzheimer's disease in memory-impaired individuals. *JAMA* **273**: 1274–1278

Petersen RC, Smith GE, Waring SC, Ivnik RJ, Tangalos EG, Kokmen E. (1999) Mild cognitive impairment: Clinical characterization and outcome. *Archives of Neurology* **56**: 303–308

Petersen RC, Stevens JC, Ganguli M, Tangalos EG, Cummings JL, DeKosky ST. (2001a) Practice parameter: Early detection of dementia: Mild cognitive impairment (an evidence-based review). Report of the Quality Standards Subcommittee of the American Academy of Neurology. *Neurology* **56**: 1133–1142

Petersen RC, Doody R, Kurz A *et al.* (2001b) Current concepts in mild cognitive impairment. *Archives of Neurology* **58**: 1985–1992

Petersen RC, Ivnik RJ, Boeve BF, Knopman DS, Smith GE, Tangalos EG. (2004) Outcome of clinical subtypes of Mild Cognitive Impairment. *Neurology* **62** (Suppl. 5): A295

Rey A. (1964) *L'examen clinique en psychologie.* Paris, Presses Universitaires de France

Riley KP, Snowdon DA, Markesbery MD. (2002) Alzheimer's neurofibrillary pathology and the spectrum of cognitive function: findings from the Nun Study. *Annals of Neurology* **51**: 567–577

Ritchie K, Leibovici D, Ledesert B, Touchon J. (1996) A typology of subclinical senescent cognitive disorder. *British Journal of Psychiatry* **168**: 470–476

Ritchie K, Artero S, Touchon J. (2001) Classification criteria for mild cognitive impairment: a population-based validation study. *Neurology* **56**: 37–42

Smith GE, Petersen RC, Ivnik RJ, Malec JF, Tangalos EG. (1996) Subjective memory complaints, psychological distress, and longitudinal change in objective memory performance. *Psychology and Aging* **11**: 272–279

Tierney MC, Szalai JP, Snow WG *et al.* (1996) Prediction of probable Alzheimer's disease in memory-impaired patients: a prospective longitudinal study. *Neurology* **46**: 661–665

Wechsler DA. (1987) *Wechsler Memory Scale-Revised.* New York, Psychological Corporation

Xu YC, Jack CR Jr, Petersen RC *et al.* (2000) Usefulness of MRI measures of entorhinal cortex vs. hippocampus in AD. *Neurology* **54**: 1760–1767

25

Treatment

ROGER BULLOCK

Life expectancy is increasing, with a consequent increase in the cognitive disorders of old age. Treating these as early as identifiable would seem an appropriate course of action. Mild cognitive impairment (MCI) represents a stage where people have the early neuropathology of dementia, particularly Alzheimer's disease (AD), but do not have sufficient symptoms to fulfil current clinical criteria. Transition to dementia is frequent, raising questions as to whether this is a new nosology or the earliest diagnosable point of the more common neurodegenerative disorders.

25.1 EPIDEMIOLOGICAL ISSUES

While the definitive description of MCI is still awaited, there is general agreement that, when it is identified in an outpatient population, it usually represents a preclinical dementia; and that appropriate intervention at this time would be relevant and valuable. MCI represents a trigger for holistic evaluation of a persons' physical and mental state, but any treatment considerations need properly defined therapeutic goals. This is important as MCI is positioned in the hinterland between preserving a state of wellness and treating a disease. The Petersen criteria (Petersen et al., 1999) try to define the MCI population with strict definitions, but in a community sample a significant proportion of MCI subjects stay stable over time, or even revert to normal cognitive scores (Ritchie et al., 2001). The Canadian study of Health and Ageing demonstrated a 1 per cent prevalence in over-65-year-olds if strict criteria were applied, rising to 3 per cent if subjective memory loss and intact activities of daily living (ADL) were not used so rigidly. Again, a third of those identified had no cognitive

impairment after follow up at 5 years (Graham et al., 1997). This non-linearity of progression is probably due to the adaptive capacity of the brain, with its continuing plasticity and many compensatory mechanisms. These issues are particularly pertinent when treatment studies are being designed.

The Petersen criteria are strict, but only produce a positive predictive value of 31 per cent, making understanding the clinical context and longitudinal reassessment essential for the individual patient. Any intervention that slows progression of dementia at this stage should lead to delay in the development of AD. In turn, this may reduce the population prevalence of severe AD, even if the benefit for the individual is less predictable. If such outcomes are not achieved, the value of such an intervention becomes less clear. Three possible treatment scenarios exist:

- *More time in MCI and mild AD, less time in moderate to severe disease* – consequently no expansion of the overall disease longevity but a longer phase of relative independence. This may increase the cost of treatment earlier in the disease, but reduce full-time care costs.
- *More time in MCI and mild AD, same time in moderate to severe.* This still leads to a longer phase of relative independence, but does not reduce the full-time care costs.
- *More time at all stages.* Preservation of independence but longer period of dependency. This increases costs at all stages and the time in residential care could actually increase.

Unless the first scenario is achieved, costs for the health and social care community could rise along with additional pharmacological costs – unless death from other causes intervenes. So, in order to adopt a universal preventative approach to MCI, an intervention needs to reduce the risk of reaching the later stages of dementia, be inexpensive, with a low risk profile, and have few side effects. Ideally, if used early enough, it should also have the potential to prevent further cognitive impairment. Examples of population initiatives include addition of folate to flour in the USA and thiamine enrichment of food in Australia, where Wernicke's encephalopathy is common.

However, the individual with MCI experiences symptoms sufficient to seek advice; and using Peterson criteria (Petersen *et al.*, 1999), may already have significant loss of cognitive ability. The goal in treatment is improvement or maintenance of this already reduced function, which for the amnestic MCI patient, is a situation akin to treating mild AD. Some individuals may improve in some aspects of cognition and function when treated at this stage; and stabilization here looks preferable to stabilization in moderate AD. However, more data are needed to understand and capture longer-term effects of current symptomatic treatments, before they can be used to treat MCI in general clinical settings. Research into what this emerging patient group actually understands and wants has to accompany this, as it is not proven that stability at this stage is any more desirable (Frank *et al.*, 2003), especially as neuropsychiatric inventory (Cummings *et al.*, 1994) scores in MCI are higher than expected – with anxiety and depression being prominent (Lysetkos *et al.*, 2002).

So current knowledge suggests a more selective prevention model is better with MCI. Here more expensive or higher risk treatments can be matched to the most appropriate individuals rather than applied across the board. With such a universal MCI definition, this application may be more difficult in practice until firmer therapeutic milestones are defined. These will remain clinical until the acceptance of robust biomarkers. Some potentially exist. For example, alteration in the ratio of different forms of the amyloid precursor protein has been described in MCI and to a greater extent in AD (Borroni *et al.*, 2003a). Cerebrospinal fluid (CSF) tau, phosphor-tau and β-amyloid are 68 per cent sensitive and 97 per cent specific at predicting MCI conversion to AD (Zetterberg *et al.*, 2003). Electrophysiological tests of olfaction appear consistent from MCI into AD (Peters *et al.*, 2003) and computerized batteries show characteristic profiles in MCI that become worse as AD criteria are reached (Dwolatsky *et al.*, 2003). Finally, volumetric magnetic resonance imaging (MRI) of regional brain areas in MCI, such as the hippocampus (Killiany *et al.*, 2000), are predictive of AD; and positron emission studies can show reduced activity in normal subjects at risk of familial AD years before clinical symptoms (Wahlund *et al.*, 1999). All these findings clearly open opportunities for early diagnosis and intervention, though it could be argued that what is being defined is the early stage of the underlying dementia, rather than a marker for MCI. These techniques are some way from the average clinic.

Cholinesterase inhibitors (ChEIs) are relatively expensive treatments with well-established side effects (Bullock, 2002). These will be prime candidates for the selective prevention model should clinical trials in MCI prove positive. Better clinical criteria may then quickly emerge, but even then, a preventative strategy may be inappropriate where either a third of those identified do not develop full dementia, or the best outcome may be to maintain an impairment, or it does not reduce any years lived free of cognitive impairment, and treatment may both increase longevity and increase costs. Difficult cost benefit decisions will have to be made – for example, by the National Institute of Clinical Excellence in the UK. Current examples of selective prevention in MCI are rare. Two examples are the specific treatment of hypertension in those with cognitive impairments and the practice in some US clinics to use non-steroidal anti-inflammatory drugs (NSAIDs) in people with first degree family histories.

25.2 PATHOPHYSIOLOGICAL MECHANISMS OF COGNITIVE IMPAIRMENT

Many factors seem to contribute to a complex cascade of events at molecular level to cause the degenerative processes that lead to MCI and dementia (Hardy and Higgins, 1992). Ageing is the predominant risk factor for which no intervention is possible, but the ageing process produces free radical damage, oxidative stress and alterations in calcium homeostasis which coincide with reduced efficacy of amyloid clearance and increasing cerebrovascular disease (Heininger, 1999). In turn, this causes synaptic damage, transmitter and receptor loss, microglial activation and inflammation, leading to neuronal death and subsequent clinical symptoms. Many of these processes are partly understood and some have putative therapeutic options, currently in development. While the licensed drugs for AD are predominantly symptomatic, new treatments may confer some protective effects. Such strategies will have the greatest impact during MCI (or perhaps even earlier).

25.3 TREATMENT STRATEGIES

25.3.1 Treating risk factors and comorbidity

The prevalence of vascular risk factors in mid-life, such as raised diastolic blood pressure, white matter hyperintensities on MRI and apolipoprotein (ApoE) ε4 genotype, relates to late-life MCI (Kivipelto *et al.*, 2001a). High systolic blood pressure and raised cholesterol levels are related to developing late-onset AD and vascular dementia (VaD) (Kivipelto *et al.*, 2001b). This contribution of vascular lesions to cognitive impairment is just becoming understood, but may explain some of the heterogeneity in MCI. Identification of these factors, at any stage, may thus impact on the clinical expression of dementia. A population strategy across primary and secondary care for hypertension detection and treatment, along with cholesterol monitoring and lowering, may not just protect from heart disease and stroke, but MCI and dementia as well.

This has already been demonstrated in normal elderly hypertensive subjects in the Syst-Eur (Forette *et al.*, 2002) and PROGRESS (Scheen, 2001) studies. Similarly, treatment with the angiotensin-converting enzyme (ACE)-inhibitor, ramipril, has improved intellectual functioning in normal elderly hypertensives (Pogosova *et al.*, 2003). If MCI was already present, treating concomitant hypertension produced a 40 per cent reduction in relative risk for dementia in a Swedish cohort (Guo *et al.*, 1999).

Statins raised particular interest when two observational studies showed their use led to large reductions in the risk of developing AD (Jick *et al.*, 2000; Wolozin *et al.*, 2000). Another large observational study in postmenopausal women correlated cognitive impairment with higher levels of low density lipoprotein and total cholesterol (Yaffe *et al.*, 2002). The mechanism of action of statins is not known, but it is independent of cholesterol levels and may be due to reduction in amyloid production, increase in ApoE ε4 and/or effects on the microvasculature (Hartmann, 2001). Also, high levels of high density lipoproteins (HDL) in late life correlate with numbers of neurofibrillary plaques and tangles (Launer *et al.*, 2001). Unfortunately, a recent study looking at statins in older people with heart disease, the PROSPER study (Shepherd *et al.*, 2002), which contained a cognitive battery, reported no effect on cognition over 3 years. However, the battery used was subject to a large learning effect and the design may not properly capture any cognitive protection. Cholesterol may play a part in the treatment equation as high levels appear to reduce the effect of ChEIs in AD (Borroni *et al.*, 2003b). Studies combining statins to ChEIs are ongoing. At present, statins cannot currently be recommended as a primary therapy, but taking them for other clinical indications probably confers additional benefit.

25.3.2 Antioxidants and oxidative stress

Oxidative stress has been proposed as a central process in various neurodegenerative disorders (Delanty and Dichter, 2000). The formation of reactive oxygen species can cause damage to lipids and induce amyloidogenesis and apoptosis, as well as increasing atheroma (Witzum, 1994). High levels of oxidative markers have been shown to be a risk factor for cognitive decline (Berr *et al.*, 2000) and reduced antioxidant activity has been demonstrated in MCI and AD (Rinaldi *et al.*, 2003). Conversely high ascorbic acid and β-carotene levels relate to improved memory performance (Perrig *et al.*, 1997). It may be that diet alone does not provide enough central activity, and that ingestion of specific free radical scavengers, such as *Ginkgo biloba* and vitamins C and E, is required (Rosler *et al.*, 1998).

Vitamin E has been studied in moderate AD (Sano *et al.*, 1997), where a delay in institutionalization was reported, but no advantages were seen in cognition or function. The 2000 IU dose used was much higher than usually given. *In vitro*, vitamin E protects nicotinic receptors from β-amyloid (Guan *et al.*, 2000), which may be relevant given that the loss of these receptors seems to correlate with the memory loss found in AD (Paterson and Nordberg, 2000). Vitamin E is already recommended in the AD practice guideline in the USA (Doody *et al.*, 2001), but perhaps less often used in Europe. It fulfils the requirement for use in a simple intervention at population level, so further studies to demonstrate its utility in MCI are needed. Currently, such a long-term study with both vitamin E and donepezil is underway in the USA (Thal, 2003).

Ginkgo biloba is one of the most used antidementia agents worldwide, from both over the counter and prescriptive routes. It has a free radical scavenging effect among other putative modes of action. Clinical trials vary, but cognition and social function have been shown to improve in MCI in one study (Le Bars *et al.*, 2002). The relative low cost and minimal side effects suggest it may have a population use, but better constructed studies will need to be performed before any recommendation can be made.

High homocysteine levels have been associated with AD (Selley, 2003), VaD (Storey *et al.*, 2003) and cognitive decline in healthy elderly individuals (McCaddon *et al.*, 2001). High levels are recognized as a marker of vitamin B_{12} and folate deficiency, both of which have also been associated with incident AD (Wang *et al.*, 2001). Oxidative stress seems to impair the metabolism of homocysteine, and it may be that only certain B_{12} supplements have any preventive effect in this circumstance, for example, glutathionylcobalamin (McCaddon *et al.*, 2002). Folate also reduces homocysteine levels and in the USA folate is already added to flour to reduce neural tube defects. This has led to a consequent reduction in population serum homocysteine levels. However, there is no evidence yet that folate administration, with or without vitamin B_{12}, has any effect on measures of cognition or mood (Malouf *et al.*, 2003). Large scale prospective studies using folate in MCI are underway in the USA.

25.3.3 Anti-inflammatory drugs

It is well established that inflammatory processes are involved in AD (Akityama *et al.*, 2000), and observational studies have shown a reduced risk of AD in long-term users of NSAIDs (Stewart *et al.*, 1997). Consequently, studies have been performed using various anti-inflammatory drugs in AD, but with mixed results (Rogers *et al.*, 1993; Scharf *et al.*, 1999). Studies of celecoxib and rofecoxib have not yet shown efficacy. This may be because one of the proposed actions of the NSAIDs is an amyloid lowering effect that may be cyclo-oxygenase independent and not present in all the NSAIDs (Weggen *et al.*, 2001). The Alzheimer's disease anti-inflammatory prevention trial (ADAPT) is looking at patients with advanced risk of AD in over 70-year-olds (Zandi and Breitner, 2001). It is using celecoxib and naproxen and is the only long-term study currently running to address how well this class works in MCI. Data suggest that ibuprofen and indomethacin have the better profile for β-amyloid lowering (Lim, 2000), and an enantiomer of flurbiprofen, which may have secretase activity, is in clinical trial for AD (Eriksen *et al.*, 2003).

Clearly no data support the primary use of NSAIDs in MCI and they have potential problems with long-term side effects. Like statins, taking them for other reasons may have additional benefits. No specific data exist for aspirin in MCI, although its action in the secondary prevention of stroke may confer similar benefits in some cases. It is not free from side effects, even at 75 mg, so more definitive work is needed before routine recommendation.

25.3.4 Oestrogen

While observational data (Tang *et al.*, 1996; Henderson *et al.*, 2000) and experimental data (Xu *et al.*, 1998; McEwen and Alves, 1999) suggest a role for oestrogen in cognitive disorders, no clinical studies have demonstrated any significant effect in AD to date (Mulnard *et al.*, 2000; Wang *et al.*, 2000). The Women's Health Initiative hormone therapy study was discontinued in 2002 because of health risks. It measured the Mini-Mental State Examination (Folstein *et al.*, 1975) in 4381 participants over a period of 7 years, finding no cognitive advantage in the oestrogen plus progestin group – and even a suggestion that they may have fared worse than placebo (Rapp *et al.*, 2003). This problem with oestrogen studies may be due to methodological issues (route of administration, length of study, dose) and the need to identify which specific oestrogen modulator will have the most beneficial effect on cognitive disorder. Clearly better studies are required but, until they are available, no data support the use of oestrogen as a primary treatment in MCI – although as with statins and NSAIDs, being on hormone replacement for other reasons may provide some cognitive advantage.

25.3.5 Nootropics

Improving memory has led to the use of drugs with non-specific actions to alter energy metabolism, cholinergic mechanisms, steroid sensitivity and excitatory amino acids (Riedel and Jolles, 1996). Piracetam has shown improvement in attention and memory in non-demented cognitively impaired elderly patients (Fioravanti *et al.*, 1991), with a second study soon to be reported – this time using the current Petersen MCI criteria. A meta-analysis of 19 studies using piracetam for cognitive impairment also showed statistical improvement versus placebo using global measures (Waegemans *et al.*, 2002). These data are not sufficient to justify the routine use of piracetam yet, even though it is commonly used in various

parts of Europe. No systematic data really support the use of any other nootropic in MCI.

25.3.6 Cholinesterase inhibitors

The cholinergic hypothesis of AD has led to the development of ChEIs (Bartus *et al.*, 1982). These are now well established in the treatment of AD. Given that a large proportion of MCI is amnestic, which is generally regarded as a precursor to AD, it is not surprising that these drugs have emerged as the likely choice to use in MCI (Jelic and Winblad, 2003). This rationale is supported by finding similar neuropathological evidence in the basal forebrain in both AD and MCI (Whitehouse *et al.*, 1981), plus radiological evidence measuring hippocampal atrophy that suggests a continuum from MCI to AD (Killiany *et al.*, 2000). However, two recent studies cast some doubt as to whether the cholinergic model holds up in MCI. First, the cholinergic deficit may appear much later in the illness (Davis *et al.*, 1999). Second, regional upregulation of choline acetyltransferase in MCI patients suggests some form of compensatory mechanism (Dekosky *et al.*, 2002). This may explain why the course through MCI is non-linear, and may give optimism that other treatment approaches at this stage may have equal benefit.

Notwithstanding this, all three currently marketed ChEIs are undergoing long-term trials in MCI. A large National Institute of Ageing study comparing donepezil, vitamin E and placebo began first (Doody *et al.*, 2001). Outcome measures include cognitive, functional and global scores. Interim analysis has confirmed the predictive value of conversion to AD using hippocampal volume and ApoE ε4. Rivastigmine is being investigated in the InDDEx study (Sramek *et al.*, 2001), where conversion to AD and a specially designed psychological battery are the primary end points. This is a 4-year study where a central committee assesses patient data when the investigators feel a patient has converted – in an attempt to standardize the end point. Baseline data analysis has shown significant scores on the NPI in this MCI patient group – particularly anxiety and depression (Feldman *et al.*, 2003). Galantamine is being evaluated versus placebo in amnestic MCI, again using traditional cognitive and functional outcomes, this time supported with volumetric MRI. A combination of delayed clinical conversion to AD and slower rates of atrophy on MRI would support a disease-modifying effect. Final results from these studies are expected in late 2005.

The trial findings will be interesting as the instruments being used are, in the main, those used in AD, and, perhaps with the exception of the clinical dementia rating (CDR) scale (Morris, 1993), their performance in MCI is not clearly understood. For example the Alzheimer Disease Assessment Scale – Cognitive Scale (ADAS-cog) (Rosen *et al.*, 1984) has a fairly flat early course, so a one-point separation from placebo may actually be clinically significant but not deemed so by licensing authorities. Additions to the ADAS-cog have been made, but no instrument has, as yet, been specifically validated for use in any individual domain or global assessment of MCI.

25.3.7 Antidepressants

With the use of Petersen criteria (Petersen *et al.*, 1999), depression excludes the use of the terminology 'MCI', as depression itself causes mild impairments in cognition. Notwithstanding this, selective serotinergic reuptake inhibitors (SSRIs) are frequently used during MCI (Devanand *et al.*, 2003), as anxiety and depression are commonly identified symptoms; and both respond to this class in the general population. The aetiology of depression at this stage is not likely to be coincidental, as most cognitively impaired patients do not report a prior history of depressive disorder (Zubenko *et al.*, 2003). Therefore treatment of the underlying condition may be the best treatment (Rabins *et al.*, 1999) – perhaps with ChEIs (Minger *et al.*, 2000). However, the best pathological post-mortem correlation with depression in AD is loss of neurones in the locus caeruleus (noradrenergic) (Zweig *et al.*, 1988), with weaker evidence of raphe neuronal loss (serotinergic) (Forstl *et al.*, 1992). These findings may not be applicable at the MCI stage, but using an antidepressant with noradrenergic as well as serotinergic effects may make a more rational choice than an SSRI alone. Apathy is also a relatively common finding in MCI and represents a key differential diagnosis of depression (Landes *et al.*, 2001). Apathy is a common finding in neuropsychiatric disorder and seems to be a marker for frontal lobe dysfunction (Cummings, 1993). Both cholinergic (Cummings and Back, 1998) and dopaminergic (Gilley *et al.*, 1991) pathways are implicated in this dysfunction, so again treatment with ChEIs may be an option (Boyle and Malloy, 2004), or perhaps dopamine stabilizing agents. One particular SSRI, sertraline, has inherent dopamine reuptake inhibition, making it a theoretically attractive option – but a combination study of donepezil and sertraline in AD did not show any advantage with the addition of sertraline (Raskind and Peskind, 2001). To date, no systematic studies have been performed with any antidepressant in MCI for depression or apathy, so any treatment is empirical, with no one antidepressant or class having been demonstrated as superior to another. Avoidance of antidepressants with anticholinergic side effects, such as tricyclics, would be practical – given the proposed cholinergic basis of several dementia subtypes.

25.3.8 Antiglutamatergic agents

Over activity of the excitatory amino acid glutamate is recognized as a cause of neurotoxicity (Dean and Lipton, 2001). For some time, strategies to block its binding site on the *N*-methyl-D-aspartate (NMDA) receptor have been tried to reduce this excitotoxicity; which is known to increase tau phosphorylation, and consequent tangle formation

(Couratier *et al.*, 1996). One NMDA receptor, memantine, has been licensed for use in moderate to severe AD (Reisberg *et al.*, 2003). It has not yet undergone studies in MCI, but suggestions of neuroprotection (Steig *et al.*, 1999) make it an obvious target. Other compounds acting on the AMPA glutamatergic receptors, as well as the NMDA, are in development, some already being considered for MCI studies.

25.3.9 Reducing medications that have intrinsic anticholinergic activity

Aside from neuroleptics, many of the commonly prescribed drugs given to older people have anticholinergic activity (Mintzer and Burns, 2000). These include warfarin, digoxin, frusemide, cimetidine and prednisolone. This anticholinergic toxicity can be measured in serum (Mulsant *et al.*, 2003) and has been shown to be a predictor of delirium (Tune, 2000) and a possible confounder in response to cholinesterase inhibitors. This is not a routine investigation yet. Chronic exposure to such toxicity is associated with poor outcomes in AD (Lu and Tune, 2003). Reversible cognitive impairments can also be induced with high levels of these anticholinergic compounds in the serum (Mulsant *et al.*, 2003). This means that as part of the review of drug treatments that occurs for any person with cognitive impairment, replacing the more anticholinergic compounds where possible with less harmful choices (for example, bumetanide instead of frusemide) is an essential step.

25.3.10 Future treatments

Whether any of the current compounds currently being studied in MCI prove to have any effect, it is likely to be mostly symptomatic. What is really needed when symptoms are minimal is an intervention that is disease modifying, either by preventing, delaying or slowing the progression of disease (Scorer, 2001). Strategies to reduce or alter amyloid production, such as secretase inhibition (Moore *et al.*, 2000), chelating agents (Finefrock *et al.*, 2003), and anti-aggregants (Gervais *et al.*, 2001) are all in development for AD, but would be sensibly employed at the MCI stage if effective. The best known study of this type involved immunization with amyloid itself (Schenk *et al.*, 1999). The trials were halted early because of side effects, but in the one case that has undergone post mortem to date, a significant reduction in the expected numbers of amyloid plaques in the brain was found (Niccoll *et al.*, 2003). However, it is by no means clear that patients in the immunization studies benefited cognitively, and further worries about the supremacy of the amyloid hypothesis comes from findings in transgenic animals that behavioural symptoms develop before amyloid deposition occurs (Moechars *et al.*, 1999). This is a reminder that intervention in tau hyperphosphorylation is also a valid treatment option, especially as tangle distribution correlates more to the AD symptomatology (Ohm *et al.*, 2003). Blockade of glycogen synthase

3-β (GSK 3-β) and cyclin dependent kinase 5 are current targets for study (Lovestone *et al.*, 1999).

However, abnormal amyloid and tau production may be the result of loss of neuronal plasticity (Mesulam, 1999). Nerve growth factor (NGF) has been postulated to regulate this plasticity by controlling neurotransmission and neuritic outgrowth (Seiler and Schwab, 1984). No definitive way has been found to effectively introduce NGF, other than through highly invasive techniques (Eriksdotter-Johnagen *et al.*, 1998). If oral compounds could produce similar effect, then this would be an avenue to explore in MCI.

25.3.11 Non-pharmacological interventions

Attention to diet and alterations in life style, for example smoking cessation and stress reduction, may have some minor effects after the MCI stage has been reached. Exercise has also been repeatedly associated with cognitive preservation (Verghese *et al.*, 2003). Both being involved in a social network (Fratiglioni *et al.*, 2000) or participating in cognitively stimulatory activity have been associated with a reduced risk of AD (Wilson *et al.*, 2002) and a slowing in the rate of cognitive decline (Coyle, 2003). One controlled study looking at memory enhancement and relaxation training for older people with MCI has shown that memory trained individuals had significantly better memory appraisals and a trend towards better recall (Rapp *et al.*, 2002). Such techniques may prove to work well in MCI, either singly or in combination with other agents. Previously, when used in AD, there seemed a point when memory training appeared to have detrimental effects – reinforcing disability rather than helping adapt to it. Targeted cognitive training could now have some positive effect, and studies to test this assumption are underway.

25.4 CONCLUSION

Early treatment opportunities in dementia, before significant losses have occurred, have to remain a long-term desire for all who work with patients with dementia. Many current and potential options are emerging as putative treatments for use in this early stage of MCI; but the main question still remains as to whether MCI is a real entity, or whether, even now, a lot of the cases being called MCI for the purpose of clinical studies are already diagnosable AD or a related disorder. Being diagnosed with dementia has dramatic social consequences in some countries, including the USA. Having a predementia anosology can resolve certain powerful political dilemmas, but then provide a difficult problem when interpreting data. Many of the MCI subjects have associated executive function abnormalities, if looked for, and when they are questioned have subtle functional changes. This satisfies the criteria for dementia and so this diagnosis may be possible against existing research criteria (American Psychiatric Association, 1994).

If this is accepted, this current crop of MCI studies aimed at treating a new indication are perhaps superfluous. What must therefore be guarded against is the continued support of an unnecessary nosology, driven by either social prejudice or the need to market an indication.

However, patients with MCI are already attending clinics, asking advice about possible treatments. Responses to such requests vary. Ethically the important thing is to do no harm, rather than feel obliged to do something that may be inappropriate. Explaining the stage of MCI to patients and allowing them to make informed choices is the best practice – bearing in mind that being told that you have a significant problem that may or may not lead to dementia is anxiety provoking in its own right. Patients need time to ask questions and must have longitudinal follow up in order to detect both progression and remission. This is a large service commitment, especially in services still trying to manage the increased numbers of mild to moderate AD.

MCI should be regarded as a potential warning of incipient brain dysfunction, and the opportunity to attempt simple preventative measures in those who come forward should not be missed. In the absence of early biomarkers, the emphasis should be preservation of cognitive wellness rather than treatment of a disease. Simple treatment options are available. Certainly lifestyle changes, including dietary advice and relaxation, can be advised; while mental and physical exercises are also non-invasive techniques that may provide benefit. Correction of any blood pressure or cholesterol abnormality is relevant at any time – whether cognitive impairment is there or not. Pharmacologically, vitamin E is currently perhaps the most appropriate drug intervention, and many US physicians are already advising its use. Further research is needed to provide clearer information regarding optimal pharmacological and non-pharmacological management of MCI.

REFERENCES

Akityama H, Berger S, Barnum S *et al.* (2000) Inflammation and Alzheimer's disease. *Neurobiological Aging* **21**: 383–421

American Psychiatric Association. (1994) *Diagnostic and Statistical Manual of Mental Disorders*, 4th edition. Washington, American Psychiatric Association

Bartus RT, Dean RL 3rd, Beer B, Lippa AS. (1982) The cholinergic hypothesis of geriatric memory dysfunction. *Science* **217**: 408–417

Berr C, Balansard B, Arnaud J *et al.* (2000) Cognitive decline is associated with systemic oxidative stress: the EVA study. Etude du Viellissement Arteriel. *Journal of the American Geriatrics Society* **48**: 1285–1291

Borroni B, Colciaghi F, Caltagione C *et al.* (2003a) Platelet amyloid precursor protein abnormalities in mild cognitive impairment predict conversion to dementia of Alzheimer type: a 2 year follow up study. *Archives of Neurology* **60**: 1740–1744

Borroni B, Pettanati C, Bordolonali T *et al.* (2003b) Serum cholesterol levels modulate long-term efficacy of ChEIs in Alzheimer's disease. *Neuroscience Letters* **343**: 213–215

Boyle P and Malloy P. (2004) Treating apathy in Alzheimer's disease. *Dementia and Geriatric Cognitive Disorders* **17**: 91–99

Bullock R. (2002) New drugs for Alzheimer's disease and other dementias. *British Journal of Psychiatry* **180**: 135–139

Couratier P, Lesort M, Sindou P *et al.* (1996) Modifications of neuronal phosphorylated tau immunoreactivity induced by NMDA toxicity. *Molecular Chemistry and Neuropathology* **27**: 259–273

Coyle JT. (2003) Use it or loose it – do effortful mental activities protect against dementia? *New England Journal of Medicine* **348**: 2489–2490

Cummings JL. (1993) Fronto-subcortical circuits and human behavior. *Archives of Neurology* **50**: 873–880

Cummings JL and Back C. (1998) The cholinergic hypothesis of neuropsychiatric symptoms in Alzheimer's disease. *American Journal of Geriatric Psychiatry* **6**: S64–S78

Cummings JL, Mega M, Gray K *et al.* (1994) The Neuropsychiatric Inventory: Comprehensive assessment of psychopathology in dementia. *Neurology* **44**: 2308–2314

Davis KL, Mohs RC, Marin D *et al.* (1999) Cholinergic markers in elderly patients with early signs of Alzheimer's disease. *JAMA* **281**: 1401–1406

Dean AL and Lipton SA. (2001) Potential and current use of *N*-Methyl-D-Aspartate (NMDA) receptor antagonists in diseases of aging. *Drugs and Aging* **18**: 717–724

Dekosky ST, Ikonomovic MD, Styren SD *et al.* (2002) Upregulation of choline acetyltransferase activity in hippocampus and frontal cortex of elderly subjects with mild cognitive impairment. *Annals of Neurology* **51**: 145–155

Delanty N and Dichter MA. (2000) Antioxidant therapy in neurologic disease. *Archives of Neurology* **57**: 1265–1270

Devanand DP, Pelton GH, Marston K *et al.* (2003) Sertraline treatment of elderly patients with depression and cognitive impairment. *International Journal of Geriatric Psychiatry* **18**: 123–120

Doody RS, Stevens JC, Beck C. (2001) Practice parameter: Management of dementia (an evidence-based review). Report of the quality standards subcommittee of the American Academy of Neurology. *Neurology* **56**: 1154–1166

Dwolatzky T, Whitehead V, Doniger GM *et al.* (2003) Validity of a novel computerized cognitive battery for mild cognitive impairment. *BMC Geriatr* **3**: 4

Eriksdotter-Johnagen M, Nordberg A, Amberla K *et al.* (1998) Intra-cerebroventricular infusion of nerve growth factor in three patients with Alzheimer's disease. *Dementia and Geriatric Cognitive Disorders* **9**: 246–257

Eriksen JL, Sagi SA, Smith TE *et al.* (2003) NSAIDs and enantiomers of flurbiprofen target γ-secretase and lower Aβ42 in vivo. *Journal of Clinical Investigation* **112**: 440–449

Feldman H, Levy AR, Hsiung GY *et al.* (2003) A Canadian cohort study of cognitive impairment and related dementias (ACCORD): study methods and baseline results. *Neuroepidemiology* **22**: 265–274

Finefrock AE, Bush AI, Doraiswamy PM. (2003) Current status of metals as therapeutic targets in Alzheimer's disease. *Journal of the American Geriatrics Society* **51**: 1143–1148

Fioravanti M, Bergamasco B, Bocola V *et al.* (1991) A multi-centre, double-blind, controlled study of piracetam vs placebo in geriatric patients with non-vascular mild-moderate impairment in cognition. *New Trends in Clinical Neuropharmacology* **5**: 27–34

Folstein MF, Folstein SE, McHugh PR. (1975) 'Mini-Mental State'. A practical method for grading the cognitive state of patients for the clinician. *Journal of Psychiatric Research* **12**: 189–198

Forette F, Seux ML, Staessen JA *et al.* (2002) The prevention of dementia with antihypertensive treatment: new evidence from the Systolic Hypertension in Europe (Syst-Eur) study. *Archives of Internal Medicine* **162**: 2046–2052

Forstl H, Burns A, Luthert P. (1992) Clinical and neuropathological correlates of depression in Alzheimer's disease. *Psychological Medicine* **22**: 877–884

Frank L, Flynn J, Bullock R *et al.* (2003) Enhancing clinical assessment of cognitive impairment with patient based functioning. Presented at the 11th Congress of the International Psychogeriatric Association. August 17–22, Chicago

Fratiglioni L, Wang L-X, Ericsson K *et al.* (2000) Influence of social network on occurrence of dementia: a community-based longitudinal study. *Lancet* **355**: 1315–1319

Gervais F, Chalifour R, Garceau D. (2001) Glycosaminoglycans mimetics: a therapeutic approach to cerebral amyloid angiopathy. *Amyloid* **8**: 28–35

Gilley DW, Wilson RS, Bennett DA *et al.* (1991) Predictors of behavioral disturbance in Alzheimer's disease. *Journal of Gerontology* **46**: 362–371

Graham JE, Rockwood K, Beattie BL *et al.* (1997) Prevalence and severity of cognitive impairment with and without dementia in an elderly population. *Lancet* **349**: 1793–1796

Guan Z, Zhang X, Nordberg A. (2000) Influence of lipid peroxidation on the nicotinic acetylcholine receptors in PC12 cells. *Neuroscience Letters* **286**: 163–166

Guo Z, Frataglioni L, Zhu L *et al.* (1999) Occurrence and progression of dementia in a community population aged 75 years and older. *Archives of Neurology* **56**: 991–996

Hardy JA and Higgins GA. (1992) Alzheimer's disease: the amyloid cascade hypothesis. *Science* **256**: 184–85

Hartmann T. (2001) Cholesterol, Aβ and Alzheimer's disease. *TINS* **24**: S45–S48

Heininger K. (1999) A unifying hypothesis of Alzheimer's disease II: Pathophysiological processes. *Human Psychopharmacology* **14**: 525–581

Henderson VW, Paganini-Hill A, Miller BL *et al.* (2000) Estrogen for Alzheimer's disease in women *Neurology* **54**: 295–301

Jelic V and Winblad B. Treatment of mild cognitive impairment: rationale, present and future strategies. *Acta Neurologica Scandinavica* **107** (Suppl. 179): 83–93

Jick H, Zornberg GL, Jick SS *et al.* (2000) Statins and the risk of dementia *Lancet* **356**: 1627–1631

Killiany RJ, Gomez-Isla T, Moss M *et al.* (2000) Use of structural magnetic resonance imaging to predict who will get Alzheimer's disease. *Annals of Neurology* **47**: 430–439

Kivipelto M, Helkala E-L, Hanninen T *et al.* (2001a) Midlife vascular risk factors and late-life mild cognitive impairment. *Neurology* **56**: 1683–1689

Kivipelto M, Helkala E-L, Laakso M *et al.* (2001b) Midlife vascular risk factors and Alzheimer's disease in later life: longitudinal, population based study. *BMJ* **322**: 1447–1451

Landes AM, Sperry SD, Strauss ME, Geldmacher DS. (2001) Apathy in Alzheimer's disease. *Journal of the American Geriatrics Society* **49**: 1700–1707

Launer LJ, White LR, Petrovitch H *et al.* (2001) Cholesterol and neuropathic markers of AD. A population-based autopsy study. *Neurology* **57**: 1477–1452

Le Bars PL, Velasco FM, Ferguson JM *et al.* (2002) Influence of the severity of cognitive impairment on the effect of the *Ginkgo biloba* extract Egb 761 in Alzheimer's disease. *Neuropsychobiology* **45**: 19–26

Lim GP. (2000) Ibuprofen suppresses plaque pathology and inflammation in a mouse model for Alzheimer's disease. *Journal of Neurosciences* **20**: 5709–5714

Lovestone S, Davis DR, Webster MT *et al.* (1999) Lithium reduces tau phosphorylation – effects in living cells and in neurones at therapeutic concentrations. *Biological Psychiatry* **45**: 995–1003

Lu CJ and Tune LE. (2003) Chronic exposure to anticholinergic medications adversely affects the course of Alzheimer's disease. *American Journal of Geriatric Psychiatry* **11**: 458–461

Lysetkos CG, Lopez O, Jones B *et al.* (2002) Prevalence of neuropsychiatric symptoms in dementia and mild cognitive impairment: results from the cardiovascular health study. *JAMA* **288**: 1475–1483

McCaddon A, Hudson P, Davies G *et al.* (2001) Homocysteine and cognitive decline in healthy elderly. *Dementia and Geriatric Cognitive Disorders* **12**: 309–213

McCaddon A, Regland B, Hudson P, Davies G. (2002) Functional vitamin B12 deficiency and Alzheimer's disease. *Neurology* **58**: 1395–1399

McEwen B and Alves S. (1999) Estrogen actions in the central nervous system. *Endocrinology Reviews* 1999; **20**: 279–307

Malouf M, Grimley EJ, Areosa SA. (2003) Folic acid with or without vitamin B12 for cognition and dementia. *Cochrane Database of Systematic Reviews* **4**: CD004514

Mesulam MM. (1999) Neuroplasticity failure in Alzheimer's disease: bridging the gap between plaques and tangles. *Neuron* **24**: 521–529

Minger SL, Esiri MM, McDonald B *et al.* (2000) Cholinergic deficits contribute to behavioral disturbance in patients with dementia. *Neurology* **55**: 1460–1467

Mintzer J and Burns A. (2000) Anticholinergic side effects of drugs in elderly people. *Journal of Royal Society of Medicine* **93**: 457–462

Moechars D, Dewachter I, Lorent K *et al.* (1999) Early phenotypic changes in transgenic mice that over express different mutants of amyloid precursor protein in brain. *Journal of Biological Chemistry* **274**: 6483–6492

Moore CL, Leatherwood DD, Diehl TS *et al.* (2000) Difluoro ketone peptidomimetics suggest a large S1 pocket for Alzheimer's gamma-secretase: implications for inhibitor design. *Journal of Medical Chemistry* **43**: 3434–3442

Morris J. (1993) The Clinical Dementia Rating (CDR): current version and scoring rules. *Neurology* **43**: 2412–2414

Mulnard RA, Cotman CW, Kawas C *et al.* (2000) Estrogen replacement therapy for treatment of mild to moderate Alzheimer Disease *JAMA* **283**: 1007–1015

Mulsant BH, Pollock BG, Kirschner M. (2003) Serum anticholinergic activity in a community-based sample of older adults: relationship with cognitive performance. *Archives of General Psychiatry* **60**: 198–203

Niccoll JA, Wilkinson D, Holmes C *et al.* (2003) Neuropathology of human Alzheimer's disease after immunization with amyloid beta peptide: a case report. *Nature Medicine* **9**: 448–452

Ohm TG, Glockner F, Distl R *et al.* (2003) Plasticity and the spread of Alzheimer's disease-like changes. *Neurochemical Research* **28**: 1715–1723

Paterson D and Nordberg A. (2000) Neuronal nicotinic receptors in the human brain. *Progress in Neurobiology* **6**: 75–111

Perrig WJ, Perrig P, Stahelen HB. (1997) The relation between antioxidants and memory performance in the old and very old. *Journal of the American Geriatrics Society* **45**: 718–724

Peters JM, Hummel T, Kratzsch T *et al.* (2003) Olfactory function in mild cognitive impairment and Alzheimer's disease: an investigation using psychophysical and electrophysiological techniques *American Journal of Psychiatry* **160**: 1995–2002

Petersen RC, Smith GE, Waring SC *et al.* (1999) Mild cognitive impairment: clinical characterization and outcome. *Archives of Neurology* **56**: 303–308

Pogosova GV, Zhidko NI, Ivanishina NS *et al.* (2003) Ramipril in elderly patients with mild and moderate hypertension. Clinical efficacy, effect on cerebral blood flow and intellectual functioning. *Kardiologia* **43**: 42–46

Rabins PV, Lysetkos CG, Steele CD. (1999) *Practical Dementia Care.* New York Oxford, University Press

Rapp S, Brenes G, Marsh AP. (2002) Memory enhancement training for older adults with mild cognitive impairment: a preliminary study. *Aging and Mental Health* **6**: 5–11

Rapp SR, Espeland MA, Shumaker SA. (2003) Effect of estrogen plus progestin on global cognitive function in postmenopausal women: the Women's Health Initiative Memory Study: a randomized controlled trial. *JAMA* **289**: 2663–2672

Raskind M and Peskind ER. (2001) Alzheimer's disease and related disorders. *Medical Clinics of North America* **85**: 803–817

Reisberg B, Doody R, Stoffler A *et al.* (2003) Memantine in moderate to severe Alzheimer's disease. *New England Journal of Medicine* **348**: 1333–1341

Riedel WJ and Jolles J. (1996) Cognition enhancers in age related cognitive decline. *Drugs and Aging* **8**: 245–274

Rinaldi P, Polidori MC, Metastasio A *et al.* (2003) Plasma antioxidants are similarly depleted in mild cognitive impairment and in Alzheimer's disease. *Neurobiological Aging* **24**: 915–919

Ritchie K, Artero S, Touchon J. (2001) Classification criteria for mild cognitive impairment. A population-based validation study. *Neurology* **56**: 37–42

Rogers J, Kirby LC, Hempelman SR *et al.* (1993) Clinical trial of indomethacin in Alzheimer's disease. *Neurology* **43**: 1609–1611

Rosen WG, Mohs RC, Davis KL. (1984) A new rating scale for Alzheimer's disease. *American Journal of Psychiatry* **141**: 1356–1364

Rosler M, Retz W, Thome J, Riederer P. (1998) Free radicals in Alzheimer's disease dementia: currently available therapeutic strategies. *Journal of Neural Transmission* **54** (Suppl.): 211–219

Sano M, Ernesto C, Thomas RG *et al.* (1997) A controlled trial of selegiline, alpha tocopherol, or both as treatment for Alzheimer's disease *New England Journal of Medicine* **336**: 1216–1222

Scharf S, Mander A, Ugoni A *et al.* (1999) A double-blind, placebo-controlled trial of diclofenac/misoprostol in Alzheimer's disease. *Neurology* **53**: 197–201

Scheen AJ. (2001) Secondary prevention of cerebrovascular accident with perindopril: the PROGRESS study. *Revue de Medicin (Liege)* **56**: 792–795

Schenk D, Barbour R, Dunn W *et al.* (1999) Immunization with amyloid-α attenuates Alzheimer disease-like pathology in the PDAPP mouse. *Nature* **400**: 173–177

Scorer CA. (2001) Preclinical and clinical challenges in the development of disease-modifying therapies for Alzheimer's disease. *DDT* **6**: 1207–1219

Seiler M and Schwab ME. (1984) Specific retrograde transport of nerve growth factor (NGF) from cortex to nucleus basalis in the rat. *Brain Research* **300**: 33–39

Selley ML. (2003) Increased concentrations of homocysteine and asymmetric dimethylarginine and decreased concentrations of nitric oxide in the plasma of patients with Alzheimer's disease. *Neurobiological Aging* **24**: 903–907

Shepherd J, Blauw GJ, Murphy MB *et al.* (2002) Pravastatin in elderly individuals at risk of vascular disease (PROSPER): a randomised controlled trial. *Lancet* **360**: 1623–1630

Sramek JJ, Veroff A, Cutler NR. (2001) The status of ongoing trials for mild cognitive impairment. *Expert Opinion in Investigative Drugs* **10**: 741–752

Steig PE, Sathi S, Warach S *et al.* (1999) Neuroprotection by the NMDA receptor-associated open-channel blocker memantine in a photothrombotic model of cerebral focal ischaemia in neonatal rat. *European Journal of Pharmacy* **375**: 115–120

Stewart WF, Kawas C, Corrada M, Metter EJ. (1997) Risk of Alzheimer's disease and duration of NSAID use. *Neurology* **48**: 626–632

Storey SG, Suryadevara V, Aronow WS, Ahn C. (2003) Association of plasma homocysteine in elderly persons with atherosclerotic vascular disease and dementia, atherosclerotic vascular disease without dementia, dementia without atherosclerotic disease and no dementia or atherosclerotic disease. *Journal of Gerontology A Biological Sciences and Medical Sciences* **58**: M1135–M1136

Tang M-X, Jacobs D, Stern Y *et al.* (1996) Effect of oestrogen during menopause on risk of Alzheimer's disease. *Lancet* **348**: 429–432

Thal L. (2003) Therapeutics and mild cognitive impairment: current status and future directions. *Alzheimer Disease and Associated Disorders* **17**: S69–S71

Tune LE. (2000) Serum anticholinergic activity levels and delirium in the elderly. *Seminar Clinics in Neuropsychiatry* **5**: 149–153

Verghese J, Lipton RB, Katz MJ *et al.* (2003) Leisure activities and the risk of dementia in the elderly. *New England Journal of Medicine* **348**: 2508–2516

Waegemans T, Wilsher CR, Danniu A *et al.* (2002) Clinical efficacy of piracetam in cognitive impairment: a meta analysis. *Dementia and Geriatric Cognitive Disorders* **13**: 217–224

Wahlund LO, Basun H, Almkvisy O *et al.* (1999) A follow up study of the family with the Swedish APP 670/671 Alzheimer's disease mutation. *Dementia and Geriatric Cognitive Disorders* **10**: 526–533

Wang PN, Liao SQ, Lui RS *et al.* (2000) Effects of estrogen on cognition, mood and cerebral blood flow in Alzheimer's disease: a controlled study. *Neurology* **54**: 2061–2066

Wang H-X, Wahlin A, Basun H *et al.* (2001) Vitamin B_{12} and folate in relation to the development of Alzheimer's disease. *Neurology* **56**: 1188–1194

Weggen S, Eriksen JL, Das P *et al.* (2001) A subset of NSAIDs lower amyloidogenic Abeta42 independently of cyclooxygenase activity. *Nature* **414**: 212–216

Whitehouse, PJ, Price DL, Clark AW *et al.* (1981) Alzheimer disease: evidence for selective loss of cholinergic neurones in the nucleus basalis. *Annals of Neurology* **10**: 122–126

Wilson RS, Mendes de Leon CF, Barnes LL *et al.* (2002) Participation in cognitively stimulating activities and risk of incipient Alzheimer's disease. *JAMA* **287**: 742–748

Witzum JL. (1994) The oxidation hypothesis of atherosclerosis. *Lancet* **344**: 793–795

Wolozin B, Kellman W, Rousseau P *et al.* (2000) Decreased prevalence of Alzheimer's disease associated with 3-hydroxy-methylglutaryl-coenzyme A reductase inhibitors *Archives of Neurology* **57**: 1439–1443

Xu H, Gouras GK, Greenfield JP *et al.* (1998) Estrogen reduces neuronal generation of Alzheimer b-amyloid peptides. *Nature Medicine* **4**: 447–451

Yaffe K, Barrett-Connor E, Lin F, Grady D. (2002) Serum lipoprotein levels, statin use, and cognitive function in older women. *Archives of Neurology* **59**: 378–384

Zandi PP and Breitner JCS. (2001) Do NSAIDs prevent Alzheimer's disease? And, if so, why? The epidemiological evidence. *Neurobiological Aging* **22**: 811–817

Zetterberg H, Wahlund LO, Blennow K. (2003) Cerebrospinal fluid markers for prediction of Alzheimer's disease. *Neuroscience Letters* **352**: 67–69

Zubenko GS, Zubenko WN, McPherson S *et al.* (2003) A collaborative study of the emergence and clinical features of the major depressive syndrome of Alzheimer's disease. *American Journal of Psychiatry* **160**: 857–866

Zweig RM, Ross CA, Hedreen JC. (1988) The neuropathology of aminergic nuclei in Alzheimer's disease. *Annals of Neurology* **24**: 233–242

PART 3

Alzheimer's disease

What is Alzheimer's disease?

HANS FÖRSTL

26.1 GENERAL

26.1.1 History

Alois Alzheimer (1898) felt that senile dementia was the most frequent neuropsychiatric disorder. Alzheimer and several other authors knew that a small proportion of patients developed signs of a 'senium praecox' (Gowers 1902). He stated: 'In some people a premature ageing or degeneration occurs, preferably affecting the central nervous system.' When Alzheimer published his famous first case of 'Alzheimer's disease' (AD) he was intrigued by the early onset of a dementia syndrome and the abundant intraneuronal neurofibrillary tangles in the patient's neocortex, which had never been seen before in a patient with such early onset of illness. In this patient, the clinical course and the neuropathological changes, particularly the neuronal loss in the superficial layers of the neocortex were excessively severe. Kraepelin (1910) decided that this presenile form of degenerative dementia with plaques and neurofibrillary tangles should bear Alzheimer's name. Initially this term was reserved for severe forms of presenile dementia with abundant plaques and neurofibrillary tangles, until a number of researchers felt that the clinical and neuropathological differences between the presenile and the senile manifestations of primary degenerative dementia were insufficient to define separate diagnostic entities (Albert, 1963; Lauter and Meyer, 1968; Corsellis, 1969). This new unitarian concept had a number of important implications. The concept of Alzheimer's disease, originally having a narrow focus, now became extended and softened. Senile dementia could no longer be accepted as the inevitable consequence of normal ageing, but became a disease. The number of patients with AD increased enormously. The economic burden and

obligation became obvious. The main risk factor was identified: age.

26.1.2 The size of the problem

Decreased mortality has led to a larger number of elderly people in our society, and decreased fertility has contributed to the higher proportion of old people. As age is the single most important demographic risk factor for AD, considerations of demographic changes are relevant for the single most important mental health problem in our ageing society. The growing importance of AD in the basic and clinical sciences is reflected by the growing number of publications. The exponential increase in publications on AD is unparalleled by research on other forms of dementia.

26.2 CLINICAL DEFINITION OF ALZHEIMER'S DISEASE

26.2.1 Diagnostic criteria

Clinically AD is a pure dementia syndrome without clinical evidence of another underlying specific disease relevant to the observed cognitive impairment. In the last decades, the cognitive paradigm of dementia has prevailed. Common elements of different diagnostic criteria for a dementia syndrome are: (1) secondary, (2) severe and (3) cognitive deficits. The deficits must not be pre-existent. They have to be severe enough to cause a significant impairment of the usual activities of daily living (ADL). This secondary impairment must not be explained by physical handicaps, but has to be related to the cognitive deficits. Most diagnostic guidelines consider amnestic deficits as a core feature of the dementia syndrome. A common and critical basic dilemma of all guidelines is the definition of clear thresholds for the distinction between near normal and already pathological cognitive problems. There is an obvious, decisive and unresolved difficulty regarding the measurement of intellectual and behavioural disturbances, which usually develop over long periods and on the basis of rather variable levels of premorbid functioning. Erkinjuntti et al. (1997) demonstrated that different diagnostic criteria yield highly inconsistent results in the definition of the dementia syndrome in elderly individuals. These differences cannot be explained exclusively by different sensitivities of the examined criteria. This general difficulty is particularly pertinent in AD where the major defining criterion is the dementia syndrome. The criteria suggested by McKhann et al. (1984), the ICD-10 (World Health Organization, 1993) and the DSM-IV criteria (American Psychiatric Association, 1994) are given in Boxes 26.1 and 26.2. The daily use of such criteria and diagnostic categories misleads us to believe that they stand for natural facts, for nosological entities. However, the authors of these operational guidelines clearly stated that they are tentative and in need of further revisions. Their major drawback is a focus on the dementia syndrome instead of the underlying neurobiological disease process. Their advantage is that they state exactly what I have to describe in this chapter.

26.2.2 Clinical symptoms

AD frequently follows a typical clinical course which reflects the underlying neuropathology. The length of the predementia phase cannot be reliably established with current clinical research tools. Theoretical considerations based on neuropathological and molecular biological findings suggest that this subclinical stage of illness extends over several decades. The clinical stages outlined in the present chapter overlap, and patients gradually progress from the mildest to the most severe manifestations of illness.

26.2.3 The predementia stages/mild cognitive impairment

Meticulous neuropsychological investigation may reveal mild cognitive impairment 5 years before the clinical diagnosis of a dementia syndrome can be established according to contemporary diagnostic standards. The pattern of the subdiagnostic difficulties includes mild impairment in acquiring new information. Other demanding cognitive tasks, including the ability to plan or to access the semantic memory store, can also be compromised causing similar cognitive problems. The differentiation between incipient AD and a reversible condition (e.g. dementia syndrome of depression)

Box 26.1 *Diagnostic criteria for research (DCR-10) for dementia in Alzheimer's disease (ICD-10: WHO, 1993)*

A. The general criteria (G1–G4) must be met.
B. There is no evidence from the history, physical examination or special investigations for any other possible cause of dementia (e.g. cerebrovascular disease, HIV disease, Parkinson's disease, Huntington's disease, normal pressure hydrocephalus), a systemic disorder (e.g. hypothyroidism, vitamin B_{12} or folic acid deficiency, hypercalcaemia), or alcohol or drug abuse.

F00.0 Dementia in Alzheimer's disease with early onset (G30.0)
1. The criteria for dementia for dementia in Alzheimer's disease (F00) must be met, and the age at onset must be below 65 years.
2. In addition, at least one of the following requirements must be met:
   (a) evidence of a relatively rapid onset and progression;
   (b) in addition to memory impairment, there must be aphasia (amnestic of sensory), agraphia, alexia, acalculia or apraxia (indicating the presence of temporal, parietal and /or frontal lobe involvement).

F00.1 Dementia in Alzheimer's disease with late onset (G30.1)
1. The criteria for dementia in Alzheimer's disease (F00) must be met and the age at onset must be 65 years or more.
2. In addition, at least one of the following requirements must be met:
   (a) evidence of a very slow, gradual onset and progression (the rate of the latter may be known only retrospectively after a course of 3 years or more);
   (b) predominance of memory impairment.
   G1 (1) over intellectual impairment
   G1 (2) (see general criteria for dementia)

F00.2 Dementia in Alzheimer's disease, atypical or mixed type (G.30.8)*

F00.9 Dementia in Alzheimer's disease, unspecified (G30.9)

*Atypical dementia, Alzheimer's type. This term and code should be used for dementias that have important atypical features or that fulfil criteria for both early- and late-onset types of Alzheimer's disease. Mixed Alzheimer's and vascular dementia is also included here

---

or benign, non-progressive memory impairment is unreliable. At the predementia stage of AD, patients do not show a significant deterioration in ADL. At this stage, individuals may take advantage of memory aids and of other supportive strategies to overcome or compensate for their cognitive deficits. The performance of complex work tasks may be

Box 26.2   *DSM-IV criteria for dementia of the Alzheimer's type (American Psychiatric Association, 1994)*

A. The development of multiple cognitive deficits manifested by both
  (1) memory impairment (impaired ability to learn new information or to recall previously learned information)
  (2) one (or more) of the following cognitive disturbances:
    (a) aphasia (language disturbance)
    (b) apraxia (impaired ability to carry out motor activities despite intact motor function)
    (c) agnosia (failure to recognize or identify objects despite intact sensory function)
    (d) disturbance in executive functioning (i.e. planning, organizing, sequencing, abstracting)
B. The cognitive deficits in criteria A1 and A2 each cause significant impairment in social or occupational functioning and represent a significant decline from a previous level of functioning.
C. The course is characterized by gradual onset and continuing cognitive decline.
D. The cognitive deficits in criteria A1 and A2 are not due to any of the following:
  (1) other central nervous system conditions that cause progressive deficits in memory and cognition (e.g. cerebrovascular disease, Parkinson's disease, Huntington's disease, subdural haematoma, normal pressure hydrocephalus, brain tumour);
  (2) systemic conditions that are known to cause dementia (e.g. hypothyroidism, vitamin B_{12} or folic acid deficiency, niacin deficiency, hypercalcaemia, neurosyphilis, HIV infection);
  (3) substance-induced conditions.

E. The deficits do not occur exclusively during the course of a delirium.
F. The disturbance is not better accounted for by another Axis I disorder (e.g. major depressive disorder, schizophrenia).

With early onset: at age 65 or below
290.11 **With delirium**: if delirium is superimposed on the dementia.
290.12 **With delusions**: if delusions are the predominant feature.
290.13 **With depressed mood**: if depressed mood (including presentations that meet full symptom criteria for a major depressive episode) is the predominant feature. A separate diagnosis of mood disorder due to a general medical condition is not given.
290.10 **Uncomplicated**: if none of the above predominates in the current clinical presentation.

With late onset: after age of 65 years
290.3   **With delirium**: if delirium is superimposed on the dementia.
290.20 **With delusions**: if delusions are the predominant feature.
290.21 **With depressed mood**: if depressed mood (including presentations that meet full symptom criteria for a major depressive episode) is the predominant feature. A separate diagnosis of mood disorder due to a general medical condition is not given.
290.0   **Uncomplicated**: if none of the above predominates in the current clinical presentation.

reduced. Patients tend to avoid difficult challenges and downplay or dissimulate their problems. In addition, non-cognitive alterations of behaviour, including social withdrawal and depressive dysphoria, may be present 5 years before a clinical diagnosis is made. Patients with more severe alterations of cerebrospinal fluid tau- and βA_4-concentration and those developing more extensive functional brain changes will convert to dementia (Riemenschneider *et al.*, 2002; Drzezga *et al.*, 2003).

26.2.4 Mild dementia stage

In most patients, a significant impairment of learning and memory is the outstanding clinical feature. In some individuals, however, aphasic or visuoconstructional deficits may prevail. Working memory, old declarative memories from the patient's earlier years and implicit memory are affected to a much lesser degree than the declarative recent memory.

Memory impairment usually interferes with various cognitive domains and usually plays a key role in the patient's difficulties with ADL. The patient's reduced ability to plan, judge and organize may not only show in complex tasks, but also in more difficult household chores (e.g. managing bank account, preparing meals). Communication may begin to suffer from shrinking vocabulary, decreasing word fluency and less precise expressive language, even though a patient may still appear eloquent, 'fluent' and even verbose on casual inspection. An impairment of object naming and semantic difficulties with word generation can be demonstrated by means of neuropsychological tests. Constructional apraxia can be revealed on drawing tasks. Spatial disorientation frequently causes major problems in driving, as patients are less capable of estimating distances and speed. Because they have an increased risk of accidents, patients with a diagnosis of AD should be carefully assessed for driving ability, regulations for which vary between countries. At the mild stage of AD, patients may still be able to live independently for most of the time, but owing to the significant cognitive difficulties in several domains, they will need support with a variety of organizational matters. If a patient wishes to remain at home, arrangements for a support system should be made at this stage before a more intensive or permanent supervision is necessary.

Non-cognitive disturbances in AD are more frequent than previously thought. Symptoms of depression may prevail in the early stage of illness (Burns et al., 1990). These emotional disturbances are typically mild and fluctuating, but also full-blown depressive episodes can occur. They may partly represent understandable emotional reactions to reduced cognitive and ADL skills or to reduced social contacts while the patient's insight is, at least, partly retained. Patients with severe depressive disturbances may show reduced cell counts in the locus caeruleus and other aminergic brain-stem nuclei (Zubenko et al., 1989; Förstl et al., 1992). A reduced dorsofrontal blood flow has been demonstrated in patients with severe apathy. Subtle impairment of complex motor tasks may remain unnoticed on standard neurological examination.

26.2.5 Moderate dementia stage

Due to the severe impairment of recent memory, patients may appear to 'live in the past'. Logical reasoning, planning and organizing significantly deteriorate at this stage. Language difficulties become more obvious as word finding difficulties, paraphasia and circumstanciality increase. Reading skills deteriorate and the comprehension of texts can be incomplete. Writing becomes increasingly insecure with an increasing number of mistakes and omissions. Patients become distractible and gradually lose insight into their condition. Longer (ideomotor) sequences of action can no longer be organized, until finally the skills of using household appliances, dressing and eating are lost. The patient's spatial disorientation increases. Cortical visual agnosia is often present and can include the inability to recognize familiar faces (prosopagnosia). One-third of patients with AD at this stage develop illusionary misidentifications and other delusional symptoms, which are triggered by their cognitive deficits but also by the underlying disease process (Reisberg et al., 1996). Up to 20 per cent of the patients develop hallucinations, mostly of visual quality, which may be associated with a particularly severe cholinergic deficit (Lauter, 1968; Perry et al., 1990). At this stage, anosognosia prevails, but residues of insight may contribute to 'catastrophic reactions' following minor distress. Patients often lose emotional control and develop temper tantrums, which may be accompanied by physical or verbal aggression. Aimless and restless activities like wandering or hoarding are common (Devanand et al., 1997).

Patients in this moderate state of illness cannot survive in the community without close supervision. They are incapable of managing financial or legal matters. Household gas or electrical appliances are a constant source of danger to patients and also their carers. Hospital or nursing home admission may be delayed or even avoided, if a closely knit support system is in

place. During this phase, there is a maximum strain on partners and other carers because of the patient's non-cognitive behavioural problems and somatic symptoms. Restlessness, aggression, disorientation and incontinence are the most frequent factors that precipitate the breakdown of family support. Sphincter control is insufficient and can be aggravated by 'pseudo-incontinence' as a consequence of spatial disorientation and clumsy handling of clothes. Many patients are at an increased risk of falls provoked by a hesitant, festinating gait and a stooped posture (Förstl et al., 1992).

26.2.6 Severe dementia stage

Specific modular cognitive deficits cannot be teased apart at that late stage of illness, when almost all cognitive functions are severely impaired. Even early biographical memories can be lost. Language is reduced to simple phrases or even single words. Patients are increasingly unable to articulate the most simplest of needs. However, many patients can receive and return emotional signals long after the loss of language skills. This emotional receptiveness has to be remembered while the patient is completely dependent on comprehensive nursing care.

Patients often misunderstand and misinterpret nursing interventions, and this may lead to aggressive reactions. Subgroups of patients may develop stereotyped motor programmes as yelling or wandering. Restlessness and aggression may also be an expression of pain or the consequence of a profoundly disturbed circadian rhythm. A large proportion of patients show extreme apathy and exhaustion. Patients need support while eating, and even the most basic motor functions (chewing and swallowing) may be impaired as an expression of extreme apraxia. Double incontinence is frequent. Other motor disturbances (e.g. rigidity and primitive reflexes) may interfere with provision of nursing support. Extrapyramidal motor symptoms are usually due to a comorbidity with Parkinson's disease. Snouting and grasping reactions are the most frequent primitive reflexes and are associated with frontal lobe atrophy. Myoclonus and epileptic seizures can be observed in a smaller proportion of patients with severe AD, but are more frequent as compared with the general elderly population. Many bedridden patients develop decubitus ulcerations, contractions and infections. Pneumonia followed by myocardial infarction and septicaemia are the most frequent causes of death in AD.

26.3 BASIC DEFINITION OF ALZHEIMER'S DISEASE

26.3.1 Neurophysiology and neuroimaging

Neither cranial computed tomography (CT) nor magnetic resonance tomography (MRT) or single photon emission computed tomography (SPECT), nor positron emission tomography (PET), not even electroencephalography (EEG) and its quantitative analysis (qEEG) are appropriate tools for diagnosing AD. Each of these methods can, however, contribute to a clinical diagnosis:

- by excluding other specific causes of dementia that are incompatible with AD, and
- by documenting functional and morphological changes that are characteristic of AD.

26.3.1.1 EEG

Hans Berger's original observation of a slowed background activity in the EEG of demented patients was repeatedly confirmed with modern quantitative methods. This slowing exceeds the changes observed in elderly individuals without cognitive changes, but is significantly less severe than in patients with reversible confusional states or other types of brain changes underlying cognitive impairment. The decrease of α power and the increase of slow θ and δ activity are correlated with the severity of illness. The dimensional complexity and the synchronicity (coherence) of the EEG signals are significantly reduced in clinically manifest AD. A statistical discrimination of patients from elderly controls can be achieved in more than 80 per cent (Besthorn et al., 1997).

26.3.1.2 SPECT AND PET

Numerous SPECT studies demonstrated a typical asymmetric temporoparietal hypoperfusion in a large proportion of patients with AD. A decrease of temporoparietal perfusion is an important sign of AD and this typical perfusion pattern represents a valuable aid for the differentiation of AD from forms of dementia with a strong vascular component and from frontal or frontotemporal brain degenerations. PET methods are possibly more sensitive for the early observation of characteristic functional changes. The correlations between reduced perfusion or reduced metabolism with cognitive deficits, stage or duration of illness are statistically significant (Bartenstein et al., 1997). Similar to qEEG, SPECT and PET allow a statistical discrimination of patients with AD from elderly controls in more than 80 per cent.

26.3.1.3 CT/MRT

The intracranial cerebrospinal fluid spaces show an age-related increase. A significant AD-associated atrophy is superimposed on this age-related effect. The corresponding decrease of brain volume is significantly correlated with the decrease of cognitive performance. As the hippocampus is an early target for neurofibrillary tangles, neuronal and gross volume loss, it should be visualized accurately at the first occasion for a thorough clinical and neuroradiological examination. The demonstration of an increasing volume loss in the mediotemporal cortex is of diagnostic importance. Similar to qEEG, SPECT and PET, planimetric and volumetric estimates of brain atrophy permit

a statistical discrimination between patients with AD and elderly controls in more than 80 per cent – which is not necessarily of great clinical importance.

26.3.2 Neuropathology

Some authors have argued that plaques and neurofibrillary tangles could also be found in the brains of non-demented persons who appeared clinically intact until their death and that their pathophysiological significance was, therefore, doubtful (e.g. Rothschild, 1937). Blessed et al. (1968) established a statistical correlation between the severity of cortical plaque depositions and the ADL and also of cognitive performance. This approach reintroduced reason, or at least commonsense, into the scientific investigation of the mind-brain relationship of dementing patients. Brun and Gustafson (1976) pointed out the typical distribution of cerebral degeneration in AD, which is usually most pronounced in the mediotemporal limbic area, the posterior inferior temporal areas, adjoining parieto-occipital lobes and posterior cingulate gyrus. The frontal lobes are less severely involved. The primary sensory projection areas are frequently spared in typical AD. Braak and Braak (1991) elaborated a topographic distribution of neurofibrillary tangles, neuritic plaques and neuropil threads, including non-demented individuals in their studies. In stages I and II, the transentorhinal cortex is affected; the neurofibrillary tangles extend into the entorhinal cortex in stages III and IV, the hemispheral isocortex shows neurofibrillary and plaque depositions in stages V and VI, when patients usually develop clinical deficits. The clinical validity of Braak and Braak's staging has been confirmed in several studies (e.g. Delacourte et al., 1998).

26.3.3 Diagnostic confirmation

According to the clinicopathological paradigm, a histopathological confirmation of clinically suspected AD is still considered the gold standard. The clinical diagnosis of AD can be confirmed by the neuropathological work-up in 80 per cent of the cases or more, similar to qEEG, SPECT, PET, CT and MRI studies. This high percentage is often mistaken as a proof of our clinical skills and may mislead to undue complacency. It must not be forgotten that the a priori probability of choosing the right diagnosis is higher than 60 per cent, simply because of the high prevalence of AD. The probability that a patient who satisfies clinical diagnostic criteria for AD will also satisfy neuropathological criteria for Alzheimer's disease is – according to Bayes' theory – directly proportional to the prevalence of AD (i.e. critical levels of plaques and neurofibrillary tangles according to standard neuropathological criteria) in the study population. In dealing with prevalent brain changes, highly sensitive – and highly unspecific – diagnostic criteria will inevitably lead to a frequent diagnostic confirmation. Numerous selection

Box 26.3   *Likelihood of dementia due to AD, shown by plaques and neurofibrillary tangles (according to Hyman and Trojanowski, 1997)*

- **Low:** Limited severity and distribution according to Braak stages I and II
- **Intermediate:** Moderate neocortical neuritic plaques and limbic neurofibrillary tangles according to Braak stages III and IV
- **High:** Frequent neocortical neuritic plaques and neurofibrillary tangles according to Braak stages V and VI

mechanisms lead to strongly biased patient samples in memory clinics and in scientific long-term studies that lead to these high, impressive validation rates. The patients have usually undergone repeated examinations; many reached a severe stage of illness before death; cases difficult to examine and with evidence of mixed pathology had been eliminated from these studies at an earlier stage. Such samples have little to do with the normal clinical situation and the diagnostic difficulties at early and mild stages of illness when diagnostic certainty is much lower. Recent studies, using operational, clinical and neuropathological criteria, have shown that the presence of Alzheimer-type changes in the brains of demented patients can be predicted with a rather high reliability (owing to their prevalence), but that the admixture of other pathologies is not infrequent (Bowler *et al.*, 1998; Holmes *et al.*, 1998). Modern neuropathological criteria (Hyman and Trojanowski 1997) do not offer a categorical 'yes-or-no' decision for the verification of AD, but yield an estimate for the likelihood that the observed plaque – and tangle counts and their distribution – explain the clinical deficits (Box 26.3).

It remains questionable whether it is appropriate for clinicians to speculate about the exclusive presence of Alzheimer-type plaques and tangles in their patients' brains, or whether it would be more adequate to aim at identifying as many treatable pathogenic cofactors as possible.

26.4 THE FUNCTIONAL NEUROANATOMY OF ALZHEIMER'S DISEASE

26.4.1 Corticocortical disconnection

Blessed *et al.* (1968) confirmed a relationship between the isocortical plaque density and the clinical deficits. This is illustrated by the severity and extension of primarily temporoparietal hypoperfusion and hypometabolism in SPECT and PET studies. Brun and Gustafson (1976) pronounced the plausible correlation between the pattern of neuropsychological deficits and the topographical pattern of the brain changes. Delacourte *et al.* (1998) observed that cognitive

deficits are inevitably associated with neurofibrillary changes in the polymodal isocortical association areas. Neurofibrillary and plaque depositions in the isocortical layers III and V are associated with a degeneration of glutamatergic pyramidal cells responsible for corticocortical and corticosubcortical projections (Pearson *et al.*, 1985; Arendt *et al.*, 1999). Up to 50 per cent of the neocortical neurones can be lost (Gomez-Isla *et al.*, 1997). This leads to a functional impairment of feedforward loops from the lower to the higher association areas, and of feedback systems from higher to lower association areas. Its cognitive consequence is an increased noise from disturbed amplification and filtering of information. A decreased EEG coherence can be considered as a neurophysiological result of this disconnection. A callosal atrophy is evidence for corticocortical axons. The cortical localization of the process can be associated with the clinical symptoms: a disruption of cortical pathways mediating visuospatial cognition is associated with constructional apraxia; damage of high order visual association areas with apperceptive agnosia.

26.4.2 Hippocampal de–afferentiation and de–efferentiation

Hyman *et al.* (1984) demonstrated an isolation of the hippocampal formation due to a cell-specific pathology in layers II and IV of entorhinal cortex and the subiculum, normally responsible for the connection with basal forebrain, thalamus, hypothalamus and association cortices. This leads to a perforant pathway destruction with consecutive glutamate depletion in the dentate gyrus (Hyman *et al.*, 1987). It is now well known that the transentorhinal followed by the entorhinal regions are early targets of neurofibrillary tangle formation and neuronal degeneration in AD (Braak and Braak, 1991; Delacourte *et al.*, 1998). Intact hippocampal pyramidal cells ('index neurones') are part of extensive hippocampal-neocortical neuronal networks and represent essential prerequisites for the storage and retrieval of declarative memories in adult individuals. Deficits of recent episodic memory are frequent presenting symptoms in AD. According to Ribot's law, recent declarative memory functions are more severely impaired than older episodic and semantic memories, which are affected in the course of illness. The volume of the amygdala-hippocampus complex is positively correlated with the performance on memory tasks and inversely correlated with the severity of dementia (Fama *et al.*, 1997, Mori *et al.*, 1997; Pantel *et al.*, 1997). There is a close association between the severity of mediotemporal lobe atrophy and hypoperfusion or hypometabolism of the temporoparietal neocortex (Lavenu *et al.*, 1997; Yamaguchi *et al.*, 1997). The severity of mediotemporal degeneration increases while the disease process extends over the isocortex. The individual contribution of the archicortical and isocortical changes to the clinical deficits are, therefore, difficult to disentangle. The situation is further complicated by severe alterations in the upper brain stem.

26.4.3 Cholinergic denervation

As explained in other chapters of this volume, the basal nucleus of Meynert and other cholinergic nuclei in the basal forebrain are the only sources of acetylcholine for the isocortex and the hippocampus. Acetylcholine in the neocortex reduces the potassium resting potential, thereby increasing neuronal excitability, and also stimulates the activity of GABAergic interneurones allowing a focused cortical excitation. In addition, acetylcholine reduces the activity of thalamic pacemaker neurones. This is how acetylcholine increases attention and allows the organized processing of information in the neocortex and limbic system (Arendt, 2002). In summary, acetylcholine reduces the resistance in hippocampo-neocortical oscillating circuits responsible for the formation and retrieval of memories. Acetylcholinesterase inhibitors temporarily reduce the resistance in these circuits.

26.4.4 Heterogeneity

There are presenile and senile, sporadic and familial forms of AD. The patients are examined at different stages of illness; and the topographic patterns – reflected by the clinical symptoms – may show some heterogeneity and deviate from the standard course of illness described above. Most of these heterogeneous patterns are not sufficiently distinctive and stable over time to warrant the definition of meaningful subtypes of AD. Few patients have been described in whom an atypical pattern of deficit, related to plaque and tangle pathology, persisted over a longer period of time, e.g. in progressive biparietal atrophy. As mentioned above, Alzheimer pathology does not protect against other forms of neuropathological change. In old age, the admixture of other pathologies, e.g. of vascular changes, Lewy bodies, etc., is not infrequent. Some neuropathological changes would be extremely difficult to detect under the cover of plaques and tangles, e.g. brain degenerations with focal cortical onset, lacking distinctive histopathology.

26.5 DIFFERENTIAL DIAGNOSES

26.5.1 What is (probably) not Alzheimer's disease

'AD' should not be considered as a synonym for normal ageing. Also, AD is not a synonym for dementia; this is often forgotten, even in diagnostic guidelines. AD is not just the clinical Alzheimer dementia syndrome, but the underlying neurodegenerative process together with its typical clinical manifestation. AD is not (only) a presenile, but also a senile form of degenerative dementia. AD is more severe than age-associated memory impairment, benign senescent forgetfulness and the like. AD is more than an amnestic syndrome, even if deficits of episodic memory may frequently represent the core symptom of AD. AD is not a confusional state, but a confusional state may represent a first transient manifestation of a subclinical cholinergic deficit and the threshold for confusional states is reduced in patients who are cholinergically challenged due to Lewy body and/or plaque and tangle pathology in the basal forebrain nuclei.

AD is different from other forms of dementia with specific features that satisfy standard clinical and neuropathological criteria, e.g. so-called vascular dementia, dementia with Lewy bodies, Pick-complex diseases and other brain degenerations with focal cortical onset and characteristic histopathological hallmarks, Creutzfeldt–Jakob disease, AIDS-related complex, Huntington's disease, alcohol-related cognitive impairment, cognitive impairment and schizophrenia, the dementia syndrome of depression or other uncommon forms dementia.

26.5.2 What may be(come) Alzheimer's disease

As mentioned earlier, patients satisfying clinical criteria for the diseases listed above may still have critical numbers of plaques and neurofibrillary tangles, and a cholinergic deficit, and may, therefore, benefit from cholinergic and other anti-dementia treatment with efficacy demonstrated for typical AD. To date, there is no method for ruling out significant numbers of plaques and neurofibrillary tangles in the patients' brains with sufficient certainty during their lifetime, but there may be features that make the presence of significant Alzheimer pathology, or comorbidity, more likely, e.g.

- a slow onset of cognitive impairment before a stroke;
- a continuous progression of dementia after treatment for normal pressure hydrocephalus;
- hippocampal atrophy;
- temporoparietal and more extensive hypoperfusion and hypometabolism (Drzezga et al., 2003);
- a family history of Alzheimer dementia;
- a molecular-genetic risk or diagnostic factor; or
- increased tau and decreased βA_4 in the cerebrospinal fluid (Riemenschneider et al., 2002).

Double pathology decreases the threshold for the manifestation of deficits. Less severe vascular changes would be required for the manifestation of dementia, if a moderate amount of plaques and neurofibrillary tangles is already present. This appears to be confirmed by observations from pivotal landmark studies (MRC-CFAS 2001; Snowdon et al., 1997). Therefore a clinical deficit unexplained by the severity and extension of a single type of specific brain changes suggests the presence of cerebral multimorbidity.

Clinically, any mild cognitive impairment, amnestic syndrome, confusional state, depression, etc. may represent an early preclinical stage of AD. Pathophysiologically, a low α power, a discrete temporoparietal hypoperfusion or hypometabolism, early molecular cerebrospinal fluid alterations may herald incipient AD. Morphologically, anyone with mild brain atrophy, any person with subthreshold counts of plaques and neurofibrillary tangles would be a candidate for AD. Genetically, asymptomatic carriers of dominant mutations or risk factors are disposed to developing AD.

26.5.3 Alzheimer–Plus

There is nearly no senile dementia without relevant Alzheimer pathology (MRC-CFAS 2001). Cognition (C) should therefore be considered as the difference between initial intellectual capability (I) and the cumulative effects of the severity (S) and extension (e) of different types of brain changes, neurofibrillary tangles (NFT), plaques (PL), Lewy bodies (LB), frontotemporal (Pi), micro- (MIC), macroangiopathic (MAC), etc.:

$$C = I - (S_{NFT} \cdot e_{NFT} + S_{PL} \cdot e_{PL} + S_{LB} \cdot e_{LB} + S_{Pi} \cdot e_{Pi} + S_{mic} \cdot e_{mic} + S_{MAC} \cdot e_{MAC} + \cdots)$$

The correlations between individual morphological features and specific symptoms are not as clear cut as in other neuropsychiatric syndromes observed in younger patients. The relationship between neuropathological changes and clinical deficits appears more fuzzy due to the variabilities of severity, extensions and admixtures (NFT – learning, declarative recent memory, hippocampal atrophy, increased tau concentrations; plaques – 'higher' neocortical neuropsychological deficits, neocortical atrophy, decreased βA_4-concentration; Lewy bodies – motivational, affective and extrapyramidal motor symptoms, pigmented nuclei pathology; Pick-complex – behavioural and language deficits, frontotemporal atrophy, tau mutations; microangiopathy – slowing, gait apraxia, leukoaraiosis; macroangiopathy – see localization and extension of lesion).

26.5.4 Future diagnostic approaches

We are, presently, concentrating our diagnostic and therapeutic efforts on the epiphenomena of AD. It is now known, that the disease process develops over many decades before it becomes clinically evident. It is hardly a rewarding exercise for patient and physician to establish the diagnosis of AD, once significant and irreversible brain changes have accrued. However, this will be the case as long as a diagnosis relies on the manifestation of a clinical dementia syndrome and does not aim at pathophysiological factors that could represent the targets of an early intervention. Cumulative incidence and morbidity suggest that everyone runs a remarkable risk of developing the symptoms of AD in old age. Therefore, risk or chance models should help to plan the timing and intensity of early interventions. Such models will include genetic, sociodemographic, somatic and environmental protective and risk factors together with the 'early' psychological and biological epiphenomena of illness (Figure 26.1). Most of these factors are discussed elsewhere in this volume. Genetic factors are currently frequently discussed. Several sociodemographic factors are of self-explanatory importance (age, life expectancy, cognitive reserve). The influence of somatic and environmental cofactors is usually disregarded because they are not considered part of the Alzheimer pathophysiology. Some of them are now getting increasing attention (oestrogen, cholesterol, cortisone; non-steroidal anti-inflammatory agents, homocysteine, vascular comorbidity). Subclinical changes that can occur in the course of the biological disease process and be discovered with special laboratory methods before the patient develops clinical symptoms can be considered as 'early epiphenomena'. These can be discrete cognitive, predominantly amnestic deficits, associated functional brain changes (Desgranges et al., 1998), discrete morphological alterations in the mediotemporal lobe (Reiman et al., 1998) and early alterations of cerebrospinal fluid. The gaps in Figure 26.1 need to be filled in the years to come in order to develop individualized risk profiles for early interventions preceding the medical manifestation of epiphenomena.

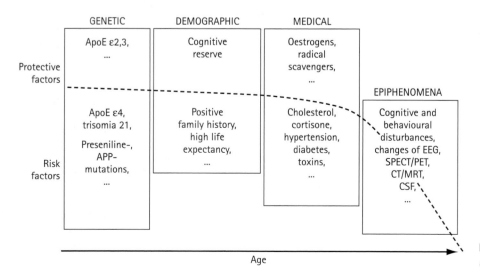

Figure 26.1 *Risk model of cognitive deterioration.*

REFERENCES

Albert E. (1963) Senile Demenz und Alzheimer – die gleiche Krankheit? *Zentralblatt für die Gesamte Neurologie und Psychiatrie.* **172**: 164

Alzheimer A. (1898) Neure Arbeiten über die Dementia senilis und die auf atherot matöser Gefässerkrankung basierenden Gehirnkrankheiten. *Monatsschrift für Psychiatrie und Neurologie* **3**: 101–115

American Psychiatric Association. (1994) *Desk Reference to the Diagnostic Criteria from DSM-IV.* APA, Washington DC, p. 85

Arendt Th. (1999) Pathologische Anatomie der Alzheimer Krankheit. In: H Förstl, H Bickel, A Kurz (eds), *Alzheimer Demenz – Grundlagen, Klinik, Therapie.* Heidelberg, Springer, pp. 87–108

Arendt T. (2002) Neuronal pathology in Alzheimer's disease. In: K Beyrenther and K Einhäuphl, (eds), *Dementia.* Shuttgart, Thiene, pp. 106–117

Bartenstein P, Minoshima S, Hirsch C *et al.* (1997) Quantitative Assessment of cerebral blood flow in patients with Alzheimer's disease by SPECT. *Journal of Nuclear Medicine* **38**: 1095–1101

Besthorn C, Zerfass R, Geiger-Kabisch C *et al.* (1997) Discrimination of Alzheimer's disease and normal aging by EEG data. *EEG and Clinical Neurophysiology* **103**: 241–248

Blessed G, Tomlinson BE, Roth M. (1968) The association between quantitative measures of dementia and of senile change in the cerebral grey matter of elderly subjects. *British Journal of Psychiatry* **114**: 797–811

Bowler JV, Munoz DG, Merskey H *et al.* (1998) Fallacies in the pathological confirmation of the diagnosis of Alzheimer's disease. *Journal of Neurology, Neurosurgery, and Psychiatry* **64**: 18–24

Braak H and Braak E. (1991) Neuropathological staging of Alzheimer-related changes. *Acta Neuropathologica* **82**: 239–259

Brun A and Gustafson L. (1976) Distribution of cerebral degeneration in Alzheimer's disease – a clinico-pathological study. *Archiv fur Psychiatrie und Nervenkrankheiten* **223**: 15–23

Burns A, Jacoby R, Levy R. (1990) Psychiatric phenomena in Alzheimer's disease. III: Disorders of mood. *British Journal of Psychiatry* **157**: 81–86

Corsellis JAN. (1969) The pathology of dementia. *British Journal of Hospital Medicine* **2**: 695–702

Delacourte A, Buée L, David JP *et al.* (1998) Lack of continuum between cerebral aging and Alzheimer's disease as revealed by PHF-tau and Aβ biochemistry. *Alzheimer's Reports* **1**: 101–110

Delacourte A, Sergeant N, Wattez A *et al.* (1998) Vulnerable neuronal subsets in Alzheimer's and Pick's disease are distinguished by their tau isoform distribution and phosphorylation. *Annals of Neurology* **43**: 193–204

Desgranges B, Baron J-C, de la Sayette V *et al.* (1998) The neural substrates of memory systems impairment in Alzheimer's disease. A PET study of resting brain glucose utilization. *Brain* **121**: 611–631

Devanand DP, Jacobs DM, Tang MX *et al.* (1997) The course of psychopathology in mild to moderate Alzheimer's disease. *Archives of General Psychiatry* **54**: 257–263

Drzezga A, Lautenschlager N, Siebner H *et al.* (2003) Cerebral metabolic changes accompanying conversion of mild cognitive impairment into Alzheimer's disease: a PET follow-up study. *European Journal of Nuclear Medicine and Molecular Imaging* **30**: 1104–1113

Erkinjuntti T, Ostbye T, Steenhuis R, Hachinski V. (1997) The effect of different diagnostic criteria on the prevalence of dementia. *New England Journal of Medicine* **337**: 1667–1674

Fama R, Sullivan ER, Shear PK *et al.* (1997) Selective cortical and hippocampal volume correlates of the Mattis Dementia Rating Scale in Alzheimer disease. *Archives of Neurology* **54**: 719–728

Förstl H, Burns A, Levy R, Cairns N, Luthert P, Lantos P. (1992) Neurological signs in Alzheimer's disease. *Archives of Neurology* **49**: 1038–1042

Gomez-Isla T, Hollister R, West H *et al.* (1997) Neuronal loss correlates with but exceeds neurofibrillary tangles in Alzheimer's disease. *Annals of Neurology* **41**: 17–24

Gowers WR (1902) A lecture on abiotrophy. *Lancet* **i**: 1003–1007

Hodges J. (1998) The amnestic prodrome of Alzheimer's disease. *Brain* **121**: 1601–1602

Holmes C, Cairns N, Lantos P, Mann A. (1998) Validity of current clinical criteria for Alzheimer's disease, vascular dementia and dementia with Lewy bodies. *British Journal of Psychiatry* **174**: 45–50

Hyman BT and Trojanowski JQ. (1997) Editorial on consensus recommendations for the postmortem diagnosis of Alzheimer disease from the National Institute on Aging and the Reagan Institute Working group on diagnostic criteria for the neuropathological assessment of Alzheimer disease. *Journal of Neuropathology and Experimental Neurology* **56**: 1095–97

Hyman BT, Van Hoesen GW, Damasio AR, Barnes CL. (1984) Alzheimer's disease: Cell-specific pathology isolates the hippocampal formation. *Science* **225**: 1168–1170

Hyman BT, Van Hoesen GW, Damasio, AR. (1987) Alzheimer's disease: Glutamate depletion in the hippocampal perforant pathway zone. *Annals of Neurology* **22**: 37–41

Kraepelin E. (1910) *Psychiatrie. Ein Lehrbuch für Studierende und Ärzte. 8. Auflage/ Bd.II/Teil1.* Leipzig, Barth, pp. 624–632

Lauter H and Meyer JE. (1968) Clinical and nosological concepts of senile dementia. In: Ch Müller and L Ciompi (eds), *Senile Dementia.* Bern/Stuttgart, Hans Huber, pp. 13–26

Lauter H. (1968) Zur Klinik und Psychopathologie der Alzheimerschen Krankheit. *Psychiatrica Clinica* **1**: 85–108

Lavenu I, Pasquier F, Leber F *et al.* (1997) Association between medial temporal lobe atrophy on CT and parietotemporal uptake decrease on SPECT in Alzheimer disease. *Journal of Neurology, Neurosurgery, and Psychiatry* **63**: 441–445

McKhann G. (1984) Clinical diagnosis of Alzheimer's disease. *Neurology* **34**: 940

MRC-CFAS. (2001) Pathological correlates of late-onset dementia in a multicentre, community-based population in England and Wales. *Lancet* **357**: 169–175

Pantel J, Schröder J, Schad LR *et al.* (1997) Quantitative magnetic resonance imaging and neurophysiological functions in dementia of the Alzheimer type. *Psychological Medicine* **27**: 221–229

Pearson RCA, Esiri MM, Hiorns RW *et al.* (1985) Anatomical correlates of the distribution of the pathological changes in the neocortex in Alzheimer disease. *Proceedings of the National Academy of Science of the United States of America* **82**: 4531–4534

Perry EK, Kerwin J, Perry RH, Blessed G, Fairbairn AF. (1990) Visual hallucinations and the cholinergic system in dementia. *Journal of Neurology, Neurosurgery, and Psychiatry* **53**: 88

Reiman EM, Uecker A, Caselli RJ *et al.* (1998) Hippocampal volumes in cognitively normal persons at genetic risk for Alzheimer's disease. The Nun study. *JAMA* **44**: 288–291

Reisberg B, Auer SR, Bonteiro I, Boksay I, Sclan SG. (1996) Behavioral disturbances of dementia: an overview of phenomenology and methodologic concerns. *International Psychogeriatrics* **8**: 169–180

Riemenschneider M, Lautenschlager N, Wagenpfeil S. (2002) Cerebrospinal fluid tau and β-Amyloid 42 proteins identify Alzheimer Disease in subjects with mild cognitive impairment. *Archives of Neurology* **59**: 1729–1734

Rothschild D. (1937) Pathologic changes in senile psychosis and their psychobiologic significance. *American Journal of Psychiatry* 757–788

Snowdon DA, Greiner LH, Mortimer JA *et al.* (1997) Brain infarction and the clinical expression of Alzheimer disease. The nun study. *JAMA* **277**: 813–817

World Health Organization. (1993) *The ICD-10 Classification of Mental and Behavioural Disorders: Diagnostic Criteria for Research.* Geneva, WHO

Yamaguchi S, Meguro K, Itoh M. (1997) Decreased cortical glucose metabolism correlates with hippocampal atrophy in Alzheimer's disease as shown by MRI and PET. *Journal of Neurology, Neurosurgery, and Psychiatry* **62**: 596–600

Zubenko GS, Moossy J, Martinez AJ, Rao GR, Koppll, Hanin I. (1989) A brain regional analysis of morphologic and cholinergic abnormalities in Alzheimer's disease. *Archives of Neurology* **46**: 634–638

27

Risk factors for Alzheimer's disease

ANTHONY F JORM

The study of risk factors for Alzheimer's disease (AD) was almost non-existent two decades ago, whereas today it is a flourishing area of research. This area is of considerable public health importance because of its potential implications for the prevention of AD by modification of risk factors.

This chapter will cover 'protection factors' as well as 'risk factors'. Although it is conventional to think of exposures in terms of increasing risk, it is sometimes more useful to invert the perspective and think of decreasing risk. We can equally validly think of a high level of factor X as increasing risk, or a low level of factor X as decreasing risk. It is simply a matter of choosing the most useful perspective. The chapter ends with a discussion of the potential for prevention through risk factor modification.

27.1 SOCIODEMOGRAPHIC FACTORS

27.1.1 Age

Old age is the most important risk factor for AD. Although the incidence rises steeply with age, there is dispute about what happens in very old age. One meta-analysis reported that incidence rises exponentially with age up to age 90 (Jorm and Jolley, 1998). These results are shown in Figure 27.1. However, another meta-analysis, involving a smaller number of studies, concluded that there is some levelling off in the rise of incidence in very old age (Gao et al., 1998). If incidence continues to rise exponentially in very old age then everybody would develop AD if they lived long enough, whereas if incidence levels off some individuals may never develop the disease over a feasible life span.

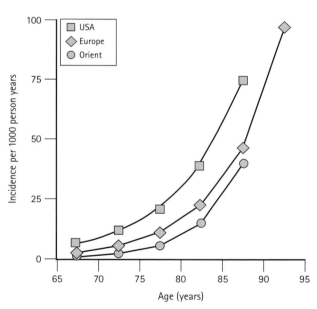

Figure 27.1 *Incidence of Alzheimer's disease across age groups: meta-analysis of data from three regions.*

27.1.2 Sex

Although many studies have reported that women have a higher prevalence of AD than men, this difference could be due to either a higher incidence or longer survival after developing the disease. Incidence studies have not presented a consistent picture. One meta-analysis found that women tend to have a higher incidence in very old age, but not in the younger old (Jorm and Jolley, 1998), whereas another concluded that women have a higher incidence overall (Gao *et al.*, 1998).

27.1.3 National and ethnic differences

If national or ethnic differences could be found, they would indicate important environmental or genetic differences. There might be major environmental differences between groups (e.g. in diet), which might not be discovered by research focusing on within-group differences. A comparison of incidence studies from different countries supports the possibility that incidence may be higher in some countries than others. One such comparison is shown in Figure 27.1. However, such effects can easily arise through methodological differences. What is needed are direct comparisons of different countries or ethnic groups using the same methodology. An important study of this sort has compared Nigerians with African Americans (Hendrie *et al.*, 2001). This study found that the incidence of AD was higher in African Americans, but the cause of the difference is not known.

27.2 FAMILIAL AND GENETIC FACTORS

27.2.1 Family history

A family history of dementia is an important risk factor. A meta-analysis of case–control studies found that risk for AD was around 3.5 times higher in individuals who had at least one first-degree relative with dementia (van Duijn *et al.*, 1991). Family history was stronger in those with early-onset AD compared with those with late-onset. Some families show an autosomal dominant pattern of inheritance for early-onset AD, but these are rare. A first-degree relative's actual percentage risk of developing AD will depend on their longevity. A large US study estimated the risk as 5 per cent up to age 70, 16 per cent up to age 80 and 33 per cent up to age 90 (Lautenschlager *et al.*, 1996).

27.2.2 Disease–causing mutations

There are a number of mutations which are sufficient in themselves to cause AD. These are mutations of the β-amyloid precursor protein gene on chromosome 21, and the presenilin genes on chromosome 1 and 14 (Lendon *et al.*, 1997). The discovery of these mutations has been of great theoretical importance for an understanding of AD disease, but from a public health perspective they account for very few cases.

27.2.3 ApoE genotype

Apolipoprotein E (ApoE) is a plasma protein involved in cholesterol transport and probably in neuronal repair. ApoE genotype alters risk for AD, but unlike the mutations discussed above, does not in itself cause the disease. This gene, on chromosome 19, has three common alleles: ε2, ε3 and ε4. The ε3 allele is the most common in the population and the ε2 allele the least common. The ε4 allele is more common in Caucasians than in Japanese. The ε4 allele increases risk in a dose-dependent manner, while the ε2 allele decreases risk. A meta-analysis of relevant studies found that ApoE genotype is an important risk factor in all ethnic groups studied (Farrer *et al.*, 1997). Among Caucasians, for example, the ε4/ε4 genotype was associated with around 15 times the risk of AD compared with the common ε3/ε3 genotype, while the ε3/ε4 genotype was associated with around three times the risk. This increased risk was found for all ages between 40 and 90 years, but the effect diminished after age 70.

27.2.4 Other genetic risk factors

There are undoubtedly other polymorphisms which affect risk for AD. Although several have been proposed, subsequent research has not always been able to replicate the initial findings. For example, many studies have looked at polymorphisms in the regulatory region of the ApoE gene, but without consistent findings.

27.2.5 Down's syndrome

Virtually all people with Down's syndrome have the neuropathological features of AD by the age of 40 years. This pathology is due to having an extra copy of the amyloid precursor protein gene which is on chromosome 21. Nevertheless, the prevalence of dementia in people with Down's syndrome is much less than 100 per cent even by age 50 (Zigman *et al.*, 1996). The reason for this discrepancy between pathology and function is not understood. One study found that men with Down's syndrome were more likely to develop dementia than women and that those with an ε4 allele were at increased risk (Schupf *et al.*, 1998).

27.3 PREMORBID COGNITIVE AND BRAIN RESERVES

27.3.1 Education

Several studies have found that less educated individuals have a higher incidence of AD or cognitive decline (Stern *et al.*, 1994; White *et al.*, 1994; Farmer *et al.*, 1995), although not all studies show this. One hypothesis to explain this association is that better educated persons are able to compensate for any cognitive decline and the diagnosis of AD or dementia is therefore delayed (Mortimer, 1988). A clinical study of regional cerebral blood flow in AD patients has supported this hypothesis. When highly educated patients were matched to less educated patients for severity of dementia, the highly educated had a greater parietotemporal perfusion deficit, implying that they were better able to compensate for the pathology (Stern *et al.*, 1992).

27.3.2 Premorbid intelligence

Education is correlated to intelligence, so it could be premorbid intelligence rather than education that is the protective factor. Indeed, one longitudinal study found that a reading vocabulary test was a better predictor of subsequent dementia than education (Schmand *et al.*, 1997). A clinical study of cerebral glucose metabolism in patients with AD showed greater hypometabolism in those with greater premorbid intelligence (Alexander *et al.*, 1997).

While the evidence on education and premorbid intelligence generally has been interpreted in terms of compensation for pathology, an epidemiological study of elderly nuns found evidence that verbal ability may directly influence AD pathology (Snowdon *et al.*, 1996). This study assessed verbal ability by analysing the autobiographies the nuns had written as young adults for density of ideas and grammatical complexity. Cognitive function was assessed approximately 58 years later and those nuns who subsequently died had a neuropathological examination. Not surprisingly, low idea density and grammatical complexity in young adulthood were associated with poorer cognitive functioning in old age. More surprising was the finding that low verbal ability early in life was related to AD pathology. Among the nuns who had died at follow up, all of those with neuropathologically confirmed AD had low verbal ability, compared with none of those without AD.

Even earlier premorbid intelligence differences have been reported in a Scottish study, which found that late-onset dementia was associated with lower intelligence test scores during childhood (Whalley *et al.*, 2000).

27.3.3 Brain reserve

The apparent protective effects of education and premorbid intelligence could be mediated by brain reserve (Schofield, 1999). Brain imaging studies have found that IQ is related to brain size and there is also some evidence that it is related to education (Jorm *et al.*, 1997). Several lines of evidence directly support the notion that brain reserve is protective. A neuropathological study found that individuals who had AD changes at autopsy, but were not demented during life, had bigger brains (Katzman *et al.*, 1988). Furthermore, individuals who have a larger brain on a scan or a larger head size appear to have a reduced risk of AD (Schofield, 1999).

27.4 MEDICAL HISTORY AND TREATMENTS

27.4.1 Head trauma

A meta-analysis of case–control studies found that a history of head trauma with loss of consciousness was associated with a doubling of risk of AD in males, but no increased risk in females (Fleminger *et al.*, 2003). Supporting a role for head trauma as a risk factor, Aβ protein can be deposited extensively in the brain following severe head injury (Roberts *et al.*, 1991). This protein is one of the pathological hallmarks of AD. Unfortunately, in most of the risk factor studies, the incidence of head trauma was assessed retrospectively using reports from relatives who may be subject to biased reporting. Most prospective studies using objective medical records of head trauma have not supported an association with AD (Fleminger *et al.*, 2003). Some research has supported the hypothesis that head trauma is only a risk factor for individuals who carry the ApoE ε4 allele (Mayeux *et al.*, 1995). However, other studies have not reported this effect.

27.4.2 Anti–inflammatory medication and arthritis

McGeer and colleagues (1990) have hypothesized that AD involves a chronic inflammatory state of the brain. They predicted that individuals taking anti-inflammatory drugs, or with diseases such as arthritis which are treated with such drugs, would be protected from AD. A meta-analysis of such studies provides some support for this prediction. Users of non-steroidal anti-inflammatory drugs (NSAIDs) were found to have 72 per cent of the risk of non-users (Etminan *et al.*, 2003). However, the appropriate dosage and duration of drug use was unclear. Randomized controlled trials of anti-inflammatory drugs are needed to confirm a preventive effect and are underway (Martin *et al.*, 2002; see also Chapter 37).

27.4.3 Oestrogen replacement

Animal studies have shown that oestrogen has multiple neuroprotective effects, including increased cerebral blood flow, stimulation of cholinergic activity, acting as a cofactor with nerve growth factors, prevention of neural atrophy and reversal of glucocorticoid damage (Burns and Murphy, 1996). Some epidemiological studies have suggested that oestrogen replacement therapy in post-menopausal women may have a protective effect. A meta-analysis pooling data from case–control and prospective studies found that oestrogen reduced the risk of AD by around 30 per cent (Yaffe *et al.*, 1998). A problem in interpreting these results is that better educated women are more likely to take oestrogen and, as discussed above, education may itself be protective. It is also possible that women tend to stop taking oestrogen if they begin to deteriorate cognitively. Randomized trials would provide the best evidence on the issue. However, data from a randomized controlled trial of oestrogen plus progestin involving over 4000 women found an increased incidence of dementia in those on medication (Shumaker *et al.*, 2003). This result has dashed the hope that oestrogen could be an important preventive intervention.

27.4.4 Vascular risk factors

AD has traditionally been thought of as separate from vascular dementia. However, in recent years, evidence has accumulated that vascular risk factors are involved. Several prospective studies show that both hypertension and diabetes increase risk for AD, although the evidence on these associations is not entirely consistent (Launer, 2002).

Another vascular risk factor receiving a lot of attention is plasma total homocysteine, which is thought to increase risk for stroke. Both case–control and prospective studies also support its role as a risk factor for AD (Morris, 2003).

Cholesterol may also have a role in AD. ApoE is the principal cholesterol carrier in the brain and, as described earlier, the ε4 allele of the ApoE gene increases risk for AD. There is some support for high cholesterol as a risk factor and for a protective effect of statins, a group of drugs that reduces cholesterol (Puglielli et al., 2003).

How these vascular risk factors increase risk is not understood. One explanation is that they cause cerebrovascular disease that summates with AD pathology to produce dementia. However, a direct involvement in AD pathology is also possible.

27.4.5 History of depression

There is a general consensus that depression may be a prodromal feature of AD, but the interest lies in whether it could also be a risk factor. A meta-analysis of case–control studies and prospective studies found that a history of depression approximately doubles the risk of developing dementia (principally AD) (Jorm, 2001). There are several potential explanations of this association, the three most likely being:

- depression is a very early prodrome of AD;
- history of depression brings forward the clinical recognition of dementing diseases by adding in additional cognitive or motivational deficits; and
- depression leads to damage to the hippocampus through excessive glucocorticoid secretion (Jorm, 2001).

27.4.6 Herpes simplex virus

A neuropathological study has found that herpes simplex virus type 1 in the brain is a risk factor for AD in individuals who carry the ApoE ε4 allele (Itzhaki et al., 1997). However, the virus was not a risk factor in individuals without the ε4 allele. The authors proposed that the virus is present in the brain in latent form and reactivates under certain conditions. ApoE genotype may affect the number of cells infected or the number of viruses released and hence the extent of any neuronal damage.

27.5 HEALTH HABITS

27.5.1 Alcohol consumption

A French prospective study found that wine drinking was protective for AD (Orgogozo et al., 1997). Risk was reduced 80 per cent in moderate drinkers compared with abstainers. Subsequent work has found a protective effect for moderate drinking of alcohol in general (Huang et al., 2002), although some work suggests the effect is greater for vascular dementia than for AD (Ruitenberg et al., 2002).

27.5.2 Smoking

The evidence on smoking as a risk factor has been inconsistent. A meta-analysis of case–control studies found a reduced risk for AD in smokers, whereas prospective studies showed a slightly increased risk (Almeida et al., 2002). Case–control studies may be affected by 'survivor bias' whereby smokers with AD are less likely to get included into studies because of early mortality.

27.6 DIET

27.6.1 Aluminium in drinking water

Early pathological research found increased concentrations of aluminium in the brains of AD cases, leading to the hypothesis that aluminium exposure plays a causative role. However, more recent research has disputed the initial finding, claiming that the aluminium was simply a contaminant in the pathologists' stains. Although aluminium exposure can produce an encephalopathy, this does not involve the pathological hallmarks of AD. Nevertheless, aluminium could play a contributing role in AD and epidemiological research on the topic has continued, centring particularly on aluminium in the water supply (Flaten, 2001). Although drinking water provides only around 2.5 per cent of dietary aluminium, the aluminium which is added as a flocculent during water treatment is in a soluble form, which might have greater bioavailability. Although the evidence is not consistent, several studies have found higher rates of AD in regions with high aluminium content in water, particularly where the water is acidic. Despite the weakness of the evidence, it might be prudent to keep the aluminium content of drinking water as low as practicable (Douglas, 1998).

27.6.2 Other dietary factors

Diet has received much less attention from researchers than many other factors. Nevertheless, there has been some interest in antioxidants as a protection factor, since these mop up free radicals, which are believed to be a source of age-related neuronal degeneration. The evidence has been rather mixed, with some studies finding that vitamins C or E might be protective, but others finding no association (Luchsinger *et al.*, 2003).

In section 27.4.4, the role of homocysteine as a risk factor was mentioned. Homocysteine is increased by low levels of folate and vitamin B_{12}, leading to the expectation that dietary factors could be important. However, the potential protective effect of increasing dietary intake of folate and B_{12} remains to be tested.

Several studies have found that fish consumption may be protective (Kalmijn *et al.*, 1997; Morris *et al.*, 2003). It has been proposed that fish in an important dietary source of *n*-3 polyunsaturated fatty acids, which are a primary component of membrane phospholipids in the brain.

Animal studies show that caloric restriction increases lifespan, presumably through decreased production of free radicals. Consistent with these findings, some epidemiological studies have found that higher caloric intake is associated either with AD or greater cognitive decline (Luchsinger *et al.*, 2002).

27.7 OCCUPATIONAL AND RECREATIONAL FACTORS

Findings on occupational hazards generally have been negative (Gun *et al.*, 1997). An exception may be exposure to electromagnetic fields. A series of case–control studies found that AD cases were more likely to have worked in occupations where exposure was high (Sobel *et al.*, 1996). These occupations involve working with electric motors very close to the body. Such occupations include carpenter, electrician, machinist and seamstress. It has been hypothesized that electromagnetic fields may upset intracellular calcium ion homeostasis which may promote the cleavage of amyloid precursor protein into $A\beta$ (Sobel and Davanipour, 1996).

There is some evidence that recreational activities may be protective. A prospective study found that reading, playing board games, playing musical instruments and dancing were protective for AD and for vascular dementia (Verghese *et al.*, 2003). It is always possible that a lower level of these activities indicates preclinical dementia, but the association was also found when subjects in a possible preclinical state were excluded. There is also evidence that having an extensive social network may protect against dementia (Fratiglioni *et al.*, 2000). Again, a preclinical effect of AD is a possibility. With recreational and social activities, a randomized controlled trial would be required to demonstrate an unequivocal protective effect.

27.8 PREVENTIVE POSSIBILITIES

Ultimately, the prevention of AD will rest on an understanding of the biological processes involved. However, even without such an understanding, public health efforts towards prevention are possible through modification of risk factors. At this stage of our knowledge there are only four risk factors that we could say are confirmed beyond reasonable doubt: old age, family history of dementia, Down's syndrome and ApoE genotype. None of these factors gives scope for preventive action through risk factor modification. Of the possible risk and protection factors reviewed above, the most relevant for preventive action are: head trauma, exposure to electromagnetic fields, anti-inflammatory medication, vascular risk factors, diet, an engaged lifestyle and education.

Prevention of head trauma is itself an important public health goal. There are already laws in many countries to require the wearing of seat belts and helmets. There are also restrictions on boxing. The possible association with AD should encourage such preventive efforts.

The research on electromagnetic fields is still in it infancy. However, it would be prudent to take action anyway. Sobel *et al.* (1996) have recommended that motors for industrial machines should be moved further from the body and be shielded by special metals.

Anti-inflammatory drugs have excited the most interest for prevention. The side effects of these drugs make them unsuitable for preventive use in the population as a whole. However, the risks may be outweighed by the potential benefits for high-risk individuals, such as those with a family history of AD. Current research, such as the Alzheimer's Disease Anti-Inflammatory Prevention Trial (ADAPT) (Martin *et al.*, 2002), will provide definitive answers.

Modification of vascular risk factors is feasible and has other potential benefits besides the prevention of AD. Antihypertensive treatment trials for the prevention of vascular diseases now generally include dementia or cognitive impairment as a secondary outcome. One trial, the Syst-Eur study, has found a preventive effect on AD (Forette *et al.*, 2002), but another trial, the SCOPE study, failed to find a preventive effect on dementia (Lithell *et al.*, 2003).

Diet provides another readily implementable approach to prevention. If homocysteine can be lowered by increasing folate intake, then food fortification could be carried out. Similarly, consumption of *n*-3 fatty acids could be encouraged through health promotion campaigns. However, randomized controlled trials of dietary interventions still need to be undertaken.

Having an engaged lifestyle is often advocated on the 'use it or lose it' principle and there is some epidemiological support for the benefits of having greater intellectual and social activity. While the evidence is not completely convincing in the absence of randomized controlled trials, there is minimal risk in a more engaged lifestyle, so encouraging such lifestyle change is justifiable.

If education and premorbid intelligence are protective, this has interesting implications for the future. Years of formal education are rising over successive cohorts in many developed countries, as are scores on IQ tests (Flynn, 1987).

Even brain weight has increased over the past century (Miller and Corsellis, 1977). These factors might lead to a lower incidence of AD in the future, although there is no evidence for a reduction in incidence over recent decades (Kokmen et al., 1988), in spite of such changes.

The effect of any successful attempt at risk factor modification would probably be to delay onset rather than to completely avoid the disease. Nevertheless, it has been estimated that even a mean delay of 1 year could produce a large reduction in the number of cases in a population (Brookmeyer et al., 1998). A delay of this magnitude may be quite feasible in the near future.

REFERENCES

Alexander GE, Furey ML, Grady CL et al. (1997) Association of premorbid intellectual function with cerebral metabolism in Alzheimer's disease: implications for the cognitive reserve hypothesis. *American Journal of Psychiatry* 154: 165–172

Almeida OP, Hulse GK, Lawrence D, Flicker L. (2002) Smoking as a risk factor for Alzheimer's disease: contrasting evidence from a systematic review of case–control and cohort studies. *Addiction* 97: 15–28

Brookmeyer R, Gray S, Kawas C. (1998) Projections of Alzheimer's disease in the United States and the public health impact of delaying disease onset. *American Journal of Public Health* 88: 1337–1342

Burns A and Murphy D. (1996) Protection against Alzheimer's disease? *Lancet* 348: 420–421

Douglas R. (1998) Alzheimer's disease, drinking water and aluminium content. *Australasian Journal on Ageing* 17: 2–3

Etminan M, Gill S, Samii A. (2003) Effect of non-steroidal anti-inflammatory drugs on risk of Alzheimer's disease: systematic review and meta-analysis of observational studies. *BMJ* 327: 128

Farmer ME, Kittner SJ, Rae DS, Bartko JJ, Regier DA. (1995) Education and change in cognitive function. The epidemiologic catchment area study. *Annals of Epidemiology* 5: 1–7

Farrer LA, Cupples LA, Haines JL et al. (1997) Effects of age, sex, and ethnicity on the association between Apolipoprotein E genotype and Alzheimer disease. *JAMA* 278: 1349–1356

Flaten TP. (2001) Aluminium as a risk factor in Alzheimer's disease, with emphasis on drinking water. *Brain Research Bulletin* 55: 187–196

Fleminger S, Oliver DL, Lovestone S, Rabe-Hesketh S, Giora A. (2003) Head injury as a risk factor for Alzheimer's disease: the evidence 10 years on; a partial replication. *Journal of Neurology, Neurosurgery, and Psychiatry* 74: 857–862

Flynn JR. (1987) Massive IQ gains in 14 Nations: What IQ test really measure. *Psychological Bulletin* 101: 171–191

Forette F, Seux ML, Staessen JA et al. and Systolic Hypertension in Europe Investigators. (2002). The prevention of dementia with antihypertensive treatment: new evidence from the Systolic Hypertension in Europe (Syst-Eur) study. *Archives of Internal Medicine* 162: 2046–2052

Fratiglioni L, Wang HX, Ericsson K, Maytan M, Winblad B. (2000) Influence of social network on occurrence of dementia: a community-based longitudinal study. *Lancet* 355: 1315–1319

Gao S, Hendrie HC, Hall KS, Hui S. (1998) The relationships between age, sex, and the incidence of dementia and Alzheimer disease. *Archives of General Psychiatry* 55: 809–815

Gun RT, Korten AE, Henderson AS et al. (1997) Occupational risk factors for Alzheimer's disease: A case–control study. *Alzheimer Disease and Associated Disorders* 11: 21–27

Hendrie HC, Ogunniyi A, Hall KS et al. (2001) Incidence of dementia and Alzheimer disease in 2 communities: Yoruba residing in Ibadan, Nigeria, and African Americans residing in Indianapolis, Indiana. *JAMA* 285: 739–747

Huang W, Qiu C, Winblad B, Fratiglioni L. (2002). Alcohol consumption and incidence of dementia in a community sample aged 75 years and older. *Journal of Clinical Epidemiology* 55: 959–964

Itzhaki RF, Lin W-R, Shang D, Wilcock GK, Faragher B, Jamieson GA. (1997) Herpes simplex virus type 1 in brain and risk of Alzheimer's disease. *Lancet* 349: 241–244

Jorm AF (2001) History of depression as a risk factor for dementia: an updated review. *Australian and New Zealand Journal of Psychiatry* 35: 776–781

Jorm AF and Jolley D. (1998) The incidence of dementia: A meta-analysis. *Neurology* 51: 728–733

Jorm AF, Creasey H, Broe GA, Sulway MR, Kos SC, Dent OF. (1997) The advantage of being broad-minded: brain diameter and neuropsychological test performance in elderly war veterans. *Personality and Individual Differences* 23: 371–377

Kalmijn S, Launer LJ, Ott A, Witteman JCM, Hofman A, Breteler MMB. (1997) Dietary fat intake and the risk of incident dementia in the Rotterdam Study. *Annals of Neurology* 42: 776–782

Katzman R, Terry R, DeTeresa R et al. (1988) Clinical, pathological, and neurochemical changes in dementia: A subgroup with preserved mental status and numerous neocortical plaques. *Annals of Neurology* 23: 138–144

Kokmen E, Chandra V, Schoenberg BS. (1988) Trends in incidence of dementing illness in Rochester, Minnesota, in three quinquennial periods, 1960–1974. *Neurology* 38: 975–980

Launer LJ. (2002) Demonstrating the case that AD is a vascular disease: epidemiologic evidence. *Ageing Research Reviews* 1: 61–77

Lautenschlager NT, Cupples LA, Rao VS et al. (1996) Risk of dementia among relatives of Alzheimer's disease patients in the MIRAGE study: what is in store for the oldest old? *Neurology* 46: 641–650

Lendon CL, Ashall F, Goate AM. (1997) Exploring the etiology of Alzheimer disease using molecular genetics. *JAMA* 277: 825–831

Lithell H, Hansson L, Skoog I et al. and SCOPE Study Group. (2003) The Study on Cognition and Prognosis in the Elderly (SCOPE): principal results of a randomized double-blind intervention trial. *Journal of Hypertension* 21: 875–886

Luchsinger JA, Tang MX, Shea S, Mayeux R. (2002) Caloric intake and the risk of Alzheimer disease. *Archives of Neurology* 59: 1258–1263

Luchsinger JA, Tang MX, Shea S, Mayeux R. (2003) Antioxidant vitamin intake and risk of Alzheimer disease. *Archives of Neurology* 60: 203–208

McGeer PL, McGeer E, Rogers J, Sibley J. (1990) Anti-inflammatory drugs and Alzheimer disease. *Lancet* 335: 1037

Martin BK, Meinert CL, Breitner JC and ADAPT Research Group. (2002) Double placebo design in a prevention trial for Alzheimer's disease. *Controlled Clinical Trials* 23: 93–99

Mayeux R, Ottman R, Maestre G et al. (1995) Synergistic effects of straumatic head injury and apolipoprotein-e4 in patients with Alzheimer's disease. *Neurology* 45: 555–557

Miller AK and Corsellis JAN. (1977) Evidence for a secular increase in human brain weight during the past century. *Annals of Human Biology* **4**: 253–257

Morris MC, Evans DA, Bienias JL *et al.* (2003) Consumption of fish and n-3 fatty acids and risk of incident Alzheimer disease. *Archives of Neurology* **60**: 940–946

Morris MS. (2003) Homocysteine and Alzheimer's disease. *Lancet Neurology* **2**: 425–428

Mortimer JA. (1988) Do psychosocial risk factors contribute to Alzheimer's disease? In: AS Henderson and JH Henderson (eds), *Etiology of Dementia of Alzheimer's Type.* Chichester, John Wiley and Sons Limited, pp. 39–52

Orgogozo JM, Dartigues JF, Lafont S *et al.* (1997) Wine consumption and dementia in the elderly: a prospective community study in the Bordeaux area. *Revue Neurologique* **153**: 185–192

Puglielli L, Tanzi RE, Kovacs DM. (2003) Alzheimer's disease: the cholesterol connection. *Nature Neuroscience* **6**: 345–351

Roberts GW, Gentlemen SM, Lynch A, Graham DI. (1991) bA4 amyloid protein deposition in brain after head trauma. *Lancet* **338**: 1422–1423

Ruitenberg A, van Swieten JC, Witteman JCM *et al.* (2002) Alcohol consumption and risk of dementia: the Rotterdam Study. *Lancet* **359**: 281–286

Schmand B, Smit JH, Geerlings MI, Lindeboom J. (1997) The effects of intelligence and education on the development of dementia. A test of the brain reserve hypothesis. *Psychological Medicine* **27**: 1337–1344

Schofield P. (1999) Alzheimer's disease and brain reserve. *Australasian Journal on Ageing*, **18**: 10–14

Schupf N, Kapell D, Nightingale B, Rodriguez A, Tycko B, Mayeux R. (1998) Earlier onset of Alzheimer's disease in men with Down syndrome. *Neurology* **50**: 991–995

Shumaker CA, Legault C, Rapp SR *et al.* and WHIMS Investigators. (2003) Estrogen plus progestin and the incidence of dementia and mild cognitive impairment in postmenopausal women: the Women's Health Initiative Memory Study: a randomized controlled trial. *JAMA* **289**: 2651–2662

Snowdon DA, Kemper SJ, Mortimer JA, Greiner LH, Wekstein DR, Markesbery WR. (1996) Linguistic ability in early life and cognitive function and Alzheimer's disease in late life. *JAMA* **275**: 528–532

Sobel E and Davanipour Z. (1996) Electromagnetic field exposure may cause increased production of amyloid beta and eventually lead to Alzheimer's disease. *Neurology* **47**: 1594–1600

Sobel E, Dunn M, Davanipour DVM, Qian Z, Chui HC. (1996) Elevated risk of Alzheimer's disease among workers with likely electromagnetic field exposure. *Neurology* **47**: 1477–1481

Stern Y, Alexander GE, Prohovnik I, Mayeux R. (1992) Inverse relationship between education and parietotemporal perfusion deficit in Alzheimer's disease. *Annals of Neurology* **32**: 371–375

Stern Y, Gurland B, Tatemichi TK, Tang MX, Wilder D, Mayeux R. (1994) Influence of education and occupation on the incidence of Alzheimer's disease. *JAMA* **271**: 1004–1010

van Duijn CM, Clayton D *et al.* (1991) Familial aggregation of Alzheimer's disease and related disorders: A collaborative re-analysis of case–control studies. *International Journal of Epidemiology* **20**: S13–S20

Verghese J, Lipton RB, Katz MJ *et al.* (2003) Leisure activities and the risk of dementia in the elderly. *New England Journal of Medicine* **348**: 2508–2516

Whalley LJ, Starr JM, Athawes R, Hunter D, Pattie A, Deary IJ. (2000) Childhood mental ability and dementia. *Neurology* **55**: 1455–1459

White L, Katzman R, Losonczy K *et al.* (1994) Association of education with incidence of cognitive impairment in three established populations for epidemiologic studies of the elderly. *Journal of Clinical Epidemiology* **47**: 363–374

Yaffe K, Sawaya G, Lieberburg I, Grady D. (1998) Estrogen therapy in postmenopausal women: Effects on cognitive function and dementia. *JAMA* **279**: 688–695

Zigman WB, Schupf N, Sersen E, Silverman W. (1996) Prevalence of dementia in adults with and without Down syndrome. *American Journal of Mental Retardation* **100**: 403–412

28

The natural history of Alzheimer's disease

JODY COREY-BLOOM AND ADAM S FLEISHER

Since the prevalence of Alzheimer's disease (AD) is expected to nearly quadruple in the next 50 years, it will undeniably continue to be an enormous public health problem in the elderly (Brookmeyer *et al.*, 1998). Knowledge of the clinical features and natural history of AD will facilitate planning in response to the increased demands on medical and social resources. In addition, this information will enable clinicians to provide patients and families with a more reliable prediction of the course of the disease. Furthermore, staging and monitoring AD is important in recruiting patients for clinical studies at definable levels of severity, and for measuring the value of interventions that may alter its course.

28.1 CLINICAL FEATURES

The diverse spectrum of symptoms of AD reflects dysfunction of widespread regions of the cerebral cortex. Symptoms begin insidiously, making it difficult to date the onset of cognitive and functional decline precisely. Progression is generally gradual and inexorable with occasional pauses; however, reliable measurement of disease progression in AD is difficult because of variability between and within subjects.

Memory loss is the cardinal and commonly presenting complaint in AD. Initially the patient has difficulty recalling new information such as names or details of conversation, while remote memories are relatively preserved. With progression, the memory loss worsens to include remote memory (Wilson *et al.*, 1983; Sullivan *et al.*, 1986; Bondi *et al.*, 1994; Cummings and Cole, 2002). Early in AD, judgement and abstraction are often impaired, suggesting involvement of the frontal lobes. Social comportment and interpersonal skills are often strikingly preserved, and may remain relatively intact long after memory and insight have been lost.

Language is frequently normal early in AD, although reduced conversational output may be noted. As dementia progresses, many patients become more recognizably aphasic. Initially this manifests as dysnomia and mild loss of fluency, with paraphasic errors and relative preservation of repetition, a pattern resembling transcortical sensory aphasia (Cummings *et al.*, 1985; Cummings and Cole, 2002). At a later stage, language is obviously dysfluent and repetition impaired; terminally, a state of near-mutism may occur (Murdoch and Chenery, 1987).

Visuospatial impairment in AD results in symptoms such as misplacing objects or getting lost, and difficulty with tasks such as recognizing and drawing complex figures (Brouwers *et al.*, 1984; Kavcic and Duffy, 2003). Difficulty with calculation (affecting skills such as handling money), apraxia and agnosia are further problems that develop in AD. Apraxia may impair activities such as operating appliances or dressing; as might be expected, more complex skills tend to break down first, while highly overlearned motor tasks (e.g. playing a musical instrument, using tools) may be retained until relatively late in the course (Rapcsak *et al.*, 1989; Helmes and Ostbye, 2002). Agnosia develops in middle to late stages of AD, and includes features such as failing to recognize family members or spouses.

Psychiatric and behavioural symptoms occur frequently in AD. Over and above a general decline of activity and interest in virtually all AD patients, depressive symptoms occur in about 25 per cent, although severe depression is uncommon (Cummings *et al.*, 1987; Rosen and Zubenko, 1991; Becker *et al.*, 1994; Cummings and Cole, 2002). The frequency of significantly depressed mood in patients with AD ranged from 0 to 87 per cent in 30 studies reviewed by Wragg and Jeste (1989) with higher rates reported from acute care facilities than in series from outpatient research sites. While many AD patients have depressive symptoms, most do not display enough features to meet DSM-IV criteria for major depressive disorders. The fact that vegetative symptoms such as sleep disturbance, weight gain, loss of libido, lack of interest and reduced motor activity are common to both AD and depression may account for the high rate of 'depression' found in some studies (Lazarus et al., 1987; Becker et al., 1994; Jost and Grossberg, 1996).

Delusions are common in AD, although they are rarely as systematized as in schizophrenia. They often have a paranoid flavour, with fears of personal harm, theft of personal property and marital infidelity. Misidentification syndromes also occur; whether these represent true delusions is unclear. The prevalence of psychotic symptoms in AD, the relationship of hallucinations and delusions to the severity of cognitive impairment, and the influence of psychosis on the rate of cognitive decline are controversial. Estimates of the prevalence of psychotic symptoms in AD range from 10 to 73 per cent, with most in the range of 28–38 per cent (Wragg and Jeste, 1989; Mega et al., 1999). Delusions have been reported in 13–75 per cent of AD patients, and hallucinations, more commonly visual than auditory, in 3–50 per cent (Mayeux et al., 1989; Becker et al., 1994; Jost and Grossberg, 1996; Cook et al., 2003). This substantial variation in frequencies is probably due to different methodologic approaches, especially in defining delusions and hallucinations, and to differences in the range of severity of AD in each series. Although psychotic symptoms may occur throughout the course of AD, they have their highest frequency at a moderate level of dementia (Drevets and Rubin, 1989).

In addition to depression and psychotic symptoms, AD patients show a wide range of behavioural abnormalities including agitation, wandering, sleep disturbances and disinhibition (Becker et al., 1994; Jost and Grossberg, 1996; Lyketsos et al., 2002). These often impose a significant burden on caregivers, and may precipitate nursing home placement. In contrast to psychotic symptoms, behavioural disturbances are more clearly associated with the degree of dementia (Teri et al., 1988). Agitation includes physical aggression, verbal aggression and non-aggressive behaviours, such as motor restlessness and pacing (Reisberg et al., 1987; Swearer et al., 1988; Burns et al., 1990; Hooker et al., 2002). Wandering behaviour affects 3–26 per cent of AD outpatients. Insomnia and sleep disturbances are inconstant features of AD and sexual disinhibition has been reported in less than 10 per cent of patients (Burns et al., 1990; Becker et al., 1994). Thus, behavioural symptoms are a pervasive and poorly understood concomitant of cognitive deterioration in AD.

Excluding mental status testing, the neurologic examination is usually normal in AD, and the presence of significant or lateralizing abnormalities often suggests other diagnoses. Primitive reflexes (snout, glabellar, grasp),

impaired graphesthesia, and an abnormal response to double simultaneous stimulation (face–hand test) are frequently encountered in AD (Galasko et al., 1990; Becker et al., 1994). Variable features, including extrapyramidal signs (rigidity and bradykinesia), gait disturbances and myoclonus may occasionally be seen early in the course of AD, and increase in prevalence with the severity of the disease (Stern et al., 1987). The frequency of extrapyramidal signs in patients with AD was as low as 12–14 per cent in some series (Galasko et al., 1990; Burns et al., 1991; Becker et al., 1994), and as high as 28–92 per cent in others (Mayeux et al., 1985; Molsa et al., 1986; Bakchine et al., 1989; Lopez et al., 2000), depending on the severity of dementia in patients who were studied. In intermediate or advanced stages of dementia, patients often develop non-specific impairment of gait and balance, leading to an increased risk of falls. Myoclonus develops late in the course of AD and longitudinal studies report an increase in its frequency during follow up (Mayeux et al., 1985; Hauser et al., 1986; Tschampa et al., 2001).

As neuronal degeneration progresses in AD, all of the above symptoms worsen, and eventually patients become uncommunicative, unable to care for themselves, walk, or maintain continence. They require total care, including feeding, and are often institutionalized.

28.2 CLINICAL UTILITY OF ASSESSING CHANGE

The course of AD and the combination of symptoms that manifest in each patient are markedly heterogeneous; however, there are several direct clinical applications of tracking change. First, in early cases of AD, where impairment is mild, documenting progression helps to confirm or establish the diagnosis of dementia. Clearly, progressive cognitive deterioration is incompatible with normal ageing, depression, delirium, or a static encephalopathy. The clinical follow up of patients who are initially classified as having AD greatly increases the accuracy of the diagnosis.

Second, progression to a greater degree than expected may prompt the physician to look for a superimposed factor that may be treatable, such as hypothyroidism, intercurrent infection, medication toxicity or depression.

Third, defining the anticipated course of AD in detail enables clinicians to provide patients and families with realistic expectations regarding the disease, and aids in making decisions for day care or institutionalization.

Longitudinal cognitive change may be fruitfully applied to several problems in clinical research. Change over time on mental status scores may be used to examine the influence of genetic/environmental factors or experimental treatment on the rate of dementia progression.

Attempts to refine the natural history of AD have used two basic methods: global staging systems and serial changes on psychometric test scores.

28.2.1 Measuring change with global staging systems

Staging systems for AD comprise information on intellectual, social and community functioning obtained by history rather than formal rating scales. Two widely used schemes are the Washington University Clinical Dementia Rating (CDR) scale (Hughes et al., 1982; Morris 1997) and the Global Deterioration Scale (GDS) (Reisberg et al., 1982, 1986), which divide AD into a succession of stages. These scales reflect an overall, indirect evaluation of cognition, primarily obtained from caregivers, rather than a direct assessment of the patient, but are able to assess the influence of cognitive loss on the ability to conduct everyday activities. They provide information about clinically meaningful function and behaviour and are less affected by the 'floor' and 'ceiling' effects commonly associated with psychometric tests.

The CDR incorporates information from patients and informants concerning six areas of mental function: memory, orientation, judgement and problem solving, community affairs, home and hobbies, and personal care. Each area is scored as $0 = $ normal, $0.5 = $ questionable, $1 = $ mild-, $2 = $ moderate-, or $3 = $ severe-impairment, and integrated to obtain an overall stage of dementia, using similar definitions of 0, 0.5, and 1–3. Interrater reliability is high, with a correlation of 0.91, and the CDR has been standardized for multicentre use (Morris, 1997). Since the CDR includes cognitive items and activities of daily living (ADL), it is not surprising that it correlates well with the cognitive Blessed Information-Memory-Concentration (BIMC) scale ($r = 0.55$) and with the ADL-based Blessed Dementia Scale (BDS) ($r = 0.53$) (Berg et al., 1988). Putting the CDR into practice, these authors followed a cohort of 43 initially mild AD patients (CDR 1) for 90 months. Over 67 per cent of patients progressed to CDR 3 (severe dementia) by 50 months, and over 80 per cent by 66 months. Many patients in this CDR 1 group reached end points: 50 per cent of patients were institutionalized by 40 months, and 80 per cent by 60 months. Thirty per cent of patients died by 40 months, and 40 per cent by 72 months. Although the CDR is clearly a useful staging instrument (Morris, 1997) and has become widely accepted in the clinical setting as a reliable and valid global assessment measure for AD, it is not as sensitive a measure of annual or short-term rate of change, as movement from one stage to the next may take several years (Storandt et al., 2002).

The GDS divides AD into a succession of seven major, clinically distinguishable stages (further subdivided into 16) ranging from normal cognition (GDS 1) to severe dementia (GDS 7) (Reisberg et al., 1982). Criteria for many of the stages combine history (initially of memory decline, later of functional impairment, progressing to loss of self-care, language and gait), and mental status examination. Stages defined by this integration of history, ADL and cognition should show high correlations with mental state screening tests: indeed, the GDS correlates well with the Mini-Mental State Examination (MMSE) ($r = 0.9$; $P < 0.001$) and the BIMC ($r = 0.8$, $P < 0.001$) (Reisberg et al., 1989). GDS stages 1 and 2 correspond to CDR 0, representing normal ageing, and GDS 3 is equivalent to CDR 0.5. In a longitudinal study, only 5 per cent of GDS 2 subjects became demented over 3–4 years, whereas 15 per cent of GDS 3 subjects progressed to more advanced stages of dementia.

The GDS has similar virtues and drawbacks to the CDR, namely difficulty in defining a natural history over periods shorter than a year or two. The primary use of these staging systems may be in research settings and in following patients longitudinally over extended periods, since the transitions from one stage to the next occur over relatively long intervals.

28.2.2 Measuring change by rate of decline on cognitive tests

As a more flexible longitudinal index of brain function, studies have measured the annual rate of change (ARC) of mental status test scores in AD. Longitudinal data exist for ARC on five mental status tests in common use: the BIMC, the MMSE, the Dementia Rating Scale (DRS), the Cambridge Cognitive Examination (CAMCOG) (Roth et al., 1986), and the Alzheimer's Disease Assessment Scale (ADAS) (Rosen et al., 1984). Unfortunately, although these rates of decline are available, their generalizability is uncertain.

Katzman et al. (1988) compared four groups of subjects with AD on the BIMC, with follow up over 1 year. These cohorts differed substantially with regard to age, education, sex and severity of dementia, and included community-dwelling and institutionalized subjects. The mean rate of change on the BIMC did not differ significantly among the four groups for subjects who initially made 24 or fewer errors (out of a possible 33). In those patients, the ARC on the BIMC was 4.4 errors per year, and did not vary with age, education or place of residence. Among demented subjects with an initial BIMC score of more than 24 errors, the rate of change was lower, presumably because the test had reached a floor. A similar overall rate of progression for the BIMC was found in a group of outpatients with AD (Ortof and Crystal, 1989). Subjects lost an average of 4.1 points per year, regardless of age of onset, duration of illness, or family history of dementia. Two further studies observed a comparable ARC in community-dwelling AD patients (Thal et al., 1988; Salmon et al., 1990). In all of these studies, the standard deviation was slightly less than the mean ARC over 1 year and the range of ARC varied widely. Significant variation in the mean ARC on the BIMC has been observed, however, by other investigators. For example, Lucca et al. (1993) noted a change of only 2.6 (± 4.9) points on the BIMC over 1 year in a group of 56 patients with AD comprising outpatients and inpatients at geriatric institutions. Using data from the California Alzheimer's Disease Diagnostic and Treatment Centers, we observed an annual rate of change of 2.8 points on the BIMC (Corey-Bloom et al., 1993).

For the MMSE, a number of studies have reported a mean ARC in AD ranging from 1.8 to 4.2 points. Of these studies, the one with the lowest ARC entered patients at a very mild stage of AD (Becker *et al.*, 1988). Studies with the highest ARC had more severely impaired subjects at entry (Yesavage *et al.*, 1988; Burns *et al.*, 1991), while the remaining studies showed an intermediate ARC (about 2.5 points per year) in patients with a moderate initial level of impairment (Uhlman *et al.*, 1986; Salmon *et al.*, 1990; Teri *et al.*, 1990; Corey-Bloom *et al.*, 1993; Aguero-Torres *et al.*, 1998; Swanwick *et al.*, 1998; Thal *et al.*, 2000; Winblad *et al.*, 2001). This illustrates that rate of change on the MMSE is affected by the severity of cognitive impairment even before the test reaches a floor.

Few studies of longitudinal cognitive change in AD have used extended follow-up periods. In a study distinguished by 7 years of follow up, Aguero-Torres *et al.* (1998) found a mean ARC of 2.8 points on the MMSE during their first period of evaluation (entry–3 years) and 3.0 points thereafter (3–7 years). Salmon *et al.* (1990) compared the BIMC, MMSE and DRS in 55 community-dwelling patients with AD over 2 years. Each subject's scores on the three tests were highly intercorrelated at entry and after 1 and 2 years. Over the study period, patients lost a mean of 3.2 points on the BIMC, 2.8 points on the MMSE and 11.4 points on the DRS per year. In general, the group declined to a greater degree on all three scales in the second year than in the first, but this was statistically significant only for the DRS. For individuals, however, the ARC of mental status scores in the first year did not predict the next year's rate of decline.

Two somewhat longer instruments, similar to the DRS, have been used for serial assessment, the CAMCOG and the ADAS. The CAMCOG is the cognitive component of the Cambridge Mental Disorders of the Elderly Examination (CAMDEX), an instrument designed for assessing dementia. It has sections testing memory, language, praxis, orientation, attention, calculation, abstraction and perception, with a maximum total score of 107. In a survey of 110 patients spanning a wide spectrum of severity of AD, Burns *et al.* found a significant decline over one year in the overall score (12.3 points), and in virtually every subsection (Burns *et al.*, 1991). Group scores for memory, orientation, attention and abstraction were close to 'floor' on initial evaluation, and declined further over 1 year. The initial mean MMSE for this group was 10 ($\pm$5.9), lower than in studies cited above, and changed by an average of 3.5 points. A more recent study by Swanwick *et al.* (1998) of 95 less demented subjects reported an annual decline on the CAMCOG of 9.4 ($\pm$9.5) points.

The ADAS includes a cognitive portion, with a maximum of 70 points, and a non-cognitive subscale scored out of 40. Kramer-Ginsberg *et al.* (1988) (and Mohs, personal communication) found an average ARC on the ADAS of 9.3 points in 60 AD patients. Yesavage *et al.* (1988) reported a similar ARC on the ADAS of 8.3 points in 30 patients with AD, and additionally noted a high intercorrelation between selected subscales of the ADAS and the MMSE. More recently, Thal *et al.* (2000) reported an ARC of 7.5 points in a larger group of 102 AD patients participating in the acetyl-L-carnitine (ALCAR)

clinical trial. It should be noted that rates of decline in clinical trials are generally lower than those reported for natural history studies, likely owing to inherent selection biases. Clinical trial participants are hand-selected with regard to concomitant comorbidities and medications, and may represent a population that tends to have better overall health care and more involved caregivers.

Unfortunately, while mean ARC for each of the above cognitive scales was reasonably consistent between studies, the standard deviations were fairly large, roughly equal to the means, indicating substantial individual variability. Some patients' scores did not decline, and even improved over 1–2 years of follow up. This variability has several possible explanations. First, AD may not progress uniformly, since patients with early dementia may enter a 'plateau' phase with relatively slow deterioration. Second, performance on these cognitive tests probably does not decline in a linear fashion. Third, test–retest variability is influenced by patients' mood, attention and motivation and many other issues that have an impact on day-to-day mental performance, adding a further element of uncertainty to ARC calculations. A fourth possibility is that a number of biological and clinical factors may modify the rate of progression of AD. These include demographic characteristics such as age at onset, gender, and education; genetic features such as apolipoprotein (ApoE) status; and clinical factors such as concomitant cerebrovascular disease, presence of psychosis or extrapyramidal signs (EPS), and use of vitamins, oestrogen, lipid lowering agents, or non-steroidal anti-inflammatory drugs.

28.3 CLINICAL PREDICTORS OF RATE OF PROGRESSION

As noted above, a number of factors have been identified that appear to affect the rate of decline in AD; however, this is a thorny issue since variables thought to have independent prognostic significance may simply be markers of the level of disease severity (Drachman *et al.*, 1990).

For example, using a large well-characterized sample of CERAD subjects, Morris *et al.* (1993) found that dementia progression may be non-linear, that rate-of-change determinations were less reliable when the observation period was 1 year or less, and that rate of progression in AD was determined by the severity of cognitive impairment: the less severe the dementia, the slower the rate of decline. Similarly, Teri *et al.* (1995), using a community-based sample of 156 probable AD patients followed for up to 5 years, found that average rate of decline in cognitive function, as measured by the MMSE and Mattis DRS, becomes more rapid as the disease progresses. This has been confirmed by a more recent study by Storandt *et al.* (2002) who, using a large cohort of mildly demented subjects, found that initial dementia severity was the most significant predictor of annual rate of progression on composite psychometric testing, with increasingly steeper slopes as severity increased. In addition, these authors found that the rates of decline were highly variable from person to person and between groups as well. There was limited evidence for any systematic predictors of cognitive decline, including combined psychometric measures.

Several studies investigating age at onset as a predictor of deterioration have reported a significant association between earlier age at onset and greater rate of cognitive or functional worsening (Lucca et al., 1993; Jacobs et al., 1994; Teri et al., 1995; Mungas et al., 2001; Backman et al., 2003). This is not supported, however, by one study of 95 subjects with AD attending an outpatient memory clinic (Swanwick et al., 1998).

Gender was not seen to influence cognitive decline in several studies of AD (Reisberg et al., 1986; Drachman et al., 1990; Burns et al., 1991; Mortimer et al., 1992; Jacobs et al., 1994; Storandt et al., 2002) but this was not the case for others that reported slower (Heston et al., 1981; Lucca et al., 1993; Aguero-Torres et al., 1998) and faster (Swanwick et al., 1998) rates of progression in men as compared with women.

Level of education has also been examined as a predictor of decline in several studies (Filley et al., 1985; Katzman et al., 1988; Drachman et al., 1990; Teri et al., 1995; Storandt et al., 2002); however, because minimally educated subjects were not included in most of these investigations, the effect of education requires further examination.

The ApoE ε4 allele is associated with both a high likelihood of developing AD and an earlier age of onset; nonetheless, there have been conflicting results with regard to the influence of ApoE genotype on the course of cognitive decline in AD. Gomez-Isla et al. (1996) in a prospective longitudinal study of 359 AD patients, found that the ApoE ε4 allele was not associated with any change in rate of progression of dementia (Gomez-Isla et al., 1996). Likewise, Growdon et al. (1996) reported that rate of decline did not vary significantly across ApoE genotype on any neuropsychological test administered to 66 probable AD patients over a span of up to 5.5 years. Kurz et al. (1996) noted no association between ε4 status and rate of cognitive decline over 3 years on the CAMCOG or MMSE in 64 clinically diagnosed AD subjects. Furthermore, Frisoni et al. (1995) reported a slower rate of progression with increasing ε4 gene dose in a retrospective examination of 62 sporadic AD patients. These latter findings were similar to those of Stern et al. (1997) who noted a slower rate of decline on the modified MMSE among patients with ApoE ε4 alleles compared with patients with other genotypes. On the other hand, Craft et al. (1998) reported an accelerated rate of decline on the DRS in ApoE ε4 homozygotes with probable AD, and Hirono et al. (2003) reported a similar accelerated rate of decline on the ADAS-cog, even after controlling for age, gender, education, test interval and baseline scores.

Concomitant cerebrovascular disease has not been shown to significantly increase rate of cognitive decline in AD (Lee et al., 2000; Storandt et al., 2002). However, one longitudinal study with autopsy follow up of 50 patients with AD and strokes, compared with 218 AD patients without strokes, showed a slight increase in rate of decline on MMSE scores in the comorbid stroke group for subjects over the age of 80 (Mungas et al., 2001).

Although it has been suggested that patients who develop EPS have a faster rate of decline, many of the earlier studies probably included patients on neuroleptics and those with dementia with Lewy bodies (DLB) (Miller et al. 1991; Mortimer et al., 1992; Chui et al., 1994; Stern et al., 1994). It is now clear that there is a pathological subset of dementia patients with α-synuclein positive cortical Lewy bodies (LBs) either in isolation or in addition to typical AD pathology (Olichney et al., 1998). A recent retrospective study by Lopez et al. (2000) compared clinical characteristics of 185 autopsy-proven AD and 60 autopsy-proven DLB subjects. These authors found no differences in rate of cognitive decline between the two, although DLB subjects developed EPS earlier (Lopez et al., 2000).

Whether neuropsychiatric symptoms superimposed on AD influence cognitive deterioration has been examined by several authors. Initial reports suggested that AD patients reached end points on a modified MMSE or BDS score more rapidly when psychotic symptoms were present (Mayeux et al., 1985; Stern et al., 1987; Drevets and Rubin 1989; Stern et al., 1990). However, these investigations did not match patients for their level of dementia. Controlling for severity of AD, several studies were unable to replicate these findings (Reisberg et al., 1986; Huff et al., 1990; Chen et al., 1991), although two additional investigations have confirmed psychosis as a robust predictor of cognitive decline (Chui et al., 1994; Stern et al., 1994). One cross-sectional study reported that AD patients with depression had more ADL impairment than those without (Pearson et al., 1989); however, other longitudinal studies found no effect of depression on rate of decline (Lopez et al., 1990; Storandt et al., 2002). Lopez et al. (1999) examined the effect of psychiatric symptoms and medications on progression in 179 mild to moderate probable AD patients, followed for a mean of 49.5 ± 27.4 months. These authors found that the presence of psychiatric symptoms and the use of psychiatric medications were associated with increased rate of functional but not cognitive decline.

Whether vitamins, oestrogen, lipid lowering agents, or non-steroidal anti-inflammatory drugs (NSAIDs) affect progression of AD is actively being investigated. High dose vitamin E has been shown to slow disease progression in a double-blind, placebo-controlled, trial of moderately severe AD patients (Sano et al., 1997). Although several observational studies have suggested that oestrogen replacement therapy may have a beneficial effect on cognitive performance in women with AD, many have substantial methodologic problems (Haskell et al., 1997; Yaffe et al., 1998). Furthermore, a recent study of the association between serum oestradiol and oestrone levels in 120 hysterectomized women taking hormone replacement therapy found no significant association between hormone levels and cognitive functioning after either

2 or 12 months of treatment (Thal *et al.*, 2003). Although large cohort analyses have demonstrated decreased prevalence of AD with use of various lipid lowering agents (Rockwood, 2002), the effect of these compounds on progression of cognitive decline in AD will only be answered by the large multicentre placebo-controlled trials currently underway. Similarly, there have been conflicting results with regard to the effect of NSAIDs on AD progression. Analysis of longitudinal changes over 1 year on measures of verbal fluency, spatial recognition and orientation revealed less decline among AD patients taking NSAIDs than among non-NSAID patients (Rich *et al.*, 1995). On the other hand, a randomized placebo-controlled trial of naproxen and rofecoxib showed no effect on cognitive decline in 351 patients with mild to moderate AD (Aisen *et al.*, 2003).

28.4 PREDICTING NURSING HOME PLACEMENT IN ALZHEIMER'S DISEASE

Most patients with AD reside in nursing homes late in the course of the illness. The interval between the diagnosis of AD and the need for institutional placement has much practical and clinical importance, but is not easy to predict. Dementia severity is usually cited as the most important predictor (Storandt *et al.*, 2002; Figure 28.1); however, behavioural symptoms such as agitation, wandering or aggression may pre-empt nursing home placement, regardless of the level of cognitive impairment. Other variables that greatly influence the decision to institutionalize a demented patient are social support and caregiver burden.

A large population-based historical cohort study by Eaker *et al.* (2002) suggests, not surprisingly, that the presence of dementia increases the overall risk of institutionalization. In their study the adjusted hazard ratio of being admitted to a nursing home for AD cases compared with controls was 5.44 (95 per cent CI 3.68, 8.05), independent of comorbid conditions.

Several studies have examined predictors of institutionalization in AD. As expected, the predictive factors are complex and vary greatly among studies. One investigation of 14 married men with AD found that urinary or faecal incontinence, inability to speak coherently and loss of skills needed for bathing and grooming were major determinants of institutionalization (Hutton *et al.*, 1985). In a 5-year study of 92 patients who developed AD before the age of 70, lower mental status scores or aphasia were more common in those who were institutionalized (Heyman *et al.*, 1987). In most instances nursing home placement occurred because the patients had become almost completely helpless and required 24-hour supervision; for 10 patients the decision was prompted by death or serious illness of their caregivers.

A prospective study of 101 initially community-dwelling AD patients found that 12 per cent with 'mild AD' were in nursing homes after 1 year, and 35 per cent after 2 years

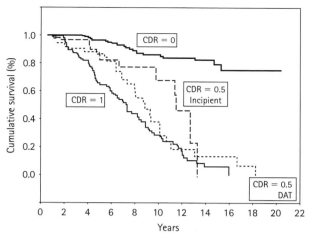

Figure 28.1 *Progression to nursing home placement in non-demented (CDR of 0) and demented (CDR 0.5 incipient, 0.5 dementia of the Alzheimer type (DAT), and CDR 1) groups. (Reproduced with permission from Storandt et al., 2002.)*

(Knopman *et al.*, 1988). For 'advanced AD', the figures were 39 per cent at 1 year and 62 per cent at 2 years. Total ADL scores were significantly related to institutionalization, while incontinence, irritability, inability to walk, wandering, hyperactivity and nocturnal behavioural problems were the leading reasons for placement cited by caregivers. The importance of disruptive behaviours such as aggressiveness, sleep disturbances and wandering have also been cited as important predictors of institutionalization among AD patients by other authors (Haupt and Kurz, 1993; Bianchetti *et al.*, 1995; Tariot *et al.*, 1995; Lopez *et al.*, 1999).

A CERAD analysis, comprising 20 university medical centres, found that the median time from enrolment to nursing home placement was 3.1 years, with significantly reduced times (2.1 years) for males who were unmarried (Heyman *et al.*, 1997). The major predictors of time to admission were measures of dementia severity upon entry into the study, including the degree of cognitive impairment, functional disability, and overall stage. Age at entry and marital status (men only) also predicted time to nursing home admission. Similar findings with regard to marital status have been reported by others (Haupt and Kurz, 1993).

Finally, a recent large multiregional, prospective study distinguished by an extremely large number of patients (n = 3944), found that specific caregiver traits (including age ≥80, low income, poor health and high perceived burden as a result of caregiving) predicted earlier placement for care recipients (Gaugler *et al.*, 2003).

28.5 SURVIVAL IN ALZHEIMER'S DISEASE

Length of survival in AD is highly variable, although an excess mortality has consistently been reported (Katzman, 1976; Jorm *et al.*, 1987; Aevarsson *et al.*, 1998). Although mean survival after symptom onset may range from 2 to >16 years, the observed survival rate among AD populations is generally significantly less than the expected rate, based on life expectancy tables (Walsh *et al.*, 1990). Depending on the study, survival at 5 years ranges from 10 to 40 per cent in different AD populations. Of course, the most favourable survival rates were seen in mild cohorts followed up in outpatient settings, with lowest survival rates reported in relatively severely demented subjects from hospital series. The median duration of survival among CERAD patients from time of study entry was 5.9 years (Heyman *et al.*, 1996), which compared favourably to the 5.3 years reported by Walsh *et al.* (1990), the 5.7 years noted by Molsa *et al.* (1986), and the 5.8 years described by Jost and Grossberg (1995). Three other studies found shorter median periods of survival of 3.4 years (Schoenberg *et al.*, 1987), 3.5 years (Barclay *et al.*, 1985), and 4.3 years (Claus *et al.*, 1998), possibly due to inclusion of more severe subjects.

The shortened survival of AD patients results from complications due to severe mental decline. Malnutrition, dehydration, pneumonia and other infections occur frequently in the terminal stages when patients are bed-bound, incontinent and unable to communicate or feed themselves. Compared with other elderly individuals, AD patients are not especially predisposed to cancer, cerebrovascular or cardiovascular disease (Molsa *et al.*, 1986).

Probably not surprisingly, the most consistent predictors of mortality in AD patients are age, gender and severity of dementia. Age was significantly associated with survival time in a large sample of patients with AD, drawn from throughout the state of California (Moritz *et al.*, 1997). Increasing age has also been related to shorter survival in several additional studies (Hier *et al.*, 1989; Walsh *et al.*, 1990; van Dijk *et al.*, 1991; Heyman *et al.*, 1996; Reisberg *et al.*, 1996; Aguero-Torres *et al.*, 1998; Claus *et al.*, 1998; Gambassi *et al.*, 1999; Ueki *et al.*, 2001). Although two reports have indicated that survival rates of patients with early-onset AD are considerably less than those of late-onset AD (Heyman *et al.*, 1987; McGonigal *et al.*, 1992), this finding has not been confirmed by others (Walsh *et al.*, 1990; Bracco *et al.*, 1994; Corder *et al.*, 1995; Bowen *et al.*, 1996; Heyman *et al.*, 1996).

Most investigators have reported shorter survival times for men than women (Schoenberg *et al.*, 1987; Berg *et al.*, 1988; Burns *et al.*, 1991; van Dijk *et al.*, 1991; Corder *et al.*, 1995; Jagger *et al.*, 1995; Molsa *et al.*, 1995; Stern *et al.*, 1995; Bowen *et al.*, 1996; Heyman *et al.*, 1996; Reisberg *et al.*, 1996; Moritz *et al.*, 1997; Claus *et al.*, 1998; Gambassi *et al.*, 1999; Lapane *et al.*, 2001; Ueki *et al.*, 2001), although this has not been the case for a few studies (Hier *et al.*, 1989; Walsh *et al.*, 1990; Becker *et al.*, 1994). Furthermore, it has been suggested by some that predictors may differ by gender. For example, Moritz *et al.* (1997) found that among men, but not women, survival times were negatively associated with selected neurological symptoms, particularly aphasia and apraxia. Among women, but not men, a history of cardiovascular conditions was associated with poorer survival. Lapane *et al.* (2001) on

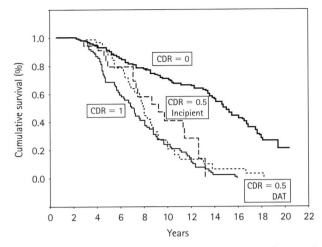

Figure 28.2   *Progression to the end point of death in non-demented (CDR of 0) and demented (CDR 0.5 incipient, 0.5 dementia of the Alzheimer type (DAT), and CDR 1) groups. (Reproduced with permission from Storandt* et al., *2002.)*

the other hand, found that the most important predictors of mortality for men were severity of dementia and the occurrence of delirium. For women, death was associated with impairment of ADL, presence of pressure sores, malnutrition and comorbidity.

Patients with more severe cognitive impairment at study entry have consistently been reported to have shorter durations of survival (Walsh *et al.*, 1990; Burns *et al.*, 1991; Evans *et al.*, 1991; Jagger *et al.*, 1995; Heyman *et al.*, 1996; Moritz *et al.*, 1997; Claus *et al.*, 1998; Ueki *et al.*, 2001; Storandt *et al.*, 2002; Figure 28.2). In addition, functional disability has been shown to decrease survival time in AD (Martin *et al.*, 1987; Bianchetti *et al.*, 1995; Heyman *et al.*, 1996; Ueki *et al.*, 2001).

Additional variables that may influence survival time in patients with AD have not been well established, including level of education (Becker *et al.*, 1994; Stern *et al.*, 1995; Geerlings *et al.*, 1997), medical comorbidity (White *et al.*, 1996; Moritz *et al.*, 1997; Aguero-Torres *et al.*, 1998; Gambassi *et al.*, 1999; Lopez *et al.*, 1999), and psychiatric or behavioural symptoms (Barclay *et al.*, 1985; Molsa *et al.*, 1986; Walsh *et al.*, 1990; Stern *et al.*, 1994; Samson *et al.*, 1996), among others.

Survival in AD appeared to be unrelated to ApoE ε4 gene dose in a study by Corder *et al.* (1995). However, Tilvis *et al.* (1998) noted increased mortality in elderly demented patients with the ε4 allele, a finding supported, at least for men, in a recent study of 92 autopsy confirmed AD cases (Dal Forno *et al.*, 2002). On the other hand, Stern *et al.* (1997) found that the presence of at least one ε4 allele was associated with a less aggressive form of AD and a decreased risk of mortality in 99 patients with probable AD followed for up to 6 years.

EPS appeared to be an important predictor of mortality in a population-based study of 198 patients with probable early-onset AD (Samson *et al.*, 1996). EPS at entry was also associated with a higher relative risk of death in 236 patients with mild AD followed semiannually by Stern *et al.* (1994).

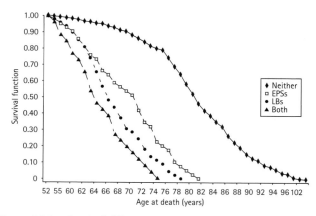

Figure 28.3 *Survival differences by the presence of extrapyramidal signs (EPSs) and Lewy bodies (LBs) from a life-table analysis. (Reproduced with permission from Haan et al., 2002.)*

A recent study of 379 AD patients found similar heightened mortality for EPS and reported that individuals with EPS were three times more likely to have LBs at autopsy (Haan *et al.*, 2002; Figure 28.3). Both EPS and LBs were associated with earlier age at death. This was not the case for a study by Lopez *et al.* (2000) who reported no differences between AD and DLB with regard to survival.

28.6 CONCLUSIONS

Despite an abundance of observations about the natural history of AD, the variability of its clinical features and rate of progression has not been explained, and the validity of 'subtypes' of AD has not been proven. Overall, the most consistent predictor of more rapid deterioration and death in AD appears to be the degree of cognitive and functional disability. Because of the relatively low prevalence of additional clinical features such as EPS, depression and psychosis at early stages of the disease, larger studies, carefully controlled for the potential confounding effect of dementia severity, are needed to clarify their effect on prognosis.

REFERENCES

Aevarsson O, Svanborg A, Skoog I. (1998) Seven-year survival rate after age 85 years: relation to Alzheimer disease and vascular dementia. *Archives of Neurology* **55**: 1226–1232

Aguero-Torres H, Fratiglioni L, Guo Z *et al.* (1998) Prognostic factors in very old demented adults: a seven-year follow-up from a population-based survey in Stockholm. *Journal of the American Geriatrics Society* **46**: 444–452

Aisen PS, Schafer KA, Grundman M *et al.* (2003) Effects of Rofecoxib and Naproxen vs placebo in Alzheimer's disease progression. *JAMA* **289**: 2819–2826

Backman L, Jones S, Small B *et al.* (2003) Rate of cognitive decline in preclinical Alzheimer's disease: The role of comorbidity. *Journals of Gerontology Series B. Psychological Sciences and Social Sciences* **58**: 228–236

Bakchine S, Lacomblez L, Palisson E *et al.* (1989) Relationship between primitive reflexes, extrapyramidal signs, reflexive apraxia, and severity of cognitive impairment in dementia of the Alzheimer type. *Acta Neurologica Scandinavica* **79**: 38–46

Barclay LL, Zemcov A, Blass JP, Sansone J. (1985) Survival in Alzheimer's disease and vascular dementias. *Neurology* **35**: 834–840

Becker J, Boller F, Lopez O *et al.* (1994) The natural history of Alzheimer's disease: description of study cohort and accuracy of diagnosis. *Archives of Neurology* **51**: 585–594

Becker JT, Huff FJ, Nebes RD *et al.* (1988) Neuropsychological function in Alzheimer's disease: pattern of impairment and rates of progression. *Archives of Neurology* **45**: 263–268

Berg L, Miller JP, Storandt M *et al.* (1988) Mild senile dementia of the Alzheimer type: 2. Longitudinal assessment. *Annals of Neurology* **23**: 477–484

Bianchetti A, Scuratti A, Zanetti O *et al.* (1995) Predictors of mortality and institutionalization in Alzheimer disease patients 1 year after discharge from an Alzheimer dementia unit. *Dementia* **6**: 108–112

Bondi M, Salmon D, Butters N. (1994) Neuropsychological features of memory disorders in Alzheimer disease. In: RD Terry, R Katzman, KL Bick (eds), *Alzheimer disease* 1st edition. Philadelphia, Lippincott-Raven Publishers, pp. 41–64

Bowen J, Malter A, Sheppard L *et al.* (1996) Predictors of mortality in patients diagnosed with probable Alzheimer's disease. *Neurology* **47**: 433–439

Bracco L, Gallato R, Grigoletto F *et al.* (1994) Factors affecting course and survival in Alzheimer's Disease. A nine-year longitudinal study. *Archives of Neurology* **51**: 1213–1219

Brookmeyer R, Gray S, Kawas C. (1998) Projections of Alzheimer's disease in the United States and the public health impact of delaying disease onset. *American Journal of Public Health* **88**: 1337–1342

Brouwers P, Cox D, Martin A, Chase T, Fedio P. (1984) Differential perceptual-spatial impairment in Huntington's and Alzheimer's dementias. *Archives of Neurology* **41**: 1073–1076

Burns A, Jacoby R, Levy R. (1990) Psychiatric phenomena in Alzheimer's disease. IV. Disorders of behavior. *British Journal of Psychiatry* **157**: 86–94

Burns A, Jacoby R, Levy R. (1991) Progression of cognitive impairment in Alzheimer's disease. *Journal of the American Geriatrics Society* **39**: 34–45

Chen JY, Stern Y, Sano M, Mayeux R. (1991) Cumulative risks of developing extrapyramidal signs, psychosis, or myoclonus in the course of Alzheimer's disease. *Archives of Neurology* **48**: 1141–1143

Chui H, Lyness S, Sobel E, Schneider L. (1994) Extrapyramidal signs and psychiatric symptoms predict faster cognitive decline in Alzheimer's disease. *Archives of Neurology* **51**: 676–681

Claus J, van Fool W, Teunisse S *et al.* (1998) Predicting survival in patients with early Alzheimer's disease. *Dementia and Geriatric Cognitive Disorders* **9**: 284–93

Cook SE, Miyahara S, Bacanu SA *et al.* (2003) Psychotic symptoms in Alzheimer disease: evidence for subtypes. *American Journal of Geriatric Psychiatry* **11**: 406–413

Corder E, Saunders A, Strittmatter W *et al.* (1995) Apolipoprotein E, survival in Alzheimer's disease patients, and the competing risks of death and Alzheimer's disease. *Neurology* **45**: 1323–1328

Corey-Bloom J, Galasko D, Hofstetter C *et al.* (1993) Clinical features distinguishing large cohorts with possible AD, probable AD, and mixed dementia. *Journal of the American Geriatrics Society* **41**: 31–37

Craft S, Teri L, Edland S *et al.* (1998). Accelerated decline in apolipoprotein E-epsilon4 homozygotes with Alzheimer's disease. *Neurology* **51**: 149–153

Cummings JL and Cole G. (2002) Alzheimer disease. *JAMA* **287**: 2335–2338

Cummings JL, Benson DF, Hill MA, Read S. (1985) Aphasia in dementia of the Alzheimer type. *Neurology* **35**: 394–397

Cummings JL, Miller B, Hill MA, Neshkes R. (1987) Neuropsychiatric aspects of multi-infarct dementia and dementia of the Alzheimer type. *Archives of Neurology* **44**: 389–393

Dal Forno G, Carson KA, Brookmeyer R *et al.* (2002) APoE genotype and Survival in Men and Women with Alzheimer's Disease. *Neurology* **58**: 1045–1050

Drachman DA, O'Donnell BF, Lew RA, Swearer JM. (1990) The prognosis in Alzheimer's disease: 'How Far' rather than 'How Fast' best predicts the course. *Archives of Neurology* **47**: 851–856

Drevets WC and Rubin EH. (1989) Psychotic symptoms and the longitudinal course of senile dementia of the Alzheimer type. *Biological Psychiatry* **25**: 39–48

Eaker ED, Vierkant RA, Mickel SF. (2002) Predictors of nursing home admission and/or death in incident Alzheimer's disease and other dementia cases compared to controls: a population-based study. *Journal of Clinical Epidemiology* **55**: 462–468

Evans DA, Smith LA, Scherr PA *et al.* (1991) Risk of death from Alzheimer's disease in a community population of older persons. *American Journal of Epidemiology* **134**: 403–412

Filley CM, Brownell H, Albert ML. (1985) Education provides no protection against Alzheimer's disease. *Neurology* **35**: 1781–1784

Frisoni G, Govoni S, Geroldi C *et al.* (1995) Gene dose of the epsilon 4 allele of apolipoprotein E and disease progression in sporadic late-onset Alzheimer's disease. *Annals of Neurology* **37**: 596–604

Galasko D, Klauber MR, Hofstetter CR *et al.* (1990) The Mini-Mental State Examination in the early diagnosis of Alzheimer's disease. *Archives of Neurology* **47**: 49–52

Gambassi G, Landi F, Lapane KL *et al.* (1999) Predictors of mortality in patients with Alzheimer's disease living in nursing homes. *Journal of Neurology, Neurosurgery, and Psychiatry* **67**: 59–65

Gaugler JE, Kane RL, Kane RA *et al.* (2003) Caregiving and institutionalization of cognitively impaired older people: utilizing dynamic predictors of change. *The Gerontologist* **43**: 219–229

Geerlings M, Deeg D, Schmand B *et al.* (1997) Increased risk of mortality in Alzheimer's disease patients with higher education? A replication study. *Neurology* **49**: 798–802

Gomez-Isla T, West H, Rebeck G *et al.* (1996) Clinical and pathological correlates of apolipoprotein E epsilon 4 in Alzheimer's disease. *Annals of Neurology* **39**: 62–70

Growdon J, Locascio J, Corkin S *et al.* (1996) Apolipoprotein E genotype does not influence rates of cognitive decline in Alzheimer's disease. *Neurology* **47**: 444–448

Haan MN, Jagust WJ, Galasko D, Kaye J. (2002) Effect of extrapyramidal and Lewy bodies on survival in patients with Alzheimer disease. *Archives of Neurology* **59**: 588–593

Haskell S, Richardson E, Horwitz R. (1997) The effect of estrogen replacement therapy on cognitive function in women: a critical review of the literature. *Journal of Clinical Epidemiology* **50**: 1249–1264

Haupt M and Kurz A. (1993) Predictors of nursing home placement in patients with Alzheimer's disease. *International Journal of Geriatric Psychiatry* **8**: 741–746

Hauser WA, Morris ML, Heston LL, Anderson VE. (1986) Seizures and myoclonus in patients with Alzheimer's disease. *Neurology* **36**: 1226–1230

Helmes E and Ostbye T. (2002) Beyond memory impairment: cognitive changes in Alzheimer's disease. *Archives of Clinical Neuropsychology* **17**: 179–193

Heston LL, Mastri AR, Anderson VE, White J. (1981) Dementia of the Alzheimer type: clinical genetics, natural history, and associated conditions. *Archives of General Psychiatry* **31**: 1085–1090

Heyman A, Wilkinson WE, Hurwitz BJ *et al.* (1987) Early-onset Alzheimer's disease: clinical predictors of institutionalization and death. *Neurology* **37**: 980–984

Heyman A, Peterson B, Fillenbaum G, Pieper C. (1996) The consortium to establish a registry for Alzheimer's disease (CERAD). Part XIV: demographic and clinical predictors of survival in patients with Alzheimer disease. *Neurology* **46**: 656–660

Heyman A, Peterson B, Cillenbaum G, Pieper C. (1997) Predictors of time to institutionalization of patients with Alzheimer's disease: the CERAD experience, part XVII. *Neurology* **48**: 1304–1309

Hier D, Warach J, Gorelick P, Thomas J. (1989) Predictors of survival in clinically diagnosed Alzheimer's disease and multi-infarct dementia. *Archives of Neurology* **46**: 1213–1216

Hirono N, Hashimoto M, Yasuda M *et al.* (2003) Accelerated memory decline in Alzheimer's disease with apolipoprotein, 4 allele. *Journal of Neuropsychiatry and Clinical Neuroscience* **15**: 354–358

Hooker K, Bowman SR, Coehlo DP *et al.* (2002) Behavioral change in persons with dementia: relationships with mental and physical health of caregivers. *Journal of Gerontology. Series B, Psychological Sciences and Social Sciences* **57**: P453–P460

Huff FJ, Belle SH, Shim YK *et al.* (1990) Prevalence and prognostic value of neurologic abnormalities in Alzheimer's disease. *Dementia* **1**: 32–40

Hughes CP, Berg L, Danziger WL *et al.* (1982) A new clinical scale for the staging of dementia. *British Journal of Psychiatry* **140**: 566–572

Hutton JT, Dippel RL, Loewenson RB *et al.* (1985) Predictors of nursing home placement of patients with Alzheimer's disease. *Texas Medicine* **81**: 40–43

Jacobs D, Sano M, Marder K *et al.* (1994) Age at onset of Alzheimer's disease: relation to pattern of cognitive dysfunction and rate of decline. *Neurology* **44**: 1215–1220

Jagger C, Clarke M, Stone A. (1995) Predictors of survival with Alzheimer's disease: a community-based study. *Psychological Medicine* **25**: 171–177

Jorm AF, Korten AE, Henderson AS. (1987) The prevalence of dementia: a quantitative integration of the literature. *Acta Psychiatrica Scandinavica* **76**: 465–479

Jost B and Grossberg G. (1995) The natural history of Alzheimer's disease: a brain bank study. *Journal of the American Geriatrics Society* **43**: 1248–1255

Jost B and Grossberg G. (1996) The evolution of psychiatric symptoms in Alzheimer's disease. *Journal of the American Geriatrics Society* **44**: 1078–1081

Katzman R. (1976) The prevalence and malignancy of Alzheimer disease: a major killer. *Archives of Neurology* **33**: 217–218

Katzman R, Brown T, Thal LJ *et al.* (1988) Comparison of rate of annual change of mental status score in four independent studies of patients with Alzheimer's disease. *Annals of Neurology* **34**: 384–389

Kavcic V and Duffy CJ. (2003) Attentional dynamics and visual perception: mechanisms of spatial disorientation in Alzheimer's disease. *Brain* **126**: 1173–1181

Knopman DS, Kitto J, Deinard S, Heiring J. (1988) Longitudinal study of death and institutionalization in patients with primary degenerative dementia. *Journal of the American Geriatrics Society* **36**: 108–112

Kramer-Ginsberg E, Mohs RC, Aryan M *et al.* (1988) Clinical predictors of course for Alzheimer patients in a longitudinal study: a preliminary report. *Psychopharmacology Bulletin* **24**: 458–462

Kurz A, Egensperger R, Haupt M *et al.* (1996) Apolipoprotein E epsilon 4 allele, cognitive decline, and deterioration of everyday performance in Alzheimer's disease. *Neurology* **47**: 440–443

Lapane KL, Gambassi G, Landi F *et al.* (2001) Gender differences in predictors of mortality in nursing home residents with AD. *Neurology* **56**: 650–654

Lazarus LW, Newton N, Cohler B *et al.* (1987) Frequency and presentation of depressive symptoms in patients with primary degenerative dementia. *American Journal of Psychiatry* **144**: 41–45

Lee J, Olichney JM, Hansen LA *et al.* (2000) Small concomitant vascular lesions do not influence rates of cognitive decline in patients with Alzheimer disease. *Archives of Neurology* **57**: 1474–1479

Lopez OL, Boller F, Becker JT *et al.* (1990) Alzheimer's disease and depression: neuropsychological impairment and progression of the illness. *American Journal of Psychiatry* **147**: 855–860

Lopez O, Wisniewski S, Becker J *et al.* (1997) Extrapyramidal signs in patients with probable Alzheimer's disease. *Neurology* **54**: 969–975

Lopez O, Wisniewski SR, Becker JT *et al.* (1999) Psychiatric medications and abnormal behavior as predictors of progression in probable Alzheimer's disease. *Archives of Neurology* **56**: 1266–1272

Lopez O, Wisniewski SR, Hamilton RL *et al.* (2000) Predictors of progression in patients with AD and Lewy bodies. *Neurology* **54**: 1774–1779

Lucca U, Comelli M, Tettamanti M *et al.* (1993) Rate of progression and prognostic factors in Alzheimer's disease: a prospective study. *Journal of the American Geriatrics Society* **41**: 45–49

Lyketsos CG, Lopez O, Jones B *et al.* (2002) Prevalence of neuropsychiatric symptoms in dementia and mild cognitive impairment: results from the cardiovascular health study. *JAMA* **288**:1475–1483

McGonigal G, McQuade CA, Thomas BM, Whalley LJ. (1992) Survival in presenile Alzheimer's and multi-infarct dementias. *Neuroepidemiology* **11**: 121–126

Martin D, Miller J, Kapoor W *et al.* (1987) A controlled study of survival with dementia. *Archives of Neurology* **44**: 1122–1126

Mayeux RT, Stern Y, Spanton S. (1985) Heterogeneity in dementia of the Alzheimer type: evidence of subgroups. *Neurology* **35**: 453–461

Mega MS, Masterman DM, O'Connor SM *et al.* (1999) The spectrum of behavioral responses to cholinesterase inhibitor therapy in Alzheimer disease. *Archives of Neurology* **56**: 1388–1393

Miller T, Tinklenberg J, Brooks J, Yesavage J. (1991) Cognitive decline in patients with Alzheimer's disease: differences in patients with and without extrapyramidal signs. *Alzheimer Disease and Associated Disorders* **5**: 251–256

Molsa P, Marttila R, Rinne U. (1995) Long-term survival and predictors of mortality in Alzheimer's disease and multi-infarct dementia. *Acta Neurologica Scandinavica* **91**: 159–164

Molsa PK, Marttila RJ, Rinne UK. (1986) Survival and cause of death in Alzheimer's disease and multi-infarct dementia. *Acta Neurologica Scandinavica* **74**: 103–107

Moritz D, Fox P, Luscombe F, Kraemer H. (1997) Neurological predictors of mortality in patients with Alzheimer disease in California. *Archives of Neurology* **54**: 878–885

Morris J. (1997) Clinical dementia rating: a reliable and valid diagnostic and staging measure for dementia of the Alzheimer type. *International Psychogeriatrics* **9** (Suppl. 1): 173–176

Morris J, Edland S, Clark C *et al.* (1993) The consortium to establish a registry for Alzheimer's disease (CERAD). Part IV. Rates of cognitive change in the longitudinal assessment of probable Alzheimer's disease. *Neurology* **43**: 2457–2465

Mortimer J, Ebbitt B, Jun S-P, Finch M. (1992) Predictors of cognitive and functional progression in patients with probable Alzheimer's disease. *Neurology* **42**: 1689–1696

Mungas D, Reed BR, Ellis WG, Jagust W. (2001) The effects of aging on rate of progression of Alzheimer disease and dementia with associated cerebrovascular disease. *Archives of Neurology* **58**: 1243–1247

Murdoch BE and Chenery HJ. (1987) Language disorders in dementia of the Alzheimer type. *Brain and Language* **31**: 122–137

Olichney JM, Galasko D, Salmon DP *et al.* (1998) Cognitive decline is faster in Lewy body variant than in Alzheimer's disease. *Neurology* **51**: 351–357

Ortof E and Crystal HA. (1989) Rate of progression of Alzheimer's disease. *Journal of the American Geriatrics Society* **37**: 511–514

Pearson JL, Teri L, Reifler BF, Raskind MA. (1989) Functional status and cognitive impairment in Alzheimer's patients with and without depression. *Journal of the American Geriatrics Society* **37**: 1117–1121

Rapcsak SZ, Croswell SC, Rubens AB. (1989) Apraxia in Alzheimer's disease. *Neurology* **39**: 664–668

Reisberg B, Ferris S, de Leon MJ, Crook T. (1982) The Global Deterioration Scale (GDS): an instrument for the assessment of primary degenerative dementia (PDD). *American Journal of Psychiatry* **139**: 1136–1139

Reisberg B, Ferris SH, Steinberg G *et al.* (1986) Longitudinal course of normal aging and progressive dementia of the Alzheimer's type: a prospective study of 106 subjects over a 3.6 year mean interval. *Progress in Neuro-Psychopharmacology and Biological Psychiatry* **10**: 571–578

Reisberg B, Borenstein J, Salob SP *et al.* (1987) Behavioral symptoms in Alzheimer's disease: phenomenology and treatment. *Journal of Clinical Psychiatry* **48**: 9–15

Reisberg B, Franssen E, Sclan SG *et al.* (1989) Stage specific incidence of potentially remediable behavioral symptoms in aging and Alzheimer disease. *Bulletin of Clinical Neurosciences* **54**: 95–112

Reisberg B, Ferris S, Franssen E *et al.* (1996) Mortality and temporal course of probable Alzheimer's disease: a 5-year prospective study. *International Psychogeriatrics* **8**: 291–311

Rich J, Rasmusson D, Folstein M. (1995) Nonsteroidal anti-inflammatory drugs in Alzheimer's disease. *Neurology* **45**: 51–55

Rockwood K. (2002) Use of lipid lowering agents, indication bias, and the risk of dementia in community dwelling elderly people. *Archives of Neurology* **59**: 223–227

Rosen J and Zubenko GS. (1991) Emergence of psychosis and depression in the longitudinal evaluation of Alzheimer's disease. *Biological Psychiatry* **29**: 224–232

Rosen WG, Mohs RC, Davis KL. (1984) A new rating scale for Alzheimer's disease. *American Journal of Psychiatry* **141**: 1356–1364

Roth M, Tym E, Mountjoy CQ *et al.* (1986) CAMDEX: a standardized instrument for the diagnosis of mental disorder in the elderly with special reference to the early detection of dementia. *British Journal of Psychiatry* **149**: 698–709

Salmon DP, Thal LJ, Butters N, Heindel WC. (1990) Longitudinal evaluation of dementia of the Alzheimer type: a comparison of three standardized mental status examinations. *Neurology* **40**: 1225–1230

Samson W, van Duijn C, Hop W, Hofman A. (1996) Clinical features and mortality in patients with early-onset Alzheimer's disease. *European Neurology* **36**: 103–106

Sano M, Ernesto C, Thomas RG *et al.* (1997) A controlled trial of selegiline, alpha-tocopherol, or both as a treatment for Alzheimer's disease. *New England Journal of Medicine* **336**: 1216–1222

Schoenberg B, Kokmen E, Okazaki H. (1987) Alzheimer's disease and other dementing illnesses in a defined United States population: incidence rates and clinical features. *Annals of Neurology* **22**: 724–749

Stern Y, Mayeux R, Sano M *et al.* (1987) Predictors of disease course in patients with probable Alzheimer's disease. *Neurology* **37**: 1649–1653

Stern Y, Hesdorffer D, Sano M, Mayeux R. (1990) Measurement and prediction of functional capacity in Alzheimer's disease. *Neurology* **40**: 8–14

Stern Y, Albert M, Brandt J *et al.* (1994) Utility of extrapyramidal signs and psychosis as predictors of cognitive and functional decline, nursing home admission and death in Alzheimer's disease. *Neurology* **44**: 2300–2307

Stern Y, Tang M, Denaro J, Mayeux R. (1995) Increased risk of mortality in Alzheimer's disease patients with more advanced educational and occupational attainment. *Annals of Neurology* **37**: 590–595

Stern Y, Brandt J, Albert M, Jacobs D *et al.* (1997) The absence of an apolipoprotein epsilon 4 allele is associated with a more aggressive form of Alzheimer's disease. *Annals of Neurology* **41**: 615–620

Storandt M, Grant EA, Miller JP, Morris JC. (2002) Rates of progression in mild cognitive impairment and early Alzheimer's disease. *Neurology* **59**: 1034–1041

Sullivan EV, Corkin S, Growden JH. (1986) Verbal and non-verbal short-term memory in patients with Alzheimer's disease and in healthy elderly subjects. *Developmental Neuropsychology* **2**: 387–400

Swanwick GRJ, Coen RF, Coakley D, Lawlor BA. (1998) Assessment of progression and prognosis in 'possible' and 'probable' Alzheimer's disease. *International Journal of Geriatric Psychiatry* **13**: 331–335

Swearer JM, Drachman DA, O'Donnell BF, Mitchell AL. (1988) Troublesome and disruptive behaviors in dementia. *Journal of the American Geriatrics Society* **36**: 784–790

Tariot P, Mack J, Patterson M *et al.* (1995) The Behavior Rating Scale for Dementia of the Consortium to establish a registry for Alzheimer's disease. *American Journal of Psychiatry* **152**: 1349–1357

Teri L, Larson EB, Reifler BV. (1988) Behavioral disturbances in dementia of the Alzheimer's type. *Journal of the American Geriatrics Society* **36**: 1–6

Teri L, Hughes JP, Larson EB. (1990) Cognitive deterioration in Alzheimer's disease: behavioral and health factors. *Journal of Gerontology* **45**: P58–P63

Teri L, McCurry S, Edland S *et al.* (1995) Cognitive decline in Alzheimer's disease: a longitudinal investigation of risk factors for accelerated decline. *Journal of Gerontology* **50A**, M49–M55

Thal LJ, Grundman M, Klauber MR. (1988) Dementia: characteristics of a referral population and factors associated with progression. *Neurology* **38**: 1083–1090

Thal LJ, Calvani M, Amato A, Carta A. (2000) A 1-year controlled trial of acetyl-l-carnitine in early-onset AD. *Neurology* **55**: 805–810

Thal LJ, Thomas RG, Mulnard R *et al.* (2003) Estrogen levels do not correlate with improvement in cognition. *Archives of Neurology* **60**: 209–212

Tilvis R, Strandberg T, Juva K. (1998) Apolipoprotein E phenotypes, dementia and mortality in a prospective population sample. *Journal of the American Geriatrics Society* **46**: 712–715

Tschampa HJ, Neumann M, Zerr I *et al.* (2001) Patients with Alzheimer's disease and dementia with Lewy bodies mistaken for Creutzfeldt–Jakob disease. *Journal of Neurology, Neurosurgery, and Psychiatry* **71**: 33–39

Uhlman RF, Larson EB, Koepsell TD. (1986) Hearing impairment and cognitive decline in senile dementia of the Alzheimer's type. *Journal of the American Geriatrics Society* **34**: 207–210

Ueki A, Shinjo H, Shimode H *et al.* (2001) Factors associated with mortality in patients with early-onset Alzheimer's disease: a five-year longitudinal study. *International Journal of Geriatric Psychiatry* **16**: 810–815

van Dijk P, Dippel D, Habbema J. (1991) Survivals of patients with dementia. *Journal of the American Geriatrics Society* **39**: 603–610

Walsh JS, Welch HG, Larson EB. (1990) Survival of outpatients with Alzheimer-type dementia. *Annals of Internal Medicine* **113**: 429–434

White H, Pieper C, Schmader K, Fillenbaum G. (1996) Weight change in Alzheimer's disease. *Journal of the American Geriatrics Society* **44**: 265–272

Wilson RS, Bacon LD, Fox JH, Kaszniak AW. (1983) Primary and secondary memory in dementia of the Alzheimer type. *Journal of Clinical Neuropsychology* **5**: 337–344

Winblad, B, Engedal, K, Soininen. H *et al.* (2001) A 1-year, randomized, placebo-controlled study of donepezil in patients with mild to moderate AD. *Neurology* **57**(3), 489–495

Wragg RE and Jeste DV. (1989) Overview of depression and psychosis in Alzheimer's disease. *American Journal of Psychiatry* **146**: 577–587

Yaffe K, Sawaya G, Lieberburg I, Grady D. (1998) Estrogen therapy in postmenopausal women: effects on cognitive function and dementia. *JAMA* **279**: 688–695

Yesavage JA, Poulsen AB, Sheikh J, Tanke E. (1988) Rates of change of common measures of impairment in senile dementia of the Alzheimer type. *Psychopharmacology Bulletin* **24**: 531–534

29

Neurochemistry of Alzheimer's disease

NICHOLAS A CLARKE AND PAUL T FRANCIS

The known neurochemistry of Alzheimer's disease (AD) has, to date, been characterized by cholinergic neurotransmission dysfunction. Human anticholinergic drug studies (Drachman and Leavitt, 1974), the demonstration of first choline acetyltransferase (ChAT) activity and then acetylcholine (ACh) deficits in people with AD (Bowen et al., 1976), and the subsequent development of the cholinesterase inhibitor (ChEI) class of drug, are now matters of historical record.

Present neurochemical understanding in AD touches, at its limits, upon how early the cholinergic deficit develops and whether it occurs in so-called mild cognitive impairment (MCI). Other basic science research, now informed by therapeutic drug use, assesses the ubiquitous glutamatergic neurotransmitter systems, the workhorse of the brain. Anatomical studies suggest interconnectivity between these two systems, but their exact role in AD will require further elucidation. Just as cholinergic and glutamatergic disruption may be additive in their effect, so may pharmacological replacement therapy be synergistic (Francis et al., 1993).

The mismetabolism of tau and amyloid proteins described elsewhere (see Chapters 31 and 32) offers the most upstream knowledge of the AD pathological cascade. Neurotransmitter deficits, neuronal loss and (aberrant) synapse proliferation and subsequent decline suggest possible windows of influence upon the disease. Refinement of neurotransmitter influence on protein mismetabolism and other cell level dysfunction is likely to follow. A recent example is the description of beneficial effects of a cholinergic agonist, specific to the muscarinic M1 receptor, upon 'healthy' amyloid precursor protein metabolism (Nitsch et al., 2000).

Recent findings with long-term ChEI treatment show delays to nursing home placements, but not time to reach a specific point of cognitive decline or death (Lopez et al.,

2002; Geldmacher et al., 2003). Future research may yet give substance to hopes that disease modification is possible by neurotransmitter manipulation in AD.

From a neurochemical standpoint ACh, glutamate, serotonin and noradrenaline are the major transmitter systems affected by AD, with relative sparing of dopamine, gamma amino butyric acid (GABA) and most peptides (Francis et al., 1993; Francis, 2003). This chapter examines both cognitive and non-cognitive (behavioural) aspects of neurotransmission, the latter also being considered to relate to structural and functional alterations in the central nervous system (CNS). Such changes are important, in part because carers find behavioural disturbances difficult to cope with, and the presence of such behaviours in AD patients often leads to the need for institutionalization. The chapter will focus on cholinergic and glutamatergic systems.

29.1 ACETYLCHOLINE

Neuropathologically, loss of neurones from the nucleus of Meynert (CH4, cholinergic nucleus) is well documented in AD, although the extent of the loss reported varies from moderate to severe, and it has been suggested that in AD cholinergic dysfunction exceeds degeneration (Perry et al., 1982). This is consistent with studies of cholinergic markers in biopsy samples from patients who had AD for approximately 3 years, where reduction in functional cholinergic measures, acetylcholine synthesis and choline uptake exceeded the reduction in ChAT activity (Francis et al., 1985).

On the basis of the above evidence, neocortical cholinergic innervation appears to be lost at an early stage of the disease. Beach and colleagues (2000) recently reported neurofibrillary tangles in the entorhinal cortex and a 20–30 per cent loss of ChAT activity in brains from patients at the earliest stages of AD, namely Braak stages I and II. However, another study using the Clinical Dementia Rating scale (CDR) suggests that the greatest reduction in markers of the cholinergic system occurs between moderate (CDR 2) and end-stage (CDR 5) disease with little change between non-demented and the moderate stage (CDR 0–2) (Davis et al., 1999). In contrast a recent study of MCI, the suggested AD prodrome, reported an increase in ChAT activity in some cortical regions (DeKosky et al., 2002). The acknowledged problems of these latter studies is that ChAT activity is not the rate-limiting step of ACh synthesis and hence there could be cholinergic dysfunction before structural loss, possibly linked to aberrant sprouting. Changes in cholinergic neurones appear to relate to aspects of cognitive function (Francis et al., 1985) as well non-cognitive behaviour (Minger et al., 2000). It has also been suggested that ACh is centrally involved in the process of conscious awareness (Perry et al., 1999), and that the variety of clinical symptoms associated with cholinergic dysfunction in AD and related disorders reflects disturbances in the conscious processing of information. There is evidence that implicit memory for example (which does not involve conscious awareness) is relatively intact in AD (Postle et al., 1996).

Nicotinic and muscarinic (M2) ACh receptors, most of which are considered to be located on cholinergic terminals, are reduced in AD (Court et al., 2001; Lai et al., 2001). Reductions in nicotinic receptors are confined to the $\alpha 4\beta 2$ subtype. The postsynaptic cholinergic system (usually present upon glutamatergic neurones) appears to be less affected, which encourages hope for therapeutic intervention. Postsynaptic muscarinic M1 receptors (Perry et al., 1990) are relatively preserved, although there may be a degree of functional uncoupling. The enzyme responsible for the breakdown of ACh, acetylcholinesterase, is reduced, perhaps in part due to a loss of cholinergic terminals, while butyrylcholinesterase activity (the function of which is not yet fully understood and which is present in extrasynaptic areas and plaques) increases.

29.1.1 Acetylcholine and cognition

A prediction of the cholinergic hypothesis is that drugs likely to potentiate this function should improve cognition in AD patients. There are a number of treatment approaches to the amelioration of the cholinergic deficit; however, the use of acetylcholinesterase inhibitors (AChEIs) is the most well-developed approach (Francis et al., 1999).

During the late 1980s and early 1990s, the first cholinomimetic compound, tacrine, underwent large-scale clinical studies and established the benefits of ChEI treatment in patients with a diagnosis of probable AD. A so-called second generation of ChEIs has been developed including donepezil, rivastigmine, metrifonate and galantamine (Francis et al., 1999). Such compounds demonstrate a clinical effect and

magnitude of benefit of at least that reported for tacrine, but with a more favourable clinical profile. Evidence has emerged from clinical trials of cholinomimetics that such drugs may improve the abnormal non-cognitive, behavioural symptoms of AD. Physostigmine, tacrine, rivastigmine and metrifonate have variously been reported in placebo-controlled trials to decrease psychotic symptoms (hallucinations and delusions), agitation, apathy, anxiety, disinhibition, pacing, aberrant motor behaviour and lack of cooperation (Cummings and Kaufer, 1996). In a recent study, muscarinic M2 receptor density was increased in the frontal cortex of AD patients with delusions and in the temporal cortex of those with hallucinations, compared with patients without psychotic symptoms. This suggests a role for M2 receptors in the psychosis of AD and may provide a rationale for treatment of behaviourally disturbed AD patients with M2 antagonists (Lai et al., 2001).

Possibly related to these findings in AD, a dementia with Lewy bodies (DLB) open label trial of rivastigmine showed almost all patients responded positively on one or more of these measures (McKeith et al., 2000). Visual hallucinations are more common in DLB, which, in turn, is associated with greater reductions in ChAT activity than observed in AD (Perry et al., 1994).

29.1.2 The cholinergic system and AD pathology

Many preclinical studies indicate that activation of cholinergic receptors influence the metabolism of one of the two key proteins involved in AD, amyloid precursor protein (APP), diverting metabolism away from the formation of amyloid (Aβ) (Nitsch, 1996; Francis et al., 1999). In support of this hypothesis two recent clinical studies showed that muscarinic M1 agonists were able to reduce cerebrospinal fluid (CSF) concentrations of Aβ (Hock et al., 2000; Nitsch et al., 2000). Furthermore, nicotinic receptor stimulation is associated with reduced plaque densities in the human brain (Court et al., 1998). These results suggest that compounds being developed for symptomatic treatment may have a serendipitous effect on the continuing emergence of pathology by reducing the production of Aβ. There is also evidence for a possible beneficial role of cholinergic neurotransmission by modulation in the generation of neurofibrillary tangles via reduced phosphorylation of tau protein. One of the primary intracellular enzymes responsible, glycogen synthase kinase-3 (GSK3) can be regulated by muscarinic activation (Sadot et al., 1996). Cholinergic neurotransmission may also be a specific target for Aβ, since it has been shown to reduce both choline uptake and ACh release in vitro (Auld et al., 1998). Furthermore, Aβ is reported to bind with high affinity to the $\alpha 7$ subtype of the nicotinic receptor, suggesting that cholinergic function through this receptor may be compromised because of high levels of (soluble) peptide in AD brains (Wang et al., 2000).

29.2 GLUTAMATE

Glutamate is the principal excitatory neurotransmitter of the brain, being used at approximately two-thirds of synapses. The majority of neurones and glia have receptors for glutamate. An integral part of protein, energy and ammonia metabolism of all cells with a high intracellular concentration, it has been difficult to distinguish the presynaptic transmitter pool of glutamate from the metabolic pool (Francis *et al.*, 1993). Considered to be the main neurotransmitter of neocortical and hippocampal pyramidal neurones, glutamate is thus involved in higher mental functions such as cognition and memory (Francis *et al.*, 1993). An important mechanism by which glutamate may contribute to learning and memory functions is via long-term potentiation (LTP) at pyramidal neurone synapses. LTP is a form of synaptic strengthening following brief, high frequency, stimulation.

Histological studies in AD indicate loss of pyramidal neurones and their synapses together with surrounding neuropil (Esiri, 1991). Corticortical and corticofugal-projecting pyramidal neurones are lost, together with those of the entorhinal and hippocampal CA1 region. Remaining neurones are subject to neurofibrillary tangle formation. Uptake of D-aspartate, a putative marker of glutamatergic nerve endings, is reduced in many cortical areas in the AD brain (Procter *et al.*, 1988).

Biochemical evidence suggests a presynaptic 'double blow' as the activity of glutamatergic neurones is heavily influenced by the cholinergic system, also dysfunctional in AD. The clinical relevance of these changes is emphasized because both glutamatergic and cholinergic dysfunction are strong correlates of cognitive decline in AD. Glutamatergic (and cholinergic) cells die over a period of years and in a very specific regional and neurochemically selective pattern (Francis *et al.*, 1993). The selectivity is intriguing, because cholinergic neurones of the basal forebrain die while those of the pons are spared; glutamatergic neurones of the frontal, temporal and parietal cortex are lost while apparently similar neurones in the motor and sensory cortex are unaffected. Factors that may lead to necrosis or apoptosis in selected groups of neurones in AD may include tangles, Aβ toxicity, microglia, free radical generation, excitotoxicity (too much or too little glutamatergic neurotransmission) and withdrawal of trophic factors. The strongest evidence suggests that most of glutamatergic pyramidal neurones die as a consequence of the presence of neurofibrillary tangles within the cytoplasm (Kowall and Beal, 1991). However, this may only account for up to 50 per cent of such cells.

Glutamate is synthesized in nerve terminals by one of several possible enzymes. First, glutamine can be converted to glutamate by the action of the mitochondrial enzyme glutaminase (Procter *et al.*, 1988); alternatively glutamate can be produced by transamination from aspartate in the cytosol. Direct measurement of glutaminase activity is unaffected in AD (Procter *et al.*, 1988). By contrast glutaminase-positive neurones are reduced in number and subject to tangle formation

(Kowall and Beal, 1991). Several groups have shown reductions in the concentration of glutamate in AD tissue and lumbar CSF (Lowe *et al.*, 1990). Although glutamate neurotransmission failure was not extensive in these studies, glutamate concentration was reduced by 14 per cent in temporal lobe biopsy samples and by 86 per cent in the terminal zone of the perforant pathway at autopsy of AD patients (Hyman *et al.*, 1987).

We have recently begun to investigate the status of the newly discovered vesicular glutamate transporters (VGLUT), VGLUT1 and VGLUT2 (Bellocchio *et al.*, 2000). These proteins are only present in the glutamatergic neurone terminals and therefore represent a useful marker of their number. Preliminary western blotting studies indicate that there is a reduction in VGLUT1 (but not VGLUT2) in the parietal cortex in AD but not in the temporal cortex (Kirvell *et al.*, 2002). However, in a different study vesicular glutamate uptake rate was lower in the temporal cortex from AD patients (Westphalen *et al.*, 2003). This lack of change in protein, but with a reduction in the protein's related activity, suggests a functional downregulation of the protein in both cases. The exact consequences of such changes remain to be determined.

Upon release into the synapse, approximately 95 per cent of glutamate is removed by glutamate transporter proteins named GLT, GLAST and EAAC. These are mainly present upon glial cells. Studies of D-aspartate binding to transporter sites in both fresh and frozen postmortem tissue reveal significant reductions in many cortical areas. However, the relevance of this measure to glutamate uptake is doubtful. Antibodies directed against the individual glutamate transporters produce conflicting data. Reduced levels of GLT protein (but not its mRNA), with normal levels of both GLAST and EAAC have been reported, not confirmed by our own studies (unpublished). Even assuming there was no reduction of transporter protein, there is considerable evidence for oxidative damage of proteins such as these glutamate transporters. This might explain the functional deficit in glutamate uptake hypothesized above (Danbolt, 2001).

Postsynaptic glutamate receptors fall into two main classes, ionotropic and metabotropic. The ionotropic subtypes, *N*-methyl-D-aspartate (NMDA) and α-amino-3-hydroxy-5-methyl-4-isoxazolepropionic acid (AMPA)/kainate subtypes have varying permeability to Na^+ and Ca^{2+} ions. The metabotropic subtypes couple to adenylyl cyclase, phospholipase C or ion channels. The ionotrophic subtypes are of particular interest given the proposed mechanism of action of the novel compound memantine on the NMDA receptor (see below). Studies have demonstrated reductions in the NMDA receptor complex in the hippocampus and neocortex.

29.2.1 Glutamate and cognition

A role for glutamate and glutamate receptors in learning and memory is widely recognized. For example NMDA antagonists impair learning and memory, while NMDA agonists and facilitators improve memory (Francis *et al.*, 1993). Likewise AMPAkines (positive modulators of AMPA receptor function) facilitate learning and memory (Lynch, 1998). Circumstantial evidence of the involvement of glutamatergic pathways includes the well-established role of structures such as the hippocampus in learning and memory. More specifically, lesions of certain glutamatergic pathways impair learning and memory. In addition, glutamate and glutamate receptors are involved in mechanisms of synaptic plasticity (LTP and long-term depression [LTD] of the synapse) which are considered to underlie learning and memory. Loss of synapses and pyramidal cell perikarya from the neocortex of AD patients correlate with measures of cognitive decline. The latter is considered to be the best evidence for a functional role of glutamatergic involvement in cognitive dysfunction in AD (Francis *et al.*, 1993).

29.2.2 The glutamatergic system and AD pathology

Excitotoxic cell death involves excess activation of receptors, leading to raised intracellular Ca^{2+} and consequent activation of a cascade of enzymes, resulting in cell death by necrosis or apoptosis (Lipton, 1999). During the 1980s it was also suggested that endogenous glutamate could accumulate and become excitotoxic, perhaps as a result of impaired clearance (as a consequence of disrupted transporter function or indirectly in conditions of reduced energy availability). There is some evidence that energy levels may be reduced in AD due to perturbed mitochondrial function (Francis *et al.*, 1993) and considerable evidence for oxidative damage of proteins including the glutamate transporter (Keller *et al.*, 1997). Others have cautioned that there is no simple relationship between raised extracellular glutamate concentrations and cell death *in vivo*. It remains possible that changes in numbers of glutamate receptors or changes in ion selectivity may lead over time to cell death. For instance the large numbers of calcium-permeable AMPA receptors present on basal forebrain cholinergic neurones may be linked to their loss in AD (Ikonomovic and Armstrong, 1996).

A further possible contribution to cell death is linked to reduced glutamatergic neurotransmission. Activation of receptors linked to phospholipase C (such as some metabotropic glutamate receptors) has been shown to increase the secretion of neuroprotective forms of APP and decrease Aβ while at the same time reducing the phosphorylation state of tau. If glutamate neurotransmission is reduced as a consequence of tangle formation, one may hypothesise that Aβ production may increase and tau become more hyperphosphorylated in neurones innervated by the affected neurone (Francis *et al.*, 1999).

29.3 INTERACTIONS BETWEEN CHOLINERGIC AND GLUTAMATERGIC SYSTEMS

It is important to remember that glutamatergic neurones of the neocortex and hippocampus are influenced by ACh through nicotinic and muscarinic receptors (Chessell and Humphrey, 1995; Dijk *et al.*, 1995). Terminals of cholinergic neurones are found in all layers of the neocortex, synapsing with pyramidal neurones in layers II/III and V (Turrini *et al.*, 2001). Both muscarinic and nicotinic receptors activate pyramidal neurones and hence facilitate glutamate release in a rat model (Chessell and Humphrey, 1995; Dijk *et al.*, 1995). It therefore follows that treatment of patients with cholinomimetics is likely to increase glutamatergic function.

29.4 TREATMENT STRATEGIES BASED ON GLUTAMATERGIC NEUROTRANSMISSION

Cholinergic stimulation is one pathway to enhancement of glutamatergic function. Other treatment strategies that more directly increase the activity of remaining glutamatergic neurones, without causing excitotoxicity, represent an important target for the symptomatic treatment of AD, and may have a disease-modifying effect. Several approaches have been tried including positive modulation of both AMPA and NMDA receptors. AMPAkines, which are considered to work by increasing the sensitivity of these receptors, are currently in clinical trial for MCI (Johnson and Simmon, 2002). Modulation of the NMDA receptor has been attempted via the glycine co-agonist site with clear indication in preclinical studies that the partial agonist d-cycloserine improved learning and memory (Myhrer and Paulsen, 1997). Clinical studies have suggested some benefit but full-scale trials have not been initiated (Schwartz *et al.*, 1996). There is currently no evidence that these drugs enhance excitotoxicity.

Perhaps the most surprising development is the success of the uncompetitive NMDA antagonist, memantine, in clinical trials in moderate and severe AD (Reisberg *et al.*, 2003). At first sight one would consider that such an approach – blockade of a receptor that would normally be activated in learning and memory – to be counterintuitive. However, there is evidence that this molecule acts like magnesium ions, able to prevent background activation of the NMDA receptor ('noise'), whilst allowing activation of this receptor for LTP formation (Francis, 2003). There is also a report of a clinical trial by Forest Laboratories Inc. (Tariot *et al.*, 2004) that shows a benefit of the addition of memantine to established treatment with a ChEI in AD patients. Since ChEIs are likely to act in part by increasing glutamate release ('signal') (Dijk *et al.*, 1995; Francis *et al.*, 1999), the benefit may be hypothesized to come from the combination of a reduction in glutamate 'noise' (by memantine) and an increase in discrete glutamate signals (donepezil) (Francis, 2003).

29.5 CONCLUSION

The changes in cholinergic neurotransmission seen in the brains of patients dying with AD provided the rationale for the development of compounds aimed at symptom relief.

Treatment of AD patients with ChEIs has confirmed the relevance of this finding. However, it has long been recognized that the major changes in AD are likely to involve the more abundant cortical glutamatergic pyramidal neurones. Hence the need for this to be addressed. Since increasing cholinergic function will also increase glutamatergic activity, there may be synergistic benefit from co-administration of drugs that target both the cholinergic system (ChEIs) and glutamatergic systems (e.g. memantine). As disease-modifying treatments become available it is likely that symptomatic therapy will continue to be required, and indeed there is evidence that such treatments may also slow disease progression.

REFERENCES

Auld DS, Kar, S, Quirion R. (1998) Beta-amyloid peptides as direct cholinergic neuromodulators: a missing link? *Trends in Neuroscience* **21**: 43–49

Beach TG, Kuo YM, Spiegel K *et al.* (2000) The cholinergic deficit coincides with A beta deposition at the earliest histopathologic stages of Alzheimer disease. *Journal of Neuropathology and Experimental Neurology* **59**: 308–313

Bellocchio EE, Reimer RJ, Fremeau RT Jr, Edwards RH. (2000) Uptake of glutamate into synaptic vesicles by an inorganic phosphate transporter. *Science* **289**: 957–960

Bowen DM, Smith CB, White P, Davison AN. (1976) Neurotransmitter-related enzymes and indices of hypoxia in senile dementia and other abiotrophies. *Brain* **99**: 459–496

Chessell IP and Humphrey PPA. (1995) Nicotinic and muscarinic receptor-evoked depolarizations recorded from a novel cortical brain slice preparation. *Neuropharmacology* **34**: 1289–1296

Court J, Martin-Ruiz C, Piggott M *et al.* (2001) Nicotinic receptor abnormalities in Alzheimer's disease. *Biological Psychiatry* **49**: 175–184

Court JA, Lloyd S, Thomas N *et al.* (1998) Dopamine and nicotinic receptor binding and the levels of dopamine and homovanillic acid in human brain related to tobacco use. *Neuroscience* **87**: 63–78

Cummings JL and Kaufer DI. (1996) Neuropsychiatric aspects of Alzheimer's disease: the cholinergic hypothesis revisited. *Neurology* **47**: 876–883

Danbolt NC. (2001) Glutamate uptake. *Progress in Neurobiology* **65**: 1–105

Davis KL, Mohs RC, Marin D *et al.* (1999) Cholinergic markers in elderly patients with early signs of Alzheimer disease. *JAMA* **281**: 1401–1406

DeKosky ST, Ikonomovic MD, Styren SD *et al.* (2002) Upregulation of choline acetyltransferase activity in hippocampus and frontal cortex of elderly subjects with mild cognitive impairment. *Annals of Neurology* **51**: 145–155

Dijk SN, Francis PT, Stratmann GC, Bowen DM. (1995) Cholinomimetics increase glutamate outflow by an action on the corticostriatal pathway: Implications for Alzheimer's disease. *Journal of Neurochemistry* **65**: 2165–2169

Drachman DA and Leavitt J. (1974) Human memory and the cholinergic system. *Archives of Neurology* **30**: 113–121

Esiri M. (1991) Neuropathology. In: R Jacoby and C Oppenheimer (eds), *Psychiatry in the Elderly*, Oxford, Oxford University Press, pp. 113–147

Francis PT. (2003) Glutamatergic systems in Alzheimer's disease. *International Journal of Geriatric Psychiatry* 18 (Suppl. 1): S15–S21

Francis PT, Palmer AM, Sims NR *et al.* (1985) Neurochemical studies of early-onset Alzheimer's disease. Possible influence on treatment. *New England Journal of Medicine* **313**: 7–11

Francis PT, Sims NR, Procter AW, Bowen DM. (1993) Cortical pyramidal neurone loss may cause glutamatergic hypoactivity and cognitive impairment in Alzheimer's disease: investigative and therapeutic perspectives. *Journal of Neurochemistry* **60**: 1589–1604

Francis PT, Palmer AM, Snape M, Wilcock GK. (1999) The cholinergic hypothesis of Alzheimer's disease: a review of progress, *Journal of Neurology Neurosurgery and Psychiatry* **66**: 137–147

Geldmacher DS, Provenzano G, McRae T, Mastey V, Ieni JR. (2003) Donepezil is associated with delayed nursing home placement in patients with Alzheimer's disease. *Journal of the American Geriatrics Society* **51**: 937–944

Hock C, Maddalena A, Heuser I *et al.* (2000) Treatment with the selective muscarinic agonist talsaclidine decreases cerebrospinal fluid levels of total amyloid beta-peptide in patients with Alzheimer's disease. *Annals of the New York Academy of Sciences* **920**: 285–291

Hyman BT, Van Hoesen GW, Damasio AR. (1987) Alzheimer's disease: glutamate depletion in the hippocampal perforant pathway zone. *Annals of Neurology* **22**: 37–40

Ikonomovic MD and Armstrong DM. (1996) Distribution of AMPA receptor subunits in the nucleus basalis of Meynert in aged humans: implications for selective neuronal degeneration. *Brain Research* **716**: 229–232

Johnson SA and Simmon VF. (2002) Randomized, double-blind, placebo-controlled international clinical trial of the Ampakine CX516 in elderly participants with mild cognitive impairment: a progress report. *Journal of Molecular Neuroscience* **19**: 197–200

Keller JN, Mark RJ, Bruce AJ *et al.* (1997) 4-hydroxynonenal, an aldehydic product of membrane lipid peroxidation, impairs glutamate transport and mitochondrial function in synaptosomes. *Neuroscience* **80**: 685–696

Kirvell SL, Fremeau RT Jr, Francis PT. (2002) *Vesicular glutamate transporter 1 in Alzheimer's disease.* Society of Neuroscience Abstracts Viewer/planner. Program No. 785.15. Washington, DC

Kowall NW and Beal MF. (1991) Glutamate-, glutaminase-, and taurine-immunoreactive neurones develop neurofibrillary tangles in Alzheimer's disease. *Annals of Neurology* **29**: 162–167

Lai MK, Lai OF, Keene J *et al.* (2001) Psychosis of Alzheimer's disease is associated with elevated muscarinic M2 binding in the cortex. *Neurology* **57**: 805–811

Lipton P. (1999) Ischemic cell death in brain neurons. *Physiological Reviews* **79**: 1431–1568

Lopez OL, Becker JT, Wisniewski S, Saxton J, Kaufer DI, DeKosky ST. (2002) Cholinesterase inhibitor treatment alters the natural history of Alzheimer's disease, *Journal of Neurology, Neurosurgery, and Psychiatry* **72**: 310–114

Lowe SL, Bowen DM, Francis PT, Neary D. (1990) Ante mortem cerebral amino acid concentrations indicate selective degeneration of glutamate-enriched neurons in Alzheimer's disease. *Neuroscience* **38**: 571–577

Lynch G. (1998) Memory and the brain: unexpected chemistries and a new pharmacology. *Neurobiology of Learning and Memory* **70**: 82–100

McKeith IG, Grace JB, Walker Z *et al.* (2000) Rivastigmine in the treatment of dementia with Lewy bodies: preliminary findings from an open trial. *International Journal of Geriatric Psychiatry* **15**: 387–392

Minger SL, Esiri MM, McDonald B *et al.* (2000) Cholinergic deficits contribute to behavioural disturbance in patients with dementia. *Neurology* 55: 1460–1467

Myhrer T and Paulsen RE. (1997) Infusion of D-cycloserine into temporal-hippocampal areas and restoration of mnemonic function in rats with disrupted glutamatergic temporal systems. *European Journal of Pharmacology* **328**: 1–7

Nitsch RM. (1996) From acetylcholine to amyloid: neurotransmitters and the pathology of Alzheimer's disease. *Neurodegeneration* **5**: 477–482

Nitsch RM, Deng M, Tennis M, Schoenfeld D, Growdon JH. (2000) The selective muscarinic M1 agonist AF102B decreases levels of total Abeta in cerebrospinal fluid of patients with Alzheimer's disease. *Annals of Neurology* **48**: 913–918

Perry RH, Candy JM, Perry EK *et al.* (1982) Extensive loss of choline acetyltransferase activity is not reflected by neuronal loss in the nucleus of Meynert in Alzheimer's disease. *Neuroscience Letters* **33**: 311–315

Perry EK, Smith CJ, Court JA, Perry RH. (1990) Cholinergic nicotinic and muscarinic receptors in dementia of Alzheimer, Parkinson and Lewy body types. *Journal of Neural Transmission-Parkinson's disease and Dementia Section* **2**: 149–158

Perry EK, Haroutunian V, Davis KL *et al.* (1994) Neocortical cholinergic activities differentiate Lewy body dementia from classical Alzheimer's disease. *NeuroReport* **5**: 747–749

Perry EK, Walker M, Grace J, Perry RH. (1999) Acetylcholine in mind: a neurotransmitter correlate of consciousness? *Trends in Neuroscience* **22**: 273–280

Postle BR, Corkin S, Growdon JH. (1996) Intact implicit memory for novel patterns in Alzheimer's disease. *Learning and Memory* **3**: 305–312

Procter AW, Palmer AM, Francis PT *et al.* (1988) Evidence of glutamatergic denervation and possible abnormal metabolism in Alzheimer's disease. *Journal of Neurochemistry* **50**: 790–802

Reisberg B, Doody R, Stoffler A, Schmitt F, Ferris S, Mobius HJ. (2003) Memantine in moderate-to-severe Alzheimer's disease. *New England Journal of Medicine* **348**: 1333–1341

Sadot E, Gurwitz D, Barg J, Behar L, Ginzburg I, Fisher A. (1996) Activation of m$_1$ muscarinic acetylcholine receptor regulates τ phosphorylation in transfected PC12 cells. *Journal of Neurochemistry* **66**: 877–880

Schwartz BL, Hashtroudi S, Herting RL, Schwartz P, Deutsch SI. (1996) D-cycloserine enhances implicit memory in Alzheimer patients. *Neurology* **46**: 420–424

Tariot PN, Farlow MR, Grossberg G, Graham SM, McDonald S, Gergel I; Memantine Study Group (2004) Memantine treatment in patients with moderate to severe Alzheimer's disease already receiving donepezil: a randomized controlled trial. *JAMA* **291**: 317–324

Turrini P, Casu MA, Wong TP, De Koninck Y, Ribeiro-da-Silva A, Cuello AC. (2001) Cholinergic nerve terminals establish classical synapses in the rat cerebral cortex: synaptic pattern and age-related atrophy. *Neuroscience* **105**: 277–285

Wang HY, Lee DHS, Dandrea MR, Peterson PA, Shank RP, Reitz AB. (2000) Beta-amyloid(1–42) binds to alpha 7 nicotinic acetylcholine receptor with high affinity – implications for Alzheimer's disease pathology. *Journal of Biological Chemistry* **275**: 5626–5632

Westphalen RI, Scott HL, Dodd PR. (2003) Synaptic vesicle transport and synaptic membrane transporter sites in excitatory amino acid nerve terminals in Alzheimer Disease. *Journal of Neural Transmission* **110**: 1013–1027

Neuropathology of Alzheimer's disease

COLIN L MASTERS

Although Alzheimer (1907) highlighted the two key histological lesions, neurofibrillary tangles (NFT) and amyloid plaques 100 years ago, recent developments in molecular biology, molecular genetics, immunohistochemistry, image analysis and protein chemistry have transformed our understanding of the pathogenesis of Alzheimer's disease (AD). For practising neuropathologists, immunohistochemistry in particular has become an essential part of the diagnostic armoury to complement the neurohistology of the common neurodegenerative conditions.

30.1 PATHOLOGY OUTSIDE THE CENTRAL NERVOUS SYSTEM

General post-mortem examination does not reveal any abnormalities outside the nervous system. Patients with AD die from terminal respiratory illness, and bronchopneumonia is most often the cause of death. Ongoing investigations have, however, revealed that subtle biochemical abnormalities may not be restricted to the brain. AD may, like a systemic illness, cause secondary changes in the cerebrospinal fluid (CSF) and peripheral blood, which reflect neuronal metabolism of the Aβ amyloid and tau proteins. As the disease progresses, the metabolic pools of Aβ and tau increase within the CSF and blood. Towards the end stages of illness, the Aβ levels may decrease as the brain acts as a metabolic 'sink' (Ritchie et al., 2003).

That sensory outposts associated with the brain undergo degeneration has been known for some time. The optic nerve

(Hinton et al., 1986) and retinal ganglion cells (Blanks et al., 1989) show degenerative changes and the anterior olfactory nucleus develops NFTs (Esiri and Wilcock, 1984). In addition, abnormalities in the processes of olfactory neurones in the nasal mucosa have been reported (Talamo et al., 1989) and tau-reactive filaments, absent from controls, have been described in the olfactory mucosa in biopsy specimens of patients with probable AD (Tabaton et al., 1991a). Deposition of Aβ in the periphery of the lens may also be linked to AD, although more studies are required to confirm this association (Goldstein et al., 2003).

30.2 MACROSCOPIC PATHOLOGY

The naked eye appearances of the brain range from unremarkable to grossly abnormal. The leptomeninges may be thickened, particularly over the convexity, and may show orange-brown areas of various sizes, indicating old, circumscribed subarachnoid haemorrhage, which most often results from amyloid (congophilic) angiopathy. The cranial nerves are normal and the large cerebral vessels in uncomplicated cases of AD have not been damaged more by atherosclerosis than expected from the patient's age. Brain weight is quite often reduced, sometimes below 1000 g. Since brain weight normally depends on the patient's age, sex and constitution, the degree of atrophy should be considered in the light of these factors. More appropriately, the severity of cerebral atrophy can be assessed by comparing the volume of the brain with the capacity of the intracranial space (Davis and Wright,

1977). A discrepancy between the findings of neuroimaging and neuropathology is not unusual: cerebral atrophy reported on computed tomography (CT) or magnetic resonance imaging (MRI) scans may not always be confirmed at post-mortem examination. Agonal changes of haemodynamics, post-mortem delay, and the effects of fixation on the brain may be responsible for this discrepancy. The normal ratio of 8:1 of total brain weight to that of the brain stem and cerebellum may decrease, indicating loss of tissue from the cerebral hemispheres. The atrophy is usually diffuse and symmetrical, although the frontoparietal region and the temporal lobes may be more severely affected than the rest of the brain (Figure 30.1). Moderate-to-severe atrophy is easy to discern: the sulci are widened and the gyri narrowed both on the outside and on coronal slices. The latter also reveal enlarged lateral ventricles with rounded angles and additional space between the hippocampi and the wall of the temporal horns. Decrease in the thickness of neocortical ribbon, apart from extreme cases of atrophy, is difficult, and may prove deceptive, to assess on naked-eye appearances. A quantitative study, however, revealed a decrease of neocortical areas of all lobes in AD, whereas in patients over the age of 80 only the temporal cortex was atrophied (Hubbard and Anderson, 1981, 1985). Reduction in cortical area may result from a decrease in the length rather than in the width of cortex, indicating loss of columns of cells and fibres perpendicular to the pial surface. A correlation appears to exist between the length, but not the thickness, of the cortical ribbon and dementia score (Duyckaerts et al., 1985). Apart from occasional small, orange-coloured old haemorrhages in the cortex, suggestive of amyloid angiopathy, uncomplicated AD usually is not associated with any other focal lesions.

30.3 HISTOLOGY, ULTRASTRUCTURE, IMMUNOCYTOCHEMISTRY AND MORPHOMETRY

The neurohistological features of AD are complex and variable. The two hallmark lesions, amyloid plaques and NFTs (Figure 30.2), are complemented by granulovacuolar degeneration, Hirano bodies, neuronal loss, abnormalities of neuronal processes and synapses, astrocytic and microglial response, and vascular changes. The white matter also may be affected (Esiri et al., 1997).

30.3.1 Amyloid plaques

The amyloid or neuritic plaque (also referred to as a 'senile' plaque) is one of the major lesions found in the AD brain, and these plaques were first described by Blocq and Marinesco in 1892. These structures, ranging in size from 50 to 200 μm (Terry, 1985), can be readily demonstrated in frozen and paraffin-embedded sections by silver impregnation methods (Figure 30.3). The lesion consists of an Aβ amyloid core with a corona of argyrophilic axonal and dendritic processes, Aβ amyloid fibrils, glial cell processes and microglial cells. Neuritic processes in the periphery of the plaque are frequently dystrophic and contain paired helical filaments, which are composed largely of ubiquinated and phosphorylated tau protein (Gonatas et al., 1967; Hanger et al., 1991). In 1927, Divry demonstrated that the core of the AD plaque contained a congophilic amyloid substance, which gave an apple green colour under polarized light. The plaque amyloid is composed of 5–10 nm filaments made up of a 40–43 amino acid (4 kDa) protein (Masters et al., 1985), and now referred to as Aβ protein.

Three types of plaque have been identified in conventional silver staining preparations: 'primitive' or 'early', 'classical' or 'mature', and 'burnt-out' or 'compact'. On the basis of light and electron microscopic studies, a three-stage evolution of the plaque has been proposed. The first stage is the

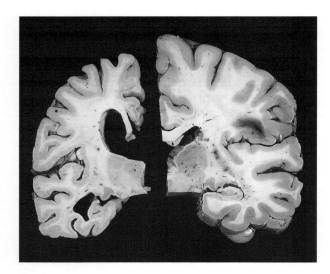

Figure 30.1 On the left, a coronal slice of the brain of a patient with severe Alzheimer's disease showing atrophy: the lateral ventricle is enlarged with rounding of its angle and there is additional space between the hippocampus and the inferior horn of the lateral ventricle. Several gyri are narrowed and the lateral fissure is widened. On the right, a slice of the right hemi-brain of a normal subject.

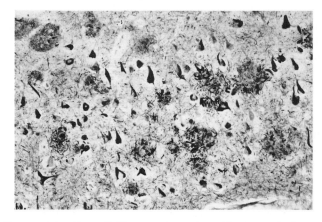

Figure 30.2 Neurofibrillary tangles and neuritic plaques in the neocortex. Modified Bielschowsky silver impregnation.

'primitive' plaque, composed of a small number of distorted neurites, largely presynaptic in origin with few amyloid fibres, astrocytic processes and the occasional microglial cell. The second stage is the 'classical' or 'mature' plaque with a dense amyloid core with a halo of dystrophic neurites, astrocytic processes and cell bodies and the occasional microglial cell. The final stage in this sequence is the 'burnt-out' plaque consisting of a dense core of amyloid (Terry *et al.*, 1981; Esiri and Morris, 1997). The relationship between dystrophic neurites, neurofibrillary degeneration and Aβ amyloid deposition is not fully understood, but the neurites and tangles appear to be downstream of Aβ accumulation. These three stages of plaque development have not been confirmed in experimental transgenic mice and therefore the temporal relationships suggested above remain speculative: it may yet transpire that the three types of plaques are independent of each other.

Studies using antibodies raised against Aβ protein have revealed the presence of a much more widespread deposition of amyloid than is visualized by traditional staining methods (Majocha *et al.*, 1988; Gentleman *et al.*, 1989; Armstrong *et al.*, 1996; Figures 30.4–30.8). Aβ immunoreactivity has been detected throughout the central nervous system including the neocortex, hippocampus, thalamus, amygdala, caudate nucleus, putamen, nucleus basalis of Meynert, mid-brain, pons, medulla oblongata, the cerebellar cortex and spinal cord (Joachim *et al.*, 1989; Ogomori *et al.*, 1989). These deposits take a variety of forms and include subpial, vascular, dysphoric, punctate or granular, diffuse, stellar, ring-with-core, and compact deposits (Ogomori *et al.*, 1989). A laminar pattern of Aβ deposits in the neocortex has been

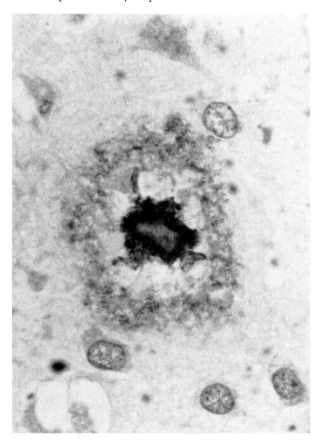

Figure 30.4 *An amyloid plaque with a dense core and corona. Aβ-amyloid immunohistochemistry.*

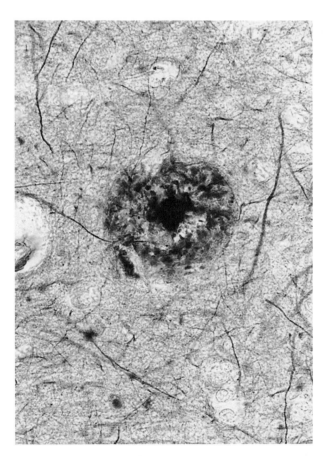

Figure 30.3 *An argyrophilic amyloid plaque in the neocortex showing a neuritic ring with an amyloid core formation. Modified Bielschowsky silver impregnation.*

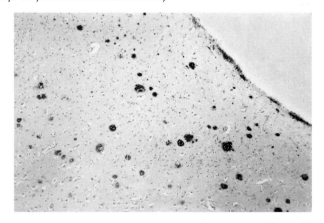

Figure 30.5 *Aβ-amyloid protein deposits in the temporal lobe of a patient with Alzheimer's disease. Several deposit morphologies can be seen. Aβ-amyloid immunohistochemistry.*

described with concentrations in layers II, III and V (Majocha *et al.*, 1988).

Aβ protein is a 38–43 residue polypeptide cleavage product of a larger precursor protein, the amyloid precursor protein (APP) (Kang *et al.*, 1987). Although most cells have the potential for producing APP, neurones and platelets express APP to high levels. Moreover, neurones process the APP with β-secretase (BACE) to a greater extent than most other cell types, and this in turn leads to the formation of full Aβ sequences. The hypothesis that Aβ deposition is an early event in the pathogenesis of AD has been given support by the presence of extracellular Aβ in diffuse plaques not associated with any neuritic change, or astrocytic involvement

(Yamaguchi *et al.*, 1991). More condensed Aβ is, however, associated with a neuritic change, reactive astrocytosis and microglial infiltration and phagocytosis. Most species of Aβ have been detected by immunohistochemistry using antibodies that recognize epitopes within the full length $A\beta_{1-42}$ or a truncated $A\beta_{1-40}$. The predominant species in sporadic AD is $A\beta_{42(43)}$ and this is found in plaques of all morphological types. Diffuse plaques contain mainly $A\beta_{42(43)}$ (Mann *et al.*, 1996a, b).

A number of other proteins co-localize with Aβ including apolipoprotein E (ApoE), a widely distributed protein involved in the transport of cholesterol. There are three common isoforms of ApoE which are encoded by three alleles, ε2, ε3

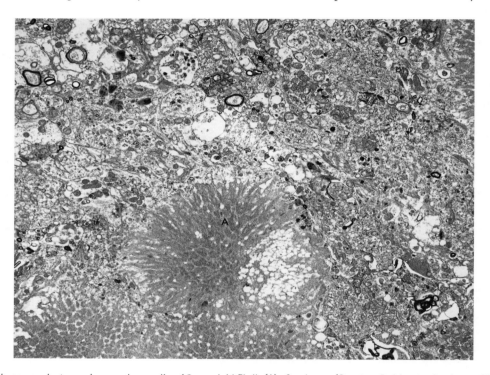

Figure 30.6 *A high-power electron micrograph revealing Aβ-amyloid fibrils (A) of a plaque. (Courtesy Dr I Janota, Institute of Psychiatry, London.)*

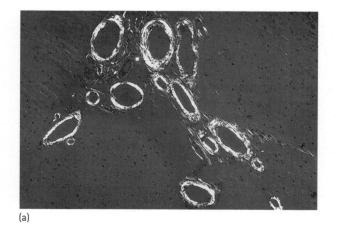

(a)

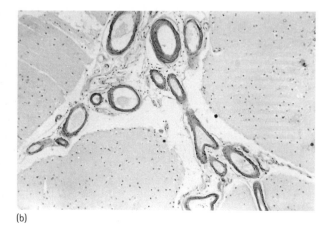

(b)

Figure 30.7 *Congophilic angiopathy. Blood vessels stained with Congo red showing birefringence under polarized light (a) and Aβ-amyloid immunohistochemistry (b).*

and ε4, and there is a strong association between the presence of the ε4 allele and the age of onset of AD. ApoE has been shown to bind to Aβ and a high proportion of Aβ and ApoE deposits tend to be co-localized. Thus, both diffuse and compact Aβ plaques may be immunolabelled by anti-Aβ and anti-ApoE antibodies (Cairns *et al.*, 1997b; Armstrong *et al.*, 1998). The presence of one or more ε4 alleles leads to both an earlier onset and a more severe Aβ amyloidosis (Roses, 1994). The relationship between Aβ and ApoE is still imperfectly understood, as ApoE knock-out mice have an increased amount of Aβ deposition on a transgenic APP background.

The plaques are also immunohistochemically positive for a number of neuroactive substances. Acetylcholinesterase, a marker of the cholinergic system, can be demonstrated within and around the neuritic elements of the corona. Many of these elements derive from cholinergic neurones in the basal forebrain, particularly the nucleus basalis of Meynert (nbM), the diagonal band of Broca and the medial septal nuclei. Several other neurotransmitters have been demonstrated in the plaque. These include substance P, neuropeptide Y, neurotensin, cholecystokinin, 5-hydroxytryptamine (5HT) and catecholamine (Walker *et al.*, 1988; Hauw *et al.*, 1991). Ubiquitin, a protein acting as a signal for degradation of abnormal proteins, is also present in intracellular neurites and NFTs (Perry *et al.*, 1987). The protease inhibitor α1-antichymotrypsin has been localized to the plaque using immunohistochemical methods (Walker *et al.*, 1988). Serum amyloid P (SAP) component is a glycoprotein complex produced in the liver, distributed in serum, and has been detected in diffuse and consolidated Aβ deposits, NFTs and neuritic degeneration (Akiyama *et al.*, 1991).

The distribution of plaques varies widely not only within architectonic units but also from one individual to another. The plaques are more numerous in associative regions of neocortex than in sensory areas and are also largest in those laminae characterized by large pyramidal neurones (Rogers and Morrison, 1985). Accumulations of Aβ protein are found in the neocortex of non-demented elderly individuals without any neurofibrillary change, suggesting that Aβ deposition precedes neurofibrillary changes. However, NFT formation has been reported in areas devoid of Aβ (Braak *et al.*, 1986; Duyckaerts *et al.*, 1988; Delaère *et al.*, 1990; Armstrong *et al.*, 1993), indicating that factors in addition to Aβ may be required to cause aggregation of tau. Tangle-bearing neurones generally project into areas with Aβ deposition, suggesting some form of retrograde transport of the toxic elements which are associated with Aβ.

30.3.2 Neurofibrillary tangles

The second histological hallmark of AD is the NFT. These are not specific to AD, since they occur in other neurodegenerative disorders, including Down's syndrome, postencephalitic parkinsonism, dementia pugilistica, amyotrophic lateral sclerosis–parkinsonism–dementia complex of Guam, subacute sclerosing panencephalitis, dementia with tangles with and without calcification, and in myotonic dystrophy (Kiuchi *et al.*,

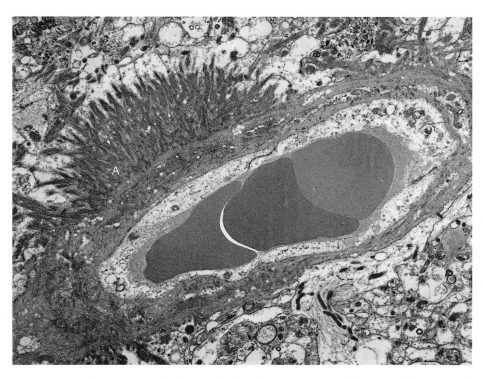

Figure 30.8   *A high-power electron micrograph showing Aβ-amyloid fibrils (A) surrounding a blood vessel: dyshoric angiopathy. (Courtesy Dr I Janota, Institute of Psychiatry, London.)*

1991). Globose NFTs also develop in progressive supranuclear palsy and sporadic motor neurone disease, but their morphology and ultrastructure differ from those seen in AD.

In AD, NFTs are common in the medial temporal structures, in the hippocampus, amygdala and parahippocampal gyrus, and they also occur throughout the neocortex and the deep grey matter including the lentiform nucleus, the nbM, the thalamus, the mamillary bodies, substantia nigra, locus caeruleus, periaqueductal grey matter, the raphé nuclei of the brain stem and the pedunculopontine nucleus.

NFTs are intracellular inclusions composed of ubiquinated and phosphorylated tau. Their configuration is determined in part by the shape of neurones in which they develop. NFTs are

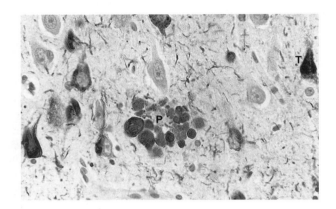

Figure 30.9   *A neuritic plaque (P) and neurofibrillary tangles (T) demonstrated by anti-tau immunohistochemistry.*

flame-shaped in pyramidal neurones, whilst in the neurones of the brain stem they assume more complex, globose forms. They can be easily discerned in histological sections stained with haematoxylin and eosin, but are best demonstrated by one of the silver impregnation techniques or with Congo red, which renders them birefringent under polarized light. They can be demonstrated by immunocytochemistry using antibodies against tau and ubiquitin (Figure 30.9).

Electron microscopy reveals the fine structural details (Figure 30.10). NFTs are mainly composed of paired helical filaments (Kidd, 1963), which in turn are formed by two filaments wound around each other. Each filament has a diameter of 10 nm with cross-over points every 80 nm, resulting in the typical periodicity of a double helix. A negative staining technique has demonstrated that each filament is composed of four protofilaments with a diameter of 3–5 nm (Wisniewski *et al.*, 1984). However, computer-assisted electron microscopy has modelled different substructures, indicating that paired helical filaments are not composed of fibrous protofilaments, as are normal neurofilaments, but are constructed from compact globular subunits, which are stacked to form the two filamentous structures of paired helical filaments (Crowther and Wischik, 1985). NFTs also contain straight filaments with an average diameter of 15 nm. These straight and the paired helical filaments may form hybrid filaments, displaying both morphologies, share surface epitopes and have identically shaped structural units. These common features indicate that paired helical and straight filaments are related and they represent only

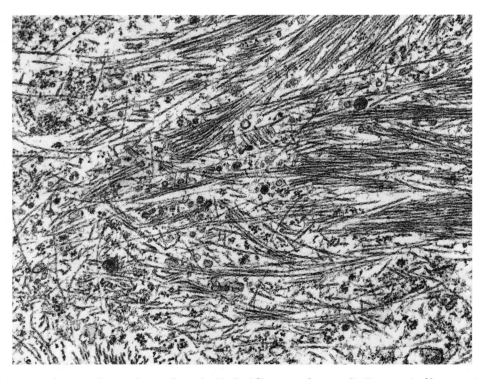

Figure 30.10   *A high-power electron micrograph revealing paired helical filaments of a neurofibrillary tangle. (Courtesy the late Professor LW Duchen, Institute of Psychiatry, London.)*

somewhat different assemblies of the same basic molecular unit (Crowther, 1991).

A major component of the NFT is a microtubule-associated protein called tau, which is involved in microtubule assembly and stabilization. In the adult human brain there are six isoforms of tau and all of these are hyperphosphorylated in AD (Hanger *et al.*, 1991; Goedert *et al.*, 1992). Antibodies that recognize specific phosphorylation-dependent epitopes may be used to identify the three sites of tau aggregation: the NFT, dystrophic neurites of plaques and neuropil threads. Phosphorylation-dependent antibodies may also be used to distinguish the taupathy in AD from other neurological disorders (Cairns *et al.*, 1997a).

Biochemically, NFTs are also seen to be composed of phosphorylated isoforms of tau, a microtubule-associated glycoprotein (Goedert *et al.*, 1988), and monoclonal antibodies can be used to quantify NFTs (Harrington *et al.*, 1991). They also contain ubiquitin, and anti-ubiquitin antibodies give strongly positive reaction with NFTs (Mori *et al.*, 1987; Perry *et al.*, 1987).

Whilst NFTs are intracytoplasmic neuronal inclusions, they may become extracellular after the neurone that contained them has vanished. These extraneuronal NFTs are most often seen in the hippocampus and entorhinal cortex in advanced disease, and both their antigenic properties and ultrastructural features differ from their intraneuronal counterparts (Tabaton *et al.*, 1991b). They are chiefly composed of straight, not paired, helical filaments and react differently with antibodies to tau and ubiquitin. A small subset of extraneuronal tangles gives positive reactions with antibodies to both tau and Aβ protein. The degradation of the NFT (the transition from intracellular to extracellular form) is a series of distinct stages involving complex molecular events that alter both the antigenicity and configuration of the tangle (Bondareff *et al.*, 1990). It is the insolubility of NFTs that is most likely to be responsible for the occurrence of extraneuronal forms (Terry, 1990). The extraneuronal NFTs may be enveloped by glial processes and eventually be internalized as part of their degradative cycle.

30.3.3 Granulovacuolar degeneration

Granulovacuolar degeneration was first described by Simchowicz (1911) in the hippocampal neurones of patients with senile dementia (Figure 30.11). Granulovacuoles are abnormal cytoplasmic structures: one or more vacuoles of 3.5 mm in diameter each contain a single granule. The electron microscope shows a dense granular core, embedded in a translucent matrix. This granular component gives a positive reaction with antibodies to tubulin (Price *et al.*, 1985), to phosphorylated epitopes of the heavy neurofilament peptide (Kahn *et al.*, 1985), to tau (Dickson *et al.*, 1987) and, in some neurones, to ubiquitin (Leigh *et al.*, 1989). A detailed immunocytochemical study has demonstrated that most epitopes of the tau molecule are sequestered in granulovacuoles

and this tau protein is antigenically similar to that found in paired helical filaments. This finding indicates that granulovacuolar degeneration in hippocampal pyramidal neurones vulnerable to neurofibrillary degeneration may offer an alternative metabolic pathway for an abnormal molecule, which contributes to the formation of both granulovacuoles and tangles (Bondareff *et al.*, 1991). Granulovacuoles are now considered to be special autophagosomes that are formed by the sequestration of electron-dense material by a two-layered membrane. Granulovacuoles are virtually restricted to the pyramidal neurones of the hippocampus and in severe AD cases the neuronal cytoplasm is replete with these abnormal structures. They also occur, much less often, in a variety of diseases, including progressive supranuclear palsy, amyotrophic lateral sclerosis–parkinsonism–dementia complex of Guam and tuberous sclerosis.

30.3.4 Hirano bodies

These abnormal structures were first described by Hirano (1965). They are most commonly seen in and amongst the pyramidal cells of the hippocampus. Hirano bodies occur in normal subjects and their frequency increases with advancing age. However, patients with AD have significantly more Hirano bodies than age-matched controls. They also occur in various neurological diseases, including Pick's disease, motor neurone disease and kuru, as well as in animals infected with kuru and scrapie (Gibson and Tomlinson, 1977). Hirano bodies stand out in sections stained with haematoxylin and eosin as bright pink, homogeneous structures that are circular in cross-section with a diameter up to 25 μm, and rectangular or spindle-shaped up to 30 μm in length in longitudinal sections. Ultrastructurally, they are composed of a complex, crystalline array of interlacing filaments forming a lattice-like or 'herring-bone' configuration (Tomonaga, 1974). They stain positively with antibodies to actin (Goldman, 1983) and immunostaining for tau has also been reported (Galloway *et al.*, 1987).

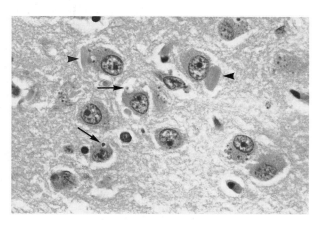

Figure 30.11 *Granulovacuolar degeneration (arrows) and Hirano bodies (arrowheads) in the pyramidal cell layer of the hippocampus. Haematoxylin and eosin.*

30.3.5 Neuronal loss

Neuronal loss is far more difficult to assess than the histological abnormalities previously described, although the decrease of particular neuronal populations is more readily accepted than in normal ageing (Terry, 1990). Whilst well-defined, neuronal groups, like the locus caeruleus, are easier to count, the cerebral cortex presents considerable technical problems. Nevertheless, it has been established that there is a significant decrease of 36–46 per cent in the concentration of large neurones, particularly from layers 3 and 5 of the neocortex (Terry et al., 1981). The loss of the large cortical neurones is age-dependent: the column of these cells is reduced in patients under 80 years of age, but appears to be normal for age in older subjects (Hubbard and Anderson, 1985). This neuronal loss, however, does not affect the neocortex evenly; it appears to be restricted to the frontal and temporal lobes, whereas the parietal and occipital regions are less involved (Mountjoy et al., 1983). The hippocampus is even more severely affected: neuronal fall-out reaches an average of 47 per cent (Ball, 1977) and the number of pyramidal neurones is reduced by 40 per cent in area H1 (Mann et al., 1985). This loss appears to correlate with the number of tangle-bearing cells, whilst the end plate and area H2 are less affected. There is also a substantial decrease of neurones in the cholinergic NbM (Whitehouse et al., 1981), in the cholinergic pedunculopontine nucleus (Jellinger, 1988), in the noradrenergic locus caeruleus (Tomlinson et al., 1981; Marcyniuk et al., 1986) and in the serotonergic raphé nuclei in the brain stem (Yamamoto and Hirano, 1985).

30.3.6 Abnormalities of neuronal processes and synapses

Neuropil threads or 'curly' fibres and dystrophic neurites have been well documented in silver-impregnated preparations developed by Gallyas (1971), but they attracted attention when it was realized that their occurrence was associated with the severity of dementia (Braak et al., 1986). Neuropil threads or curly fibres are slender, short structures found in the neuropil of the cortex. Dystrophic neurites, some of which contribute to the formation of plaques, also appear as somewhat contorted, thread-like structures in these preparations. These abnormal neurites are likely to be a heterogeneous population of dendrites and axons (Tourtellotte and Van Hoesen, 1991). Their ultrastructural and immunocytochemical features are strikingly similar to those of NFTs, indicating that they also originate from the altered neuronal cytoskeleton. Neuropil threads immunostain with antibodies to tau (Kowall and Kosik, 1987; Probst et al., 1989) and to ubiquitin (Joachim et al., 1987). Electron microscopy has revealed that they are often in dendrites and contain straight filaments of 14–16 nm in diameter in addition to paired helical filaments (Tabaton et al., 1989; Yamaguchi et al., 1990b). Moreover, they are often in the dendrites of those nerve cells

that contain NFTs in their cell body (Braak and Braak, 1988). There is increasing evidence that their distribution is more closely associated with NFTs than with plaques. In addition to abnormal neurites, there are quantitative changes: the terminal segments of dendrites of pyramidal cells in layer 2 of the parahippocampal gyrus are fewer and shorter than in normal adult brains (Buell and Coleman, 1979). Considerable decrease of synapses also occurs and this loss is likely to contribute to the development of the disease (Davis et al., 1987). Moreover, immunocytochemical quantification of synaptophysin, a protein localized in presynaptic terminals, revealed an average decrease of 50 per cent in the density of the granular neuropil immunoreaction in the parietal, temporal and mid-frontal cortex (Masliah et al., 1989). In the electron microscope, some presynaptic terminals were distended and contained altered synaptic organelles, including swollen vesicles and dense bodies, similar to those seen in dystrophic neurites. These latter structures gave positive staining with antibodies to synaptophysin and immunoreactivity was mainly localized to the outer membranes of synaptic vesicles and dense bodies. This finding lends further support to the view that progressive synaptic derangements occurs in the neocortex of AD (Masliah et al., 1991).

30.3.7 Glial changes

Astrocytes can be readily observed immunohistochemically by using an antibody to glial fibrillary acidic protein (GFAP; see Figure 30.12). Both NFTs and plaques have been found to be more prevalent in the pyramidal cell-rich layers II, III and V than in other laminae (Mann et al., 1985; Majocha et al., 1988; Braak et al., 1989) and both have been associated with patterns of gliosis in AD (Beach et al., 1989; Itagakai et al., 1989; Cairns et al., 1992) where perivascular gliosis is prominent throughout the cerebrum. In AD extensive gliosis has a laminar pattern in the neocortex, but there does not appear to be an AD-specific pattern of subcortical gliosis (Beach and McGeer, 1988; Beach et al., 1989). In addition to NFTs, plaques and dystrophic neurites, reactive astrocytosis is associated with degenerating neurones in AD. In the pathogenesis of the plaque it appears as though Aβ deposition is an early event preceding gliosis (Yamaguchi et al., 1990a).

It has been proposed by Probst et al. (1987) that microglial cells, normally associated with phagocytosis, are a possible source of Aβ in AD. The presence of major histocompatibility complex (MHC) class II antigens on reactive microglia in association with plaques in AD is indicative of an immune response, although the significance of such expression on the cell surfaces of reactive microglial cells is uncertain. Reactive microglial cells have been found in association with diffuse Aβ deposits and, more frequently, with compact cores of plaques (Itagakai et al., 1989). Leukocyte common antigen and complement receptors, including the cell adhesion molecules, the β-2 integrins, have been localized on microglial

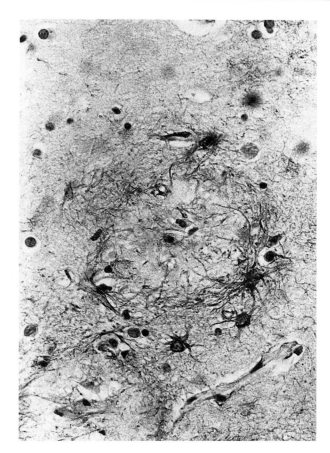

Figure 30.12 *Astrocyte cell bodies and processes encircling a plaque. Glial fibrillary acidic protein immunohistochemistry.*

cells around plaques (Akiyama and McGeer, 1990). These data are consistent with a phagocytic role for microglia and provide evidence for an inflammatory response of brain tissue in AD (see Chapter 33).

30.3.8 Vascular abnormalities

When stained with the dye Congo red, cerebral blood vessels containing amyloid appear apple green under polarized light. Pantelakis (1954) called this deposition congophilic angiopathy (see Figure 30.7, p. 396). These congophilic changes affect leptomeningeal and cortical arterioles, and occasionally intracortical capillaries and venules. The parieto-occipital cortex is usually more affected than that in the frontal and temporal lobes and the change is most easily identified in the striate cortex in the occipital lobe. The brain stem and cerebellar cortex are less frequently affected.

Vascular amyloid is now known to be the same protein as the Aβ amyloid found in plaques. Although vascular amyloid is frequently present in AD, it may be absent even when there are abundant plaques and parenchymal deposits. Occasionally, Aβ appears to extend from the vessel wall into the surrounding cerebral tissue; this is referred to as dysphoric angiopathy (or the drusige Entartung of Scholz). This is commonly seen

in lamina III of the striate cortex and adjacent occipital cortex, occasionally in Ammon's horn and in the cerebellum (Hauw *et al.*, 1991).

Two forms of familial cerebral amyloid angiopathy or hereditary cerebral haemorrhage with amyloidosis have been identified. In both the Dutch (Levy *et al.*, 1990) and Icelandic forms there is an autosomal dominant form of inheritance. Patients suffer from recurrent cerebral haemorrhages that lead to an early death (before 40 years of age in Icelandic patients, and between 50 and 60 years in Dutch patients). The amyloid fibrils in patients with hereditary cerebral haemorrhage with amyloidosis – Icelandic type (HCHWA-I) are made up of cystatin C, a degradation product of a larger protease inhibitor. In the Dutch patients (HCHWA-D) the amyloid fibrils are composed of a 39 amino acid peptide homologous to Aβ protein found in amyloid angiopathy in AD, Down's syndrome, sporadic cerebral amyloid angiopathy (CAA) and normal ageing. Mutations in the Aβ coding sequence in these families proved to be seminal for understanding the role of Aβ in AD pathogenesis.

30.3.9 White matter changes

Although the degenerative process in AD primarily affects the grey matter, the white matter may not be spared. CT scans may show areas of hypodensity. The precise pathological substrate remains controversial. Since amyloid angiopathy is often part of AD, it is possible that the white matter changes result mainly from vascular causes. Symmetrical, incomplete infarctions of the white matter histologically correspond to partial loss of myelin sheaths, axons and oligodendrocytes. These changes are accompanied by mild astrocytosis and macrophage response, whilst there is hyaline fibrosis of small vessels. Cavitating infarctions do not develop and this white matter damage, which occurs in the absence of hypertensive vascular degeneration, is thought to be caused by hypoperfusion (Brun and England, 1986). However, severe loss of cortical neurones may also contribute to fibre loss and consequent pallor of white matter.

30.4 FAMILIAL ALZHEIMER'S DISEASE

AD is a disease primarily of old age and it is difficult to determine the proportion of genetic cases as many family members will die before expressing the disease. Familial forms of AD with multiple affected individuals are rare and account for probably fewer than 5 per cent of AD cases. Mutations in the APP gene and two related genes, presenilin-1 (PS1) and presenilin-2 (PS2), account for the majority of early-onset autosomal dominant cases of familial AD (Goate *et al.*, 1991; Lamb, 1997). Although clinical features may differ between families, the neuropathological features are not markedly different between familial Alzheimer's disease (FAD) and early-onset sporadic cases (Davies, 1986). However, prominent

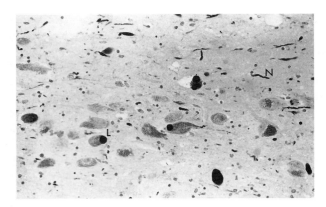

Figure 30.13 *Lewy bodies (L) and dystrophic neurites (N) in the midbrain of a patient who died with familial Alzheimer's disease with the APP717 valine-isoleucine mutation. (α-Synuclein immunohistochemistry.)*

cerebellar plaques and Aβ deposition have been reported in familial cases (Iseki *et al.*, 1990; Struble *et al.*, 1991; Fukutani *et al.*, 1996, 1997). Computerized methods of image analysis have been used to more accurately define the pathological phenotype of AD. Using these techniques, differences in Aβ load have been reported. Mann *et al.* (1996a, b) have shown that both APP and PS mutations lead to measurable increases in Aβ load.

In those cases with an early onset, below 65 years of age, the duration of illness tends to be shorter, and the density of NFTs and plaques is often greater, than in sporadic, late-onset patients. Cortical and brain stem Lewy bodies may coexist with AD in APP (Lantos *et al.*, 1992) and PS mutation patients (Figure 30.13). It is now known that the Lewy body and dystrophic neurites of Parkinson's disease and dementia with Lewy bodies contain the protein α-synuclein (Spillantini *et al.*, 1997). Familial and sporadic forms of AD may also be found in combination with cerebrovascular disease. Rare sporadic cases of AD have been found in combination with other neurodegenerative disorders including Pick's disease, Creutzfeldt–Jakob disease, motor neurone disease and progressive supranuclear palsy.

30.5 PATHOGENESIS

The aetiology and pathogenesis of AD are not fully understood. Although many risk factors have been proposed, the evidence for most of these is weak except for age, family history and ApoE genotype. A genetic contribution to the aetiology of AD has received strong support in the last few years and it is likely that more genes (such as LRP, α_2M and IDE) will be associated with the disease. In the more common non-familial, sporadic cases, and in discordant monozygotic twins, environmental factors may be important in the aetiology.

The discovery of mutations in the APP and PS genes, all of which lead to over-production of Aβ or preferential production of a long 42-amino acid form of Aβ, has confirmed the central role of APP and Aβ deposition in the pathogenesis of AD (Goate *et al.*, 1991; Lamb, 1997). Deposition of Aβ appears to be an early event in both AD and Down's syndrome and precedes the development of plaques, NFTs, microgliosis and astrocytosis (Rozemuller *et al.*, 1989). The amyloid deposits characteristic of AD, 42–43 amino acid Aβ fragments, are the abnormal proteolytic cleavage products of APP. It is known that Aβ has both toxic (Yanker *et al.*, 1989) and trophic (Whitson *et al.*, 1989) effects on neurones in culture, which may relate to plaque and NFT formation.

Metal ions such as aluminium have been implicated as an environmental toxic agent in the pathogenesis of AD, since it has toxic effects on neurones in culture and its accumulation in renal patients is known to be encephalopathic. Accumulations of aluminosilicates in the central region of the core of plaques and within neurones containing NFTs have been reported (Candy *et al.*, 1986). Another environmental factor implicated in Aβ deposition is head trauma. Roberts *et al.* (1991) showed that in a series of patients suffering sustained head injury, there were extensive deposits of Aβ in the neocortex, suggesting that severe head injury can trigger Aβ deposition in a few days. Whether these patients would have gone on to develop AD is unknown.

Although varying amounts of Aβ with a range of morphologies may be found in cognitively normal elderly individuals, it is quantitatively much more severe and cyto-architectonically defined in AD (Majocha *et al.*, 1988; Cairns *et al.*, 1991). The importance of overexpression of APP and its abnormal cleavage product, Aβ, in the pathogenesis of AD has been demonstrated by recent transgenic mouse models (Borchelt *et al.*, 1998). Transgenic mice expressing the full length human APP develop Aβ deposits similar in morphology to those found in AD, but as noted above, differing somewhat in their human 'subtype' counterparts. These animal models will be useful for testing anti-amyloid drugs.

30.6 NEUROPATHOLOGY AND CLINICAL FINDINGS

Alzheimer first suggested a correlation between the presence of NFTs, plaques and dementia in 1906. Roth *et al.* (1966) and Wilcock and Esiri (1982) demonstrated that elderly patients' mental test scores correlated with the neuropathological lesions characteristic of AD. Many other neuropathological and neurochemical changes (Zubenko *et al.*, 1991) have been associated with AD and the accuracy of clinical diagnosis ranges from 43 to 87 per cent (Boller *et al.*, 1989; Jellinger *et al.*, 1990) and, in one sample of 26 cases, 100 per cent (Morris *et al.*, 1988). Conversely, inaccuracy in the ante-mortem diagnosis of AD is common, and for this reason, post-mortem examination remains an essential component of AD research. An accurate differential diagnosis is made difficult by the problems of distinguishing between mild dementia and the cognitive changes of normal ageing ('mild cognitive impairment') – the earliest clinically recognizable form of AD.

Although not all studies have produced positive findings, there is general agreement that cases with earlier onset, shorter duration of illness and greater cognitive impairment have more cortical plaques, whereas late-onset cases, which take a milder course, tend to show less cortical change (Bowen *et al.*, 1979; Hansen *et al.*, 1988). High correlations were observed between cognitive performance and plaque counts in brain biopsies from dementing patients examined earlier in the course of illness (Mann *et al.*, 1986, 1988; Neary *et al.*, 1986). Plaques and NFTs were detected in 38 (75 per cent) of 51 unselected non-demented patients who died between the ages of 55 and 64 years (Ulrich, 1985). These lesions were consistently found in the entorhinal cortex, the hippocampus, or both, suggesting that this region is a site of origin of the lesions. A morphometric analysis of cerebral slices by de la Monte (1989) showed that patients with 'preclinical' AD had shrinkage of white matter comparable to that found in AD, yet the cortical areas were normal, suggesting that white matter degeneration is an intrinsic component of AD. In clinical AD there was global cerebral atrophy of both cortex and white matter. Neuronal death in patients with AD is closely associated with extensive synapse loss in the neocortex, and this has been correlated with cognitive impairment (Terry *et al.*, 1991). Measures of the morphological substrates of brain function frequently show an overlap between AD and control groups (Coleman and Flood, 1987). There does not appear to be a consistent relationship between the pattern of vascular amyloid and the distribution of plaques. Neither is there a correlation between vascular amyloid and dementia (Mountjoy *et al.*, 1982). More recent studies have confirmed that the Aβ amyloid *per se* is probably not the best indicator of severity of disease – rather, the soluble Aβ, which are a prelude to plaque formation, show a closer correlation with the degree of neurodegeneration (McLean *et al.*, 1999).

30.7 DIAGNOSTIC PROBLEMS AND CRITERIA

Despite the fact that the neurohistological abnormalities of AD have been established, the neuropathological diagnosis is not always straightforward (Cruz-Sanchez *et al.*, 1995). There are several reasons to explain this problem.

First, the histopathology of AD is complex and the various abnormalities, previously described, when severe and extensive enable a diagnosis to be made. However, there are considerable differences from case to case, and this histological heterogeneity of disease presents the most formidable difficulties for the neuropathologist. The severity and distribution of any of the histological lesions may vary considerably and are influenced by the age and genetic background of the patient, amongst other factors. Quantitative morphometry and neurochemistry have supported the view that AD is not a uniformly diffuse disorder: morphological abnormalities and neurochemical deficits tend to be more severe and more

extensive in younger patients. There may be subtle differences in the pathology of familial and sporadic cases, and atypical cases exist both in the familial and sporadic forms.

Second, although there are several histological abnormalities in AD, only Aβ deposition approaches a level of specificity, since many of these lesions occur in normal ageing and in other diseases of the nervous system.

Third, AD may be associated with other diseases, most commonly with vascular disease and rarely with other neurodegenerative disorders.

For these reasons, it is important to establish a set of neuropathological or neurochemical criteria. Although several attempts have been made, no universally accepted criteria exist for the neuropathological diagnosis of AD. A Working Party, convened by the Medical Research Council in the United Kingdom, offered only minimal criteria for sampling and examination of AD tissues (Wilcock *et al.*, 1989). An attempt has been made to define AD in terms of hippocampal pathology. Based on quantitative morphometry, it was suggested that more than 20 tangle-bearing neurones per mm^3 and fewer than 5600 neurones per mm^3 should be diagnostic (Ball *et al.*, 1985). This threshold, however, has proven too low and would include 30 per cent of mentally normal elderly people (Anderson and Hubbard, 1985). A North American panel of neuropathologists has recommended age-adjusted plaque and tangle counts. In patients under 50, plaques and tangles in excess of 2–5 per mm^2 in the neocortex should secure the diagnosis of AD. Between 60 and 65 years, there should be more than 8 plaques per mm^2, between 66 and 75 years more than 10 and over the age of 75, more than 15. In the first two age groups, some neurofibrillary tangles may be found, but in the last group these may not be necessary for diagnosis (Khachaturian, 1985). The value of these criteria has, however, been diminished by the statement that these figures can be revised downwards by as much as 50 per cent in the presence of positive clinical history of AD.

A survey of the practical application of these criteria has revealed considerable variations in the use of criteria and the methods of examination (Wisniewski *et al.*, 1989). A European Multicentre Study found that subjective assessment currently was more reliable to compare cases from different laboratories, since quantitative values are greatly influenced by the neurohistological technique employed (Duyckaerts *et al.*, 1990).

The most widely used protocol for neuropathological assessment is that developed by the Task Force of the Consortium to Establish a Registry for AD (CERAD). This takes clinical findings into consideration, and neuropathological criteria for 'definite', 'probable' and 'possible' AD are proposed (Mirra *et al.*, 1991). This system is based on a semi-quantitative assessment of plaque scores. The presence or absence of tangles does not enter into the formal assessment. The more recent National Institute on Aging and Reagan Institute (NIA-RI) criteria require both semiquantitative measures of plaque and tangle distribution and additional sampling (Geddes *et al.*, 1997; Hyman and Trojanowski,

1997). A change from previous criteria is the opinion that any Alzheimer lesions should be considered as pathological even when they appear to be incidental. By acknowledging that a spectrum of changes exists within AD, these criteria may prove more successful than previous ones (Geddes *et al.*, 1997; Hyman and Trojanowski, 1997).

In the final analysis, it is likely that a combination of morphologic and biochemical assays will yield a set of criteria through which a secure diagnosis of AD will be made. Current indications are that blood, CSF and brain tissue levels of Aβ (soluble, insoluble), tau and β-secretase (BACE) may provide a more practical method for the diagnosis and therapeutic monitoring of AD (McLean *et al.*, 1999; Holsinger *et al.*, 2002, 2004).

This chapter was originally written by Peter Lantos and Nigel Cairns and appeared as chapter 37 in the second edition of Dementia. It was updated by Colin Masters for this third edition.

REFERENCES

Akiyama H and McGeer PL. (1990) Brain microglia constitutively express β-2 integrins. *Journal of Immunology* **30**: 81–93

Akiyama H, Yamada T, Kawamata T, McGeer PL. (1991) Association of amyloid P component with complement proteins in neurologically diseased brain tissue. *Brain Research* **548**: 349–352

Alzheimer A. (1907) Über eine eigenartige Erkrankung der Hirnrinde. *Allgemeine Zeitschrift für Psychiatrie* **64**: 146–148

Anderson JM and Hubbard BM. (1985) Definition of Alzheimer's disease. *Lancet* **1**: 408

Armstrong RA, Myers D, Smith CUM. (1993) The spatial patterns of β/4 deposit subtypes in Alzheimer's disease. *Acta Neuropathologica* **86**: 36–41

Armstrong RA, Cairns NJ, Myers D *et al.* (1996) A comparison of β-amyloid deposition in the medial temporal lobe in sporadic Alzheimer's disease, Down's syndrome and normal elderly brains. *Neurodegeneration* **5**: 35–41

Armstrong RA, Cairns NJ, Lantos PL. (1998) The spatial pattern of β-amyloid (Ab) deposits in Alzheimer's disease patients is related to apolipoprotein genotype. *Neuroscience Research Communications* **22**: 99–106

Ball MJ. (1977) Neuronal loss, neurofibrillary tangles and granulovacuolar degeneration in the hippocampus with ageing brain and senile dementia: a quantitative study. *Acta Neuropathologica* **37**: 111–118

Ball MJ, Fisman M, Hachinski V *et al.* (1985) A new definition of Alzheimer's disease: a hippocampal dementia. *Lancet* **1**: 14–16

Beach TG and McGeer EG. (1988) Lamina-specific arrangement of astrocytic gliosis and senile plaques in Alzheimer's disease visual cortex. *Brain Research* **473**: 357–361

Beach TG, Walker R, McGeer EG. (1989) Patterns of gliosis in Alzheimer's disease and aging cerebrum. *Glia* **2**: 420–436

Blanks JC, Hinton DR, Sadun AA, Miller, CA. (1989) Retinal ganglion cell degeneration in Alzheimer's disease. *Brain Research* **501**: 364–372

Blocq P and Marinesco G. (1892) Sur les lesions et la pathogénie de l'epilepsie dite essentielle. *Semaine Medicale* **12**: 445–446

Boller F, Lopez OL, Moossy J. (1989) Diagnosis of dementia: clinicopathologic correlations. *Neurology* **39**: 76–79

Bondareff E, Wischik CM, Novak M *et al.* (1990) Molecular analysis of neurofibrillary degeneration in Alzheimer's disease. *American Journal of Pathology* **137**: 711–723

Bondareff W, Wischik CM, Novak M, Roth M. (1991) Sequestration of tau by granulovacuolar degeneration in Alzheimer's disease. *American Journal of Pathology* **139**: 641–647

Borchelt DR, Woing PC, Sisodia SS, Price DL. (1998) Transgenic mouse models of Alzheimer's disease and amyotrophic lateral sclerosis. *Brain Pathology* **8**: 735–757

Bowen DM, Spillane JA, Curzon G *et al.* (1979) Accelerated ageing or selective neuronal loss as an important cause of dementia? *Lancet* **1**: 11–14

Braak H and Braak E. (1988) Neuropil threads occur in dendrites of tangle-bearing nerve cells. *Neuropathology and Applied Neurobiology* **14**: 39–44

Braak H, Braak E, Grundke-Iqbal I, Iqbal K. (1986) Occurrence of neuropil thread, in the senile human brain and in Alzheimer's disease: a third location of paired helical filaments outside of neurofibrillary tangles and neuritic plaques. *Neuroscience Letters* **65**: 351–355

Braak H, Braak E, Kalus P. (1989) Alzheimer's disease areal and laminar pathology in the occipital isocortex. *Acta Neuropathologica* **77**: 494–506

Brun A and England E. (1986) A white matter disorder in dementia of the Alzheimer type: a pathoanatomical study. *Annals of Neurology* **19**: 253–262

Buell SJ and Coleman PD. (1979) Dendritic growth in the aged human brain and failure of growth in senile dementia. *Science* **206**: 854–856

Cairns NJ, Chadwick A, Luthert PJ, Lantos PL. (1991) β-Amyloid protein load is relatively uniform throughout neocortex and hippocampus in elderly Alzheimer's disease patients. *Neuroscience Letters* **129**: 115–118

Cairns NJ, Chadwick A, Luthert PJ, Lantos PL. (1992) Astrocytosis, βA4-protein deposition and paired helical filament formation in Alzheimer's disease. *Journal of the Neurological Sciences* **112**: 68–75

Cairns NJ, Atkinson PF, Hanger DP *et al.* (1997a) Tau protein in the glial cytoplasmic inclusions of multiple system atrophy can be distinguished from abnormal tau in Alzheimer's disease. *Neuroscience Letters* **230**: 49–52

Cairns NJ, Fukutani Y, Chadwick A *et al.* (1997b) Apolipoprotein E, β-amyloid (Aβ), phosphorylated tau and apolipoprotein E genotype in Alzheimer's disease. *Alzheimer Research* **3**: 109–114

Candy JM, Oakley AE, Klinowski J *et al.* (1986) Aluminosilicates and senile plaque formation in Alzheimer's disease. *Lancet* **1**: 354–357

Coleman PD and Flood DG. (1987) Neuron numbers and dendritic extent in normal aging and Alzheimer's disease. *Neurobiology of Aging* **8**: 521–545

Crowther RA. (1991) Straight and paired helical filaments in Alzheimer's have a common structural unit. *Proceedings of the National Academy of Sciences of the United States of America* **88**: 2288–2292

Crowther RA and Wischik CM. (1985) Image reconstruction of the Alzheimer paired helical filament. *EMBO Journal* **4**: 3661–3665

Cruz-Sánchez FF, Ravid R, Cuzner ML. (1995) *Neuropathological Diagnostic Criteria for Brain Banking.* Oxford, IOS Press

Davies P. (1986) The genetics of Alzheimer's disease: a review and a discussion of the implications. *Neurobiology of Aging* **7**: 459

Davis CA, Mann DMA, Sumpter PQ, Yates PO. (1987) A quantitative morphometric analysis of the neuronal and synaptic content of the frontal and temporal cortex in patients with Alzheimer's disease. *Journal of the Neurological Sciences* **78**: 151–164

Davis PJM and Wright EA. (1977) A new method for measuring cranial cavity volume and its application to the assessment of cerebral atrophy at autopsy. *Neuropathology and Applied Neurobiology* **3**: 341–358

Delaère P, Duyckaerts C, Masters C *et al.* (1990) Large amounts of neocortical βA4 deposits without neuritic plaques nor tangles in a psychometrically assessed, non-demented person. *Neuroscience Letters* **116**: 87–93

de la Monte SM. (1989) Quantitation of cerebral atrophy in preclinical and end-stage Alzheimer's disease. *Annals of Neurology* **25**: 450–459

Dickson DW, Ksiezak-Reding H, Davies P, Yen SH. (1987) A monoclonal antibody that recognizes a phosphorylated epitope in Alzheimer neurofibrillary tangles, neurofilaments and tau proteins immunostains granulovacuolar degeneration. *Acta Neuropathologica* **73**: 254–258

Divry P. (1927) Etude histo-chimique des plaques séniles. *Journal Belge de Neurologie et de Psychiatrie* **27**: 643–657

Duyckaerts C, Hauw J-J, Piette F *et al.* (1985) Cortical atrophy in senile dementia of the Alzheimer type is mainly due to a decrease in cortical length. *Acta Neuropathologica* **66**: 72–74

Duyckaerts C, Delaère P, Poulain V *et al.* (1988) Does amyloid precede paired helical filaments in the senile plaques? A study of 15 cases with graded intellectual status in aging and Alzheimer's disease. *Neuroscience Letters* **91**: 354–359

Duyckaerts C, Delaère P, Hauw J-J *et al.* (1990) Rating of the lesions in senile dementia of the Alzheimer type: a concordance between laboratories. A European multicenter study under the auspices of EURAGE. *Journal of the Neurological Sciences* **97**: 295–323

Esiri MM and Morris JH. (1997) *The Neuropathology of Dementia.* Cambridge, Cambridge University Press

Esiri MM and Wilcock GK. (1984) The olfactory bulbs in Alzheimer's disease. *Journal of Neurology, Neurosurgery, and Psychiatry* **47**: 56–60

Esiri MM, Hyman BT, Beyreuther K, Masters CL. (1997) Ageing and dementia. In: DI Graham, PL Lantos (eds), *Greenfield's Neuropathology*, 6th edition, Vol. II. London, Arnold, pp. 153–233

Fukutani Y, Cairns NJ, Rossor MN, Lantos PL. (1996) Purkinje cell loss and astrocytosis in the cerebellum in familial and sporadic Alzheimer's disease. *Neuroscience Letters* **214**: 33–36

Fukutani Y, Cairns NJ, Rossor MN, Lantos PL. (1997) Cerebellar pathology in sporadic and familial Alzheimer's disease including APP 717(val-ile) mutation cases: a morphometric investigation. *Journal of the Neurological Sciences* **149**: 177–184

Galloway PG, Perry G, Kosik KS, Gambetti P. (1987) Hirano bodies contain tau protein. *Brain Research* **403**: 337–340

Gallyas F. (1971) Silver staining of Alzheimer's neurofibrillary changes by means of physical development. *Acta Morphologica Academiae Scientifica Hungarica* **19**: 1–8

Geddes JW, Tekirian TL, Soultanian NS *et al.* (1997) Comparison of neuropathologic criteria for the diagnosis of Alzheimer's disease. *Neurobiology of Aging* **18** (Suppl. 4): S99–S105

Gentleman SM, Bruton C, Allsop D *et al.* (1989) A demonstration of the advantages of immunostaining in the quantification of amyloid plaque deposits. *Histochemistry* **92**: 355–358

Gibson PH and Tomlinson BE. (1977) Numbers of Hirano bodies in the hippocampus of normal and demented people with Alzheimer's disease. *Journal of the Neurological Sciences* **33**: 199–206

Goate A, Chartier-Harlin MC, Mullan M *et al.* (1991) Segregation of a missense mutation in the amyloid precursor protein gene with familial Alzheimer's disease. *Nature* **349**: 704–706

Goedert M, Wischik CM, Crowther RA *et al.* (1988) Cloning and sequencing of the cDNA encoding a core protein of the paired helical filament of Alzheimer's disease: identification as the microtubule-associated protein tau. *Proceedings of the National Academy of Sciences of the United States of America* **85**: 4051–4055

Goedert M, Spillantini MG, Cairns NJ, Crowther RA. (1992) Tau proteins of Alzheimer paired helical filaments; abnormal phosphorylation of all six isoforms. *Neuron* **8**: 159–168

Goldman JE. (1983) The association of actin with Hirano bodies. *Journal of Neuropathology and Experimental Neurology* **42**: 146–152

Goldstein LE, Muffat JA, Cherny RA *et al.* (2003) Cystolic beta-amyloid deposition and supranuclear cataracts in lenses from people with Alzheimer's disease. *Lancet* **361**: 1258–1265

Gonatas NK, Anderson A, Vongelista I. (1967) The contribution of altered synapses in the senile plaque: an electronmicroscopic study in Alzheimer's dementia. *Journal of Neuropathology and Experimental Neurology* **26**: 25–39

Hanger DP, Brion J-P, Gallo J-M *et al.* (1991). Tau in Alzheimer's disease and Down's syndrome is insoluble and abnormally phosphorylated. *Biochemical Journal* **275**: 99–104

Hansen LA, De Teresa R, Davies P, Terry RD. (1988) Neocortical morphometry, lesion counts, and choline acetyltransferase levels in the age spectrum of Alzheimer's disease. *Neurology* **38**: 48–55

Harrington CR, Mukaetova-Ladinska EB, Hills R *et al.* (1991) Measurement of distinct immunochemical presentations of tau protein in Alzheimer's disease. *Proceedings of the National Academy of Sciences of the United States of America* **88**: 5842–5846

Hauw J-J, Duyckaerts C, Delaere P. (1991) Alzheimer's disease. In: S Duckett (ed.), *The Pathology of the Aging Nervous System.* London, Lea and Febiger, pp. 113–147

Hinton DR, Sadun AA, Blanks JC, Miller CA. (1986) Optic nerve degeneration in Alzheimer's disease. *New England Journal of Medicine* **315**: 485–487

Hirano A. (1965) Pathology of amyotrophic lateral sclerosis. In: DC Gajdusek, CJ Gibbs Jr, M Alpers (eds), *Slow, Latent and Temperate Virus Infections.* Washington DC, Government Printing Office, pp. 23–26

Holsinger RMD, McLean CA, Beyreuther K, Masters CL, Evin G. (2002) Increased expression of the amyloid precursor β-secretase in Alzheimer's disease. *Annals of Neurology* **51**: 783–786

Holsinger RMD, Mclean CA, Collins SJ, Masters CL, Evin G. (2004) Increased β-secretase activity in cerebrospinal fluid of Alzheimer's disease subjects. *Annals of Neurology* **55**: 898–899

Hubbard BM and Anderson JM. (1981) A quantitative study of cerebral atrophy in old age and senile dementia. *Journal of the Neurological Sciences* **50**: 135–145

Hubbard BM and Anderson JM. (1985) Age-related variations in the neuron content of the cerebral cortex in senile dementia of Alzheimer type. *Neuropathology and Applied Neurobiology* **11**: 369–382

Hyman BT and Trojanowski JQ. (1997) Editorial on consensus recommendations for the postmortem diagnosis of Alzheimer disease from the National Institute on Aging and the Reagan Institute Working Group on diagnostic criteria for the neuropathological assessment of Alzheimer's disease. *Journal of Neuropathology and Experimental Neurology* **56**: 1095–1097

Iseki E, Matsushita M, Kosaka K *et al.* (1990) Morphological characteristics of senile plaques in familial Alzheimer's disease. *Acta Neuropathologica* **80**: 227–232

Itagakai S, McGeer PL, Akiyama H *et al.* (1989) Relationship of microglia and astrocytes to amyloid deposits of Alzheimer's disease. *Journal of Neuroimmunology* **24**: 173–182

Jellinger K. (1988) The pedunculopontine nucleus in Parkinson's disease, progressive supranuclear palsy and Alzheimer's disease. *Journal of Neurology, Neurosurgery, and Psychiatry* **51**: 540–543

Jellinger K, Danielczyk W, Fischer P, Gabriel E. (1990) Clinicopathological analysis of dementia disorders in the elderly. *Journal of the Neurological Sciences* **95**: 239–258

Joachim CL, Morris JH, Selkoe DJ, Kosik KS. (1987) Tau epitopes are incorporated into a wide range of lesions in Alzheimer's disease. *Journal of Neuropathology and Experimental Neurology* **46**: 611–622

Joachim CL, Morris JH, Selkoe DJ. (1989) Diffuse senile plaques occur commonly in the cerebellum in Alzheimer's disease. *American Journal of Pathology* **135**: 309–319

Kahn J, Anderton BH, Probert A *et al.* (1985) Immunohistological study of granulovacuolar degeneration using monoclonal antibodies to neurofilaments. *Journal of Neurology, Neurosurgery, and Psychiatry* **48**: 924–926

Kang J, Lemaire HG, Unterbeck A *et al.* (1987) The precursor of Alzheimer's disease amyloid A4 protein resembles a cell-surface receptor. *Nature* **325**: 733–736

Khachaturian ZS. (1985) Diagnosis of Alzheimer's disease. *Archives of Neurology* **42**: 1097–1104

Kidd M. (1963) Paired helical filaments in electron microscopy of Alzheimer's disease. *Nature* **197**: 192–193

Kiuchi A, Otsuka N, Namba Y *et al.* (1991) Presenile appearance of abundant neurofibrillary tangles without senile plaques in the brain in myotonic dystrophy. *Acta Neuropathologica* **82**: 1–5

Kowall NW and Kosik KS. (1987) Axonal disruption and aberrant localization of tau protein characterize the neuropil pathology of Alzheimer's disease. *Annals of Neurology* **22**: 639–643

Lamb BT. (1997). Presenilins, amyloid-β and Alzheimer's disease. *Nature Medicine* **3**: 28–29

Lantos PL, Luthert PJ, Hanger D *et al.* (1992) Familial Alzheimer's disease with the amyloid precursor protein position 717 mutation and sporadic Alzheimer's disease have the same cytoskeletal pathology. *Neuroscience Letters* **137**: 221–224

Leigh PN, Probst A, Dale GE *et al.* (1989) New aspects of the pathology of neurodegenerative disorders as revealed by ubiquitin antibodies. *Acta Neuropathologica* **79**: 61–72

Levy E, Carman MD, Fernandez-Madrid IJ *et al.* (1990) Mutation of the Alzheimer's disease amyloid gene in hereditary cerebral hemorrhage, Dutch type. *Science* **248**: 1124–1126

Majocha RE, Benes FM, Reifel JL *et al.* (1988) Laminar-specific distribution and infrastructural detail of amyloid in the Alzheimer's disease cortex visualized by computer-enhanced imaging of epitopes recognized by monoclonal antibodies. *Proceedings of the National Academy of Sciences of the United States of America* **85**: 6182–6186

Mann DMA, Yates PO, Marcynink B. (1985) Some morphometric observations in the cerebral cortex and hippocampus in presenile Alzheimer's disease, senile dementia of Alzheimer type and Down's syndrome in middle age. *Journal of the Neurological Sciences* **69**: 139–159

Mann DMA, Yates PO, Marcyniuk B. (1986) A comparison of nerve cell loss in cortical and subcortical structures in Alzheimer's disease. *Journal of Neurology, Neurosurgery, and Psychiatry* **49**: 310–312

Mann DMA, Yates PO, Marcyniuk B *et al.* (1988) The progression of the pathological changes of Alzheimer's disease in frontal and temporal neocortex examined both at biopsy and at autopsy. *Neuropathology and Applied Neurobiology* **14**: 177–195

Mann DMA, Iwatsubo T, Cairns NJ *et al.* (1996a) Amyloid β protein (Aβ) deposition in chromosome 14-linked Alzheimer's disease: predominance of Aβ$_{42(43)}$. *Annals of Neurology* **40**: 149–156

Mann DMA, Iwatsubo T, Ihara Y *et al.* (1996b) Predominant deposition of amyloid-β$_{42(43)}$ in plaques in cases of Alzheimer's disease and hereditary cerebral hemorrhage associated with mutations in the amyloid precursor protein gene. *American Journal of Pathology* **148**: 1257–1266

Marcyniuk B, Mann DMA, Yates PO. (1986) The topography of cell loss from locus ceruleus in Alzheimer's disease. *Journal of the Neurological Sciences* **76**: 335–345

Masliah E, Terry RD, DeTeresa RM, Hansen LA. (1989) Immunohistochemical quantification of the synapse-related protein synaptophysin in Alzheimer disease. *Neuroscience Letters* **103**: 234–239

Masliah E, Hansen L, Albright T *et al.* (1991) Immunoelectron microscopic study of synaptic pathology in Alzheimer's disease. *Acta Neuropathologica* **81**: 428–433

Masters CL, Simms G, Weinman NA, Multhaup G, McDonald BL, Beyreuther K. (1985) Amyloid plaque core protein in Alzheimer disease and Down syndrome. *Proceedings of the National Academy of Sciences of the United States of America* **82**: 4245–4249

McLean CA, Cherny RA, Fraser FW *et al.* (1999) Soluble pool of Aβ as a determinant of severity of neurodegeneration in Alzheimer's disease. *Annals of Neurology* **46**: 860–866

Mirra SS, Heyman A, McKeel D *et al.* (1991) The consortium to establish a registry for Alzheimer's disease (CERAD). Part II. Standardization of the neuropathologic assessment of Alzheimer's disease. *Neurology* **41**: 479–486

Mori H, Kondo J, Ihara Y. (1987) Ubiquitin is a component of paired helical filaments in Alzheimer's disease. *Science* **235**: 1641–1644

Morris JC, McKeel DW, Fulling K *et al.* (1988) Validation of clinical diagnostic criteria for Alzheimer's disease. *Annals of Neurology* **24**: 17–22

Mountjoy CQ, Tomlinson BE, Gibson PH. (1982) Amyloid senile plaques and cerebral blood vessels. A semi-quantitative investigation of a possible relationship. *Journal of the Neurological Sciences* **57**: 89–103

Mountjoy CQ, Roth M, Evans NJR, Evans HM. (1983) Cortical neuronal counts in normal elderly controls and demented patients. *Neurobiology of Aging* **4**: 1–11

Neary D, Snowden JS, Bowen DM *et al.* (1986) Neuropsychological syndromes in presenile dementia due to cerebral atrophy. *Journal of Neurology, Neurosurgery, and Psychiatry* **49**: 163–174

Ogomori K, Kitamoto T, Tateishi J *et al.* (1989) β-Protein amyloid is widely distributed in the central nervous system of patients with Alzheimer's disease. *American Journal of Pathology* **134**: 243–251

Pantelakis S. (1954) Un type particulier d'angiopathie sénile du système nervaux central: l'angiopathie congophile. Topographie et fréquence. *Monatsschrift für Psychiatrie und Neurologie* **128**: 219–256

Perry G, Friedman R, Shaw G, Chau V. (1987) Ubiquitin is detected in neurofibrillary tangles and senile plaque neurites of Alzheimer's disease brains. *Proceedings of the National Academy of Sciences of the United States of America* **84**: 3033–3036

Price DL, Stuble RG, Altschuler RJ *et al.* (1985) Aggregation of tubulin in neurons in Alzheimer's disease. *Journal of Neuropathology and Experimental Neurology* **44**: 366

Probst A, Brunnschweiler H, Lautenschlager C, Ulrich J. (1987) A special type of senile plaque, possibly an initial stage. *Acta Neuropathologica* **74**: 133–141

Probst A, Anderton BH, Brion J-P, Ulrich J. (1989) Senile plaque neurites fail to demonstrate anti-paired helical filament and anti-microtubule associated protein-tau immunoreactive proteins in the absence of neurofibrillary tangles in the neocortex. *Acta Neuropathologica* **77**: 430–436

Ritchie CW, Bush AI, Mackinnon A *et al.* (2003) Metal-protein attenuation with iodochlorhydroxyquin (clioquinol) targeting Aβ amyloid deposition and toxicity in Alzheimer disease: a pilot phase 2 clinical trial. *Archives of Neurology* **60**: 1678–1691

Roberts GW, Gentleman SM, Lynch A, Graham DI. (1991) βA4 amyloid protein deposition in brain after head trauma. *Lancet* **338**: 1422–1423

Rogers J and Morrison JH. (1985) Quantitative morphology and laminar distribution of senile plaques in Alzheimer's disease. *Journal of Neuroscience* **5**: 2801–2808

Roses AD. (1994). Apolipoprotein E affects the rate of Alzheimer's disease expression: β amyloid burden is a secondary consequence dependent on ApoE genotype and duration of disease. *Journal of Neuropathology and Experimental Neurology* **53**: 429–437

Roth M, Tomlinson BE, Blessed G. (1966) Correlations between scores for dementia and counts of 'senile plaques' in cerebral grey matter of elderly subjects. *Nature* **209**: 109–110

Rozemuller JM, Eikelenboom P, Stam FC *et al.* (1989) A4 protein in Alzheimer's disease: primary and secondary cellular events in extracellular amyloid deposition. *Journal of Neuropathology and Experimental Neurology* **48**: 674–691

Simchowicz T. (1911) Histologische Studien über die Senile Demenz. *Histologische und Histopathologische Arbeiten* **4**: 267–444

Spillantini MG, Schmidt ML, Lee VM *et al.* (1997) α-Synuclein in Lewy bodies. *Nature* **388**: 839–840

Struble RG, Polinsky RJ, Hedreen JC *et al.* (1991) Hippocampal lesions in dominantly inherited Alzheimer's disease. *Journal of Neuropathology and Experimental Neurology* **50**: 82–94

Tabaton M, Mandybur TI, Perry G *et al.* (1989) The widespread alteration of neurites in Alzheimer's disease may be unrelated to amyloid deposition. *Annals of Neurology* **26**: 771–778

Tabaton M, Cammarata S, Mancardi GL *et al.* (1991a) Abnormal tau-reactive filaments in olfactory mucosa in biopsy specimens of patients with probable Alzheimer's disease. *Neurology* **41**: 391–394

Tabaton M, Cammarata S, Mancardi G *et al.* (1991b) Ultrastructural localization of β-amyloid, tau, and ubiquitin epitopes in extracellular neurofibrillary tangles. *Proceedings of the National Academy of Sciences of the United States of America* **88**: 2098–2102

Talamo BR, Ruder RA, Kosik KS *et al.* (1989) Pathological changes in olfactory neurons in patients with Alzheimer's disease. *Nature* **337**: 736–739

Terry RD. (1985) Alzheimer's disease. In: RL Davis and DM Robertson (eds), *Textbook of Neuropathology*. Baltimore, Williams and Wilkins, pp. 824–841

Terry RD. (1990) Normal aging and Alzheimer's disease: growing problems. In: PA Cancilla, FS Vogel, N Kaufman (eds), *Neuropathology. International Academy of Pathology Monograph*. Baltimore, Williams and Wilkins, pp. 41–54

Terry RD, Peck A, DeTeresa R, Schechter R, Horoupian DS. (1981) Some morphometric aspects of the brain in senile dementia of the Alzheimer type. *Annals of Neurology* **10**: 184–192

Terry RD, Masliah E, Salmon DP *et al.* (1991) Physical basis of cognitive alterations in Alzheimer's disease: synapse loss is the major correlate of cognitive impairment. *Annals of Neurology* **30**: 572–580

Tomlinson BE, Irving D, Blessed G. (1981) Cell loss in the locus ceruleus in senile dementia of Alzheimer type. *Journal of the Neurological Sciences* **49**: 419–428

Tomonaga M. (1974) Ultrastructure of Hirano bodies. *Acta Neuropathologica* **28**: 365–366

Tourtellotte WG and Van Hoesen GW. (1991) The axonal origin of a subpopulation of dystrophic neurites in Alzheimer's disease. *Neuroscience Letters* **129**: 11–16

Ulrich J. (1985) Alzheimer changes in nondemented patients younger than sixty-five: possible early stages of Alzheimer's disease and senile dementia of the Alzheimer type. *Annals of Neurology* **17**: 273–277

Walker LC, Kitt CA, Cork LC *et al.* (1988) Multiple transmitter systems contribute neurites to individual senile plaques. *Journal of Neuropathology and Experimental Neurology* **47**: 138–144

Whitehouse PJ, Price DL, Clark AW *et al.* (1981) Alzheimer's disease: evidence for selective loss of cholinergic neurons in the nucleus basalis. *Annals of Neurology* **10**: 122–126

Whitson JS, Selkoe DJ, Cotman CW. (1989) Amyloid β protein enhances the survival of hippocampal neurons *in vitro. Science* **243**: 1488–1490

Wilcock GK and Esiri MM. (1982) Plaques, tangles and dementia. *Journal of the Neurological Sciences* **56**: 343–356

Wilcock GK, Hope RA, Brooks DN *et al.* (1989) Recommended minimum data to be collected in research studies on Alzheimer's disease. *Journal of Neurology, Neurosurgery, and Psychiatry* **52**: 693–700

Wisniewski HM, Merz PA, Iqbal K. (1984) Ultrastructure of paired helical filaments of Alzheimer's neurofibrillary tangle. *Journal of Neuropathology and Experimental Neurology* **43**: 643–656

Wisniewski HM, Rabe A, Zigman W, Silverman W. (1989) Neuropathological diagnosis of Alzheimer's disease. *Journal of Neuropathology and Experimental Neurology* **48**: 606–609

Yamaguchi H, Nakazato Y, Hirai S, Shoji M. (1990a) Immunoelectron microscopic localization of amyloid β protein in the diffuse plaques of Alzheimer-type dementia. *Brain Research* **508**: 320–324

Yamaguchi H, Nakazato Y, Shoji M *et al.* (1990b) Ultrastructure of the neuropil threads in the Alzheimer brain: their dendritic origin and accumulation in the senile plaques. *Acta Neuropathologica* **80**: 368–374

Yamaguchi H, Nakazato Y, Shoji M *et al.* (1991) Ultrastructure of diffuse plaques in senile dementia of the Alzheimer type: comparison with primitive plaques. *Acta Neuropathologica* **82**: 13–20

Yamamoto T and Hirano A. (1985) Nucleus raphe dorsalis in Alzheimer's disease: neurofibrillary tangles and loss of large neurons. *Annals of Neurology* **17**: 573–577

Yanker BA, Dawes LR, Fisher S *et al.* (1989) Neurotoxicity of a fragment of the amyloid precursor associated with Alzheimer's disease. *Science* **245**: 417–420

Zubenko GS, Moossy J, Martinez J *et al.* (1991) Neuropathologic and neurochemical correlates of psychosis in primary dementia. *Archives of Neurology* **48**: 619–624

31

Role of tau protein in neurodegenerative dementias

ELIZABETA B MUKAETOVA-LADINSKA

Neurodegenerative dementias are characterized by an insidious onset of memory and personality changes that follow a progressive course over at least a 6-month period in the absence of acute medical, psychiatric and/or neurological diseases. Numerous factors may increase the risk for their development: advanced age, genetic predisposition, gender, low educational level, various environmental factors (e.g. head injury, exposure to aluminium, pesticides, electromagnetic field) and altered autoimmune mechanism. A consistent feature of the neurodegenerative process, highly correlated with the extent of cognitive impairment, is the presence of neurofibrillary pathology (neurofibrillary tangles (NFTs), dystrophic neurites and neuritic plaques; see Plate 8).

Immunohistochemical studies have identified a number of proteins that are present within neurofibrillary pathology. Neurofilament proteins, actin, ubiquitin, vimentin, amyloid protein (Aβ), microtubule associated protein 2 and tau protein have been found within NFTs (Plate 8). The term 'taupathies' has now been introduced to refer to a rather heterogeneous group of neurodegenerative disorders attributable to characteristic filamentous tau deposits and/or altered tau processing (Box 31.1).

The discovery of numerous tau protein mutations in frontotemporal lobe dementia and parkinsonism linked to chromosome 17 (FTDP-17) provides further proof of the central role of tau abnormalities in the aetiology of neurodegenerative disorders and its importance for the dementia syndrome. This chapter will address the normal function of tau protein, mechanisms of its aggregation into intracellular filamentous structures found in taupathies, biochemical and genetic characteristics of taupathies, tau protein diagnostic advances and therapeutic developments for prevention of tau aggregation.

31.1 TAU PROTEIN: STRUCTURE AND BIOLOGICAL ROLE

Tau protein is a family of hydrophilic, heat-stable and soluble microtubule-associated proteins (MAPs). Its major functions include stabilization of microtubules (MTs), stimulation of MT polymerization, and suppression of MT dynamics and, together with MAP1B, tau may regulate axonal elongation and neuronal migration. Tau protein is predominantly expressed within neurones and axons of the central and peripheral nervous system, and, albeit at low level, is also found in astrocytes, oligodendrocytes and neuronal nuclei. Its mRNA is also present in non-neuronal tissue, including heart, kidney, liver, muscles, pancreas, testis and fibroblasts. In progressive supranuclear palsy (PSP), frontotemporal dementia (FTD), severe Alzheimer's disease (AD), animal models of taupathies and ganglion cell tumours, tau protein is also overtly expressed in glial cells, in particular oligodendrocytes.

The human gene encoding tau protein (MAPT) is located on chromosome 17 (17q21) and consists of 16 exons. Alternative RNA splicing of exons 2, 3 and 10 in the adult human brain results in six different tau isoforms (see Plate 9). These contain:

- an acidic N-terminal domain (containing zero, 0N; one, 1N; or two, 2N; 29 amino acid N-terminal inserts, due

Box 31.1 *Taupathies: conditions with presence of neurofibrillary pathology and/or altered processing of tau protein*

- Ageing
- Argyrophilic grain dementia (diffuse and limbic forms)*
- Alzheimer's disease
- Amyotrophic lateral sclerosis/parkinsonism-dementia complex of Guam
- Corticobasal degeneration*
- Creutzfeldt–Jakob disease
- Dementia pugilistica
- Dementia with motor neurone disease-type inclusions*
- Diffuse neurofibrillary tangles with calcification
- Down's syndrome
- Frontal leukoencephalopathy with white matter glial tau deposits
- Frontotemporal lobe degeneration:*
  - frontotemporal lobe dementia with parkinsonism linked to chromosome 17 (including familial multiple system taupathy with presenile dementia, palidopontonigral degeneration, progressive subcortical gliosis)
  - frontotemporal lobe dementia linked to chromosome 3
  - Pick's disease
- Gerstmann–Straussler–Scheinker syndrome
- Hallervorden–Sptaz disease
- Head trauma
- Hippocampal sclerosis dementia with taupathy
- Lewy body variant of Alzheimer's disease
- Multiple system atrophy
- Myotonic dystrophy
- Niemann–Pick disease
- Postencephalitic parkinsonism
- Primary progressive aphasia*
- Prion protein cerebral amyloid angiopathy
- Progressive supranuclear palsy*
- Recessive taupathy with acute respiratory failure
- Sporadic or familial 'tau-less' taupathy (dementia lacking distinctive histopathology [DLDH])*
- Subacute sclerosing panencephalitis
- Tangle-predominant Alzheimer's disease

*Pick's complex denoting overlap between 3R and 4R, and tau-less taupathies. (Modified according to Kertesz, 2003.)

to alternative splicing of exons 2 and 3) that interacts with plasma membrane and associates with phospholipase C-γ;
- a proline-rich middle domain; and
- a C-terminal domain (encoded by exons 9–12) containing three or four tandem repeats (3R and 4R, respectively, formed by alternative splicing of exon 10: referred to as the 'microtubule-binding domain').

These isoforms consist of 352–441 amino acids, with an apparent molecular weight ranging from 45 to 65 kDa.

Exons 4A, 6 and 8 are not characteristic for the human brain mRNA: human mRNA containing either exon 6 or 8 has not been described, whereas mRNA containing exon 4A is found only in the larger human, rodent and bovine peripheral isoform of tau protein. This higher molecular weight tau protein ('big tau') is expressed as a result of alternative splicing and inclusion of the large exon 4A in the N-terminal portion of the tau protein molecule, with an extra 254 amino acid insert (Goedert *et al.* 1992). In the adult rat brain, almost all neurones extending processes into the peripheral neuronal system express 'big tau', except for the bipolar neurones of the olfactory, vestibular and spiral ganglia. Retinal ganglion cells are the only central nervous system (CNS) neurones whose processes remain entirely within the CNS, which express high levels of 'big tau'.

The expression of the different tau isoforms is developmentally regulated. In the embryonic brain, only the shortest of the six isoforms (0N3R) is expressed. In the adult human brain, all six isoforms are present and the 4R isoforms are predominant in the adult human and rodent brain. However, even in adulthood, not all six tau isoforms are present in all neuronal cell lines. Thus, tau mRNAs containing exon 10 are not found in the granular cells of the dentate gyrus (Goedert *et al.*, 1989).

31.1.1 Role of tau protein in MT assembly and tubulin polymerization

Tau, MAP1 and MAP2 proteins regulate the assembly of microtubules. Tau protein binds to spectrin and actin filaments, and can serve as a linker of MTs to other cytoskeletal components such as neurofilaments. It can also interact with various cytoplasmic organelles, including plasma membrane and mitochondria.

Tau protein binds to the α- and β-tubulin subunits via 3- or 4- repeat domains, promoting the formation of microtubules (see Plate 10). The 4R tau binds to the MT $\approx$3-fold more strongly than 3R tau, and confers the ability to assemble MT more effectively than 3R tau. Two isoforms of five tandem repeat tau protein have been described in chicken brain, and they have the greatest ability to promote MT assembly (Yoshida and Goedert, 2002).

The most potent MT-binding site to induce MT polymerization is the region between MT tandem repeats 1 and 2 corresponding to 274–281 amino acids. This region is unique to the 4R tau, and contributes to the 40-fold tubulin binding difference between 3R and 4R tau alone. The MT-binding region of tau protein also binds to both RNA and residues 250–298 of presenilin 1 (PS1). This region of PS1 is also involved in the binding of GSK3β. Since the MT-binding region can also inhibit protein phosphatase 2A (PP2A) activity by competing for binding tau protein at the MT-binding domains, this region may be involved in regulating the extent of post-translational modification of the tau protein (e.g. phosphorylation).

31.2 TAU AGGREGATION AND FORMATION OF FILAMENTOUS STRUCTURES IN TAUPATHIES

Intracellular filamentous structures present in various tau-pathies are polymers of the repeat region of tau protein:

- paired helical filaments (PHFs), ultrastructural components of NFTs, dystrophic neurites and neuritic plaques consist of double helical stack filaments, with a longitudinal spacing between crossovers of 65 and 80 nm and a width between 10–15 nm and 27–34 nm;
- straight filaments (SFs), measuring 10–15 nm in width; and
- twisted-ribbon-like filaments with an irregular periodicity of 90–130 nm (found in some familial dementias, e.g. familial progressive subcortical gliosis, cortical basal degeneration [CBD], familial multiple system taupathy).

Although full-length recombinant tau protein does not aggregate in physiological conditions, at high concentrations and/or low pH, it can aggregate with the MT-binding fragment. Similarly, tau protein can form oligomers upon binding to MTs *in vitro*. The hexapeptide interaction motif at the *C*-terminal end of the tau protein molecule (^{306}VQIVYK^{311}) within the R3 MT domain (encoded by exon 11) and its related hexapeptide (^{275}VQIINK^{280}) within the R2 (encoded by exon 10) are able to assemble into thin filaments without a helical appearance, and these filaments can nucleate PHFs from full-length tau. Furthermore, point mutations within this hexapeptide prevent tau aggregation (von Bergen *et al.*, 2001). The repeat region of the tau protein alone can assemble into filaments by forming a β sheet structure. This finding has been confirmed for both native filaments and filaments assembled *in vitro* from expressed wild and mutant tau proteins. Similarly, fibrillization of recombinant tau can be induced by treatment with various agents, including phospho-transferases, polyanionic compounds and fatty acids. However, under similar conditions other proteins also tend to show PHF-like assemblies *in vitro*, e.g. the *C*-terminal end of amyloid protein precursor (APP) and α1-antichymotrypsin.

The *N*-terminal tau domain is not able to form filaments, and it appears to have an inhibitory effect on the formation of tau aggregates. This is further confirmed by the fact that 'big' tau, the isoform found in the peripheral nervous system containing the longest *N*-terminal domain, does not form filamentous aggregates.

Several putative mechanisms for the formation of intra-cellular filaments, including PHFs and SFs, have been suggested:

- proteolytic processing of tau protein;
- mechanisms that detach or decrease the association of tau protein from the MT-binding site;
- mutations in the MAPT gene; and
- enhancement of tau aggregation by the presence of other proteins.

31.2.1 Proteolytic processing of tau protein

Peptides containing little more than the MT-binding region of the tau protein molecule are capable of polyamine-induced self-assembly *in vitro*. Furthermore, NFTs in neurodegenerative disorders contain *N*- and/or *C*-terminally truncated tau protein. Although the *C*-terminal end of the tau protein molecule inhibits polymerization *in vitro*, this inhibitory effect is eliminated following activation of various caspases, and only then can the self-assembly of tau protein occur.

Aggregation of tau protein requiring only the *C*-terminal truncation downstream of the MT-binding region of the protein molecule has been pursued in this model, based upon the molecular findings that tau protein extracted from PHFs is truncated at the *C*-terminal end (Glu391; Wischik *et al.* 1988) (Plate 10). Monoclonal antibodies raised against this site immunolabel PHFs that are stripped of their 'fuzzy coat' (the *N*- and the *C*-terminal portion of the tau protein molecule). The remaining MT-binding region in this model is considered sufficient to promote self-assembly with other tau MT domains, based on its self-propagating properties. Namely, the truncated tau aggregate generated after the first binding (or 'digestion' cycle) is able to bind full-length tau protein, even with increased affinity. This self-propagation cycle has been demonstrated *in vitro* using tau bound to a solid phase (Wischik and Harrington, 2000). Anionic surfaces presented as micelles or vesicles may well serve to nucleate this type of tau fibrillization. In this model, phosphorylation of tau protein does not enhance tau–tau binding but rather inhibits binding by 24–50-fold.

C-terminal caspase cleavage of the tau protein at Asp421 has 67 per cent more and 10-fold faster polymerization than the full-length tau protein. Furthermore, caspase cleavage and truncation at Asp421 is also observed in Aβ-treated neurones. This may provide a link between amyloid deposition and the neurofibrillary changes in AD.

31.2.2 Post-translational modification of tau protein: role of phosphorylation

Post-translational modifications are important for the physiological activity of tau protein, and contribute to pathological assembly of the protein into intraneuronal or glial tau pathology. Such modifications include phosphorylation, glycosylation, acetylation and nitration. Nitrated tau aggregates are present in various taupathies, including AD, Down's syndrome (DS), CBD, PSP, Pick's disease and FTDP-17. The extent of *O*-glycosylation is equal to the extent of serine/threonine (Ser/Thr) phosphorylation of the tau protein molecule, suggesting a role both in modulating tau protein function and the formation of PHFs.

Of 79 putative tau phosphorylation sites, at least 30 have been identified. These residues are predominantly outside the MT-binding region with the exception of six phosphorylation sites located in R1-R4: Ser262(R1), Ser285(R1-R2 interrepeat),

Table 31.1 *Phosphorylated and proteolytic sites of the tau protein in fetal and adult human brain and various proposed stages of tangle development. (According to Wischik et al., 1988; Jicha et al., 1997; Brion et al., 1999; Buée, 2000; Augustinack et al., 2002; Lauckner et al., 2003)*

Tangle stages	Phosphorylation and truncation sites of tau protein
Fetal and adult human brain	pSer199, pSer202, pThr205, pThr231, pSer262, pSer396, pSer404
Pre-tangles	pThr153, pSer199/pS202/pThr205, pThr231, pSer262, pSer396, pSer404, pSer409, pSer422
Intracellular NFTs	pSer46, pThr175/pThr181, pSer199, pSer202, pSer214, pSer262/pSer356, pS396/pSer404, pSer422
Extracellular NFTs	pSer199/pSer202/pThr205, pThr212/pSer214, pSer396/pSer404, Glu391 truncation
Glial/astrocytic tau filaments and NFTs	pSer199/pSer202/pThr205, pSer262/pSer356, pSer396/pSer404

Glu, glutamine; NFTs, neurofibrillary tangles; Ser, serine; Thr, threonine

---

Box 31.2 *Protein kinases, phosphatases and modulators of tau phosphorylation involved in regulating (de)phosphorylation of the tau protein molecule in normal ageing and dementia*

Proline-directed kinases (Ser–Pro and Thr–Pro sites)
- Glycogen synthase kinase-3 (GSK-3)
- Cyclin-dependent kinase-5 (cdk5)
- Protein kinase A (PKA)
- Mitogen-activated kinases
- Microtubule-affinity-regulating kinases (MARK)

Tyrosine-directed kinases
- Tyrosine kinase fyn
- MAP kinases (stress-activated kinases)
- Phospho-JNK (c-jun NH_2-terminal kinase)
- p38
- Extracellular signal-regulated kinase 1 (ERK-1)
- ERK-2

Protein phosphatases (Ser/Thr sites)
- Protein phosphatase 1 (PP1)
- PP2A
- PP2B
- PP2C

Modulators of tau phosphorylation
- Pin1 (prolyl isomerase binding to Thr231 and isomerizing Pro232)
- Cholesterol

Ser305(R2-R3 interrepeat), Ser324(R3) and Ser352 and Ser356(R4). The extent of phosphorylation of tau protein is inversely associated with attachment to the MT network, especially when phosphorylated at sites Ser214 and Ser262. Phosphorylation outside the MT-binding region also influences MT assembly, reducing the tau-tubulin binding affinity (Plate 10).

Although tau protein hyperphosphorylation is considered to facilitate and induce self-assembly of each of the six tau isoforms into PHFs and SFs (see Plate 11), the same sites of tau phosphorylation are also present in fetal and native adult human tau protein (Table 31.1). Thus, phosphorylated Ser199 (pSer199) is expressed in the hippocampus in childhood, in neurones vulnerable to neurodegeneration in young adults, in early and late stages of AD, and in other neurodegenerative disorders with neurofibrillary pathology. Similarly, other tau phosphorylated sites (pSer202, pThr205, pSer262: pSer396, and pSer404) are found in fetal, adult human and AD brain tissue. In addition to pSer199 and pSer202, diffuse intra-neuronal accumulation of pSer409 and pSer422 is present in the so-called 'pretangle' stage of tau aggregates (Table 31.1; Plate 11). pSer262 is the only site in the first repeat of tau that is phosphorylated. pSer262 neither alters the binding affinity of tau to MT nor abolishes the MT-binding, regardless of the phosphorylation state of flanking domains.

31.2.2.1 PROTEIN KINASES AND PHOSPHATASE INHIBITORS

Up-regulation of protein kinases and down-regulation of phosphatase inhibitor activities are both implicated in the abnormal phosphorylation of the tau protein molecule in neurodegenerative disorders (Box 31.2).

Numerous protein kinases are involved in both the physiological and pathological phosphorylation of tau protein. Thus, GSK3β is involved in developmental Wnt signalling (important for proper axis formation during embryonic development), and it also phosphorylates tau at the same sites that are phosphorylated in AD. Similarly, exposure of cortical and primary neuronal cultures to amyloid protein induces GSK3β activity (Takashima *et al.*, 1998). This activity is also regulated by other protein kinases, e.g. protein kinase B (PKB) that inactivates GSK3β. The increase in PKB levels corresponds with an increase in total tau protein levels.

Different protein kinases phosphorylate tau protein at different sites (Table 31.2), and can influence tau-MT-binding. MAPK and GSK proline-directed kinases phosphorylate most Ser-Pro and Thr-Pro motifs in the regions flanking the MT repeat domain of tau protein, and these phosphorylated sites have little effect on tau-MT interactions. In contrast, MARK and PKA phosphorylate several sites within the MT-binding repeats including Ser262, Ser324 and Ser356. These sites, along with pSer214 (phosphorylated by PKA only), strongly decrease affinity of tau for MTs and inhibit filament formation. Similarly, Rho kinase tau phosphorylation leads to decreased activity of tau in promoting MT assembly. Intraneuronal cdc2 accumulation appears to progress the deposition of pSer202/pThr205 tau sites and suggests that cdc2

Table 31.2   *Implication of protein kinases and phosphatase inhibitors in phosphorylation of the tau protein molecule. MAPK family includes SAPK/JNK-P, p38-P, MAPK/ERK-P. MAPK family and GSK3β are present in neuronal populations and also in some astrocytes and oligodendrocytes. In addition to these kinases, Rho kinase phosphorylates tau at Thr245, Thr377, Ser409 and also phosphorylates Ser262 to some extent, and leads to decreased activity of tau to promote MT assembly (Amano et al., 2003). PKA and GSK3β also phosphorylate additional sites (Adapted from Tseng et al., 1999, Bennecib et al., 2000; Tomizawa et al., 2001; Ferrer et al., 2002, 2003; Rank et al., 2002).*

Protein kinases/phosphatase inhibitors	Thr181	Ser202	Thr205	Ser208/210	Ser214	Thr231	Ser235	Ser262	Ser396/404	Ser422
MAPK	✓	✓						✓	✓	✓
PKA					✓		✓	✓		
GSK-3β		✓			✓	✓	✓	✓	✓	
TPK-II						✓				
TTK				✓						
Cdc2		✓	✓			✓	✓			
Cdk5									✓	
↓PP1		✓*						✓**	✓*	
↓PP2A		✓						✓**	✓	✓

*PP1 up-regulates the phosphorylation at these sites indirectly by regulating the activities of GSK3β, cdk5 and cdc2
**Decreased activity of PP2A and PP1 promotes CaMKII activity and leads to phosphorylation of this site and Ser356
TTK, tau-tubulin kinase; TPK, tau-protein kinase

is involved in the abnormal phosphorylation of tau and consequent aggregation into PHFs at an early stage (Pei *et al.*, 2002).

Various protein kinases are differentially expressed in tau deposits in neurones and glial cells in the taupathies (Ferrer *et al.*, 2001). Thus, MAPK/ERK-P has been detected in a subset of neurones and glial cells bearing phosphorylated tau deposits, but rarely in NFTs; p38-P immunoreactivity in a majority of tangle-bearing neurones (in AD, PSP and CBD), pretangle neurones, astrocytes and coiled bodies (in PSP and CBD), neuritic plaque corona in AD, Pick's bodies in Pick's disease; SAPK/JNK-P immunoreactivity in neurones and in glial cells that accumulate tau aggregates in AD, Pick's disease, PSP and CBD; CaM kinase II is selective for neurones but not glial cells.

Protein phosphatases rapidly dephosphorylate tau protein (Box 31.2). Their activity is developmentally regulated and counterbalances the action of protein kinases. Reduction of protein phosphatase activities is linked to the formation of PHF-tau. Phosphatases are associated directly (PP2A) or indirectly (e.g. PP1 via tau protein) with microtubules. In neurodegenerative disorders, particularly AD, the levels of expression of protein phosphatase mRNA and activity of the enzymes are substantially depleted in brain areas harbouring the highest density of tau pathology.

31.2.3   Mutations in the MAPT gene

Alterations in tau genotype have been extensively investigated with respect to their contribution to the development of neurodegenerative dementias. The extended tau haplotypes H1 and H2 (referring to contiguous polymorphisms in exons 1, 7 and 13 and in intron 9), covering the entire human tau gene, are associated with various neurodegenerative disorders. Thus H1 haplotype is overrepresented in PSP, FTDP-17 and, more inconsistently, in CBD, Parkinson's disease and AD, but not in amyotrophic lateral sclerosis. In contrast,

the H2 haplotype is associated with FTD with fluent, anomic aphasia. The tau gene haplotypes have a synergistic effect on apolipoprotein E (ApoE) ε2 and ε4 alleles, and can significantly increase the risk for AD and FTD (Short *et al.*, 2002). Although the over-representation of H1 haplotype seems to be characteristic for the 4R taupathies, this is not the case for argyrophilic grain disease (AGD).

The discovery of mutations in the MAPT gene in frontotemporal lobe dementia linked to chromosome 17 consolidated the evidence about the importance of tau protein pathology alone in generating a dementia syndrome. To date, various missense, deletion, silent and intronic mutations in the MAPT gene have been identified in both familial and sporadic forms of dementia. The mutations are localized in exons 1, 9–13 and in introns 9–11 (Table 31.3). Overall, the frequency of tau mutations in non-AD taupathies is relatively low (on average 6 per cent), and is increased in familial forms of taupathies (11–33 per cent; Poorkaj *et al.*, 2001).

31.2.3.1   EFFECT OF TAU MUTATIONS ON TAU–MICROTUBULE BINDING

It has been suggested that altered tau properties owing to mutations can lead to an increase in unbound MT mutant tau isoforms in the neuronal cytoplasm, and increase the ability of tau to self-aggregate into filament structures. Indeed, the majority of missense mutations impair the ability of tau protein to bind and polymerize microtubules, irrespective of posttranslational modifications. However, a non-significant impact of tau missense mutations upon tau–microtubule interactions has also been reported. These inconsistent findings may reflect differences in various tau mutations with respect to their ability to bind to microtubules, promote MT assembly and bundle MTs. Thus, some mutations (e.g. G272V or P301L) have more subtle effects on MTs in comparison to V337M or R406W, especially since the former two mutations are present in 3R but

Table 31.3 *Tau protein mutations, clinical phenotypes and their effect upon tau protein properties*

Mutations	Clinical phenotypes	Tau properties
Exon 1: R5H; R5L	PSP FTDP-17	Decreased tau binding to MT Increased tau fibrillation Neuronal and glial inclusions
Intron4: E4+39	PSP	Not described
Exon9: K257T; I260V; L266V; G272V	Pick's disease Pick-like disease FTDP-17	Decrease in MT assembly Tau positive Pick's body-like inclusions. Filaments contain 3R and 4R tau (predominantly 3R)
Intron 9: E9+33	Familial FTD	Not described Altered alternative splicing of tau protein
Exon 10: N279K; ΔK280; L284L; N296H; N296N; ΔN296; P301L; P301S; S305N; S305S	PPND PSP FTDP-17 AD CBD PSP/CBD	Decreased tau ability to bind to MT Inclusions consisting of twisted ribbons of 4R tau isoforms in neurons and glia
Intron 10: E10+3; E10+11; E10+12; E10+13; E10+14; E10+16; E10+19; E10+29; E10+33	FTDP-17 PSP CBD Familial MSA Familial PSG	Increase in exon 10 inclusions, except for E10+19 and E10+29, where there is decrease
Exon 11: L315R; S320Y; S320F	Pick's disease	Decrease in MT assembly Pick's body inclusions Filaments contain 3R and 4R (absence of 0N3R isoform)
Intron 11: E11+34	AD	Not described
Exon12: V337M; E342V; S352L*; K369I	FTDP-17 Pick's disease	Decrease in MT assembly Neuronal pathology identical to AD or similar to PD Decreased phosphorylation of tau protein Accelerated filament formation 4R tau isoforms (with exception of V337M and K369I mutations that have 3R filaments)
Exon13: G389R; R406W	Pick's disease PSP	Decrease in MT assembly Pick-body like inclusions Straight and twisted filaments R406W alters tau susceptibility for phosphorylation 3R and 4R tau

*Recessive taupathy with acute respiratory failure
PPND, palidopontonigral degeneration; PSG, progressive subcortical gliosis

not in 4R tau, suggesting that the effect of tau mutations on microtubules is site- and isoform-dependent. In addition, mutations affecting the alternative splicing of exon 10 (N279K, delK280, L284L, N296N, S305S, S305N and intronic mutations proximal to the 5'-splice site of exon 10) alter the ratio of tau mRNA with or without exon 10 (E10+/E10−). All but one of these splicing mutations (delK280) and two tau mutations in the intronic sequence following the stem loop structure in exon 10 (E10+19 and E10+29) cause an increase in the proportion of 4R tau, and reduce the level of 3R isoforms. These three mutations result in an increase in 3R tau, decrease in 4R and decrease in MT assembly.

The diverse effects of tau mutations may account for the different clinical and pathological phenotypes in the various taupathies, especially the heterogeneous FTDP-17 disorders. In support of this is the example of clinical and biochemical

diversity of three tau mutations in the same codon (N296) in exon 10 of the MAPT gene. Two mutations, N296N and N296H are associated with similar autosomal dominant FTDP-17-like phenotypes with age of onset in the mid-50s. In contrast, the third mutation (delN296) gives rise to atypical PSP in individuals homozygous for the mutation, whereas in heterozygotic individuals the phenotype is similar to idiopathic Parkinson's disease. The N296N mutation increases the inclusion of exon 10 in tau mRNA and therefore increases the ratio of 4R/3R tau protein. The N296H mutation, however, causes increased splicing out of exon 10: reduces the ability of tau to promote tubulin polymerization and increases tau aggregation (Grover *et al.*, 2002).

delN296 has no or very little effect on splicing, but since asparagine at position 296 is key to disruption of the MT-binding region, delN296 causes a large reduction in the ability of tau to promote MT assembly (delN296>N296H). Its effect on tau filament formation appears to be inconsistent, with both increased (delN296>N296H) and no effect reported on the self-aggregation of tau into filaments.

Some of the mutations in exons 9 and 12 (e.g. K257T, G272V, V337M and K369I) also stimulate the heparin-induced assembly of filaments *in vitro*. Two mutations within exon 10, P301L and P301S cause the same effect. These two mutations lead to neuronal and glial pathology with narrow, twisted and ribbon-like filaments composed of 4R tau, similar to those found in PSP (Spillantini *et al.*, 1998). Transgenic mice expressing tau containing the G272V mutation develop oligodendroglial fibrillary lesions consisting of both straight and twisted filaments, associated with phosphorylation of tau protein at Ser202/Thr205 sites (Götz *et al.*, 2001a). Ultrastructural differences in the spacing of microtubules have been reported for the mutation V337M in exon 12 using transfected cells and transgenic mice. In the latter, tau aggregates form in the hippocampus, and MT are lost in degenerating neurones.

Correlations between genotype and phenotype have now been described for FDTP-17. Mutations within exon 10 and the intron following exon 10 result in filamentous neuronal and glial tau pathology. In exon 10 mutations, the tau filaments are narrow twisted ribbons consisting predominantly of 4R tau isoforms, whereas in the case of intronic mutations, the filaments are wide twisted ribbons, formed exclusively from 4R tau isoforms. Missense mutations outside exon 10 lead to predominantly neuronal pathology with PHFs and SFs consisting of all six tau isoforms (Spillantini *et al.*, 1997).

31.2.3.2 TAU MUTATIONS AND TAU PROTEIN PHOSPHORYLATION

Mutations in tau protein also affect its phosphorylation. Thus, decreased phosphorylation is found at Ser202/Thr205 and Ser396/Ser404 sites in neuroblastoma cell lines transfected with 0N4R tau isoforms carrying the missense mutations P301L, V337M and R406W. The integrity of microtubules is not affected, but intracellular tau protein levels are increased with all mutations. Additional studies on *in vitro* phosphorylation of wild type 2N4R tau and mutant forms (P301L, V337M and R406W) by GSK3β found alteration in the extent of phosphorylation in P301L or V377M tau in comparison to R406W tau. The latter mutation decreases phosphorylation at various tau sites. These phosphorylation sites are similar to those in V337M mutation, except for the Ser396/Ser404 site which is increased in the latter mutation.

These *in vitro* results differ from the tau phosphorylation status in brain tissue from some FTDP-17 individuals. Thus, the Sarcosyl-insoluble fraction of R406W tau extracted from brain tissue of a FTDP-17 case is highly phosphorylated in contrast to the soluble R406W tau that is less phosphorylated than wild-type tau. On the other hand, P301L and P301S transgenic mice brains exhibit a higher degree of tau phosphorylation at numerous sites in Sarcosyl and acid-extractable fractions and filaments (Götz *et al.*, 2001b).

31.2.4 Facilitation of tau aggregation in the presence of other proteins

Tau aggregation can be facilitated by co-incubation of the tau protein with other proteins. Thus, co-incubation with sulphated glycosaminoglycans in close to physiological conditions will result in tau assembly only when tau protein is present at 40–100 times higher than physiological concentrations. Similarly, thrombin induces rapid tau protein hyperphosphorylation, and this is related to p44/42 mitogen activated protein kinase activation.

31.2.4.1 HEPARIN AND TAU AGGREGATION

A short segment of tau located in the third MT-binding domain (residues 317–335) is probably the minimal segment of that region able to grow into filaments *in vitro* in the presence of heparin. The 1/2R peptides corresponding to either N- or C-terminal halves of this segment are unable to form filaments. The C-terminal domain contains a sequence spanning from residues 391–407 that grows into filaments *in vitro*, irrespective of whether it is incubated with heparin (Pérez *et al.*, 2001).

31.2.4.2 Aβ AND TAU AGGREGATION

Positive correlation between amyloid deposits and tangles has been demonstrated in various neuropathological studies for both AD and DS, although the sites of initiation of these two distinct neuropathological features are different (Braak and Braak, 1991). However, some of the taupathies (including CBD, PSP, senile dementia with tangles, FTDP-17) do not exhibit amyloid pathology.

Transgenic animals with amyloid protein precursor (APP) and presenilin proteins 1 and 2 (PS1 and PS2) carrying pathogenic mutations have been used to address the relationship between altered amyloid protein processing and tau aggregates. Thus, Tg2576 mice (with APP695 K595N/M596L mutation), as well as having a substantial degree of brain amyloid deposition, have phosphorylated tau protein within some dystrophic neurites of senile plaques. The major kinase for tau phosphorylation is GSK3β, although a smaller contribution from GSK3α, cdk5 and MAPK has also been noted. This suggests that brain amyloidosis has a potential role in inducing taupathy. However, such findings are not consistent. Although elderly transgenic mice with the London mutation (APP V717F) exhibit amyloid plaques and develop hyperphosphorylated tau restricted to dystrophic neurites only, they do not develop filamentous PHF structures. Similar findings have been reported for other APP transgenic models, including the Swedish mutation alone (codon 670/671), APP V717I mutation or the two combined. This indicates that transgenic APP models alone, despite the over expression of APP by 7-fold, are only able to recapitulate the early cytoskeletal changes present in preclinical AD. Furthermore, not all APP mutations have an effect on the phosphorylation state of tau. Thus, the AD-causative V642I mutation of APP results in the secretion of $A\beta_{42}$, in the presence of unaltered levels of phosphorylated tau protein.

The characteristic AD phenotype (plaques and tangles) develops only in transgenic animals that express both APP and tau proteins mutations. Thus, in Lewis et al. (2001) animal model, crossbreeding Tg2576 transgenic mice (which usually develop amyloid deposits by 9–12 months of age) with hemizygous JNPL3 mice (over expressing P301L tau mutation and developing tangle formation by 6 months of age) results in the development of amyloid and tau protein deposits. Likewise, when $A\beta_{42}$ fibrils are injected in the somatosensory cortex and hippocampus in mice expressing tau carrying the P301L mutation, there is a 5-fold increase in neurofibrillary changes in neurones which project into injection sites, and an increase in the level of phosphorylated tau (Götz et al., 2001c). Increased phosphorylation of tau protein also occurs in rat brain after injection with $A\beta_{25-35}$.

Tissue culture studies provide further evidence of a link between the processing of APP and tau protein. Thus cultured hippocampal neurones from wild-type and human tau transgenic mice treated with fibrillar $A\beta$ degenerate, in contrast to tau knockout neurones. The $A\beta_{1-42}$ promotes aggregation of tau protein in vitro in a dose-dependent manner. This $A\beta$ mediated aggregated tau serves as a substrate for tau kinase II (TPKII), leading to an 8-fold increase in TPK-II dependent tau phosphorylation containing pThr231 (Rank et al., 2002). The carboxyl-terminal end of APP has also been shown to be involved in induction of tau phosphorylation by increasing GSK3β activity.

31.2.4.3 PRESENILINS AND TAU AGGREGATION

Presenilin 1 (PS1, residues 250–298) binds to both tau and GSK3β. PS1 point mutations that cause AD (C263R and P264L) result in an increased ability of PS1 to bind to GSK3β and increase its tau-directed kinase activity, resulting in hyperphosphorylation of tau protein (Takashima et al., 1998). In AD, PS1 mutations may promote neuritic dystrophy and tangle formation by interfering with Notch1 signalling and enhancing pathological changes in tau.

The strongest evidence that PS1 contributes to tau phosphorylation comes from studies exploring PS1 mutations in association with $A\beta$, in both in vitro studies and transgenic animal models. Thus, in cultures treated with $A\beta$, PS1 mutations M146V and I143T significantly increase neuritic dystrophy and AD-like changes in tau such as hyperphosphorylation, release from MTs, and increased tau protein levels. In transgenic mice with Swedish APP (K670N, M671L) and PS1 M146L gene mutations, hyperphosphorylation of the tau protein lags behind the accumulation of $A\beta$ deposits and is manifested by punctate intraneuronal deposits and dystrophic neurites in the cortex and hippocampus (Kurt et al., 2003). Transgenic mice carrying both the Swedish APP mutation and PS1 P264L mutation develop neurites containing phosphorylated tau, and this correlates with activation of MAP kinase pathways (Savage et al., 2002). Mice transgenic for

both human tau and PS1 M146L mutation also produce an increase in tau phosphorylation similar to that which occurs in transgenic mice carrying human tau, suggesting that the presenilin mutations alone may not be sufficient to induce neurofibrillary pathology. Similarly, I143T and G384A PS1 mutations in vitro do not increase tau phosphorylation.

31.2.4.4 α-SYNUCLEIN AND TAU AGGREGATION

The C-terminal end of α-synuclein can bind to the MT-binding region of the tau protein, and can stimulate the protein kinase A-catalysed phosphorylation of tau protein at Ser262 and Ser356 residues. Furthermore, high concentrations of tubulin inhibit the tau-α-synuclein binding. These findings suggest that α-synuclein modulates tau phosphorylation and indirectly affects the stability of axonal MTs.

31.2.4.5 APOLIPOPROTEIN E AND TAU AGGREGATION

ApoE plays a role in lipid metabolism and in humans is represented by three isoforms (ApoE2, ApoE3 and ApoE4, corresponding to three alleles, ε2, ε3 and ε4, respectively). Although ApoE is a glial protein, it is also found in a small number of cortical neurones, restricted to cell body and proximal dendrites. In AD, a small number of neurones devoid of NFTs contain ApoE diffuse cytoplasmic accumulation. ApoE is also found in some tangle-bearing neurones, predominantly in extracellular NFTs.

The ε4 allele of ApoE gene is a strong susceptibility factor for some of the taupathies, including AD, DLB, Pick's disease and CBD. However, in other taupathies, including the tangle-only form of AD ('senile dementia with tangles') and AGD, there is a low prevalence of the ApoE ε4 allele or an increase in the ε2 allele when compared with age-matched or AD subjects. This inconsistent association of ApoE ε4 allele with taupathies mirrors the findings regarding ApoE ε4 allele influence on neurofibrillary pathology. Thus no differences, and an increase in neurofibrillary pathology burden (tangles and neuritic plaques) and phosphorylated tau have been described in ApoE ε4 allele carriers (Mukaetova-Ladinska et al., 1997).

Previous studies have failed to demonstrate ApoE influence upon tau phosphorylation, leading to the conclusion that ApoE intraneuronal accumulation may be secondary in tangle-bearing neurones in response to repair processes induced by tangle-associated neuronal damage. However, isoform-specific interactions of ApoE with tau may regulate intraneuronal tau metabolism and alter the rate of filamentous formation and/or the extent of phosphorylation. Flaherty et al. (1999) tested the effects of ApoE isoforms (E2, E3 and E4) on tau phosphorylation in brain microtubule fractions and found that ApoE attenuates tau hyperphosphorylation in the fractions, but the pattern was indistinguishable for the different isoforms. Binding studies with fragments of ApoE demonstrate that the tau-binding region of ApoE3 corresponds to its receptor-binding domain and is distinct from the region that binds lipoprotein particles or $A\beta$ peptide. ApoE fragments, especially the truncated ApoE4 (Delta 272–299), can induce tangle-like intraneuronal inclusions containing phosphory-lated tau and high molecular weight neurofilaments.

The influence of ApoE and its isoforms upon tau aggregation has been explored further in animal studies. Transgenic mice expressing human ApoE4 isoform have impaired axonal transport, axonal degeneration and hyperphosphorylated tau protein in their brains. Kobayashi *et al.* (2003) examined the effect of specific isoforms using transgenic 'knock-in' (KI) mice. There were no significant differences in levels of tau phosphorylation between ApoE3-KI and ApoE4-KI mouse hippocampi. Selective up-regulation of pSer235 and pSer413 and decrease at pSer202/pThr205 and pThr205, with an increase in protein level of tau protein kinase I/glycogen synthase kinase 3β (TPKI/GSK3β) and extracellular signal-regulated kinase 2 (ERK2) were demonstrated for ApoE4-KI mice, when compared with ApoE3-KI mice. However, ApoE-deficient mice which show learning and memory impairments also exhibit hyperphosphorylation localized *N*-terminally to the MT-binding domain of tau (Genis *et al.*, 2000).

31.3 TAU PROTEIN: PATHOLOGICAL AND BIOCHEMICAL CHANGES IN NEURODEGENERATION

31.3.1 Tau pathology in ageing

Intraneuronal tau aggregates are characteristic for the ageing human and primate brain. However, these changes are not unique to the brain tissue and NFTs and 'curly fibres' can also be found in other organs, including liver, pancreas, ovary, testis and thyroid in elderly individuals with AD. The frequency of neuro-fibrillary pathology, especially NFTs, increases with age. Thus, it is estimated that nearly half of people over the age of 50 years and all the elderly over 75 years will exhibit NFTs restricted predominantly to the medial temporal lobe. A community-based neuropathological study conducted in elderly people in the UK (70–103 years at death) found NFTs in 61 per cent of the elderly with dementia and 34 per cent of non-demented individuals (Neuropathology Group of the Medical Research Council Cognitive Function and Ageing Study [MRC CFAS], 2001).

31.3.2 Comparative pathology in taupathies

The clinical manifestations of the taupathies differ due to involvement of specific neuroanatomical domains and distinct neuropathological and molecular substrates. More extensive and widespread tau pathology, including numerous NFTs, neuritic plaques and dystrophic neurites in various allo- and neocortical areas, is commonly found in AD, elderly DS individuals and in some individuals with DLB. In general the development of NFTs is initiated in the medial temporal lobe areas, particularly the α-layer of the entorhinal cortex, and then progresses via the hippocampal area back to the pre-α layer of the entorhinal cortex (corresponding to

Braak stages [BST] 1 and 2). More pronounced tangle pathology in entorhinal and transentorhinal cortex (BST 3 and 4) follows before its appearance in neocortical areas, including primary sensory and striate areas (BST 5 and 6) (Braak and Braak, 1991). The most affected neocortical areas in AD are the temporal and parietal neocortex, followed by the frontal and occipital lobes (Mukaetova-Ladinska *et al.*, 1993). Widespread neurofibrillary pathology in AD correlates with the severity of cognitive impairment and non-cognitive changes (Mukaetova-Ladinska *et al.*, 2000).

In PSP, CBD and multiple system atrophy (MSA), the development of neurofibrillary pathology within neurones, and oligodendroglia in the case of MSA, is initiated within the subcortical ganglia and centres including basal ganglia, sub-thalamus, brain stem (PSP), cerebellar nuclei and substantia nigra (CBD, MSA), and white matter (MSA). Neocortical areas are relatively spared or even intact. Similar findings have been described for frontal lobe dementia, especially FTDP-17. The subcortical location of tau pathology in these disorders contributes to slow cognitive decline and impaired attentional control and frontal 'executive' function.

Tau aggregates in the form of tangles are also found in glial cells in some of the taupathies (e.g. FTDP-17, PSP, severe stages AD) and they contain phosphorylated tau, both as diffuse aggregates and within tangle formation. Tau protein also accumulates in astrocytes in PSP (referred to as 'tufted' astro-cytes). In AGD, the argyrophilic grains are tau-immunoreactive comma-shaped structures.

Cerebellar neurones in general have substantially less tau protein than neurones in other cortical and medial temporal lobe areas (Mukaetova-Ladinska *et al.*, 1993). However, in some forms of neurodegenerative dementia, e.g. PSP and CBD, 'doughnut'-shaped structures, positive to tau protein, are found in the molecular layers of the cerebellum (in up to 46 per cent of PSP and 29 per cent of CBD patients).

31.3.3 Tau protein incorporation in neurofibrillary pathology

The pattern of incorporation of tau protein into neurofibrillary pathology, especially tangles, undergoes three putative stages:

1. pre-tangles, characterized by non-fibrillar punctate cytoplasmic and dendritic accumulations;
2. intraneuronal tangles, containing fibrillar tau positive structures; and
3. extracellular NFTs ('ghost tangles') when the PHFs remain present in the neuropil once the neuronal cell membrane has been disrupted (see Plate 12).

The sequence of these events includes phosphorylation of various sites of the tau protein molecule, followed by proteolytic cleavage at both the *N*- and the *C*-terminal end, resulting in a 'protease-resistant PHF core' (Table 31.1 p. 411). In advanced stages of AD in particular, astrocytes also contain NFTs. Aggregates of phosphorylated tau are found in the astrocytes in various taupathies, including Pick's disease, but

Colour plates

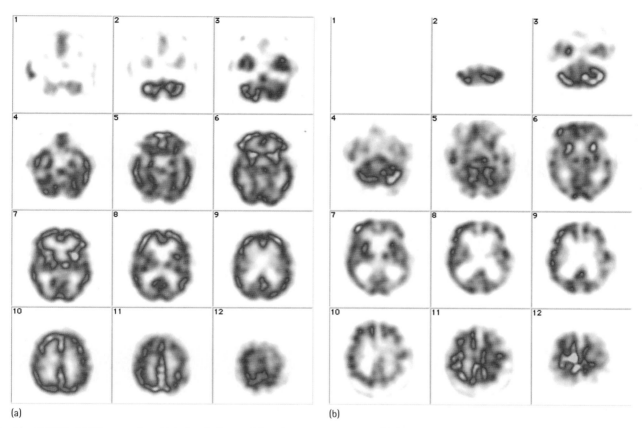

Plate 1 *HMPAO-SPECT scans of an Alzheimer's disease (a) and a vascular dementia (b) patient.*

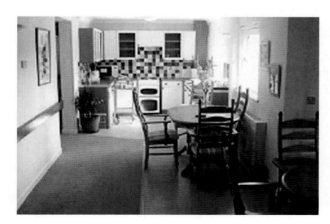

Plate 2 *Dining room, Drumry House, Glasgow.*

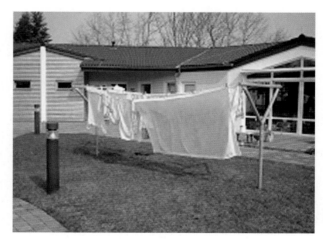

Plate 3 *Washing line, Clara Zetkin Home, Brandenburg.*

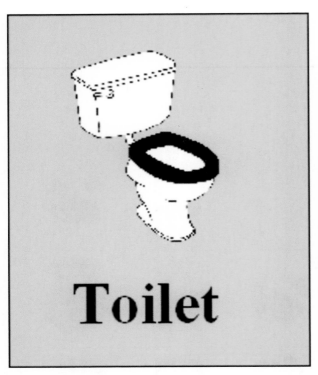

Plate 4   *One of the most effective signs: words and a picture (Wilkinson et al., 1995).*

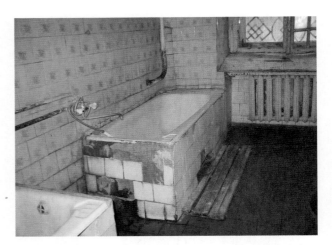

Plate 6   *Bathroom on an old age psychiatry ward somewhere in the former USSR. Note (a) the obvious state of dilapidation; (b) more than one tub (in fact there were three) negates privacy; (c) baths are against the wall preventing nurses from being either side of a disabled patient; (d) such a bathroom is typical of thousands in the region.*

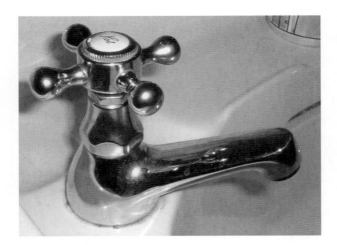

Plate 5   *A cross-head tap is much easier to understand.*

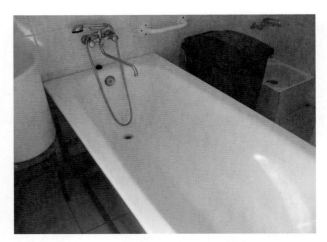

Plate 7   *Money was raised by the Geneva Initiative on Psychiatry for refurbishment of the old age psychiatry ward in the same hospital depicted in Plate 6. The architect was brought to the UK to visit facilities there. This bathroom with a single tub accessible from both sides was the first fruit of his visit.*

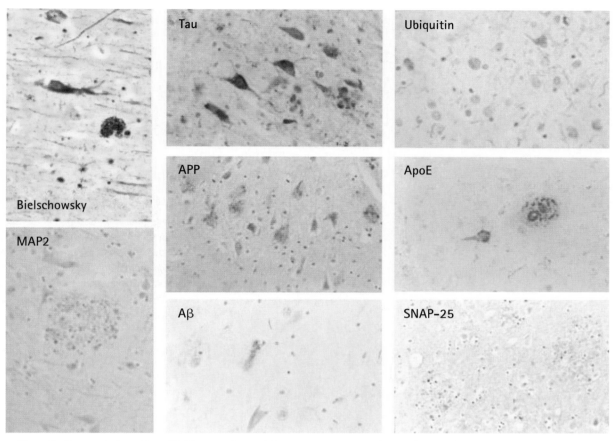

Plate 8 *Neurofibrillary pathology. Neurofibrillary tangles and plaques are seen on sections stained with Bielschowsky silver. Various proteins, including tau, APP, amyloid, synaptic proteins (SNAP-25, synaptophysin), ubiquitin, MAP2, apolipoprotein E also are found within various neurofibrillary structures (tangles, plaques and dystrophic neuritis).*

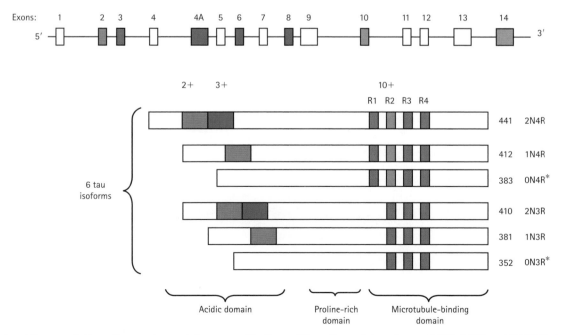

Plate 9 *Schematic presentation of human tau protein gene and isoforms. Alternative splicing of exons 2 (E2), 3 (E3) and 10 (E10) give rise to six isoforms containing 352–441 amino acids. The microtubule repeat binding region is labelled with R1–R4.*
* Fetal tau protein isoforms.

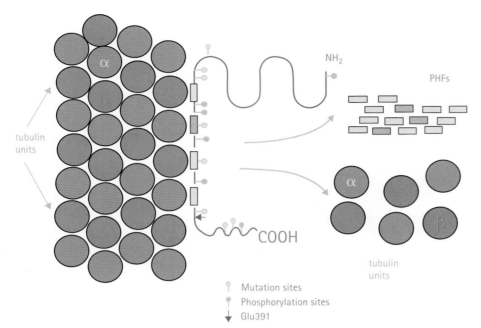

Plate 10 *Binding of tau protein to microtubules. Tau protein binds to α- and β-tubulin subunits via the microtubule-binding region. Phosphorylation and C-terminal end truncation of the tau protein molecule, as well as tau mutations leading to detachment of the protein from the microtubules and assembly into PHFs. Note that the schematic presentation does not reflect all known phosphorylation and mutation sites.*

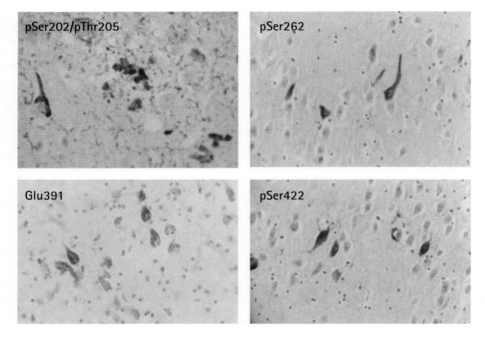

Plate 11 *Phosphorylated and truncated tau protein within neurofibrillary pathology.*

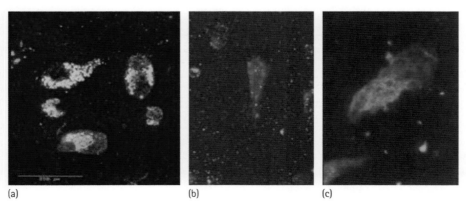

Plate 12 *Stages of tangle development: (a) pre-tangle; (b) intracellular tangles and (c) extracellular tangles.*

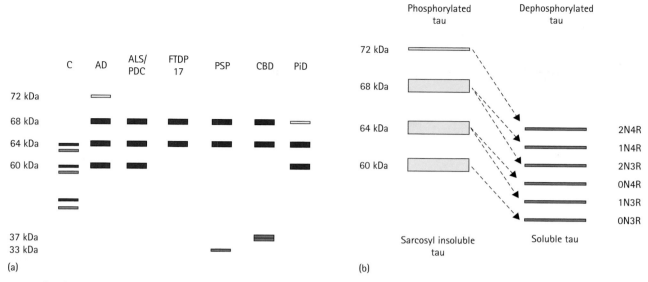

Plate 13 (a, b) *Schematic presentation of western blot patterns in taupathies. (a) Sarcosyl insoluble tau preparations in neurodegenerative disorders are characterized by distinct tau profiles, that depend upon the expression of different tau isoforms, the extent of their phosphorylation, as well as differences in the N-terminal proteolytic cleavage (in the case of PSP and CBD). (b) Upon dephosphorylation, the Sarcosyl insoluble phosphorylated bands resolve into six bands corresponding to the six tau isoforms found in soluble tau preparation. This pattern is also characteristic for the control brain.*

Abbreviations: AD, Alzheimer's disease; ALS/PDC, amyotrophic lateral sclerosis and Parkinson dementia complex; C, control; CBD, corticobasal degeneration; FTDP-17, fronto-temporal lobe dementia and parkinsonism linked to chromosome 17; PiD, Pick's disease; PSP, progressive supranuclear palsy

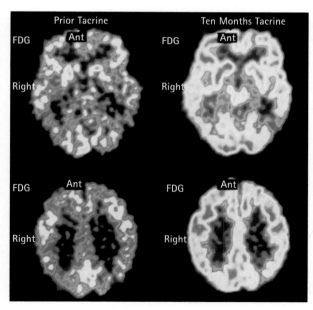

Plate 14 *PET scans before and after tacrine.*

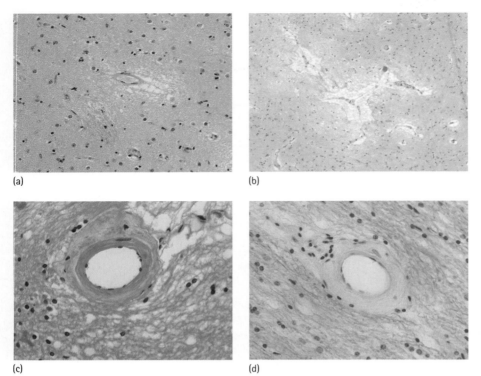

(a)

(b)

(c)

(d)

Plate 15 *Pathological lesions associated with small vessel disease. (a) and (b), small infarcts and several ischaemic foci of two different sizes in the basal ganglia of a 70-year-old man with cognitive impairment. Since the lesion is only visible by microscopic examination, it is hence a microinfarct, which could resolve into a cyst or a lacune. (c) and (d), hyalinized vessels with perivascular rarefaction in the white matter of a 70-year-old man with VaD and 60-year-old woman with CADASIL. Moderate gliosis in the surrounding region is also evident in both cases. Magnification bar: a, b = 500 μm; c, d = 100 μm.*

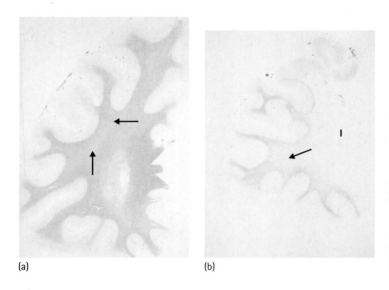

(a)

(b)

Plate 16 *White matter lesions visualized by conventional histopathological staining. (a) and (b), white matter pathology in the frontal lobes of a 75-year-old man and 80-year-old woman diagnosed with VaD. (a) Rarefaction in deep white matter (arrows) with sparing of U-fibres. (b) Regions of severe demyelination (arrow) perifocal to the infarct (I).*

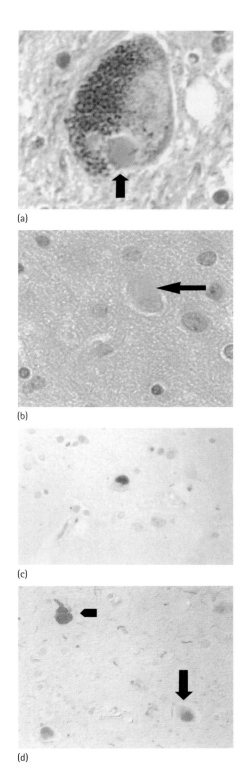

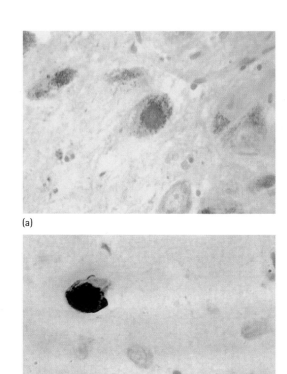

Plate 18 *(a) Substantia nigra neurone containing an α-synuclein reactive Lewy body in the centre of the neuromelanin cluster. (b) α-Synuclein reactive cortical Lewy body. Cortical Lewy bodies and brainstem Lewy bodies frequently stain as an outer halo only with α-synuclein antibodies.*

Plate 17 *(a) Typical subtantia nigra Lewy body with eosinophilic core and clear halo (arrow). (b) Cortical Lewy bodies are much less distinct and lack a well-defined halo (arrow). (c) Anti-ubiquitin antibodies allow more ready identification of cortical Lewy bodies in most cases. (d) In a case with mixed cortical Lewy bodies (arrow) and neurofibrillary tangles (arrowhead), the distinction between these lesions depends on the quality of the ubiquitin staining, especially the fine granular staining of cortical Lewy bodies.*

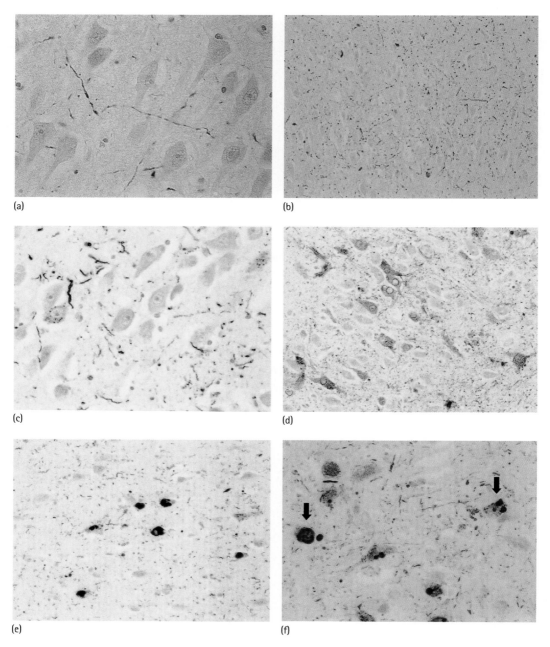

Plate 19 *(a) Scanty Lewy neurites in hippocampal sector CA2 reactive to ubiquitin. (b) DLB patient with abundant ubiquitin reactive neuritic change in CA2. (c) Lewy neurites are strongly reactive for α-synuclein (CA2 sector). (d) In many cases, both neurites and CA2 neurones show reactivey to some phosphorylated tau epitopes (e.g. tau-2). The neuronal staining is frequently diffuse and granular and does not form neurofibrillary tangles. (e) Neocortical Lewy bodies and Lewy neurites reactive for α-synuclein in a case of DLB. (f) Substantia nigra Lewy bodies (arrows) and Lewy neurites are morphologically indistinguishable in DLB and Parkinson's disease.*

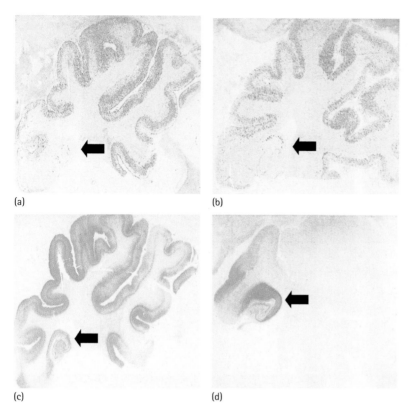

(a)

(b)

(c)

(d)

Plate 20 *(a, c) Alzheimer's disease patient.
(b, d) Dementia with Lewy bodies 'common form' patient.
The two cases show similar intensity and distribution of
βA 4 staining (a, b) throughout the temporal lobes,
including the hippocampal formation (arrows). The lamina
of plaques in the dentate molecular layer is clearly visible,
especially in the DLB tissue. The Alzheimer's disease patient
shows intense staining for PHF-tau (c) in the whole of the
temporal neocortex and hippocampus. BY contrast,
PHF-tau staining in DLB (d) is confined to the CA1 sector
of the hippocampus and part of the entorhinal cortex.*

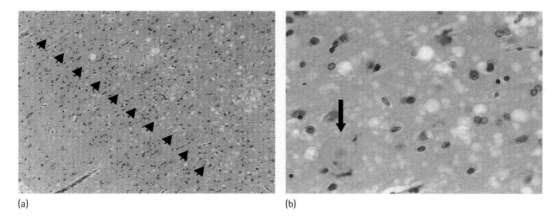

(a)

(b)

Plate 21 *Microvacuolation in the temporal cortex. This patient shows an extreme degree of vacuolar degeneration of the neuropil sufficient to
raise a suspicion of a prion disorder. Creutzfeldt-Jakob disease was excluded by prion immunocytochemistry. At low power (a) the changes are
most marked in cortical layer 3 (above the arrowheads). At higher power (b) amyloid plaques (arrow) typical of Alzheimer's disease are present.
This case showed widespread cortical Lewy body formation.*

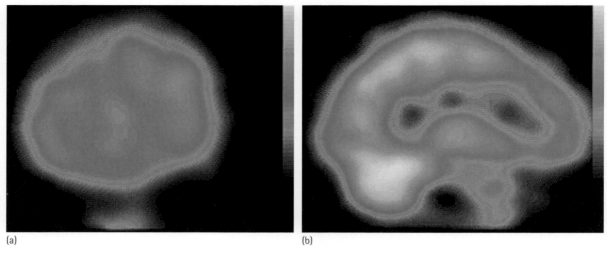

(a)

(b)

Plate 22 *SPECT scan of patient with FTD. The coronal (a) and sagittal (b) views show marked reduction in uptake of tracer in the anterior cerebral hemispheres.*

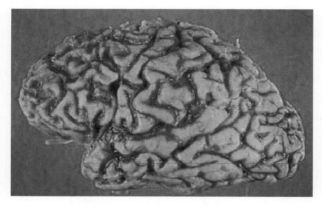

Plate 23 *The brain in FTLD. The whole brain shows severe frontotemporal atrophy.*

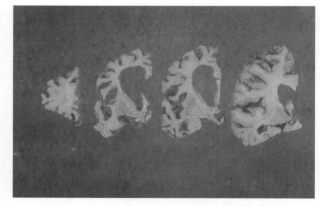

Plate 24 *The brain in FTLD. On coronal section frontotemporal atrophy is accompanied by dilatation of the lateral ventricle and atrophy of the corpus striatum.*

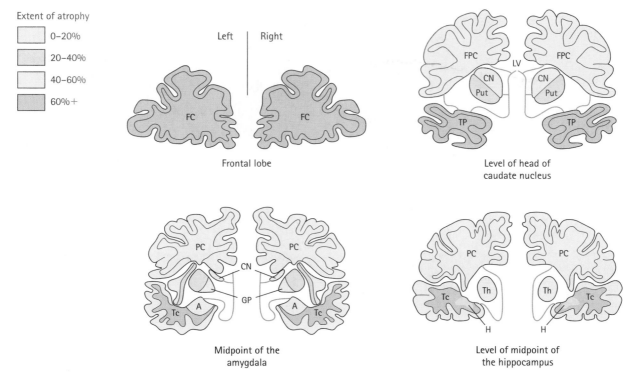

Extent of atrophy

- 0–20%
- 20–40%
- 40–60%
- 60%+

Left | Right

FC — FC

Frontal lobe

FPC — FPC
LV
CN / Put — CN / Put
TP — TP

Level of head of
caudate nucleus

PC — PC
CN
GP
Tc — A — A — Tc

Midpoint of the
amygdala

PC — PC
Tc — Th — Th — Tc
H — H

Level of midpoint of
the hippocampus

Plate 25   *The brain in FTLD. The distribution of atrophy is illustrated diagrammatically.*

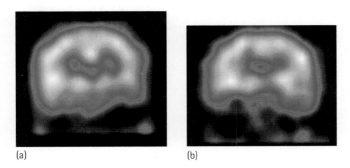

(a)   (b)

Plate 27   *SPECT scans of two patients with semantic dementia
showing abnormal uptake of tracer in the temporal lobes, in one case
(a) especially on the left side and in the other case (b) on the right.*

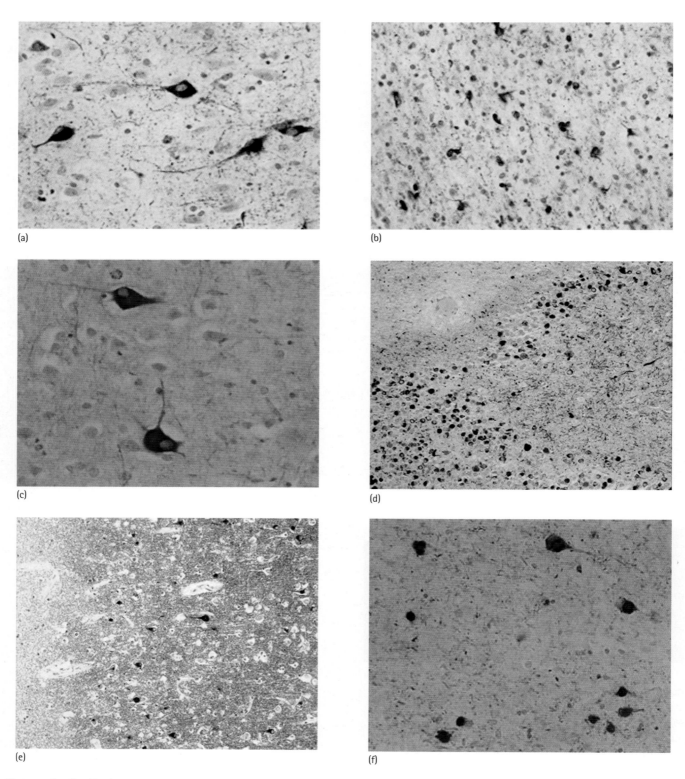

Plate 26 (a–f) *Tau immunopathology in FTLD. In FTDP-17 associated with + 16 splice site mutation (a, b) – there are numerous tau-immunoreactive neurones (a) and glial cells (b) in which the aggregated tau is present as amorphous deposits or tangle-like structures. Numerous tau-immunoreactive swollen cells are present (c). In FTDP-17 associated with Q336R mutation the aggregated tau is present as rounded inclusions (Pick bodies) within neurones of the cerebral cortex (d) and hippocampus dentate gyrus (e) that are similar in appearance to those seen in sporadic FTLD with Pick-type histology (f). Swollen cells similar to those in + 16 mutation (c) are also present (not shown).*

not frontotemporal lobar degeneration. In FTDP-17, straight filaments appear to be phosphorylated at Ser202/Thr205 and Ser212/Thr214 sites (G372V mutation; Götz et al., 2001a). Certain tau phosphorylation sites (e.g. Ser202/Thr205 and phosphorylation at [159]PPGQK[163] site), together with truncation at Glu391 within the NFTs, have now been associated with neuronal apoptosis.

31.3.4 3R/4R tau isoforms in taupathies

The comparative biochemistry of taupathies points to differences in post-translational modifications and isoform content of tau protein (see Plate 13a). Additional changes also appear as the disease progresses. In general, in sporadic taupathy, 3R and 4R tau isoforms accumulate in AD, 3R in Pick's disease, and 4R in PSP, CBD, AGD and FTDP-17. In familial taupathies, mutations that affect the splicing of exon 10 accumulate 4R tau and phenotypically mimic CBD/PSP, while the majority of others simulate an NFT-predominant form of dementia.

Immunoprobes have been raised against cognate regions for the 3R and 4R tau isoforms, corresponding to the amino acid sequences deriving from the junction of exons 9 and 11 and exon 10, respectively (de Silva et al., 2003). This has led to determination of specific distribution of 3R and 4R tau proteins in the human brain, both in normal ageing and neurodegenerative disorders. Although initial studies found an absence of 4R tau mRNA in dentate fascia neurones in the adult human brain in AD and PSP, tangle-bearing neurones in this region contain 4R tau isoforms (de Silva et al., 2003). 4R tau isoforms are also present in the astrocytic tau inclusions in Pick's disease, pre-tangles, NFTs, astrocytic plaques, tufted astrocytes, coiled bodies and argyrophilic threads in PSP and CBD, and argyrophilic grains.

In AD, all six tau isoforms are subjected to phosphorylation and are incorporated into PHFs, resulting in a tau triplet at 60, 64 and 68 kDa and a minor band at 72 kDa detected by immunoblotting (see Plate 13b). In Pick's disease, only phosphorylated 3R isoforms assemble into filaments and there is a tau doublet at 60 and 64 kDa with a minor band at 68 kDa, whereas in PSP and CBD, phosphorylated 4R tau isoform aggregates provide the 64 and 68 kDa bands. Arai et al. (2004) reported additional, shorter amino-terminally cleaved tau of 33 kDa in PSP and a doublet of 37 kDa in CBD (Plate 13b). In the familial multiple system taupathy 64, 68 and a minor 72 kDa band are present, and contain predominantly 4R tau isoforms (Spillantini et al., 1997). AGD is characterized by 4R tau isoform aggregates: in BST 1 it contains 64 and 68 kDa and a minor 72 kDa band, whereas by BST 2 and 3 there is an additional minor 60 kDa band (Tolnay et al., 2002).

31.3.5 Comparative biochemistry of taupathies

In ageing, there is a gradual loss of the soluble, axonally bound tau protein that occurs in the absence of significant neurofibrillary or amyloid pathology. In contrast, in AD and

DS the loss of soluble tau protein is more pronounced than in elderly controls. This tau loss is accompanied by significant increase in insoluble, PHF-derived tau protein (Mukaetova-Ladinska et al., 1993) (Figure 31.1a). This is not the case for DLB or Parkinson's disease: in these two disorders there is a slight decrease in soluble tau protein, but the levels of insoluble tau (truncated at Glu391 or phosphorylated at Ser202/Thr205) are similar to those found in age-matched controls (Harrington et al. 1994). Only when DLB and AD are matched for extent of neurofibrillary pathology by Braak stages does the level of phosphorylated and PHF-tau become identical in these two disorders (Figure 31.1b).

Phosphorylation of tau protein appears to occur quite late in the disease progression as judged by phosphorylated Ser202/Thr205 site in soluble tau fraction (corresponding to BST 6), whereas in the Sarcosyl-insoluble fraction various phosphorylated tau sites are detected relatively early on, together with C-terminal truncation of the tau protein (Mukaetova-Ladinska et al., 2000) (Figure 31.1c). The use of quantitative biochemistry has been useful in detecting very subtle tau changes at molecular level in the absence of obvious pathology, e.g. tau-less taupathy characterized by loss of soluble tau protein only (Zhukareva et al., 2002).

31.4 TAU PROTEIN AS A CEREBROSPINAL FLUID MARKER FOR DEMENTIA

Cerebrospinal fluid (CSF) has been extensively investigated as a target for developing clinically sensitive and specific diagnostic tools to differentiate between and aid the clinical diagnosis of neurodegenerative disorders. Various proteins and enzymes involved in neurodegenerative disorders have been investigated as CSF markers. The most consistent findings are those of increased CSF tau and a decrease in $A\beta_{1-42}$ protein levels in early and incipient AD which differentiate this disease from age-associated memory impairment, depression, and other types of dementia. However, there are also reports that tau (total and/or phosphorylated) and $A\beta_{1-42}$ measures may not differentiate between various dementia syndromes in the clinical setting. Furthermore, a subgroup of cognitively impaired individuals with a post mortem confirmed AD exhibited a CSF tau protein content similar to that of cognitively intact subjects (Clark et al., 2003). Inconsistency between the findings may be attributable to ApoE genotype, since it has been demonstrated that ApoE ε4 allele carriers have a higher level of CSF-tau concentrations (Tapiola et al., 2000). However, not all studies have confirmed this.

31.4.1 CSF total tau protein

CSF total tau protein (t-tau) is now considered to be a marker for axonal damage and neuronal degeneration, whereas the presence of phosphorylated tau protein (p-tau) reflects

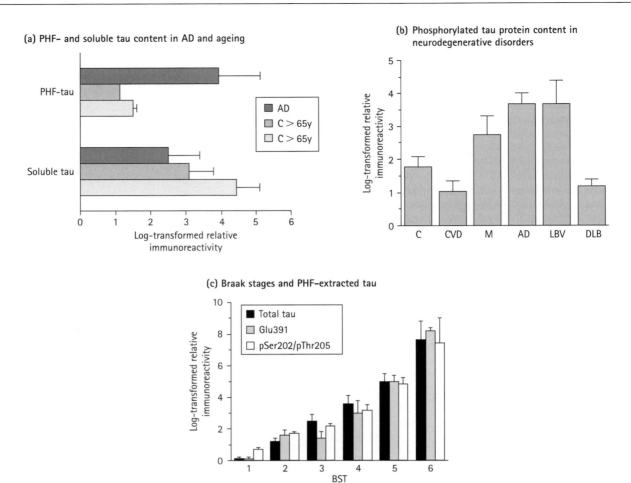

Figure 31.1   *Comparative tau biochemistry. (a) Loss of soluble tau and increase in PHF-tau in AD. In AD, there is significant loss of soluble tau (P = 0.001) and an increase in PHF-tau (P = 0.0001) compared with both young and elderly controls. (b) Increase in phosphorylated Sarcosyl insoluble tau is present in AD, LBV and mixed type of dementia, but not DLB or CVD (ANOVA: F = 2.72, P = 0.035). (c) With increase in Braak stage, there is a progressive increase in PHF-extracted tau, including total PHF-extracted tau, truncated PHF-tau at Glu391 and Sarcosyl insoluble phosphorylated tau (pSer202/pThr205 sites). Tau measures: soluble tau, Ab 7.51; PHF-tau, mAb 423 (a); Sarcosyl insoluble, phosphorylated tau, mAb AT8 (b); Glu391 truncated tau, mAb 423; phosphorylated tau, mAb AT8; total tau, mAb 7.51 (c). AD, Alzheimer's disease; BST, Braak stages; C, control; CVD, cerebrovascular dementia; DLB, dementia with Lewy bodies; LBV, Lewy body variation of AD; M, mixed type dementia.*
* P ≤ 0.05. (Figures adapted after Mukaetova-Landinska et al., 1993, 1996 (a); Mukaetova-Ladinska et al., 2000 (b), and Harrington et al., 1994 and Mukaetova-Ladinska et al., 2000 (c).)

neurofibrillary pathology. Overall, CSF t-tau protein increases as a function of age and in AD, there is up to 3-fold increase in CSF t-tau protein level in comparison to elderly controls (Frank *et al.*, 2003) (Table 31.4). Familial forms of AD (e.g. PS1 A431V mutation) also have an increase in t-tau, and a modest increase in t-tau protein has been found in FTDP-17 with P301L and G272V tau mutations. Age-dependent reference values for t-tau protein measurements have now been established: for subjects 21–50 years old at <300 pg/mL; for age 51–70 years at <450 pg/mL; and 70–93 years at <500 pg/mL (Buerger *et al.*, 1999). In AD, the cut-off value of CSF tau at 375 pg/mL has 59.1 per cent sensitivity and 89.5 per cent specificity for the diagnosis of AD (Shoji *et al.*, 2002).

Increased CSF t-tau is also found in vascular dementia, DLB, Creutzfeldt–Jakob disease, normal pressure hydrocephalus, vitamin B_{12} deficiency encephalopathy, stroke (transient increase in t-tau level) and traumatic brain injury with diffuse axonal damage. In contrast subcortical forms of dementia, including Parkinson's disease, PSP, CBD and alcoholic dementia are not usually associated with an increase in t-tau level (Table 31.4).

In mild dementia, CSF t-tau levels are significantly higher in the majority of AD subjects when compared with normal ageing. Progression of cognitive decline has been shown to be closely linked to elevation of t-tau in some cross-sectional clinical studies (Hampel *et al.*, 2003). However, longitudinal

Table 31.4   *CSF tau protein measures in various neurodegenerative disorders*

Tau protein	Disease	Sensitivity (%)	Specificity (%)	Authors
t-tau	AD↑	91.2	95.0	Arai *et al.*, 1997
		63	89	Kahle *et al.*, 2000
		88	96	Kapaki *et al.*, 2003
				Sunderland *et al.*, 2003
				Gomez-Tortosa *et al.*, 2003
				Ganzer *et al.*, 2003
	AD↑(PS1 A431V)			Matsushita *et al.*, 2002
	FTD↑	90	77	Riemenschneider *et al.*, 2002
				Fabre *et al.*, 2001
	FTD↔			Sjögren *et al.*, 2000
	FTD (P301L and G272V)↑			Rosso *et al.*, 2003
	CBD↑	81.5	80	Urakami *et al.*, 1999
				Urakami *et al.*, 2001
	CJD↑	92	97	Van Everbroeck *et al.*, 2002
	PSP↔			Urakami *et al.*, 1999
	DLB↔			Tschampa *et al.*, 2001
				Kanemaru *et al.*, 2000
	DLB↑			Arai *et al.*, 1997
	Semantic dementia↑			Anderson *et al.*, 2000
	MS↔			Jimenez-Jimenez *et al.*, 2002
	Depression↔			Andreasen *et al.*, 1999
	TBI↑↓			Franz *et al.*, 2003
t-tau and AD7C-NTP PThr181	AD↑	63	93	Kahle *et al.*, 2000
	AD↑			Nagga *et al.*, 2002
				Parnetti *et al.*, 2001
	FTD↓			Pasquier *et al.*, 2003
	FTD (P301L and G272V)↔			Rosso *et al.*, 2003
	DLB↔			Parnetti *et al.*, 2001
t-tau and pThr181 pSer199	Sch↔			Schönknecht *et al.*, 2003
	AD↑	85.2	85	Urakami *et al.*, 2003
	PS1 A431V AD↑			Matsushita *et al.*, 2002
	Atypical CBD↑			Ohara *et al.*, 2002
pThr231	AD↑	90.2	80	Buerger *et al.*, 2002
				de Leon *et al.*, 2002
				Mitchell and Brindle, 2003
	MCI↑			de Leon *et al.*, 2002
pSer199 and pThr231	Depression↔			Mitchell and Brindle, 2003
C- and N-cleaved tau	TBI↑			Zemlan *et al.*, 2002; Chatfield *et al.*, 2002

TBI, traumatic brain injury

studies have failed to confirm these findings (Tapiola *et al.*, 2000). In subarachnoid haemorrhage, an increased level of t-tau has been correlated with both injury severity and unfavourable clinical outcome (Kay *et al.*, 2003).

31.4.2 CSF phosphorylated tau protein

Several quantitative assays using immunoprobes against phosphorylated sites of tau protein have now been developed to assess the extent of phosphorylation of tau protein in CSF: pThr181, pSer199, pThr231, and assays based on two phosphorylation tau sites: pThr231/pSer235 and pSer396/pSer404.

pSer199 is positively correlated with t-tau, appears to be elevated in CSF in both sporadic and familial forms of AD and can be used to discriminate between AD and other forms of dementia. pThr181 level is also increased in AD in comparison to FTD, vascular dementia, Parkinson's disease, acute stroke and control subjects, and may be a useful discriminator between AD and DLB (Table 31.5).

pThr231 appears to be an early marker of pathology in AD, preceding the formation of PHFs, and the CSF measurements confirm it as a highly sensitive marker for AD (90.2 per cent sensitivity level in comparison to t-tau; both markers have specificity of 92.3 per cent) (Buerger *et al.*, 2002). pThr231 distinguishes AD from FTD and major depression

Table 31.5   *Use of total and phosphorylated tau protein markers in CSF to discriminate between neurodegenerative disorders. (Modified from Riemenschneider et al., 2002; Schönknecht et al., 2003 and Hampel et al., 2003, 2004)*

Total tau and phosphorylation tau sites	Improved diagnosis/ Differential diagnosis
t-tau	Progressive MCI versus stable MCI AD versus vascular dementia and major depression
pThr181	AD versus DLB
pSer199	AD versus other dementias
pThr231	Progression of MCI to AD AD versus FTD and major depression
pSer396/pSer404	AD versus vascular dementia

(Table 31.5). Furthermore, CSF pThr231, but not t-tau, is increased in minimal cognitive impairment (MCI) and correlates with cognitive decline and conversion from MCI to AD, but not with severity of dementia (Buerger *et al.*, 2002). Assays based on pThr231/Ser235 identify a higher level of phosphorylated tau in MCI subjects, and seem able to differentiate MCI subjects who later develop AD from memory 'complainers' (Arai *et al.*, 2000). In the course of AD progression, the pThr231 level tends to decline in contrast to an unaltered t-tau level (Hampel *et al.*, 2001). Hampel *et al.* (2003) suggested that the decline in CSF pThr231 might be explained by the incorporation of pThr231 into PHFs.

Overall, a review of current literature supports the role of CSF p-tau in improving early diagnosis of dementia and in aiding differential diagnoses (Hampel *et al.*, 2003, 2004). Although reduction in CSF Aβ_{42} and increase in t-tau have high sensitivity and specificity in discriminating AD from controls, the specificity compared with other dementias is moderate. The combination of CSF p-tau with other CSF markers may improve the accuracy of diagnosis. Thus, in DLB, a decrease of Aβ_{42} with unchanged levels of tau protein in CSF was found, and an increase in p-tau combined with a decrease in Aβ makes an AD diagnosis more accurate. (Papassotiropoulos *et al.*, 2003). The cut-off points of 444 pg/mL for CSF Aβ_{42} and 195 pg/mL for CSF p-tau gave a sensitivity and specificity of 92 per cent and 89 per cent respectively, to distinguish AD patients from controls.

31.4.3   MMSE correlation with CSF tau measurements

Although most studies have found an increase in both total and phosphorylated tau in AD, the association of these changes with disease duration remains controversial. An absence of correlation with cognitive decline (Gomez-Tortosa *et al.*, 2003) and an increase with dementia severity (Arai *et al.*, 1997) have been reported. Non-significant elevation of CSF-tau has also been detected in non-symptomatic carriers of APP (KN670/671ML, E693G) and PS1 (M146V, H163Y) mutations. These findings suggest that CSF-tau protein levels are altered before the onset of symptoms, and may help identify MCI patients who will progress to AD. This has been confirmed in two recent studies, in which the MCI group which progressed to AD had particularly high levels of t-tau and p-tau compared with the MCI patients who progressed to non-AD dementias, and to the MCI group which did not show progression.

Correlative biochemico-neuroradiological studies have reported that both CSF t-tau and p-tau levels correlate with ventricular widening on MRI brain scans over a 16-month period, suggesting that CSF-tau levels reflect the intensity of the disease process: the higher the tau level, the more rapid is progression of the disease (Wahlund and Blennow, 2003). Interestingly, ventriculoperitoneal shunt treatment in subjects with probable AD results in stable or improved cognitive functioning and a decrease in levels of CSF-tau.

31.4.4   CSF tau measurements and treatment

The use of cholinesterase inhibitors (ChEIs) and other novel therapeutic interventions currently being developed may potentially use monitoring CSF biomarkers for diagnostic and outcome purposes. To date a limited number of studies have addressed the CSF-tau changes in relation to available antidementia therapeutic compounds. Treatment with a vitamin B$_{12}$–B$_6$–folate combination does not result in significant changes in the levels of CSF-tau in MCI individuals. Cholesterol-lowering treatment with simvastatin (20 mg/day for 12 weeks) reduces α-secretase cleaved APP (sAPP) and β-sAPP, with unaltered levels of t-tau, p-tau and Aβ_{42} (Sjögren *et al.*, 2003), suggesting that simvastatin acts directly on the processing of APP, but not tau protein, by inhibiting both the α- and the β-secretase pathways.

A limited number of studies have described monitoring CSF-tau in dementia subjects treated with ChEIs. The results suggest that use of ChEIs does not change the level of CSF-tau protein over 1–2 years' treatment. Thus, 1 year's treatment with rivastigmine does not alter CSF-tau levels, in contrast to a significant increase seen in tacrine-treated and untreated AD patients. These changes were mainly present in ApoE ε4 carriers (Stefanova *et al.*, 2003). Similar results of unchanged t-tau and p-tau following treatment with donepezil, rivastigmine, galantamine and metrifonate have been reported. This would suggest that the ChEIs may be modifying the course of the AD process by stalling the progression of neurofibrillary pathology and neuronal loss. This remains to be confirmed neuropathologically.

31.5 THERAPY FOR TAUPATHIES

Since tau protein incorporation within various filamentous structures results in highly protease-resistant insoluble products, and leads eventually to neuronal cell death, the goals of any tau-directed therapy will need to be prevention of their formation and/or dissolving these structures once they are formed. In light of the complexity of altered tau protein metabolism and the non-uniform neuropathological phenotype in neurodegenerative dementias, it seems appropriate to search for a key step that is shared by the different mechanisms which lead to tau pathology-driven dementia.

31.5.1 Decreasing tau protein phosphorylation

Two of the most promising pharmacological therapeutic approaches for treatment of neurodegeneration at present are the development of drugs that can:

- inhibit sequestration of both normal and hyperphosphorylated tau protein into insoluble aggregates, and
- reverse or modify the hyperphosphorylation of tau and correct the existing protein phosphorylation/dephosphorylation imbalance.

The problem with this approach is finding sufficient specificity for treatment without affecting other essential cellular functions reliant on cellular signalling mechanisms.

The use of mood stabilizers for symptomatic treatment of agitation seems to have some neuroprotective effect in terms of inhibiting apoptosis and slowing of neurofibrillary formation. It seems to do this by inhibiting tau protein hyperphosphorylation. Lithium ions interact with the Mg^{2+} binding site of GSK3β and inhibit activity of the enzyme. This decreases the extent of tau phosphorylation without affecting neuronal morphology. Lithium can also protect, both *in vitro* and *in vivo*, against Aβ toxicity and can inhibit neuronal tau hyperphosphorylation induced by Aβ.

GSK3β selective inhibitors that compete with the ATP-binding site of the enzyme (e.g. SB216763 and SB415286) have been explored for their therapeutic potential. Another GSK3-specific inhibitor (AR-A014418) *in vitro*, does not suppress the activity of another 26 kinases, including cdk2 and cdk5. It inhibits tau phosphorylation in tissue culture models over-expressing 4R tau, protects against cell death via blocking P13/PKB signalling pathway and also inhibits Aβ-mediated neurodegeneration.

p38 mitogen-activated protein kinase and cdk5 are also explored as therapeutic targets for therapeutic interventions in AD. Another group of kinases, the CLK family, has been demonstrated as involved in regulating the use of exon 10: even when regulatory elements of this exon contain mutations. These kinases cause exon 10 to be skipped by influencing specific changes in pre-mRNA processing pathways. Changes in the phosphorylation of splicing factors might serve as a therapeutic target in familial forms of taupathy over-expressing 4R tau, as is the case in FTDP-17 or AGD.

31.5.2 Inhibition of tau polymerization

The process of tau aggregation represents a potential target for developing therapeutic agents that inhibit the high affinity tau-tau binding interaction. Furthermore, targeting the MT-binding region of the tau molecule may also reverse the proteolytic stability of insoluble tau filaments. Wischik and Harrington (2000) reported a concentration-dependent untwisting of PHFs by methylene blue that led to their disappearance. They also identified diaminophenothiazines that were able to inhibit tau-tau aggregation *in vitro*.

31.5.3 Stabilizing microtubules

Another possibility for tau-targeted interventions may involve developing agents that will stabilize the MTs, alter signalling events in neurones and/or modulate MT properties (e.g. via cytosolic complexes, involving Arl2, cofactor D and protein phosphatase 2A). One of the candidates could be Pin1 (peptidyl prolyl cis/trans isomerase), which binds to phosphorylated tau proteins (pThr231 site). Pin1 may also be able to restore the ability of hyperphosphorylated tau proteins to polymerize MTs. Stabilization of MTs may be one of the earliest stages in prevention of overt neurodegenerative changes, since both the ageing and neurodegenerative processes cause a reduction in the number of MTs and in their assembly. Pin1 is also involved in neurones re-embarking on the cell cycle, which may be another therapeutic target.

31.5.4 Amyloid route

The relationship between Aβ deposition and tau protein aggregation remains unclear. Although previous hypotheses suggested that these two processes are independent, recent data suggest that there may be an interaction between the two pathological processes. $Aβ_{25-35}$ neurotoxicity leads to hyperphosphorylation of the tau protein molecule, and similarly inhibition of phosphatases resulting in hyperphosphorylated tau contributes to development of amyloid deposits. The formation of PHF-like filaments in tissue culture can be induced by aggregated $Aβ_{42}$ synthetic peptide, with pSer422 preventing this PHF-like aggregation. Oral and subcutaneous administration of small molecular weight glycosaminoglycans, e.g. heparin C3, have been shown to decrease the extent of tau hyperphosphorylation in animals, without affecting the cholinergic brain system.

31.5.5 Neurotrophin route

The 'antinerve growth factor transgenic mice' (Capsoni et al., 2000) outlines the influence of neurotrophins in development of AD-type pathology. This mouse model develops neuronal cell loss, phosphorylated and insoluble tau and NFTs, suggesting that neurotrophins mediate the neurodegenerative process. Regulation of neurotrophin activity may not only have impact on the onset and progression of the disease process, but be used for the development of treatments for prevention of tau-aggregation and hyperphosphorylation. Calorie restriction and diet may also have an impact on the latter via increasing the levels of neurotrophins, specifically brain-derived neurotrophic factor (BDNF) and neurotrophin-3 (NT-3). FGF (fibroblast growth factor-2) in a dose-dependent manner increases the expression of tau and its level of phosphorylation and increases GSK3 levels, but reduces MAP2 expression (Tatebayashi et al., 2003).

31.5.6 The future

Small interfering RNA (siRNA) has some therapeutic promise in relation to silencing dominantly acting disease genes, especially if mutant alleles can be targeted selectively, e.g. single-nucleotide polymorphism or disease mutation. Using two *Drosophila* models (one with mutant R406W and V337M tau [Wittmann et al., 2001], and the other a wild-type tau protein [Jackson et al., 2002]), it was demonstrated that the formation of tau pathology is a late event, a byproduct rather than an early cause of neuronal cell loss. Tau expressed in these two models may interact with an important neuro-developmental pathway, the Wnt pathway, which may be of potential importance for therapeutic interventions directed at non-overt preclinical stages of dementia.

31.6 CONCLUSIONS

Although the relationship between tau and other neuropathological markers associated with the neuropathology of dementia still remains somewhat controversial, there is no doubt that tau pathology alone can contribute to the development of dementia syndromes. The discovery of the tau protein mutations that cause dementia supports the latter. Furthermore, these mutations shed light on a more complex picture of tau function, post-translational modifications and interactions with MTs and aggregation. Molecular epidemiology demonstrates alterations in tau protein metabolism in a dynamic context: age-associated decline of tau protein is followed by incorporation of the tau protein into PHFs and filamentous structures, leading to further depletion of axonally bound tau protein. These biochemical changes, in turn, are closely linked to the appearance of clinical symptoms of dementia.

One of the major problems in testing any therapeutic approach targeted towards altered tau processing is the lack of adequate animal or cell models that truly reflect neurodegenerative disease. The novel transgenic tau animal models alone, or those coupled with the APP and PS1 mutations,

represent the best attempts at recapitulating the abnormal pathology of neurodegenerative dementias. These animal models and organotypic slice cultures seem promising as disease model systems to test novel therapeutic agents aimed at arresting the formation of insoluble tau aggregates.

REFERENCES

Amano M, Kaneko T, Maeda A et al. (2003) Identification of tau and MAP2 as novel substrates of Rho-kinase and myosin phosphatase. *Journal of Neurochemistry* **87**: 780–790

Andersen C, Fabre SF, Östberg P et al. (2000) Tau protein in cerebrospinal fluid from semantic dementia patients. *Neuroscience Letters* **294**: 155–158

Andreasen N, Minthon L, Clarberg A et al. (1999) Sensitivity, specificity, and stability of CSF-tau in AD in a community-based patient sample. *Neurology* **53**: 1488–1494

Arai H, Higuchi S, Sasaki H. (1997) Apolipoprotein E genotyping and cerebrospinal fluid tau protein: implications for the clinical diagnosis of Alzheimer's disease. *Gerontology* **43** (Suppl. 1): 2–10

Arai H, Ishiguro K, Ohno H et al. (2000) CSF phosphorylated tau protein and mild cognitive impairment: a prospective study. *Experimental Neurology* **166**: 201–203

Arai T, Ikeda K, Akiyama H et al. (2004) Identification of amino-terminally cleaved tau fragments that distinguish progressive supranuclear palsy from corticobasal degeneration. *Annals of Neurology* **55**: 72–79

Augustinack JC, Schneider A, Mandelkow EM, Hyman BT. (2002) Specific tau phosphorylation sites correlate with severity of neuronal cytopathology in Alzheimer's disease. *Acta Neuropathology (Berlin)* **103**: 26–35

Bennecib M, Gong CX, Grundke-Iqbal I, Iqbal K. (2000) Role of protein phosphatase-2A and -1 in the regulation of GSK-3: cdk5 and cdc2 and the phosphorylation of tau in rat forebrain. *FEBS Letters* **485**: 87–93

Braak H and Braak E. (1991) Neuropathological staging of Alzheimer-related changes. *Acta Neuropathologica (Berlin)* **82**: 239–259

Brion JP, Tremp G, Octave JN. (1999) Transgenic expression of the shortest human tau affects its compartmentalization and its phosphorylation as in the pretangle stage of Alzheimer's disease. *American Journal of Pathology* **154**: 255–270

Buée L, Bussière T, Buée-Scherrer V et al. (2000) Tau protein isoforms, phosphorylation and role in neurodegenerative disorders. *Brain Research. Brain Research Reviews* **33**: 95–130

Buerger K, Padberg F, Nolde T et al. (1999) CSF tau protein discriminates between Alzheimer's disease, major depression and healthy controls in young old, but not in old old. *Neuroscience Letters* **277**: 21–24

Buerger K, Teipel SJ, Zinkowski R et al. (2002) CSF tau protein phosphorylated at threonine 231 correlates with cognitive decline in MCI subjects. *Neurology* **59**: 627–629

Capsoni S, Ugolini G, Comparini A et al. (2000) Alzheimer-like neurodegeneration in aged antinerve growth factor transgenic mice. *Proceedings of the National Academy of Sciences of the United States of America* **97**: 6826–6831

Chatfield DA, Zemlan FP, Day DJ, Menon DK. (2002) Discordant temporal patterns of S100 β and cleaved tau protein elevation after head injury: a pilot study. *British Journal of Neurosurgery* **16**: 471–476

Clark CM, Xie S, Chittams J et al. (2003) Cerebrospinal fluid tau and βamyloid: How well do these biomarkers reflect autopsy-confirmed dementia diagnosis? Archives of Neurology 60: 1696–1702

de Leon MJ, Segal S, Tarshish CY et al. (2002) Longitudinal cerebrospinal fluid tau load increases in mild cognitive impairment. Neuroscience Letters 333: 183–186

de Silva R, Lashley T, Gibb G et al. (2003) Pathological inclusion bodies in taupathies contain distinct complements of tau with three and four microtubule-binding repeat domains as demonstrated by new specific monoclonal antibodies. Neuropathology and Applied Neurology 29: 288–302

Fabre SF, Forsell C, Viitanen M et al. (2001) Clinic-based cases with frontotemporal dementia show increased cerebrospinal fluid tau and high apolipoprotein E ε4 frequency, but no tau gene mutations. Experimental Neurology 168: 413–418

Ferrer I, Blanco R, Carmona M, Puig B. (2001) Phosphorylated mitogen-activated protein kinase (MAPK/ERK-P), protein kinase of 38 kDa (p38-P), stress-activated protein kinase (SAPK/JNK-P), and calcium/calmodulin-dependent kinase II (CaM kinase II) are differentially expressed in tau deposits in neurones and glial cells in taupathies. Journal of Neural Transmission 108: 1397–1415

Ferrer I, Barrachina M, Puig B. (2002) Glycogen synthase kinase-3 is associated with neuronal and glial hyperphosphorylated tau deposits in Alzheimer's disease, Pick's disease, progressive supranuclear palsy and corticobasal degeneration. Acta Neuropathology (Berlin) 104: 583–591

Ferrer I, Pastor P, Rey MJ et al. (2003) Tau phosphorylation and kinase activation in familial taupathy linked to deln 296 mutation. Neuropathology and Applied Neurobiology 29: 23–34

Flaherty D, Lu Q, Soria J, Wood JG. (1999) Regulation of tau phosphorylation in microtubule fractions by apolipoprotein E. Journal of Neuroscience Research 56: 271–274

Frank RA, Galasko D, Hampel H et al. (2003) Biological markers for therapeutic trials in Alzheimer's disease. Proceedings of the biological markers working group; NIA initiative on neuroimaging in Alzheimer's disease. Neurobiological Aging 24: 521–536

Ganzer S, Arlt S, Schoder V et al. (2003) CSF-tau CSF-Aβ1–42: ApoE-genotype and clinical parameters in the diagnosis of Alzheimer's disease: combination of CSF-tau and MMSE yields highest sensitivity and specificity. Journal of Neural Transmission 110: 1149–1160

Genis I, Chen Y, Shohami E, Michaelson DM. (2000) Tau hyperphosphorylation in apolipoprotein E-deficient and control mice after closed head injury. Journal of Neuroscience Research 60: 559–564

Goedert M, Spillantini MG, Jakes R et al. (1989) Multiple isoforms of human microtubule-associated protein tau: sequences and localization in neurofibrillary tangles of Alzheimer's disease. Neuron 3: 519–526

Goedert M, Spillantini MG, Crowther RA. (1992) Cloning of a big tau microtubule associated protein characteristic for the peripheral nervous system. Proceedings of the National Academy of Sciences of the United States of America 89: 1983–1987

Gomez-Tortosa E, Gonzalo I, Fanjul S et al. (2003) Cerebrospinal fluid markers in dementia with Lewy bodies compared with Alzheimer disease. Archives of Neurology 60: 1218–1222

Götz J, Tolnay M, Barmettler R et al. (2001a) Oligodendroglial tau filament formation in transgenic mice expressing G272V tau. European Journal of Neuroscience 13: 2131–2140

Götz J, Chen F, Barmettler R, Nitsch RM. (2001b) Tau filament formation in transgenic mice expressing P301L tau. Journal of Biological Chemistry 276: 529–534

Götz J, Chen F, van Dorpe J, Nitsch RM. (2001c) Formation of neurofibrillary tangles in P301L tau transgenic mice induced by Aβ42 fibrils. Science 293: 1491–1495

Grover A, DeTure M, Yen S-H, Hutton M. (2002) Effects on splicing and protein function of three mutations in codon N296 of tau in vitro. Neuroscience Letters 323: 33–36

Hampel H, Buerger R, Kohnken R et al. (2001) Tracking of Alzheimer's disease progression with CSF tau protein phosphorylated at threonine 231. Annals of Neurology 49: 545–546

Hampel H, Goernitz A, Buerger K. (2003) Advances in the development of biomarkers for Alzheimer's disease: from CSF total tau and $A\beta_{1-42}$ proteins to phosphorylated tau protein. Brain Research Bulletin 61: 243–253

Hampel H, Buerger K, Zinkowski R et al. (2004) Measurement of phosphorylated tau epitopes in the differential diagnosis of Alzheimer disease: a comparative cerebrospinal fluid study. Archives of General Psychiatry 61: 95–102

Harrington CR, Perry RH, Perry EK et al. (1994) Senile dementia of Lewy body type and Alzheimer type are biochemically distinct in terms of paired helical filaments and hyperphosphorylated tau protein. Dementia 5: 215–228

Jackson GR, Wiedau-Pasoz M, Sang T-K et al. (2002) Human wild-type tau interacts with wingless pathway components and produces neurofibrillary pathology in Drosophila. Neuron 34: 506–519

Jicha GA, Lane E, Vincent I et al. (1997) A conformation- and phosphorylation-dependent antibody recognizing the paired helical filaments of Alzheimer's disease. Journal of Neurochemistry 69: 2087–2095

Jimenez-Jimenez FJ, Zurdo JM, Hernanz A et al. (2002) Tau protein concentrations in cerebrospinal fluid of patients with multiple sclerosis. Acta Neurologica Scandinavica 106: 351–354

Kahle PJ, Jakowec M, Teipel SJ et al. (2000) Combined assessment of tau and neuronal thread protein in Alzheimer's disease. Neurology 54: 1068–1069

Kanemaru K, Kameda N, Yamanouchi H. (2000) Decreased CSF amyloid β42 and normal tau levels in dementia with Lewy bodies. Neurology 54: 1875–1876

Kapaki E, Paraskevas GP, Zalonis I, Zournas C. (2003) CSF tau protein and β-amyloid (1–42) in Alzheimer's disease, diagnosis: discrimination from normal ageing and other dementias in the Greek population. European Journal of Neurology 10: 119–128

Kay A, Petzhold A, Kerr M et al. (2003) Temporal alterations in cerebrospinal fluid amyloid β-protein and apolipoprotein E after subarachnoid hemorrhage. Stroke 34: e240–e243

Kertesz A. (2003) Pick's complex and FTDP-17. Movement Disorders 18 (Suppl. 6): S57–S62

Kobayashi M, Ishiguro K, Katoh-Fukui Y et al. (2003) Phosphorylation state of tau in hippocampus of apolipoprotein E4 and E3 knock-in mice. NeuroReport 14: 699–702

Kurt MA, Davies DC, Kidd M et al. (2003) Hyperphosphorylated tau and paired helical filament-like structures in the brains of mice carrying mutant amyloid precursor protein and mutant presenilin-1 transgenes. Neurobiological Disease 14: 89–97

Lauckner J, Frey P, Geula C. (2003) Comparative distribution of tau phosphorylated at Ser_{262} in pre-tangles and tangles. Neurobiological Aging 24: 767–776

Lewis J, Dickson DW, Lin W-L et al. (2001) Enhanced neurofibrillary degeneration in transgenic mice expressing mutant tau and APP. Science 293: 1487–1491

Matsushita S, Arai H, Okamura N et al. (2002) Clinical and biomarker investigation of a patient with a novel presenilin-1 mutation (A431V) in the mild cognitive impairment stage of Alzheimer's disease. Biological Psychiatry 52: 907–910

Mitchell A and Brindle N. (2003) CSF phosphorylated tau – does it constitute an accurate biological test for Alzheimer's disease? International Journal of Geriatric Psychiatry 18: 407–411

MRC CFAS (Neuropathology Group of the Medical Research Council Cognitive Function and Ageing Study) (2001) Pathological correlates of late-onset dementia in a multicentre, community-based population in England and Wales. Lancet 357: 169–175

Mukaetova-Ladinska EB, Harrington CR, Roth M, Wischik CM. (1993) Biochemical and anatomical redistribution of tau protein in Alzheimer's disease. American Journal of Pathology 143: 565–578

Mukaetova-Ladinska EB, Harrington CR, Roth M, Wischik CM. (1996) Alterations in tau protein metabolism during normal ageing. Dementia 7: 95–103

Mukaetova-Ladinska EB, Harrington CR, Roth M, Wischik CM. (1997) Presence of the apolipoprotein E type ε4 allele is not associated with neurofibrillary pathology or biochemical changes to tau protein. Dementia and Geriatric Cognitive Disorders 8: 288–295

Mukaetova-Ladinska EB, Garcia-Sierra F, Hurt J et al. (2000) Staging of cytoskeletal and β-amyloid changes in human isocortex reveals biphasic synaptic protein response during progression of Alzheimer's disease. American Journal of Pathology 157: 623–636

Nagga K, Gottfries J, Blennow K, Marcusson J. (2002) Cerebrospinal fluid phospho-tau, total tau and β-amyloid(1–42) in the differentiation between Alzheimer's disease and vascular dementia. Dementia and Geriatric Cognitive Disorders 14: 183–190

Ohara S, Tsuyuzaki J, Oide T et al. (2002) A clinical and neuropathological study of an unusual case of sporadic taupathy. A variant of corticobasal degeneration? Neurocscience Letters 330: 84–88

Papassotiropoulos A, Streffer JR, Tsolaki M et al. (2003) Increased brain β-amyloid load, phosphorylated tau, and risk of Alzheimer disease associated with an intronic CYP46 polymorphism. Archives of Neurology 60: 29–35

Parnetti L, Lanari A, Amici S et al. (2001) Phospho-Tau International Study Group. CSF phosphorylated tau is a possible marker for discriminating Alzheimer's disease from dementia with Lewy bodies. Phospho-Tau International Study Group. Neurological Sciences 22: 77–78

Pasquier F, Fukui T, Sarazin M et al. (2003) Laboratory investigations and treatment in frontotemporal dementia. Annals of Neurology 54: S32–S35

Pei J-J, Braak H, Gong C-X et al. (2002) Up-regulation of cell division cycle (cdc) 2 kinase in neurons with early stage Alzheimer's disease neurofibrillary degeneration. Acta Neuropathologica (Berlin) 104: 369–376

Pérez M, Arrasate M, Montejo de Garcini E et al. (2001) In vitro assembly of tau protein: mapping the regions involved in filament formation. Biochemistry 40: 5983–5991

Poorkaj P, Grossman M, Steinbart E et al. (2001) Frequency of tau gene mutations in familial and sporadic cases of non-Alzheimer' dementia. Archives of Neurology 58: 383–387

Rank RB, Pauley AM, Bhattacharya K et al. (2002) Direct interaction of soluble human recombinant tau protein with Aβ$_{1-42}$ results in aggregation and hyperphosphorylation by tau protein kinase II. FEBS Letters 514: 263–268

Riemenschneider M, Wagenpfeil S, Diehl J et al. (2002) Tau and Aβ42 protein in CSF of patients with frontotemporal degeneration. Neurology 58: 1585–1586

Rosso SM, Van Herpen E, Pijnenburg YA et al. (2003) Total tau and phosphorylated tau 181 levels in cerebrospinal fluid of patients with frontotemporal dementia due to P301L and G272V tau mutations. Archives of Neurology 60: 1209–1213

Savage MJ, Lin YG, Ciallella JR et al. (2002) Activation of c-Jun N-terminal kinase and p38 in an Alzheimer's disease model is associated with amyloid deposition. Journal of Neuroscience 22: 3376–3385

Schönknecht P, Hempel A, Hunt A et al. (2003) Cerebrospinal fluid tau protein levels in schizophrenia. European Archives of Psychiatry and Clinical Neurosciences 253: 100–102

Shoji M, Matsubara E, Murakami T et al. (2002) Cerebrospinal fluid tau in dementia disorders: a large multicenter study by a Japanese study group. Neurobiology and Aging 23: 363–370

Short RA, Graff-Radford NR, Adamson J et al. (2002) Differences in tau and apolipoprotein E polymorphism frequencies in sporadic frontotemporal lobar degeneration syndromes. Archives of Neurology 59: 611–615

Sjögren M, Rosengren L, Minthon L et al. (2000) Cytoskeleton proteins in CSF distinguish frontotemporal dementia from AD. Neurology 54: 1960–1964

Sjögren M, Gustafsson K, Syversen S et al. (2003) Treatment with simvastatin in patients with Alzheimer's disease lowers both α- and β-cleaved amyloid precursor protein. Dementia and Geriatric Cognitive Disorders 16: 25–30

Spillantini MG, Goedert M, Crowther RA et al. (1997) Familial multiple system taupathy with presenile dementia: a disease with abundant neuronal and glial tau filaments. Proceedings of the National Academy of Sciences of the United States of America 94: 4113–4118

Spillantini MG, Crowther RA, Kamphorst W et al. (1998) Tau pathology in two Dutch families with mutations in the microtubule-binding region of tau. American Journal of Pathology 153: 1359–1363

Stefanova E, Blennow K, Almkvist O et al. (2003) Cerebral glucose metabolism, cerebrospinal fluid-β-amyloid$_{1-42}$ (CSF-Aβ$_{42}$), tau and apolipoprotein E genotype in long-term rivastigmine and tacrine treated Alzheimer disease (AD) patients. Neuroscience Letters 338: 159–163

Sunderland T, Linker G, Mirza N et al. (2003) Decreased β-amyloid$_{1-42}$ and increased tau levels in cerebrospinal fluid of patients with Alzheimer disease. JAMA 289: 2094–2103

Takashima A, Murayama M, Murayama O et al. (1998) Presenilin 1 associates with glycogen synthase kinase-3β and its substrate. Proceedings of the National Academy of Sciences of the United States of America 95: 9637–9641

Tapiola T, Pirttilä T, Mikkonen M et al. (2000) Three-year follow-up of cerebrospinal fluid tau, β amyloid 42 and 40 concentrations in Alzheimer's disease. Neuroscience Letters 280: 119–122

Tatebayashi Y, Lee MH, Li L et al. (2003) The dentate gyrus neurogenesis: A therapeutic target for Alzheimer's disease. Acta Neuropathologica (Berlin) 105: 225–232

Tolnay M, Sergeant N, Ghestem A et al. (2002) Argyrophilic grain disease and Alzheimer's disease are distinguished by their different distribution of tau protein isoforms. Acta Neuropathologica (Berlin) 104: 425–434

Tomizawa K, Amori A, Ohtake A et al. (2001) Tau-tubulin kinase phosphorylates tau at Ser-208 and Ser-210: sites found in paired helical filament-tau. FEBS Letters 492: 221–227

Tschampa HJ, Schulz-Schaeffer W, Wiltfang J *et al.* (2001) Decreased CSF amyloid β42 and normal tau levels in dementia with Lewy bodies. *Neurology* **56**: 576

Tseng H-C, Lu Q, Henderson E, Graves D. (1999) Phosphorylated tau can promote tubulin assembly. *Proceedings of the National Academy of Sciences of the United States of America* **96**: 9503–9508

Urakami K, Mori M, Wada K *et al.* (1999) A comparison of tau protein in cerebrospinal fluid between corticobasal degeneration and progressive supranuclear palsy. *Neuroscience Letters* **252**: 127–129

Urakami K, Wada K, Arai H *et al.* (2001) Diagnostic significance of tau protein in cerebrospinal fluid from patients with corticobasal degeneration or progressive supranuclear palsy. *Journal of the Neurological Sciences* **183**: 95–98

Urakami K, Ito N, Arai H *et al.* (2003) The measurement of phosphorylated tau in human cerebrospinal fluid as a diagnostic marker for Alzheimer's disease. *Seishin Shinkeigaku Zasshi – Psychiatria et Neurologia Japonica* **105**: 393–397

von Bergen M, Barghorn S, Li L *et al.* (2001) Mutations of tau protein in frontotemporal dementia promote aggregation of paired helical filaments by enhancing local β-structure. *Journal of Biological Chemistry* **276**: 48165–48174

Van Everbroeck B, Green AJ, Vanmechelen E *et al.* (2002) Phosphorylated tau in cerebrospinal fluid as a marker for Creutzfeldt-Jakob disease. *Journal of Neurology, Neurosurgery, and Psychiatry* **73**: 79–81

Wahlund LO and Blennow, K. (2003) Cerebrospinal fluid biomarkers for disease stage and intensity in cognitively impaired patients. *Neuroscience Letters* **339**: 99–102

Wischik CM, Novak M, Thogersen HC *et al.* (1988) Isolation of a fragment of tau derived from the core of the paired helical filament of Alzheimer Disease. *Proceedings of the National Academy of Sciences of the United States of America* **85**: 4506–4510

Wischik CM and Harrington CR. (2000) The role of tau protein in the neurodegenerative dementias. In: J O'Brien, D Ames, A Burns (eds), *Dementia*. London: Arnold, pp. 461–492

Wittmann CW, Wsolek MF, Shulman JM *et al.* (2001) Taupathy in Drosophila: neurodegeneration without neurofibrillary tangles. *Science* **293**: 711–714

Yoshida H and Goedert M. (2002) Molecular cloning and functional characterization of chicken brain tau: isoforms with up to five tandem repeats. *Biochemistry* **41**: 15203–15211

Zemlan FP, Jauch EC, Mulchahey JJ *et al.* (2002) C-tau biomarker of neuronal damage in severe brain injured patients: association with elevated intracranial pressure and clinical outcome. *Brain Research* **947**: 131–139

Zhukareva V, Sundarraj S, Mann D *et al.* (2003) Selective reduction of soluble tau proteins in sporadic and familial frontotemporal dementias: An international follow-up study. *Acta Neuropathologica (Berlin)* **105**: 469–476

32

Role of Aβ amyloid in the pathogenesis of Alzheimer's disease

CRAIG W RITCHIE, CATRIONA MCLEAN, KONRAD BEYREUTHER AND COLIN L MASTERS

The details of the molecular neuropathology of Alzheimer's disease (AD), from the amyloid precursor protein (APP) through to the production of amyloid Aβ, plaque formation, neurodegeneration and to final neuronal death is discussed in this chapter. This process, like Alexander's Gordian knot, has been scrutinized over the last two decades with the hope now that a decisive therapeutic incision is not too distant. Points in the biochemical pathway that may be amenable to therapeutic intervention are highlighted.

The theory that Aβ amyloid underlies the neurodegenerative changes in AD is currently pre-eminent (Figure 32.1). Integral to this thesis is the presumed neurotoxicity of Aβ. This peptide is the main constituent of the amyloid plaque, one of the characteristic pathological features of AD. It is also found in vessel walls as a congophilic amyloid angiopathy (Glenner and Wong, 1984; Masters et al., 1985). Neurofibrillary changes are also major features in the brains of patients with AD. Tau protein, a microtubule-associated protein, is ubiquinated, phosphorylated and accumulates as neurofibrillary tangles (NFTs) and dystrophic neurites (Kosik et al., 1986; Wood et al., 1986). The link between Aβ accumulation and tau-associated NFTs remains unknown, although NFTs appear to be downstream of the events that surround Aβ accumulation in the AD brain.

The biogenesis of Aβ from APP and putative mechanisms for its neurotoxicity, together with factors such as apolipoprotein E (ApoE) and α2-macroglobulin (α2M), which may interact with Aβ and affect its clearance from the brain, is the focus of this chapter. Recent and more detailed reviews on these subjects can be found elsewhere (Blacker and Tanzi, 1998; Hardy et al., 1998; Multhaup et al., 1998; Price et al., 1998; Lansbury, 1999; Scheper et al., 1999; Butterfield, 2002, 2003; Citron, 2002; Lahiri et al., 2002; Suh and Checler, 2002; Walsh et al., 2002; Atwood et al., 2003; Bertram and Tanzi, 2004).

32.1 Aβ AMYLOID ACCUMULATION AND PLAQUE DEVELOPMENT

One of the two characteristic microscopic features of AD is the accumulation of Aβ amyloid in plaques of varying morphology. These are extracellular or perivascular congophilic deposits of aggregated Aβ with a high content of β-pleated sheet secondary structure. The amyloid plaque itself is the end result of a process of Aβ oligomerization, fibril formation, aggregation, and precipitation occurring in several stages, with each stage potentially having a different impact on surrounding neurones. Initially it is postulated that a soluble species of Aβ forms oligomers that may represent the toxic species (McLean et al., 1999). The oligomers may then aggregate into protofibrillar structures, which may first be seen as precipitates in diffuse amyloid plaques; this progresses

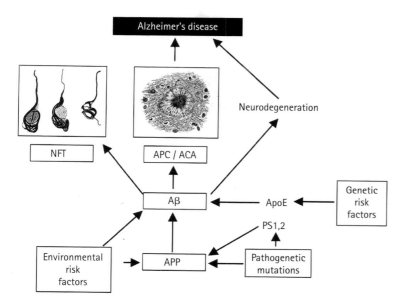

Figure 32.1   *The amyloidocentric pathway that leads to Alzheimer's disease proceeds from the proteolytic processing of the amyloid β precursor protein (APP) into the Aβ amyloid. The amyloid forms visible plaques (amyloid plaque cores, APC; amyloid congophilic angiopathy, ACA). The relationship between Aβ and neurofibrillary tangle (NFT) formation remains unclear. The mechanisms that underly the basic neurodegenerative changes in Alzheimer's disease are also uncertain. This pathway is subject to modulation by environmental and genetic factors at various points.*

with dystrophic neurite formation both within the neuropil and around dense crystalloid precipitates of amyloid cores. Following this, an intermediate stage is reached where the plaque increases in complexity before a final stage of a non-neuritic 'burned out' or 'end-stage plaque' is reached.

In AD, processing of APP creates a high ratio of $A\beta_{42}$ ('long' Aβ of 42 amino acids) to $A\beta_{40}$ ('short' Aβ of 40 amino acids). These processes are discussed later in this chapter. The more insoluble long Aβ is the primary constituent of the amyloid plaque. However, immunocytochemical techniques have demonstrated that diffuse plaques contain not only $A\beta_{42}$ but also $A\beta_{40}$ and, in a small proportion of plaques (most of which have a dense amyloid core), $A\beta_{(16-40/42)}$ (the p3 fragment) (Dickson, 1997). Perivascular amyloid identified in the congophilic angiopathies predominantly consists of $A\beta_{40}$ (Suzuki *et al.*, 1994; Barelli *et al.*, 1997).

Plaque morphology also varies as a function of topographic location. Smaller granular deposits are seen in the deep grey matter nuclei, and linear streaks occur in the molecular layer of the cerebellum. The morphology of the amyloid plaque therefore varies depending upon both location and stage of development.

The number of amyloid plaques at post mortem does not correlate well with the severity of clinical disease (McKee *et al.*, 1991; Morris *et al.*, 1991; Terry *et al.*, 1991; Berg *et al.*, 1998). However, plaque formation may correlate with the degree of neuronal injury as identified by the cellular pro-apoptotic response as measured by the TUNEL technique (Sheng *et al.*, 1998). The poor correlation may also be explained in part by a process of growth and resolution of plaques with the establishment of a plateau phase for plaque production (Hyman and Tanzi, 1992). There is also an emerging view that the soluble $A\beta_{42}$ load may be more closely related to clinical severity (McLean *et al.*, 1999), whether or not the $A\beta_{42}$ exists as an oligomer or complexed to other proteins (Lorenzo and Yanker,

1994; Howlett *et al.*, 1995). A major argument raised by opponents of the amyloid theory is that individuals can have numerous plaques but no clinical cognitive impairment. This may be countered by the observation, as will be elaborated below, that Aβ, whilst being the crucial factor in inducing neurodegeneration in AD, will only act upon compromised cells, such compromise appearing, for example, in the form of age-related oxidative stress (Lockhart *et al.*, 1994). Furthermore, Aβ and the plaque are components within a very complex biological system that relies on numerous other pathological processes before AD develops clinically. These processes are mediated by both genetic and environmental risk factors.

The damage caused by the soluble, aggregated or fibrillar Aβ may induce a reactive astrocytic and microglial 'inflammatory' response. Aβ may interact with metal ions, including iron, zinc and copper. These interactions in turn may lead to the production of neurotoxic free radicals, contributing to the load of reactive oxygen species generated by microglia. Overall, the AD brain is under considerable oxidative stress; these aspects of neurotoxicity of Aβ are discussed in more detail below.

32.2 GENETIC EVIDENCE FOR THE ROLE OF Aβ IN ALZHEIMER'S DISEASE

The most convincing support for the central role of Aβ and APP in the pathogenesis of AD is that all of the known fully penetrant autosomal dominant gene mutations that cause early-onset AD lead to an increase of $A\beta_{42}$ production (Table 32.1). Mutations in the APP gene itself lead to the development of aberrant APP that is preferentially processed to produce an increase in the $A\beta_{42:40}$ ratio. All causative APP mutations identified to date occur in proximity to the Aβ domain of the protein. Similarly, multiple mutations in the two presenilin genes have a dramatic effect on the $A\beta_{42:40}$ ratio.

Table 32.1 *Pathogenic mutations that cause Alzheimer's disease*

Mutations	Mechanism of action	Effect
APP gene dosage or aberrant regulation		
Down's syndrome (trisomy 21)	Upregulation of APP gene promoter up to 5–6-fold	Increased total Aβ
Pathogenic APP gene mutations		
APP codons:		
670/671 ('Swedish')	Increase β-secretase cleavage	Excess total Aβ production
692 and 693 ('Dutch and Flemish')	Decrease α-secretase activity?	Resultant increase in β- and γ-activity with consequent increased total Aβ
715 ('French')	Affects γ-secretase activity	Increased amounts of Aβ p3 fragment
717 ('London')	Altered γ-secretase activity	Increased ratio of $A\beta_{42:40}$
723 ('Australian')	Affects γ-secretase activity	Increased ration of $A\beta_{42:40}$
Pathogenic PS1, 2 gene mutations		
More than 70 point or missense mutations and exon deletion mutations	Direct or indirect alteration of γ-secretase	Increased ratio of $A\beta_{42:40}$

32.3 AMYLOID PRECURSOR PROTEIN

The APP is a transmembrane protein that is found in most cell types including neuronal and glial cells (Figure 32.2). It is especially enriched in the alpha-granule of platelets. The APP gene is located on chromosome 21 (Kang *et al.*, 1987). The pathogenic APP mutations account for less than 5 per cent of all cases of AD inherited in an autosomal dominant manner.

The precise physiological function of APP is unknown, though no doubt is complex and possibly related to synaptic plasticity, repair and regeneration. The structural domains suggest that it may have a role in cell–cell (synapse) or cell–matrix interactions (neurite stabilization). In the platelet, APP has been shown to be involved in inhibition of platelet aggregation via an effect on arachidonic acid metabolism (Henry *et al.*, 1998). There is also evidence to suggest that APP is affected by metal ion binding, calcium levels and heparin binding. APP has also been associated with cell proliferation and neurite outgrowth in response to nerve growth factor (Milward *et al.*, 1992; Small *et al.*, 1994; Yankner, 1996). Other *in vitro* experiments have suggested that a deficiency of APP renders cells more susceptible to a variety of neurotoxic insults.

32.4 APP PROCESSING BY α-, β- AND γ-SECRETASES

APP exists in three major isoforms of 695, 751 and 770 amino acids. The 695-amino-acid isoform (APP695) is predominantly expressed in neurones (Kang *et al.*, 1987; Tanzi *et al.*, 1987). The APP751 and APP770 isoforms are predominantly expressed in peripheral tissues and astrocytes (Golde *et al.*, 1990; Kang and Müller-Hill, 1990). APP is synthesized in the endoplasmic reticulum and is then transported through the Golgi apparatus to the cell surface. In its transmembrane orientation (as shown in Figure 32.2) it undergoes proteolytic cleavage to produce Aβ. The half-life of APP is short and is processed by at least two pathways (α- and β-/γ-secretase activities). In peripheral cells, α-secretase activity predominates, cleaving the Aβ domain of APP at position 16/17. This leads to the production of soluble ectodomain protein sAPPα (Evin *et al.*, 1994). The soluble ectodomains of APP (both sAPPα and sAPPβ) do not aggregate and do not participate in plaque formation. α-Secretase activity leaves in the membrane a small carboxyl-terminal fragment which undergoes further processing. The α-secretase activity may be sequence non-specific and act on several other transmembrane proteins. Furthermore, recent work has identified a disintegrin and metalloprotease (ADAM), as being a potent effector of α-secretase activity (Lammich *et al.*, 1999). Increase of ADAM-10 expression and activity may theoretically be effective as a treatment for AD.

Aβ therefore exists in several forms depending on the site of cleavage by as yet largely undefined α-, β- or γ-secretases. The length of the Aβ fragment varies depending on the site of cleavage leading to a product between 39 and 43 amino acids in length. The N-terminal 28 residues are from the extracellular portion of APP, and the 11–15 C-terminal residues are derived from the transmembrane domain. It is the $A\beta_{42}$ which is considered to be the more insoluble and toxic moiety and is a product of γ-secretase cleavage of the APP molecule. β- and γ-secretase activity involves cleavage of APP at sites corresponding to positions 1 (β-secretase) and 40 or 42 (γ-secretase) of the Aβ fragment, releasing the insoluble amyloidogenic peptide $A\beta_{(1–40/42)}$ commonly referred to as $A\beta_{42}$. Determination of the identity of γ-secretase could have important therapeutic implications. Recent evidence suggests an intimate relationship between PS1 and γ-secretase, and there is increasing evidence that the active sit of γ-secretase lies within the transmembrane domains of the PS molecule (De Strooper *et al.*, 1999; Struhl and Greenwald, 1999; Wolfe *et al.*, 1999; Ye *et al.*, 1999). The macromolecular complex which constitutes γ-secretase activity is presently discerned as >400 kDa in

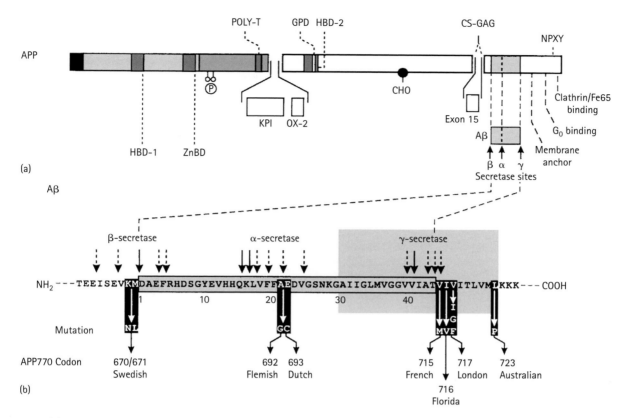

Figure 32.2   *(a) The structural domains of APP are schematically shown. Within the large extracellular ectodomain there are heparin-binding sites (HBD-1,2), metal-binding sites (ZnBD), growth-promoting domains (GPD), carbohydrate-attachment sites (CHO; CS-GAG), and alternatively spliced exons (KPI, OX2, exon 15). The shorter cytoplasmic domain has interacting motifs for G_0 protein, clathrin (NPXY) and the Fe65 family of proteins. (b) The Aβ (juxtatransmembrane and transmembrane) domains are shown in more detail. The β-, α- and γ-secretase sites are shown, with the major cleavage sites indicated by unbroken arrows. The critical pathogenic mutations are shown to be clustered near the secretase sites (see also Table 32.1).*

mass, and contains at least three other molecules: Aph1, Pen2 and nicastrin (Iwatsubo, 2004). Active development of inhibitors of γ-secretase has progressed at a radical pace, and the results of clinical trials are expected soon.

32.5 APP MUTATIONS AND Aβ PRODUCTION

The various APP mutations inevitably produce increased ratios of $A\beta_{42}$ through a variety of mechanisms (Table 32.1). The mutations at codons 670/671 (the 'Swedish' mutation), increase β-secretase cleavage and lead to an overall excess amyloid production (Cai *et al.*, 1993). Mutations at codon 717 (the 'London' mutation), 715 (the 'French' mutation), 716 (the 'Florida' mutation) and 723 (the 'Australian' mutation) act at the γ-secretase site, increasing the ratio of $A\beta_{42:40}$ (Suzuki *et al.*, 1994; Brooks *et al.*, 1995; Eckman *et al.*, 1997; Ancolio *et al.*, 1999; Kwok *et al.*, 2000). Mutations at 692 and 693 (the 'Dutch' and 'Flemish' mutations) are either associated with α-secretase activity, presumably leading to a decrease in this pathway with a resultant increase in β- and γ-activity (Haass *et al.*, 1994) or yield a mutant Aβ peptide

with enhanced toxicity or propensity to aggregation. In Down's syndrome (trisomy 21), where there is an extra copy of the APP gene, there is a similar increase in the overall levels of $A\beta_{42}$ (Teller *et al.*, 1996).

It is necessary to elucidate the mechanisms that regulate the activity of the secretase enzymes involved in APP metabolism, as a greater understanding of these processes will aid the development of therapeutic interventions. One factor that may predict which form of cleavage is utilized is cell type, with glial cells and neurones (both differentiated and undifferentiated) producing different isoforms of APP (Haass *et al.*, 1991; Baskin *et al.*, 1992; Hung *et al.*, 1992). Another factor that influences the cleavage pathway may be the release of APP by protein kinase C (PKC), which leads to a predominance of the α-secretase pathway (Caporaso *et al.*, 1992; Gillespie *et al.*, 1992; Sinha and Lieberburg, 1992). Of interest, PKC mediated α-secretase activity may be induced by neurotransmitters and other first-messenger ligands (Buxbaum *et al.*, 1992; Lahiri *et al.*, 1992; Nitsch *et al.*, 1992). If these first and second messenger pathways prove to directly influence the production of $A\beta_{42}$, then these systems could provide another target for pharmacological intervention.

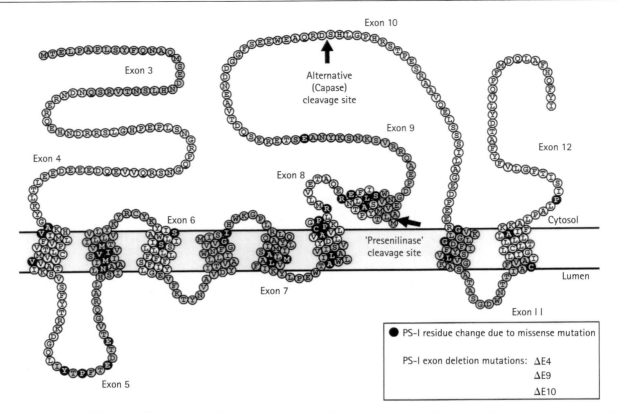

Figure 32.3 *A model of the presenilin 1 molecule. The multiple mutations that cause early-onset Alzheimer's disease are seen to cluster in the transmembrane domains and in proximity to the normal 'presenilinase' cleavage site. The cytosolic loop between transmembrane domains 6 and 7 may play a critical role in γ-secretase activity.*

32.6 PRESENILINS 1 AND 2

The PS1 gene is located on chromosome 14 and PS2 on chromosome 1. In the brain, PS1 is found in both neurones and glia. It has a multipass transmembrane orientation (Figure 32.3). PS2 expression in the pancreas and muscle exceeds other sites including the brain (Rogaev, 1998). The presenilin molecules undergo cleavage by unidentified mechanisms to yield *N*- and *C*-terminal fragments. The functions of PS1 and PS2 are unknown, though it has been proposed that they may have a role in signalling pathways from plasma membranes to the cell nucleus during cell differentiation, or they may play a role in receptor trafficking and protein recycling.

A link between PS mutations and Aβ production has been confirmed as an increased ratio of $A\beta_{42:40}$ is noted in transfected cell lines and transgenic mice expressing mutant forms of PS1 (Borchelt *et al.*, 1996; Citron *et al.*, 1996; Duff *et al.*, 1996; Lemere *et al.*, 1996). Knock-out PS1 cells lose γ-secretase activity, consistent with the concept of PS harbouring the active γ-secretase site (De Strooper *et al.*, 1998). Furthermore, patients and at-risk individuals with PS mutations have increased ratios of $A\beta_{42:40}$ (Scheuner *et al.*, 1996). PS1 may have an anti-apoptotic activity (Roperch *et al.*, 1998) and mutations in PS1 may sensitize neuronal cells to apoptosis

by disruption of intracellular calcium levels (Keller *et al.*, 1998).

In summary, all the identified genotypes in autosomal dominant AD have, as their common denominator, an increase in the production of $A\beta_{42}$. This observation suggests a direct causal relationship between $A\beta_{42}$ and the development of AD.

32.7 Aβ AND NEUROTOXICITY

Despite the above evidence that an increase in the proportion of $A\beta_{42}$ is a common end point for all the autosomal dominant mutations that lead to AD, the exact mechanism of underlying $A\beta_{42}$ and neuronal degeneration remains unclear (Box 32.1).

Aβ has been shown to be directly neurotoxic to hippocampal neurones that are particularly sensitive to oxidative stress and are affected first in the spread of AD throughout the cerebral cortex. While some authors have been unable to demonstrate neurotoxicity of Aβ when it exists in an immature, non-fibrillar, amorphous aggregate (Lorenzo and Yanker, 1994), there is now an emerging consensus that the smaller oligomeric aggregates of Aβ, in association with factors such as metal ions, constitute the principal forms of the toxic Aβ species. Aβ can potentiate the neuronal insult of excitatory amino acids (Koh *et al.*, 1990), oxidative stress (Lockhart *et al.*, 1994) and glucose deprivation (Copani *et al.*, 1991). This may explain why the cumulative exposure of the ageing brain to other risk factors renders it more vulnerable to the toxic effects of Aβ. Aβ has also been shown *in vitro* to cause plasma membrane lipid peroxidation, impairment of ion motive ATPases, glutamate uptake and uncoupling of γ-protein linked receptors (Behl *et al.*, 1994; Butterfield *et al.*, 1994; Hensley *et al.*, 1994; Mark *et al.*, 1996). These pathological processes may contribute to a loss of intracellular calcium homeostasis that has been reported in cultured neurones (Mattson *et al.*, 1993). Aβ, when introduced into neuronal cultures, leads to a gradual increase in intracellular calcium, though this activity is not affected by the addition of either calcium channel blockers or chelating agents (Lorenzo and Yanker, 1994; Whitson and Appel, 1995). Aβ may also impair redox activity in mitochondria, leading to the production of free radicals (Shearman *et al.*, 1994). Cellular damage mediated by Aβ is inhibited by vitamin E (Behl *et al.*, 1992). This supports the above observation that a free-radical-based process, mediated by Aβ, leads to neuronal damage and that this process, *in vitro*, can be inhibited by antioxidants. The use of antioxidants in the treatment of AD has been investigated clinically in recent years and some clinical efficacy has been shown with vitamin E (Sano *et al.*, 1997). Preliminary trials with compounds which target the redox-active metal binding sites on Aβ have yielded encouraging results (Ritchie *et al.*, 2003).

32.8 APOLIPOPROTEIN E, α2-MACROGLOBULIN AND OTHER GENETIC MODIFIERS OF ENVIRONMENTAL RISK IN ALZHEIMER'S DISEASE

32.8.1 Apolipoprotein E

ApoE isoforms represent a major genetic susceptibility factor for sporadic AD, affecting all people over the age of 60 years. It is the first of what may prove to be a multiple set of genetic risk factors that have the potential to modify any putative environmental risk factor.

The ApoE gene, located on chromosome 19, was the first polymorphic gene to be associated with a complex disease using positional cloning strategies. The ApoE gene products vary depending upon the inherited pair of polymorphic alleles. There are three allelic varieties ε2, ε3 and ε4. ApoE is a

glycoprotein of 299 amino acids that is a normal constituent of plasma and cerebrospinal fluid (CSF) lipoprotein particles. The physiological function of the protein is to mediate cholesterol uptake, storage, transport and metabolism. There is a binding site for Aβ present near the *C*-terminus of the ApoE molecule (Wisniewski *et al.*, 1993). ApoE is a component of the VLDL and HDL complexes involved in cellular uptake and metabolism of cholesterol (Mahley, 1988). ApoE is normally upregulated and released from astrocytes following neuronal injury and not only affects lipid metabolism following this trauma, but may also complex with VLDL to increase neurite outgrowth and synaptogenesis. However, the different ApoE genotypes differentially affect this process. Individuals carrying the ε4 allele have a decreased capacity for compensatory neurite outgrowth and synaptogenesis following neuronal injury (Poirier, 1994).

It has also been demonstrated that individuals with at least one ε4 allele develop greater numbers of neuritic plaques (Olichney *et al.*, 1996) irrespective of whether or not they have clinical AD (Rebeck *et al.*, 1993; Schmechel *et al.*, 1993; Polvikoski *et al.*, 1995). ApoE ε4 also complexes with Aβ, whereas ApoE ε3 does not have the same affinity, thus promoting protofibril formation, which, as has been alluded to already, may be the immediate neurotoxic product in AD. A model therefore exists that outlines the interaction between Aβ and ApoE which explains why the latter exists as one of many contributing genetic risk factors to the development of AD. At the very least, it links the metabolism of cholesterol into the Aβ-mediated pathway of AD causation.

Not only is the genotype that an individual carries relevant as a risk factor for AD, but variations in ApoE levels may also be an important factor in predicting disease onset. The promoter of ApoE that regulates the synthesis of the lipoprotein is polymorphic. The allelic variants at −491 (Bullido *et al.*, 1998), −427 (Artiga *et al.*, 1998) and −219 (Lambert *et al.*, 1998) of the ApoE promoter region, when homozygous, may be associated with increased risk of AD, and a combination of the adverse alleles of the promoter and coding regions confer even greater risk of developing AD (Artiga *et al.*, 1998).

Clinically, possession of the ε4 allele increases the risk of developing AD at any particular age. In individuals who are ε4 heterozygotes, there is an approximate doubling of risk and for those that are homozygous for ε4 the risk is increased by a factor of between 6 and 8 (National Institute on Aging/Alzheimer's Association Working Group, 1996). Possession of an ε4 allele may lead to an earlier age of onset (Blacker *et al.*, 1997; Burlinson *et al.*, 1998) and there may be an even greater risk of developing AD in females who carry the ε4 allele (Poirier *et al.*, 1993; Payami *et al.*, 1994; Duara *et al.*, 1996). There are, however, conflicting reports regarding the rate of decline associated with different genotypes. The ApoE ε2 allele may confer protection against the development of AD (Corder *et al.*, 1994; Myers *et al.*, 1996).

The ε4 allele also confers additional risk of developing AD in those patients who have suffered strokes (Slooter *et al.*, 1997), though other authors, in smaller studies, have failed to replicate this finding (Burlinson *et al.*, 1998). Other cerebral insults such as head injuries have been associated with increased Aβ deposition in patients who carry an ε4 allele (Nicoll *et al.*, 1995). Determining the ApoE status of a patient may be of value in aiding the diagnosis of AD where there is already a high clinical suspicion of the condition. However, there may only be a marginal increase in diagnostic accuracy (American College of Medical Genetics/American Society of Human Genetics Working Group on Apolipoprotein E and Alzheimer's Disease, 1995; National Institute on Aging/ Alzheimer's Association Working Group, 1996). In isolation, knowledge of the ApoE genotype of any given individual lacks the sensitivity, specificity or positive predictive value to be useful as a screening tool.

32.8.2 α2-Macroglobulin, low density lipoprotein receptor-related protein and insulin degrading enzyme

Whilst the ApoE gene was the first polymorphic marker to be identified as a genetic modifier of risk for AD, other candidate genetic loci are being investigated, including α2-macroglobulin (α2M), a protease inhibitor found in association with amyloid plaques in AD. The gene for α2M is located on chromosome 12: binds Aβ with high affinity, and may influence fibril formation and the toxicity of Aβ *in vitro* (Hughes *et al.*, 1998). The activity of α2M has also been associated with low density lipoprotein receptor-related protein (LRP1). Both α2M and LRP1 are upregulated following neuronal injury (Lopes *et al.*, 1994). Furthermore, α2M is thought to mediate Aβ degradation via endocytosis through LRP1 (Narita *et al.*, 1997). As ApoE and APP are also ligands of LRP1, it is postulated that different isoforms of ApoE and α2M may interact differentially and competitively for this system, affecting the clearance of Aβ.

Several investigators have now shown that, like ApoE, different LRP1 genotypes are associated with the development of AD (Kang *et al.*, 1997; Hollenbach *et al.*, 1998), mediated possibly through an increase in Aβ burden. α2M genotypes, unlike ApoE genotypes, have seemingly no effect on the age of onset in AD (Liao *et al.*, 1998). The odds ratio for AD associated with the γ/γ α2M genotype was shown to be 1.77 (1.16–2.70, $P < 0.01$) and in combination with ApoE γ4 was 9.68 (3.91–24.0, $P < 0.001$). In the same study, there was no increased risk of AD demonstrated in heterozygotic individuals with γ/γ genotype, and stratification of the sample based on the presence or absence of the ApoE γ4 allele demonstrated a similar overrepresentation of the γ/γ genotype in both strata (Liao *et al.*, 1998). This finding was demonstrated in a population-based study. This initial work suggests that the α2M γ/γ genotype may increase the risk of developing AD, that this risk is independent of the effects of ApoE γ4, and that the risks are additive and substantial. The studies to date require further replication and the effect requires demonstration in different populations in a similar manner to studies defining the risks associated with ApoE γ4. If future studies do conclude that α2M is an independent risk factor

for AD, then predictive testing considering both genes (and also including genotyping of the ApoE promoter regions) could be developed with much higher positive predictive values than those demonstrated with ApoE testing alone.

Whole genome search strategies (Blacker *et al.*, 2003; Ertekin-Taner *et al.*, 2004) have yielded other 'hot spots' of interest, the most intriguing of which is that on chromosome 10, close to the insulin degrading enzyme (IDE) locus. Attempts to identify IDE as a risk factor have so far failed, but it remains an attractive candidate for its demonstrated role in promoting the clearance of Aβ from the brain (Farris *et al.*, 2004).

32.9 INTERVENTIONS

Being able to determine the risk that a given individual has of developing AD late in life has few clinical implications at present. As proven disease-modifying treatments for AD do not exist, the main benefit of defining a population at high risk of developing AD is to identify a cohort for clinical trials of drugs with a postulated preventative or significant disease-modifying action.

Current therapeutic interventions for AD operate far downstream from the postulated initial toxicity of Aβ$_{42}$. Their efficacy is dependent upon augmenting the activity of surviving cholinergic neurones; the cholinesterase inhibitors (donepezil, galantamine) have shown only modest effect on clinical progression of AD and have no demonstrable disease-modifying effect. To prevent neuronal damage and clinical impairment, effective therapies must either affect the initial production of Aβ$_{42}$ from APP or mediate its toxicity or clearance. Specific interventions may therefore target inhibition of γ-secretase, upregulate the α-secretase pathway, influence the phosphorylation state of the APP molecule, chelate metal ions, scavenge free radicals, affect the postulated overactivation of microglial cells in response to amyloid deposition or a combination of these. These actions may, if the amyloid theory is correct, decrease Aβ$_{42}$ production and amyloid plaque formation, protect neurones from the postulated neurotoxic effects of this system or aid clearance of Aβ$_{42}$ from the brain.

32.10 CONCLUSIONS

This chapter has highlighted the complexity and intricacies of the various systems that tie Aβ to the neuronal degeneration of AD. Intensive investigation of these biochemical systems has elucidated several potential targets for rational therapeutic intervention. The test of the amyloid theory will be in the examination of interventions that modulate the production and accumulation of Aβ$_{42}$, initially in mice before human trials take place. In preparation for these trials, defining a high-risk population based on genetic risk factors will continue with the hope that more effective disease-modifying drugs will be available for trial in the not too distant future.

REFERENCES

American College of Medical Genetics/American Society of Human Genetics Working Group on ApoE and Alzheimer disease. (1995) Statement on use of Apolipoprotein E testing for Alzheimer's disease. *JAMA* **274**: 1627–1629

Ancolio K, Dumanchin C, Barelli H *et al.* (1999) Unusual phenotypic alteration of β-amyloid precursor protein maturation (βAPP) by a new Val-715 to met βAPP-770 mutation responsible for probable early-onset Alzheimer's disease. *Proceedings of the National Academy of Sciences of the United States of America* **96**: 4119–4124

Artiga MJ, Bullido MJ, Frank A *et al.* (1998) Risk for Alzheimer's disease correlates with transcriptional activity of the ApoE gene. *Human Molecular Genetics* **7**: 1887–1892

Atwood CS, Obrenovich ME, Liu TB *et al.* (2003) Amyloid-β a chameleon walking in two worlds: a review of the trophic and toxic properties of amyloid-β. *Brain Research Reviews* **43**: 1–16

Barelli H, Lebeau A, Vizzavona J *et al.* (1997) Characterization of new polyclonal antibodies specific for 40 and 42 amino acid-long amyloid β peptides: their use to examine the cell biology of presenilins and the immunohistochemistry of sporadic Alzheimer's disease and cerebral amyloid angiopathy cases. *Molecular Medicine* **3**: 695–707

Baskin F, Rosenberg R, Davis RM. (1992) Morphological differentiation and proteoglycan synthesis regulate Alzheimer amyloid precursor protein processing in PC-12 and human astrocyte cultures. *Journal of Neuroscience Research* **32**: 274–279

Behl C, Davis J, Cole GM, Schubert D. (1992) Vitamin E protects nerve cells from amyloid β protein toxicity. *Biochemical and Biophysical Research Communications* **186**: 944–950

Behl C, Davis JB, Lesley R, Schubert D. (1994) Hydrogen peroxide mediates amyloid β protein toxicity. *Cell* **77**: 817–827

Berg L, McKeel DW, Miller P *et al.* (1998) Clinicopathologic studies in cognitively healthy aging and Alzheimer disease. Relation of histologic markers to dementia severity, age, sex, and apolipoprotein E genotype. *Archives of Neurology* **55**: 326–335

Bertram L and Tanzi RE. (2004) Alzheimer's disease: one disorder, too many genes? *Human Molecular Genetics* **13**: R135–R141

Blacker D and Tanzi RE. (1998) The genetics of Alzheimer's disease. Current status and future prospects. *Archives of Neurology* **55**: 294–296

Blacker D, Haines JL, Rodes L *et al.* (1997) ApoE4 and age at onset of Alzheimer's Disease: the NIMH genetics initiative. *Neurology* **48**: 139–147

Blacker D, Bertram L, Saunders AJ *et al.* (2003) Results of a high-resolution genome screen of 437 Alzheimer's disease families. *Human Molecular Genetics* **12**: 23–32

Borchelt DR, Thinakaran G, Eckman CB *et al.* (1996) Familial Alzheimer's disease-linked presenilin 1 variants elevate Aβ-1-42/1–40 ratio *in vitro* and *in vivo*. *Neuron* **17**: 1005–1013

Brooks WS, Martins RN, Devoecht J *et al.* (1995) A mutation in codon 717 of the amyloid precursor protein gene in an Australian family with Alzheimer's disease. *Neuroscience Letters* **199**: 183–186

Bullido MJ, Artiga MJ, Recuero M *et al.* (1998) A polymorphism in the regulatory region of ApoE associated with risk of Alzheimer's dementia. *Nature Genetics* **18**: 69–71

Burlinson S, Burns A, Mann D, Pickering-Brown S, Owen. F. (1998) Effect of apolipoprotein E status on clinical features of dementia. *International Journal of Geriatric Psychology* **13**: 177–185

Butterfield DA, Hensley K, Harris M, Mattson M, Carney J. (1994) β-Amyloid peptide free radical fragments initiate synaptosomal lipoperoxidation in a sequence-specific fashion: implications to Alzheimer's disease. *Biochemical and Biophysical Research Communications* **200**: 710–715

Butterfield DA. (2002) Amyloid β-peptide (1–42)-induced oxidative stress and neurotoxicity: implications for neurodegeneration in Alzheimer's disease brain. A review. *Free Radical Research* **36**: 1307–1313

Butterfield DA. (2003) Amyloid β-peptide (1–42)-associated free radical-induced oxidative stress and neurodegeneration in Alzheimer's disease grain: mechanisms and consequences. *Current Medicinal Chemistry* **10**: 2651–2659

Buxbaum JD, Oishi M, Chen HI *et al.* (1992) Cholinergic agonists and interleukin 1 regulate processing and secretion of the Alzheimer β/A4 amyloid protein precursor. *Proceedings of the National Academy of Sciences of the United States of America* **89**: 10075–10078

Cai XD, Golde TE, Younkin SG. (1993) Release of excess amyloid β protein from a mutant amyloid β protein precursor. *Science* **259**: 514–516

Caporaso GL, Gandy SE, Buxbaum JD. (1992) Protein phosphorylation regulates secretion of Alzheimer β/A4 amyloid precursor protein. *Proceedings of the National Academy of Sciences of the United States of America* **89**: 3055–3059

Citron M, Diehl TS, Gordon G *et al.* (1996) Evidence that the 42- and 40-amino acid forms of amyloid β protein are generated from the β-amyloid precursor protein by different protease activities. *Proceedings of the National Academy of Sciences of the United States of America* **93**: 13170–13175

Citron M. (2002) Alzheimer's disease: treatments in discovery and development. *Nature Neuroscience* **5**: 1055–1057

Copani A, Koh J, Cotman CW. (1991) β-Amyloid increases neuronal susceptibility to injury by glucose deprivation. *Neuropharmacology and Neurotoxicology* **2**: 763–765

Corder EH, Saunders AM, Risch NJ *et al.* (1994) Protective effect of apolipoprotein E type 2 allele for late onset Alzheimer's disease. *Nature Genetics* **7**: 180–184

De Strooper B, Saftig P, Craesaerts K *et al.* (1998) Deficiency of presenilin-1 inhibits the normal cleavage of amyloid precursor protein. *Nature* **391**: 387–390

De Strooper B, Annaert W, Cupers P *et al.* (1999) A presenilin-1-dependent γ-secretase-like protease mediates release of Notch intracellular domain. *Nature* **398**: 518–522

Dickson DW. (1997) The pathogenesis of senile plaques. *Journal of Neuropathology and Experimental Neurology* **56**: 321–339

Duara R, Barker WW, Lopez-Alberola R *et al.* (1996) Alzheimer's disease: interaction of apolipoprotein E genotype, family history of dementia, gender, education, ethnicity and age of onset. *Neurology* **46**: 1575–1579

Duff K, Eckman C, Zehr C *et al.* (1996) Increased amyloid-β 42(43) in brains of mice expressing mutant presenilin 1. *Nature* **383**: 710–713

Eckman CB, Mehta ND, Crook R *et al.* (1997) A new pathogenic mutation in the APP gene (I716V) increases the relative proportion of Aβ 42(43). *Human Molecular Genetics* **6**: 2087–2089

Ertekin-Taner N, Allen M, Fadale D *et al.* (2004) Genetic variants in haplotype block spanning IDE are significantly associated with plasma Aβ42 levels and risk for Alzheimer disease. *Human Mutation* **23**: 334–342

Evin G, Beyreuther, K, Masters, CL. (1994) Alzheimer's disease amyloid precursor protein (AβPP): proteolytic processing, secretases and βA4 amyloid production. *International Journal of Experimental and Clinical Investigation* **1**: 263–280

Farris W, Mansourian S, Leissring MA *et al.* (2004) Partial loss-of-function mutations in insulin-degrading enzyme that induce diabetes also impair degradation of amyloid β protein. *American Journal of Pathology* **164**: 1425–1434

Gillespie SL, Golde TE, Younkin SG. (1992) Secretory processing of the Alzheimer amyloid β/A4 protein precursor is increased by protein phosphorylation. *Biochemical and Biophysical Research Communications* **187**: 1285–1290

Glenner GG and Wong CW. (1984) Alzheimer's disease: initial report of the purification and characterization of a novel cerebrovascular amyloid protein. *Biochemical and Biophysical Research Communications* **120**: 885–890

Golde TE, Estus S, Usiak M, Younkin LH, Younkin SG. (1990) Expression of β amyloid protein precursor mRNAs: recognition of a novel alternatively spliced form and quantitation in Alzheimer's disease using PCR. *Neuron* **4**: 253–267

Haass C, Hung AY, Selkoe DJ. (1991) Processing of β-amyloid precursor protein in microglia and astrocytes favors an internal localization over constitutive secretion. *Journal of Neuroscience* **11**: 3783–3793

Haass C, Hung AY, Selkoe DJ, Teplow DB. (1994) Mutations associated with a locus for familial Alzheimer's disease result in alternative processing of amyloid β protein precursor. *Journal of Biological Chemistry* **269**: 17741–17748

Hardy J, Duff K, Gwinn Hardy K, Perez-Tur J, Hutton M. (1998) Genetic dissection of Alzheimer's disease and related dementias: amyloid and its relationship to tau. *Nature Neuroscience* **1**: 355–358

Henry A, Li QX, Galatis D *et al.* (1998) Inhibition of platelet activation by the Alzheimer's disease amyloid precursor protein. *British Journal of Haematology* **103**: 402–415

Hensley K, Carney JM, Mattson MP *et al.* (1994) A model for β-amyloid aggregation and neurotoxicity based on free radical generation by the peptide: relevance to Alzheimer disease. *Proceedings of the National Academy of Sciences of the United States of America* **91**: 3270–3274

Hollenbach E, Ackerman S, Hyman BT, Rebeck GW. (1998) Confirmation of an association between a polymorphism in exon 3 of the low-density lipoprotein receptor-related protein gene and Alzheimer's disease. *Neurology* **50**: 1905–1907

Howlett DR Jennings KH, Lee DC *et al.* (1995) Aggregation state and neurotoxic properties of Alzheimer beta-amyloid peptide. *Neurodegeneration* **4**: 23–32

Hughes SR, Khorkova O, Goyal S *et al.* (1998) α2-Macroglobulin associates with β-amyloid peptide and prevents fibril formation. *Proceedings of the National Academy of Sciences of the United States of America* **95**: 3275–3278

Hung AY, Koo EH, Haass C, Selkoe DJ. (1992) Increased expression of β-amyloid precursor protein during neuronal differentiation is not accompanied by secretory cleavage. *Journal of Biological Chemistry* **268**: 22956–22959

Hyman BT and Tanzi RE. (1992) Amyloid, dementia and Alzheimer's disease. *Current Opinion in Neurology and Neurosurgery* **5**: 88–93

Iwatsubo T. (2004) The γ-secretase complex: machinery for intramembrane proteolysis. *Current Opinion in Neurobiology* **14**: 379–383

Kang DE, Saitoh T, Chen X *et al.* (1997) Genetic association of the low-density lipoprotein receptor-related protein gene (LRP), an apolipoprotein E receptor, with late onset Alzheimer's disease. *Neurology* **49**: 56–61

Kang J and Müller-Hill B. (1990) Differential splicing of Alzheimer's disease amyloid A4 precursor RNA in rat tissues: preA4695 mRNA is predominantly produced in rat and human brain. *Biochemical and Biophysical Research Communications* **166**: 1192–1200

Kang J, Lemaire H, Unterbeck A *et al.* (1987) The precursor of Alzheimer's disease amyloid A4 protein resembles a cell-surface receptor. *Nature* **325**: 733–736

Keller JN, Guo Q, Holtsberg FW, Brucekeller AJ, Mattson MP. (1998) Increased sensitivity to mitochondrial toxin-induced apoptosis in neural cells expressing mutant presenilin-1 is linked to perturbed calcium homeostasis and enhanced oxyradical production. *Journal of Neuroscience* **18**: 4439–4450

Koh J, Yang LL, Cotman CW. (1990) β-Amyloid protein increases the vulnerability of cultured cortical neurons to excitotoxic damage. *Brain Research* **533**: 315–320

Kosik KS, Joachim CL, Selkoe DJ. (1986) Microtubule-associated protein tau (τ) is a major antigenic component of paired helical filaments in Alzheimer disease. *Proceedings of the National Academy of Sciences of the United States of America* **83**: 4044–4048

Kwok JBJ, Li QX, Hallup M *et al.* (2000) Novel Leu 723 pro amyloid precursor protein mutation increases amyloid β42 (43) peptide levels and induces apoptosis. *Annals of Neurology* **47**: 249–253

Lahiri DK, Nall C, Farlow M. (1992) The cholinergic agonist carbachol reduces intracellular β-amyloid precursor protein in PC 12 and C6 cells. *Biochemistry International* **28**: 853–860

Lahiri DK, Farlow MR, Greig NH, Sambamurti K. (2002) Current drug targets for Alzheimer's disease treatment. *Drug Development Research* **56**: 267–281

Lambert JC, Pasquier F, Cottel D *et al.* (1998) A new polymorphism in the ApoE promoter associated with risk of developing Alzheimer's dementia. *Human Molecular Genetics* **7**: 533–540

Lammich S, Kojro E, Postina R *et al.* (1999) Constitutive and regulated α-secretase cleavage of Alzheimer's amyloid precursor protein by a disintegrin metalloprotease. *Proceedings of the National Academy of Sciences of the United States of America* **96**: 3922–3927

Lansbury PT Jr. (1999) Evolution of amyloid: what normal protein folding may tell us about fibrillogenesis and disease. *Proceedings of the National Academy of Sciences of the United States of America* **96**: 3342–3344

Lemere CA, Lopera F, Kosik KS *et al.* (1996) The E280A presenilin 1 Alzheimer mutation produces increased Aβ42 deposition and severe cerebellar pathology. *Nature Medicine* **2**: 1146–11450

Liao A, Nitsch RM, Greenberg SM *et al.* (1998) Genetic association of an α2-macroglobulin (Val 1000 Ile) polymorphism and Alzheimer's disease. *Human Molecular Genetics* **7**: 1953–1956

Lockhart BP, Benicourt C, Junien JL, Privat A. (1994) Inhibitors of free radical formation fail to attenuate direct β-amyloid(25–35) peptide-mediated neurotoxicity in rat hippocampal cultures. *Journal of Neuroscience Research* **39**: 494–505

Lopes MB, Bogaev CA, Gonias SL, Vandenberg SR. (1994) Expression of α2-macroglobulin receptor/low density lipoprotein receptor-related protein is increased in reactive and neoplastic glial cells. *FEBS Letters* **338**: 301–305

Lorenzo A and Yanker BA. (1994) β-Amyloid neurotoxicity requires fibril formation and is inhibited by Congo red. *Proceedings of the National Academy of Sciences of the United States of America* **91**: 12243–12247

McKee AC, Kosik KS, Kowall NW. (1991) Neuritic pathology and dementia in Alzheimer's disease. *Annals of Neurology* **30**: 156–165

McLean CA, Cherney RA, Fraser FW *et al.* (1999) Soluble pool of Aβ as a determinant of severity of neurodegeneration in Alzheimer's disease. *Annals of Neurology* **46**: 860–866

Mahley RW. (1988) Apolipoprotein E: cholesterol transport protein with expanding role in cell biology. *Science* **240**: 622–630

Mark RJ, Blanc EM, Mattson MP. (1996) Amyloid β-peptide and oxidative cellular injury in Alzheimer's disease. *Molecular Neurobiology* **12**: 211–224

Masters CL, Simms G, Weinman NA *et al.* (1985) Amyloid plaque core protein in Alzheimer disease and Down syndrome. *Proceedings of the National Academy of Sciences of the United States of America* **82**: 4245–4249

Mattson MP, Cheng B, Culwell AR *et al.* (1993) Evidence for excitoprotective and intraneuronal calcium-regulating roles for secreted forms of the β-amyloid precursor protein. *Neuron* **10**: 243–254

Milward E, Papadopoulos R, Fuller SJ *et al.* (1992) The amyloid protein precursor of Alzheimer's disease is a mediator of the effects of nerve growth factor on neurite outgrowth. *Neuron* **9**: 129–137

Morris JC, McKeel DW, Storandt M *et al.* (1991) Very mild Alzheimer's disease: informant-based clinical psychometric and pathologic distinction from normal aging. *Neurology* **41**: 469–478

Multhaup G, Masters CL, Beyreuther K. (1998) Oxidative stress in Alzheimer's disease. *Alzheimer's Reports* **1**: 147–154

Myers R, Schaeter EJ, Wilson PW *et al.* (1996) Apolipoprotein E4 association with dementia in a population based study: the Framingham study. *Neurology* **46**: 673–677

Narita M, Holtzman DM, Schwartz AL, Bu GJ. (1997) α2-Macroglobulin complexes with and mediates the endocytosis of β-amyloid peptide via cell surface low-density lipoprotein receptor-related protein. *Journal of Neurochemistry* **69**: 1904–1911

National Institute on Aging/Alzheimer's Association Working Group. (1996) Apolipoprotein E genotyping in Alzheimer's disease. *Lancet* **347**: 1091–1095

Nicoll J, Roberts GW, Graham D. (1995) Apolipoprotein E ε4 allele is associated with deposition of amyloid following head injury. *Nature Medicine* **1**: 135–137

Nitsch RM, Slack BE, Wurtman RJ, Growdon JH. (1992) Release of Alzheimer amyloid precursor derivatives stimulated by activation of muscarinic acetylcholine receptors. *Science* **258**: 304–307

Olichney JM, Hansen LA, Galasko D *et al.* (1996) The apolipoprotein E ε4 allele is associated with increased neuritic plaques and cerebral amyloid angiopathy in Alzheimer's disease and Lewy body variant. *Neurology* **47**: 190–196

Payami H, Montee KR, Kaye JA *et al.* (1994) Alzheimer's disease, apolipoprotein ε4, and gender. *JAMA* **271**: 1316–1317

Poirier J. (1994) Apolipoprotein E in CNS models of CNS injury and in Alzheimer's disease. *Trends in Neuroscience* **17**: 525–530

Poirier J, Davignon J, Bouthillier D *et al.* (1993) Apolipoprotein E polymorphism and Alzheimer's disease. *Lancet* **342**: 697–699

Polvikoski T, Sulkava R, Haltia M *et al.* (1995) Apolipoprotein E, dementia and cortical deposition of β-amyloid protein. *New England Journal of Medicine* **333**: 1242–1247

Price DL, Sisodia SS, Borchelt DR. (1998) Genetic neurodegenerative diseases: the human illness and transgenic models. *Science* **282**: 1079–1083

Rebeck GW, Reiter JS, Strickland DK, Hyman BT. (1993) Apolipoprotein E in sporadic Alzheimer's disease: allelic variation and receptor interactions. *Neuron* **11**: 575–580

Ritchie CW, Bush AI, Mackinnon A *et al.* (2003). Metal-protein attenuation with iodochlorhydroxyquin (clioquinol) targeting Aβ amyloid deposition and toxicity in Alzheimer's disease: a pilot phase 2 clinical trial. *Archives Neurology* **60**: 1685–1691

Rogaev EI. (1998) Presenilins – discovery and characterization of the genes of Alzheimer's disease. *Molecular Biology* **32**: 58–69

Roperch JP, Alvaro V, Prieur S *et al.* (1998) Inhibition of presenilin 1 expression is promoted by p53 and p21waf-1 and results in apoptosis and tumor suppression. *Nature Medicine* **4**: 835–838

Sano M, Ernesto C, Thomas RG *et al.* (1997) A controlled trial of selegiline, alpha-tocopherol, or both as treatment for Alzheimer's disease. *New England Journal of Medicine* **336**: 1216–1222

Scheper W, Annaert W, Cupers P, Saftig P, De Strooper B. (1999) Function and dysfunction of the presenilins. *Alzheimer's Reports* **2**: 73–81

Scheuner D, Eckman C, Jensen M *et al.* (1996) Secreted amyloid β-protein similar to that in the senile plaques of Alzheimer's disease is increased *in vivo* by the presenilin 1 and 2 and APP mutations linked to familial Alzheimer's disease. *Nature Medicine* **2**: 864–870

Schmechel DE, Saunders AM, Strittmatter WJ *et al.* (1993) Increased amyloid β-peptide deposition in cerebral cortex as a consequence of apolipoprotein E genotype in late-onset Alzheimer's disease. *Proceedings of the National Academy of Sciences of the United States of America* **90**: 9649–9653

Shearman MS, Ragan CI, Iversen LL. (1994) Inhibition of PC12 cell redox activity is a specific, early indicator of the mechanism of β-amyloid-mediated cell death. *Proceedings of the National Academy of Sciences of the United States of America* **91**: 1470–1474

Sheng JG, Zhou XQ, Mrak RE, Griffin WS. (1998) Progressive neuronal injury associated with amyloid plaque formation in Alzheimer's disease. *Journal of Neuropathology and Experimental Neurology* **57**: 714–717

Sinha S and Lieberburg I. (1992) Normal metabolism of the amyloid precursor protein (APP). *Neurodegeneration* **1**: 169–175

Slooter AJC, Tang MX, van Duijn CM *et al.* (1997) Apolipoprotein E ε4 and the risk of dementia with stroke (a population based investigation). *JAMA* **277**: 818–821

Small DH, Nurcombe V, Reed G *et al.* (1994) A heparin-binding domain in the amyloid protein precursor of Alzheimer's disease is involved in the regulation of neurite outgrowth. *Journal of Neuroscience* **14**: 2117–2127

Struhl G and Greenwald I. (1999) Presenilin is required for activity and nuclear access of notch in Drosophila. *Nature* **398**: 522–524

Suh Y and Checler HF. (2002) Amyloid precursor protein, presenilins, and α-synuclein: molecular pathogenesis and pharmacological applications in Alzheimer's disease. *Pharmacological Reviews* **54**: 469–525

Suzuki N, Iwatsubo T, Odaka A *et al.* (1994) High tissue content of soluble beta 1–40 is linked to cerebral amyloid angiopathy. *American Journal of Pathology* **145**: 452–460

Tanzi RE, Gusella JF, Watkins PC *et al.* (1987) Amyloid β protein gene: cDNA, mRNA distribution and genetic linkage near the Alzheimer locus. *Science* **235**: 880–884

Teller JK, Russo C, DeBusk LM *et al.* (1996) Presence of soluble amyloid β-peptide precedes amyloid plaque formation in Down's syndrome. *Nature Medicine* **2**: 93–95

Terry RD, Masliah E, Salmon DP *et al.* (1991) Physical basis of cognitive alterations in Alzheimer's disease: synapse loss is the major correlate of cognitive impairment. *Annals of Neurology* **30**: 572–580

Walsh D, Klyubin MI, Fadeeva JV, Rowan MJ, Selkoe DJ. (2002) Amyloid-beta oligomers: their production, toxicity and therapeutic inhibition. *Biochemical Society Transactions* **30**: 552–557

Whitson JS and Appel SH. (1995) Neurotoxicity of Aβ-amyloid protein *in vitro* is not altered by calcium channel blockade. *Neurobiology of Aging* **16**: 5–10

Wisniewski T, Golabek A, Matsubara E, Ghiso J, Frangione B. (1993) Apolipoprotein E: binding to soluble Alzheimer's β-amyloid. *Biochemical and Biophysical Research Communications* **192**: 359–365

Wolfe MS, Xia W, Ostaszewski BL *et al.* (1999) Two transmembrane aspartates in presenilin-1 required for presenilin endoproteolysis and γ-secretase activity. *Nature* **398**: 513–517

Wood JG, Mirra SS, Pollock NJ, Binder LI. (1986) Neurofibrillary tangles of Alzheimer disease share antigenic determinants with the axonal microtubule associated protein tau τ. *Proceedings of the National Academy of Sciences of the United States of America* **83**: 4040–4043

Yankner BA. (1996) Mechanisms of neuronal degeneration in Alzheimer's disease. *Neurology* **16**: 921–932

Ye Y, Lukinova N, Fortini ME. (1999) Neurogenic phenotypes and altered Notch processing in Drosophila presenilin mutants. *Nature* **398**: 525–529

33

Vascular factors in Alzheimer's disease

ROBERT STEWART

The growing recognition of vascular factors in Alzheimer's disease (AD) has challenged preconceived ideas about the nature of dementia. Assumptions about AD and vascular dementia as distinguishable clinical disorders have been steadily eroded as the large overlap between assumed underlying pathology and observed clinical syndromes has become increasingly evident. In neuropathological research, the focus on neuritic plaques and neurofibrillary tangles as the hallmarks of 'Alzheimer pathology' is challenged by an increasing body of research highlighting associated abnormalities in the vasculature. Developments in neuroimaging have been a mixed blessing. The ability to detect more minor levels of vascular disturbance is undoubtedly useful in investigating causal pathways and a long way on from relying on clinical evidence of cerebral infarction. However, detectable 'abnormalities' now include a larger proportion that are coincidental rather than causal, particularly in older age groups.

33.1 CHALLENGES FOR RESEARCH

A major obstacle for research in this area has been the assumption that AD and vascular dementia are discrete disorders at a pathological and clinical level. This assumption arose, one suspects, because of a need for clinicians to assign diagnoses rather than because of any supportive evidence. The authors of the seminal post-mortem studies in the 1960s and 1970s recognized that people with dementia could have Alzheimer pathology, could have cerebral infarction or could have both. Mixed dementia was retained in all subsequent diagnostic systems but received little or no research attention. Research instead focused on AD, using clinical and pathological

diagnostic criteria, which excluded potentially mixed disease because of the higher interrater agreement attained by using a narrow syndrome definition. Vascular factors in AD became a difficult area to research because AD could only be diagnosed in the absence of vascular factors.

A more fundamental challenge to understanding the role of vascular factors in AD is the limited interface between epidemiological and biological research. Epidemiological research investigates associations between potential risk factors and a specified disorder, accepting that causal processes in between may not be measurable in the population. These causal processes can be represented as a 'black box' between exposure and outcome. Biological research on the other hand focuses on potential causal processes within the 'box'. However, in the absence of tissue biopsies (which are impractical in dementia research), findings at a molecular or cellular level cannot be linked directly to clinical symptoms/syndromes observed in life. Because of this lack of connection, AD has become in effect two disorders – one a process of nerve cell death with particular features at a cellular level that can only be observed at autopsy, the second a clinical disorder characterized by its symptoms and clinical course. AD the pathological disorder is likely to be have been present for a decade or two before AD the clinical disorder becomes apparent. However, large numbers of people with significant levels of AD pathology show no clinical evidence of dementia (Neuropathology Group of the Medical Research Council Cognitive Function and Ageing Study, 2001). Diagnostic criteria for AD as a clinical disorder attempt to predict the presence of AD pathology by the time of death (McKhann et al., 1984). However, these criteria poorly reflect mixed disease (Holmes et al., 1999), which will become increasingly common with population ageing.

The role of vascular factors in AD may therefore be considered from two perspectives. One concerns the association between vascular disease, vascular risk factors and risk of AD as a clinically defined syndrome. The second concerns vascular abnormalities associated with Alzheimer pathology. These will be considered separately before research findings are described which may link the strands together.

33.2 VASCULAR FACTORS AND CLINICAL ALZHEIMER'S DISEASE

The most commonly used criteria for 'probable' AD require that other potential causes of dementia are not present. There is obviously a strong subjective element involved in deciding what represents a sufficient potential 'cause', an issue which has become steadily more problematic with increasingly sophisticated techniques for identifying mild degrees of comorbidity (and with ageing populations where significant comorbidity is to be expected). An inevitable byproduct of this classification system is that AD samples tend to be relatively healthy, and it is not surprising that several early case–control studies found similar or lower levels of vascular risk factors.

33.2.1 Associations between vascular risk factors and AD

Progress only began to be made when studies began to use screened community samples and applied more broad definitions of AD, allowing people with comorbid cerebrovascular disease to be included if this was not clearly causal. There is now a substantial body of prospective epidemiological research supporting a role for vascular risk factors in the aetiology of AD. Identified risk factors include large vessel atherosclerosis as estimated by carotid ultrasound or the ankle:brachial blood pressure index (Hofman et al., 1997), conventional risk factors for cerebrovascular disease such as hypertension (Skoog et al., 1996b; Kivipelto et al., 2001), type 2 diabetes (Brayne et al., 1998; Ott et al., 1999) and atrial fibrillation (Ott et al., 1997), as well as conventional cardiovascular risk factors such as raised cholesterol levels (Notkola et al., 1998; Kivipelto et al., 2001) and smoking (Ott et al., 1998). They also include risk factors such as raised homocysteine levels (Clarke et al., 1998; Seshadri et al., 2002) and insulin resistance (Kuusisto et al., 1997) and protective factors such as moderate alcohol intake (Ruitenberg et al., 2002) and increased physical activity (Yoshitake et al., 1995; Laurin et al., 2001) where other causal pathways may be involved, but whose associations with AD may have a vascular component.

33.2.2 Effects of dementia on vascular risk factors

Despite strong associations with cerebrovascular disease, associations between hypertension and dementia (including AD) proved remarkably difficult to demonstrate for some time. Raised blood pressure in mid-life is associated with later cognitive impairment and dementia (Elias et al., 1993; Launer et al., 1995). However, this has tended only to be apparent in studies with follow-up periods of 10 years or more. Studies with shorter follow up often find no association (Posner et al., 2002), and cross-sectional studies frequently show associations between dementia and low rather than high blood pressure (Guo et al., 1996). Skoog's analysis of a cohort with 15-year follow-up data found that participants with AD had raised systolic blood pressure at the start of the study but lower blood pressure by the time dementia had developed (Skoog et al., 1996b). This does not appear to be accounted for by antihypertensive treatment since randomized trials of these agents show no deleterious effects on cognition (Prince et al., 1996; Forette et al., 1998). It is therefore likely that there are metabolic changes associated with early dementia, which account for this reversal of association. These illustrate a further difficulty with investigating vascular risk factors since AD cannot be assumed to be a 'passive' outcome but instead may influence the exposures in question. Weight loss occurs in early dementia (Barrett-Connor et al., 1996; Nourhashemi et al., 2003) as well as declining blood pressure. The extent to which these processes influence other vascular risk factors, such as cholesterol levels, insulin resistance and glucose tolerance, has not been adequately investigated. However, there are obvious implications for prevention and treatment.

33.2.3 Interactions with ApoE genotype

Several studies have investigated the role of apolipoprotein E (ApoE) genotype in the relationship between vascular risk factors and AD. The ApoE ε4 allele was first recognized for its associations with cholesterol metabolism, and has been found at least in some studies to be associated with stroke (Margaglione et al., 1998; McCarron et al., 1999). However, there is no evidence to date that cholesterol levels or other vascular factors substantially explain the well established association between ε4 and AD (Slooter et al., 1999; Prince et al., 2000). The focus instead has shifted to investigating interactions between vascular factors and ε4 as risk factors, although findings remain conflicting and difficult to synthesise. A preliminary finding from one community study was that vascular disease was more strongly associated with AD in the presence of ApoE ε4 (Hofman et al., 1997). Subsequent findings from later examinations in the same study did not support this interaction (Slooter et al., 1999), although other studies have reported similar interactions (Johnston et al., 2000). For some vascular risk factors, ε4 interactions have been found in the opposite direction. Insulin resistance and smoking, for example, have been found to be more strongly associated with AD in people without ε4 (Kuusisto et al., 1997; Ott et al., 1998). Because interactions tend not to be reported as absent, it is difficult at present to exclude publication bias as an explanation for these results.

33.2.4 The role of clinical stroke

An important question arising is the extent to which associations between vascular risk factors and AD are explained by cerebral infarction. Most of the studies cited above have, in secondary analyses, divided AD cases into those with and without clinical evidence of cerebrovascular disease and most have found that associations remain in the less mixed group. An exception may be atrial fibrillation, which appears to be particularly associated with AD co-occurring with stroke (Ott et al., 1997). The association between stroke itself and AD is almost impossible to investigate because of the way in which AD is defined. However, there have been important findings which question the extent to which the two are separable:

- The majority of people developing dementia after stroke do so in the absence of further clinical infarction (Tatemichi et al., 1994).
- Post-stroke dementia frequently follows an AD-like clinical course (Kokmen et al., 1996).
- Post-stroke dementia is frequently associated with evidence of prestroke cognitive decline (Hénon et al., 2001).
- Cognitive impairment is a risk factor for later first onset of stroke (Ferucci et al., 1996).
- Post-stroke dementia is associated with an increased risk of stroke recurrence (Moroney et al., 1997).

For dementia associated with stroke, these findings suggest that the stroke episode itself, although undoubtedly having an impact on cognitive function, may frequently occur in the context of more insidious and gradual decline. This may reflect comorbid AD in a substantial number of cases.

33.3 VASCULAR FACTORS AND ALZHEIMER'S DISEASE PATHOLOGY

Epidemiological research therefore supports a role for conventional vascular risk factors in the aetiology of clinical AD. Parallel neurobiological research has suggested that vascular processes may be an important feature of AD at a pathological level.

33.3.1 Cerebral amyloid angiopathy

Traditionally research into the role of amyloid in AD has focused on its deposition in parenchymal neuritic plaques. However, other pathology associated with the disorder has long been recognized. Cerebral amyloid angiopathy (CAA) describes the deposition of β-amyloid, amongst other proteins, in the walls of cortical vessels. CAA increases with age and is particularly common in AD (Yamada, 2000). It is also recognized to be a risk factor for cerebrovascular disorders such as small and large vessel haemorrhage, leukoencephalopathy and infarction, and is a feature of some familial early-onset dementia syndromes. CAA is therefore a feature of AD

but also a potential cause of cognitive decline in its own right. This was demonstrated in a recent autopsy follow up of a large and well-characterized community population, which found a strong and synergistic relationship between 'conventional' AD pathology and CAA on cognitive function in life (Pfeiffer et al., 2002). The effect of CAA on cognitive function was apparent in those with clinical AD and so was not fully explained by overt cerebrovascular disease, suggesting that it may underlie some of the gradual decline traditionally attributed to parenchymal pathology. The mechanism has yet to be elucidated through which small vessel abnormalities may result in neurodegeneration. However, further support is provided by a study that found blood vessels isolated from the brains of people with AD were neurotoxic in vitro (Grammas et al., 1999).

33.3.2 Microangiopathy

A growing body of evidence suggests that vascular abnormalities in AD are not restricted to arterial and arteriolar amyloid deposition, but are also seen in cerebral microvessels and capillaries. Microangiopathic changes include basement membrane thickening and collagen accumulation (Farkas et al., 2000), as well as smooth muscle cell irregularities, endothelial degeneration and other abnormalities (Kalaria and Skoog, 2002). The underlying causal pathways have yet to be established but might include oxidative stress or blood–brain barrier dysfunction secondary to AD pathology itself or secondary to a common underlying risk factor (Kalaria and Skoog, 2002). Microangiopathy may itself exacerbate AD through effects on the microcirculation, compromising the normal removal of neurotoxic β-amyloid (de la Torre and Mussivand, 1993; Preston et al., 2003), and could also exacerbate the cell damage associated with comorbid cerebascular disease (Stewart, 1998).

33.4 WHITE MATTER LESIONS AND ALZHEIMER'S DISEASE

Neuroimaging findings lie somewhere between epidemiology and pathology in AD research since associations are investigated with the clinical disease but inferences are made regarding underlying pathological processes. White matter hyperintensities (WMH) on magnetic resonance imaging (MRI) are frequently found in association with AD, although they are by no means a characteristic feature. The pathological processes underlying WMH have not been definitely established, at least in part because of methodological difficulties involved in linking neuroimaging appearances observed in life with post-mortem findings some time later. Arteriosclerotic changes are often seen in association with white matter alterations, and ischaemia due to small vessel occlusion or hypoperfusion may underlie the dysmyelination and neuronal loss also observed. However, blood–brain barrier disturbance and transient episodes of cerebral oedema may also underlie

WMH (Pantoni and Lammie, 2002). Vascular amyloid deposition has been considered as a possible factor accounting for white matter changes in AD, and both CAA and WMH are found in combination in a rare genetic syndrome (Haan et al., 1990). However, white matter changes have generally not been found to be associated with vascular amyloid in groups with dementia (Erkinjuntti et al., 1996).

Whatever the precise pathology, there is reasonable epidemiological evidence to suggest that WMH represent subclinical cerebrovascular disease in many cases. WMH have been consistently found to be associated with conventional risk factors for cerebrovascular disease such as hypertension (Breteler et al., 1994b; Liao et al., 1997; Dufouil et al., 2001), smoking (Liao et al., 1997), hypercholesterolaemia (Breteler et al., 1994b) and atherosclerosis (Bots et al., 1993). There is also a reasonable body of evidence to suggest that, at a population level, they are associated with worse cognitive function (Breteler et al., 1994a; Kuller et al., 1998), in people both with and without dementia (Skoog et al., 1996a). However, a focus on population-level associations in large studies runs the risk of glossing over considerable individual heterogeneity. WMH are common findings in older populations and may be present at an apparently severe degree without detectable evidence of cognitive impairment (Fein et al., 1990). WMH appear to be associated with dementia, although findings have been less consistent than for studies of cognitive function (Smith et al., 2000; Piguet et al., 2003). More specific associations with AD are less easy to establish because of variation in the way in which diagnostic criteria are applied and in the extent to which WMH are considered as excluding AD. What can at least be claimed with reasonable confidence is that WMH are frequently present in people with clinical AD (if only because both are common and age-associated) and that they represent comorbid cerebrovascular disease in many cases.

33.5 CAUSAL LINKS BETWEEN VASCULAR DISEASE AND ALZHEIMER'S DISEASE

The neuropathological findings summarized above suggest that vascular abnormalities are a feature of AD pathology and may be important in its clinical expression. White matter hyperintensities in AD may or may not be a marker of these particular pathological features but do suggest the involvement of vascular processes because of well-recognized associations with risk factors for cerebrovascular disease. The next question to consider concerns pathways that might explain the association observed in life between vascular risk factors and AD.

33.5.1 Links at a pathological level

Various pathways have been proposed, which may explain an association between AD and vascular risk factors and which relate to links at the level of pathological processes. These will be summarized.

- *Ischaemic injury and amyloid deposition*: β-amyloid production appears to be a non-specific response to cerebral trauma but has been described in particular in the hippocampi of rodents after severe but transient ischaemia (Kogure and Kato, 1993), providing a potential link between ischaemia/infarction and AD pathology.
- *Inflammation*: There is growing recognition that inflammatory processes are important in mediating cerebral damage following stroke (Emsley and Tyrrell, 2002). Inflammation is also an important feature of AD pathology (Halliday et al., 2000), and might conceivably underlie links between the two processes.
- *The blood–brain barrier*: Increased permeability of the blood–brain barrier has been found in association with transient ischaemia (Pluta et al., 1996), and this has been suggested to underlie both perivascular amyloid deposition and white matter changes (Tomimoto et al., 1996).
- *Abnormal protein glycation*: Advance glycation end products, metabolic oxidation products associated with diabetes and hyperglycaemia (Vlassara et al., 1992) have also been found in association with neurofibrillary tangles and neuritic plaques in AD (Dickson, 1997). These may underlie, at least in part, the association between diabetes and AD that does not appear to be entirely mediated through cerebrovascular disease (Stewart and Liolitsa, 1999).

33.5.2 Links at a cognitive level

The mechanisms above suggest that vascular factors may directly influence the pathological processes that are believed to underlie AD. However, clinical AD might still be 'caused' without any direct interaction at a pathological level but instead by interaction in clinical manifestations. Alzheimer pathology develops slowly, possibly over as long a period as 20 years. The chance of someone developing dementia depends a great deal on the extent to which a given level of pathology affects cognition and on the extent to which a person can compensate for this. Alzheimer pathology begins in the hippocampus and manifests in its early stages as declining memory function. Mild levels of cerebrovascular disease on the other hand would be expected to exert most damage on deep white matter and on fronto-subcortical connections. The consequent disruption of executive functions such as selective attention and mental flexibility may be enough to 'unmask' early AD that might not otherwise have become apparent for several years. Vascular factors may therefore accelerate the age of onset of clinical AD.

33.5.3 Links at a functional level

The 'onset' of dementia is defined, at least in research settings, as the point where declining cognitive function starts to interfere with daily functioning. This is not an entirely satisfactory definition of 'incidence' since it involves a considerable degree of subjective judgement on the part of the participant, their family and the research worker. It also assumes a process that can be isolated from all the other factors influencing daily functioning in older people. A given level of cognitive impairment may be more likely to be classified as problematic if daily function is already impaired – for example because of motor system impairment owing to cerebrovascular disease. Or, from the opposite perspective, a person in good physical health may be able to sustain a greater degree of cognitive decline before this can be said to be problematic.

33.5.4 Evidence for these causal links

The hypothetical causal pathways summarized above suggest that vascular factors might act directly to increase the progression of AD pathology, or alternatively they might lower the threshold (cognitive or functional) at which clinical dementia manifests for a given degree of neurodegeneration. These two processes can be tested empirically since they predict different associations between vascular factors and neuropathological findings. Clinicopathological studies that have investigated cerebrovascular pathology as an exposure have tended to support the second mechanism. Cerebrovascular disease and AD overlap substantially in community-derived samples and are clearly not in themselves sufficient to cause dementia since either pathology can be severe with no evidence of dementia in life (Neuropathology Group of the Medical Research Council Cognitive Function and Ageing Study, 2001). However, AD pathology has not in general been found to be more severe in the presence of cerebrovascular disease. Instead, women with mild Alzheimer pathology in the Nun Study were found to be more likely to have had dementia in life if cerebral infarction was also present (Snowdon et al., 1997). The OPTIMA study in Oxford similarly found that cognitive function had been most impaired in people with early Alzheimer pathology if cerebrovascular disease was also present (Esiri et al., 1999), suggesting an effect on cognitive rather than functional reserve.

Findings to date for detectable levels of cerebrovascular disease therefore suggest that this acts to 'cause' AD through reducing the pathological threshold for clinical dementia. However, findings for certain vascular risk factors suggest that there may also be effects on AD pathology itself. A post-mortem study of people without dementia found higher senile plaque counts in those with coronary artery disease (Sparks et al., 1990) and higher neurofibrillary tangle counts in those with previous hypertension (Sparks et al., 1995). Neuropathological follow-up studies in a cohort of Japanese-American men have found higher levels of AD pathology associated with increased mid-life blood pressure (Petrovitch et al., 2000) and diabetes (Peila et al., 2002). These findings differ from those for cerebrovascular disease and suggest either that vascular risk factors influence AD pathology through different mechanisms. Alternatively it is possible that cerebrovascular disease and AD pathology are associated with

higher levels of mortality in combination, diluting their association in older cohorts.

33.5.5 Common underlying factors

Associations between vascular factors and AD need not imply direct causal links between the two but might, at least in part, arise from common underlying processes. ApoE genotype has been considered in this respect although, as discussed earlier, has not been found to explain substantially the co-occurrence of cerebrovascular disease and AD. Both AD and cerebrovascular disease are 'disorders of ageing', i.e. they become more common with increased age. However, 'ageing' as a process is not synonymous with increased chronological age and there is substantial individual variation in the physiological changes that occur in the transition from mid- to late life. 'Ageing' is likely to be influenced by a variety of factors, both genetic and acquired. Many of these are unknown, e.g. genetic factors common to diseases of ageing. Others may be unquantifiable, e.g. lifetime exposure to oxidative stress. Dementia is conventionally stressed as a disorder distinct from 'normal ageing'. However, it is likely that there are processes that mediate general vulnerability to ageing processes whether these are experienced in the brain parenchyma or in the vasculature.

A more specific factor that might link both vascular factors and AD is insulin resistance. This is recognized to be important in underlying the clustering of vascular risk factors such as hypertension, type 2 diabetes mellitus and hypercholesterolaemia (Reaven, 1988), all of which have been found to be associated with AD as summarized above. However, insulin levels themselves in theory could have direct effects on cognitive function. Insulin receptors are dense in the hippocampus (Marks et al., 1991). Their role in hippocampal function is not understood, but increased levels of insulin have been found to inhibit hippocampal synaptic activity in vitro (Palovcik et al., 1984). Insulin has also been found to reduce choline acetyltransferase activity (Brass et al., 1992), a key factor in the cognitive impairment associated with AD, and there are links which can be made between insulin growth factor-1 and the enzyme pathways which regulate tau protein phosphorylation – and hence neurofibrillary tangle formation (Stewart and Liolitsa, 1999). Insulin resistance has been found to be associated independently with AD in a population study (Kuusisto et al., 1997) but mediating pathways for this have yet to be established.

33.5.6 Direction of cause and effect

Since vascular risk factors emerge in mid-life and a considerable period before AD incidence begins to increase, it is generally assumed that any causal processes are directed from the vascular risk factor to AD. However, this does not exclude adverse effects of AD on the vasculature at a later stage. Links at a pathological level between vascular factors and AD may be complex and bi-directional. For example, hypertension might cause small vessel disease and, consequently, cerebral ischaemia or infarction. This might in turn precipitate deposition of both parenchymal and vascular amyloid causing neuronal loss. However, the presence of vascular abnormalities independently associated with co-occurring AD might also increase the extent of ischaemia and neurodegeneration associated with arteriosclerotic disease. Vascular factors might therefore be both a cause and a consequence of AD. At a clinical level, it is likely that worsening cognitive function owing to early AD may have adverse effects on risk for vascular disease, particularly through difficulties with adherence to treatment regimes from declining memory function (Rost *et al.*, 1990). Surprisingly this has received scant attention despite the frequent co-occurrence of AD and common vascular risk factors such as hypertension and type 2 diabetes.

33.6 IMPLICATIONS

This chapter has focused on evidence for the involvement of vascular factors in AD, and on processes that might underlie these associations. Clearly there are potentially important implications for prevention and treatment of dementia. A reduction in vascular risk across a population would in theory reduce the risk of later dementia, whether vascular risk factors were acting on AD pathology or reducing cognitive/functional reserve. However, 'treatment' of AD (i.e. reducing cognitive/functional decline) through modifying vascular risk would only be effective if there are direct effects on neurodegenerative processes. Observational evidence to date has not demonstrated clear associations between co-occurring cerebrovascular disease and progression of dementia, although there has been little research in this area (Lee *et al.*, 2000; Mungas *et al.*, 2001). A commonly neglected implication concerns the care of people with dementia. In terms of clinical care, people with AD will commonly have disorders such as hypertension or diabetes, which require pharmacotherapy and medical review. Neurodegenerative processes themselves may have effects on factors such as blood pressure and body composition, altering susceptibility to drug effects and side effects, and requiring close attention. In terms of formal and informal social care, people with AD will often also have clinically apparent cerebrovascular disease, which may already be affecting non-cognitive areas of functioning, increasing the level of support required. Vascular factors may have an important impact on quality of life for people with AD and their caregivers regardless of whether relationships with AD reflect cause, effect or coincidence. However, this aspect of the interface has received scant attention to date.

REFERENCES

Barrett-Connor E, Edelstein SL, Corey-Bloom J, Wiederholt WC. (1996) Weight loss precedes dementia in community-dwelling older adults. *Journal of the American Geriatrics Society* **44**: 1147–1152

Bots ML, van Swieten JC, Breteler MM *et al.* (1993) Cerebral white matter lesions and atherosclerosis in the Rotterdam Study. *Lancet* **341**: 1232–1237

Brass BJ, Nonner D, Barrett JN. (1992) Differential effects of insulin on choline acetyltransferase and glutamic acid decarboxylase activities in neuron-rich striatal cultures. *Journal of Neurochemistry* **59**: 415–4124

Brayne C, Gill C, Huppert FA *et al.* (1998) Vascular risks and incident dementia: results from a cohort study of the very old. *Dementia and Geriatric Cognitive Disorders* **9**: 175–180

Breteler MMB, van Amerongen NM, van Swieten JC *et al.* (1994a) Cognitive correlates of ventricular enlargement and cerebral white matter lesions on magnetic resonance imaging. *Stroke* **25**: 1109–1115

Breteler MMB, van Swieten JC, Bots ML *et al.* (1994b) Cerebral white matter lesions, vascular risk factors, and cognitive function in a population-based study: the Rotterdam Study. *Neurology* **44**: 1246–1252

Clarke R, Smith D, Jobst K, Refsum H, Sutton L, Ueland PM. (1998) Folate, vitamin B12, and serum total homocysteine levels in confirmed Alzheimer disease. *Archives of Neurology* **55**: 1449–1455

de la Torre JC and Mussivand T. (1993) Can disturbed brain microcirculation cause Alzheimer's disease? *Neurological Research* **15**: 146–153

Dickson DW. (1997) The pathogenesis of senile plaques. *Journal of Neuropathology and Experimental Neurology* **56**: 321–339

Dufouil C, de Kersaint-Gilly A, Besançon *et al.* (2001) Longitudinal study of blood pressure and white matter hyperintensities. *Neurology* **56**: 921–926

Elias MF, Wolf PA, D'Agostino RB, Cobb J, White LR. (1993) Untreated blood pressure level is inversely related to cognitive functioning: the Framingham study. *American Journal of Epidemiology* **138**: 353–364

Emsley HCA and Tyrrell PJ. (2002) Inflammation and infection in clinical stroke. *Journal of Cerebral Blood Flow and Metabolism* **22**: 1399–1419

Erkinjuntti T, Benavente O, Eliasziw M *et al.* (1996) Diffuse vacuolization (spongiosis) and arteriosclerosis in the frontal white matter occurs in vascular dementia. *Archives of Neurology* **53**: 325–332

Esiri MM, Nagy Z, Smith MZ, Barnetson L, Smith AD. (1999) Cerebrovascular disease and threshold for dementia in the early stages of Alzheimer's disease. *Lancet* **354**: 919–920

Farkas E, De Jong GI, De Vos RA, Jansen Steur EN, Luiten PG. (2000) Pathological features of cerebral cortical capillaries are doubled in Alzheimer's disease and Parkinson's disease. *Acta Neuropathologica* **100**: 395–402

Fein G, Van Dyke C, Davenport L *et al.* (1990) Preservation of normal cognitive functioning in elderly subjects with extensive white-matter lesions of long duration. *Archives of General Psychiatry* **47**: 220–223

Ferucci L, Guralnik JM, Salive ME *et al.* (1996) Cognitive impairment and risk of stroke in the older population. *Journal of the American Geriatrics Society* **44**: 237–241

Forette F, Seux M-L, Staessen JA *et al.* (1998) Prevention of dementia in randomised double-blind placebo-controlled Systolic Hypertension in Europe (Syst-Eur) trial. *Lancet* **352**: 1347–1351

Grammas P, Moore P, Weigel PH. (1999) Microvessels from Alzheimer's disease brains kill neurons *in vitro*. *American Journal of Pathology* **154**: 337–342

Guo Z, Viitanen M, Fratiglioni L, Winblad B. (1996) Low blood pressure and dementia in elderly people: the Kungsholmen project. *BMJ* **312**: 805–808

Haan J, Roos RA, Algra PR, Lanser JB, Bots GT, Vegter-Van der Vlis M. (1990) Hereditary cerebral haemorrhage with amyloidosis–Dutch type. Magnetic resonance imaging findings in 7 cases. *Brain* **113**: 1251–1267

Halliday G, Robinson SR, Shepherd C, Kril J. (2000) Alzheimer's disease and inflammation: a review of cellular and therapeutic mechanisms. *Clinical and Experimental Pharmacology and Physiology* **27**: 1–8

Hénon H, Durieu I, Guerouaou D, Lebert F, Pasquier F, Leys D. (2001) Poststroke dementia: incidence and relationship to prestroke cognitive decline. *Neurology* **57**: 1216–1222

Hofman A, Ott A, Breteler MMB *et al.* (1997) Atherosclerosis, apolipoprotein E, and prevalence of dementia and Alzheimer's disease in the Rotterdam Study. *Lancet* **349**: 151–154

Holmes C, Cairns N, Lantos P, Mann A. (1999) Validity of current clinical criteria for Alzheimer's disease, vascular dementia and dementia with Lewy bodies. *British Journal of Psychiatry* **174**: 45–50

Johnston JM, Nazar-Stewart V, Kelsey SF, Kamboh MI, Ganguli M. (2000) Relationships between cerebrovascular events, APoE polymorphism and Alzheimer's disease in a community sample. *Neuroepidemiology* **19**: 320–326

Kalaria RN and Skoog I. (2002) Pathophysiology: overlap with Alzheimer's disease. In: T Erkinjuntti and S Gauthier (eds), *Vascular Cognitive Impairment*. London, Martin Dunitz, pp. 145–166

Kivipelto M, Helkala E-L, Laakso MP *et al.* (2001) Midlife vascular risk factors and Alzheimer's disease in later life: longitudinal, population based study. *BMJ* **322**: 1447–1451

Kogure K and Kato H. (1993) Altered gene expression in cerebral ischemia. *Stroke* **24**: 2121–2127

Kokmen E, Whistman JP, O'Fallon WM, Chu CP, Beard CM. (1996) Dementia after ischemic stroke: a population-based study in Rochester, Minnesota (1960–1984) *Neurology* **19**: 154–159

Kuller LH, Shemanski L, Manolio T *et al.* (1998) Relationship between ApoE, MRI findings, and cognitive function in the Cardiovascular Health Study. *Stroke* **29**: 388–398

Kuusisto J, Koivisto K, Mykkänen L *et al.* (1997) Association between features of the insulin resistance syndrome and Alzheimer's disease independently of apolipoprotein E4 phenotype: cross sectional population based study. *BMJ* **315**: 1045–1049

Launer LJ, Masaki K, Petrovitch H, Foley D, Havlik RJ. (1995) The association between midlife blood pressure levels and late-life cognitive function. *JAMA* **274**: 1846–1851

Laurin D, Verreault R, Lindsay J, MacPherson K, Rockwood K. (2001) Physical activity and risk of cognitive impairment and dementia in elderly persons. *Archives of Neurology* **58**: 498–504

Lee J-H, Olichney JM, Hansen LA, Hofsetter CR, Thal LJ. (2000) Small concomitant vascular lesions do not influence rates of cognitive decline in patients with Alzheimer disease. *Archives of Neurology* **57**: 1474–1479

Liao D, Cooper L, Cai J *et al.* (1997) The prevalence and severity of white matter lesions, their relationship with age, ethnicity, gender, and cardiovascular disease risk factors: the ARIC study. *Neuroepidemiology* **16**: 149–162

McCarron MO, Delong D, Alberts MJ. (1999) ApoE genotype as a risk factor for ischemic cerebrovascular disease. *Neurology* **53**: 1308–1311

McKhann G, Drachman D, Folstein M, Katzman R, Price D, Stadlan EM. (1984) Clinical diagnosis of Alzheimer's disease. Report of the NINCDS-ADRDA Work group under the auspices of the Department of Health and Human Services Task Force on Alzheimer's Disease. *Neurology* **34**: 939–944

Margaglione M, Seripa D, Gravina C *et al.* (1998) Prevalence of apolipoprotein E alleles in healthy subjects and survivors of ischemic stroke. *Stroke* **29**: 399–403

Marks JL, King MG, Baskin DG. (1991) Localisation of insulin and type 1 IGF receptors in rat brain by *in vitro* autoradiography and in situ hybridisation. *Advances in Experimental Medical Biology* **293**: 459–470

Moroney JT, Bagiella E, Tatemichi TK, Paik M, Stern Y. (1997) Dementia after stroke increases the risk of long-term stroke recurrence. *Neurology* **48**: 1317–1325

Mungas D, Reed BR, Ellis WG, Jagust WJ. (2001) The effects of age on rate of progression of Alzheimer disease and dementia with associated cerebrovascular disease. *Archives of Neurology* **58**: 1243–1247

Neuropathology Group of the Medical Research Council Cognitive Function and Ageing Study. (2001) Pathological correlates of late-onset dementia in a multicentre, community-based population in England and Wales. *Lancet* **357**: 169–175

Notkola I-L, Sulkava R, Pekkanen J *et al.* (1998) Serum total cholesterol, apolipoprotein E 4 allele, and Alzheimer's disease. *Neuroepidemiology* **17**: 14–20

Nourhashemi F, Deschamps V, Larrieu S, Letenneur L, Dartigues J-F, Barberger-Gateau P. (2003) Body mass index and incidence of dementia: the PAQUID study. *Neurology* **60**: 117–119

Ott A, Breteler MMB, de Bruyne MC, van Harskamp F, Grobbee DE, Hofman A. (1997) Atrial fibrillation and dementia in a population-based study. *Stroke* **28**: 316–321

Ott A, Slooter AJC, Hofman A *et al.* (1998) Smoking and the risk of dementia and Alzheimer's disease in a population-based cohort study: the Rotterdam Study. *Lancet* **351**: 1840–1843

Ott A, Stolk RP, van Harskamp F, Pols HAP, Hofman A, Breteler MMB. (1999) Diabetes mellitus and the risk of dementia. *Neurology* **53**: 1937–1942

Palovcik RA, Philips MI, Kappy MS, Raizada MK. (1984) Insulin inhibits pyramidal neurons in hippocampal slices. *Brain Research* **309**: 187–191

Pantoni L and Lammie A. (2002) Cerebral small vessel disease: pathological and pathophysiological aspects in relation to vascular cognitive impairment. In: T Erkinjuntti and S Gauthier (eds), *Vascular Cognitive Impairment*. London, Martin Dunitz, pp. 115–133

Peila R, Rodriguez BL, Launer LJ. (2002) Type 2 diabetes, APoE gene, and the risk for dementia and related pathologies: the Honolulu-Asia Aging Study. *Diabetes* **51**: 1256–1262

Petrovitch H, White LR, Izmirilian G *et al.* (2000) Midlife blood pressure and neuritic plaques, neurofibrillary tangles, and brain weight at death: the Honolulu Asia Aging Study. *Neurobiology of Aging* **21**: 57–62

Pfeiffer LA, White LR, Ross GW, Petrovich H, Launer LJ. (2002) Cerebral amyloid angiopathy and cognitive function: the HAAS autopsy study. *Neurology* **58**: 1587–1588

Piguet O, Ridley L, Grayson DA *et al.* (2003) Are MRI white matter lesions clinically significant in the 'old-old'? Evidence from the Sydney Older Persons Study. *Dementia and Geriatric Cognitive Disorders* **15**: 143–150

Pluta R, Barcikowski M, Janusezewski S, Misicka A, Lipowski AW. (1996) Evidence of blood–brain barrier permeability/leakage for circulating human Alzheimer's -amyloid-(1–42)-peptide. *NeuroReport* **7**: 1261–1265

Posner HB, Tang M-X, Luchsinger J, Lantigua R, Stern Y, Mayeux R. (2002) The relationship of hypertension in the elderly to AD, vascular dementia, and cognitive function. *Neurology* **58**: 1175–1181

Preston SD, Steart PV, Wilkinson A, Nicoll JA, Weller RO. (2003) Capillary and arterial cerebral amyloid angiopathy in Alzheimer's disease: defining the perivascular route for the elimination of amyloid beta from the human brain. *Neuropathology and Applied Neurobiology* **29**: 106–117

Prince MJ, Bird AS, Blizard RA, Mann AH. (1996) Is the cognitive function of older patients affected by antihypertensive treatment? Results from 54 months of the Medical Research Council's treatment trial of hypertension in older adults. *BMJ* **312**: 801–804

Prince M, Lovestone S, Cervilla J *et al.* (2000) The association between ApoE and dementia is mediated neither by vascular disease nor its risk factors in an aged cohort of survivors with hypertension. *Neurology* **54**: 397–402

Reaven GM. (1988) Role of Insulin resistance in human disease. *Diabetes* **37**: 1595–1607

Rost K, Roter D, Quill T, Bertakis K. (1990) Capacity to remember prescription drug changes: deficits associated with diabetes. *Diabetes Research and Clinical Practice* **10**: 183–187

Ruitenberg A, van Swieten JC, Witteman JCM *et al.* (2002) Alcohol consumption and risk of dementia: the Rotterdam Study. *Lancet* **359**: 281–286

Seshadri S, Beiser A, Selhub J *et al.* (2002) Plasma homocysteine as a risk factor for dementia and Alzheimer's disease. *New England Journal of Medicine* **346**: 476–483

Skoog I, Berg S, Johansson B, Palmertz B, Andreasson L-A. (1996a) The influence of white matter lesions on neuropsychological functioning in demented and non-demented 85-year-olds. *Acta Neurologica Scandinavica* **93**: 142–148

Skoog I, Lernfelt B, Landahl S *et al.* (1996b) 15-year longitudinal study of blood pressure and dementia. *Lancet* **347**: 1141–1145

Slooter AJC, Cruts M, Ott A *et al.* (1999) The effect of APoE on dementia is not through atherosclerosis: the Rotterdam Study. *Neurology* **53**: 1593–1595

Smith CD, Snowdon DA, Wang H, Markesbery WR. (2000) White matter volumes and periventricular white matter hyperintensities in aging and dementia. *Neurology* **54**: 838–842

Snowdon DA, Greiner LH, Mortimer JA, Riley KP, Greiner PA, Markesbery WR. (1997) Brain infarction and the clinical expression of Alzheimer disease. *JAMA* **277**: 813–817

Sparks DL, Hunsaker JC, Scheff SW, Kryscio RJ, Henson JL, Markesbery WR. (1990) Cortical senile plaques in coronary artery disease, aging and Alzheimer's disease. *Neurobiology of Aging* **11**: 601–607

Sparks DL, Scheff SW, Liu H, Landers TM, Coyne CM, Hunsaker JC. (1995) Increased incidence of neurofibrillary tangles (NFT) in non-demented individuals with hypertension. *Journal of the Neurological Sciences* **131**: 162–169

Stewart R. (1998) Cardiovascular factors in Alzheimer's disease. *Journal of Neurology, Neurosurgery, and Psychiatry* **65**: 143–147

Stewart R and Liolitsa D. (1999) Type 2 diabetes mellitus, cognitive impairment and dementia. *Diabetic Medicine* **16**: 93–112

Tatemichi TK, Paik M, Bagiella E *et al.* (1994) Risk of dementia after stroke in a hospitalised cohort: results of a longitudinal study. *Neurology* **44**: 1885–1891

Tomimoto H, Akiguchi I, Suenaga T *et al.* (1996) Alterations of the blood–brain barrier and glial cells in white-matter lesions in cerebrovascular and Alzheimer's disease patients. *Stroke* **27**: 2069–2074

Vlassara H, Fuh H, Makita Z, Krungkrai S, Cerami A, Bucala R. (1992) Exogenous advanced glycosylation end products induce complex vascular dysfunction in normal animals: a model for diabetic and aging complications. *Proceedings of the National Academy of Sciences of the United States of America* **89**: 12043–12047

Yamada M. (2000) Cerebral amyloid angiopathy: an overview. *Neuropathology* **1**: 8–22

Yoshitake T, Kiyohara Y, Kato I *et al.* (1995) Incidence and risk factors of vascular dementia and Alzheimer's disease in a defined elderly Japanese population: the Hisayama Study. *Neurology* **45**: 1161–1168

Genetics of Alzheimer's disease

MARGIE SMITH

Major advances in our understanding of the pathogenesis of Alzheimer's disease (AD) have come from molecular studies of patients with autosomal dominant early-onset AD (EOAD). Mutations in the amyloid protein precursor (APP) and presenilin genes (PS1 and PS2) located on chromosomes 21:14 and 1 respectively exert their effect in a fully penetrant manner. More recently, studies of late-onset AD (LOAD) have led to the determination of a number of possible risk loci. On the basis of these studies it has been postulated that the pathogenesis of LOAD is probably multifactorial. Continued research in this complex area of the genes and proteins involved in AD will help establish a logical basis for therapeutics and management.

34.1 MOLECULAR GENETICS OF EARLY–ONSET ALZHEIMER'S DISEASE

34.1.1 Mutations in the APP gene

The APP gene was implicated as a potential locus for AD mutations on the basis of four main intersecting lines of evidence. First, it is well known that individuals with Downs's syndrome (trisomy 21) develop the pathological lesions of AD by the fourth decade. This evidence implied a relationship between chromosome 21 and AD pathology (Mann *et al.*, 1984, 1989). Second, a 40–42 amino acid proteolytic peptide (Aβ) of the full length APP is a major constituent of senile plaques (Masters *et al.*, 1985; Goldgaber *et al.*, 1987; Kang *et al.*, 1987). Genetic linkage studies have shown an additional line of evidence for linkage to a locus associated with EOAD in the region of chromosome 21 containing the APP gene (St George-Hyslop *et al.*, 1987; Goate *et al.*, 1989). Finally, a missense mutation (APP E693Q) was identified in the Aβ region

of the APP gene characterized by hereditary cerebral haemorrhage with amyloidosis of the Dutch type (HCHWA-D) (Levy *et al.*, 1990; Kamino *et al.*, 1992). This is a rare disorder caused by severe βA4 amyloid deposition in meningeal and cerebral microvessels (Levy *et al.*, 1990; Van Broeckhoven *et al.*, 1990). It has recently been shown that E693G mutation causes AD by increasing amyloid β-protofibril formation and decreasing amyloid β levels in plasma and conditioned media (Nilsberth *et al.*, 2000). Three different mutations have now been reported at codon 693: the 'Dutch' mutation (Glu22Gln), the Arctic Glu22Gly mutation and 'Italian' mutation (Glu22Lys). Peptides of the wild-type 'Dutch' and 'Italian' variants were made and their cytotoxic effects were evaluated in human cerebral endothelial cells in culture. The effect of each mutation was different under these conditions, the E22Q peptide exhibiting the highest content of beta-sheet formation and aggregation properties. In contrast the 'Dutch' variant peptide induced apoptosis of cerebral endothelial cells. These results indicate that a change in amino acid at position 22 confers distinct structural properties on the peptides that affect the onset of the inexorable disease process (Miravalle *et al.*, 2000). After the initial finding of the E693Q mutation, a sequence variation affecting the valine at codon 717 (position 46 relative to the βA4 sequence) was found to be associated with the EOAD phenotype. At least 13 families worldwide have been identified with a V717I mutation, conferring an age of onset for AD in the mid-fifties (Goate *et al.*, 1991; Hardy *et al.*, 1991; Naruse *et al.*, 1991; Fidani *et al.*, 1992; Sorbi *et al.*, 1993, 1995; Brooks *et al.*, 1995; Campion *et al.*, 1996, 1999; Matsumura *et al.*, 1996; Finckh *et al.*, 2000). A 'mixed' phenotype of AD and/or severe cerebral amyloid angiopathy is caused by a mutation (A692G) at the βA4 residue 21 adjacent to the E693Q HCHWA-D (Hendriks *et al.*, 1992). This finding provided supporting evidence for the hypothesis that HCHWA-D and AD are pathological variants of the same disease, being associated with a phenotype of AD or other βA4 amyloidosis related disorders. A double mutation (K670N and M671L) in a large Swedish EOAD kindred with a mean age of onset of 55 years was identified (Mullan *et al.*, 1992). More recently four other APP mutations have been identified the Austrian (Thr714Ile) (De Jonghe *et al.*, 2000), Florida (Ile716Val) (Eckman *et al.*, 1997), French (Val715Met) (Ancolio *et al.*, 1999) and Australian (Leu723Pro) (Kwok *et al.*, 2000a).

The Swedish mutation was the first APP mutation for which a direct effect on βA4 processing could be demonstrated (Mullan *et al.*, 1992). This double point mutation (the 'Swedish' mutation) Lys670Met and Asp671Leu is upstream of the β-secretase cleavage site and results in a 5–8-fold increase in the formation of both $A\beta_{40}$ and $A\beta_{42}$ (Citron *et al.*, 1992). Two single point mutations at amino acid 717: (the 'London' mutation Val717Ile; and the 'Indiana' mutation Val717Phe) are adjacent to the γ-secretase site and specifically increase the production of $A\beta_{42}$ (Suzuki *et al.*, 1994), which is known to form insoluble amyloid fibrils (Selkoe, 1994). Synthetic peptides containing the HCHWA mutation show accelerated fibril formation (Wisniewski *et al.*, 1991). The majority of APP mutations molecular effect is to increase $A\beta_{42}$ production (Hardy, 1997); however, overexpression of the Val715Met mutation in human HEK293 cells and murine neurones reduces the total Aβ production and increases the recovery of the physiologically secreted product, APPα. It was thought that some cases of familial AD may be associated with a reduction of in the overall production of Aβ but could be caused by increased production of truncated forms of Aβ ending at the 42 position (Ancolio *et al.*, 1999).

Whilst APP mutations identified to date do not contribute to LOAD, it is possible that genetic variability within the promoter contributes to the risk of developing AD (Wavrant-De Vrieze *et al.*, 1999).

34.1.2 Mutations in the PS1 gene

After the initial finding of an EOAD locus on chromosome 21 it became apparent that the majority of EOAD kindreds did not show linkage to chromosome 21 (Schellenberg *et al.*, 1988; Tanzi *et al.*, 1987; Van Broeckhoven *et al.*, 1987; St George-Hyslop *et al.*, 1990). The PS1 gene was identified in 1995 through positional cloning strategies. Five mutations were identified in eight of 14 pedigrees analysed (Sherrington *et al.*, 1995). All the mutations occurred within highly conserved domains of the PS1 protein as shown by comparison to the murine homologue that provides supporting evidence that these mutations are indeed pathogenic. Not all mutations occur at residues that are conserved between PS1 and PS2. The PS1 gene was previously denoted as the S182 or AD3 locus; 133 mutations have been detected in the PS1 gene (they can be viewed at the following website: http://molgen-www.uia.ac.be/)

The age of onset of AD due to PS1 mutations is accelerated; however, variability in age onset is observed. The M139V and

M146V mutations have an age onset around 40 years (Clark *et al.*, 1995; Van Broeckhoven, 1995), whereas for kindreds identified with the E280 and C410Y mutations the age of onset is between 45 and 50 (Clark *et al.*, 1995; Sherrington *et al.*, 1995); the Ala409Thr mutation has an onset of 85 years (Aldudo *et al.*, 1999). EOAD linked to chromosome 14 is estimated to account for 70 per cent of all EOAD pedigrees (St George-Hyslop *et al.*, 1992; Van Broeckhoven *et al.*, 1992).

The phenotype of PS1 mutations is heterogeneous. It was initially thought that the only difference between AD and EOAD was the earlier age of onset (Sherrington *et al.*, 1995); however, there are five reports of AD associated with spastic paraparesis (SP) of the lower limbs. The brain pathology in one kindred was described as unique with large plaques lacking the classical core of amyloid fibrils. The term 'cotton wool' was coined by virtue of their size and appearance (Crook *et al.*, 1998). PS1 mutations associated with SP include a small deletion in exon 4 (DeltaI83/M84) (Steiner *et al.*, 2001), an insertion of six nucleotides in the coding region of exon 5 (from TAC to TTTATATAC) between amino acids K155 and Y156, point mutations in the coding region of exon 8 (Val261Phe) (Farlow *et al.*, 2000) and (Arg278Thr) (Kwok *et al.*, 1997), a point mutation in the splice acceptor consensus of intron 8 resulting in in-frame skipping of exon 9 and an amino acid change at the splice junction of exon 8 and exon 10 (g.58304G > A, c.869–955del) (Sato *et al.*, 1998; Kwok *et al.*, 2000b), (g.58304G > T, c.869–955del) (Perez-Tur *et al.*, 1995; Hutton *et al.*, 1996; Kwok *et al.*, 1997; Kwok *et al.*, 2000b) and large genomic deletions (g.56305–62162del) (Kwok *et al.*, 1997; Smith *et al.*, 2001) identified in an Australian kindred and (g.56681–61235) the Delta9Finn kindred (Crook *et al.*, 1998). Interestingly a point mutation in the splice donor consensus site of intron 4 resulting in three different transcripts with a single-codon insertion, partial and complete deletion of exon 4 respectively, the latter two resulting in a frame-shift and premature stop codon (g.23024delG, c.338–339insTAC, c.170–338del, c.88–338del) (Tysoe *et al.*, 1998) is not associated with spastic paraparesis. It was hypothesized that this mutation leads to AD through haplo insufficiency of full length PS1. This is in direct contrast to other PS1 mutations, which are thought to confer a 'toxic' gain of function in which $A\beta_{42}$ secretion is selectively increased (Tysoe *et al.*, 1998). Other phenotypes associated with EOAD are frontotemporal features (Raux *et al.*, 2000), myoclonic seizures (Ezquerra *et al.*, 1999), and a psychiatric disorder (Tedde *et al.*, 2000).

Mutations are located throughout the PS1 protein; however, their distribution may not be random. Mutations tend to occur at residues conserved between PS1 and PS2 and as such the majority are in transmembrane domains. Specifically the cluster of mutations in transmembrane 1: 2, 3, 4, and 6 line up on one side of the α-helix. This helical face may be important for the interaction with other transmembrane proteins (Clark *et al.*, 1995). It has been suggested that disruption of the helical faces impairs presenilin function so that more $A\beta_{42}$ is produced (Hardy and Crook, 2001). The majority of PS1 mutations cluster in exon 8, which is close to the cleavage site. If this is a functional domain then disruption of its function may be critical to pathogenicity. The clustering of APP mutations around the α-secretase, β-secretase, and γ-secretase sites lead to different molecular mechanisms; however, the final outcome is the same.

The normal biological and pathological functions of PS1 are poorly understood; however, there is ample evidence for a role of PS1 in the proteolytic processing of APP and in Notch processing (Wolfe *et al.*, 1999). PS1 is endoproteolytically cleaved between amino acids 291 and 299 resulting in a *N*-terminal fragment of 30 kDa and a *C*-terminal fragment of 18 kDa (Thinakaran *et al.*, 1996). The proteolytic cleavage site is located in that part of PS1 encoded by exon 9; therefore the delta 9 mutant does not undergo cleavage and accumulates as full length PS1 (Thinakaran *et al.*, 1996). Conversely, the efficiency of processing is not affected by missense mutations in AD brains (Hendriks *et al.*, 1997), in brains of transgenic mice (Duff *et al.*, 1996), and in transfected cells (Borchelt *et al.*, 1996). Cells transfected with PS1 mutants (M146V, A246G, A260V, G384, C410T) have impaired proteolysis (Mercken *et al.*, 1996) and in lymphocytes of mutation carriers (Takahashi *et al.*, 1999). There is no correlation between different PS1 mutations, age onset and Aβ$_{42\,(43)}$ production in transfected embryonic kidney cells (Mehta *et al.*, 1998).

34.1.3 Mutations in the PS2 gene

Directly after the identification of the PS1 cDNA sequence, 'expressed sequence tags' (ESTs) were described with considerable homology to two different segments within the PS1 open reading frame (T03796). Cloning of the full-length cDNA of this corresponding gene, mapped to chromosome 1 enabled the identification of missense mutations in cDNAs in affected Volga-German subjects (Levy-Lahad *et al.*, 1995). Evidence of the physical genome mapping of PS2 on chromosome 1q42.1 was performed using fluorescence *in-situ* hybridization (Tokano *et al.*, 1997). The majority of kindreds analysed exhibited the N141I missense mutation thereby identifying a founder effect. EOAD onset in these kindreds generally occurs later than in EOAD kindreds linked to chromosome 14 but with a broader range of age at onset from 54.8 ± 8.4 The mean duration of disease is 11.3 ± 4.6 years and mean age at death approximately 66 years. Clinically kindreds with PS1 mutations have a more aggressive disease than those with PS2 mutations (Lampe *et al.*, 1994). The wide variation in age of onset indicates that other genetic and or environmental factors influence the age of onset. Nonpenetrance over the age of 80 years has also been observed (Sherrington *et al.*, 1996). The penetrance is over 95 per cent for PS2 kindred; however, presymptomatic individuals harbouring the mutation over the age of 80 may escape disease. A total of 15 kindreds have been identified with a PS2 mutation. The majority of these mutations are localized to exons 5, 7 and 12 of the PS2 gene.

The exon 5 T122P mutation is highly penetrant unlike the previously reported PS2 mutations N141I and M239V (Levy-Lehad *et al.*, 1995). Consistent with the variable penetrance of the N141I and M239V mutations, the M239I mutation has associated phenotypic variability with some affected having an earlier onset and more severe course than the index case (Finckh *et al.*, 2000).

34.2 RISK FACTORS AND CANDIDATE GENES

The study of LOAD is in its infancy, with risk loci on chromosomes 6, 9, 10 and 12 having been identified. With the recent completion of the human genome project putative genes that map to a region of linkage can be identified. This strategy should identify new genetic risk factors. However, none of the numerous studies involving more than 100 candidate genes have revealed convincing evidence for any predisposing risk alleles (Finckh, 2003) other than apolipoprotein E (ApoE).

34.2.1 ApoE as a risk factor

Analysis has shown that that the ApoE locus cannot account for all the genetic risk associated with sporadic early and late-onset forms of AD (Templeton, 1995). The association of ApoE with LOAD has been studied extensively (Saunders, 2000). Polymorphisms within the ApoE promoter region correlate with increased transcriptional activity of the ApoE gene *in vitro*. Association studies of ApoE polymorphisms suggest that the -491 A/T genotype, the -491AA genotype, the -219 T/G, the -427 C/T genotype and the Th1/E47cs genotype increase the risk of developing AD. Not surprisingly results from other groups show positive, and partial association of ApoE polymorphisms and increased risk of developing AD (Bullido *et al.*, 1998). Recently sequence haplotype variation in 5.5 Kb of genomic DNA encompassing the whole of the ApoE locus and adjoining flanking regions in 96 individuals from four populations: 22 single nucleotide polymorphisms and 31 distinct haplotypes were identified (Fullerton *et al.*, 2000). Significantly seven of these polymorphisms were located upstream of exon 1 with the potential to alter transcription.

34.2.2 Candidate genes on chromosome 12

In 1997 a complete genomic screen identified linkage to a locus on chromosome 12 in a 36 cM region between markers D12S373 and D12S390. Other chromosomes of interest were 4, 6 and 20 (Pericak-Vance *et al.*, 1997). Two other linkage studies using independent LOAD cases provided supporting evidence for a locus on chromosome 12 (Rogaeva *et al.*, 1998; Wu *et al.*, 1998). However, Wu *et al.* (1998) were unable to confirm the precise location. A follow-up study of the families reported by Pericak-Vance *et al.* (1997) which controlled for family size, the presence of an ApoE ε4 allele, and presence of dementia with Lewy bodies found that linkage to chromosome 12 was stronger in families with the affected individuals lacking an ApoE ε4 allele and having a diagnosis of dementia with Lewy bodies (Scott *et al.*, 2000). The highest LOD score was observed in affected individuals whose ApoE genotype did not contain an ε4 allele. This region may therefore harbour a new late-onset gene with reduced dependence on the ε4 allele. This finding suggests that LOAD is genetically complex involving many genes in addition to ApoE.

34.2.2.1 LOW-DENSITY LIPOPROTEIN RECEPTOR

Two candidate genes within the region of linkage to chromosome 12 have been identified, the α_2-macroglobulin gene (A2M) and the low density lipoprotein receptor-related protein (LRP). LRP has been shown to be a multiligand endeictic receptor that mediates the internalization and degradation of ligands. LRP and its ligands, A2M, ApoE, and Kunitz protease containing isoforms of β-APP (Kang *et al.*, 1997) are all genetically associated with AD. A2M is a multifunctional binding protein that is thought to be involved in the degradation and clearance of Aβ (Borth, 1992). Kang *et al.* (1997) investigated the role of ApoE as a ligand for three receptors, the low density lipoprotein receptor (LDL-R), very low density lipoprotein receptor (VLDL-R) and LRP. This study aimed to determine if there was an association between these receptors and Alzheimer's disease (AD). An association between a silent polymorphism in exon 3 (C766T) within the LRP gene and AD was significant after corrections were made for multiple testing. The association was not found to be significant when the effects of known risk factors for AD were applied. When the ApoE ε4 was applied the effect of LRP no longer reached statistical levels of significance. It was concluded that LRP although being a candidate gene may be a minor risk factor and that independent verification on a large number of samples was required. One other LRP polymorphism, a tetranucleotide repeat has been thought to be associated with AD.

Associations between AD and these two polymorphisms are controversial with some groups reporting an association whilst others have found no significant association (Lendon *et al.*, 1997; Lambert *et al.*, 1999; Bertram *et al.*, 2000a; Kang *et al.*, 1997; 2000). Recently Kang *et al.* (2000) provided the first *in vivo* evidence that the LRP pathway may modulate Aβ deposition by regulating the removal of soluble Aβ.

34.2.2.2 α_2-MACROGLOBULIN

A2M is a ligand for LRP, an abundant pan-protease inhibitor that is found immunohistochemically in neuritic plaques and has been implicated in the binding, degradation, and clearance of Aβ (Borth, 1992). Association studies have been performed using two polymorphisms in the A2M gene, a 5 bp intronic insertion/deletion at the splice acceptor site of exon 18 (Matthijis and Marynen, 1991) and a missense mutation (Val1000Ile). Association studies have yielded conflicting results with reports of positive (Dodel *et al.*, 2000; Verpillat *et al.*, 2000) and negative associations (Gibson *et al.*, 2000; Koster *et al.*, 2000). It is possible that A2M deletion

polymorphism's genetic contribution accounts for a small fraction of AD cases.

34.2.3 Chromosome 9

The initial genomic screens reported linkage to regions of chromosomes 4, 6, 12, and 20 (Pericak-Vance *et al.*, 1997); however, in a second genomic screen using over 466 families, the highest LOD score was to a region on chromosome 9 (Pericak-Vance *et al.*, 2000). Independent genomes scan for LOAD also reported linkage to the same region (Kehoe *et al.*, 1999).

34.2.4 Chromosome 6

Linkage analysis by two independent groups (Pericak-Vance *et al.*, 1997; Kehoe *et al.*, 1999) showed evidence of linkage to chromosome 6. Three markers of interest on chromosome 6 were observed: D6S1004, D6S1019 and D6S391 (Pericak-Vance *et al.*, 1997). Kehoe *et al.* (1999) reported a multipoint peak located part way between that reported by Pericak-Vance *et al.* (1997) at D61018. In a later screen using 2-point linkage analysis on chromosome 6, linkage was found but not in this region (Pericak-Vance *et al.*, 2000). Linkages to several markers flanking the tumour necrosis factor locus have recently been reported. However, linkage was only observed in ApoE ε kindred (Collins *et al.*, 2000). This latter finding indicates the complexity of LOAD genotyping with some susceptibility genes being modulated by the ApoE status of the individual.

34.2.5 Chromosome 10

There is increasing evidence that for one or more susceptibility loci on chromosome 10 (Bertram *et al.*, 2000b; Ertekin-Taner *et al.*, 2000; Majores *et al.*, 2000; Myers *et al.*, 2000; Pericak-Vance *et al.*, 2000). The largest genomic scan to date was performed in a quest to find the remaining AD genes using 446 families (730 affected sib-pairs). The data were further stratified into an autopsy-confirmed subset of 199 families. Significantly the autopsy confirmed subset had an MLS of 4.31 on chromosome 9. Parametric and non-parametric linkage analysis was used (Pericak-Vance *et al.*, 2000). Recent studies have suggested that insulin-degrading enzyme (IDE) in neurones and microglia degrades Aβ. Parametric and non-parametric linkage analysis of 435 AD families found that seven genetic markers on chromosome 10 map near the IDE gene. Significant linkage for adjacent markers (D10S1671, D10S583, D10S170 and D10S566) was most pronounced in late-onset kindred (Bertram *et al.*, 2000b). A two-stage genome-wide screen was performed using sibling pairs with LOAD and an age of onset greater than 65 years. Non-parametric analysis stratified by the presence or absence of ApoE ε4 alleles provided evidence of a LOAD susceptibility locus on chromosome 10, close to marker D10S1211. This locus was found to modify the risk for AD independently of the ApoE genotype.

34.3 DIAGNOSTIC GENETIC TESTING FOR ALZHEIMER'S DISEASE

The identification of three genes causative for EOAD, APP and recently PS1 and PS2 raises the question of the role for genetic testing in AD. A consensus statement discussing the ethical aspects of the clinical introduction of genetic testing for AD concluded, 'except for autosomal dominant early-onset families, genetic testing in asymptomatic individuals is unwarranted'. Predictive testing for EOAD was offered in research settings following the identification of APP mutations on chromosome 21 using established Huntington's disease guidelines (Lennox *et al.*, 1994). The experience of three individuals belonging to a Swedish kindred with early-onset autosomal dominant AD was documented. Only three members of this large kindred proceeded with predictive testing, indicating a low demand for testing. One individual who was found to harbour the mutation reacted with depressive and suicidal feelings whilst the other two subjects expressed relief (Lannfelt *et al.*, 1995).

The ApoE gene, which confers some susceptibility to late-onset AD, has high commercial potential but the sensitivity and specificity of the test is low. An asymptomatic individual with an $\varepsilon 4$ allele will not necessarily develop AD. However, testing for ApoE $\varepsilon 4$ maybe useful as an aid for the diagnosis of individuals presenting with AD. Use of ApoE genetic testing as a diagnostic adjunct in patients already presenting with dementia may prove useful, but it remains under investigation. The premature introduction of genetic testing and possible adverse consequences 'are to be avoided' (Post *et al.*, 1997). Athena Neurosciences in 1996 introduced the Admark ApoE Genetic Test 'for greater certainty in differential diagnosis of AD'. The requesting physician must sign a consent stating that the individual has dementia prior to ApoE genotyping being performed.

Predictive testing is performed when a known family mutation has been identified in at least one other affected family member. Pretest assessment and counselling involves obtaining an accurate pedigree, neurological examination (not compulsory) and psychological appraisal. This is critical to understanding the individual's ability to cope with the results of the test. EOAD contributes less than 5 per cent of all AD cases; therefore there is no logical reason to perform genetic testing beyond this small cohort.

34.4 CONCLUSION

Genetic studies of EOAD have had a significant impact on our understanding of the pathogenesis of AD that in turn has led to research into diagnostic and therapeutic strategies and the availability of predictive testing of EOAD families. However, as people with EOAD represent only 5 per cent of all those with AD, some of the focus of genetic research has now shifted towards LOAD. Currently in LOAD, there appears to be a complex interplay of many risk factors, much as is seen in other pathogenic processes such as atherosclerosis. The current complexity of this area undermines the role for risk factor testing in LOAD. Understanding this genetic interplay is pivotal and likely to be the focus of genetic research in the next decade.

REFERENCES

Aldudo J, Bullido MJ, Valdivieso F. (1999) DGGE method for the mutational analysis of the coding and proximal promoter regions of the Alzheimer's disease presenilin-1 gene: two novel mutations. *Human Mutation* **14**: 433–439

Ancolio K, Dumanchin C, Barelli H *et al.* (1999) Unusual phenotypic alteration of beta amyloid precursor protein (betaAPP) maturation by a new Val-715>Met betaAPP-770 mutation responsible for probable early-onset Alzheimer's disease. *Proceedings of the National Academy of Science of the United States of America* **96**: 4119–4124

Bertram L, Blacker D, Crystal A *et al.* (2000a) Candidate genes showing no evidence for association or linkage with Alzheimer's disease using family-based methodologies. *Experimental Gerontology* **35**: 1353–1361

Bertram L, Blacker D, Mullin K *et al.* (2000b) Evidence for genetic linkage of Alzheimer's disease to chromosome 10q. *Science* **290**: 2302–2303

Borchelt DR, Thinakaran G, Eckman CB *et al.* (1996) Familial Alzheimer's disease-linked presenilin 1 variants elevate Aβ1–42/1–40 ratio *in vitro* and in vivo. *Neuron* **17**: 1005–1013

Borth W. (1992) Alpha 2-macroglobulin, a multifunctional binding protein with targeting characteristics. *FASEB Journal* **6**: 3345–3353

Brooks WS, Martins RN, De Voecht J *et al.* (1995) A mutation in codon 717 of the amyloid precursor protein in an Australian family with Alzheimer's disease. *Neuroscience Letters* **199**: 183–186

Bullido MJ, Artiga MJ, Recuero M *et al.* (1998) A polymorphism in the regulatory region of APoE associated with risk for Alzheimer's dementia. *Nature Genetics* **18**: 69–71

Campion D, Brice A, Hannequin D *et al.* (1996) No founder effect in three novel Alzheimer's disease families with APP 717 Val > Ile mutation. *Journal of Medical Genetics* **33**: 661–664

Campion D, Dumanchin C, Hannequin D *et al.* (1999) Early-onset autosomal dominant Alzheimer's disease: prevalence, genetic heterogeneity, and mutation spectrum. *American Journal of Human Genetics* **65**: 664–670

Citron M, Oltersdorf T, Haass C *et al.* (1992) Mutation of the beta-amyloid precursor protein in familial Alzheimer's disease increases β-protein production. *Nature* **360**: 672–674

Clark RF, Hutton M, Fuldner RA *et al.* (1995) The structure of the presenilin 1 gene and identification of six novel mutations in early onset AD families. *Nature Genetics* **11**: 219–222

Collins JS, Perry RT, Watson B *et al.* (2000) Association of a haplotype for tumour necrosis factor in siblings with late-onset Alzheimer's disease: the NIMH Alzheimer Disease Genetics Initiative. *American Journal of Medical Genetics* **96**: 823–830

Crook R, Verkkoniemi A, Perez-Tur J *et al.* (1998) A variant of Alzheimer's disease with spastic paraparesis and unusual plaques due to deletion of exon 9 of presenilin. *Nature Medicine* **4**: 452–455

De Jonghe C, Kumar-Singh S, Cruts M *et al.* (2000) Unusual Aβ amyloid in Alzheimer's disease due to an APP T7141 mutation at the γ42-secretase site. *Neurobiology of Aging* (Suppl. 1): S200

Dodel RC, Du Y, Bales KR et al. (2000) Alpha2 macroglobulin and the risk of Alzheimer's disease. Neurology 54: 438–442

Duff K, Eckman C, Zehr C et al. (1996) Increased amyloid-beta42(43) in brains of mice expressing mutant presenilin 1. Nature 383: 710–713

Eckman CB, Mehta ND, Crook R et al. (1997) A new pathogenic mutation in the APP gene (I716V) increases the relative proportion of A beta 42(43) Human Molecular Genetics 12: 2087–2089

Ertekin-Taner N, Graff-Radford N, Younkin LH et al. (2000) Linkage of plasma Abeta42 to a quantitative locus on chromosome 10 in late-onset Alzheimer's disease pedigrees. Science 290: 2303–2304

Ezquerra M, Carnero C, Blesa R et al. (1999) A presenilin 1 mutation (Ser169Pro) associated with early-onset AD and myoclonic seizures. Neurology 52: 566–570

Farlow MR, Murrell JR, Hulette CM et al. (2000) Hereditary lateral sclerosis and Alzheimer disease associated with mutation at codon 261 of the presenilin 1 (PS1) gene. Neurobiology of Aging 21 (Suppl.): S62

Fidani L, Rooke K, Chartier-Harlin M et al. (1992) Screening for mutations in the open reading frame and promoter of the β-amyloid precursor protein in familial Alzheimer's disease: identification of a further family with APP Val->Ile. Human Molecular Genetics 1: 165–168

Finckh U. (2003) The future of genetic association studies in Alzheimer disease. Journal of Neural Transmission 110: 253–266

Finckh U, Muller-Thomsen T, Mann U et al. (2000) High prevalence of pathogenic mutations in patients with early-onset dementia detected by sequence analyses of four different genes. American Journal of Human Genetics 66: 110–117

Fullerton SM, Clark AG, Weiss KM et al. (2000) Apolipoprotein E variation at the sequence haplotype level: implications for the origin and maintenance of a major human polymorphism. American Journal of Human Genetics 67: 881–900

Gibson AM, Singleton AB, Smith G et al. (2000) Lack of association of the alpha2-macroglobulin locus on chromosome 12 in AD. Neurology 54: 433–438

Goate A, Haynes AR, Owen MJ et al. (1989) Predisposing locus for Alzheimer disease on chromosome 21. Lancet 1: 352–355

Goate A, Chartier HM, Mullan M et al. (1991) Segregation of a missense mutation in the amyloid precursor protein gene with familial Alzheimer's disease. Nature 349: 704–706

Goldgaber D, Lerman MI, McBride OW. (1987) Characterisation and chromosomal localization of a cDNA encoding brain amyloid of Alzheimer disease on chromosome 21. Science 235: 877–880

Hardy J. (1997) Amyloid, the presenilins and Alzheimer's disease. Trends in Neuroscience 20: 154–159

Hardy J and Crook R. (2001) Presenilin mutations line up along transmembrane α-helices. Neuroscience Letters 306: 203–205

Hardy J, Mullan M, Chartier-Harlin MC et al. (1991) Molecular classification of Alzheimer's disease. Lancet 337: 1342–1343

Hendriks L, van Duijn C, Cras P et al. (1992) Presenilin dementia and cerebral haemorrhage linked to a mutation at condon 692 of the B-amyloid precursor protein gene. Nature Genetics 1: 218–221

Hendriks L, Thinakaran G, Harris CL et al. (1997) Processing of presenilin 1 in brains of patients with Alzheimer's disease and controls. NeuroReport 8: 1717–1721

Hutton M, Busfield F, Wragg M et al. (1996) Complete analysis of the presenilin 1 gene in early onset Alzheimer's disease. NeuroReport 7: 801–805

Kamino K, Orr HT, Payami H et al. (1992) Linkage and mutational analysis of familial Alzheimer disease kindreds for the APP gene region. American Journal of Human Genetics 51: 998–1014

Kang J, Lemaire HG, Unterbeck A et al. (1987) The precursor of Alzheimer disease amyloid A4 protein resembles a cell surface receptor. Nature 325: 733–736

Kang DE, Saitoh T, Chen X et al. (1997) Genetic association of the low-density lipoprotein receptor-related protein gene (LRP), an apolipoprotein E receptor, with late-onset Alzheimer's disease. Neurology 49: 56–61

Kang DE, Pietrzik CU, Baum L et al. (2000) Modulation of amyloid beta-protein clearance and Alzheimer's disease susceptibility by the LDL receptor-related protein pathway. Journal of Clinical Investigation 106: 1159–1166

Kehoe P, Wavrant-De Vrieze F, Crook R et al. (1999) A full genome scan for late onset Alzheimer's disease. Human Molecular Genetics 8: 237–245

Koster MN, Dermaut B, Cruts M et al. (2000) The alpha2-macroglobulin gene in AD: a population-based study and meta-analysis. Neurology 55: 678–684

Kwok JB, Taddei K, Hallupp M et al. (1997) Two novel (M233T and R278T) presenilin-1 mutations in early-onset Alzheimer's disease pedigrees and preliminary evidence for association of presenilin-1 mutations with a novel phenotype. NeuroReport 8: 1537–1542

Kwok JBJ, Li Q-X, Hallup M et al. (2000a) Novel Leu723Pro amyloid precursor protein mutation increases amyloid beta42(43) peptide levels and induces apoptosis. Annals of Neurology 47: 249–253

Kwok JBJ, Smith MJ, Brooks WS et al. (2000b) Variable presentation of Alzheimer's disease and/or spastic paraparesis phenotypes in pedigrees with a novel PS-1 exon 9 deletion or exon 9 splice acceptor mutations. Neurobiology of Aging 21 (Suppl.): S25

Lambert JC, Chartier-Harlin MC, Cottel D et al. (1999) Is the LDL receptor-related protein involved in Alzheimer's disease? Neurogenetics 2: 109–113

Lampe TH, Bird TD, Nochlin D et al. (1994) Phenotype of chromosome 14-linked familial Alzheimer's disease in a large kindred. Annals of Neurology 36: 368–378

Lannfelt H, Axelman K, Lilius L, Basun H. (1995) Genetic counseling of a Swedish Alzheimer family with amyloid precursor protein mutation. American Journal of Human Genetics 56: 332–335

Lendon CL, Talbot CJ, Craddock NJ et al. (1997) Genetic association studies between dementia of the Alzheimer's type and three receptors for apolipoprotein E in a Caucasian population. Neuroscience Letters 222: 187–190

Lennox A, Karlinsky H, Meschino W et al. (1994) Molecular genetic predictive testing for Alzheimer disease: deliberations and preliminary recommendations. Alzheimer Disease and Associated Disorders 8: 126–147

Levy E, Carman MD, Fernandez-Madrid IJ et al. (1990) Mutation of the Alzheimer's disease amyloid gene in hereditary cerebral hemorrhage, Dutch Type. Science 248: 1124–1126

Levy-Lahad E, Wijsman EM, Nemens E et al. (1995) A familial Alzheimer's disease locus on chromosome 1. Science 269: 970–973

Majores M, Bagli M, Papassotiropoulos A et al. (2000) Allelic association between the D10S1423 marker and Alzheimer's disease in a German population. Neuroscience Letters 289: 224–226

Mann DMA, Yates PO, Marcyniuk B. (1984) Alzheimer's presenile dementia, senile dementia, of the Alzheimer type, and Down's syndrome in middle age form a continuum of pathologic changes. Neuropathology and Applied Neurobiology 10: 188–207

Mann DM, Brown A, Prinja D et al. (1989) An analysis of the morphology of senile plaques in Down's syndrome patients of different ages using immunocytochemical and lectin histochemical techniques. Neuropathology and Applied Neurobiology 15: 317–329

Masters CL, Simms G, Weinman NA *et al.* (1985) Amyloid plaque core protein in Alzheimer disease and Down syndrome. *Proceedings of the National Academy of Sciences of the United States of America* **82**: 4245–4249

Matsumura Y, Kitamura E, Miyoshi K *et al.* (1996) Japanese siblings with missense mutation (717Val > Ile) in amyloid precursor protein of early-onset Alzheimer's disease. *Neurology* **46**: 1721–1723

Matthijis G and Marynen P. (1991) A deletion polymorphism in the human alpha-2-macroglobulin (A2M) gene. *Nucleic Acids Research* **19**: 5102

Mehta ND, Refolo LM, Eckman C *et al.* (1998) Increased Abeta42(43) from cell lines expressing presenilin 1 mutations. *Annals of Neurology* **43**: 256–258

Mercken M, Takahashi H, Honda T *et al.* (1996) Characterisation of human presenilin 1 using *N*-terminal specific monoclonal antibodies: evidence that Alzheimer mutations affect proteolytic processing. *FEBS Letters* **389**: 297–303

Miravalle H, Tokuda T, Chiarle R *et al.* (2000) Substitutions at codon 22 of Alzheimer's A-beta peptide induce diverse conformational changes and apoptotic effects in human cerebral endothelial cells. *Journal of Biological Chemistry* **275**: 27110–27116

Mullan M, Crawford F, Axelman K *et al.* (1992) A pathogenic mutation for probable Alzheimer's disease in the APP gene at the *N*-terminus of β-amyloid. *Nature Genetics* **1**: 345–347

Myers A, Holmans P, Marshall H *et al.* (2000) Susceptibility locus for Alzheimer's disease on chromosome 10. *Science* **290**: 2304–2305

Naruse S, Igarashi S, Aoki K *et al.* (1991) Mis-sense mutation Val to ILE in exon 17 of amyloid precursor protein in Japanese familial Alzheimer's disease. *Lancet* **337**: 978–979

Nilsberth C, Westlind-Danielsson A, Eckman CB *et al.* (2000) The Arctic mutation (E693G) causes Alzheimer's disease through a novel mechanism: increased amyloid β protofibril formation and decreased amyloid β levels in plasma and conditioned media. *Neurobiology of Aging* **21** (Suppl. 1): S58

Perez-Tur J, Froelich S, Prihar G *et al.* (1995) A mutation in Alzheimer's disease destroying a splice acceptor site in the presenilin-1 gene. *NeuroReport* **7**: 297–301

Pericak-Vance MA, Bass MP, Yamaoka LH *et al.* (1997) Complete genomic screen in late-onset familial Alzheimer's disease: evidence for a new locus on chromosome 12. *JAMA* **278**: 1237–1241

Pericak-Vance MA, Grubber J, Bailey LR *et al.* (2000) Identification of novel genes in late-onset Alzheimer's disease. *Experimental Gerontology* **35**: 1343–1352

Post SG, Whitehouse PJ, Binstock RH *et al.* (1997) The Clinical Introduction of Genetic Testing for Alzheimer Disease. *JAMA* **277**: 832–836

Raux G, Gantier R, Thomas-Anterion C *et al.* (2000) Dementia with prominent frontotemporal features associated with L113P presenilin 1 mutation. *Neurology* **55**: 1577–1579

Rogaeva E, Premukumar S, Song Y *et al.* (1998) Evidence for an Alzheimer disease susceptibility locus on chromosome 12 and for further locus heterogeneity. *JAMA* **280**: 614–618

St George-Hyslop PH, Tanzi RE, Polinsky RJ *et al.* (1987) The genetic defect causing familial Alzheimer disease maps on chromosome 21. *Science* **235**: 885–859

St George-Hyslop PH, Haines JL, Farrer LA *et al.* (1990) Genetic linkage studies suggest that Alzheimer's disease is not a single homogenous disorder. *Nature* **347**: 194–197

St George-Hyslop PH, Haines J, Rogaev E *et al.* (1992) Genetic evidence for a novel familial Alzheimer's disease locus on chromosome 14. *Nature Genetics* **2**: 330–234

Sato S, Kamino K, Miki T *et al.* (1998) Splicing mutation of presenilin-1 gene for early-onset familial Alzheimer's disease. *Human Mutation* (Suppl. 1): S91–S94

Saunders AM. (2000) Apolipoprotein E and Alzheimer's disease: an update on genetic and functional analyses. *Journal of Neuropathology and Experimental Neurology* **59**: 751–758

Schellenberg GD, Bird TD, Wijsman EM *et al.* (1988) Absence of linkage of chromosome 21q21 markers to familial Alzheimer's disease. *Science* **241**: 1507–1510

Scott WK, Grubber JM, Conneally PM *et al.* (2000) Fine mapping of the chromosome 12 late-onset Alzheimer disease locus: potential genetic and phenotypic heterogeneity. *American Journal of Human Genetics* **66**: 922–932

Selkoe D. (1994) Cell biology of the amyloid beta-protein precursor and the mechanism of Alzheimer's disease. *Annual Review of Cell Biology* **10**: 373–403

Sherrington R, Rogaev EI, Liang Y *et al.* (1995) Cloning a gene bearing missense mutations in early-onset familial Alzheimer's disease. *Nature* **375**: 754–760

Sherrington R, Froelich S, Sorbi S *et al.* (1996) Alzheimer's disease associated with mutations in presenilin 2 is rare and variably penetrant. *Human Molecular Genetics* **5**: 985–988

Smith MJ, Kwok JBJ, McLean CA *et al.* (2001) Variable phenotype of Alzheimer's disease with spastic paraparesis. *Annals of Neurology* **49**: 125–129

Sorbi S, Nacmias B, Forleo P *et al.* (1993) APP717 and Alzheimer's disease in Italy. *Nature Genetics* **4**: 10

Sorbi S, Nacmiass B, Forleo P *et al.* (1995) Epistatic effect of APP717 mutation and apolipoprotein E genotype in familial Alzheimer's disease. *Annals of Neurology* **38**: 124–127

Steiner H, Revesz T, Neumann M *et al.* (2001) A pathogenic presenilin-1 deletion causes aberrant Ab42 Production in the absence of congophilic amyloid plaques. *Journal of Biological Chemistry* **276**: 7233–7239

Suzuki N, Cheung TT, Cai XD *et al.* (1994) An increased percentage of long amyloid β protein secreted by familial amyloid β protein precursor (β APP717) mutants. *Science* **264**: 1336–1340

Takahashi H, Mercken M, Honda T *et al.* (1999) Impaired proteolytic processing of presenilin-1 in chromosome 14-linked familial Alzheimer's disease patient lymphocytes. *Neuroscience Letters* **260**: 121–124

Tanzi RE, St George-Hyslop PH, Haines JL *et al.* (1987) The genetic defect in familial Alzheimer's disease is not tightly linked to the amyloid β-protein gene. *Nature* **329**: 156–157

Tedde A, Forleo P, Nacmias B *et al.* (2000) A presenilin 1 mutation (Leu392Pro) in a familial AD kindred with psychiatric symptoms at onset. *Neurology* **55**: 1590–1591

Templeton AR. (1995) A cladistic analysis of phenotypic associations with haplotypes inferred from restriction endonucleases mapping or DNA sequencing. V. Analysis of case/control sampling designs: Alzheimer's disease and apolipoprotein E locus. *Genetics* **140**: 403–409

Thinakaran G, Borchelt DR, Lee MK *et al.* (1996) Endoproteolysis of presenilin 1 and accumulation of processed derivatives in vivo. *Neuron* **17**: 181–190

Tokano T, Sahara N, Yamanouchi Y, Mori H. (1997) Assignment of Alzheimer's presenilin-2 (PS-2) gene to 1q42.1 by fluorescence in situ hybridisation. *Neuroscience Letters* **221**: 205–207

Tysoe C, Whittaker J, Xuereb J *et al.* (1998) A Presenilin-1 truncating mutation is present in two cases with autopsy-confirmed early-onset Alzheimer disease. *American Journal of Human Genetics* **62**: 70–76

Van Broeckhoven C. (1995) Presenilins and Alzheimer's disease. *Nature Genetics* **11**: 230–232

Van Broeckhoven C, Genthe AM, Vandenberghe A *et al.* (1987) Failure of familial Alzheimer's disease to segregate with the A4-amyloid gene in several European families. *Nature* **329**: 153–155

Van Broeckhoven C, Hann J, Bakker E *et al.* (1990) Amyloid beta protein precursor gene and hereditary cerebral hemorrhage with amyloidosis (Dutch). *Science* **248**: 1120–1122

Van Broeckhoven C, Backhovens H, Cruts M *et al.* (1992) Mapping of a gene predisposing to early-onset Alzheimer's disease to chromosome 14q24.3. *Nature Genetics* **2**: 335–339

Verpillat P, Bouley S, Hannequin D *et al.* (2000) Alpha2-macroglobulin gene and Alzheimer's disease: confirmation of association by haplotypes analyses. *Annals of Neurology* **48**: 400–402

Wavrant-De Vrieze F, Crook R, Holmans P *et al.* (1999) Genetic variability at the amyloid-beta precursor protein locus may contribute to the risk of late-onset Alzheimer's disease. *Neuroscience Letters* **269**: 67–70

Wisniewski T, Ghiso J, Frangione B. (1991) Peptides homologous to the amyloid protein of Alzheimer's disease containing a glutamine for glutamic acid substitution have accelerated amyloid fibril formation. *Biochemical and Biophysical Research Communications* **179**: 1247–1254

Wolfe MS, Xia W, Moore CL *et al.* (1999) Peptidomimetic probes and molecular modeling suggest Alzheimer's γ-secretases are intramembrane-cleaving aspartyl proteases. *Biochemistry* **38**: 4720–4727

Wu WS, Holmans P, Wavrant-DeVrieze F *et al.* (1998) Genetic studies on chromosome 12 in late-onset Alzheimer's disease. *JAMA* **280**: 619–622

35

Transgenic mouse models of Alzheimer's disease

SIMON P BROOKS AND STEPHEN B DUNNETT

The purpose of this chapter is to review the recent developments in the field of transgenic (Tg) mouse models of Alzheimer's disease (AD). The Tg models were a great leap forward for scientists and the technology is still in its infancy, but already double and even triple Tg models of disorders have been developed that seek to recapitulate the primary core symptoms of diseases in a single model. This chapter will review the progress that has been made with Tg models of AD, initially looking at advances gained from using the single Tg models, and later at the very recent developments of double and triple Tg models.

35.1 DISEASE AETIOLOGY

The aetiology of the early-onset familial AD (EOFAD) can be simply defined as being genetic, the causes being mutations in either the amyloid precursor protein (APP) gene or in the presenilin 1 (PS1) or 2 (PS2) genes which reside on chromosomes 21, 14 and 1 respectively (Blanquet *et al.*, 1987; Goldgaber *et al.*, 1987; Levy-Lahad *et al.*, 1995; Sherrington *et al.*, 1995). Age of onset in EOFAD can begin as early as 35 years of age and disease progression is extremely rapid, resulting in death at around 7 years after the initial diagnosis. In contrast late-onset AD is essentially of unknown origin although over 40 per cent of patients possess the apolipoprotein E (ApoE) ε4 allele, compared with 15 per cent in the general population. However, there is no evidence to suggest that ApoE ε4 is a causative factor in late-onset AD, despite the finding that it decreases the age of onset from on average 84 years of age to 68 (Corder *et al.*, 1993) and has been found

to accelerate plaque formation (Baum *et al.*, 2000). Tg models that over express the ApoE ε4 gene do not develop neurofibrillary tangles or plaques and generally lack AD pathology, the only factor that links them to AD is the finding that there appears to be hyperphosphorylation of tau (see below) in these animals (Tesseur *et al.*, 2000). In light of these findings, we will not focus on the ApoE ε4 models of late-onset AD but on EOFAD and associated animal models of the core pathological biomarkers of AD, the neuritic plaques and neurofibrillary tangles. The genetic nature of EOFAD makes it accessible to recapitulation through the creation of transgenic animals that carry one of the human mutations.

35.2 CELLULAR PATHOLOGY OF ALZHEIMER'S DISEASE

35.2.1 The amyloid precursor protein, presenilins and plaque formation

One of the core pathologies that defines AD is the presence of insoluble deposits of peptide that over time form into abnormal plaques. These plaques are comprised of deposits of amyloid peptide, which have been created through the cleaving of the 110–130 kDA APP by a specific class of protease, the secretases (Kang *et al.*, 1987). The amyloid peptide found in the plaques of AD brains consists mainly of the 40–42-residue β-amyloid peptides (Glenner and Wong 1984; Masters *et al.*, 1985), which accumulate to form neurotoxic aggregations (Selkoe, 2001) that are hypothesized to be responsible for neuronal degeneration and dementia (Dahlgren *et al.*, 2002).

It is believed that the presenilin mutations (PS1 and PS2), that are known to be involved in EOFAD, cause dysregulation of APP. It has been reported that patients with PS1 mutations have greater number of $A\beta_{42}$ plaques compared with patients with the other forms of the disease (Mann *et al.*, 1996) suggesting that PS1 mutations preferentially increase $A\beta_{42}$ peptide production. PS1 has been shown to reduce amyloid peptides 5-fold, whereas the mutated PS1 increases the production of amyloid peptides in a way that induces an increase in ratio between $A\beta_{42}$ and $A\beta_{40}$ by selectively increasing $A\beta_{42}$ production. It is believed that the presenilins regulate amyloid production through an interaction with secretase proteomes, but no evidence is available as to how this interaction occurs. However, it seems that β secretase cleaves APP to create β-CTFs (c-terminal fragments) which then get truncated by γ-secretase creating $A\beta$ and it may be that the presenilins interfere with this process (see Sato *et al.*, 1997).

Both the plaques and neurofibrillary tangles (see below) identified in the brains of demented people have a well characterized distribution within the hippocampus and neocortex (Tomlinson *et al.*, 1970; Corsellis, 1976) although tangles have been identified in subcortical regions (Ishii, 1966; Tomlinson *et al.*, 1981; Whitehouse *et al.*, 1982).

35.2.2 Neurofibrillary tangles (NFTs)

NFTs are neuronal inclusions of paired helical filaments (PHFs) comprising hyperphosphorylated and ubiquinated tau protein (Goedert *et al.*, 1995; Buee *et al.*, 2000). The exact role of tau protein in the brain is not fully understood but it appears to be a structural component of the neuronal cytoskeleton. Mutations in the gene on chromosome 17 that encode tau induces the formation of NFTs in another dementia, namely frontotemporal dementia with parkinsonism linked to chromosome 17 (FTDP-17). This disease is characterized by dementia in the absence of amyloid plaques and tau mutations have been found to cause NFTs and cell death (Clark *et al.*, 1998; Goedert *et al.*, 1998; D'Souza, 1999).

35.2.3 Cholinergic deficit

Whilst changes in several neurotransmitter systems have been identified in AD (see Dunnett, 1994) the most consistent and profound neurotransmitter disturbance in AD is a cholinergic deficit (Coyle *et al.*, 1982; Geula and Mesulam, 1994; Procter *et al.*, 1996) which correlates with the degree of dementia (Perry *et al.*, 1978; Bierer *et al.*, 1995) and with the density of amyloid plaques (Perry *et al.*, 1978; Geula and Mesulam, 1994). A more recent study has found that cholinergic loss better reflects tangle density (Geula *et al.*, 1998) than plaque density. The importance of the cholinergic system in AD is highlighted through the use of cholinomimetic compounds to treat the symptoms of AD (Parnetti *et al.*, 1997), although pharmacokinetic factors have largely limited their widespread usefulness.

35.3 THE INFLUENCE OF BACKGROUND STRAIN AND MOUSE SEX

Factors other than the transgene can influence the characteristics of any given mouse model of AD. Three factors of particular note are:

- the background strain on which the transgenic line is developed and subsequently backcrossed or maintained;
- the sex of the animal; and
- the specific promotor that has been used to drive the neuronal expression of the transgene.

With regards to background strains, an excellent review by Hsiao (1998) draws attention to differences in mortality rates between inbred C57BL/6j mice that had had the TG2576 transgene array transferred to them and the greatly reduced mortality rate when the host mice contained alleles from the SJL strain. Strain variation also produced changes in the behavioural manifestation of the disease progression between the latter cross-strain (C57BL/6j × SJL) and FVB/N mice, with the FVB/N mice exhibiting neophobia and thigmotaxic behaviour and the C57BL/6j × SJL mice showing no behavioural abnormalities prior to death (see Hsiao, 1998).

Sex differences have been identified in APP transgenic mice resulting in an increased plaque load in female Tg2576 mice compared with age-matched males carrying the same transgene (Callahan *et al.*, 2001). A study by Park and colleagues (2003) did not find an initial sex difference in the Tg2576 mice, but the administration of lovastatin (which lowers plasma cholesterol) did produce sex specific effects on levels of $A\beta$, which were found to be significantly elevated in only the female mice. However, human sex differences have been found in studies in human AD with women being reported to be more susceptible than males to the disease (Molsa *et al.*, 1982), so it is not surprising that these apparent differences can be reflected in the mouse models.

35.4 TRANSGENIC MOUSE MODELS WITH APP MUTATIONS

35.4.1 APP transgenics

The first Tg mouse model to show deposits and plaques with a regional distribution similar to that for AD was created by Kawabata *et al.* (1991). This particular mouse expressed human mutant APP *C*-terminal fragments. Since this time several different lines of enquiry have produced a number of mutant mouse lines that over-express different mutant genes. The most prominent and most researched of these mouse models are the APP models of AD that are usually designed to express human mutant APP and reliably produce animals with neuritic plaques in the cerebral cortex and hippocampus. Specific APP mutations are named after the place of origin of the kindred families predisposed to AD in humans. Some transgenic models are based on over-expression of the normal human APP, but the more effective Tg models involve the transfer of a mutant allele into the Tg mouse, for example, the Swedish mutation in the Tg2576 transgenic line. The most widely used APP mutations are the Swedish, Indiana, London, Dutch and Flemish mutations. In this review, the different mutations will be addressed as APP/Swe, APP/Ind, APP/Lon, APP/Dut and APP/Fle respectively. See the summary table (Table 35.1, pp. 456–457) for a general overview of some of the specific differences between the more commonly used APP mice.

In 1991 it was discovered that injections of Aβ into the rat neocortex or hippocampus resulted in the formation of plaque-like structures complete with neuritic degeneration (Kowell et al., 1991) and that a memory deficit was produced in mice by injecting the same protein intraventricularly (Flood et al., 1991). These findings coupled with publication of the mouse genome, led directly to the development of Tg APP mice that were designed to express high levels of human mutant APP, with the hope of producing β-amyloid plaques in the mouse brain with both the temporal and spatial patterning of AD.

35.4.2 APP expression and histology of APP mice

The APP/Ind mouse with the V717 human mutation (Games et al., 1995) expressed a 10-fold higher expression of mutant human Aβ in the Tg mouse brains than found in previous models. The expression of human mutant Aβ was under the control of the PDGF (platelet derived growth factor) promoter and hence was preferentially regionalized by neurones of the cortex, hippocampus, hypothalamus and cerebellum in the Tg animals. Interestingly, levels of APP in the thalamus of homozygotic mice were higher than levels of APP in the hippocampus of the heterozygotic animals, yet the heterozygotic animals showed marked hippocampal pathology whereas the homozygotes showed relatively little thalamic pathology (Johnson-Wood et al., 1997). Compared with 4-month old animals, 8-month animals showed an 8-fold increase in Aβ levels, and a 400-fold increase by 18 months of age in the cortex. In the hippocampus at 8 months old the increase was 17-fold, and at 18 months 500-fold (Johnson-Wood et al., 1997) illustrating the progressive nature of the disease-like pathology in these animals.

Plaques were found to be present at 4 month of age. Aggregate size was roughly 20 μm in diameter, which increased up to around 150 μm at 8 months of age (Johnson-Wood et al., 1997), confirming previous findings by Games et al. (1995). By 10 months of age many large Aβ deposits were found throughout the frontal and cingulate cortex and the molecular layers of the hippocampus, especially the dentate gyrus. Chen et al. (2000) characterized plaque formation in limbic regions of the APP/Ind mutations and found very few plaques were present in the hippocampal formation at 9 months of age, but by 16 months plaque density was higher

especially in layers II and III of the entorhinal cortex, in the molecular layer of the dentate gyrus, and in striatum molecular lacunosum of area CA1. By 21 months plaques were present throughout the hippocampus, in the cingulate cortex, the insular dorsal cortex to the rhinal fissure and entorhinal cortex. No plaques were present in control mice. Synaptic and dendritic density were reduced in the molecular layer of the hippocampal dentate gyrus, as found with the synaptophysin and the dendritic marker MAP-2 (Games et al., 1995).

The Tg2576 mice (Hsiao et al., 1996) carrying the Swedish mutation are very widely used and have also been well characterized. The Swedish mutation mice show a similar pathology to the Indiana mutation mice with general increase in amyloid in hippocampus and cortex (Callahan et al., 2001). They show Aβ deposits in the brain at 9–11 months (Hsiao et al., 1996). A problem with these models is that they do not reflect the temporal or spatial pattern produced by endogenous APP. However, a genomic model has been developed recently (R1.40) that uses a copy of the Swedish mutant APP that is expressed with the endogenous human promoter. This model has Aβ deposits by 14 months (Lamb et al., 1997; Lamb et al., 1999; Kulnane and Lamb, 2001). R1.40 mice express high levels of CTFα and β and APP in brain tissue in contrast to Wild-type (Wt) brains that express high levels of APP, low levels of CTFα and no CTFβ (Lehman et al., 2003). Therefore the Swedish mutation increases CTFβ production through the secretase-β pathway (Lehman et al., 2003).

In the APP/Swe, mice the hippocampus showed the highest brain proportion of CTFβ of all brain areas studied with the cortex showing an intermediate level (Lehman et al., 2003). Aβ40 was also exhibited at significantly higher levels in the hippocampus than any other brain region. At 13.5 months these mice exhibited abundant Aβ deposits in the striatum, dentate gyrus and hippocampus (Hsiao et al., 1996; Callahan et al., 2001; Sigurdsson et al., 2001). These deposits were primarily made up of Aβ42 (63 per cent in younger animals and 70 per cent in older animals) (Kulnane and Lamb, 2001). R1.40 mice showed almost nothing in the hippocampus until 22 months when deposits were present in the same regions as for Tg2576 (Lehman et al., 2003). As in humans, most Aβ deposits stain for Aβ42 with a subset staining for Aβ40

In the olfactory bulb both models showed low to moderate levels of Aβ by 22 months, and in the cerebellum APP was significantly higher in the APP/Swe animals but Aβ42 levels were not different (Lehman et al., 2003). No tau deposits or NFTs were found but there was evidence of tau phosphorylation (Kulnane and Lamb, 2001).

A fourth APP mouse is called the London mouse (APP/Lon). At 17–22 months of age these mice exhibited amyloid plaques that were concentrated in the frontal cortex layers IV–VI, in the hippocampus, the amygdala and entorhinal cortex (Bronfman et al., 2000). In the hippocampus plaques were found in the subiculum primarily but also the striatum radiatum, and the CA1 and CA3 regions. Thioflavin-S staining confirmed the amyloid nature of the plaques (Bronfman et al., 2000).

A comparative study of the APP/Swe and APP/Lon mutated mice by Moechars et al. (1999) found considerable strain variations. In all of the old APP/Lon mice and 50 per cent of the old APP/Swe mice amyloid deposits and neuritic plaques were detected, being most abundant in the hippocampus and the cortex. In APP/Swe mice the deposits were fewer but larger (130 μm) and located in the primary olfactory cortex and amygdala. There was preferential staining for $A\beta_{40}$ in the APP/Swe mice and $A\beta_{42}$ in the APP/Lon mice (Moechars et al., 1999). Deposits were absent in Wt mice. Plaques appeared to be similar to those found in AD brains, but no NFTs were found although an epitope typical for hyperphosphorylated tau was detected in dystrophic neurites associated with amyloid plaques. All Tg APP mice had a higher mortality rate during the first year (21–72 per cent) compared with Wt (4.3 per cent) mice (Moechars et al., 1999).

In the Flemish and Dutch mutations (APP/Fle and APP/Dut) only relatively minor histological changes were apparent, such as spongiosis of the neuropil in the frontal cortical regions and the parahippocampal and cerebellar areas (Kumar-Singh et al., 2000). The use of a GFAP antibody detected glial activation in the cerebral cortex, cerebellar and limbic areas including the hippocampus. Neuronal expression of mutant APP was greatest in cortical layers II, IV and V, which were also areas where neurones were found to contain condensed nuclei. High APP levels were also found in the pyramidal layer of the hippocampus, olfactory bulbs, basal pontine nucleus and the cranial nerve nuclei (Kumar-Singh et al., 2000). A similar profile was found for the APP/RK mouse (Moechars et al., 1999) that failed to develop plaques despite large increases in APP expression in the cortex, amygdala, striatum and the hippocampal pyramidal layer and the granular cells of the dentate gyrus.

Although the above mice were designed to carry a mutant APP allele the temporal and spatial profile of amyloid deposition and plaque development can vary markedly between transgenic lines and mouse strains.

Creating a Tg mouse that contains two familial AD mutations (Swe/Ind) had the effect of inducing an early onset of amyloid deposition and plaque development in mice at around 16 weeks of age (Mucke et al., 2000; Christi et al., 2001) with plaques developing in the molecular layer of the dentate gyrus and the deeper layers of the neocortex (Mucke et al., 2000). These mice have been reported to show spatial learning deficits at 3 months of age (Janus et al., 2000) and an enhanced startle response and a reduction in PPI before the plaques were identified (McCool et al., 2003).

35.4.3 Cholinergic transmission in the APP mice

There is evidence to suggest that there are ongoing changes in the cholinergic neurones in AD mice. A decreased density of SYN-IR sensitive presynaptic terminals has been found in the hippocampus that precedes plaque formation in APP mice (Games et al., 1995; Hsia et al., 1999). Twelve-month old

APP/Ind mice show AChE-immunoreactive dystrophic fibres in the vicinity of amyloid plaques (Sturchler-Pierrat et al., 1997). In contrast, Gau et al. (2002) found no differences in four cholinergic markers (VAChT, SDHACU, ChAT, AChE) between Tg and Wt APP/Ind mice across three age groups (14, 18 and 23 months) despite ongoing amlyoidogenesis. In 17–22-month-old London mutation mice AChE fibres are reorganized in the hippocampus and amyloid plaques are surrounded by dystrophic AChE-positive fibres. Also an increased density of AChE fibres in the CA1 region of the hippocampus and dentate gyrus of 17–22-month-old APP/Lon mice was found, suggesting compensatory sprouting (see Bronfman et al., 2000). Extensive cholinergic differentiation was found in the subiculum of aged APP/Lon mice (about 60 per cent reduction in AChE staining) and in some amyloid plaques AChE staining appeared in the core whilst around most plaques AChE fibres appeared distorted (Bronfman et al., 2000). However, no changes in the total AChE activity were found in the hippocampus, frontal or parietal cortex areas (Bronfman et al., 2000). It has been suggested that, because behavioural deficits precede amyloid deposition, it may be that soluble Aβ peptides have a detrimental effects on cellular function even prior to plaque formation (Hsia et al., 1999).

35.4.4 Electrophysiology in the APP mice

In electrophysiological studies, APP mice have been shown to exhibit interesting responses to glutamate challenges and widespread but subtle changes in glutamatergic function. In APP/Lon mice Masliah et al. (2000) found decreased binding and affinity for aspartate uptake and a decrease in expression of EAAT1 and 2 (glutamate transporters). The authors suggest that an increased APP expression disturbs astroglial transport of excitatory amino acids leading to increased susceptibility to glutamate toxicity. APP has been reported to perform a role in neurotrophic and neuroprotective activity in cell culture (Masliah et al., 1996) and in vivo (Masliah et al., 1998; Mucke et al., 1994). APP has also been shown to be protective against glutamate toxicity in the Tg mouse (Masliah et al., 1997). In AD similar findings have been found, that glial glutamate transport is decreased (Cowburn et al., 1988; Masliah et al., 1996; Li et al., 1997). Hence in APP mice an increased APP expression disrupts normal functioning of the glutamate transporter system, possibly through amyloid β peptide-mediated inhibition (Harris et al., 1996), resulting in an increased risk of excitotoxicity (Masliah et al., 2000).

APP mice showed disparity between reaction to kainate and NMDA challenges. Kainate had an LD50 of 28 mg/kg and 32 mg/kg for the APP/Fle and /Dut mice respectively whereas Wt mice were not affected at 32 mg/kg. In contrast NMDA had an LD50 of 70 mg/kg in the Wt mice and the LD50 ranged between 160 and 200 mg/kg in the Tg mice suggesting an decreased sensitivity to NMDA excitation (Kumar-Singh et al., 2000). These findings together with

Table 35.1 *Key features of the most commonly used Tg APP mouse lines*

Familial transgene	Line	Mouse strain	cDNA	APP mutation	Promoter	Reference	Major pathology	Functional deficits
	1	B6/D2	C-TF	None	human Thy-1	Kawabata *et al.,* 1991	8 months – plaques, tangles, dystrophic neurites in corex, hippocampus and amygdala	NR
Wild type	NSE: β-APP751	JU	751	None	NSE: β-APP751	Quon *et al.,* 1991	Cortical and hippocampal β-amyloid deposits	NR
	MTA4	B6 x LT/Sv	695	None	hMTII	Beer *et al.,* 1991	↑ APP expression in pyramidal and Purkinje cells	Hypoactivity and motor deficits
Dutch	APP/Du/	FVB/N	695	E693Q	Mouse Thy-1	Kumar-Singh *et al.,* 2000	No amyloid deposits. Glial reaction, apoptosis with extensive spongiosis	8 weeks ↑ agitation + bouts of wild running. 6 months ↑ aggression + some seizures. Premature death
Flemish	APP/Fl/	FVB/N	695	A692G	Mouse Thy-1	Kumar-Singh *et al.,* 2000	No amyloid deposits. Glial reaction, apoptosis with extensive spongiosis	8 weeks ↑ agitation + bouts of wild running. 6 months ↑ aggression + some seizures. Premature death
Indiana	Line 109	SWx (B6/D2)	695, 751, 770	V717F M671L +	PDGF	Games *et al.,* 1995	6 months – Aβ deposits. Plaques became present in hippocampus, corpus callosum and cortex associated with distorted neurites	3 months – reference, working and operant memory deficits ↑ freezing + sterotypy. From 6 months – object recognition deficits
London	APP/Ld/2	FVB/Nx(B6)	695	V642I	Mouse Thy-1	Moechars *et al.,* 1999	13 months – amyloid plaques in hippocampus and cortex. Reactive astrocytes and microglia, plus dystrophic neurites	8 weeks ↑ agitation. 3 months ↓ ambulation, ↑ anxiety, spatial navigation deficits. 6 months some seizures

Swedish	Tg 2576	B6/SJL x (B6)	695	K670N-M671L	Hamster prion	Hsiao et al., 1996	9–11 months – amyloid deposits in hippocampus and cortex later developing in the striatum	9–10 months spatial memory and spontaneous alternation deficits
	APP 14	B6D2 x (B6)	751	K670N-M671L	Human Thy-1	Andrä et al., 1996	No pathology up to 2 years	NR
	APP 23	B6D2 x (B6)	751	K670N-M671L	Mouse Thy-1	Sturchler-Pierrat et al., 1997	6 months – APP deposits in neocortex and hippocampus that form plaques. Tau hyperphosphorylation. Distorted neurites and inflammatory response	
Swedish	APP/Sw/1	FVB/N	770	K670N-M671L	Mouse Thy-1	Moechars et al., 1999	18–25 months – some amyloid deposits and neuritic plaques in the olfactory bulb and amygdala	12–17 weeks – ↑ neophobia
Swe/Ind	TgCRND8	C3H/B6	695	K670N-M671L V717F	Hamster Prion	Janus et al., 2000	From 3 months – amyloid plaques in cortex and hippocampus	3 months – spatial learning deficits
Swe/Lon	APP 22	B6D2F1 x (B6)	751	K670N-M671L V717I	Human Thy-1	Sturchler-Pierrat et al., 1997	18 months – APP deposits in neocortex and hippocampus that form plaques. Tau hyperphosphorylation. Distorted neurites and inflammatory response	NR
Swe/Lon/ Ind	PDGFβ-APP$_{695}$SDL	NR	695	K670N-M671L + V717I + E693Q	PDGFβ	Wirths et al., 2001	19 months – onset of neuropil plaque deposition	NR

Key to mouse strain abbreviations: B6, C57BL/6j; D2, DBA/2; B6D2F1 x (B6), for example, denotes a C57BL/6j first generation cross with DBA/2 strain which is then backcrossed (denoted with parenthesis) onto a C57BL/6j background; C-Tf, C-Terminal Fragment reports that suggest no evidence for apoptosis in the APP mice are suggestive of a down-regulation in the number of NMDA receptors, which may contribute to the cognitive decline in some of these mouse strains. Moechars *et al.* (1999) found that LTP was significantly decreased after tetanic stimulation in APP/Lon mice of 5–7 months old in CA1 region of the hippocampus and that these mice were also less sensitive to an NMDA challenge than non-transgenic mice at 3–4 months of age but more sensitive to kainite (Moechars *et al.*, 1999).

35.4.5 Behavioural changes in the APP mice

As a general rule of thumb the APP Tg mice have been shown to develop both reactive and cognitive deficits that appear to worsen over time. Of interest though is the finding that behavioural deficits can precede plaque formation, or, in the case of the APP/Dut and APP/Fle mice, behavioural deficits are present in the absence of plaque formation.

APP/Ind mice have been found to show cognitive deficits in the form of reference memory errors on a radial arm maze task from 3 months of age and the object recognition task from 5 months in the homozygote animals and 9–10 months in the heterozygote animals (Dodart *et al.*, 1999). Complementary results were also obtained in a water maze task in mice of 13 months old (Chen *et al.*, 2000), although no deficits were found in the object recognition task. In addition, Dodart *et al.* (1999) also ran operant tasks consisting of 15-minute daily session for 5 days in which the mice had to press a lever and then travel around a 5-cm long partition to acquire the reward; 21 days later the mice were retested on a single session for retention. The results confirmed that at 3 months of age Wt mice performed better (produced more reinforced bar presses) than Tg mice.

APP/Lon mice have been reported to exhibit an increased fear response as measured by freezing behaviour, which increased from 0 per cent at 7–9 weeks to 35 per cent at 17–30 weeks of age (Moechars *et al.*, 1998). At 3–6 months of age these mice were impaired at the acquisition of a hidden platform water maze task but not the cued (visual) platform task when compared with non-Tg littermates. Likewise the Tg animals performed poorly in the probe task 24 hours later, spending significantly less time in the target quadrant, and producing significantly less platform crossings than non-Tg animals. These deficits preceded plaque formation (Moechars *et al.*, 1998).

Interestingly both the APP/Dut and the APP/Fle mutation have been shown to develop behavioural deficits that are characteristic of AD, but in the absence of APP deposits (Kumar-Singh *et al.*, 2000). These mice also have an increased mortality rate as over the first 180 days of life only 3 per cent of Wt mice died compared with 8 and 16 per cent of the APP/Fle and APP/Dut Tg mice respectively with no obvious signs of illness. In roughly 15 per cent of the mice that survived for longer than 18 months, seizures developed that were unrelated to the APP transgene expression. Mice

were normal up to 8 weeks of age, then started to show increased reactivity to an open environment, aggression towards other mice, and signs of emotionality, such as hyperactivity and increased aggression, which are correlated with expression level of the transgene. Thus, for example, around 33 per cent of Flemish and 44 per cent of Dutch Tg mice residents attacked in the first minute of contact compared with none of the Wt mice, and overall 78 and 83 per cent of mice attacked within the 3 minutes allotted compared with 11 per cent of the Wt mice (Kumar-Singh *et al.*, 2000). APP/RK Tg mice have also been shown to exhibit increased aggression relative to the WT mice (see also Moechars *et al.*, 1996).

35.5 TRANSGENIC β-CTF MOUSE MODELS

35.5.1 β-CTF mice

Different mouse models have also been developed to express the amyloidogenic human APP carboxy terminal fragment (Nalbantaglu *et al.*, 1997; Berger-Sweeney *et al.*, 1999; Rutten *et al.*, 2003). Taken generally, these mice express high levels of β-CTFs (Rutten *et al.*, 2003), hippocampal cell loss (Nalbantaglu *et al.*, 1997) and degeneration (Berger-Sweeney *et al.*, 1999) in the cortex and hippocampus, but fail to develop neuritic plaques. These mice show increased immunoreactivity for Aβ that became stronger and more prevalent with age.

35.5.2 Behaviour in the β-CTF mouse models

Behaviourally, the Tg animals over-expressing the CTFs of APP exhibited cognitive deficits when placed in the water maze, but were not impaired at a visually cued platform tasks (Nalbantaglu *et al.*, 1997; Berger-Sweeney *et al.*, 1999). The cognitive deficit in these mice may be related to an abnormality in LTP generation that has been found in these animals (Nalbantaglu *et al.*, 1997).

35.6 TRANSGENIC MOUSE MODELS OF TAU MUTATIONS

35.6.1 Tau mice

Mice expressing the tau mutation were developed to look at a group of disorders where these mutations caused cell death in man. The principal disease that underlies the tau pathologies is FTDP-17, for which patients carry at least one mutation of the tau gene. Probably the most well characterized mutations of the tau gene are the P301L and P301S variants but animal models for other mutations of the tau gene have been developed including V337M, and R406W.

Studies using mice with mutations at position 301 on the tau gene have found tau expressed in the cerebellum, hippocampus, thalamus, hypothalamus, spinal cord, brain stem fimbria fornix, amygdala, striatum, olfactory bulb and cortex. (Lewis *et al.*, 2000; Götz *et al.*, 2001; Allen *et al.*, 2002). In the hippocampus CA1 cells were found to be affected but not CA3 cells (Götz *et al.*, 2001) and in the CA1 pyramidal neurones human tau was present in axons but also in cell bodies and apical dendrites. Phosphorylated tau was found in the hippocampus and cortex (Götz *et al.*, 2001). Allen *et al.* (2002) reported that temporal cortex layers II, IV and V showed most cortical reactivity to tau-reactive antibodies. Somatodendritic tau immunoreactivity thought to represent pre-tangles had a wider distribution in the brain, including cortex (especially piriform and entorhinal) hippocampus and basal ganglia. The tangles at the ultrastructural level was comprised of filaments which were straight (10–30 nm diameter) but others had a twisted ribbon appearance (Lewis *et al.*, 2000). Ribbon-like filaments were also found by Allen *et al.* (2002) but were of a smaller size of between 5 and 15 nm, and a small number of AD-like paired helical filaments with a cross-over spacing of about 70–80 nm were also identified. In 11-month-old tau-expressing mice with the V337M human mutation the expressed mutant protein was found in the hippocampal regions CA1, 2 and 3 in cell bodies and dendrites. The tau was of paired-helical type, and made from phosphorylated tau. In the hippocampus, mutant tau was expressed at 70 per cent of the expression of endogenous tau as compared with 10 per cent of whole brain tau (Tanemura *et al.*, 2002). In these mice atrophied and misshaped cells were found, similar to those seen in human AD brains (Ginsberg *et al.*, 1997).

In contrast, both the P301L and the P301S mice show motor deficits associated with a 48–49 per cent reduction in motor neurones in the brain stem and gliosis in the anterior horns (Lewis *et al.*, 2000 and Allen *et al.*, 2002 respectively). Gliosis and co-localized NFTs were found in neurones in the brain stem, diencephalons, basal telencephalon and spinal cord in the P301L mice (Lewis *et al.*, 2000).

Transgenic mice expressing the shortest tau isoform (T44) have also been generated (Ishihara *et al.*, 2001). In 18-month-old animals, staining of filamentous lesions in cortical neurones was similar to that seen in AD and stained for Congo red and Gallyas silver suggesting that the older animals have Aβ in their lesions (Ishihara *et al.*, 2001) as in AD. These filamentous lesions were found primarily in the hippocampus, entorhinal cortex and amygdala, less in the neocortex, and not at all in the spinal cord (Ishihara *et al.*, 2001). As in AD, intraneuronal inclusions in the old Tg mice were ubiquinated. The inclusions in the older mice (24 months) contained exclusively straight tau filaments. The Tau aggregates in the Tg animals were insoluble whereas in the Wt mice 90 per cent of endogenous tau was soluble (Ishihara *et al.*, 2001).

Mice that express human R406W tau have also been developed (Tatebayashi *et al.*, 2002) and at 5 months old exhibit mutant tau prominently in the hippocampus (17.8 per cent of endogenous tau) followed by the neocortex (17 per cent), olfactory bulb (14.3 per cent), the striatum (14.1 per cent) and the thalamus (7.59 per cent). Mutant tau was recorded only at trace level in the cerebellum, mid-brain and the spinal cord (Tatebayashi *et al.*, 2002).

35.6.2 Behaviour in transgenic tau mice

Behavioural disturbances in the P301L and P301S tau mice are largely motor in nature, developing in heterozygotes at 6.5 months and homozygotes at 4.5 months of age (Lewis *et al.*, 2000). Phenotypical changes include lack of body extension during tail elevation and spontaneous back paw clenching whilst standing, delayed righting reflex and rope grasping, weak limbs and dystonic posture, reduction in body weight, and an increase in docility. These animals also developed a neurological phenotype characterized by muscle weakness and tremor (Allen *et al.*, 2002). These motor disturbances are uncharacteristic of AD and are reflective of the spinal cord cell loss (Lewis *et al.*, 2000; Allen *et al.*, 2002).

In contrast the R406W mice at 16–23 months of age exhibited largely cognitive abnormalities. In tests for cued and contextual fear responses Tg mice showed less freezing after foot shock during the conditioning phase and after a 48-hour delay with a cue in a different context. Mortality was higher in the Tg animals (Tatebayashi *et al.*, 2002). A deficit in prepulse inhibition response was found (Tatebayashi *et al.*, 2002) but the motor deficits were not as pronounced as in the P301 mice.

35.7 TRANSGENIC MOUSE MODELS WITH PRESENILIN MUTATIONS

A second route for inducing an increase in Aβ$_{42}$ has been through the development of PS1 mutant mice (Borchelt *et al.*, 1996; Duff *et al.*, 1996). Patients with PS1 mutations associated with AD have greater number of Aβ$_{42}$ plaques compared with patients with the sporadic disease (Mann *et al.*, 1996). Signs of apoptosis and neurodegeneration have been reported in PS1 mice (Chui *et al.*, 1999) and, as would be expected, there is an increased expression of diffuse Aβ$_{42}$ in the brain (Duff *et al.*, 1996; Schuener *et al.*, 1996). However, PS1 mutant mice do not form Aβ deposits (Borchelt *et al.*, 1996; Duff *et al.*, 1996; Holcomb *et al.*, 1999; Barrow *et al.*, 2000) suggesting that Aβ levels do not reach the necessary threshold to start forming aggregates (McGowen *et al.*, 1999). Consequently these single mutation PS1 mouse were soon surpassed by the use of these mice in double Tg mouse models as it was found that the PS1 transgene potentiates the deposition of Aβ in APP mice (Borchelt *et al.*, 1997; Holcomb *et al.*, 1998).

35.8 DOUBLE TRANSGENIC (DTg) MOUSE MODELS

35.8.1 APP/PS1 double transgenic mice

Double Tg mice carrying an APP mutation and a PS1 mutation have by now been well characterized and show that the addition of the PS1 mutation increases amyloid deposition and plaque formation at an earlier time point in the animals life than the single APP mutation alone.

When PS1 × APP/Swe mouse lines were created the PS1 control mice failed to develop an AD pathology but the DTg mice developed large numbers of fibrillar Aβ deposits in the cerebral cortex and hippocampus earlier in life than the pure APP/Swe littermates (Holcomb et al., 1998; Gordon et al., 2002). Plaque number (per mm^2) was found to be highest in the visual cortex at 54 weeks of age (132 ± 11.3) and lowest in the entorhinal cortex at (101.1 ± 13.1), although the cingulate cortex and the entorhinal cortex had the highest mean plaque area at 54 weeks of age (≈300 μm^2) (Wengenack et al., 2000). Plaques appear near to the mid-line and spread laterally and ventrally through the cortex over time (Wengenack et al., 2000). Roughly a 41 per cent increase in Aβ$_{42(43)}$ was found at 6 weeks in double versus single APP Tg mice. Congo red and thioflavin-S showed Aβ deposits in cortex and hippocampus in all DTg mice at 13–16 weeks of age, but this was absent in APP/Swe mice, and these deposits increased with age from 5 per section to 77 per section in 24–32 week old mice (Holcomb et al., 1998). Importantly, amyloid deposition occurs primarily in the cortex and hippocampus whilst the subcortical regions were almost amyloid free, and generally plaque number and amyloid burden increased with age and appeared to be relatively stable between individuals (Wengenack et al., 2000). In addition 8-month-old APPSwe/PS1 double Tg mice showed a decrease in the number of vesicular acetylcholine transporter (VACh-T)-immunoreactive synapses in the frontal cortex, which were reduced in size in the hippocampus (Wong et al., 1999).

These APP/PS1 mice have been reported to have behavioural deficits on both cognitive (Holcomb et al., 1998; Holcomb et al., 1999) and motor tests (Holcomb et al., 1999) by 9 months of age. A study by Puoliväli and colleagues (2002) showed that the age-dependent impairment in water maze performance in these DTg mice correlates with the total amount of Aβ in the hippocampus at a stage when the amyloid deposits cover less than 1 per cent of the hippocampal volume.

In a study by Wirths and colleagues (2001), mice with the human PS1 mutation (M146L) were crossed with a mouse line carrying three APP mutations (Swe, Dut, and Lon) to create a single mouse line. Onset of plaque deposition was 8 months, whilst the onset of neuropil deposits in single Tg mice was at 19 months (Wirths et al., 2001). These double Tg mice expressed an almost 2-fold increase in Aβ relative to the other control mouse lines (Blanchard et al., 2003). Aβ accumulation was detected at 2–4 months of age with the order of deposition as follows: subiculum and dorsal CA1, entorhinal cortex, the rest of hippocampus, and then cortex (Blanchard et al., 2003). Human AD brain sections that were used for comparable analysis showed strong APP expression in pyramidal neurones in the hippocampus, neocortex, and in neuritic plaques. Aβ staining showed extracellular staining in aged AD brains but there was no evidence of neuronal staining. In DTg mice APP was found throughout the cortex and hippocampus at all ages and in the neuritic component of plaques.

Aβ staining was only found in some young animals (8 months old) extracellularly, but was present in all mice intraneuronally at this time point in hippocampal pyramidal cells and granular cells of the dentate gyrus and cortical pyramidal cells (Wirths et al., 2001). In aged DTg mice this intraneuronal staining was virtually absent, but extracellular Aβ deposits were found that were indistinguishable from plaques in PM human brain (Wirths et al., 2001).

A recent paper using APP/Ind × PS1 mutant mice examined these mice for signs of tau immunoreactivity and found that these DTg mice at 8–12 weeks of age showed Aβ deposits with no tau immunoreactivity, but at 24 weeks old the DTg mice exhibited plaques throughout the cortex and hippocampus, and tau labelling confined to areas exhibiting heavy Aβ load, primarily the parietal, cingulate and temporal cortex, but occasionally hippocampus (Kurt et al., 2003). Immunogold labelling revealed hyperphosphorylated tau epitopes in some dystrophic neurites in 24-month-old DTg mice. There was also evidence of straight filaments (10–12 nm wide) in some 8-month-old mice, with one mouse showing single and paired helical filaments (Kurt et al., 2003). The importance of this paper is that it clearly demonstrates that these DTg APP/PS1 mice develop tau pathology in addition to plaques and it shows that tau pathology comes later than plaques but that it is associated with them.

There is relatively little information regarding functional deficits in the APP/PS1 double mutation mice, although a cross-strain Tg2576 × PS1 line have been found to exhibit increased locomotor activity and decreased spontaneous alternation in a Y-maze by 6 months of age when compared with non-Tg and PS1 mice, but did not differ on the spontaneous alternation task from APP (Tg2576) mice until 9 months of age (Holcomb et al., 1999). None of the mice strains in the latter study exhibited spatial learning deficits in a water maze test.

35.8.2 Other double mutation mouse models

Increased plaque burden can also be induced in APP mice by creating DTg mice that express an APP mutation and human AChE. The mean estimated plaque burden for these mice was 40 per cent higher in 12-month-old doubly transgenic mice than in the APP/Swe mice controls (Rees et al., 2003). In a recent study of a PS1/Tau double mutation mouse (Boutajangout et al., 2002) expression of PS1 with tau was not sufficient to produce neurofibrillary tangles even in neurones co-expressing an accumulation of the human mutant tau isoform.

35.9 TRIPLE TRANSGENIC (TTg) MOUSE MODELS

TTg mouse models are still relatively scarce. Of greatest interest to AD research are models that attempt to draw together both the plaque and the NFT pathologies into a single model, as in the human condition, but TTg mice have been developed to examine the role of genes in a single feature of AD pathology.

A TTg model has been developed that was designed to over-express cdk5 and p35 in tau mice (Van den Haute *et al.*, 2001) in an effort to increase tau phosphorylization. However, no increased phosphorylation was found, in contrast to the double Tg P301L X p25 mice that did produce increased phosphorylation (Noble *et al.*, 2003).

At least two mouse lines have been successfully created that develop plaques and NFTs. The presenilin PS1 (M146V) mutation and the APP/Swe mutation have been inserted in to Tg mice expressing mutant P301L tau (Oddo *et al.*, 2003). These mice progressively developed tangles and plaques as did a similar mouse line developed by Oddo *et al.* (2003). These latter mice were Dtg APP/Swe X tau P301L crossed with PS1 M146V knock-in mice. Aβ deposition was found to precede tau pathology. Pathological sequence was interneuronal Aβ immunoreactivity in cortical areas, followed by extracellular Aβ deposits, especially in the frontal cortex (layers IV and V). By 15 months of age posterior cortical areas were affected as were some limbic regions. MC1 staining (which detects conformational changes in tau) and AT8 became apparent at 12 months of age. Tau deposits became increasingly evident in the CA1 cells of the hippocampus followed by cortex (Oddo *et al.*, 2003).

35.10   CONCLUSIONS

The ultimate goal of Tg models of disease is to provide a therapeutic platform on which to test new compounds and novel therapeutic approaches for curing disease.

Traditionally drug therapies in humans with AD have focused on augmenting the existing (but diminishing) cholinergic neurotransmission through the use of cholinomimetic and acetylcholinesterase-inhibiting compounds (Christie *et al.*, 1981; Davis and Mohs, 1982). While this approach is still widely used, it has a limited success rate (≈40 per cent) and is only useful in mild and moderate AD patients (Levy, 1994) and is a disease management strategy rather than a preventative cure. One of the major advantages to come from the development of transgenic animal models of AD is their use in drug trials for novel therapeutic compounds and strategies. In recent years Aβ immunization has been reported to reduce plaque number and improve memory deficits in Tg animals (Janus *et al.*, 2000; Morgan *et al.*, 2000; and see Hirschfield and Hawkins, 2003, for a review) and has inadvertently stimulated a re-examination of the role of amyloid in AD (see Bishop and Robinson, 2002, for a review). Other compounds such as the antioxidant *Ginkgo biloba* have also been found to reverse spatial learning deficits in Tg2576 mice without changing plaque burden or soluble Aβ levels (Stackman *et al.*, 2003). Alternative approaches to drug

therapies such as the use of viral vectors to stimulate an immune response have now been used. An adeno-associated virus vaccine expressing the cholera toxin B subunit and an Aβ fusion protein has recently been reported to reverse memory deficits and reduce Aβ deposition in APP London mice (Zhang *et al.*, 2003). Transgenic mice may also prove to be useful to trial novel neural transplant approaches for AD.

So whilst Tg technology is still relatively young, the development of mouse models that incorporate more than a single gene are bringing scientists ever closer to complete models of diseases and as such they represent a significant breakthrough in our search for a cure for diseases such as AD.

REFERENCES

Allen B, Ingram E, Takao M *et al.* (2002) Abundant tau filaments and nonapoptotic neuro-degeneration in transgenic mice expressing human P301S tau protein. *Journal of Neuroscience* **22**: 9340–9351

Andrä K, Abramowski D, Duke M *et al.* (1996) Expression of APP in transgenic mice: a comparison of neuron-specific promoters. *Neurobiology and Aging* **17**: 183–190

Barrow PA, Empson RM, Gladwell CM *et al.* (2000) Functional phenotype in transgenic mice expressing mutant human presenilin-1. *Neurobiological Disease* **7**: 119–126

Baum L, Chen L, Ng HK, Pang CP. (2000) Apolipoprotein E isoforms in Alzheimer's disease pathology and etiology. *Microscopy Research and Technique* **50**: 278–281

Berger-Sweeney J, McPhie DL, Arters JA *et al.* (1999) Impairments in learning and memory accompanied by neurodegeneration in mice transgenic for the carboxyl-terminus of the amyloid precursor protein. *Molecular Brain Research* **66**: 150–162

Bierer LM, Haroutunian V, Gabriel S *et al.* (1995) Neurochemical correlates of dementia severity in Alzheimer's disease relative importance of the cholinergic system. *Journal of Neurochemistry* **64**: 749–760

Bishop GM and Robinson SR. (2002) The amyloid hypothesis: let sleeping dogmas lie? *Neurobiology and Ageing* **23**: 1101–1105

Blanchard V, Moussaoui S, Czech C *et al.* (2003) Time sequence of maturation of dystrophic neurites associated with AB deposits in APP/PS1 transgenic mice. *Experimental Neurology* **184**: 247–263

Blanquet V, Goldgaber D, Turleau C *et al.* (1987) In situ hybridization of the beta amyloid protein (APP) cDNA to the vicinity of the interface of 21q21 and q22 in normal and Alzheimer's disease individuals. *Cytogenetics and Cell Genetics* **46**: 582

Borchelt DR, Ratovitski T, van Lare J *et al.* (1997) Accelerated amyloid deposition in the brains of transgenic mice coexpressing mutant presenilin 1 and amyloid precursor protein. *Neuron* **19**: 939–945

Borchelt DR, Thinakaran CB, Eckman MK *et al.* (1996) Familial Alzheimer's disease-linked presenilin 1 variants elevate Ab1-42/1–40 ratio in vitro and in vivo. *Neuron* **17**: 1005–1013

Boutajangout A, Leroy K, Touchet N *et al.* (2002) Increased tau phosphorylation but absence of formation of neurofibrillary tangles in mice double transgenic for human tau and Alzheimer's mutant (M146L) presenilin-1. *Neuroscience Letters* **318**: 29–33

Bronfman FC, Moechars D, Van Leuvan F. (2000) Acetylcholinesterase-positive fiber differentiation and cell shrinkage in the septohippocampal pathway of aged amyloid precursor protein London mutant transgenic mice. *Neurobiological Disease* **7**: 152–168

Buee L, Bussiere T, Buee-Scherrer V *et al.* (2000) Tau protein isoforms, phosphorylation and role in neurodegenerative disorders. *Brain Research Review* **33**: 95–130

Callahan MJ, Lipinski WJ, Bian F. (2001) Augmented senile plaque load in aged female b-amyloid precursor protein transgenic mice. *American Journal of Pathology* **158**: 1173–1177

Chen G, Chen KS, Knox J *et al.* (2000) A learning deficit related to age and b-amyloid plaques in a mouse model of Alzheimer's disease. *Nature* **408**: 975–979

Christi MA, Yang DS, Janus C *et al.* (2001) Early-onset amyloid deposition and cognitive deficits in transgenic mice expressing a double mutant form of amyloid precursor protein 695. *Journal of Biological Chemistry* **276**: 21562–21570

Christie JE, Shering A, Ferguson J *et al.* (1981) Physostigmine and arecoline: effects of intravenous infusions in Alzheimer's presenile dementia. *British Journal of Psychiatry* **138**: 46–50

Chui D-H, Tanahashi H, Ozawa K *et al.* (1999) Transgenic mice with Alzheimer's presenilin 1 mutations show accelerated neurodegeneration without amyloid plaque formation. *Nature Medicine* **5**: 560–564

Clark LN, Poorkaj P, Wszolek Z *et al.* (1998) Pathogenic implications of mutations in the tau gene in pallido-ponto-nigral degeneration and relayed neurodegenerative disorders linked to chromosome 17. *Proceedings of the National Academy of Sciences of the United States of America* **95**: 13103–13107

Corder EH, Saunders AM, Strittmatter WJ *et al.* (1993) Gene dose of apolipoprotein E type 4 allele and the risk of Alzheimer's disease in late onset families. *Science* **261**: 921–923

Corsellis JAN. (1976) Ageing and dementias. In: W Blackwood and JAN Corsellis (eds), *Greenfield's Neuropathology*, 3rd edition. London, Arnold, pp. 796–848

Cowburn R, Hardy J, Roberts P *et al.* (1988) Presynaptic and postsynaptic glutamatergic function in Alzheimer's disease. *Neuroscience Letters* **86**: 109–113

Coyle JT. (1982) Excitatory amino acid neurotoxins. In: LL Iversen, SD Iversen, SH Snyder (eds.), *Handbook of Psychopharmacology Volume 15: New Techniques in Psychopharmacology*. New York, Plenum Press, pp. 237–269

D'Souza I, Poorkaj P, Hong M *et al.* (1999) Missense and silent tau gene mutations cause frontotemporal dementia with parkinsonism-chromosome 17 type, by affecting multiple alternative RNA splicing regulatory elements. *Proceedings of the National Academy of Sciences of the United States of America* **96**: 5598–5603

Dahlgren KN, Manelli AM, Stine Jr WB *et al.* (2002) Oligomeric and fibrillar species of amyloid-b peptides differentially affect neuronal viability. *Journal of Biological Chemistry* **277**: 3590–3598

Davis KL and Mohs R. (1982) Enhancement of memory processes in Alzheimer's disease with multiple dose intravenous physostigmine. *American Journal of Psychiatry* **139**: 1421–1424

Dodart J-C, Meziane H, Mathis C *et al.* (1999) Behavioural disturbance in transgenic mice overexpressing the V717F β-amyloid precursor protein. *Behavioural Neuroscience* **113**: 982–990

Duff K, Eckman C, Zehr C *et al.* (1996) Increased amyloid-b42 (43) in brains of mice expressing mutant presenilin 1. *Nature* **383**: 710–713

Dunnett SB. (1994) Animal models of Alzheimer's disease. In: A Burns, R Levy (eds), *Dementia*, 1st edition. London, Chapman and Hall, pp. 239–265

Flood JF, Morley JE, Roberts E. (1991) Amnestic effects in mice of four synthetic peptides homologous to amyloid B-protein from patients with Alzheimer's disease. *Proceedings of the National Academy of Sciences of the United States of America* **88**: 3363–3366

Games D, Adams D, Alessandrini R *et al.* (1995) Alzheimer type neuropathology in transgenic mice overexpressing V717F beta-amyloid precursor protein. *Nature* **373**: 523–527

Gau J-T, Steinhilb ML, Kao T-C *et al.* (2002) Stable β-secretase activity and presynaptic cholinergic markers during progressive central nervous system amyloidogenesis in Tg2576 mice. *American Journal of Pathology* **160**: 731–738

Geula C and Mesulam MM. (1994) Cholinergic systems and related neuropathological predilection patterns in Alzheimer's disease. In: RD Terry, R Kaltzman, KL Bick (eds), *Alzheimer's Disease*. New York, Raven Press, pp. 263–291

Geula C, Mesulam MM, Saroff DM *et al.* (1998). Relationship between plaques, tangles and loss of cortical cholinergic fibres in Alzheimer's disease. *Journal of Neuropathology and Experimental Neurology* **57**: 63–75

Ginsberg SD, Crino PB, Lee VM *et al.* (1997) Sequestration of RNA in Alzheimer's disease neurofibrillary tangles and senile plaques. *Annals of Neurology* **41**: 200–209

Glenner GG and Wong CW. (1984) Alzheimer's disease: initial report on the purification and characterization of a novel cerebrovascular amyloid protein. *Biochemical and Biophysical Research Communications* **120**: 885–890

Goedert M, Spillantini MG, Jakes R *et al.* (1995) Molecular dissection of the paired helical filament. *Neurobiological Aging* **16**: 325–334

Goedert M, Crowther RA, Spillantini MG. (1998) Tau mutations cause frontotemporal dementias. *Neuron* **21**: 955–958

Goldgaber D, Lerman MI, McBride OW *et al.* (1987) Characterization and chromosomal location of a cDNA encoding brain amyloid of Alzheimer's disease. *Science* **235**: 877–880

Gordon MN, Holcomb LA, Jantzen PT *et al.* (2002) Time course of the development of Alzheimer-like pathology in the doubly transgenic PS1 + APP mouse. *Experimental Neurology* **173**: 183–195

Götz J, Chen F, Barmettler R *et al.* (2001) Tau filament formation in transgenic mice expressing P301L tau. *Journal of Biological Chemistry* **265**: 529–234

Harris ME, Wang Y, Pedigo Jr NW *et al.* (1996) Amyloid β peptide (25–35) inhibits Na+-dependent glutamate uptake in rat hippocampal astrocyte cultures. *Journal of Neurochemistry* **67**: 277–286

Hirschfield GM and Hawkins PN. (2003) Amyloidosis: new strategies for treatment. *International Journal of Biochemical Cell Biology* **35**: 1608–1613

Holcomb L, Gordon M, McGowen E *et al.* (1998) Accelerated Alzheimer-like phenotype in transgenic mice carrying both mutant amyloid precursor protein and presenilin 1 transgenes. *Nature Medicine* **4**: 97–100

Holcomb LA, Gordon MN, Jantzen P *et al.* (1999) Behavioural changes in transgenic mice expressing both amyloid precursor protein and presenilin-1 mutations: lack of association with amyloid deposits. *Behavioural Genetics* **29**: 177–185

Hsia AY, Masliah E, McConlogue L *et al.* (1999) Plaque-independent disruption of neural circuits in Alzheimer's disease mouse models. *Proceedings of the National Academy of Sciences of the United States of America* **96**: 3228–3233

Hsiao K. (1998) Transgenic mice expressing Alzheimer amyloid precursor proteins. *Experimental Gerontology* **33**: 883–889

Hsiao K, Chapman P, Nilsen S *et al.* (1996) Correlative memory deficits, Aβ elevation, and amyloid plaques in transgenic mice. *Science* **274**: 99–102

Ishihara T, Zhang B, Higuchi M *et al.* (2001) Age-dependent induction of congophilic neurofibrillary tau inclusions in tau transgenic mice. *American Journal of Pathology* **158**: 555–562

Ishii T. (1966) Distribution of Alzheimer's neurofibrillary changes in the brain stem and hypothalamus of senile dementia. *Acta Neuropathologica* 6:181–187

Janus C, Pearson J, McLaurin J *et al.* (2000) AB peptide immunization reduces behavioural impairment and plaques in a model of Alzheimer's disease. *Nature* **408**: 979–982

Johnson-Wood K, Lee W, Motter R *et al.* (1997). Amyloid precursor protein processing an dAB42 deposition in a transgenic mouse model of Alzheimer disease. *Proceedings of the National Academy of Sciences of the United States of America* **94**:1550–1555

Kang J, Lemaire H-G, Unterbeck JM *et al.* (1987) The precursor of Alzheimer's disease amyloid A4 protein resembles a cell surface receptor. *Nature* **325**: 733–736

Kawabata S, Higgins GA, Gordon JW. (1991) Amyloid plaques, neurofibrillary tangles and neuronal loss in brains of transgenic mice overexpressing a C-terminal fragment of human amyloid precursor protein. *Nature* **354**: 476–578

Kowell NW, Beal MF, Busciglio J *et al.* (1991) An in vivo model for the neurodegenerative effects of β-amyloid and protection by substance P. *Proceedings of the National Academy of Sciences of the United States of America* **88**: 7247–7251

Kumar-Singh S, Dewachter I, Moechars D *et al.* (2000) Behavioural disturbances without amyloid deposits in mice overexpressing human amyloid precursor protein with Flemish (A692G) or Dutch (E693Q) mutation. *Neurobiological Disease* 7: 9–22

Kurt MA, Davies DC, Kidd M *et al.* (2003) Hyperphosphorylated tau and paired helical filament-like structures in the brains of mice carrying mutant amyloid precursor protein and mutant presenilin-1 transgenes. *Neurobiological Disease* **14**: 89–97

Kulnane LS and Lamb BT. (2001) Neuropathological characterization of mutant amyloid precursor protein yeast artificial chromosome transgenic mice. *Neurobiology of Disease* 8: 982–992

Lamb BT, Call LM, Slunt HH *et al.* (1997) Altered metabolism of familial Alzheimer's disease-linked amyloid precursor protein variants in yeast artificial chromosome transgenic mice. *Human Molecular Genetics* 6: 1535–1541

Lamb BT, Bardel KS, Shapiro-Kulnane LS *et al.* (1999) Amyloid production and deposition in mutant amyloid precursor protein and presenilin-1 yeast artificial chromosome transgenic mice. *Nature Neuroscience* 2: 695- 697

Lehman EJH, Shapiro-Kulnane L, Lamb BT. (2003) Alterations in β-amyloid production and deposition in brain regions of two transgenic models. *Neurobiological Aging* 24: 645–653

Levy R. (1994) Cholinergic treatment of Alzheimer's disease. In: A Burns and R Levy (eds), *Dementia*, 1st edition. London, Chapman and Hall, pp. 511–518

Levy-Lahad E, Wijsman EM, Nemens E *et al.* (1995) A familial Alzheimer's disease locus on chromosome 1. *Science* **269**: 970–973

Lewis J, McGowen E, Rockwood J *et al.* (2000) Neurofibrillary tangles, amyotrophy and progressive motor disturbance in mice expressing mutant (P301L) tau protein. *Nature Genetics* **25**: 402–405

Li S, Mallory M, Alford M *et al.* (1997) Glutamate transporter alterations in Alzheimer's disease are possibly associated with abnormal APP. *Journal of Neuropathology and Experimental Neurology* **56**: 901–911

McCool MF, Varty GB, Del Vecchio RA *et al.* (2003) Increased auditory startle response and reduced prepulse inhibition of startle in transgenic mice expressing a double mutant form of amyloid precursor protein. *Brain Research* **994**: 99–106

McGowen E, Sanders S, Iwatsbo T *et al.* (1999) Amyloid phenotype characterization of Transgenic mice overexpressing both mutant amyloid precursor protein and mutant presenilin 1 transgenes. *Neurobiology of Disease* **6**: 231–244

Mann DM, Iwatsubo T, Cairns NJ *et al.* (1996) Amyloid beta protein (Aβ) deposition in chromosome 14-linked Alzheimer's disease: Predominance of Aβ-42(43). *Annals of Neurology* **40**: 149–156

Masliah E, Alford M, Salmon D *et al.* (1996) Deficient glutamate transport is associated with neurodegeneration in Alzheimer's disease. *Annals of Neurology* **40**: 759–766

Masliah E, Westland CE, Rockenstein EM *et al.* (1997) Amyloid precursor proteins protect neurones of transgenic mice against acute and chronic excitotoxic injuries in vivo. *Neuroscience* **78**: 135–141

Masliah E, Raber J, Alford M *et al.* (1998) Amyloid protein precursor stimulates excitatory amino acid transport: implications for roles in neuroprotection and pathogenesis. *Journal of Biological Chemistry* **273**: 12548–12554

Masliah E, Alford M, Mallory M *et al.* (2000) Abnormal glutamate transport function in mutant amyloid precursor protein transgenic mice. *Experimental Neurology* **163**: 381–387

Masters CL, Simms G, Weinman NA *et al.* (1985) Amyloid plaque core protein in Alzheimer's disease and Down syndrome. *Proceedings of the National Academy of Sciences of the United States of America* **82**: 4245–4249

Moechars D, Lorent K, De Strooper B *et al.* (1996) Expression in brain of amyloid precursor protein mutated in the a-secretase site causes disturbed behaviour, neuronal degeneration and premature death in transgenic mice. *EMBO Journal* **15**: 1265–1274

Moechars D, Lorent K, Dewachter I *et al.* (1998) Transgenic mice expressing an α-secretion mutant of the amyloid precursor protein in the brain develop a progressive CNS disorder. *Behaviour and Brain Research* **95**: 55–64

Moechars D, Dewachter I, Lorent K *et al.* (1999) Early phenotypic changes in transgenic mice that overexpress different mutants of myeloid precursor protein in brain. *Journal of Biological Chemistry* **274**: 6483–6492

Molsa PK, Marttila RJ, Rinne UK. (1982) Epidemiology of dementia in a Finnish population. *Acta Neurologica Scandinavica* **65**: 541–552

Morgan D, Diamond DM, Gottschall PE *et al.* (2000) AB peptide vaccination prevents memory loss in an animal model of Alzheimer's disease. *Nature* **408**: 982–985

Mucke L, Masliah E, Yu G-Q *et al.* (2000) High-level neuronal expression of AB1-42 in wild-type human amyloid protein precursor transgenic mice: synaptotoxicity without plaque formation. *Journal of Neuroscience* **20**: 4050–4058

Mucke LE, Masliah E, Johnson WB *et al.* (1994) Synaptotrophic effects of human amyloid b protein precursors in the cortex of transgenic animals. *Brain Research* **666**: 151–167

Nalbantaglu J, Tirado-Santiago G, Lahsaini A *et al.* (1997) Impaired learning and LTP in the mice expressing the carboxy terminus of the Alzheimer amyloid precursor protein. *Nature* **387**: 500–505

Noble W, Olm V, Takata K *et al.* (2003) Cdk5 is a key factor in Tau aggregation and tangle formation in vivo. *Neuron* **38**: 555–565

Oddo S, Caccamo A, Shepherd JD *et al.* (2003) Triple-transgenic model of Alzheimer's disease with plaques and tangles, Intracellular AB and synaptic dysfunction. *Neuron* **39**: 409–421

Park IH, Hwang EM, Hong HS. (2003) Lovastatin enhances AB production and senile plaque deposition in female Tg2576 mice. *Neurobiological Aging* **24**: 637–643

Parnetti L, Senin U, Mecocci P. (1997) Cognitive enhancement therapy for Alzheimer's disease. *Drugs* **56**: 752–768

Perry EK, Tomlinson BE, Blessed G. (1978) Correlation of cholinergic abnormalities with senile plaques and mental test scores in senile dementia. *BMJ* **2**: 1457–1459

Procter AW. (1996) Neurochemical correlates of dementia. *Neurodegeneration* 5: 403–407

Puoliväli J, Wang J, Heikkinen T *et al.* (2002) Hippocampal AB-42 levels correlate with spatial memory deficit in APP and PS1 double transgenic mice. *Neurobiological Disease* 9: 339–347

Quon D, Wang Y, Catalono R *et al.* (1991) Formation of beta-amyloid protein deposits in brains of transgenic mice. *Nature* 352: 239–241

Rees T, Hammond PI, Soreq H *et al.* (2003). Acetylcholinesterase promotes beta-amyloid plaques in cerebral cortex. *Neurobiological Aging* 24: 777–787

Rutten BPF, Wirths O, Van de Berg WDJ *et al.* (2003) No alterations of hippocampal neuronal number and synaptic bouton number in a transgenic mouse model expressing the B-cleaved C-terminal APP fragment. *Neurobiological Disease* 12: 110–120

Sato M, Kawarabayashi T, Shoji M *et al.* (1997) Neurodegeneration and gliosis in transgenic mice over-expressing a carboxy-terminal fragment of Alzheimer amyloid-beta protein precursor. *Dementia and Geriatric Cognitive Disorders* 8: 269–307

Scheuner D, Eckman C, Jensen M *et al.* (1996) Secreted amyloid b protein similar to that seen in senile plaques in Alzheimer's disease is increased in vivo by the presenilin 1 and 2 and APP mutations linked to familial Alzheimer's disease. *Nature Medicine* 2: 864–870

Selkoe DJ. (2001) Alzheimer's disease: genes, proteins and therapy. *Physiological Review* 81: 741–766

Sherrington R, Rogaev EI, Liang Y *et al.* (1995) Cloning of a gene bearing missense mutations in early-onset familial Alzheimer's disease. *Nature* 375: 754–760

Sigurdsson ME, Scholtzova H, Mehta PD *et al.* (2001) Immunization with a nontoxic/nonfibrillar amyloid-β homologous peptide reduces Alzheimer's disease-associated pathology in transgenic mice. *American Journal of Pathology* 159: 439–447

Stackman RW, Eckenstein F, Frei B *et al.* (2003) Prevention of age-related spatial memory deficits in a transgenic moue model of Alzheimer's disease by chronic *Ginkgo biloba* treatment. *Experimental Neurology* 184: 510–520

Sturchler-Pierrat C, Abramowski D, Duke M *et al.* (1997) Two amyloid precursor protein transgenic mouse models with Alzheimer's disease-like pathology. *Proceedings of the National Academy of Sciences of the United States of America* 94:13287–13292

Tanemura K, Murayama M, Akagi T *et al.* (2002) Neurodegeneration with tau accumulation in a transgenic mouse expressing V337M human tau. *Journal of Neuroscience* 22: 133–141

Tatebayashi Y, Miyasaka T, Chui D-H *et al.* (2002) Tau filament formation and associative memory deficit in aged mice expressing mutant (R406W) human tau. *Proceedings of the National Academy of Sciences of the United States of America* 99: 13896–13901

Tesseur I, Van Dorpe J, Spittaels K *et al.* (2000) Expression of human apolipoprotein E4 in neurones causes hyperphosphorylation of protein tau in the brains of transgenic mice. *American Journal of Pathology* 156: 951–964

Tomlinson BE, Blessed G, Roth M. (1970) Observations on the brains of demented old people. *Journal of the Neurological Sciences* 1: 205–242

Tomlinson BE, Irving D, Blessed G. (1981) Cell loss in the locus caeruleus in senile dementia of Alzheimer type. *Journal of the Neurological Sciences* 49: 419–428

Van den Haute C, Spittaels K, Van Dorpe J *et al.* (2001) Coexpression of human cdk5 and its activator p35 with human protein tau in neurones in brain of triple transgenic mice. *Neurobiological Disease* 8: 32–44

Wengenack TM, Whelan S, Curran GL *et al.* (2000) Quantitative histological analysis of amyloid deposition in Alzheimer's double transgenic mouse brain. *Neuroscience* 101: 939–944

Whitehouse PJ, Price DL, Struble RG *et al.* (1982) Alzheimer's disease and senile dementia: loss of neurons in the basal forebrain. *Science* 215: 1237–1239

Wirths O, Multhaup G, Czech C *et al.* (2001) Intraneural AB accumulation precedes plaque formation in b-amyloid precursor protein and presenilin-1 double transgenic mice. *Neuroscience Letters* 306: 116–120

Wong TP, Bebeir T, Duff K *et al.* (1999) Reorganisation of cholinergic terminals in the cerebral cortex and hippocampus of transgenic mice carrying mutated presenilin-1 and amyloid precursor protein transgenes. *Journal of Neuroscience* 19: 2706–2716

Zhang J, Xiobing W, Chuan Q *et al.* (2003) A novel recombinant adeno-associated virus vaccine reduces behavioural impairment and β-amyloid plaques in a mouse model of Alzheimer's disease. *Neurobiological Disease* 14: 365–379

36

How effective are cholinergic therapies in improving cognition in Alzheimer's disease?

DAVID G WILKINSON

Nearly 10 years after the dramatic success of L-dopa therapy for Parkinson's disease, it seemed that a similar treatment approach for Alzheimer's disease (AD) may be on the horizon when substantial presynaptic cholinergic abnormalities were found in the post-mortem brains of affected individuals (see Chapter 29). The results so far have been relatively modest which may not be surprising if we reconsider that these were rather overoptimistic and unrealistic expectations. First, even quite marked cholinergic loss is not necessarily associated with cognitive impairment. For instance, studies of Parkinson's disease show that choline acetyltransferase (ChAT) loss is more severe in patients with dementia than in those without, despite the fact that plaque densities are similar (Perry et al., 1985). While this supports the cholinergic hypothesis, the fact that ChAT levels are also reduced in non-demented patients appears to challenge this. Olivopontocerebellar atrophy (OPCA) also presents an interesting conundrum. For example, in one pedigree the patients show a 40–50 per cent reduction in ChAT levels in temporal and frontal cortex, 20–40 per cent decrements in hippocampus and degeneration of the nucleus basalis of Meynert (nbM), but no evidence of dementia (Kish et al., 1990). One possible interpretation of these data would be to suggest that the importance of forebrain acetylcholine (ACh) in cognition and memory may have been overestimated. By extrapolation then, the cognitive deficits occurring as a direct result of loss of ACh may be quite subtle, so it is perhaps not surprising that cognitive benefits resulting from increasing ACh levels are small. What is becoming clear is that the cholinergic deficit seen in any chronic brain disease may be the result of a variety of insults, rather than the cause of a specific condition like AD.

There are, of course as well as cholinergic deficits, numerous other neurotransmitter deficits in AD, notably in noradrenaline (NA), 5-hydroxytryptamine (5HT), gamma-aminobutyric acid (GABA), glutamate, somatostatin, neuropeptide Y and corticotrophin releasing factor (CRF) (see Rosser, 1988 for review), all or any of which may possibly limit the potential therapeutic effect of increasing ACh levels. We also now have data on drugs affecting other neurotransmitters, which have shown improvements in cognition in AD, one of which, memantine, has been licensed for use in moderate and severe AD (Reisberg et al., 2003).

36.1 CHOLINERGIC TREATMENTS AND THEIR ASSESSMENT

The fact that cholinomimetics have some effects on cognition is, of course, some validation of the presence of a cholinergic deficit. However, of the many treatment approaches only cholinesterase inhibitors (ChEIs) have been consistently able to produce statistically significant improvements in cognitive test results. Some other strategies may have proved unsuccessful because it has been difficult to attain therapeutic doses owing to unacceptable associated side effects, whereas in others this may indicate a flaw in the hypothesis or the lack of appropriate measures of change. The measurement of such subtle changes in cognition has posed a considerable problem in a disease which, by definition, should be relentlessly deteriorating, though in practice can still fluctuate considerably from month to month, and even year to year (Holmes and Lovestone, 2003).

36.2 TREATMENT STRATEGIES

36.2.1 ACh precursors and releasing agents

One of the first treatment strategies was an attempt to increase ACh production by precursor loading. However, there is really no demonstrable shortage of choline or lecithin in the brain and repeated studies have failed to produce positive results (see Becker et al., 1988 for review), although a Cochrane review of mixed dementias suggested some evidence of positive effect in the short term for choline (Fioravanti and Yanagi, 1998).

A number of drugs have been regarded as ACh releasers. This mode of action is often inferred, largely owing to an inability to demonstrate other actions, although a few pyridine derivatives that are predominantly potassium channel blocking agents appear genuinely in this class. There have been at least two UK phase III studies of ACh releasers, both of which were potassium channel blockers. Linopirdine (DUP 996) showed no advantage over placebo and was later found to have a releasing effect on ACh only in the presence of high potassium concentrations, suggesting a limited use *in vivo*. The other, besipirdine (HP749), was a selective M-channel blocker (a potassium channel inactivated by muscarinic agonists) and was found not to be an effective ACh releaser and trials have been unremarkable.

36.2.2 ACh agonists

The lack of response to ACh precursors and releasing agents has to some degree been mirrored at the other side of the synapse when one looks directly at acting ACh agonists. Whilst precursor loading and cholinesterase inhibition are inevitably dependent on intact presynaptic neurones, the finding that at least two subtypes of central cholinergic receptors were not changed in post-mortem AD brain (Palacios et al., 1986) led to the obvious step of trying to stimulate them directly.

Early attempts with compounds like arecoline, pilocarpine, bethanecol, oxotremorine and RS86, some of which needed to be given by intrathecal infusion, were abandoned due to short half-lives and the central and peripheral side effects. There are now a number of orally active selective muscarinic agonists that have reached clinical trials but, despite initial therapeutic optimism, results have been disappointing.

36.2.2.1 XANOMELINE

Xanomeline is an M1- and M4-selective agonist and the first to show a significant though modest treatment effect on cognition as measured by the ADAS-cog (Bodick et al., 1997). This was the first trial of an M1 agonist to report a cognitive improvement but what was perhaps more interesting was the reported improvement in behaviour, including decreases in hallucinations, agitation, vocal outbursts, delusions, suspiciousness and mood swings. Unfortunately, because of unacceptable side effects (nausea, vomiting and fainting), the oral preparation has been dropped, though phase II trials using transdermal patches are underway, in the hope of eliminating the troublesome metabolite produced in the gut and thought to be responsible for the side effects. The improvements seen in non-cognitive symptoms have led some to postulate its use as an antipsychotic (Mirza et al., 2003).

36.2.2.2 OTHER MUSCARINIC AND NICOTINIC AGONISTS

Sabcomeline (SB202026), a partial agonist functionally selective for M1 receptors, has a lower affinity for the M2 and M3 sites, which are thought to mediate side effects. A significant improvement on ADAS-cog was seen in a randomized placebo-controlled trial in 364 patients over 14 weeks, but showed a non-statistically significant improvement in CIBIC-plus (Kumar and Orgogozo, 1996).

Milameline is a partial agonist with equal affinity for M1 and M2 receptors. Lack of cognitive efficacy caused the cessation of phase III studies, even though, anecdotally, it seems to have had some beneficial non-cognitive effects.

Talsaclidine, a functionally selective M1 receptor agonist, and AF102B, have both shown small improvements in ADAS-cog and some claim that they may influence amyloid production. This is based on the fact that stimulation of M1 receptors has been shown to increase the 'normal' processing of amyloid precursor protein (APP) through the α-secretase pathway (Nitsch et al., 1992). It may be for this reason that further development of M1 agonists persists, though tolerability appears to be a common limiting factor.

Nicotinic agonists, often thought to be too toxic, are arousing interest, particularly as galantamine, a cholinesterase inhibitor also stimulates nicotinic receptors through allosteric modulation. However, there are only a few such drugs in trials at the preclinical/phase I stage.

36.2.3 Cholinesterase inhibitors

Acetylcholinesterase inhibitors (AChEIs) have shown consistent efficacy and to date are the only class of cholinomimetics to have gained regulatory approval for treating AD. At present four compounds have gained licences – tacrine (Cognex), donepezil (Aricept), rivastigmine (Exelon) and galantamine (Reminyl) – with a number of others in development (see Table 36.1).

The clinical development of cholinesterase inhibitors (ChEIs) for the treatment of AD started nearly 20 years ago with intravenous administration of physostigmine. The results were encouraging and clearly showed cognitive improvement in AD but the short duration of action and side effects meant it was not suitable for clinical use.

36.2.4 Tacrine (Cognex)

The paper by Summers et al. (1986) reporting a trial of tacrine (tetrahydroaminoacridine or THA), although by current standards judged to be very flawed, ignited the blue touch paper and set the AD research community alight, in an attempt to replicate or refute his findings. Numerous trials

Table 36.1   *Summary of clinical trial data: the effect of AChEIs on ADAS-cog (ITT)*

Drug	Author	No. on active treatment	Dose (mg/day)	Duration of study (weeks) ITT analysis	Placebo/active difference on ADAS-cog points	Difference from baseline
Tacrine	Farlow *et al.* (1992)	37	80	12	3.8	
	Knapp *et al.* (1994)	238	160	30	4.1	
Eptastigmine	Canal and Imbimbo (1996a, 1996b)	83	45	25	4.7	
Donepezil	Rogers *et al.* (1998)	152	5	24	2.5	0.7
	Rogers and Friedhoff (1998)	150	10	24	2.9	1.0
	Burns *et al.* (1999)	273	10	24	2.92	1.2
Rivastigmine	Corey-Bloom *et al.* (1998)	231	6–12	26	3.8	−0.3
	Rösler *et al.* (1999)	243	6–12	26	1.6	+0.26
Metrifonate	Cummings *et al.* (1998)	111	30–60	12	2.9	0.75
	de Jongh (1998)	1290	60–80	26	3.8	1.8
Galantamine	Wilkinson and Murray (2001)	54	30	12	3.3	1.8
	Wilcock *et al.* (2000)	218	32	26	4.1	1.7
	Raskind *et al.* (2000)	423	24/32	26	3.7	1.7

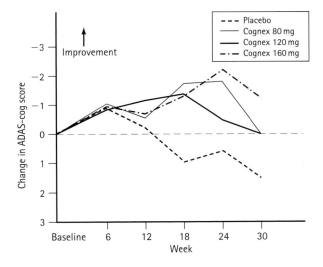

Figure 36.1   *ADAS-cog change from baseline in patients completing 30 weeks of tacrine trial. (Data from: Knapp* et al., *1994.)*

took place (e.g. Davis *et al.*, 1992) but the definitive study was the one by Knapp *et al.* (1994), which tested the compound at higher doses than earlier trials and for a longer period, as a result of the Food and Drug Administration (FDA) request for positive evidence on cognition for 6 months. This was a 30-week trial at a time when studies had usually been only of 6 or 12 weeks' duration. Since then the 24–30-week trial has now become standard. What the Knapp study showed was that at high doses, 160 mg/day, there were statistically significant improvements over placebo in ADAS-cog, CIBI and MMSE; that the improvements started to wane after a few months and that placebo patients steadily declined (Figure 36.1). However, what also became clear was that poor tolerability and side effects would limit the usefulness of the drug.

Tacrine was developed as an analeptic and originally used in anaesthesia to potentiate suxamethonium and to alleviate

post-anaesthetic delirium. It is a reversible inhibitor of both acetyl- and butyryl-cholinesterase (BuChE) and requires dosing four times a day. The major side effect was a liver transaminitis, subsequently found to be of little clinical significance in that it resolved on stopping the drug and 80 per cent of patients could be rechallenged with no recurrence. However, combined with the gastrointestinal side effects, this meant that 70 per cent of patients on the 160 mg/day were unable to complete the 30-week study, and as only 27 per cent of those achieved a >4 point improvement on the ADAS-cog, this meant that in fact only about 10 per cent of patients started on tacrine gained a significant benefit over the 7.5-month period. Clearly this figure could be raised by rechallenging those with transaminitis but this is contentious and off-putting for patient and clinician alike. Further evidence from PET scanning on patients before and after treatment with tacrine seemed to demonstrate considerable improvement in brain metabolism, suggesting a functional change that mirrored clinical findings (Plate 14).

36.2.5 Physostigmine and eptastigmine

The race subsequently started to find more acceptable alternatives to tacrine. Early trial results with a long-acting sustained-release preparation of physostigmine suggested similar efficacy with better tolerability than tacrine. As with earlier physostigmine preparations, although there seemed to be no liver problems, nausea remained an issue. A larger study, unfortunately with a complicated enrichment protocol, showed small improvements. The improved cognition occurred only in patients who had also shown a response in a prestudy, dose-titration phase. It had a short, 6-week, double-blind phase and the effect size at the end point was 1.75 points on the ADAS-cog scale (Thal *et al.*, 1997).

Whilst a lot of the early work on AChEIs took place with physostigmine, its short action and poor tolerability prevented it from becoming an acceptable treatment and as yet it is not licensed. The heptyl analogue of physostigmine, eptastigmine, was found to be more stable, longer lasting, if less potent, and significantly less toxic than the former. In phase III studies it has shown typical AChEI efficacy in terms of improvement in ADAS-cog. One study by Canal and Imbimbo (1996a) showed an effect size of 4.7 points over 25 weeks, which is as good a response as any seen in studies to date. Clinical development, however, has been slow and one company withdrew after a neutropenia developed in two patients (Enz, 1998). There is some suggestion that this drug may be of particular benefit in the middle to late stages of the disease (Canal and Imbimbo, 1996b). A review of the data has been published by Braida and Sala (2001).

36.2.6 Metrifonate

This old drug was for years the mainstay of treatment for bilharzia because of its cholinergic effects. It is in itself, a simple organophosphorus compound, relatively inactive, but it is slowly hydrolysed to dichlorvos in the body, a potent irreversible AChEI. Its slow metabolism and permanent inactivation of the enzyme mean once daily dosing is more than adequate, indeed weekly dosing is used in tropical medicine. Another feature of metrifonate is that, as well as having a completely different mode of action from the other AChEIs, it has excellent tolerability and a rather different range of side effects including rhinitis, leg muscle cramps and diarrhoea. Unfortunately, axial and proximal muscle weakness had been noted in a number of patients in the US, severe enough to cause respiratory failure in a few patients and the trial programme has been halted. Like the other AChEIs it did demonstrate cognitive improvement in AD. Pooled data from US studies (Figure 36.2) showed an effect size of 3.8 ADAS-cog points with an improvement over baseline of 1.8 points, the latter comparable with the best in its class (de Jongh, 1988). The European MALT study (Dubois *et al.*, 1999) showed similar efficacy on cognition, significant changes in behaviour and function and, for the first time in a placebo-controlled study, significant improvements

in carer burden (Shikiar *et al.*, 2000). Because of side effects, however, this drug is unlikely to be studied further.

36.2.7 Donepezil (Aricept)

Donepezil has had the greatest impact so far on the treatment of AD. It was licensed and subsequently cleared for marketing in the US in November 1996 and in the UK in March 1997. It has a high oral bioavailability, is unaffected by food, and has a long plasma half-life of 70 hours permitting once daily dosing. It has almost total plasma protein binding and is a highly selective reversible inhibitor of AChE. It is 10 times less potent than physostigmine but this has not diminished its efficacy in terms of benefits on cognitive function, global assessment and activities of daily living (Burns *et al.*, 1999). The three pivotal placebo-controlled studies all showed an improvement in cognition over baseline at the end of 6 months of around 1 point on the ADAS-cog with an end point effect size over placebo of just under 3 points (Figure 36.3). There have been two 1 year-long placebo-controlled studies that have shown an advantage for long-term treatment both in preservation of cognition (Winblad *et al.*, 2001) and function (Mohs *et al.*, 2001). A third study provided 1-year data for donepezil comparing the rates of cognitive decline after 1 year in patients with probable AD treated with donepezil and those who remained untreated (Doody *et al.*, 2001). Cognitive decline, based on change from baseline in Mini-Mental State Examination (MMSE) scores, was significantly slower in patients treated with donepezil compared with untreated patients ($P = 0.007$). However, it is important to note that the MMSE may not be the most accurate index of the rate of cognitive decline (Goldblum *et al.*, 1994). In fact in the Aricept Withdrawal and Rechallenge Study (AWARE) it was clear that, even in the 30 per cent of patients initially showing no apparent benefit on open label donepezil treatment (often based on MMSE), significant treatment benefits were observed in

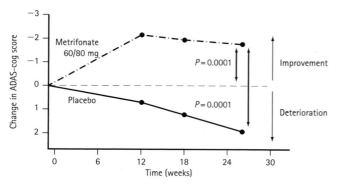

Figure 36.2   *ADAS-cog change from baseline in patients completing 26-week metrifonate trial (pooled data, USA). (Data from de Jongh, 1998.) Patients were those who completed double-blind treatment.* P < 0.05 *(relative to placebo).*

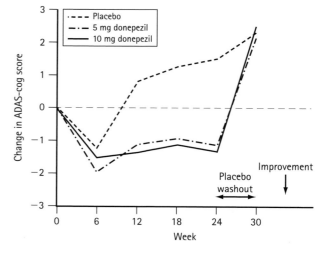

Figure 36.3   *ADAS-cog change from baseline in patients completing 30 weeks of donepezil study. (Data from Rogers et al., 1998.)*

those continuing treatment versus those switching to placebo (Triau *et al.*, 2003) suggesting it may not be an adequate measure of response.

Long-term follow-up studies seem to suggest (although without a placebo group it is only a suggestion) that the cognitive advantage over placebo is maintained for up to 2 years (Rogers and Friedhoff, 1998), and perhaps even longer (Rogers *et al.*, 2000).

There is now clear evidence from clinical practice that changes in behavioural or non-cognitive symptoms are also a feature of response to donepezil (Gauthier *et al.*, 2002). Whether one regards these effects as separate from the cognitive improvement is a moot point but there is now a large body of evidence demonstrating clear cognitive effects with clinical relevance and extremely good tolerability in very mild, mild to moderate, and severe AD (Rogers and Friedhoff, 1998; Feldman *et al.*, 2001; Seltzer *et al.*, 2003). Naturalistic studies in clinical practice have confirmed these effects and it is clear that the 10 mg dose confers greater efficacy than 5 mg, with tolerability being no different from placebo levels if the dose titration from 5–10 mg is left for 4–6 weeks (Matthews *et al.*, 2000).

36.2.8 Rivastigmine (Exelon)

A carbamate derivative of physostigmine, rivastigmine, which is licensed for the symptomatic treatment of mild to moderate AD, has effects like those of eptastigmine. It does not inactivate ACh by the usual microsomal activity but by attaching a carbamyl residue, which means that, although it has a half-life of 2 hours, cholinesterase inhibition in the brain is thought to last for up to 10 hours. It is therefore classed as a pseudo-irreversible inhibitor and is highly specific for AChE.

The phase III clinical trials indicate broadly similar levels of efficacy to donepezil, although direct comparisons are not possible. For example, in one study the effect size of 3.8 ADAS-cog points is largely made up of deterioration in the placebo group and there is very little improvement over baseline scores (Figure 36.4). The trial was said to include a less

selected population with the placebo group deteriorating at a greater and more naturalistic rate than normally seen in trial patients. These data provide a classical example of why, however tempting it is to do so, it is bad science to compare the results of different trials even if protocols are similar, because trial populations vary so much. In this instance we have to accept that the treatment effect size, of 3.8 ADAS-cog points, however construed, is a clinically significant finding.

Of course, the corollary to the increased rate of decline in the placebo group in this trial is that it could indicate an unusual lack of placebo response. A marked placebo response, is a persistent feature of most other trials. In one phase III study of rivastigmine, for instance, only 16 per cent of placebo patients were better or no worse at 6 months, a much lower percentage than in any other trial (Corey-Bloom *et al.*, 1998). This, considered with the fact that 20 per cent of the high dose group had improved by 7 points or greater on the ADAS-cog, suggests the effect size was a genuine reflection of efficacy in a worsening group of patients (Figure 36.5).

A recent meta-analysis was conducted to show the effects of rivastigmine over 5 years compared with the projected cognitive decline of untreated patients over the same period. Rivastigmine data came from open-label extensions of four 6-month, randomized, placebo-controlled trials. Treatment was continued for up to 5 years with open-label rivastigmine (up to 12 mg/day) and appeared to prevent decline to severe dementia (MMSE <10 points) by at least 2 years compared with the estimated levels of decline, although the few left at the end of the study could arguably be seen as rather atypical patients. These studies, also available for other drugs, are of course not hard evidence, but do suggest a long-term effect (Small *et al.*, 2003).

The main drawbacks of rivastigmine are its short half-life, the consequent twice daily dosing, and the necessity for a slow titration to minimize the cholinergic side effects. The trial data suggest these are not severe but include nausea, vomiting and anorexia. Rivastigmine has also been linked to improvements in non-cognitive symptoms demonstrated by

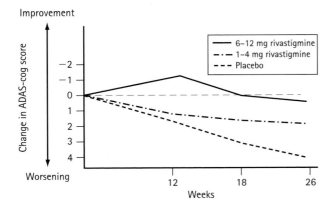

Figure 36.4 *ADAS-cog change from baseline (ITT) in patients completing 26 weeks of rivastigmine study (Data from Corey-Bloom et al., 1998).*

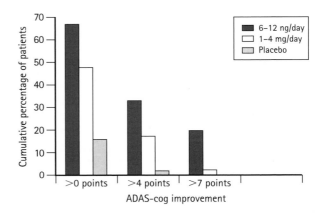

Figure 36.5 *ADAS-cog change from baseline in patients completing 26 weeks of rivastigmine trial (Data from Corey-Bloom et al., 1998).*

the results of a study in patients with dementia with Lewy bodies, which showed that scores on the 10-point Neuropsychiatric Inventory (NPI) were significantly better ($P = 0.01$) after 20 weeks for those on rivastigmine compared with placebo (McKeith *et al.*, 2000).

36.2.9 Galantamine (Reminyl)

The last of the major AChEIs to be licensed for the treatment of mild to moderate AD is by no means the least interesting. Like physostigmine and codeine, this compound is a natural alkaloid and shares with them the potential to allosterically potentiate submaximal nicotinic responses induced by ACh, and competitive agonists. It may well be that this nicotinic effect is the reason why the AChEIs are more effective than other cholinomimetics. Allosteric potentiating ligands like galantamine could therefore enhance nicotinic transmission under conditions of reduced secretion or increased degradation of ACh, or where the ACh sensitivity of nicotinic ACh receptors is reduced. This may well mean they will have a preventive and corrective action on impaired nicotinic transmission and may have more than a symptomatic effect on AD itself (Schrattenholz *et al.*, 1996).

Studies so far have demonstrated consistent evidence of cognitive improvement. An American study with 636 patients showed an effect size of 3.7 points on the ADAS-cog with improvement of 1.7 points from baseline at 6 months (Raskind *et al.*, 2000). An international study showed an effect size of 4.1 points on ADAS-cog, again with improvement over baseline of 1.7 points at 6 months (Wilcock *et al.*, 2000). The data from the US open label continuation study indicate maintenance of this benefit with no decrement from baseline a year later (Lilienfield and Parys, 2000). Both studies also showed improvements in the global assessment and functional ability.

What is worth noting in many of these trials is the proportion of patients who show quite marked improvements in cognition. In a phase II study of galantamine, 10 per cent of patients on the 30 mg dose of galantamine showed an improvement of 15 points or greater on the ADAS-cog after 12 weeks (Wilkinson and Murray, 2001). No placebo patients ever show this kind of response and this is echoed in other AChEI trials (Figure 36.6).

Galantamine, like all AChEIs, does have tolerability problems unless titrated slowly and, as expected, the side effects are predominantly gastrointestinal. It is, however, over 90 per cent bioavailable so can be given with food. It is a competitive, reversible and specific inhibitor of ACh, with a half-life of about 8 hours. It needs to be given twice daily and has an optimal dose of around 24 mg daily. There are no long-term data from placebo-controlled trials of galantamine but open label continuation studies, now extending to 4 years claim, as with the other AChEIs, that despite a tendency to cognitive decline in the long term there is an advantage to continued treatment compared with the expected decline in patients without treatment.

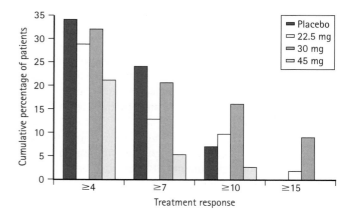

Figure 36.6   *ADAS-cog change from baseline in patients completing 12-week galantamine trial. (Data from Wilkinson and Murray 2001.)*

36.2.10 Comparative studies

All the currently available AChEIs seem to have similar cognitive effects with none showing mean improvements on the ADAS-cog of greater than 5 points in 6-month controlled trials. This may be the limit of their efficacy but without comparative studies in the same population it is impossible to make judgements about the relative importance of each compound. Unfortunately, because the differences between the drugs will be small, comparative studies would require enormous numbers to demonstrate statistical significance, consequently to run double-blind trials would be very expensive with the risk of showing no advantage for the company involved.

There equally would be little point in funding such trials by independent bodies unless there were vast differences in cost. Three comparative studies have been conducted for marketing reasons and are all somewhat limited by being open label, albeit with blinded raters. Two sponsored by the makers of donepezil comparing it against rivastigmine and galantamine had similar designs and were run to compare the recommended dosing regimes and tolerability. The first, a 12-week comparison between donepezil and rivastigmine, showed no difference between the two drugs on cognition but many fewer patients were able to be titrated up to the recommended maximum doses of rivastigmine with consequently significantly more gastrointestinal side effects overall compared with donepezil. Unsurprisingly, both clinicians and carers preferred donepezil with its better side effect profile, simpler titration and once daily dosing (Wilkinson *et al.*, 2002).

The second study, between donepezil and galantamine, was also of only 12 weeks duration, which meant that the maximum dose of galantamine was only reached in the last month compared with 2 months for the donepezil group. Tolerability, whilst still in favour of donepezil, was much more acceptable in the galantamine group. However, significant advantages were demonstrated for donepezil over its comparator in cognition and function and may represent a function of the short duration of the study (Jones *et al.*, 2004).

The third study, sponsored by the makers of galantamine, was somewhat different. Hoping to show some evidence of disease modification as a result of its proposed nicotinic effects, the researchers enrolled a somewhat more severe group (MMSE 9–18) for 1 year and used computerized tests of attention in some centres. They used an activity of daily living scale as the primary outcome measure and this showed no difference between the groups. There were no significant differences in the secondary outcomes of MMSE ADAS-cog, NPI or caregiver burden; however, a subanalysis of those enrolled with MMSE scores from 12–18 did show an advantage on MMSE, one of the secondary outcomes, for the galantamine group (Wilcock *et al.*, 2003). The discrepancy between the two studies of donepezil and galantamine underlines the very small differences between the drugs in relation to outcomes, with all three compounds having broadly similar effects. This was a confirmation of the pivotal trial data with the drugs being separated only by their different side effect profiles and dosing regimes.

36.3 CONCLUSION

This review of the available data on the cognitive effects of all the current cholinomimetic treatments shows that only the AChEIs have a clear statistical and clinical advantage over placebo. The clinical utility may be even greater if one looks at behavioural change, one area where other classes of drug (e.g. M1 agonists) have also shown some positive effects. The averaged outcomes from placebo-controlled studies conceal the fact that, while some patients show little benefit, others show considerable improvements (>15 points on ADAS-cog). Unfortunately, however, all studies to date suggest that predicting response is not possible before treatment starts. The effect appears to be maintained over a number of months and, while it does fade in those who have responded, the advantage over placebo may remain for a number of years. As efficacy fades it may be possible to maintain the cognitive benefits by increasing the dose of AChEIs, as long as the drug is tolerated.

What is not clear is whether intermittent treatment, allowing restitution of neurotransmitter and receptor sensitivity, will sustain the cognitive improvement, a claim made, but as yet unsubstantiated, for rivastigmine, the AChEI with the shortest half life. The numerous interactions with, and modulation of, cholinergic function by other neurotransmitters may explain why cholinomimetics seem to have a ceiling effect and the combination of cholinergic and other strategies may yet show a synergistic effect. One study adding memantine to donepezil in moderately severe AD has shown promise, although a similar study in mild to moderate AD has not (Hartmann and Mobius, 2003; Tariot *et al.*, 2003). Clearly work on oxidative stress, the inflammatory response,

modification of APP processing, tau phosphorylation, the effects of excitatory amino acids and the ion channels will all come to bear on the treatment of AD in due course. However, AChEIs have shown clear clinical benefits in cognition and behaviour and will be the cornerstone of pharmacological treatment in AD for some years to come.

REFERENCES

Becker R, Giacobini E, Elbe R *et al.* (1988) Potential pharmacotherapy of Alzheimer's disease. A comparison of various forms of physostigmine administration. *Acta Neurologica Scandinavica* **77**: 19–22

Bodick NC, Offen WW, Levey AL *et al.* (1997) Effects of xanomeline, a selective muscarinic receptor agonist, on cognitive function and behavioural symptoms in Alzheimer's disease. *Archives of Neurology* **54**: 465–475

Braida D and Sala M. (2001) Eptastigmine: ten years of pharmacology, toxicology, pharmacokinetic, and clinical studies. *CNS Drug Review* **7**: 369–386

Burns A, Rossor M, Hecker J *et al.* for the International Donepezil Study Group. (1999) The effects of donepezil in Alzheimer's disease – results from a multinational trial. *Dementia and Geriatric Cognitive Disorders* **10**: 237–244

Canal I and Imbimbo BP. (1996a) Clinical trials and therapeutics: relationship between pharmacodynamic activity and cognitive effects of eptastigmine in patients with Alzheimer's disease. *Clinical Pharmacology and Therapeutics* **15**: 49–59

Canal I and Imbimbo BP. (1996b) Relationship between pharmacodynamic activity and cognitive effects of eptastigmine in patients with Alzheimer disease. *Clinical Pharmacology and Therapeutics* **60**: 218–228

Corey-Bloom J, Anand R, Veach J. (1998) A randomised trial evaluating the efficacy and safety of ENA 713 (rivastigmine tartrate), a new acetylcholinesterase inhibitor, in patients with mild to moderately severe Alzheimer's disease. *International Journal of Geriatric Psychopharmacology* **1**: 55–65

Cummings JL, Cyrus PA, Bieber MD *et al.* (1998) Metrifonate treatment of the cognitive deficits of Alzheimer's disease. *Neurology* **50**: 1214–1221

Davis KL, Thal LJ, Camzu ER *et al.* (1992) A double-blind placebo-controlled multicentre study of tacrine for Alzheimer's disease. The Tacrine Collaborative Study Group. *New England Journal of Medicine* **327**: 1253–1259

de Jongh P. (1998) *Clinical development of metrifonate: an overview of cognitive and global outcomes. Collegium Internationale Neuro-Psychopharmacologium.* Glasgow, Bayer AG

Doody RS, Dunn JK, Clark CM *et al.* (2001) Chronic donepezil treatment is associated with slowed cognitive decline in Alzheimer's disease. *Dementia and Geriatric Cognitive Disorders* **12**: 295–300

Dubois B, McKeith I, Orgogozo J, Collins O, Meulien D. (1999) A multicentre, randomized, double-blind, placebo-controlled study to evaluate the efficacy, tolerability and safety of two doses of metrifonate in patients with mild-to-moderate Alzheimer's disease: the MALT study. *International Journal of Geriatric Psychiatry* **14**: 973–982

Enz A. (1998) Classes of drugs. In: S Gauthier (ed.), *Pharmacotherapy of Alzheimer's Disease.* London, Martin Dunitz

Farlow M, Gracon SI, Hershey LA et al. (1992) A controlled trial of tacrine in Alzheimer's disease. JAMA 268: 2523–2529

Feldman H, Gauthier S, Hecker J et al. (2001) A 24-week, randomized, double-blind study of donepezil in moderate to severe Alzheimer's disease. Neurology 57: 613–621

Fioravanti M and Yanagi M. (1998) CDP-choline in the treatment of cognitive and behavioural disturbances associated with chronic cerebral disorders of the aged. (Cochrane Review) In: The Cochrane Library, Issue 2. Oxford: Update Software

Gauthier S, Feldman H, Hecker et al. (2002) Efficacy of donepezil on behavioral symptoms in patients with moderate to severe Alzheimer's disease. International Psychogeriatrics 14: 389–404

Goldblum MC, Tzortzis C, Michot JL, Panisset M, Boller F. (1994) Language impairment and rate of cognitive decline in Alzheimer's disease. Dementia 5: 334–338

Hartmann S and Mobius HJ. (2003) Tolerability of memantine in combination with cholinesterase inhibitors in dementia therapy. International Clinical Psychopharmacology 18: 81–85

Holmes C and Lovestone S. (2003) Long-term cognitive and functional decline in late onset Alzheimer's disease: therapeutic implications. Age and Ageing 32: 200–204

Jones RW, Soininen H, Hager K et al. (2004) A multinational, randomised, 12-week study comparing the effects of donepezil and galantamine in patients with mild to moderate Alzheimer's disease. International Journal of Geriatric Psychiatry 19: 58–67

Kish SJ, Distefano LM, Dozic S et al. (1990) [3H]Vesamicol binding in human brain cholinergic deficiency disorders. Neuroscience Letters 117: 347–352

Knapp MJ, Knopman DS, Soloman PR et al. (1994) A 30 week randomized controlled trial of high dose tacrine in patients with Alzheimer's disease. JAMA 271: 985–991

Kumar R and Orgogozo J. (1996) Efficacy and safety of SB202026 as a symptomatic treatment for Alzheimer's disease. Neurobiology of Aging 17: 161

Lilienfield S and Parys W. (2000) Galantamine: additional benefits to patients with Alzheimer's disease. Dementia and Geriatric Cognitive Disorders 11 (Suppl. 1): 19–27

McKeith I, Del Ser T, Spano et al. (2000) Efficacy of rivastigmine in dementia with Lewy bodies: a randomised, double-blind, placebo-controlled international study. Lancet 16: 2031–2036

Matthews HP, Korby J, Wilkinson DG, Rowden J. (2000) Donepezil in Alzheimer's Disease: eighteen months results from Southampton Memory Clinic. International Journal of Geriatric Psychiatry 15: 713–720

Mirza NR, Peters D, Sparks RG. (2003) Xanomeline and the antipsychotic potential of muscarinic receptor subtype selective agonists CNS Drug Review 9: 159–186

Mohs RC, Doody RS, Morris JC et al. (2001) A 1-year, placebo-controlled preservation of function survival study of donepezil in AD patients. Neurology. 14: 481–488

Nitsch RM, Slack BE, Wurtman RJ et al. (1992) Release of Alzheimer's amyloid precursor derivatives stimulated by activation of muscarinic acetylcholine receptors. Science 258: 304–307

Palacios JM, Cortes R, Probst A et al. (1986) Mapping of subtypes of muscarinic receptors in the human brain with receptor autoradiographic techniques. Trends in Pharmacological Sciences 6: 56–60

Perry EK, Curtis M, Candy JM et al. (1985) Cholinergic correlates of cognitive impairment in Parkinson's disease: comparisons with Alzheimer's disease. Journal of Neurology, Neurosurgery, and Psychiatry 48: 413–421

Raskind MA, Peskind ER, Wessel T, Yuan W. (2000) Galantamine in AD a 6-month randomized, placebo-controlled trial with a 6-month extension. Neurology 54: 2261–2268

Reisberg B, Doody R, Stoffler A, Schmitt F, Ferris S, Mobius HJ. (2003) Memantine in moderate-to-severe Alzheimer's disease. New England of Medicine 3: 1333–1341

Rogers S and Friedhoff L. (1998) Long-term efficacy and safety of donepezil in the treatment of Alzheimer's disease: an interim analysis of the results of a US multicentre open label extension study. European Neuropsychopharmacology 8: 67–75

Rogers SL, Farlow MD, Doody RS et al. (1998) A 24 week, double-blind, placebo-controlled trial of donepezil in patients with Alzheimer's disease. Neurology 50: 136–145

Rogers SL, Doody RS, Pratt RD, Leni JR. (2000) Long-term efficacy and safety of donepezil in the treatment of Alzheimer's disease: final analysis of a US multicentre open-label study. European Neuropsychopharmacology 10: 195–203

Rösler M, Anand R, Cicin-Sain A et al. (1999) Efficacy and safety of rivastigmine in patients with Alzheimer's disease: international randomised controlled trial. BMJ 318: 633–640

Rosser M. (1988) In: LL Iversen, SD Iversen, SH Snyder (eds), Handbook of Psychopharmacology, Vol. 20. New York, Plenum Press, pp. 107–130

Schrattenholz A, Pereira EF, Roth U, Weber KH, Albuquerque EX, Maelicke A. (1996) Agonist responses of neuronal nicotinic acetylcholine receptors are potentiated by a novel class of allosterically acting ligands. Molecular Pharmacology 49: 1–6

Seltzer B, Zolnouni P, Nunez M et al. (2003) Donepezil treatment benefits in early stage Alzheimer's disease. Journal of the American Geriatrics Society 51: S100; P170

Shikiar R, Shakespeare A, Sagnier P, Wilkinson D et al. (2000) The impact of Metrifonate therapy on caregivers of patients with Alzheimer's disease: results from the MALT clinical trial. Journal of the American Geriatrics Society 48: 268–274

Small G, Mendiondo M, Quarg P, Spiegel R. (2003) Efficacy of rivastigmine treatment in Alzheimer's disease over 5 years. Poster presentation: International College of Neuro-Psychopharmacology, Puerto Rico

Summers WK, Majovski LV, Marsh GM, Tachiki K, Kling A. (1986) Oral tetrahydroauminoacridine in long-term treatment of senile dementia, Alzheimer type. New England Journal of Medicine 315: 1241–1245

Tariot P, Farlow M, Grossberg G et al. (2003) Memantine/donepezil dual therapy is superior to placebo/donepezil therapy for treatment of moderate to severe Alzheimer's disease. 11th IPA Congress, Chicago, PB-089

Thal LJ, Swartz G, Samo M et al. (1997) A multicenter double-blind study of controlled-release physostigmine for the treatment of symptoms secondary to Alzheimer's disease. Neurology 47: 1389–1395

Triau E, Heun R, Holub R et al. (2003) Cognition is physicians' main indicator of treatment efficacy in Alzheimer's disease patients. European Psychopharmacology 13: (Suppl. 4) S406–P4.051

Wilcock G, Lilienfeld S, Gaens E. (2000) Efficacy and safety of galantamine in patients with mild to moderate Alzheimer's disease: a multi-centre randomised controlled trial. BMJ 321: 1–7

Wilcock G, Howe I, Coles H and members of the GAL-GBR-2 study group. (2003) A long-term comparison of galantamine and donepezil in the treatment of Alzheimer's disease. *Drugs and Aging* **20**: 777–789

Wilkinson D and Murray J. (2001) Galantamine: a randomised, double blind, dose-finding trial in patients with Alzheimer's disease. *International Journal of Geriatric Psychiatry* **16**: 852–857

Wilkinson D, Passmore P, Bullock R *et al.* (2002) A multinational, randomized, 12-week comparative study of donepezil and rivastigmine in patients with mild to moderate Alzheimer's disease. *International Journal of Clinical Practice* **56**: 441–446

Winblad B, Engedal K, Soininen H *et al.* (2001) Donepezil enhances global function, cognition and activities if daily living compared with placebo in a one-year, double blind trial in patients with mild-to-moderate Alzheimer's disease. *Neurology* **57**: 489–496

37

Non-cholinergic therapies of dementia

LON S SCHNEIDER

Until recently cholinesterase inhibitors (ChEIs) have been the only approved treatments for Alzheimer's disease (AD). Recently memantine was approved by European, North American and other regulators for the treatment of moderate to severe dementia of the Alzheimer's type. There continue to be no approved treatments in Europe and North America for other dementias, although several trials suggest the feasibility for ChEIs for the vascular dementias (Erkinjuntti *et al.*, 2002; Black *et al.*, 2003; Wilkinson *et al.*, 2003) or dementia with Lewy bodies (McKeith *et al.*, 2000).

In addition there are a range of medications, vitamins or herbs, not explicitly approved for Alzheimer's disease or dementia, that have potential usefulness, that have not been clearly demonstrated in clinical trials to be efficacious, but that can either be prescribed by physicians or purchased by patients. These medications include piracetam, extract of *Ginkgo biloba*, selegiline, vitamin E, multiple B vitamins and the HMG-CoA reductase inhibitors (statins). Notably, medications such as oestrogens and anti-inflammatories have been advocated by some in the recent past, but now need reconsideration in the light of current clinical trials showing no evidence and potential cognitive worsening with these drugs (Aisen *et al.*, 2003b; Rapp *et al.*, 2003; Visser *et al.*, 2003).

37.1 PREVENTION OF DEMENTIA

From a public health point of view, preventing the onset of AD is more important than the treatment of dementia after it develops. In this respect interventions that might decrease the risk of dementia such as reducing blood pressure to prevent cerebrovascular disease, the use of lipid lowering drugs,

or reducing homocysteine with B vitamins will be discussed in this chapter. Other considerations in prevention include improving diet, ceasing smoking, improving exercise, effectively treating diabetes mellitus, and preventing head injury. However, these 'preventative' measures are non-specific for dementia and have salutary effects on a range of conditions.

There is direct clinical trials evidence that vitamins and trace elements supplementation improves cognitive function in elderly subjects who may or may not have had dementia. For example, 86 older subjects were randomized to a 1-year trial of placebo or a supplement containing various vitamins and elemental metals. In this small trial performed in India there were improvements on memory, long-term retrieval, category fluency and digit span, as well as a rather marked improvement on Mini-Mental State Exam (MMSE) scores. However, generalizing such findings to other populations may be difficult considering that diagnosis and baseline nutritional status may be factors in the response, and notably MMSE scores were low in this middle-class Indian cohort, averaging 21–15 (Chandra, 2001). Nevertheless, this trial points to the potential that a variety of non-specific health or physiological interventions could have salutary effects on cognition.

37.2 POTENTIAL NON-CHOLINERGIC STRATEGIES FOR ALZHEIMER'S DISEASE

ChEIs are the only medications currently approved in the US for treating mild to moderate AD. The use of ChEIs for the management of the cognitive and behavioural symptoms of AD is reviewed elsewhere in this book. The overall effectiveness of ChEIs, modest at best, is manifested generally as stabilization of cognitive symptoms over 6 months to 1 year compared with the continuing cognitive decline in placebo-treated patients. Additionally, only a minority of patients treated benefit over those 6 months. As such, clinicians regularly encounter requests for information on other potential treatments including over-the-counter medications, herbal remedies, vitamins and agents approved for other indications or those which are available only outside the US.

Since the goals of treatment can range from symptomatic improvement to slowing symptom progression, or even to delaying the onset of dementia, potential benefits must be weighed carefully against adverse-effect risks. Moreover, it is particularly important to weigh treatment options with patients diagnosed with mild cognitive impairment (MCI) since only 8–15 per cent of these MCI patients develop dementia on an annual basis, while nearly 40 per cent do not appear to progress to AD and indeed may no longer display any cognitive impairment at 2-year follow up (Larrieu et al., 2002). Some potential or emerging treatment options based on available clinical data are discussed below (see Table 37.1).

37.2.1 Homocysteine reduction and vitamin E

Elevated levels of homocysteine (HC) may contribute to cardiovascular disease (Wilcken and Dudman, 1989; Bellamy and McDowell, 1997), cognitive impairment (Lehmann et al., 1999) and dementia (Seshadri et al., 2002). Plasma concentrations of HC rise when its metabolism to methionine or cysteine is impaired, which may occur under a number of circumstances including natural ageing. Increased plasma levels of HC are associated with damage to vascular endothelial cells (Wilcken and Dudman, 1989) and increased risk for thrombosis (Bellamy and McDowell, 1997), possibly through lipid peroxidation (Voutilainen et al., 1999) and release of endothelium-derived relaxing factor causing vasodilatation (Stamler et al., 1993). More relevant to AD, HC also potentiates the neurotoxic effects of Aβ in vitro, in hippocampal neurones (Ho et al., 2001; Kruman et al., 2002) through an unknown mechanism. It is therefore possible that reducing levels of HC would lead to cognitive benefits in people with cerebrovascular disease or AD, possibly by delaying the onset of dementia, or improving cognitive function. HC plasma levels can be reduced by as much as 30 per cent using a regimen of B vitamins (e.g. B_{12} 1 mg/day, B_6 25 mg/day, and folic

Table 37.1 *Non-cholinergic approaches for the treatment of AD*

Agent*	Possible mode of action	Status
Vitamins B_6, B_{12}, folate therapy	Combination may lower homocysteine (HC) levels. Elevated HC may raise risks for cardiovascular disease and AD	Unproven effects. Observational studies show decreases in incidence of AD. Clinical trial is ongoing
Vitamin E or selegiline	Antioxidant effects may be neuroprotective	In a single trial each was effective at delaying clinical progression of moderate to severe AD patients, but not effective for improving cognition (Sano et al., 1997). One trial of vitamin E (compared to donepezil and placebo) for MCI is underway
Oestrogens	Have neurotrophic properties; enhances NGF, synaptogenesis, increase acetylcholine	New evidence is largely negative; no evidence for cognitive improvement; risks outweigh benefits. May be worse than placebo (Mulnard et al., 2000; Rapp et al., 2003). Should not be used for treating or preventing dementia or cognitive impairment
Non-steroidal anti-inflammatory drugs (NSAIDs)	Anti-inflammatory mechanism may be neuroprotective	Clinical trials results in AD and MCI generally are negative (Scharf et al., 1999; Van Gool et al., 2001; Aisen et al., 2003b; Visser et al., 2003). One prevention trial ongoing
HMG-CoA reductase inhibitors (statins)	Inhibits the production of cholesterol, modulates APP processing	Observational studies show decreases in incidence of AD. Two large cardiovascular trials did not show cognitive effects in elderly. At least one ongoing trial in AD
Ginkgo biloba	Possible anti-oxidant and other mechanisms, could be neuroprotective	Some clinical trials in AD are positive. One prevention trial (GEMS) is ongoing
Memantine	NMDA-receptor antagonist; anti-glutamate effects, may protect against calcium-induced neurotoxicity	Clinical trials in moderate to severe AD are positive. Trials in mild to moderate AD are ongoing. Approved for moderately severe to severe AD in EU, Canada and US

*Except for memantine none of the agents is approved for AD in the EU or North America

acid 5 mg/day) and a placebo-controlled clinical trial is underway to determine whether such a regimen will slow the rate of cognitive decline in AD (Aisen *et al.*, 2003a).

37.2.2 Antioxidants

The antioxidant effects of vitamin E (α-tocopherol) might have an impact on reducing clinical progression of illness. In the prototypical antioxidant trial (Sano *et al.*, 1997), vitamin E, selegiline (a monoamine oxidase inhibitor relatively selective for the MAO-B subtype at doses of 10 mg/day) or their combination in moderate to severe AD patients was associated with a delay in either nursing home placement and the loss of activities of daily living, supporting a protective effect for the treatments. Interestingly, despite the delay in the progression of functional impairment, no significant effect on cognition was observed. Further investigation is warranted, including studies in earlier stages of AD and in MCI. At present, a multicentre trial comparing vitamin E and donepezil in MCI patients is ongoing: http://adcs.ucsd.edu/MCI_Protocol.htm.

37.2.3 Anti-inflammatories

Markers of inflammation in the brains of AD patients suggest a potential therapeutic benefit of anti-inflammatory use (Aisen and Davis, 1994; Breitner, 1996; Aisen, 2000). Epidemiological studies with non-steroidal anti-inflammatory drugs (NSAIDs) have indicated that these agents may be potentially effective for reducing the incidence or delaying the onset of AD (Rich *et al.*, 1995; McGeer and McGeer, 1996; in t' Veld *et al.*, 2001). Yet, barring one exception (Rogers *et al.*, 1993), randomized, placebo-controlled studies of NSAIDs in AD patients have failed to show a clinical benefit (Scharf *et al.*, 1999; Aisen 2000; Van Gool *et al.*, 2001; Aisen *et al.*, 2003a, b).

A recently completed 1-year multicentre, placebo-controlled trial involving 351 participants tested the potential of either the cox-2 inhibitor rofecoxib or the non-selective NSAID naproxen to slow the progressive cognitive decline that is characteristic in patients with mild to moderate AD (Aisen *et al.*, 2003b). In this study, there was no difference in change of ADAS-cog score in patients treated with either NSAID compared with the placebo group, indicating that anti-inflammatory drugs may not be effective in slowing cognitive decline in mild to moderate AD.

To investigate the effect of NSAIDs in delaying the onset of AD, an ongoing multisite trial (the Alzheimer's Disease Anti-inflammatory Prevention Trial, ADAPT) (Martin *et al.*, 2002) is enrolling over 2500 patients aged 70+ years with a family history of dementia to be randomized to treatment with naproxen, celecoxib, or placebo, and followed for 5–7 years. Another trial will evaluate subjects 'at risk' for developing AD for short-term effects of ibuprofen on beta-amyloid$_{1-42}$ (Aβ) levels in cerebrospinal fluid, which may be an early biomarker for AD. Results from these and similar trials will be required to assess adequately the clinical benefit of NSAID use in AD.

37.2.4 HMG–CoA reductase inhibitors (statins)

Emerging evidence suggests that cholesterol lowering and the use of HMG-CoA reductase inhibitors may impact the development or progression of AD possibly because cholesterol levels modulate the enzymatic processing of amyloid precursor protein (APP) and the production of Aβ, a main component of neuritic plaques in AD brain (Refolo *et al.*, 2000). Cholesterol-fed rabbits demonstrate increased levels of Aβ in the brain, and hypercholesterolaemia induced by a high cholesterol diet results in increased levels of Aβ in the CNS (Sparks *et al.*, 1994, 1995). Furthermore, simvastatin administration *in vitro* reduces intra- and extracellular Aβ levels in neuronal cultures (Fassbender *et al.*, 2001).

Observational studies of patient databases have demonstrated that lovastatin- or pravastatin-treated patients have a 60–73 per cent lower prevalence of AD (Wolozin *et al.*, 2000) and an analysis of a UK clinical practice database suggests a markedly reduced risk for dementia in patients taking statins compared with case-matched controls (Jick *et al.*, 2000). In a case–control analysis of the Canadian Study of Health and Aging, statin use was associated with reduced risk for AD as well (Rockwood *et al.*, 2002).

Large clinical trials, however, thus far have not supported statin use for improving cognition or prevention of dementia. A randomized placebo-controlled trial of pravastatin (the PROSPER study) in 5804 subjects aged 70–82 years with histories or risk factors for vascular disease reported favourable cardiovascular outcomes but no significant effect on cognitive function or disability during the average 3.2 year follow-up period (Shepherd *et al.*, 2002). Further, a randomized, placebo-controlled trial of the effect of simvastatin on cardiovascular outcomes in a subgroup of patients aged 70+ years (n = 5806), demonstrated no significant difference in the proportion of patients with cognitive impairment or in the incidence of dementia over the average 5-year follow-up period (Heart Protection Study Collaborative, 2002).

One placebo-controlled clinical trial randomized 44 AD patients to placebo or simvastatin 80 mg/day for 26 weeks, reporting both reduced CSF Aβ and less decline on MMSE in patients on simvastatin (Simons *et al.*, 2002). An ongoing clinical trial of 400 patients with mild to moderate AD will evaluate the effects of simvastatin in slowing the clinical decline of AD patients.

37.2.5 *Ginkgo biloba*

The ability of an extract from the leaves of *Ginkgo biloba* to improve cognitive function in AD patients is the subject of ongoing work. Preclinical evidence suggests the components in *Ginkgo* might have neuroprotective effects, including scavenging of oxygen free radicals, protection of membranes against lipid peroxidation, inhibition of Aβ formation and aggregation, and protection against Aβ toxicity, as well as putative anti-apoptotic effects via inhibition of caspase-3 activation (Luo *et al.*, 2002). A number of clinical studies support the relatively common use in some European countries of *Ginkgo biloba* as a cognitive enhancer (Weitbrecht and Jansen, 1986; Mancini, 1993; Hofferberth, 1994; Kanowski *et al.*, 1996; Le Bars *et al.*, 1997; Maurer *et al.*, 1997; Birks *et al.*, 2002). However, a clear role for *Ginkgo biloba* either as a symptomatic agent or as prevention for AD has not been determined.

A 52-week, placebo-controlled, double-blind trial of 309 patients with either AD or vascular dementia demonstrated that 120 mg/day standardized *Ginkgo biloba* extract (EGb 761) conferred a statistically significant improvement on ADAS-cog scores compared with placebo, indicating a stabilization of cognitive decline (Le Bars *et al.*, 1997). The results of this trial are controversial since it included a mixed patient population of AD and vascular dementia, and very little deterioration was observed in the placebo group compared with other AD trials of similar length.

A Cochrane meta-analysis also supports a positive effect of *Ginkgo biloba* (Birks *et al.*, 2002). Interestingly, studies in normal elderly subjects have been contradictory (Mix and Crews, 2002; Solomon *et al.*, 2002), presenting a confusing picture for *Ginkgo biloba* extract use, perhaps partly owing to variations in dose, duration and methodological issues such as lack of blinding. It is speculative that *Ginkgo biloba* extract may be more effective in the cognitively impaired, where it is typically used, than in healthy subjects.

A 6-month placebo-controlled trial of two doses of *Ginkgo biloba* extract, EGb 761, 240 mg/day and 120 mg/day, in patients with mild to moderate AD has been completed. A 5-year placebo-controlled, randomized trial of approximately 3000 subjects aged 75+ years (the GEMS trial), funded by the US National Institute for Complementary and Alternative Medication (NICAM), is currently underway to evaluate *Ginkgo biloba* in prevention of AD. Another prevention study, also sponsored by the US National Institutes of Health, is underway to determine the effect of 240 mg/day EGb 761 in preventing (or delaying) the conversion of 200 healthy subjects 85 years or older to MCI. Results of these trials will lead to a better understanding of a role for *Ginkgo biloba* extract as a potential AD therapeutic agent.

37.2.6 NMDA–receptor antagonism

Part of the consequent pathology in AD involves neurotoxicity; overstimulation of NMDA receptors by glutamate has been implicated as a cause of neurotoxicity (Greenamyre *et al.*, 1988). Inhibiting the excitotoxic impact of glutamate is problematic, since its normal action on its various receptors is necessary for learning and memory. In preclinical studies, a non-competitive NMDA-receptor antagonist, memantine, protected against the effects of glutamate and calcium-mediated neurotoxicity due to influx of calcium (Parsons *et al.*, 1999).

It has been available in Germany for the treatment of Parkinson's disease and various other neurological disorders since 1982, and was approved in 2002 by the European Union and in 2003 by the FDA for treating moderately severe to severe AD. Memantine's effects appear subtler than a range of NMDA antagonists that have not proven to be clinically successful.

37.2.6.1 MECHANISM OF ACTION

Memantine is an open channel blocker that does not have appreciable activity until increased glutamate levels trigger the receptor and cause the ion channel to open. Then it enters the channel and occupying a site 'downstream', preventing calcium influx and preventing the depolarization/hyperactivation of the neurone. Since it is cleared from its site of action quickly, memantine might provide partial blocking of the channel depending on intrasynaptic levels of glutamate. As glutamate increases, causing channels to open, memantine appears to block more. As glutamate decreases, memantine blocks less, allowing greater neuronal activity. In some respects memantine can be viewed as a modulator of glutamatergic activity (Rogawski and Wenk, 2003).

37.2.6.2 PHARMACOKINETICS

The absorption of memantine is not affected by food intake; bioavailability is 100 per cent. Plasma protein binding is 45 per cent and peak plasma concentrations occur 3–7 hours after oral intake. It is widely distributed and rapidly diffuses across the blood–brain barrier. The majority of the parent compound (57–82 per cent) is excreted unchanged in the urine; there is minimum hepatic metabolism; elimination half-life ($t_{1/2}$) is 60–80 hours. There are potential interactions with hydrochlorothiazide resulting in a potentially reduced diuretic effect. There are no known interactions with ChEIs (Namenda prescribing information, Forest Laboratories Inc., 2003).

37.2.6.3 CLINICAL TRIALS

The effect of memantine on cognition generally has been positive in clinical trials (Gortelmeyer and Erbler 1992; Winblad and Poritis 1999; Wilcock *et al.*, 2000; Larrieu *et al.*, 2002; Aisen *et al.*, 2003b; Reisberg *et al.*, 2003) (Table 37.2). Memantine (20 mg/day) was investigated for the treatment of moderate to severe AD in a 28-week placebo-controlled trial of 252 patients (Reisberg *et al.*, 2003). The decline of cognitive function, as measured by the change in Severe Impairment Battery (SIB) score, was lessened in memantine patients compared with the deterioration observed in placebo patients (Figure 37.1).

A 26-week randomized, placebo-controlled trial of memantine in moderate to severe AD also showed greater improvement in cognition, global assessment and function compared with placebo (Tariot *et al.*, 2004). In this trial memantine or placebo was administered double-blinded to

Table 37.2 *Placebo-controlled trials of memantine*

Authors	Dose (mg/day)	N	Diagnosis/severity	Length (weeks)	Main measures
Gortelmeyer and Erbler, 1992	20	88	Mild to moderate dementia	6	SCAG, GBS ($P < 0.05$)
Reisberg *et al.*, 2003; MRZ-9605	20	252	Moderate to severe AD	28	SIB ($P < 0.05$) ADCS-ADL ($P = 0.02$) CIBIC+ ($P = 0.06$)
Winblad and Poritis, 1999; MRZ-9403	10	167	Severe dementia, AD and vascular	12	CGI-C ($P < 0.001$) BGP ($P = 0.02$)
Wilcock *et al.*, 2002; MRZ-9202	20	548	Mild to moderate vascular dementia	28	ADAS-cog ($P < 0.05$) CGI-C (NS)
Orgogozo *et al.*, 2002; MRZ-9408	20	288	Mild to moderate vascular dementia	28	ADAS-cog ($P < 0.05$) CIBIC+ (NS)
Tariot *et al.*, 2004; MEM-MD-02	20	404	Moderate to severe on donepezil	24	SIB ($P < 0.0001$) ADCS-ADL ($P < 0.03$) CIBIC+ ($P < 0.03$)

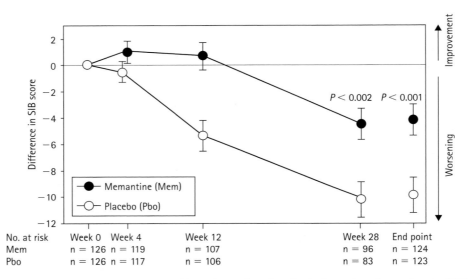

Figure 37.1   *Memantine in moderate to severe AD patients. Mean change from baseline in Severe Impairment Battery (SIB) score ($\pm$ SE) in the observed-cases analysis is shown for each time point, and for the end point using a last observation carried forward analysis (Reisberg* et al., *2003).*

patients who had been maintained on stable doses of donepezil for at least 6 months. In fact, the average time on donepezil was approximately 2.5 years, with nearly 90 per cent on donepezil for over 1 year before being randomized. Notably, the placebo-treated patients, i.e. patients who continued on donepezil throughout the 6 months of the trial, continued to decline at a rather rapid rate, suggesting that memantine substantially stabilized symptoms over this short period of time, while any effect of the cholinesterase inhibitor may have been lost previously or overcome by the disease course.

Additionally, in nursing home patients with severe dementia (MMSE < 10), probably either AD or vascular dementia, memantine showed significant improvement over placebo in a 12-week trial as measured by global and functional measures (Winblad and Poritis, 1999).

There have been two trials in patients with vascular dementia (Orgogozo *et al.*, 2002; Wilcock *et al.*, 2002). These patients tended to have ischaemic vascular dementia. In these trials there were salutary effects on cognition using the ADAS-cog and adverse events were mild (Orgogozo *et al.*, 2002; Wilcock *et al.*, 2002). Lastly, at least three clinical trials assessing the efficacy of memantine in mild to moderate AD have been completed but not published. News releases from Forest Laboratories and Lundbeck in January 2004 stated that one of two placebo-controlled trials in patients not on ChEIs was statistically significantly in favour of memantine.

37.2.6.4 ADVERSE EFFECTS

Adverse events were noticeable in the moderate to severe monotherapy trial (Reisberg *et al.*, 2003) in that agitation was less frequent in patients on memantine without there being significant increases in other adverse events. In the memantine add-on trial (Tariot *et al.*, 2004), confusion, generally rated as mild, occurred four times more frequently in the memantine group, and headache twice as frequently. Of note gastrointestinal symptoms were less frequent with diarrhoea or faecal incontinence occurring half as frequently in the memantine group, suggesting that the actions of memantine may mitigate some of the cholinergic effects of donepezil.

37.3 SUMMARY

Of the treatments discussed only *Ginkgo biloba* extract (EGb 761) and memantine have a measure of regulatory approval. Memantine is specifically approved for moderate to severe AD. The evidence base for both these treatments is better developed. By contrast there is insufficient evidence to inform clinical practice on the use of homocysteine reduction or statins for either the treatment of dementia or its prevention. The evidence is also insufficient for vitamin E. There has been only one underpowered clinical trial assessing vitamin E effects in moderate to severe Alzheimer's disease that showed analysis-dependent results for either vitamin E alone or vitamin E combined with selegiline. The trial had substantial dropouts over the several year follow up and, importantly, there is no clear effect on improvement of cognition. Although not detailed in this chapter, the evidence for the use of selegiline is somewhat greater including the vitamin E trial and earlier short-term trials in elderly individuals with non-specific dementias or cognitive impairment.

The use of hormone replacement therapy, specifically oestrogens or oestrogens combined with a progestin, cannot be endorsed. In fact the bulk of the evidence is that their use is associated with greater cognitive impairment in people with AD and are not effective in preventing or delaying the onset of dementia. Similarly, overall, anti-inflamatories have not been shown to be effective and in fact may be harmful in patients who have AD. One true prevention trial is ongoing, however, and may provide information on its preventative uses (Martin *et al.*, 2002).

In view of memantine's effects in moderate to severe patients (typically patients with MMSEs < 15 or so) and with some suggestion of potential efficacy in heterogeneous vascular dementia, it may be considered as a symptomatic treatment. Clinical considerations involve either using it alone, perhaps in people who had been on ChEIs in the past and who are either intolerant or who found the medication not effective, or using it in patients who are being maintained on ChEIs for rather long periods. At the moment there is no evidence on whether memantine should be started prior to or simultaneously with a cholinesterase inhibitor, whether the two treatments together are better than either one alone.

Dosing is fairly straightforward with a titration to 10 mg b.i.d. over the course of 3 weeks. Adverse events appear

particularly mild with memantine; however, post-introductory experiences and further clinical trials will allow for better estimates.

REFERENCES

Aisen PS. (2000) Anti-inflammatory therapy for Alzheimer's disease: implications of the prednisone trial. *Acta Neurologica Scandinavica* **176** (Suppl.): 85–89

Aisen PS and Davis KL. (1994) Inflammatory mechanisms in Alzheimer's disease: implications for therapy. *American Journal of Psychiatry* **151**: 1105–1113

Aisen PS, Egelko S, Andrews H *et al.* (2003a) A pilot study of vitamins to lower plasma homocysteine levels in Alzheimer disease. *American Journal of Geriatric Psychiatry* **11**: 246–249

Aisen PS, Schafer KA, Grundman M *et al.* (2003b) Effects of rofecoxib or naproxen vs placebo on Alzheimer disease progression: a randomized controlled trial. [comment]. *JAMA* **289**: 2819–2826

Bellamy MF and McDowell IF. (1997) Putative mechanisms for vascular damage by homocysteine. *Journal of Inherited Metabolic Disease* **20**: 307–315

Birks J, Grimley Evans J, Van Dongen M. (2002) *Ginkgo biloba* for dementia and cognitive impairment [Protocol]. *Cochrane Database of Systematic Reviews* 2

Black S, Román GC, Geldmacher DS *et al.* (2003) Efficacy and tolerability of donepezil in vascular dementia: positive results of a 24-week, multicenter, international, randomized, placebo-controlled clinical trial. *Stroke* **34**: 2323–2330

Breitner JC. (1996) Inflammatory processes and antiinflammatory drugs in Alzheimer's disease: a current appraisal. *Neurobiology of Aging* **17**: 789–794

Chandra RK. (2001) Effect of vitamin and trace-element supplementation on cognitive function in elderly subjects. *Nutrition* **17**: 709–712

Erkinjuntti T, Kurz A, Gauthier S *et al.* (2002) Efficacy of galantamine in probable vascular dementia and Alzheimer's disease combined with cerebrovascular disease: a randomised trial. *Lancet* **359**: 1283–1290

Fassbender K, Simons M, Bergmann C *et al.* (2001) Simvastatin strongly reduces levels of Alzheimer's disease beta-amyloid peptides A beta 42 and A beta 40 *in vitro* and in vivo. *Proceedings of the National Academy of Sciences of the United States of America* **98**: 5856–5861

Gortelmeyer R and Erbler H. (1992) Memantine in the treatment of mild to moderate dementia syndrome. A double-blind placebo-controlled study. *Arzneimittel-Forschung* **42**: 904–913

Greenamyre JT, Maragos WF, Albin RL *et al.* (1988) Glutamate transmission and toxicity in Alzheimer's disease. *Progress in Neuropsychopharmacology and Biological Psychiatry* **12**: 421–430

Heart Protection Study Collaboration. (2002) MRC/BHF Heart Protection Study of cholesterol lowering with simvastatin in 20 536 high-risk individuals: a randomized placebo-controlled trial. *Lancet* **360**: 7–22

Ho PI, Collins SC, Dhitavat S *et al.* (2001) Homocysteine potentiates beta-amyloid neurotoxicity: role of oxidative stress. *Journal of Neurochemistry* **78**: 249–253

Hofferberth B. (1994) The efficacy of EGb 761 in patients with senile dementia of the Alzheimer type, a double-blind, placebo-controlled study on different levels of investigation. *Human Psychopharmacology* **9**: 215–222

In t' Veld BA, Ruitenberg A, Hofman A *et al.* (2001) Nonsteroidal antiinflammatory drugs and the risk of Alzheimer's disease. *New England Journal of Medicine* **345**: 1515–1521

Jick H, Zornberg GL, Jick SS et al. (2000) Statins and the risk of dementia. Lancet **356**: 1627–1631 [erratum appears in Lancet (2001) **357**: 562]

Kanowski S, Herrmann WM, Stephan K et al. (1996) Proof of efficacy of the ginkgo biloba special extract EGb 761 in outpatients suffering from mild to moderate primary degenerative dementia of the Alzheimer type or multi-infarct dementia. Pharmacopsychiatry **29**: 47–56

Kruman II, Kumaravel TS, Lohani A et al. (2002) Folic acid deficiency and homocysteine impair DNA repair in hippocampal neurons and sensitize them to amyloid toxicity in experimental models of Alzheimer's disease. Journal of Neuroscience **22**: 1752–1762

Larrieu S, Letenneur L, Orgogozo JM et al. (2002) Incidence and outcome of mild cognitive impairment in a population-based prospective cohort. Neurology **59**: 1594–1599

Le Bars PL, Katz MM, Berman N et al. (1997) A placebo-controlled, double-blind, randomized trial of an extract of Ginkgo biloba for dementia. North American EGb Study Group. JAMA **278**: 1327–1332

Lehmann M, Gottfries CG, Regland B. (1999) Identification of cognitive impairment in the elderly: homocysteine is an early marker. Dementia and Geriatric Cognitive Disorders **10**: 12–20

Luo Y, Smith JV, Paramasivam V et al. (2002) Inhibition of amyloid-beta aggregation and caspase-3 activation by the Ginkgo biloba extract EGb761. Proceedings of the National Academy of Sciences of the United States of America **99**: 12197–1202

McGeer PL and McGeer EG. (1996) Anti-inflammatory drugs in the fight against Alzheimer's disease. Annals of the New York Academy of Sciences **777**: 213–220

McKeith I, Del Ser T, Spano P et al. (2000) Efficacy of rivastigmine in dementia with Lewy bodies: a randomised, double-blind, placebo-controlled international study. Lancet **356**: 2031–2036

Mancini M. (1993) Clinical and therapeutic effects of ginkgo biloba extract vs. placebo in senile dementia or artheriosclerotic origin. Gazzetta Medica Italiana **152**: 69–80

Martin BK, Meinert CL, Breitner JC et al. (2002) Double placebo design in a prevention trial for Alzheimer's disease. Controlled Clinical Trials **23**: 93–99

Maurer K, Ihl R, Dierks T et al. (1997) Clinical efficacy of Ginkgo biloba special extract EGb 761 in dementia of the Alzheimer type. Journal of Psychiatric Research **31**: 645–655

Mix JA and Crews WD Jr. (2002) A double-blind, placebo-controlled, randomized trial of Ginkgo biloba extract EGb 761 in a sample of cognitively intact older adults: neuropsychological findings. Human Psychopharmacology **17**: 267–277

Mulnard RA, Cotman CW, Kawas C et al. (2000) Estrogen replacement therapy for treatment of mild to moderate Alzheimer disease: a randomized controlled trial. Alzheimer's Disease Cooperative Study. JAMA **283**: 1007–1015

Orgogozo JM, Rigaud AS, Stoffler A et al. (2002) Efficacy and safety of memantine in patients with mild to moderate vascular dementia: a randomized, placebo-controlled trial (MMM 300). Stroke **33**: 1834–1839

Parsons CG, Danysz W, Quack G. (1999) Memantine is a clinically well tolerated N-methyl-D-aspartate (NMDA) receptor antagonist – a review of preclinical data. Neuropharmacology **38**: 735–767

Rapp SR, Espeland MA, Shumaker SA et al. (2003) Effect of estrogen plus progestin on global cognitive function in postmenopausal women: the Women's Health Initiative Memory Study: a randomized controlled trial. JAMA **289**: 2663–2672

Refolo LM, Malester B, LaFrancois J et al. (2002) Hypercholesterolaemia accelerates the Alzheimer's amyloid pathology in a transgenic mouse model. Neurobiology of Disease **7**: 321–331

Reisberg B, Doody R, Stoffler A et al. (2003) Memantine in moderate-to-severe Alzheimer's disease. New England Journal of Medicine **348**: 1333–1341

Rich JB, Rasmusson DX, Folstein MF et al. (1995) Nonsteroidal anti-inflammatory drugs in Alzheimer's disease. Neurology **45**: 51–55

Rockwood K, Kirkland S, Hogan DB et al. (2002) Use of lipid-lowering agents, indication bias, and the risk of dementia in community-dwelling elderly people. Archives of Neurology **59**: 223–227

Rogawski M and Wenk G. (2003) The neuropharmacological basis for the use of memantine in the treatment of Alzheimer's disease. CNS Drug Reviews **9**: 275–308

Rogers J, Kirby LC, Hempelman SR et al. (1993) Clinical trial of indomethacin in Alzheimer's disease. Neurology **43**: 1609–1611

Sano M, Ernesto C, Thomas RG et al. (1997) A controlled trial of selegiline, alpha-tocopherol, or both as treatment for Alzheimer's disease. The Alzheimer's Disease Cooperative Study. New England Journal of Medicine **336**: 1216–1222

Scharf S, Mander A, Ugoni A et al. (1999) A double-blind, placebo-controlled trial of diclofenac/misoprostol in Alzheimer's disease. Neurology **53**: 197–201

Seshadri S, Beiser A, Selhub J et al. (2002) Plasma homocysteine as a risk factor for dementia and Alzheimer's disease. New England Journal of Medicine **346**: 476–483

Shepherd J, Blauw GJ, Murphy MB et al. (2002) Pravastatin in elderly individuals at risk of vascular disease (PROSPER): a randomized controlled trial. Lancet **360**: 1623–1630

Simons M, Schwarzler F, Lutjohann D et al. (2002) Treatment with simvastatin in normocholesterolemic patients with Alzheimer's disease: A 26-week randomized, placebo-controlled, double-blind trial. Annals of Neurology **52**: 346–350

Solomon PR, Adams F, Silver A et al. (2002) Ginkgo for memory enhancement: a randomized controlled trial. JAMA **288**: 835–840

Sparks DL, Scheff SW, Hunsaker JC 3rd et al. (1994) Induction of Alzheimer-like β-amyloid immunoreactivity in the brains of rabbits with dietary cholesterol. Experimental Neurology **126**: 88–94

Sparks DL, Liu H, Gross DR et al. (1995) Increased density of cortical apolipoprotein E immunoreactive neurons in rabbit brain after dietary administration of cholesterol. Neuroscience Letters **187**: 142–144

Stamler JS, Osborne JA, Jaraki O et al. (1993) Adverse vascular effects of homocysteine are modulated by endothelium-derived relaxing factor and related oxides of nitrogen. Journal of Clinical Investigation **91**: 308–318

Tariot PN, Farlow MR, Grossberg GT et al. (2004) Memantine treatment in patients with moderate to severe Alzheimer disease already receiving donepezil: a randomized controlled trial. JAMA **291**: 317–324

Van Gool WA, Weinstein HC, Scheltens P et al. (2001) Effect of hydroxychloroquine on progression of dementia in early Alzheimer's disease: an 18-month randomized, double-blind, placebo-controlled study. Lancet **358**: 455–460 [erratum appears in Lancet 2001 **358**: 1188]

Visser H, Thal L, Ferris S et al. (2003) A randomized, double-blind, placebo-controlled study of rofecoxib in patients with mild cognitive impairment. 42nd Annual Meeting of the ACNP, San Juan, Puerto Rico

Voutilainen S, Morrow JD, Roberts LJ 2nd et al. (1999) Enhanced in vivo lipid peroxidation at elevated plasma total homocysteine levels. Arteriosclerosis, Thrombosis and Vascular Biology **19**: 1263–1266

Weitbrecht WU and Jansen W. (1986) [Primary degenerative dementia: therapy with Ginkgo biloba extract. Placebo-controlled double-blind and comparative study]. Fortschritte der Medizin **104**: 199–202

Wilcken DE and Dudman NP. (1989) Mechanisms of thrombogenesis and accelerated atherogenesis in homocysteinaemia. *Haemostasis* **19** (Suppl. 1): 14–23

Wilcock GK, Lilienfeld S, Gaens E. (2000) Efficacy and safety of galantamine in patients with mild to moderate Alzheimer's disease: multicentre randomized controlled trial. Galantamine International-1 Study Group. *BMJ* **321**: 1445–1449

Wilcock G, Mobius HJ, Stoffler A. (2002) A double-blind, placebo-controlled multicentre study of memantine in mild to moderate vascular dementia (MMM 500). *International Clinical Psychopharmacology* **17**: 297–305

Wilkinson D, Doody R, Helme R *et al.* (2003) Donepezil in vascular dementia: a randomized, placebo-controlled study. *Neurology* **61**: 479–486

Winblad B and Poritis N. (1999) Memantine in severe dementia: results of the 9M-Best Study (Benefit and efficacy in severely demented patients during treatment with memantine). *International Journal of Geriatric Psychiatry* **14**: 135–146

Wolozin B, Kellman W, Ruosseau P *et al.* (2000) Decreased prevalence of Alzheimer disease associated with 3-hydroxy-3-methyglutaryl coenzyme A reductase inhibitors. *Archives of Neurology* **57**: 1439–1443

38

Treatments for behavioural and psychological symptoms in Alzheimer's disease and other dementias

LOUIS PROFENNO, PIERRE TARIOT, REBEKAH LOY AND SALEEM ISMAIL

Merriam *et al.* (1988) asserted that Alzheimer's disease (AD) is 'the most widely encountered cause of psychiatric pathology associated with a specific neuropathological substrate'. This is consistent with phenomenological studies and literature reviews, which generally converge on the conclusion that roughly 90 per cent of patients with dementia will develop significant behavioural problems at some point in the course of illness (Tariot and Blazina, 1993). The 'behavioural and psychological signs and symptoms of dementia' (Finkel *et al.*, 1996) do not typically meet criteria for discrete psychiatric disorders. They do, however, tend to occur in clusters of signs and symptoms that may vary among patients and over time (Tariot and Blazina, 1993). Examples of these clusters are provided in Table 38.1, based upon a review of published studies regarding psychopathological changes in dementia that was performed in 1993. With experience, these clusters of signs and symptoms can be both predicted and recognized, and can be used as guideposts in the selection of appropriate therapy.

This chapter will focus on agitation, which Cohen-Mansfield and Billig (1986) defined as 'inappropriate verbal, vocal, or motor activity unexplained by apparent needs or confusion'. Cohen-Mansfield and Billig (1986) empirically categorized agitated behaviours into three key groups:

- disruptive but not aggressive (e.g. attempts to leave, robes and disrobes, repeated complaints or questions);

Table 38.1 *Summary of literature regarding psychopathology of dementia* (per cent of patients affected among studies reviewed)*

	Range	Median
1. Disturbed affect/mood	0–86	19
2. Disturbed ideation	10–73	33.5
3. Altered perception		
• Hallucinations	21–49	28
• Misperceptions	1–49	23
4. Agitation		
• Global	10–90	44
• Wandering	0–50	18
5. Aggression		
• Verbal	11–51	24
• Physical	0–46	14.3
• Resistive/uncooperative	27–65	44
6. Anxiety	0–50	31.8
7. Withdrawn/passive behaviour	21–88	61
8. Vegetative behaviours		
• Sleep	0–47	27
• Diet/appetite	12.5–77	34

*Adapted from Tariot and Blazina, 1993

- socially inappropriate (e.g. disrobing or urinating in public); and
- aggressive (e.g. physical, such as hitting or slapping, or verbal, such as obscenities or name-calling).

As Table 38.1 indicates, half or more of patients with dementia will show some feature of agitation at some point in the course of illness.

38.1 A RATIONAL APPROACH

This chapter proposes a systematic general approach to the evaluation and management of agitation that is based on an elaboration of prior work (Leibovici and Tariot, 1988; Tariot et al., 1995a; Tariot, 1996, 1999; Tariot and Schneider, 1998; Loy et al., 1999); key aspects are described below:

- *Define target symptoms.* Review the available evidence and delineate the patient's behaviour pattern, e.g. 'wanders without an apparent destination, calls out repeatedly, bites and kicks during care'.
- *Establish or revisit medical diagnoses.* It is almost a truism in geriatrics that delirium is a frequent cause of incident agitation, and must always be suspected. Common culprits include respiratory or urinary infections, dehydration, occult trauma, electrolyte disturbances, or side effects of medications. Such medical problems should be treated specifically and the patient monitored carefully, ideally without the need for other medications.
- *Establish or revisit neuropsychiatric diagnoses.* It is also possible that the disturbed behaviour may reflect a long-standing, recurrent, or new onset discrete psychiatric disorder. When a specific disorder is identified, it should be specifically treated and monitored.
- *Assess and reverse aggravating factors.* Examples might include deficits in hearing or vision, or an environment that is too dark, noisy, or cold. Disrupted daily routines may present a remediable factor. It is important to look hard for environmental triggers.
- *Adapt to specific cognitive deficits.* Some patients may be able to respond to verbal reassurance and redirection, whereas others may not. Pain or distress may need to be inferred from behaviour or facial expression. Some may need constant environmental cueing to organize their behaviour. It is important to identify each patient's cognitive strengths and weaknesses, attempting to capitalize on residual strengths and avoid weaknesses.
- *Identify relevant psychosocial factors.* It can be easy to overlook the fact that a patient with dementia may be suffering anxiety, sadness, denial, or fury in response to major and minor life events. In some long-term care facilities, for instance, moving from one unit to another can be associated with perceived loss of status as well as contact with familiar people. It is easy to overlook this as a precipitant of 'agitation'.
- *Educate caregivers.* Caregivers can learn that change in behaviour usually has meaning, and that the behaviours can occur in discernible patterns. This helps caregivers interact in a more supportive manner. In the process, caregivers can be taught to employ essential behaviour management principles, learning, for instance, that their own behaviour is a major determinant of the patient's behaviour. Caregivers can be trained to identify common triggers as well as consequences of agitated behaviour, and work with health professionals to attempt to minimize the triggers and maximize more positive circumstances.

If the behavioural disturbance is grossly aggressive or disruptive, and frankly dangerous, it may be necessary to use antipsychotics or benzodiazepines on an emergency basis, preferably by mouth but sometimes parenterally. In rare cases, hospitalization is needed. Once the emergency is under control, it is imperative to pay attention to the basics outlined above.

38.2 DEVELOPMENT OF THE PSYCHOBEHAVIOURAL METAPHOR

For persisting non-emergent problems where non-pharmacological interventions have been exhausted, we adopt an approach that begins with a definition of a target symptom pattern that is at least roughly analogous to a drug-responsive syndrome. We refer to this as the 'psychobehavioural metaphor' (Leibovici and Tariot, 1988). We then match the dominant target symptoms (the metaphor) to the most relevant drug class. For example, in the case of a verbally and physically agitated patient who is also irritable, negative, has become socially withdrawn, and appears dysphoric, we might well first undertake a trial of an antidepressant. Conversely, if the patient showed 'agitation' in the context of increased motor activity, loud and rapid speech, and lability of affect, we might consider early use of a mood stabilizer. The 'aggressive' patient whose hostile actions are associated with delusions is likely to be treated first with an antipsychotic. Although this approach to drug selection is face-valid, there is limited empirical support for it thus far (Devanand, 2000; Lyketsos et al., 2000; Tariot et al., 2001a, 2002a; De Deyn et al., 2003). Thus, the validity of the approach that we have endorsed for some years, and that reflected in most consensus guidelines (Rabins et al., 1997; Alexopoulos et al., 1998; Doody et al., 2001), has not been established empirically.

The approach adopted in this chapter more or less reflects the position of the American Geriatrics Society and American Association for Geriatric Psychiatry consensus statement (2003) with respect to the use of target symptoms to guide selection of drug class. We emphasize selection of a medication with at least some empirical evidence of efficacy and with the highest likelihood of tolerability and safety. We observe some general rules such as starting with low doses and escalating slowly, assessing target symptoms as well as toxicity, and discontinuing the medication if it is harmful or ineffective. Even when a medication is helpful at subtoxic doses, an empirical trial is often performed in reverse and the patient monitored for recurrence of the problem. This type of approach is actually mandated in the nursing home setting in the USA by Federal regulations created in 1987. Sometimes several medications need to be tried in series before a successful one is identified; sometimes combinations are warranted; sometimes no medication is found that is helpful. We hold the view that best practice includes routine use of cholinesterase inhibitors in most patients with AD as well as certain other dementias, meaning that psychotropic use occurs against this backdrop. The recent emergence of memantine as an antidementia agent will mean that a substantial proportion of patients may receive psychotropics in addition to this, alone or in combination with cholinesterase inhibitors, as well. The trials conducted with these agents were aimed toward obtaining regulatory approval and not informing clinical practice regarding issues such as the advantages or disadvantages of one agent versus the other for relief of behavioural symptoms, or of using psychotropics in combination with these agents. Practice will outstrip evidence for the foreseeable future.

38.3 SPECIFIC CLASSES OF PSYCHOTROPICS

The remainder of this chapter reviews the most relevant classes of agents and specific agents within those classes, focusing on information from about the last 5 years and on older studies that remain as crucial guides to practice. Much of the older literature was reviewed previously in the prior edition of this textbook (Rosenquist *et al.*, 2000); this chapter builds on that as well as some of our earlier work (Tariot, 1999, Loy *et al.*, 1999, Profenno and Tariot, 2004). Table 38.2 provides an overview of individual agents and typical starting doses proposed, based upon a mixture of data and clinical experience.

38.4 CONVENTIONAL ANTIPSYCHOTICS

Within the context of the 'metaphor' approach, antipsychotics would be used first for treatment of agitation that included psychotic features (Tables 38.3 and 38.4). In reality, antipsychotics have been used and studied in patients with a wide range of psychopathology. There are two main classes of antipsychotics: so-called conventional antipsychotics and the newer atypical agents. Prior reviews of the conventional agents have concluded that the effects of these agents were consistent but modest, and that no single agent was better than another (Wragg and Jeste, 1989; Schneider *et al.*, 1990).

Lanctot *et al.* (1998) performed a meta-analysis including some studies that were less rigorous than those included in the Schneider *et al.* (1990) meta-analysis. These authors also concluded that type and potency of agent did not influence response. They reported an average therapeutic effect (antipsychotic versus placebo) of 26 per cent, with placebo response rates ranging from 19 to 50 per cent. Side effects were reported to occur more often on drug than placebo (mean difference 25 per cent). These meta-analyses did not include five more recent studies (Devenand *et al.*, 1998;

Table 38.2 *Selected current pharmacological treatments for agitation in dementia**

Drug and class	Suggesting starting** and (maximal) daily dose (mg/day)
Antipsychotics	
Traditional:	
• Haloperidol	0.25–0.5 (2–4)
• Thioridazine	12.5–25 (50–100)
• Thiothixene	0.5–1 (2–4)
Atypical:	
• Clozapine	6.25–12.5 (25–100)
• Olanzapine	2.5 (5–10)
• Quetiapine	25 (50–200)
• Risperidone	0.5 (1–2)
• Aripiprazole	5 (15)
• Ziprasidone	unknown
Anxiolytics and sedatives	
Benzodiazepines:	
• Alprazolam	0.5 (1–2)
• Lorazepam	0.5 (2–4)
• Oxazepam	10 (40–60)
Non–benzodiazepines:	
• Zolpidem	2.5 (5)
• Buspirone	10 (30–60)
Antidepressants	
• Trazodone	25–50 (200–300)
SSRIs:	
• Citalopram	10 (20)
• Fluoxetine	10 (20)
• Sertraline	25–50 (100–200)
Anticonvulsants	
• Carbamazepine	50–100 (300–500)
• Divalproex	125–375 (500–1500)
β–blockers	
• Propranolol	20 (50–100)
Others	
• Selegiline	10
• Oestradiol/progesterone	0.625/2.5

* Adapted from Loy *et al.*, 1999
** Suggestions are based on published data as well as anecdotal experience, and should be regarded accordingly

De Deyn *et al.*, 1999; Allain *et al.*, 2000; Teri *et al.*, 2000; Tariot *et al.*, 2002a). The data from these newer studies generally conform to the results of the meta-analyses.

Reviews regarding conventional agents cite side effects including akathisia, parkinsonism, tardive dyskinesia, sedation, peripheral and central anticholinergic effects, postural hypotension, cardiac conduction defects and falls (Lanctot *et al.*, 1998). Most of these data come from short-term controlled trials; evidence regarding long-term safety is generally lacking. Data available from other elderly populations, however, indicate that caution is warranted. For instance, rates of tardive dyskinesia are 5–6-fold greater in older than in younger populations after treatment with conventional agents (Jeste

Table 38.3 *Conventional antipsychotics*

Study	Diagnosis	N	Design	Dose (mg/day); duration	Response	Adverse effects
Haloperidol						
Schneider et al., 1990	Dementia	252 (in 7 DB, PC trials in primary dementia)	Meta-analysis of 33 neuroleptic trials	2.5–4.6, haloperidol; 3–8 weeks	Little benefit beyond placebo across all neuroleptics; average effect 18% greater than placebo	Not reported
Devanand et al., 1998	AD	71	Randomized DB, PC, parallel group	2–3 or 0.5–0.75; 6 weeks	Decreased psychosis, aggression, agitation with higher dose only, 55–60% response versus 25–35% low dose response versus 25–30% placebo	Moderate–severe EPS at high dose (20%)
Christensen and Benfield, 1998	Organic mental syndrome	48	Randomized cross-over to alprazolam	Mean 0.64; 6 weeks	No difference between treatments on CGI, CAG	None seen at this low dose
De Deyn et al., 1999	AD, vascular, mixed	344	Randomized, MC DB, parallel group risperidone or placebo	Mean 1.2; 13 weeks	Significantly greater improvement for haloperidol versus placebo on BEHAVE-AD and CMAI, decreased physical and verbal aggression (72% risperidone versus 69% haloperidol versus 61% placebo on BEHAVE-AD)	EPS 22%, somnolence (18% haloperidol versus 4% placebo)
Allain et al., 2000	AD, VaD, mixed	306	Randomized MC, DB, PC, parallel group	100–300 tiapride or 2–6 haloperidol; 21 days	Significantly improved CGI and MOSES irritability/aggressiveness subscore for both drugs compared to placebo, no differences between drugs	Less EPS with tiapride than haloperidol
Teri et al., 2000	AD	149	Randomized DB, PC, parallel group	1.8 haloperidol, 200 trazodone, or behaviour management techniques; 16 weeks	Reduced agitation not significantly different between treated and placebo groups	Less EPS with behaviour management techniques
Tariot et al., 2002a	Probable AD with psychosis	284	Randomized, PC, DB versus quetiapine (n = 94 on haloperidol)	Mean 1.89; 8 weeks	No change in psychosis, some decrease in agitation	EPS, sedation

AD, Alzheimer's disease; BEHAVE-AD, Behavioral Pathology in Alzheimer's Disease Rating Scale; CGI, Clinical Global Impression; CMAI, Cohen–Mansfield Agitation Inventory; DB, double-blind; EPS, extrapyramidal symptoms; MC, multicentre; MOSES, Multidimensional Observation Scale for Elderly Subjects; PC, placebo-controlled; SCAG, Sandoz Clinical Assessment–Geriatric Scale; VaD, vascular dementia *et al.*, 1995). For practical purposes, side effects typically guide selection of these agents when they are used in patients with dementia. A clinical issue that is of particular importance is dementia with co-occurring extrapyramidal disorders such as dementia with Lewy bodies, where occasional extraordinary sensitivity to conventional agents is seen (Ballard *et al.*, 1998). For all these reasons, atypical antipsychotics may have special utility in patients with dementia. This may account for the enthusiasm expressed by 'experts' toward use of atypicals in this population (Alexopoulos *et al.*, 1998).

38.5 ATYPICAL ANTIPSYCHOTICS

These are listed in Table 38.4.

38.5.1 Clozapine

Only anecdotes and case reports are available; none is new since our previous chapter was written. Individual patients showed partial improvement in agitation or psychosis, whereas others developed side effects including sedation and anticholinergic effects. Whilst not mentioned specifically in these reports, agranulocytosis and seizures have been reported in other populations, the former requiring regular haematological testing for months. Dose-response issues are unresolved. In using this medication, we err on the side of caution by starting at 6.25 or 12.5 mg/day. Based on the relative lack of motor toxicity encountered with clozapine, a case can be made to select this agent preferentially in patients with dementia and extrapyramidal disorders. However, in view of the lack of information regarding dose-response, the risk of side effects in the elderly and the lack of controlled data regarding efficacy and tolerability, most clinicians are likely to choose from among the newer atypical agents first.

38.5.2 Risperidone

The earliest exploratory studies indicated that doses in the range of 0.5–2 mg/day might be best tolerated, with dose-related risk of motor toxicity (especially in patients with extrapyramidal disorders). Sedation, peripheral oedema, and orthostatic hypotension were sometimes reported. Use of risperidone can result in increased prolactin levels in other populations, although the clinical significance of this in patients with dementia is uncertain. We do not routinely check serum prolactin levels, and would only take action in response to elevated levels associated with symptoms associated with its use (e.g. galactorrhoea in women, sexual dysfunction in men) or with symptoms indicative of a possible hypothalamic tumour (e.g. diplopia). The earlier open trials and case series indicated that risperidone may decrease agitation, aggression or psychosis in patients with dementia, spawning more definitive trials. Three large multicentre trials of risperidone

have been completed in nursing home patients with relatively severe dementia (De Deyn *et al.*, 1999; Katz *et al.*, 1999; Brodaty *et al.*, 2003).

In the aggregate, these risperidone studies comprise the largest placebo-controlled, multicentre studies ever conducted of any form of treatment for agitation or aggression associated with dementia. A conservative interpretation of the available evidence would be that the efficacy of risperidone is roughly equivalent to that of haloperidol. The tolerability of risperidone appears to be better, with low to moderate risk of dose-related parkinsonism and sedation and numerically higher rates of peripheral oedema and sedation in patients treated with risperidone versus placebo. As more data have emerged from the large clinical trials with risperidone, there has been more opportunity to examine possible side effects that might not be discernible in single clinical trials.

In October 2002, HealthCanada issued a letter to healthcare professionals stating that risperidone use may be associated with cerebrovascular events in elderly patients with dementia (Wooltorton, 2002). In April 2003, the FDA issued a similar warning of cerebrovascular events with risperidone in patients with dementia and noted that risperidone has not been shown to be safe or effective in treating dementia-related psychosis.

38.5.3 Olanzapine

Recent studies suggest benefit of olanzapine in treating agitation in patients with dementia. A 6-week, randomized, parallel-group, multicentre study of olanzapine in 206 nursing home residents with dementia and agitation and/or psychosis has been completed using fixed doses of 5, 10 and 15 mg/day versus placebo (Street *et al.*, 2000). In patients receiving 5 and 10 mg/day, significant improvement in agitation and aggression compared with placebo was seen, and patients receiving 5 mg/day also demonstrated significant improvement compared with placebo in broader assessments of psychopathology. Sedation and postural instability were observed at all doses in at least 25 per cent of subjects. Some of the patients from this trial received follow-up open-label, flexible-dose treatment for 18 weeks; results were consistent with the findings from an earlier paper (Street *et al.*, 2001).

Meehan *et al.* (2002) studied acute treatment of agitation with intramuscular olanzapine in 272 inpatients or nursing home residents with AD and/or vascular dementia. Olanzapine was found to be superior to placebo in treating agitation at 2 and 24 hours. Adverse events were not significantly different between groups. At present, this formulation has not been marketed in the US.

However, a cautionary note is warranted when considering using this agent in patients with dementia. In January 2004, Eli Lilly issued a warning of increased incidence of cerebrovascular adverse events in patients with dementia who were treated with olanzapine.

Table 38.4 *Atypical antipsychotics*

Study	Diagnosis	N	Design	Dose (mg/day): duration	Response	Adverse effects
Olanzapine						
Satterlee et al., 1995	AD	238	Randomized MC, PC, DB	1–8; 8 weeks	No benefit versus placebo	None reported versus placebo
Street et al., 2000	AD, moderate-severe	206	Randomized, MC, PC, DB, parallel group	5, 10 and 15; 6 weeks	Decreased agitation, delusions, hallucinations on NPI-NH at 5 and 10 (but not 15) mg/day versus placebo	Dose-dependent sedation, abnormal gait
Street et al., 2001	AD	105	Open as f/u to previous 6-week DB trial	Flexible 5–15; 18 weeks	Significantly improved agitation and other symptoms by NPI/NH and other scales	Somnolence, accidental injury, rash
Meehan et al., 2002	AD, VaD, or mixed with acute agitation	272	Randomized, MC, PC, DB	IM 5, 2.5, or 1 lorazepam; 2 hours and prn x 2	Decreased agitation at 2 and 24 hours within 20 hours	No significant difference between placebo and any active treatment
Quetiapine						
Tariot et al., 2000a	Various psychotic disorders	184	Open, MC	12.5–800 (median 137.5); 52 weeks	Significant decreases in BPRS total and CGI severity	Somnolence (31%), accidental injury (24%), dizziness (17%)
Scharre and Chang, 2002	AD	10	Open	50–150 (mean = 100): 12 weeks	Improved NPI for delusions and agitation or aggression	Drowsiness (40%), weight gain (40%)
Davis and Baskys, 2002	DLB	10	Open	25–150 (50 mg modal); 12 weeks	Significant reduction in total NPI and agitation subscales of NPI and BPRS	No significant increase in EPS
Tariot et al., 2002a	Probable AD with psychosis	284	Randomized, DB, PC versus haloperidol (n = 91 on quetiapine)	Mean 100; 8 weeks	No change in psychosis, some decrease in agitation	Sedation
Risperidone						
Herrmann et al., 1998	AD, vascular, Lewy body	22	Case reports	Mean 1.5; 1 week–10 months	Improvement CGI (17)	EPS (11), sedation (1), drooling (1)
Lavretsky and Sultzer, 1998	AD, vascular, PD, PSP, mixed	15	Open (concurrent psychotropics allowed)	0.5–3; 9 weeks	Decreased agitation (in all 15)	Sedation (5), akathisia (1)

(Continued)

Table 38.4 (Continued)

Study	Diagnosis	N	Design	Dose (mg/day); duration	Response	Adverse effects
Risperidone						
De Deyn et al., 1999	AD, vascular, mixed dementia	344	Randomized MC, DB, parallel group versus placebo or haloperidol	Mean 1.1; 13 weeks	Decreased physical and verbal aggression (72% risperidone versus 69% haloperidol versus 61% for placebo)	EPS not different from placebo, somnolence (12% risperidone versus 4% placebo)
Katz et al., 1999	AD, vascular, mixed dementia	625	Randomized MC, PC, DB, parallel group (lorazepam, benztropine and chloral hydrate allowed PRN)	0.5, 1.0, 2.0; 12 weeks	Dose-dependent decrease in aggression and psychosis, significant at 1 and 2 (but not 0.5) mg/day	Somnolence, EPS 21% (on 2 mg/day, compared to 12% on placebo), mild peripheral oedema in some
Brodaty et al., 2003	AD, VaD, mixed	345	Randomized, MC, PC, DB	Mean 1.0; 12 weeks	Significant reductions in CMAI total aggression score and BEHAVE-AD aggressiveness	Somnolence, UTI

AD, Alzheimer's disease; BEHAVE-AD, Behavioral Pathology in Alzheimer's Disease Rating Scale; CMAI, Cohen-Mansfield Agitation Inventory; DB, double-blind; EPS, extrapyramidal symptoms; DLB, Dementia with Lewy bodies; MC, multicentre; NPI-NH, Neuropsychiatric Inventory – Nursing Home version; PC, placebo-controlled; PD, Parkinson's disease; PSP, progressive supranuclear palsy; UTI, urinary tract infection; VaD, vascular dementia

38.5.4 Quetiapine fumarate

Two open trials and a case series with quetiapine within a dose range of 25–800 mg/day suggested possible behavioural benefits for agitation (Tariot *et al.*, 2000a; Davis and Baskys, 2002; Scharre and Chang, 2002). A 10-week multicentre placebo-controlled trial of quetiapine versus haloperidol was conducted in elderly nursing home patients with psychosis that was operationally defined. These criteria were implemented prior to the development of clinical criteria for the psychosis of AD proposed recently (Jeste and Finkel, 2000). This trial is notable in that it may have been the first large placebo-controlled study of antipsychotics in patients with dementia selected because of the presence of psychotic symptoms. The results from the analysis of the subgroup (n = 284) with AD have been presented in abstract form (Tariot *et al.*, 2002a) and a manuscript is under review. Flexible doses of the medication were permitted; the mean daily dose of haloperidol was 2 mg/day at end point, while that of quetiapine was about 120 mg/day. None of the treatment groups differed with respect to reduction in measures of psychosis, which was the primary outcome of the trial, whereas there was evidence of reduced agitation on some measures with both haloperidol and quetiapine treatment but not placebo. Tolerability of quetiapine was superior to that of haloperidol. A more critical review of the data will be possible once the trial results are published.

The broad dose range in which quetiapine has shown efficacy means that clinicians should titrate the dose upward to find the optimally effective range for a given individual. Because a high-dose study of quetiapine in dogs showed evidence of cataract formation, appropriate evaluation for this is recommended at present (e.g. via slit lamp examination or direct ophthalmoscopy). A causal link has not been shown in humans, and it is worth noting that a similar recommendation has been made for other psychotropics (e.g. carbamazepine, thioridazine). Definitive studies conducted in humans should resolve the issue of whether this caution is necessary.

38.5.5 Ziprasidone and aripiprazole

There are no geriatrics-specific studies of ziprasidone in the elderly and none in patients with dementia. Results from a placebo-controlled trial of aripiprazole in 208 outpatients meeting new clinical criteria for psychosis of AD (Jeste and Finkel, 2000) have been presented in abstract form (De Deyn *et al.*, 2003). The medication was generally well tolerated, with numerically more frequent sedation in the active treatment group. The primary outcome, a measure of psychosis, did not show a difference between drug and placebo, although there was some behavioural benefit on secondary measures. A better understanding of this trial will be possible after the results are published.

38.5.6 Atypicals: summary

The data indicate that atypical antipsychotics as a class are likely better tolerated than typical antipsychotics and at least as efficacious. There appear to be modest differences within the class of atypicals in terms of effectiveness, but the significance of these differences is unclear. The Clinical Antipsychotic Trials of Intervention Effectiveness (CATIE) protocol for AD, a trial developed in collaboration with the National Institute of Mental Health (NIMH), will be the first head-to-head study of these agents in dementia patients. This 36-week placebo-controlled study compares the effectiveness of the atypical antipsychotics olanzapine, quetiapine and risperidone, as well as citalopram, for psychosis and agitation occurring in outpatients with AD (Schneider *et al.*, 2001).

At present, there are only limited data regarding the long-term safety and efficacy of these agents. Jeste *et al.* (2000) recently reported a cumulative incidence rate for tardive dyskinesia of 2.6 per cent in 330 patients with dementia treated openly with risperidone (mean dose about 1 mg/day) for a median of 273 days. This figure is much lower than that reported in older people treated with conventional agents (Jeste *et al.*, 1995), and is consistent with data reported in a recent prospective longitudinal study of risperidone and haloperidol in older subjects with mixed psychiatric disorders (Jeste *et al.*, 1999). There are, however, no placebo-controlled data addressing these issues, and no studies employing withdrawal manoeuvres.

Evidence of increased incidence of cerebrovascular accidents in patients with dementia who have been treated with two members of this class of medications, i.e. risperidone and olanzapine, suggests need for increased caution in selecting and using this class of medication in patients with dementia. A preliminary meta-analysis of clinical trials of atypical antipsychotics in dementia by Schneider and Dagerman (2003) suggests a trend for death to be associated with randomization to any antipsychotic. It is possible that patients with existing cerebrovascular disease, or with risk factors, might be most susceptible. However, this has yet to be definitively addressed with studies designed to assess side effects or efficacy as a function of baseline medical condition. All in all, the risk/benefit ratio of any treatment must be borne in mind: the risk of not treating a morbid complication of the illness has to be weighed against the small perceived or real risk of active treatment. That is, if an alternative agent is to be used, how convincing are the data about its safety and efficacy?

38.6 BENZODIAZEPINES

According to the 'metaphor' approach adopted in this chapter, we would consider these agents first for patients with prominent anxiety. Since features of anxiety and depression overlap extensively in any case, and particularly in patients with dementia, many physicians opt to use an antidepressant rather than a benzodiazepine if medication is needed. Benzodiazepines have been used for agitation associated with dementia, in several studies that have been reviewed previously (Patel and Tariot, 1991; Loy *et al.*, 1999). Most of these showed, on average, a reduced level of agitation with short-term therapy. There have been very few studies in the past 10 years, none of which was placebo-controlled. In the aggregate, as reviewed in the previous version of this chapter, these studies suggest that agitation associated with anxiety, sleep problems and motor tension might be most likely to respond. Some of the earlier studies in which benzodiazepines were compared with traditional antipsychotics suggested that antipsychotics might be superior.

Prior reviews indicate that side effects occur commonly with benzodiazepines, including sedation, ataxia, falls, confusion, anterograde amnesia, lightheadedness, paradoxical agitation, as well as tolerance and withdrawal syndromes (Patel and Tariot, 1991). It is because of this safety profile that we reserve use of benzodiazepines for situational disturbances, such as dental procedures, for as-needed use, or situations where routine use has been attempted and found to be convincingly safe. Drugs such as lorazepam and oxazepam tend to be selected first because they have straightforward metabolism and relatively short half-lives.

38.7 BUSPIRONE

There have been no randomized, placebo-controlled, double-blind studies of this agent. Reduced agitation has been reported in some open trials that we have summarized previously (Loy *et al.*, 1999; Rosenquist *et al.*, 2000), using doses in the range of 10–60 mg/day. The medication has the advantage of generally good tolerability, with the exception of headache, nervousness and dizziness in a modest percentage of patients. There is no evidence regarding tolerance or paradoxical effects in this population.

38.8 ANTIDEPRESSANTS

These are listed in Tables 38.5 and 38.6.

We would consider using this class of agents first in patients with agitation accompanied by evidence of depressive features as described in the introduction. There is some evidence linking impulsivity to disordered serotonergic function (Coccaro, 1996), lending support to the use of serotonergic agents. They have also probably been more widely assayed because of their good tolerability profile and widespread use in other psychiatric disorders.

Trazodone was one of the first studied (Table 38.5). There has been only one published double-blind, placebo-controlled study, showing no relative benefit of trazodone over haloperidol or placebo in outpatients with dementia and agitation (Teri *et al.*, 2000). The trial also included a non-blinded behaviour management arm; this also showed no relative benefit. Among the non-placebo-controlled studies, doses typically reported ranged from 50 to 400 mg/day, occasionally higher. Irritability, anxiety, restlessness and depressed affect have been reported to improve, along with sleep disturbance. Reported side effects have included sedation, orthostatic hypotension and delirium. The most rigorous among these compared trazodone (mean dose about 220 mg/day) with haloperidol (mean dose 2.5 mg/day) (Sultzer *et al.*, 1997). Agitation improved equally in both patient groups, although tolerability was reported to be better in the trazodone group. The Expert Consensus Guideline (Alexopoulos *et al.*, 1998) favours use of trazodone to treat sleep disturbance primarily, relegating it to second- or-third-line use for 'mild' agitation. A typical starting dose would be 25 mg/day, with maximum doses usually of 100–250 mg/day.

Table 38.5 *Antidepressants*

Study	Diagnosis	N	Design	Dose (mg/day); duration	Response	Adverse effects
Trazodone						
Sultzer *et al.*, 1997	Dementia	28	Randomized DB parallel haloperidol	50–250; 9 weeks	Decreased agitation for both; trazodone better for verbal aggression, oppositional and repetitive behaviours	Sedation (1), imbalance (1); one-third; fewer dropouts in trazodone group
Teri *et al.*, 2000	AD	149	Randomized DB, PC, parallel group	1.8 haloperidol, 200 trazodone, or behaviour management techniques; 16 weeks	Reduced agitation not significantly different between treated and placebo groups	Less EPS with behaviour management techniques

AD, Alzheimer's disease; DB, double blind; EPS, extrapyramidal symptoms; PC, placebo-controlled

Data regarding selective serotonin reuptake inhibitors (SSRIs) are summarized in Table 38.6. Nyth and Gottfries (1990) performed a review of controlled studies of citalopram, which suggest some beneficial behavioural effects. Results from two open trials support this conclusion (Ragneskog *et al.*, 1996; Pollock *et al.*, 1997).

Recently, a double-blind, placebo-controlled study compared citalopram and perphenazine with placebo in patients with various dementia diagnoses, probable AD and dementia with Lewy bodies being the more common diagnoses, who had at least one symptom of psychosis or behavioural disturbance: 85 hospitalized patients were treated after 3 days of dose escalation with doses of 20 mg/day citalopram or 0.1 mg/kg/day of perphenazine for up to 14 days. Both citalopram and perphenazine demonstrated significant improvement compared with placebo for agitation, lability and psychosis. Side effects were similar in the three treatment groups (Pollock *et al.*, 2002).

Table 38.6 *Antidepressants: selective serotonin reuptake inhibitors*

Study	Diagnosis	N	Design	Dose (mg/day); duration	Response	Adverse effects
Citalopram						
Nyth and Gottfries, 1990	AD, vascular	98	DB, PC	10–30; 4 weeks	Decreased emotional blunting, confusion, irritability, anxiety, mood, restlessness	Confusion (2), dizziness (1), sedation (1)
Nyth *et al.*, 1992	Dementia (29)	149	DB, PC	10–30; 6 weeks	Decreased anxiety, fear-panic, depressed mood in all	Tiredness (18), problem concentrating (9), apathy (8), dizziness (7), sedation (11), tension (11)
Ragneskog *et al.*, 1996	AD (55), vascular dementia (30), alcoholic dementia (5), NOS (3)	123	Open, 2 centres	20–40; 1–12 months	Decreased CGI or GBS for irritability, depression (60%), restlessness, anxiety	Tiredness (15); dizziness (14); drowsiness, sleep disturbances, restlessness (4), aggression (3), anxiety (2)
Pollock *et al.*, 1997	AD	15	Open	20; 2 weeks	Decreased agitation, hostility, delusions, disinhibition	Dropouts from nausea (1), myoclonus (1)
Pollock *et al.*, 2002	Inpatient AD, VaD, mixed, or other not specified	85	Randomized DB, PC, parallel group	20 citalopram or 6.5 mean perphenazine, up to 17 days	Significantly improved agitation for citalopram versus placebo	Similar scores among all groups
Fluoxetine						
Auchus and Bissey-Black, 1997	AD	15	DB, PC parallel group versus haloperidol	20; 6 weeks	Neither more effective than placebo for agitation	Anxiety, nervousness, confusion, tremor
Sertraline						
Burke *et al.*, 1997	AD, NOS dementia	19	Chart review	50; variable duration (10/11 AD; 4/8 NOS)	Improved on CGI	None reported
Paroxetine						
Ramadan *et al.*, 2000	AD or VaD	15	Open	10–40; 3 months	Verbal agitation reduced	Weight gain (5), diarrhoea (1), worsened EPS (1)

AD, Alzheimer's disease; CGI, Clinical Global Impression; DB, double-blind; GBS, Gottfried–Bråne–Steen; NOS, not otherwise specified; PC, placebo-controlled; VaD, vascular dementia

No benefit of administration has been reported yet for fluoxetine or fluvoxamine, and only anecdotes have been published regarding other serotonergic agents (e.g. sertraline), all suggesting possible benefit at least in individual patients. Gastrointestinal distress, loss of appetite and weight, sedation, insomnia, sexual dysfunction and occasional paradoxical agitation can occur with serotonergic agents, although, as a group, they tend to be well tolerated. Results from large placebo-controlled studies will be critical to clarify the optimal role of this class of agents.

38.9 ANTICONVULSANTS

These are listed in Tables 38.7 and 38.8.

We might consider use of anticonvulsants first in patients with features of mania, as well perhaps in those with prominent impulsivity, lability, or episodic aggression. Evidence regarding these agents was summarized previously: we will review it briefly here.

Chambers et al. (1982) performed an 8-week cross-over study of carbamazepine in 19 women with mild agitation who also received antipsychotics: this brief report was negative. Tariot et al. (1994) performed a 12-week placebo-controlled pilot cross-over study of carbamazepine in 25 patients, showing encouraging effects on agitation and not other aspects of psychopathology. A more recent confirmatory parallel group study of 6 weeks' duration in 51 patients also found a significant reduction in agitation using a mean dose of 300 mg/d (Tariot et al., 1998). Tolerability in these studies was generally good, with evidence of sedation and ataxia (Tariot et al., 1995b).

A 6-week, randomized, double-blind, placebo-controlled, parallel group trial of carbamazepine 100 mg q.i.d. was conducted in 21 patients with probable AD with agitation and mild psychotic or mood disturbances who had failed previous treatment with antipsychotics (Olin et al., 2001). Secondary analysis suggested improvement in agitation-related symptoms. Adverse events were reported as mild. Side effects seen in other populations, such as rashes, sedation, haematologic abnormalities, hepatic dysfunction and altered electrolytes, would be more likely to be evident with widespread use of carbamazepine in the elderly (Tariot et al., 1995b). Further, it has considerable potential for significant drug–drug interactions. The carbamazepine studies provide evidence to support the concept that anticonvulsants have anti-agitation efficacy. The question of whether alternative agents may be equally or more effective, or at least safer and better tolerated, remains open.

Valproic acid, also available as the enteric-coated derivative, divalproex sodium, is approved by the US FDA for treatment of acute mania associated with bipolar disorder. There are at present 18 case reports or case series in patients with dementia addressing efficacy, safety and tolerability (Tariot, 2004). There was wide variation in the daily dose (240–4000 mg/day) and plasma levels of valproate (14–107 µg/mL); approximately two-thirds of patients showed clinically evident improvement in agitation, chiefly reported in descriptive terms. Side effects were consistent with Package Insert information. The preliminary data suggested that valproate may be effective and safe for the treatment of agitation associated with dementia and supported further studies.

The first randomized, placebo-controlled, parallel group study of this agent was 6 weeks in duration (Porsteinsson et al., 2001). The 'best dose' of divalproex sodium (mean = 826 mg/day, mean level 46 µg/day) was assessed in 56 nursing home residents with dementia complicated by agitation. The primary measure of agitation showed a nearly significant reduction with valproate versus placebo. Serious adverse events occurred at a rate of 10 per cent in both the drug and placebo groups, with milder side effects occurring more frequently in the drug group, chiefly consisting of sedation,

Table 38.7 *Anticonvulsants: carbamazepine*

Study	Diagnosis	N	Design	Dose (mg/day); duration	Response	Adverse effects
Tariot et al., 1994	AD, VaD	25	Cross-over PC (some other psychotropics permitted)	300 modal; 5 weeks	Decreased agitation (16 versus 4 placebo)	Tics (1), sedation
Tariot et al., 1998	Dementia	51	Randomized PC (no psychotropics except chloral hydrate as needed)	300 modal; 6 weeks	Improved on CGI (20/26); also improved on OAS, BPRS, BRSD	Ataxia (9 vs. 3 placebo), disorientation (4 versus 0 placebo), tics (1), sedation
Olin et al., 2001	AD	21	Randomized, DB, PC	388; 6 weeks	Improved BPRS hostility item	Diarrhoea more common with active treatment

AD, Alzheimer's disease; BPRS, Brief Psychiatric Rating Scale; BRSD, CERAD Behavioral Rating Scale for Dementia; DB, double-blind; OAS, Overt Aggression Scale; PC, placebo-controlled; VaD, vascular dementia gastrointestinal distress, and ataxia, typically rated as mild, and the expected decrease in average platelet count (about 20 000/mm^3). Forty-six of these participants were subsequently treated for 6 weeks in an open fashion with clinically optimal doses of divalproex sodium (range 250–1500 mg/day, mean 851 mg/day) (Porsteinsson et al., 2003). The results confirmed and extended those from the placebo-controlled phase of the trial.

A randomized, double-blind, placebo-controlled, cross-over study of valproate 480 mg/day for 3 weeks was conducted in patients with dementia and aggressive behaviour (Sival et al., 2002). No significant differences in aggressive behaviour in this short-term trial were seen between placebo and active treatments according to the primary outcome measure. However, there was a trend to improvement in measures of aggression that correlated with serum valproate levels, and sodium valproate showed significant effects on restless, melancholic and anxious behaviours, interpreted as generally consistent with anti-agitation results seen previously, as well as trends for improvement for dependent and suspicious

behaviours. There were no drug-placebo differences in rate or type of adverse events.

A multicentre, randomized, placebo-controlled, 6-week, study of divalproex sodium conducted in 172 nursing home residents with dementia and agitation who also met criteria for secondary mania incorporated an aggressive dosing and titration protocol resulting in a target dose of 20 mg/kg/day for 10 days (Tariot et al., 2001a). This titration rate and dose resulted in sedation in about 20 per cent of the drug-treated group and a relatively high dropout rate, leading to premature discontinuation of the study (n = 100 completers). There were no significant drug–placebo differences in change in manic features, but there was a significant effect of drug on agitation. Sedation occurred in 36 per cent of the drug group versus 20 per cent of the placebo group, and mild thrombocytopenia occurred in 7 per cent of the drug group and none of the placebo treated patients.

The results from this trial were used to amend the Package Insert information, cautioning against use of similar doses and/or titration rates in the elderly. If valproate is used, the

Table 38.8 *Anticonvulsants: divalproex*

Study	Diagnosis	N	Design	Dose (mg/day); plasma level (μg/mL); Duration	Response	Adverse effects
Herrmann, 1998	AD, LB, vascular dementia	16	Open	750–2500 (mean = 1331); mean level = 459 μM; 5–34 weeks	Improved on CMAI, BEHAVE-AD (11)	Sedation, ataxia, diarrhoea (1)
Kunik et al., 1998	Dementia	13	Retrospective review (concurrent BDZs, antipsychotics)	500–1750 (mean = 846); mean level = 48; duration variable	Decreased physical not verbal agitation and aggression on CMAI (10)	None reported; drug interaction with phenytoin noted (1)
Porsteinsson et al., 2001	AD, vascular dementia, mixed dementia	56	Randomized PC (no psychotropics except chloral hydrate as needed)	375–1375 (mean = 826); mean level = 45; 6 weeks	Decreased agitation by BPRS and CGI	Sedation and nausea, vomiting or diarrhoea
Tariot et al., 2001a	AD and/or vascular dementia with secondary mania	172	Randomized, DB, PC, parallel-group	1000 median	Significant improvement on CMAI verbal agitation subscale	Somnolence, thrombocytopenia
Sival et al., 2002	AD, vascular dementia, other and mixed dementia	42	Randomized, DB, PC, cross-over	480; mean level = 41; 3 weeks active treatment	No change in aggressive behaviour compared to placebo	Small increase in incidence of adverse events compared to placebo
Porsteinsson et al., 2003	AD, vascular dementia, mixed dementia	46	Open extension	250–1500 (mean = 851); mean level = 47; 6 weeks	Decreased agitation by BPRS and CGI	Fall, sedation, and nausea, vomiting or diarrhoea

AD, Alzheimer's disease; BPRS, Brief Psychiatric Rating Scale; CGI, Clinical Global Impression; CMAI, Cohen-Mansfield Agitation Inventory; DB, double-blind; LB, Lewy body; PC, placebo-controlled available evidence would suggest a starting dose of about 125 mg p.o. b.i.d., increasing by 125–250 mg increments every 5–7 days, with a maximal dose determined by clinical response, or where there is uncertainty, a serum level of about 60–90 μg/mL. In our hands, the typical target dose is about 10–12 mg/kg/day. The usefulness of the new once-daily extended release formulation is not established in this population.

There are no controlled studies of which we are aware of the newer anticonvulsants including lamotrigine, gabapentin and topiramate. There are a few case reports and case series suggest benefit with gabapentin (Regan and Gordon, 1997; Hawkins et al., 2000; Herrmann et al., 2000; Roane et al., 2000; Megna et al., 2002).

There are emerging biological data addressing the mechanism of action of mood stabilizers suggesting in particular that lithium and valproate, but not other agents, may have clinically relevant neuroprotective properties (Manji et al., 2000; Tariot et al., 2002b). Further understanding of these issues may differentiate among available agents and also lead to the identification of new targets for therapy.

38.10 SELEGILINE

Also known as L-deprenyl, selegiline relatively selectively inhibits monoamine oxidase (MAO) type B at doses up to 10 mg/day, while non-selectively inhibiting MAO A and B at higher doses. It has primarily been used in the treatment of motor dysfunction patients with Parkinson's disease but there are a surprising number of clinical reports in patients with dementia. In many cases, the agent was looked at as a possible disease modifier or cognition-enhancing agent, rather than as treatment for behaviour per se. In a meta-analysis, Tolbert and Fuller (1996) reported that all uncontrolled studies of this agent in dementia that addressed behavioural changes indicated beneficial behavioural effects of selegiline, whilst two of the five double-blind, placebo-controlled studies reported somewhat positive behavioural effects. A different meta-analysis of 11 randomized placebo-controlled double-blind trials found that four trials indicated positive behavioural effects (Birks and Flicker, 1998). Since the overall evidence of behavioural efficacy is limited, selegiline is not likely to be a first, or even second, choice for the treatment of agitation. Its role as a neuroprotective agent or cognitive enhancer in dementia has yet to be fully clarified.

38.11 β–ADRENERGIC RECEPTOR BLOCKERS

This class of agents has not been subject to rigorous study. Most of the evidence comes from open trials conducted more than 10 years ago (Rosenquist et al., 2000). Doses used are typically below 100 mg/day for propranolol.

Adverse reactions of β-blockers include bradycardia, hypotension, potential worsening of congestive heart failure or asthma, reduced adrenergic response to hypoglycaemia in patients with diabetes, sedation, increased confusion, psychosis, depression and increased atrioventricular block. It is unclear what role this class of medication has in the treatment of agitation associated with dementia at this point. If it is to be attempted at all, we would argue that it should occur only after safer and more conventional therapies have failed, and only with careful monitoring for side effects.

38.12 LITHIUM

There are no controlled studies of this agent for agitation in dementia; there are at most some case series published in the 1980s (Rosenquist et al., 2000). The limited literature suggests that occasional patients showed improvement, but toxicity was common, including worsening of extrapyramidal syndromes, ataxia and confusion. Since the therapeutic index is so narrow, we find it hard to justify using this agent in a patient lacking a syndromal diagnosis of bipolar disorder. Even then, we are more inclined to use anticonvulsants first. If we choose lithium, close monitoring is in order.

38.13 CHOLINERGIC THERAPIES

We completed a previous review of studies with cholinergic therapies (Rosenquist et al., 2000).

As summarized by Cummings (2000), there is mounting evidence that cholinergic agents, especially cholinesterase inhibitors, may have modest clinically relevant psychotropic effects in some patients with dementia. For the most part, the studies were not designed to address behavioural outcomes as the primary goal. A prospective clinical trial of metrifonate versus placebo found modest reduction in average neuropsychiatric symptoms in the drug group versus placebo group (Morris et al., 1998). A retrospective analysis of two 26-week double-blind, placebo-controlled multicentre trials of metrifonate found a behavioural effect size of 15 per cent, with significant improvement observed in measures of agitation/aggression and aberrant motor behaviour as well as hallucinations, dysphoria and apathy (Raskind et al., 1999; Cummings et al., 2001). Although these data support the potential behavioural impact of cholinergic treatment, development of metrifonate has been abandoned because of toxicity.

Tariot et al. (2000b) showed reduced incidence of neuropsychiatric symptoms on drug versus placebo in outpatients who generally lacked psychopathology at baseline in a 5-month study of galantamine. A secondary analysis of behavioural data from a 6-month, placebo-controlled trial of donepezil in nursing home residents with probable AD complicated by behavioural symptoms showed reduced agitation (Tariot et al., 2001b). In a case series, 28 patients with AD treated with donepezil 5 mg/day for 1 month followed by a mean dose of 10 mg/day for 5 months showed improvement in symptoms of agitation (Paleacu *et al.*, 2002).

38.14 MEMANTINE

Memantine is a non-competitive inhibitor of *N*-methyl-*D*-aspartate (NMDA) receptors that may permit normal memory formation but blocks their excitotoxic activation (Winblad *et al.*, 2002). The FDA recently approved memantine for treatment of moderate to severe AD. A placebo-controlled study of memantine 10 mg/day for 3 months in patients with severe dementia showed significant clinical improvements in memantine-treated patients (Winblad and Poritis, 1999). In a more recent double-blind, placebo-controlled study, 252 patients with moderate to severe AD were randomized to treatment with memantine 20 mg/day or placebo for 7 months (Reisberg *et al.*, 2003). There were significant improvements among memantine-treated patients in the primary global and functional end points. The behavioural data indicated a trend to less worsening in memantine-treated patients in psychopathology, without agitation effects. Agitation was more common as an adverse event in the placebo group.

38.15 HORMONAL THERAPY

There are no definitive studies of hormonal agents, which are sometimes used when more conventional therapies fail. The available literature was summarized previously (Rosenquist *et al.*, 2000). The anecdotal evidence is by no means conclusive, and only suggests that these agents might occasionally be helpful. Controlled studies would be extremely useful.

38.16 SUMMARY

Humane treatment of patients with dementia includes vigorously addressing the kinds of behavioural and psychological signs and symptoms that are likely to occur. The main emphasis should be on non-pharmacological approaches, including carefully investigating for possible delirium and searching hard for social or environmental interventions that capitalize on the patient's residual strengths. It is indeed this process of attempting to 'find what works' that makes treatment in this population so fascinating, as well as challenging.

Psychotropics should be reserved for cases where other, simpler interventions have been attempted and deemed inadequate. We advocate a target symptom-based approach, which matches the most salient target symptoms to a relevant drug class. Although there is no compelling empirical support for this approach, it has the advantage of being face-valid and

logical, which are reassuring features when one is a consultant in a confusing situation.

Much of the available data do in fact indicate that antipsychotics as a group can show benefit for agitation associated with psychotic features. Further, evidence also is mounting that this class of agents may also show benefit for agitation or aggression not associated with psychotic features. As indicated, the side effects of the typical antipsychotics are protean. The data are emerging regarding safety and potentially greater effectiveness of atypical antipsychotics. The available literature regarding non-antipsychotic medication includes antidepressants, anticonvulsants, anxiolytics and a variety of other agents with less foundation. As data accrue regarding these therapeutic approaches, we will have a clearer sense of exactly how and when they should be deployed. In the meantime, clinicians are obliged to deal as thoughtfully as possible with patients on a case-by-case basis, attempting first and foremost to avoid toxicity of therapies intended to help.

REFERENCES

Alexopoulos GS, Silver JM, Kahn DA, Frances A, Carpenter D. (1998) Treatment of agitation in older persons with dementia. *Postgraduate Medicine* (April), 1–88

Allain H, Dautzenberg PH, Maurer K, Schuck S, Bonhomme D, Gerard D. (2000) Double blind study of tiapride versus haloperidol and placebo in agitation and aggressiveness in elderly patients with cognitive impairment. *Psychopharmacology (Berlin)* **148**: 361–366

American Geriatrics Society; American Association for Geriatric Psychiatry. (2003) Consensus statement on improving the quality of mental health care in US. nursing homes: management of depression and behavioral symptoms associated with dementia. *Journal of American Geriatrics Society* **51**: 1287–298

Auchus AP and Bissey-Black C. (1997) Pilot study of haloperidol, fluoxetine, and placebo for agitation in Alzheimer's disease. *Journal of Neuropsychiatry and Clinical Neurosciences* **9**: 591–593

Ballard C, Grace J, McKeith I, Holmes C. (1998) Neuroleptic sensitivity in dementia with Lewy bodies and Alzheimer's disease. *Lancet* **351**: 1032–1033

Birks J and Flicker L. (1998) The efficacy and safety of selegiline for the symptomatic treatment of Alzheimer's disease: a systematic review of the evidence (Cochrane review). *Cochrane Library*, Issue 2. Oxford, Update Software

Brodaty H, Ames D, Snowdon J *et al.* (2003) A randomized placebo-controlled trial of risperidone for the treatment of aggression, agitation, and psychosis of dementia. *Journal of Clinical Psychiatry* **64**: 134–143

Burke WJ, Dewan V, Wengel SP, Roccaforte WH, Nadolny GC, Folks DG. (1997) The use of selective serotonin reuptake inhibitors for depression and psychosis complicating dementia. *International Journal of Geriatric Psychiatry* **12**: 519–525

Chambers CA, Bain J, Rosbottom R, Ballinger BR, McLaren S. (1982) Carbamazepine in senile dementia and overactivity – a placebo controlled double blind trial. *IRCS Medical Science* **10**: 505–506

Christensen DB and Benfield WR. (1998) Alprazolam as an alternative to low-dose haloperidol in older, cognitively impaired nursing facility patients. *Journal of the American Geriatrics Society* **46**: 620–625

Coccaro EF. (1996) Neurotransmitter correlates of impulsive aggression in humans. *Annals of the New York Academy of Sciences* **794**: 82–89

Cohen-Mansfield J and Billig N. (1986) Agitated behaviors in the elderly. I. A conceptual review. *Journal of the American Geriatrics Society* **34**: 711–721

Cummings JL. (2000) Cholinesterase inhibitors: a new class of psychotropic compounds. *American Journal of Psychiatry* **157**: 4–16

Cummings JL, Nadel A, Masterman D, Cyrus PA. (2001) Efficacy of metrifonate in improving the psychiatric and behavioral disturbances of patients with Alzheimer's disease. *Journal of Geriatric Psychiatry and Neurology* **14**: 101–108

Davis P and Baskys A. (2002) Quetiapine effectively reduces psychotic symptoms in patients with Lewy body dementia: an advantage of the unique pharmacological profile? *Brain and Aging* **2**: 49–53

De Deyn PP, Rabheru K, Rasmussen A *et al*. (1999) A randomized trial of risperidone, placebo, and haloperidol for behavioral symptoms of dementia. *Neurology* **53**: 946–955

De Deyn PP, Jeste DV, Auby P *et al*. (2003) Aripiprazole in dementia of the Alzheimer's type. Poster presented at 16th Annual Meeting of American Association for Geriatric Psychiatry, March

Devanand DP, Marder K, Michaels KS *et al*. (1998) A randomized, placebo-controlled, dose-comparison trial of haloperidol for psychosis and disruptive behaviors in Alzheimer's disease. *American Journal of Psychiatry* **155**: 1512–1520

Devanand DP. (2000) Depression in dementia. In: N Qizilbash, L Schneider, H Chui *et al*. (eds), *Evidence-based dementia: A practical guide to diagnosis and management*. Oxford, Blackwell Science Ltd

Doody RS, Stevens JC, Beck C. (2001) Practice parameter: management of dementia (an evidence-based review) Report of the Quality Standards Subcommittee of the American Academy of Neurology. *Neurology* **56**: 1154–1166

Finkel SI, Costa e Silva J, Cohen G, Miller S, Sartorius N. (1996) Behavioral and psychological signs and symptoms of dementia: a consensus statement on current knowledge and implications for research and treatment. *International Psychogeriatrics* **8** (Suppl. 3): 497–500

Hawkins JW, Tinklenberg JR, Sheikh JI, Peyser CE, Yesavage JA. (2000) A retrospective chart review of gabapentin for the treatment of aggressive and agitated behavior in patients with dementias. *American Journal of Geriatric Psychiatry* **8**: 221–225

Herrmann N. (1998) Valproic acid treatment of agitation in dementia. *Canadian Journal of Psychiatry* **43**: 69–72

Herrmann N, Rivard MF, Flynn M, Ward C, Rabheru K, Campbell S. (1998) Risperidone for the treatment of behavioral disturbances in dementia: a case series. *Journal of Neuropsychiatry and Clinical Neurosciences* **10**: 220–223

Herrmann N, Lanctot K, Myszak M. (2000) Effectiveness of gabapentin for the treatment of behavioral disorders in dementia. *Journal of Clinical Psychopharmacology* **20**: 90–93

Jeste DV and Finkel SI. (2000) Psychosis of Alzheimer's disease and related dementias. Diagnostic criteria for a distinct syndrome. *American Journal of Geriatric Psychiatry* **8**: 29–34

Jeste DV, Caligiuri MP, Paulsen JS *et al*. (1995) Risk of tardive dyskinesia in older patients. A prospective longitudinal study of 266 outpatients. *Archives of General Psychiatry* **52**: 756–765

Jeste DV, Lacro JP, Bailey A, Rockwell E, Harris MJ, Caligiuri MP. (1999) Lower incidence of tardive dyskinesia with risperidone compared with haloperidol in older patients. *Journal of the American Geriatrics Society* **47**: 716–719

Jeste DV, Okamoto A, Napolitano J, Kane JM, Martinez RA. (2000) Low incidence of persistent tardive dyskinesia in elderly patients with dementia treated with risperidone. *American Journal of Psychiatry* **157**: 1150–1155

Katz I, Jeste DV, Mintzer JE, Clyde C, Napolitano J, Brecher M. (1999) Comparison of risperidone and placebo for psychosis and behavioral disturbances associated with dementia: a randomized, double-blind trial. *Journal of Clinical Psychiatry* **60**: 107–115

Kunik ME, Puryear L, Orengo CA, Molinari V, Workman RH Jr. (1998) The efficacy and tolerability of divalproex sodium in elderly demented patients with behavioural disturbances. *International Journal of Geriatric Psychiatry* **13**: 29–34

Lanctot KL, Best TS, Mittmann N, Liu BA, Oh PI, Einarson TR, Naranjo CA. (1998) Efficacy and safety of neuroleptics in behavioral disorders associated with dementia. *Journal of Clinical Psychiatry* **59**: 550–561

Lavretsky H and Sultzer D. (1998) A structured trial of risperidone for the treatment of agitation in dementia. *American Journal of Geriatric Psychiatry* **6**: 127–135

Leibovici A and Tariot PN. (1988) Agitation associated with dementia: a systematic approach to treatment. *Psychopharmacology Bulletin* **24**: 49–53

Loy R, Tariot PN, Rosenquist K. (1999) Alzheimer's disease: behavioral management. In: IR Katz, D Oslin, MP Lawton (eds), *Annual Review of Gerontology and Geriatrics: Psychopharmacologic Interventions in Late Life*. Volume 19, pp. 136–194

Lyketsos CG, Sheppard JM, Steele CD *et al*. (2000) Randomized, placebo-controlled, double-blind clinical trial of sertraline in the treatment of depression complicating Alzheimer's disease: initial results from the Depression in Alzheimer's Disease study. *American Journal of Psychiatry* **157**: 1686–1689

Manji HK, Moore GJ, Chen G. (2000) Lithium up-regulates the cytoprotective protein Bcl-2 in the CNS in vivo: a role for neurotrophic and neuroprotective effects in manic depressive illness. *Journal of Clinical Psychiatry* **61** (Suppl. 9): 82–96

Meehan KM, Wang H, David SR *et al*. (2002) Comparison of rapidly acting intramuscular olanzapine, lorazepam, and placebo: a double-blind, randomized study in acutely agitated patients with dementia. *Neuropsychopharmacology* **26**: 494–504

Megna JL, Devitt PJ, Sauro MD, Dewan MJ. (2002) Gabapentin's effect on agitation in severely and persistently mentally ill patients. *Annals of Pharmacotherapy* **36**: 12–16

Merriam AE, Aronson MK, Gaston P, Wey SL, Katz I. (1988) The psychiatric symptoms of Alzheimer's disease. *Journal of the American Geriatrics Society* **36**: 7–12

Morris JC, Cyrus PA, Orazem J, Mas J, Bieber F, Ruzicka BB, Gulanski B. (1998) Metrifonate benefits cognitive, behavioral, and global function in patients with Alzheimer's disease. *Neurology* **50**: 1222–1230

Nyth AL and Gottfries CG. (1990) The clinical efficacy of citalopram in treatment of emotional disturbances in dementia disorders. A Nordic multicentre study. *British Journal of Psychiatry* **157**: 894–901

Nyth AL, Gottfries CG, Lyby K *et al*. (1992) A controlled multicenter clinical study of citalopram and placebo in elderly depressed patients with and without concomitant dementia. *Acta Psychiatrica Scandinavica* **86**: 138–145

Olin JT, Fox LS, Pawluczyk S, Taggart NA, Schneider LS. (2001) A pilot randomized trial of carbamazepine for behavioral symptoms in treatment-resistant outpatients with Alzheimer's disease. *American Journal of Geriatric Psychiatry* **9**: 400–405

Paleacu D, Mazeh D, Mirecki I, Even M, Barak Y. (2002) Donepezil for the treatment of behavioral symptoms in patients with Alzheimer's disease. *Clinical Neuropharmacology* **25**: 313–317

Patel S and Tariot PN. (1991) Pharmacologic models of Alzheimer's disease. *Psychiatric Clinics of North America* 14: 287–308

Pollock BG, Mulsant BH, Sweet R *et al.* (1997) An open pilot study of citalopram for behavioral disturbances of dementia. Plasma levels and real-time observations. *American Journal of Geriatric Psychiatry* 5: 70–78

Pollock BG, Mulsant BH, Rosen J *et al.* (2002) Comparison of citalopram, perphenazine, and placebo for the acute treatment of psychosis and behavioral disturbances in hospitalized, demented patients. *American Journal of Psychiatry* 159: 460–465

Porsteinsson AP, Tariot PN, Erb R *et al.* (2001) Placebo-controlled study of divalproex sodium for agitation in dementia. *American Journal of Geriatric Psychiatry* 9: 58–66

Porsteinsson AP, Tariot PN, Jakimovich LJ, Kowalski N, Holt C, Erb R, Cox C. (2003) Valproate therapy for agitation in dementia: open-label extension of a double-blind trial. *American Journal of Geriatric Psychiatry* 11: 434–440

Profenno LA and Tariot PN. (2004) Pharmacologic management of agitation in Alzheimer's disease. *Dementia and Geriatric Cognitive Disorders* 17: 65–77

Rabins P, Blacker D, Bland W *et al.* and the American Psychiatric Association Work Group on Alzheimer's Disease and Related Dementias. (1997) Practice guideline for the treatment of patients with Alzheimer's disease and other dementias of late life. *American Journal of Psychiatry* 154: 1–39

Ragneskog H, Eriksson S, Karlsson I, Gottfries CG. (1996) Long-term treatment of elderly individuals with emotional disturbances: an open study with citalopram. *International Psychogeriatrics* 8: 659–668

Ramadan FH, Naughton BJ, Bassanelli AG. (2000) Treatment of verbal agitation with a selective serotonin reuptake inhibitor. *Journal of Geriatric Psychiatry and Neurology* 13: 56–9

Raskind MA, Cyrus PA, Ruzicka BB, Gulanski BI. (1999) The effects of metrifonate on the cognitive, behavioral, and functional performance of Alzheimer's disease patients. Metrifonate Study Group. *Journal of Clinical Psychiatry* 60: 318–325

Regan WM and Gordon SM. (1997) Gabapentin for behavioral agitation in Alzheimer's disease. *Journal of Clinical Psychopharmacology* 17: 59–60

Reisberg B, Doody R, Stöffler A, Schmitt F, Ferris S, Möbius HJ, for the Memantine Study Group. (2003) Memantine in moderate-to-Severe Alzheimer's Disease. *New England Journal of Medicine* 348: 1333–1341

Roane DM, Feinberg TE, Meckler L, Miner CR, Scicutella A, Rosenthal RN. (2000) Treatment of dementia-associated agitation with gabapentin. *Journal of Neuropsychiatry and Clinical Neuroscience* 12: 40–43

Rosenquist K, Tariot P, Loy R. (2000) Treatments for behavioural and psychological symptoms in AD and other dementias. In: J O'Brien, D Ames, A Burns (eds), *Dementia*. London: Edward Arnold, pp. 571–602

Satterlee WG, Reams SG, Burns PR, Hamilton S, Tran PV, Tollefson GD. (1995) A clinical update in olanzapine treatment in schizophrenia and in elderly Alzheimer's disease patients. *Psychopharmacology Bulletin* 31: Abstract.

Scharre DW and Chang SI. (2002) Cognitive and behavioral effects of quetiapine in Alzheimer's disease patients. *Alzheimer Disease and Associated Disorders* 16: 128–130

Schneider L and Dagerman K. (2003) Meta-analysis of atypical antipsychotics for dementia patients: balancing efficacy and adverse events. Abstract II-69, *NCDEU 43rd Annual Meeting 5/27–30* [Unpublished, www.nimh.nih.gov./ncdeu/index.cfm]

Schneider LS, Pollock VE, Lyness SA. (1990) A metaanalysis of controlled trials of neuroleptic treatment in dementia. *Journal of the American Geriatrics Society* 38: 553–563

Schneider LS, Tariot PN, Lyketsos CG *et al.* (2001) National Institute of Mental Health Clinical Antipsychotic Trials of Intervention Effectiveness (CATIE): Alzheimer disease trial methodology. *American Journal of Geriatric Psychiatry* 9: 346–360

Sival RC, Haffmans PM, Jansen PA, Duursma SA, Eikelenboom P. (2002) Sodium valproate in the treatment of aggressive behavior in patients with dementia–a randomized placebo controlled clinical trial. *International Journal of Geriatric Psychiatry* 17: 579–585

Street JS, Clark WS, Gannon KS *et al.* (2000) Olanzapine treatment of psychotic and behavioral symptoms in patients with Alzheimer disease in nursing care facilities: a double-blind, randomized, placebo-controlled trial. The HGEU Study Group. *Archives of General Psychiatry* 57: 968–976

Street JS, Clark WS, Kadam DL *et al.* (2001) Long-term efficacy of olanzapine in the control of psychotic and behavioral symptoms in nursing home patients with Alzheimer's dementia. *International Journal of Geriatric Psychiatry* 16 (Suppl. 1): S62–70

Sultzer DL, Gray KF, Gunay I, Berisford MA, Mahler ME. (1997) A double-blind comparison of trazodone and haloperidol for treatment of agitation in patients with dementia. *American Journal of Geriatric Psychiatry* 5: 60–69

Tariot PN. (1996) Treatment strategies for agitation and psychosis in dementia. *Journal of Clinical Psychiatry* 57 (Suppl. 14): 21–29

Tariot PN. (1999) Treatment of agitation in dementia. *Journal of Clinical Psychiatry* 60 (Suppl. 8): 11–20

Tariot PN. (2004) Valproate use in neuropsychiatric disorders in the elderly. *Psychopharmacology Bulletin* 37: 116–128

Tariot PN and Blazina L. (1993) The psychopathology of dementia. In: J Morris J (ed.), *Handbook of Dementing Illnesses*. New York, Marcel Dekker Inc, pp. 461–475

Tariot PN and Schneider LS. (1998) Nonneuroleptic treatment of complications of dementia: applying clinical research to practice. In: JC Nelson (ed.), *Geriatric Psychopharmacology*. New York, Marcel Dekker Inc, pp. 427–453

Tariot PN, Erb R, Leibovici A *et al.* (1994) Carbamazepine treatment of agitation in nursing home patients with dementia: a preliminary study. *Journal of the American Geriatrics Society* 42: 1160–1166

Tariot PN, Schneider LS, Katz IR. (1995a) Anticonvulsant and other non-neuroleptic treatment of agitation in dementia. *Journal of Geriatric Psychiatry and Neurology* 8 (Suppl. 1): S28–S39

Tariot PN, Frederiksen K, Erb R *et al.* (1995b) Lack of carbamazepine toxicity in frail nursing home patients: a controlled study. *Journal of the American Geriatrics Society* 43: 1026–1029

Tariot PN, Erb R, Podgorski CA *et al.* (1998) Efficacy and tolerability of carbamazepine for agitation and aggression in dementia. *American Journal of Psychiatry* 155: 54–61

Tariot PN, Salzman C, Yeung PP, Pultz J, Rak IW. (2000a) Long-term use of quetiapine in elderly patients with psychotic disorders. *Clinical Therapeutics* 22: 1068–1084

Tariot PN, Solomon PR, Morris JC, Kershaw P, Lilienfled S, Ding C, and the Galantamine USA-10 Study Group. (2000b) A 5-month, randomized placebo-controlled trial of galantamine in AD. *Neurology* 54: 2269–2276

Tariot PN, Schneider L, Mintzer J *et al.* (2001a) Safety and tolerability of divalproex sodium for the treatment of signs and symptoms of mania in elderly patients with dementia: results of a double-blind, placebo-controlled trial. *Current Therapeutic Research* 62: 51–67

Tariot PN, Cummings JL, Katz IR *et al.* (2001b) A randomized, double-blind, placebo-controlled study of the efficacy and safety of donepezil in patients with Alzheimer's disease in the nursing home setting. *Journal of the American Geriatrics Society* **49**: 1590–1599

Tariot P, Schneider L, Katz I, Mintzer J, Street J. (2002a) Quetiapine in nursing home residents with Alzheimer's dementia and psychosis. *American Journal of Geriatric Psychiatry* **10** (March/April supplement): 93

Tariot PN, Loy R, Ryan JM, Porsteinsson A, Ismail S. (2002b) Mood stabilizers in Alzheimer's disease: symptomatic and neuroprotective rationales. *Adverse Drug Delivery Reviews* **54**: 1567–1577

Teri L, Logsdon RG, Peskind E *et al.* (2000) Treatment of agitation in AD: a randomized, placebo-controlled clinical trial. *Neurology* **55**: 1271–1278

Tolbert SR and Fuller MA. (1996) Selegiline in treatment of behavioral and cognitive symptoms of Alzheimer disease. *Annals of Pharmacotherapy* **30**: 1122–1129

Winblad B and Poritis N. (1999) Memantine in severe dementia: results of the 9M-Best Study (Benefit and efficacy in severely demented patients during treatment with memantine). *International Journal of Geriatric Psychiatry* **14**: 135–146

Winblad B, Mobius HJ, Stoffler A. (2002) Glutamate receptors as a target for Alzheimer's disease–are clinical results supporting the hope? *Journal of Neural Transmission* **62** (Suppl.): 217–225

Wooltorton E. (2002) Risperidone (Risperdal): increased rate of cerebrovascular events in dementia trials. *Canadian Medical Association Journal* **167**: 1269–1270

Wragg RE and Jeste DV. (1989) Overview of depression and psychosis in Alzheimer's disease. *American Journal of Psychiatry* **146**: 577–587

A predominantly psychosocial approach to behaviour problems in dementia: treating causality

MICHAEL BIRD

This chapter describes an approach to behaviour problems in dementia and concentrates on identifying both the causes of the behaviour in the individual case, and why it is defined as a problem. It begins with a conceptual discussion. Section 39.2 outlines the variables that must be assessed in order to uncover the causes of the problem. Section 39.3 discusses treatment options, including three case studies by way of illustration. Finally, there is a short conclusion on the nature of psychosocial approaches and their relationship with psychopharmacology.

39.1 CONCEPTUAL BACKGROUND: THE NATURE OF CHALLENGING BEHAVIOUR

Over the last decade, what may be called the *behaviour syndrome – standard therapy model* has predominated in the psychogeriatric literature. This model sees the person with dementia as the identified patient and the behaviour as the syndrome to be treated, usually with a standardized treatment such as antipsychotic medication.

The conceptual basis of this model underpins and can be seen in the large number of classification instruments where a named behaviour is the syndrome, or where behaviours are clustered into broader syndromes. Examples are: 'Pacing up and down' from the Dementia Behaviour Disturbance Scale (Baumgarten *et al.*, 1990); 'cognitive abulia' in the BEHAV-AD (Reisberg *et al.*, 1989); or, 'irritability/lability' in the Neuropsychiatric Inventory (Cummings *et al.*, 1994). It can also be seen in the many journal articles appearing each year advocating a standard and usually pharmacological treatment for a mysterious syndrome called 'agitation'. Though agitation does have a meaning in psychiatry, it is often used indiscriminately in dementia research for just about any behaviour that causes problems, and is therefore clinically meaningless.

Standardized treatments for specific behaviours or syndromes are not the focus of this chapter, which is based on a different conceptualization of problem behaviour in dementia. This assumes that, regardless of its nature, the behaviour is actually the end symptom of multiple and case-specific biopsychosocial causality. Rather than simply trying to suppress or manage the symptom, the behaviour, treatment in most cases is much more effectively targeted at causality. Causality will be idiosyncratic to the case, and will include not only causes of behaviour but also why it is perceived as a problem. Treatment may be directed at the person with dementia and/or family carers or care staff. This model is supported by two broad classes of evidence and a controlled clinical trial:

- Though brain impairment associated with dementia is usually a necessary condition for behaviour which may be seen as 'challenging', the same behaviour in different cases will usually be caused by an interaction of that impairment with many case-specific factors. These factors can include medical/physical problems, the environment – including the way care is carried out, mental illness or personal history. For example, many factors can contribute to vocal disruption in dementia, including pain or understimulation (e.g. Cohen-Mansfield and Werner, 1997), overstimulation (e.g. Meares and Draper, 1999), anxiety (e.g. Hallberg *et al.*, 1993), the nature of social interaction with care staff (Edberg *et al.*, 1995), post-traumatic stress disorder (Bird *et al.*, 2002) or hallucinations (Tsai *et al.*, 1996).

- There is abundant evidence that factors other than the behaviour determine whether it is seen as a problem. An obvious example is wandering, which may only be classified as problem behaviour where there is no perimeter fence. However, many other factors influence emotional response to patient behaviour, for example depression in home carers (e.g. Hinchliffe *et al.*, 1995), and organizational or staff variables in residential care (Baillon *et al.*, 1996; Moniz-Cook *et al.*, 2000). Bird *et al.* (2002) found that different care staff exposed to the same behaviour by the same patient exhibited great variability in distress levels about the behaviour (ranging from none to very high). There was also strikingly low agreement amongst senior staff about severity of the problems caused by these residents.

So, what constitutes 'challenging' behaviour is often determined by the eye of the beholder; any definition must therefore include the effects of the behaviour. The definition used for this chapter is 'any behaviour associated with the dementing illness which causes distress or danger to the person with dementia or others, or is a manifestation of distress' (Bird *et al.*, 1998).

If this conceptualization is correct, it follows that there is no easily defined syndrome based on the behaviour, nor a standard treatment. The nature of the behaviour does not even predict whether intervention is required. Where intervention is required because the behaviour is a manifestation of distress or is causing significant distress, treatment will be mainly directed at causes, including the reasons why it causes distress.

Support for the effectiveness and efficacy of this approach may be found in a controlled trial by Bird *et al.* (2002), where a small clinical team treated a series of cases (n = 44) of behavioural disturbance, many severe, and concentrated on causality. There was a 43 per cent post-intervention reduction in frequency of the main referred behaviour, with the effect still evident 3 months later. Interventions were predominantly psychosocial, but medication was used as an adjunct in a significant minority of cases. In a few cases it was the primary modality, for example where the cause was depression or pain or distressing hallucinations. There was no relationship between the nature of the behaviour and the type of treatment. The interventions required initial time-intensive engagement (a mean of 5.5 visits per case) while the case was assessed and a tailored treatment package devised and implemented. However, overall, they took no more clinical visits than a control group (n = 22), which used the more usual predominantly pharmacological approach. Both groups produced equivalent improvements in behaviour and carer/nursing staff emotional response, but the causality-focused approach had far fewer medication changes, drug side effects, and hospitalizations for the behaviour.

39.2 ASSESSMENT

If challenging behaviour is the end product of an interaction between many case-specific variables, multidimensional assessment is essential. Each case must be approached with questions rather than preconceived answers in the form of standard treatments. Multiple sources of information are required, in particular the people who know the patient best. In nursing homes it is essential to include hands-on care staff, often ignored, as well as more senior staff and family. Another essential source is the person with dementia, using direct discussion where possible, focused attention (for example, to the content of screaming), and behavioural observation. The primary assessment questions may be encapsulated under the questions below.

39.2.1 Is the behaviour causing distress or danger to the patient or others?

If the behaviour is a manifestation of distress by the patient, there is clearly an obligation to treat regardless of whether it is causing distress to others. If it is not a manifestation of distress and it is not causing distress or danger, the behaviour, by definition, is not 'challenging', and not a legitimate target for clinicians. Bizarre behaviour is not necessarily the same as challenging behaviour. A common example is benign hallucinations or delusions (Peisah and Brodaty, 1994), though investigation may be necessary to determine whether these phenomena are symptoms of treatable physical illness, especially if there is relatively sudden onset. However, there are many other behaviours associated with dementia that are often classified as aberrant or agitated, such as pacing or repeatedly sorting clothing, where it is essential to first assess whether it is a problem for anybody. 'Treating' a behaviour simply because it challenges the clinician's perception of what is normal risks producing non-benign outcomes, especially with the side effects associated with psychotropic medication (Katona, 2001).

Even if there is distress amongst carers or nursing staff, it is important to discover who is distressed, and the source and severity of that distress, in order to determine whether home carer or nursing staff concerns are a more appropriate target than the behaviour (see Section 39.3, pp. 502–503).

39.2.2 What is the patient actually doing, and what is the context?

Labels like agitation carry almost no clinical information. It is essential to determine what the person with dementia is actually doing to cause distress, and the context in which it occurs (when, where, or to whom?). Even the term aggression carries little information. It could range from frequent dangerous physical violence to occasional verbal abuse or innocuous pushing away, in which case dealing with carer concerns is likely to predominate in any intervention. The context even of severe aggressive behaviour could range from a response to hallucinations (Tsai *et al.*, 1996) to its very common occurrence during intimate personal care in nursing homes (Bridges-Parlet *et al.*, 1994; Bird *et al.*, 2002), though even here it often occurs only with some staff.

39.2.3 Aetiology – what is causing or exacerbating the behaviour?

Beyond the brain impairment itself, important within-patient variables include past history and character, pattern of cognitive and sensory impairment, physical health and comfort, and mental health. External variables are the vast complex of physical and social phenomena that form the patient's immediate world. The role of assessment is to develop evidence-based hypotheses about the factors that produce the behaviour and, of those, which are realistically adjustable. The following comments provide only a flavour of the critical importance of this information.

39.2.3.1 WITHIN-PATIENT VARIABLES

The most common adjustable patient characteristics relate to medical/physical problems, including pain or discomfort, constipation, drug interactions and infections (Peisah and Brodaty, 1994; Cohen-Mansfield and Werner, 1999; Bird *et al.*, 2002). Depression can also precipitate behaviour problems, and must be assessed (Menon *et al.*, 2001). For example, Elmståhl *et al.* (1998) reported that nursing home residents with dementia who were depressed or in physical pain were more likely to be on antipsychotics than the appropriate medication. Though interventions for these phenomena will be primarily medical, psychosocial methods can be used as adjuncts (see Case 2 in Section 39.3, pp. 504–505).

Beyond this, even non-adjustable factors such as past history can provide vital information when an intervention is planned. For example, learning that a woman who screamed and was violent during bathing was a probably manifesting panic based on known premorbid trauma helped staff to change their approach and largely eliminate the behaviour (Woods and Bird, 1998). In Case 1 below (Section 39.3, pp. 503–504), learning that a resident resisting personal care suffered from obsessive-compulsive disorder related to cleanliness meant that the behaviour was unlikely to change, so the intervention was directed at improving staff skills and confidence.

39.2.3.2 EXTERNAL VARIABLES

Many texts concentrate on the physical environment in dementia care (e.g. Day *et al.*, 2000) and it can be an important causal and, by adjustment, ameliorating factor in challenging behaviour. This applies to either the presence or absence of stimuli. For example, incontinence has been reduced by visual, auditory or situational cues (Hanley, 1986; Bird *et al.*, 1995);

screaming by room relocation (Meares and Draper, 1999); wandering by visual barriers (Hussian and Brown, 1987); and self-harm by removal of cues precipitating it (Bird *et al.*, 1998). The patient described in the previous paragraph who screamed in the bathroom because of panic could have her hair washed without incident in a local salon (Woods and Bird, 1998).

It is, however, more often the care environment that is critical in assessment. The association between violence and care interactions has already been noted. In other examples, Cohen-Mansfield and colleagues (1992) found a relationship between disturbed behaviour and staff schedules; Edberg *et al.* (1995) showed that the nature of nurse–patient interactions was associated with vocal disruption; Rogers *et al.* (2000) that carer practices increased patient dependence; and Schnelle *et al.* (1999) that night-time disturbance occurred because staff behaviour woke residents up.

These findings are unsurprising. Most people with dementia live, by necessity, in dependent and dynamic relationships either at home or in institutions. What the patient does and feels affects carers, whose actions and emotions in turn affect the patient. Assessment must therefore include the way care is carried out. Even if carer practices are not causing the behaviour, it is often easier to change what they are doing than patient behaviour direct. Working with home or institutional carers to adapt their attitudes and approach predominated in the intervention study by Bird *et al.* (2002) (see Appendix at the end of the chapter, p. 507).

39.2.4 What realistically can be done? Case-specific constraints and possibilities

Detailed assessment of causality frequently suggests obvious solutions – for example, alleviating loneliness by having someone socialize with the resident several hours a day. However, interventions must also be feasible. To do this, the final key component of assessment is to determine the constraints and potentialities of the situation on the ground. This involves both the person with dementia and the care environment in which the intervention must take place.

39.2.4.1 PATIENT POSSIBILITIES

Assessment of residual capacity of the person with dementia is essential. For example, highly structured counselling is possible in early dementia (e.g. Teri, 1994; Woods and Bird, 1998); learning to respond to cues is still possible in the moderate stages (Bird, 2001). Conversely, assessment may show that nothing can be done directly with the patient because he or she is too impaired or too difficult, or because the behaviour is not going to change.

Formal neuropsychological assessment can provide guidance, but a more direct method is behavioural experiment. For example, operant conditioning was used in a case of gross sexual assault of female staff during showering because, though it is often ineffective in dementia, assessment showed some insight and a capacity to learn simple associations (Bird *et al.*, 1998). The experiment of having a novel 'no nonsense' nurse shower the patient showed that the behaviour was at least partially under his control, and a further experiment that the reinforcer for abstaining from assault (reading the newspaper with a carer) was genuinely pleasurable.

The number of visual cues one sees in nursing homes that are illegible even to the young cognitively intact clinician underlines how rarely assessing the patient's capacity to respond to an intervention is considered before it is put in place. Cues are useless in dementia unless the patient can see them, learn to attend to them and, having done so, remember what they mean and, having done that, act on them (Bird, 2001).

39.2.4.2 ENVIRONMENTAL POSSIBILITIES

Assessment in order to become familiar with the possibilities and limitations of the care environment is equally essential. For example, with a fit younger patient whose violent behaviour was partially related to 'living in this prison' (a nursing home with no outside access), it was necessary to engage a volunteer to take him out jogging because assessment showed clearly that staff were insufficiently motivated to perform this task regularly (Bird *et al.*, 2002). In Case 3 (Section 39.3, pp. 505–506), provision of care at timed intervals was implemented as part of the intervention with a woman who shouted and pressed the buzzer frequently. It was only attempted because assessment showed flexible organization and because staff were sufficiently motivated to carry it out. This would not have been possible in a nursing home with a rigid structure, nor in one where management regarded psychotropic medication as the universal panacea.

As this implies, part of the assessment must include capacity for change within a given care setting. To assess this, clinicians must rely on clinical judgement. For example, depression or anger in home carers often inhibits them from looking at behaviour objectively. The author's rough rule of thumb is that, if even minimal objectivity is impossible, an intervention requiring a change in carer behaviour is not possible until carer distress is addressed. In residential facilities, the closer the institution approximates the acute hospital medical model, the more difficult it will be to implement non-pharmacological interventions. In certain facilities only a masochist would attempt complex psychosocial interventions, though sometimes even a small core of committed staff is sufficient to start the ball rolling. The clinician must look for flexibility of approach and the presence of, or potential to develop, some kind of dementia literacy. In this respect, an empathic understanding of how the patient experiences the world is more important than theoretical knowledge of brain-behaviour relationships.

There is a small but growing literature on the problems of gaining compliance from staff in undertaking psychosocial interventions in residential dementia care (e.g. Schnelle *et al.*, 1998), though it remains an unresolved issue (Allen-Burge *et al.*, 1999).

39.3 INTERVENTIONS

39.3.1 Carer distress as the clinical target

As already discussed, the emotional response of those exposed to a behaviour is often the most important factor in determining whether intervention is required. Restricting treatment to the behaviour alone is, therefore, an absurd limitation of options. In a significant minority of cases, addressing carer concerns is sufficient. Beyond this, even if patient behaviour change is necessary, the most common method will probably involve working with home carers or nursing staff to change their attitude or approach (see Appendix, p. 507). Interventions aimed at carer or care staff attitudes or practices require the same rapport as normal psychotherapy though, in institutions, multiple staff of varying levels of skill, insight, flexibility and motivation makes the task more complex. Equally, as in one-to-one psychotherapy, if carer/care staff concerns are not at least listened to, there can be little rapport and little chance of compliance. Work in progress (Edberg and Bird, 2003), involving focus groups of staff in a number of countries, suggests that, in aged care institutions, listening to and responding to staff distress remains relatively rare.

At least two intervention studies that have included a strong psychosocial component and carer measures (Hinchliffe *et al.*, 1995; Bird *et al.*, 2002), have shown a relationship between reduced problem behaviour and alleviation of carer distress, but causal direction is impossible to attribute. In both studies, in some situations carer distress was alleviated such that, though the behaviour remained, it ceased to be seen as a significant problem (see Case 1 below).

It is often necessary to reduce carer distress before attempting an intervention requiring their input. For example, it was necessary to work first on the anger of a home carer whose confrontational response to her husband's obsessive toileting was exacerbating the problem (Bird, 2003). Emotional support, education on dementia, and learning that her husband was genuinely anxious enabled her to respond with empathy, physical comfort and gentle assertion – reducing the behaviour to more manageable proportions and improving her own mental health.

Many factors influence whether carers or care staff are distressed by patient behaviour. Known examples include: appraisal – not the reality – of physical threat (Rodney, 2000); nursing home organizational factors (Baillon *et al.*, 1996); interpretation of the behaviour (Harvath, 1994); depression in carers (Hinchliffe *et al.*, 1995; Teri, 1997); low dementia literacy (Hagen and Sayers, 1995); level of support provided (Moniz-Cook *et al.*, 2000); and morale and attitude to care (Jenkins and Allen, 1998).

These are variables which can be addressed directly. Though controlled clinical intervention studies are astonishingly rare within the vast home carer burden literature, a few structured support and education programmes have demonstrated clear benefits, including more effective management of behaviour problems and concomitant delayed entry into residential care (Teri, 1999). In institutions, programmes that have addressed staff attitude and care practices have produced not only improved staff morale (Berg *et al.*, 1994) but also: reduced problem behaviour (Hagen and Sayers, 1995; Rovner *et al.*, 1996; Bird *et al.*, 2002); reduced patient dependence (Baltes *et al.*, 1994); reduced patient anxiety and depression (Bråne *et al.*, 1989); improved staff–patient cooperation and therefore reduced problems in personal care (Edberg *et al.*, 1996); and reduced use of physical restraint and antipsychotic drugs (Ray *et al.*, 1993; Levine *et al.*, 1995).

So, there is abundant evidence that the clinician called to 'treat' a case of challenging behaviour who ignores carer distress about that behaviour as the primary clinical target, or as a critical ancillary to dealing with the behaviour, is working with a grossly circumscribed repertoire; 20 per cent of cases reported by Bird *et al.* (2002) were ameliorated without addressing patient behaviour.

39.3.2 Addressing the causes of the behaviour

When physical/medical or mental health contributory factors that can be treated pharmacologically have been addressed, and where the intervention requires more than addressing carer/care staff distress, the clinician must develop a psychosocial package that addresses other causes.

The literature on psychosocial approaches was plagued for many years by scarcely believable assertions, uncontaminated by evidence, of benefits from various generic or proprietary therapies. More recently, there has been movement in a scientific direction. For example, the first controlled trial of aromatherapy, undertaken by a prestigious psychogeriatric team in the UK has now been published. It showed positive effects of massage with melissa oil on generalized agitation (Ballard *et al.*, 2002).

Opie *et al.* (1999) remains one of the best literature reviews of psychosocial approaches. The majority of the 44 studies incorporated had study designs classified as 'weak' but effects were consistent and strong enough for the reviewers to advocate a strong coordinated research effort.

Examples are:

- 'white noise' (waterscape sounds) reducing verbal disruption in that proportion of the subjects who would tolerate headphones (Burgio *et al.*, 1996);
- social interaction reducing verbal disruption (Cohen-Mansfield and Werner, 1997);
- bright light reducing nocturnal disturbance (Colenda *et al.*, 1997) or motor restlessness (Haffmans *et al.*, 2001);
- music tailored to the patient's tastes reducing generalized agitation (Gerdner and Swanson, 1993) or physical aggression (Clark *et al.*, 1998);
- social stimulation reducing physical aggression (Wystanski, 2000);

- personalized tapes made by family members reducing agitation (Woods and Ashley, 1995);
- cued recall of more adaptive behaviour for a variety of problems (Bird, 2001; Bird *et al.*, 1995) and
- cue cards for repetitive questions (Bird *et al.*, 1995; Bourgeois *et al.*, 1997).

As these example show, most research evaluating psychosocial interventions has followed the same *behaviour syndrome – standard treatment* conceptualization as pharmacological research, though it tends to focus more at the level of treatments for specific behaviour. It is valuable because it adds more techniques to the tool-kit, in the same way as drug trials suggest formulations that can be applied with minimal risk to the patient. These generic or behaviour-specific techniques are especially useful where there is no identifiable cause of the behaviour, or there are no other options and the behaviour is still significantly distressing.

However, standardized interventions are not the focus of this chapter. If the cause of vocal disruption is treatable pain, treatable infection, or treatable depression, rote application of baroque music or white noise or melissa oil, though potentially less harmful, is as ludicrous and unprofessional as rote prescription of antipsychotic medication. If disturbed sleep/wake cycles are caused by nurses waking patients at night, training staff to exhibit common sense is likely to be more relevant than bright-light therapy.

39.3.3 Three case studies

In the controlled trial by Bird *et al.* (2002), by far the most common psychosocial interventions, apart from alleviating carer/care staff distress, were not the application of standardized interventions. They were to change the care practices and responses of carers/care staff or the environmental features that were contributing to the behaviours or exacerbating them to unmanageable proportions. These methods are summarized in the Appendix (p. 507). Brief descriptions of the psychosocial and/or pharmacological interventions for all cases undertaken in the trial can be found in the study report.

Three cases from the trial are reported here to give a more general flavour of the causality-based approach described in this chapter. Behaviour intensity measures (duration or frequency) reported in Figure 39.1 are based on direct observation and recording. Validated staff response measures reported are:

- individual staff stress caused by the behaviour;
- individual ability to cope with the patient's behaviour; and
- problem severity assessing overall degree of disruption to the facility.

39.3.3.1 CASE 1

L, 87 years, had progressive dementia of undiagnosed aetiology. She had lived in a hostel since well before onset of

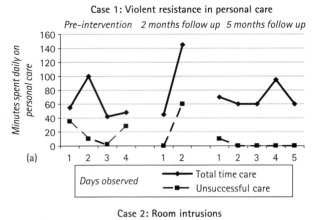

Case 1: Violent resistance in personal care

Pre-intervention   2 months follow up   5 months follow up

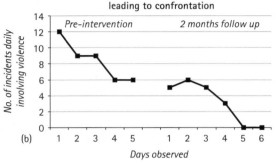

Case 2: Room intrusions
leading to confrontation

Pre-intervention   2 months follow up

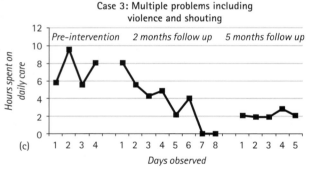

Case 3: Multiple problems including
violence and shouting

Pre-intervention   2 months follow up   5 months follow up

Figure 39.1 (a–c) *Pre- and post-intervention behaviour intensity outcomes of three typical cases.*

impairment and was much loved by senior staff. She was dysphasic and not testable on the Mini-Mental State Exam (MMSE) of Folstein *et al.* (1985). She was in the moderate range on the Clinical Dementia Rating (CDR) of Morris (1993). Otherwise pleasant and easy to manage, she was referred for violent resistance and swearing and yelling during toileting and showering. Low-dose antipsychotic medication had been tried by the general practitioner but it resulted in chronic unsteadiness and a severe fall. Most staff had given up, leaving her personal care for two older staff, who could usually accomplish the task using a mix of chocolate bribes and knowing when to back off or be assertive (i.e. dementia-specific nursing skills). Because L was doubly incontinent, she sometimes had to wait for several hours covered in urine and faeces until one of the experts came on.

At assessment, we followed up on a statement by L's 93-year-old sister: 'She's always been as mad as a hatter'. It became clear that L had suffered most of her life from obsessive-compulsive disorder related to cleanliness. Though she had been in the hostel for 15 years, no member of staff knew this. We assessed the chances of care staff knowing, understanding and applying all L's rituals as nil and the behaviour, accordingly, as unlikely to change. We discussed the situation with staff and, though L was clearly appropriate for nursing home placement, they were adamant they wanted to keep her. The intervention therefore consisted of the two experts showing the others how they undertook personal care and, equally important, providing encouragement to keep going. Figure 39.1a shows no decrease in the total amount of staff time taken to provide personal care to L, but a decrease after 2 months and a total cessation after 5 months of unsuccessful attempts (i.e. where staff gave up). They all now felt confident to accomplish the task. Though mean stress scores did not decline because L continued to resist, the mean coping score post-intervention reflected significantly increased personal self-efficacy. The hostel manager downgraded the problem from severe to moderate on the problem severity scale.

In this case, the cause of the behaviour was known, but nothing could be done to change it. The task was always likely to be stressful but part of the reason it was a problem was a sense of hopelessness and lack of support for staff. The intervention addressed this. The staff regarded it as a success and they were able to realize their wish of continuing to care for L.

39.3.3.2 CASE 2

P, 84 years, lived in an excellent nursing home. She scored 7 on the MMSE and was graded in the severe range on the CDR. She was referred for barging into other resident's rooms and 'tidying up', including stripping or making beds still occupied by other residents. Fights and confrontations were common. Family history showed that she had always been a busy well-organized person, and somewhat bossy. P was easy to move on in the morning but became increasingly disturbed as the day progressed, physically resisting or directly assaulting staff trying to redirect her. Escalation of her behaviour through the day was put down to 'sundowning', a syndrome like many others in dementia that simply labels a pattern of behaviour but does not explain it. Discussions with staff suggested that, if she could be induced to take a rest in the middle of the day, problems were minimal. Perusal of her medical notes revealed both a hip and knee reconstruction, and later in the day she could clearly be seen grimacing when using the affected leg.

The primary cause of the behaviour therefore was escalating pain, interacting with her premorbid character. However, because of cognitive impairment, it did not occur to P to rest; the worse the pain, the busier the she became. She was only on analgesics 'as required'.

The intervention was systematic pharmacological and psychosocial pain relief. For the psychosocial component we tried a bath in the middle of the day to relax her limbs but this created more problems than it solved because P had strong opinions on when one should be bathed. However, once they understood the cause and what was required, the staff developed their own intervention. This was to place a water chair in the staff room and invite P to their 'meeting' over the 2 hours when they took turns to have lunch. Exhausted, she would quickly fall asleep, often for more than an hour. The behaviour dropped from 8.4 room intrusions daily involving physical confrontation to 2.86 (Figure 39.1b). She was also easier to redirect. We were unable to obtain valid frequency data at 5-month follow up as P was bed-bound at that time and easily manageable but, once she was active again, the problem did not resume. Mean staff stress levels dropped from very high to the middle of the scale and senior staff downgraded problem severity from extreme to mild. There was no movement on the coping measure.

39.3.3.3 CASE 3

K was an 82-year-old woman of non-English speaking background who was causing major problems in a nursing home. She could no longer walk following a severe stroke and also because she had refused all physiotherapy. One member of staff was experiencing symptoms of post-traumatic stress disorder, including nightmares about K, and agency staff refused to come to the nursing home if they had to care for her. Because of language problems, she could not validly be tested with the MMSE. CDR assessment placed her in the mild range of cognitive impairment. She was referred for:

- violent resistance in personal care, especially dangerous because she was a very large woman, and staff had been injured transferring her to the shower trolley;
- pressing the buzzer and calling out hundreds of times a day;
- assaulting staff and other residents;
- refusing to let other residents be in her room, though she was in a shared room;
- having physical fights with her daughters, one at least of whom was in the nursing home from early morning to late at night;
- refusing to be attended by anybody other than the director of nursing or a current favourite;
- family aggressively and frequently demanding that someone do something for their mother.

Staff distress was manifested as fear, resentment and anger, frustration and helplessness. It was caused by a strong sense of duty of care, unawareness of their own rights, lack of knowledge about K, and lack of appreciation of the level of family guilt for not looking after their mother. The behaviour was caused by abdominal pain, anger that she was in the nursing home rather than being cared for by her family, fear in bed-to-commode or shower trolley transfers, feeling that she had lost control of all aspects of her life, family conflict whilst in the nursing home, and, possibly, depression.

The intervention was to, first, hold a meeting at which every staff member attended, including those off-duty, where we allowed them to air their considerable distress in a non-judgemental atmosphere. A consensus decision was taken about the limits of acceptable behaviour. Staff were also given a lot of information about K's remarkable life by two of her daughters, and we facilitated a discussion about how she might be feeling. We held a separate meeting with the family to discuss their concerns, establish rapport, and also to advise them that part of the intervention would involve them paying for a single room.

Thereafter, we devised a programme collaboratively with staff for each feature of her behaviour. For morning care, staff were not to struggle with K. If she resisted they were to make her safe and comfortable, and withdraw showing no anger and promising to come back when she felt better. They practised safe bed transfers with each other, and practised looking and sounding calm even if they did not feel it. When she did finally comply, they were to provide positive reinforcement in the form of effusive thanks and massage after the shower. When she called out and pressed the buzzer repeatedly, it was usually because she was in pain. Staff would go to her three times to relieve the pain as much as possible, then explain on the fourth visit that they could do no more, and would come back at an agreed interval. A staff member was delegated to be K's carer each shift so that the job was rotated. They were given count-down timers to ensure that they did attend her at roughly the agreed time. The buzzer was disconnected but registered on personal pagers carried by staff. K was given regular rather than as-required pain relief, and antidepressants were also tried, though they had no discernable effect. The family were advised that they could only attend between 11.00 and 17.00 hours. This clearly relieved them.

The intervention began formally on a specified day, and staff had access to telephone support for the first week thereafter. This was especially important for the first 2 days when K sat for several hours covered in faeces and urine but refusing to be showered. Figure 39.1c shows that, at 2-month follow up, time devoted to personal care of K had dropped from a mean of 7.3 staff hours a day to 4.8; at 5-month follow up it was 2.2 hours a day. This was still excessive but staff were extremely happy about their achievement. Staff stress associated with K dropped from the maximum to the middle of the scale, and the coping measure showed modest but consistent improvement. Senior staff downgraded problem severity from extreme to moderate. Occasional booster sessions were required for staff but K remained manageable until she died.

Most of this intervention addressed the causes both of staff distress and the behaviour. Putting K in a single room and ensuring that the family were not present when morning and evening care took place reduced factors that significantly exacerbated the problem. K learned that she could trust the staff to come at regular intervals and did not need to continuously press the buzzer or shout, and that it was in any case a waste of time doing so. Control of when she was showered and toileted was returned to her. Staff learned that they were not alone in their feelings about K, and that they did not have to stay when being assaulted and shouted at, so they too were in control of the situation. They learned a lot more about K and were able to see her point of view, and respect her and be less angry. Anger on both sides was further reduced because relations between staff and K improved dramatically. This was partly because staff attended her at timed intervals rather than when they were exasperated or frightened, so they were calmer and interactions were less confrontational. Anger was also reduced by the massage, initially conceived as reinforcement for compliance. It is almost impossible to give or receive massage in an agitated state, and it became an important social interaction between K and staff, where they learned more about each other.

39.4 CONCLUSION

The multifactorial nature of behaviour problems, in aetiology and other contextual variables that determine treatment choice, make the *behaviour syndrome – standard treatment* model completely inappropriate for psychosocial interventions. It is probably not particularly useful for pharmacological approaches either. The development and evaluation of standard techniques, pharmacological and psychosocial, is important but only as a means of adding to the tool-kit from which the health worker can select the most appropriate combination of techniques after holistic assessment – not before it. Unfortunately, both clinical experience and the high rate of inappropriate prescribing for behaviour problems suggests that many clinicians think only of answers, often in a kind of scattergun approach. If enough pellets are fired, something may hit the target.

It is essential to go into a case with a bagful of questions before even beginning to consider what the answer may be. For a given behaviour in a given case, these answers will be selected from an astonishingly diverse range, entirely dependent on the information uncovered by assessment. For a screaming case, for example, the range might include but certainly not be restricted to:

- doing nothing about the behaviour and instead addressing carer issues;
- transferring the patient to a facility sensible enough to have a sound-proof room or installing double-glazing;
- changing rosters so that only certain nurses perform intimate personal care;
- transmitting soothing sounds through headphones;
- engaging a volunteer to sit holding the patient's hand;
- or adjusting medication, for example rationalizing polypharmacy or prescribing antidepressants, analgesics or antipsychotics.

So, psychosocial and pharmacological approaches are not mutually exclusive; both need to form part of the tool-kit.

The relationship between them is not one of competition. According to the conceptualization presented in this chapter, recommendations to always use psychosocial methods first (e.g. Peisah and Brodaty, 1994; Herrmann, 2001) are incorrect, and are in any case infinitely more honoured in the breach than the observance. Studies such as the randomized controlled trial of Teri *et al.* (2000), where antipsychotics, antidepressants, and behavioural treatment were compared for treatment of challenging behaviour, though methodologically sound, are asking the wrong questions. The question is not whether one treatment is superior to the other. The question is: what combination of methods, psychosocial and/or pharmacological, which can realistically be implemented on the ground, will best address the causes of the referred problem – including why it is a problem.

Trials for such a conceptualization, where there is no easily labelled syndrome based on the behaviour and no easily identified standard treatment, require development of methodologies that fit the phenomena. Trials where a standard treatment is applied to a diffuse range of behaviours labelled as 'agitation', though they have merit in adding to the therapeutic tool-kit, may be regarded as an example of making the phenomena fit the methodology.

Results of studies that have grappled with this issue and applied and measured case-specific interventions (e.g. Hinchliffe *et al.*, 1995; Bird *et al.*, 2002; Opie *et al.*, 2002) do, however, beg the question as to why there is such an imbalance in favour of psychopharmacology, in particular antipsychotics. In our trial, we used a predominantly psychosocial approach directed at causality, and obtained equivalent reductions in behaviour and carer/staff distress at no more time per case, and less costs in medications, side effects, and hospitalizations, than a group where treatment was primarily pharmacological and directed at the behaviour (Bird *et al.*, 2002).

Although there has been some decline in antipsychotic use in the USA (Svarstad *et al.*, 2001) following publication of the Beers criteria (Beers, 1997) and legislation to enforce them, the predominant use of antipsychotics for challenging behaviours in dementia continues (e.g. Dhalla *et al.*, 2002; Sloane *et al.*, 2002; van Reekum *et al.*, 2002). This is despite abundant evidence of only moderate efficacy at best, high risks of side effects (e.g. Lanctot *et al.*, 1998; Katona, 2001), and risks of missing pharmacologically treatable causes of behaviour such as pain, infections or depression (Nygaard *et al.*, 1994; Peisah and Brodaty, 1994; Elmståhl *et al.*, 1998; Menon *et al.*, 2001). In some cases, antipsychotics may be the treatment of choice, for example where hallucinations are causing distress and neuroleptic malignant syndrome is not present, or where there is simply no other alternative.

Usually, however, there are alternatives and they are much more likely to be visible when the clinician looks beyond the behaviour to its causes. When there is a focus on causality, psychosocial methods are much more likely to come into play. Unfortunately, despite frequent calls for more research into psychosocial alternatives or adjuncts to psychopharmacology for behaviour problems in dementia (e.g. Teri *et al.*, 2000; Herrmann, 2001; Margallo-Lana *et al.*, 2001), the research effort remains fragmented. It is largely undertaken by a finite number of enthusiasts around the world, largely dependent upon charitable and government grants because, by definition, psychosocial research is never going to be funded by the pharmaceutical industry.

APPENDIX

Examples of psychosocial methods used in a case series (n = 44) where they were the primary modality (Bird *et al.*, 2002). Seventy-five per cent of interventions took place in residential care facilities and, for most cases, several methods were combined:

A. Working primarily with carers/nurses (categories in order of frequency of use)

1) *Changing nursing care practices to fit the problem*
Examples: Increasing sensitivity in intimate personal care; letting patient sleep to natural waking time; not waking patient at night even when wet; structured patient-specific activity at key times; selection of a 'specialized team' for care of certain patients.

2) *Attitude change*
Examples: Presentation of the patient as a person as well as a problem (often includes history and accomplishments); education in the fact that behaviour usually has identifiable causes, and what those causes might be in this particular case; reframing behaviour in the context of the disease.

3) *Education in basic dementia care skills*
Examples: Going with the flow wherever possible and avoiding confrontation and logic; minimizing abrupt or noisy approaches to the patient; 'going slow is quicker'; planning excursions ahead (including location and appropriateness of public toilets), learning to read signs of patient emotional arousal

4) *Changing the physical or social environment (other than changing carer practices)*
Examples: Restricting means to undertake the behaviour; decreasing social interaction at known trouble times (e.g. meals); hiding or restricting access to cues that precipitate the behaviour; music at strategic times.

5) *Support*
Examples: Supportive counselling, cognitive-behavioural therapy, or referral to carer agencies to do this; listening to and validating care staff distress; validation what carers/care staff are already doing; showing carers/care staff that they have rights too.

6) *Others*
Examples: Differential reinforcement (only three stroke-related cases; not normally effective in dementia); personal electronic sensor to alert staff that a patient has wandered; negotiating limits for a family where visits are exacerbating the behaviour.

B. Working with the patient direct

1) *Dealing with physiological precipitants of behaviour*
Examples: Managing physical discomfort (especially pain) more systematically; close monitoring of fluid intake and prompt response to urinary tract infections; reducing patient's alcohol intake.

2) *Using spared memory*
Using spaced retrieval and fading cues to teach patient to associate tangible cues with desired behaviour; having only toilet lit at night and all other doors closed.

3) *Direct negotiation and discussion of issues with patient*
Three cases only of mild impairment, but backed up by simple large-print letter to be read repeatedly by patient and carer and/or large-letter cue cards in strategic places (e.g. back of toilet door).

REFERENCES

Allen-Burge R, Stevens AB, Burgio LD. (1999) Effective behavioural interventions for decreasing dementia-related challenging behavior in nursing homes. *International Journal of Geriatric Psychiatry* **14**: 213–232

Baillon S, Scothern G, Neville PG, Boyle A. (1996) Factors that contribute to stress in care staff in residential homes for the elderly. *International Journal of Geriatric Psychiatry* **11**: 219–226

Ballard CG, O'Brien JT, Reichelt K, Perry EK. (2002) Aromatherapy as a safe and effective treatment for the management of agitation in severe dementia: the results of a double-blind placebo-controlled trial with Melissa. *Journal of Clinical Psychiatry* **63**: 553–558

Baltes MM, Neumann EM, Zank S. (1994) Maintenance and rehabilitation of independence in old age: an intervention program for staff. *Psychology and Aging* **9**: 179–188

Baumgarten M, Becker R, Gauthier S. (1990) Validity and reliability of the Dementia Behaviour Disturbance Scale. *Journal of the American Geriatrics Society* **38**: 221–226

Beers MH. (1997) Explicit criteria for determining potentially inappropriate medication use by the elderly. *Archives of International Medicine* **157**: 1531–1536

Berg A, Hansson UW, Hallberg IR. (1994) Nurses' creativity, tedium and burnout during one year of clinical supervision and implementation of individually planned nursing care: comparisons between a ward for severely demented patients and a similar control ward. *Journal of Advanced Nursing* **20**: 742–749

Bird M. (2001) Behavioural difficulties and cued recall of adaptive behaviour in dementia: experimental and clinical evidence. *Neuropsychological Rehabilitation* **11**: 357–375

Bird M. (2003) Psychiatric and behavioural problems: psychosocial approaches. In: KT Mulligan, M Van der Linden, AC Juillerat (eds), *The Clinical Management of Early Alzheimer's Disease: A Handbook.* Mahwah, New Jersey, Lawrence Erlbaum Associates, pp. 143–168

Bird M, Alexopoulos P, Adamowicz J. (1995) Success and failure in five case studies: use of cued recall to ameliorate behaviour problems in senile dementia. *International Journal of Geriatric Psychiatry* **10**: 5–11

Bird M, Llewellyn-Jones R, Smithers H et al. (1998) Challenging behaviours in dementia: a project at Hornsby/Ku-ring-gai Hospital. *Australian Journal on Ageing* **17**: 10–15

Bird M, Llewellyn-Jones R, Smithers H, Korten A. (2002) *Psychosocial Approaches to Challenging Behaviour in Dementia: A Controlled Trial.* Canberra, Commonwealth Department of Health and Ageing

Bourgeois M, Burgio L, Schulz R *et al.* (1997) Modifying repetitive verbalizations of community-dwelling patients with AD. *The Gerontologist* **37**: 30–39

Bråne G, Karlsson I, Kihlgren M, Norberg A. (1989) Integrity-promoting care of demented nursing home patients: psychological and biochemical changes. *International Journal of Geriatric Psychiatry* **4**: 165–172

Bridges-Parlet S, Knopman D, Thompson T. (1994) A descriptive study of physically aggressive behaviour in dementia by direct observation. *Journal of the American Geriatrics Society* **42**: 192–197

Burgio L, Scilley K, Hardin J *et al.* (1996) Environmental 'White Noise': an intervention for verbally agitated nursing home residents. *Journals of Gerontology: Psychological Sciences* **51B**, P364–P373

Clark ME, Lipe AW, Bilbrey M. (1998) Use of music to decrease aggressive behaviours in people with dementia. *Journal of Gerontological Nursing* **24**: 10–17

Cohen-Mansfield J and Werner P. (1997) Management of verbally disruptive behaviours in nursing home residents. *Journals of Gerontology* **52A**: M369–M377

Cohen-Mansfield J and Werner P. (1999) Longitudinal predictors of non-aggressive agitated behaviours in the elderly. *International Journal of Geriatric Psychiatry* **14**: 831–844

Cohen-Mansfield J, Marx M, Werner P, Freedman L. (1992) Temporal patterns of agitated nursing home residents. *International Psychogeriatrics* **4**: 197–206

Colenda C, Cohen W, McCall W, Rosenquist P. (1997) Photo-therapy for patients with Alzheimer's disease with disturbed sleep patterns: results of a community-based pilot study. *Alzheimer Disease and Associated Disorders* **11**: 175–178

Cummings J, Mega M, Gray K *et al.* (1994) The Neuropsychiatric Inventory: comprehensive assessment of psychopathology in dementia. *Neurology* **44**: 2308–2314

Day K, Carreon D, Stump C. (2000) The therapeutic design of environments for people with dementia: a review of the empirical research. *The Gerontologist* **40**: 397–416

Dhalla IA, Anderson GM, Mamdani MM *et al.* (2002) Inappropriate prescribing before and after nursing home admission. *Journal of the American Geriatrics Society* **50**: 995–1000

Edberg AK and Bird M. (2003) Strain in nursing care of people with dementia from a transcultural perspective. *International Psychogeriatrics* **15** (Suppl. 2): 31–32

Edberg AK, Nordmark Å, Sandgren Å, Hallberg IR. (1995) Initiating and terminating verbal interaction between nurses and severely demented patients regarded as vocally disruptive. *Journal of Psychiatric and Mental Health Nursing* **2**: 159–167

Edberg AK, Hallberg IR, Gustafson L. (1996) Effects of clinical supervision on nurse-patient cooperation quality. *Clinical Nursing Research* **5**: 127–149

Elmståhl S, Stenberg I, Annerstedt L, Ingvad B. (1998) Behavioural disturbances and pharmacological treatment of patients with dementia in family caregiving: a 2-year follow-up. *International Psychogeriatrics* **10**: 239–252

Folstein M, Anthony JC, Parked I *et al.* (1985) The meaning of cognitive impairment in the elderly. *Journal of the American Geriatrics Society* **33**: 228–235

Gerdner L and Swanson E. (1993) Effects of individualized music on confused and agitated elderly patients. *Archives of Psychiatric Nursing* **7**: 284–291

Haffmans PMJ, Sival RC, Lucius SAP *et al.* (2001) Bright light therapy and melatonin in motor restless behaviour in dementia: a placebo-controlled study. *International Journal of Geriatric Psychiatry* **16**: 106–110

Hagen B and Sayers D. (1995) When caring leaves bruises: the effects of staff education on resident aggression. *Journal of Gerontological Nursing* **21**: 7–16

Hallberg IR, Edberg AK, Nordmark Å, Johnsson K. (1993) Daytime vocal activity in institutionalised severely demented patients identified as vocally disruptive by nurses. *International Journal of Geriatric Psychiatry* **8**: 155–164

Hanley I. (1986) Reality orientation in the care of the elderly patient with dementia: three case studies. In: I Hanley and M Gilhooly (eds), *Psychological Therapies for the Elderly.* London, Croom Helm, pp. 65–79

Harvath T. (1994) Interpretation and management of dementia-related behaviour problems. *Clinical Nursing Research* **3**: 7–26

Herrmann N. (2001) Recommendations for the management of behavioural and psychological symptoms of dementia. *Canadian Journal of the Neurological Sciences* **28**: S96–S107

Hinchliffe AC, Hyman IL, Blizard B, Livingston G. (1995) Behavioural complications of dementia – can they be treated? *International Journal of Geriatric Psychiatry* **10**: 839–847

Hussian RA and Brown DC. (1987) Use of a two dimensional grid pattern to limit hazardous ambulation in demented patients. *Journal of Gerontology* **5**: 558–560

Jenkins H and Allen C. (1998) The relationship between staff burnout/distress and interactions with residents in two residential homes for older people. *International Journal of Geriatric Psychiatry* **13**: 466–472

Katona CLE. (2001) Psychotropics and drug interactions in the elderly patient. *International Journal of Geriatric Psychiatry* **16**: S86–S90

Lanctot KL, Best TS, Mittmann N *et al.* (1998) Efficacy and safety of neuroleptics in behavioural disorders associated with dementia. *Journal of Clinical Psychiatry* **59**: 550–561

Levine JM, Marchello V, Totolos E. (1995) Progress toward a restraint-free environment in a large academic nursing facility. *Journal of the American Geriatrics Society* **43**: 914–918

Margallo-Lana M, Swann A, O'Brien J *et al.* (2001) Prevalence and pharmacological management of behavioural and psychological symptoms amongst dementia sufferers living in care environments. *International Journal of Geriatric Psychiatry* **16**: 39–44

Meares S and Draper B. (1999) Treatment of vocally disruptive behaviour of multi-factorial aetiology. *International Journal of Geriatric Psychiatry* **14**: 285–290

Menon AS, Gruber-Baldini AL, Hebel JR *et al.* (2001) Relationship between aggressive behaviours and depression among nursing home residents with dementia. *International Journal of Geriatric Psychiatry* **16**: 139–146

Moniz-Cook E, Woods R, Gardiner E. (2000) Staff factors associated with perception of behaviour as 'challenging' in residential and nursing homes. *Aging and Mental Health* **4**: 48–55

Morris JC. (1993) The Clinical Dementia Rating (CDR): current version and scoring rules. *Neurology* **43**: 2412–2414

Nygaard HA, Brudvik E, Juvik OB *et al.* (1994) Consumption of psychotropic drugs in nursing home residents: a prospective study in patients permanently admitted to a nursing home. *International Journal of Geriatric Psychiatry* **9**: 387–391

Opie J, Rosewarne R, O'Connor DW. (1999) The efficacy of psychosocial approaches to behaviour disorders in dementia: a systematic literature review. *Australian and New Zealand Journal of Psychiatry* **33**: 789–799

Opie J, Doyle C, O'Connor DW. (2002) Challenging behaviours in nursing home residents with dementia: a randomized controlled trial of multidisciplinary interventions. *International Journal of Geriatric Psychiatry* **17**: 6–13

Peisah C and Brodaty H. (1994) Practical guidelines for the treatment of behavioural complications of dementia. *Medical Journal of Australia* **161**: 558–564

Ray W, Taylor J, Meador K *et al.* (1993) Reducing antipsychotic drug use in nursing homes: a controlled trial of provider education. *Archives of Internal Medicine* **22**: 713–721

Reisberg B, Fransson E, Sclan S *et al.* (1989) Stage-specific incidence of potentially remediable behavioral symptoms in aging and Alzheimer's disease: a study of 120 patients using the BEHAV-AD. *Bulletin of Clinical Neurosciences* **54**: 95–112

Rodney V. (2000) Nurse stress associated with aggression in people with dementia: its relationship to hardiness, cognitive appraisal and coping. *Journal of Advanced Nursing* **31**: 172–180

Rogers JC, Holm MB, Burgio LD *et al.* (2000) Excess disability during morning care in nursing home residents with dementia. *International Psychogeriatrics* **12**: 267–282

Rovner B, Steele C, Folstein M. (1996) A randomized trial of dementia care in nursing homes. *Journal of the American Geriatrics Society* **44**: 7–13

Schnelle J, Cruise P, Rahman A, Ouslander J. (1998) Developing rehabilitative behavioral interventions for long-term care: technology transfer, acceptance, and maintenance issues. *Journal of the American Geriatrics Society* **46**: 771–777

Schnelle JF, Alessi CA, Al-Samarrai NR *et al.* (1999) The nursing home at night: effects of an intervention on noise, light and sleep. *Journal of the American Geriatrics Society* **47**: 430–438

Sloane PD, Zimmerman SI, Brown LC *et al.* (2002) Inappropriate medication prescribing in residential care/assisted living facilities. *Journal of the American Geriatrics Society* **20**: 1001–1011

Svarstad BL, Mount JK, Bigelow W. (2001) Variations in the treatment culture of nursing homes and responses to regulations to reduce drug use. *Psychiatric Services* **52**: 666–672

Teri L. (1994) Behavioral treatment of depression in patients with dementia. *Alzheimer Disease and Associated Disorders* **8**: 66–74

Teri L. (1997) Behavior and caregiver burden: behavioral problems in patients with Alzheimer disease and its association with caregiver distress. *Alzheimer Disease and Associated Disorders* **11**: S35–S38

Teri L. (1999) Training families to provide care: effects on people with dementia. *International Journal of Geriatric Psychiatry* **14**: 110–119

Teri L, Logsdon RG, Peskind E *et al.* (2000) Treatment of agitation in AD. *Neurology* **55**: 1271–1278

Tsai S-J, Hwang J-P, Yang C-H, Liu K-M. (1996) Physical aggression and associated factors in probable Alzheimer disease. *Alzheimer Disease and Associated Disorders* **10**: 82–85

van Reekum R, Clarke D, Conn D *et al.* (2002) A randomized, placebo-controlled trial of the discontinuation of long-term antipsychotics in dementia. *International Psychogeriatrics* **14**: 197–210

Woods B and Bird M. (1998) Non-pharmacological approaches to treatment. In: G Wilcock, R Bucks, K Rockwood (eds), *Diagnosis and Management of Dementia: A Manual for Memory Disorders Teams.* Oxford, Oxford University Press, pp. 311–331

Woods P and Ashley J. (1995) Stimulated presence therapy: using selected memories to manage problem behaviours in Alzheimer's disease patients. *Geriatric Nursing* **16**: 9–14

Wystanski M. (2000) Assaultive behaviour in psychiatrically hospitalized elderly: a response to psychosocial stimulation and changes in pharmacotherapy. *International Journal of Geriatric Psychiatry* **15**: 582–585

40

Psychological approaches for the management of cognitive impairment in Alzheimer's disease

ANNE UNKENSTEIN

There is currently no curative medical treatment available to reverse the cognitive impairment that occurs in Alzheimer's disease (AD). A psychological approach aims to promote the best possible quality of life for both people with AD and their carers, by offering positive, individualized and effective management. With the growing emphasis on early diagnosis of dementia, there are increasing opportunities to provide psychological interventions from the earliest stages of AD. This chapter outlines factors influencing the choice of practical management strategies, discusses assessment and feedback and describes specific techniques for managing cognitive impairment in the early, middle and late stages of AD.

40.1 FACTORS INFLUENCING MANAGEMENT OF COGNITIVE IMPAIRMENT IN ALZHEIMER'S DISEASE

Each person who has AD is unique. The way the person presents results from a complex interaction of brain disease, personality, biography, health and social psychology (Kitwood, 1993). Each person needs to be treated as an individual. An approach that might prove successful for one person may prove ineffective for another (Woods and Bird, 1999). There is no single correct approach to the management of cognitive impairment in AD. The help that is relevant can vary considerably.

There is a great deal of variation in cognitive function in AD according to the stage of dementia and different patterns of brain pathology. AD does not necessarily imply global impairment of brain function. There will nearly always be some retained abilities. It is important to identify these cognitive strengths and use them positively. Interventions can draw on retained skills in order to bypass weaknesses.

Cognitive impairment is just one aspect of AD. People with this disease also experience changes in behaviour, emotional control, personality and self-care. These changes need to be taken into account when working on strategies for cognitive impairment. A team approach with agreement about realistic goals and consistent strategies is recommended. Carers need to be included in management planning. Wherever the person with AD lives, carers will be involved. They may be relatives, friends, neighbours or health professionals.

Not all of the person's symptoms are directly due to brain disease. People with AD are very sensitive to their physical and psychological environment. The first diagnosis of dementia is often made when a person experiences a change to his/her usual environment such as the death of a spouse or moving to a new house. It is important to be aware of environmental factors that can be altered in order to enhance cognitive function.

Health factors can exacerbate any cognitive impairment. Sensory impairment, especially of vision and hearing, can adversely affect cognitive function. People with AD commonly experience anxiety, distress and depression. Confusion can also be increased during acute or chronic illness and with any physical discomfort or pain. Alcohol, some medications and fatigue may cause transient exaggeration of cognitive impairment (Robinson et al., 2001). It is necessary to be alert to any superimposed health problems and to control these to help people maintain maximum function.

Progressive decline in cognitive function is characteristic of AD. Management strategies need to be flexible and adapted over time. Assessment at regular intervals will allow for the development of realistic expectations. The aim of any strategies employed is to maintain as high a level of function as possible by helping the individual to better utilize remaining function.

40.2 ASSESSMENT

A thorough assessment is required in order to design an individualized approach to management of cognitive impairment. This should include assessment of the person's medical and psychological status and assessment of cognition. Assessment of the person's health is important, as there may be additional treatable medical conditions.

It is beneficial to interview the carers to gain information about the person's personality, interests, home environment and the history of events leading up to the assessment. Information about strategies that the carers have already tried and their willingness to provide support can also be gathered.

A neuropsychological assessment provides a basis for individual intervention. It allows for a focus on strengths by outlining abilities that remain unaffected, and also outlines areas of cognitive impairment to be managed. Serial neuropsychological assessment can be used to monitor progression of symptoms over time. It can provide an objective viewpoint to the carers and to the person with AD with regard to the progression of symptoms. Part of the assessment is to check the attitude of the person to their symptoms, as this will influence choice of strategies.

The assessment phase will identify the problem but it is important to go beyond this phase for better management of cognitive impairment. It is beneficial to share the information gathered with the person with AD and the carers.

40.3 FEEDBACK

A feedback session following assessment can serve many purposes. It provides information about how the disease is affecting various aspects of cognitive function in order to improve understanding. Whilst it is important to acknowledge areas of loss, a positive approach can be maintained by highlighting what the person can still do.

The carers are often the people who provide ongoing management of the person with cognitive impairment. Feedback can empower carers by acknowledging the success they have had with strategies that they have already tried. It can also provide emotional support and practical help and assistance. Carers can access a great deal of general information about AD (e.g. Tappen 1997; Kuhn 2003). However, specific information that is more relevant to their particular situation can be provided in a feedback session.

Feedback can be given to carers alone or including the person with dementia where appropriate. A description of the person's cognitive strengths and weaknesses is given. This information is then used to help carers make sense of behaviour that otherwise would seem to suggest that the person is purposefully being annoying. For example, by outlining the different types of memory and how each is affected, it becomes easier to understand why a person can recall information from their remote past but not what was said two minutes ago. Furthermore, if carers know that the person has memory impairment they are more likely to understand why the person persistently repeats the same question or forgets to pass on a phone message. It can be reinforced that this is not something that is done deliberately. Behaviour is thus reinterpreted as related to brain disease and not purposeful or intended. This information is also useful when it comes to management of cognitive impairment. For example, if carers know that forgetfulness is due to memory loss from brain disease they are more likely to understand that the person is unlikely to learn by repetition. They are also more likely to use strategies that avoid reliance on intact memory ability.

A feedback session offers an opportunity to ask the person with dementia and the carers how the cognitive problems manifest themselves in everyday life. This information can be used to make strategies realistic and relevant to the life of the person with dementia (Wilson, 1995).

A written reminder of what was discussed during the feedback session can be useful. Both the person with dementia and the carers may forget what was discussed, especially if they are just coming to terms with the diagnosis.

An initial discussion of strategies to help manage cognitive impairment can be included in a feedback session. The types of strategies employed will vary according to the person's individual situation and the stage of AD.

40.4 EARLY STAGE – MEMORY STRATEGIES

In early stage AD the most significant cognitive impairment is in memory function. Impairment of new learning is most prominent, including acquisition and retention of new information. At this stage, people with AD may forget what you have just told them, forget where they have put something, repeat the same thing as if they haven't said it before or have difficulty learning how to use something new.

At this stage the person often remains aware of cognitive losses and may be motivated to seek methods to compensate for them. The person is usually living in the family home. Initial strategies therefore focus on the individual with increasing involvement of family carers over time. The aim is to maintain as much independence as possible. Family members and friends need to avoid taking over responsibilities too soon.

Many of the strategies that are used by people experiencing normal memory change with ageing are useful at this stage (see Sargeant and Unkenstein, 2001, for a detailed description of memory strategies). It is important to ask people whether they are already using any memory aids before explaining the use of memory strategies. People should be encouraged to draw on strategies that they have used in the past. They will be more likely to use strategies if they are already familiar with them (Kotler-Cope and Camp, 1990). Everyone has different preferences. For instance, some people like to use diaries whilst others prefer a noticeboard.

People need not just one technique, but a whole range of strategies. It is important to find out the typical things a person tends to forget and work out some strategies that will suit these specific situations and be usable for that person. Strategy use will vary according to differing interests, lifestyles and home environments. A home visit is sometimes useful to help tailor strategies to particular situations.

The emphasis is on practical compensatory techniques rather than attempting to restore lost cognitive function by direct retraining. People with early AD and their relatives and friends often ask if repetitive practice is helpful. Attempting to reteach lost skills can unnecessarily confront the person with an experience of repeated failure and there is no evidence that specific training improves memory in general (Bird, 2000).

A more practical approach is to avoid challenging the person's lost memory function. For example, rather than asking a question that relies on intact memory function such as 'What show did you watch on television last night?', rephrase the question to 'Did you enjoy the show that you watched last night?' If people become repetitious it may be best to try distracting them with another topic of conversation. Enhancing familiarity is also beneficial. Developing a regular routine and doing things at a set time of the day or week will reduce the load on memory.

Memory strategies can be thought of as internal or external. Internal strategies involve some form of internal mental manipulation, for example, mentally retracing one's steps to remember where an object was left. External strategies involve using some sort of external aid, for example a note pad for writing a list, or a diary. They can also involve making changes to the environment, for instance, having designated locations in which to store particular items.

Internal strategies focus on enhancing encoding and retrieval processes. The emphasis is on making more efficient use of current cognitive capacity. A motivated individual may employ simple internal strategies in the early stage of AD. These strategies typically involve one of three main features: focusing attention, adding meaning to the information to be remembered, or reducing the amount of information to be remembered. Simple internal strategies such as ensuring understanding, associating new information with information that is known well and visualization may be useful for motivated individuals in the earliest stages of AD.

Internal strategies or mnemonic techniques can also be quite complex. Well known mnemonic techniques include the method of loci and peg word systems. These techniques require training and considerable remaining cognitive capacity including new learning and motivation for success.

Even in the early stage of AD, people usually do not have the motivation or learning ability required to use these techniques (Camp and McKitrick, 1992). More recently, researchers have investigated the use of other learning methods for those with AD. With specific training techniques it has been shown that people with AD can learn new information under certain conditions. See De Vreese et al. (2001) and Grandmaison and Simard (2003) for a review of the efficacy of memory stimulation in AD.

External strategies aim to compensate for memory impairment by reducing the demand on a person's memory. They are generally easier to use and more suitable for everyday remembering than internal strategies. They may involve written reminders, storage of objects in specially designated places, technical memory devices and reminders from other people.

Written reminders assist with remembering locations of objects, a task that has to be done, appointments, shopping items, messages, names and instructions. Calendars, diaries, notebooks, notepads, noticeboards, sticky notes and computers are all useful. Having a pen or pencil attached reduces the load on memory even further. Such written aids should not only be readily visible and accessible but should also be in close proximity to the to-be-remembered activity. For example, a shopping list pad on refrigerator door, or instructions for how to operate a piece of equipment permanently displayed on that equipment.

External memory strategies can assist with orientation in early stage AD. It is helpful to mark off the days as they pass on a calendar, or use a flip-top desk calendar and turn each day over as it passes. Newspapers can also serve as prompts. Clocks should be positioned in places where they are readily seen and ideally should have day and date built in.

Storing objects in specially designated places can help with remembering the location of objects, a task that has to be done or something to be taken out. For example, keys can be stored near the front door of the house. This makes it easy to pick up the keys when leaving the house and to get into the habit of putting them back when returning.

Leaving objects in visible locations can act as a reminder to do something. Medications can be left somewhere obvious in the kitchen if they are to be taken with meals. A special place near the front door, such as a hall table, can be used to put objects that are to be taken out with a person.

A useful storage device for managing medications is a dosette box. The box is divided into compartments that relate to the day of the week or time of the day into which a set number of tablets can be placed. The box has to be filled at weekly or other intervals, but it is simple to use and lets people know whether they have taken the necessary tablets.

Basic alarms are useful to help people remember something they have to do. A common example is an oven timer used as a reminder to turn the oven off. Many household objects have built in memory aids. For instance, many telephones have a system that enables storage of frequently used numbers that can then be dialled by pressing only one appropriately labelled button. Automatic shut-off devices on electrical and gas appliances, such as stovetops, kettles or lights can be installed. These devices will turn the power off after a period of time if the appliances are left on accidentally. More complex electronic memory aids can be useful for motivated and insightful individuals but may require training to know how to operate them. They usually rely on other cognitive processes remaining intact and may not suit the person with even early AD.

Reminders from other people can provide an excellent memory back-up system. Family members can provide telephone reminders or leave notes in a regular and prominent location. Reminders need to be specific. For example, a note saying 'back in 5 minutes' does not provide enough information. The person with AD needs to know at what time the person will return (Twining, 1991).

40.5 MIDDLE STAGE – WORKING WITH CARERS

In middle stage AD people experience increasing memory loss, language difficulties and specific disorders such as apraxia. They may be unable to function independently outside the home and require increasing assistance with tasks of personal care. They could be living in their own home or supported accommodation. By this stage the person's insight into their cognitive losses usually has diminished.

With little awareness of their difficulties and increased cognitive impairment, it becomes difficult to work on strategies with the person with AD alone. The management of cognitive impairment therefore becomes focused on working in collaboration with family members or other carers. Carers know the person best and often come up with strategies that work well for that person. Carers can provide reminders for the person, encourage the person to use external memory aids and make appropriate changes to the environment. Without this assistance the person is unlikely to make use of memory strategies. By this stage strategies for other areas of cognitive impairment are also required. Providing support and information to the carers can help to further tailor strategies to make them suit the individual's current cognitive strengths and weaknesses.

Carers will need to become increasingly involved in the use of external memory strategies and can assist with setting up a designated 'memory centre' in a visible location in the home environment (Sargeant and Unkenstein, 2001). Here the carer could hang a whiteboard on which the day, date and daily schedule is written or a clock with the day and date on it. A pin board next to this can be used to display other important information. The carer may need to keep reminding the person to check the memory centre. Carers can also develop 'communication books'. For this a notebook is left in a special location where visitors can write messages. The person can be encouraged to check this book regularly as a reminder of who has visited recently.

These strategies are a form of reality orientation, an approach that emphasizes the use of external cues and structures to assist the person in maintaining contact with the environment (see Woods, 2002 and Spector *et al.*, 2000a for a review of reality orientation). An individual approach to reality orientation is required. Carers can help identify to which realities the person needs or desires to be oriented.

Carers can continue to encourage a regular routine of familiar activities. Sudden unexplained changes or unfamiliar activities could cause the person distress (Tappen, 1997). Carers can help the person focus on activities that are familiar and based on previous interests, such as gardening, walking the dog or other household tasks. Drawing on the continued strength of procedural and lifetime memories can provide meaningful activity. Carers at accommodation facilities can find out about the person's past likes, dislikes, lifestyle and life interests from family members. This information and any old photos available can be recorded in a book that can be used as a cue for discussion and reminiscence (see Spector *et al.*, 2000b for a review of reminiscence).

A familiar environment will reduce the demand on the person's memory. Unnecessary changes such as rearranging furniture should be avoided. If changes have to be made, they should be introduced slowly, with explanation.

Carers may need assistance with strategies for other areas of cognitive impairment. For example, the person at this stage may experience apraxia, an inability to carry out routine patterns of voluntary movement. A common problem caused by apraxia is difficulty with dressing. Helping the carer to understand that a person can sometimes dress automatically, but has difficulty when the movement comes under conscious control is useful. To remove the degree of voluntary focus from the action, avoid giving the person direct instructions about performing the task. Specific techniques include distracting the person's attention from the task, imitation, laying the clothes out in the order in which the person likes to put them on and giving reassurance and praise for each successful step. See Holden (1995) for strategies for other specific cognitive disorders.

40.6 LATER STAGE – ENVIRONMENTAL ADAPTATION

In the later stages of AD people experience marked confusion and widespread cognitive disturbance. Most people with this stage of AD are living in supported accommodation with professional carers. Strategies for management of cognitive impairment need to be focused more heavily on the environment in which the person is living. Adaptations are made to the environment rather than expecting the individual to change. Visiting the person's residence allows one to observe environmental cues, how they might best be used and/or changed and how new ones might be introduced (Kapur, 1995).

At this stage people become dependent on their environment to support them. Making adaptations to the environment can enhance people's feelings of security and help them cope with their confusion and disorientation. When people first move into a new residence there is often a settling in period. An unfamiliar and new environment can increase confusion. It helps to make the environment as familiar as possible. Familiar possessions, such as photos, objects and furniture can be put in the person's room.

A routine and daily timetable should be emphasized. Orientation information or cues can lessen confusion. For example, having access to a window helps a person to tell the time of the day and the weather. A good sensory environment with adequate light is important. Making each part of a large place unique in some way is useful for orientation to the environment. Colour and furniture can highlight difference. Smaller spaces are less confusing than large.

Clear labelling throughout the accommodation facility can further lessen confusion. Direction can be marked on the floor or walls with coloured lines or arrows. Individual rooms can be clearly labelled. Large uppercase print with black against white is often best for older people (Kapur, 1995). Pictures may be more easily understood than written labels. For example, a picture of a toilet on the toilet doors. Carers can wear name badges, with their first name only, that are large enough to read. People will require continued instruction as to how to use these orientation aids.

To maximize cognitive function it helps to simplify the environment to avoid the person becoming overwhelmed. If there is excessive stimulation then confusion may be exacerbated. It helps to remove distractions, keep noise levels down and not have too many people around (Robinson *et al.*, 2001).

It is often difficult to communicate with the individual with this stage of dementia. Using an empathic, validating approach that displays respect and sensitivity to feelings can help to ensure understanding.

40.7   CONCLUSION

Better management of cognitive impairment in AD using a psychological approach is just one part of the challenge to maintain maximum function throughout the course of the illness (Kitwood, 1993). For any symptom of the disease, the first step involves investigating what may be causing the person to present in that particular way. Multidisciplinary assessment will establish whether there are any environmental factors that can be altered or health factors that can be treated in order to enhance the individual's function. Effective management strategies that are relevant to the stage of AD and other individual variables can be developed using a collaborative approach involving the person with dementia, carers and health professionals.

REFERENCES

Bird M. (2000) Psychosocial rehabilitation for problems arising from cognitive deficits in dementia. In: RD Hill *et al. Cognitive Rehabilitation in Old Age.* Oxford, Oxford University Press, pp. 249–269

Camp CJ and McKitrick LA. (1992) Memory interventions in Alzheimer-type dementia populations: methodological and theoretical issues. In: RL West and JD Sinnott (eds), *Everyday Memory and Ageing: Current Issues, Research and Methodology.* New York, Prager, pp. 155–172

De Vreese LP, Neri M, Fioravanti M, Belloi L, Zanetti O. (2001) Memory and rehabilitation in Alzheimer's disease: a review of progress. *International Journal of Geriatric Psychiatry* 16: 794–809

Grandmaison E and Simard M. (2003) A critical review of memory stimulation programs in Alzheimer's disease. *Journal of Neuropsychiatry and Clinical Neuroscience* 15: 130–144

Holden U. (1995) *Ageing, Neuropsychology and the 'New' Dementias.* London, Chapman and Hall

Kapur N. (1995) Memory aids in the rehabilitation of memory disordered patients. In: AD Baddeley, BA Wilson, FN Watts (eds), *Handbook of Memory Disorders.* Chichester, John Wiley and Sons Ltd, pp. 533–556

Kitwood T. (1993) Person and process in dementia. *International Journal of Geriatric Psychiatry* 8: 541–545

Kotler-Cope S and Camp CJ. (1990) Memory interventions in aging populations. In: E Lovelace (ed.), *Aging and Cognition: Mental Processes, Self-awareness and Interventions.* North Holland, Elsevier Science Publications, pp. 231–261

Kuhn D. (2003) *Alzheimer's Early Stages: First Steps for Family, Friends and Caregivers.* Alameda, CA, Hunter House

Robinson A, Spencer B, White L. (2001) *Understanding Difficult Behaviours. Some Practical Suggestions for Coping with Alzheimer's Disease and Related Illnesses.* Ann Arbor, MI, The Alzheimer's Program, Eastern Michigan University

Sargeant D and Unkenstein A. (2001) *Remembering Well: How Memory Works and What to Do When it Doesn't.* St Leonards, NSW, Allen and Unwin

Spector A, Orrell M, Davies S, Woods B. (2000a) Reality orientation for dementia (Cochrane Review). In: *The Cochrane Library,* Issue 2. Oxford, Update Software.

Spector A, Orrell M, Davies S, Woods B. (2000b) Reminiscence therapy for dementia (Cochrane Review). In: *The Cochrane Library,* Issue 2. Oxford, Update Software.

Tappen RM. (1997) *Interventions for Alzheimer's Disease: A Caregivers Complete Reference.* Baltimore, Health Professions Press, Inc

Twining C. (1991) *The Memory Handbook: A Practical Guide to Understanding and Managing Early Dementia.* Bicester, Winslow Press

Wilson BA. (1995) Management and remediation of memory problems in brain-injured adults. In: AD Baddeley, BA Wilson, FN Watts (eds), *Handbook of Memory Disorders.* Chichester, John Wiley and Sons Ltd, pp. 451–479

Woods B. (2002) Reality orientation: a welcome return? *Age and Ageing* 31: 155–156

Woods B and Bird M. (1999) Non-pharmacological approaches to treatment. In: G Wilcock, R Bucks, K Rockwood (eds), *Diagnosis and Management of Dementia: a Manual for Memory Disorders Teams.* Oxford, Oxford University Press, pp. 311–331

41

Prevention of Alzheimer's disease

NITIN B PURANDARE, CLIVE BALLARD AND ALISTAIR BURNS

Primary prevention of Alzheimer's disease (AD) is the ultimate goal of therapeutic intervention. The prevalence of dementia would be reduced by 50 per cent if risk reduction strategies were successful in delaying the onset of dementia by 5 years (Jorm et al., 1987). Our selective review focuses on four key areas that are particularly amenable to therapeutic intervention: control of risk factors for cerebrovascular disease, anti-inflammatory drugs, anti-oxidants, and increasing functional neuronal capacity.

41.1 CONTROL OF RISK FACTORS FOR CEREBROVASCULAR DISEASE

41.1.1 Hypertension

41.1.1.1 EPIDEMIOLOGICAL EVIDENCE

Epidemiological studies have established hypertension in mid-life (systolic and diastolic) as a risk factor for AD and vascular dementia (VaD) in later life (Guo et al., 2001; Peila et al., 2001, Murray et al., 2002). The Honolulu Asia Aging Study (HAAS) followed over 3500 Japanese-American men over 25 years, and found hypertension to increase the risk of dementia by 4–5-fold in those who were never treated with antihypertensives. The risk was greatest in those with systolic hypertension and apolipoprotein E (ApoE) ε4-allele after controlling for other risk factors (odds ratio, OR = 13.0) (Peila et al., 2001). In HAAS the OR for dementia in patients with systolic hypertension and ApoE ε4 decreased from 13.0 to 1.9 in those receiving antihypertensives. Murray et al. (2002) followed 1900 African-Americans over 5 years and found use of antihypertensives to be associated with 38 per cent (OR = 0.62) reduction in incident AD and VaD.

41.1.1.2 RANDOMIZED CONTROLLED TRIALS

Six randomized controlled trials (RCTs) of antihypertensives have been published with cognition and or dementia as one of the outcomes (see Table 41.1). Earlier trials using diuretics or beta-blockers did not demonstrate a lower risk of incident dementia (Applegate et al., 1994; Prince et al., 1996). The results of more recent trials using calcium channel blockers (Syst-Eur trial: Forette et al., 1998 and 2002) or angiotensin-converting enzyme (ACE) inhibitors (HOPE trial: Bosch et al., 2002; PROGRESS trial: Tzourio et al., 2003) have been mixed but more encouraging. The Syst-Eur trial (Forette et al., 1998) reported that nitrendipine (calcium channel blocker) reduced the risk of AD by 50 per cent over 2 years. The PROGRESS (2003) trial, which included both normotensive and hypertensive patients with previous history of cerebrovascular disease, found a significant reduction in stroke related dementia in patients treated with perindopril (ACE inhibitor) as the main antihypertensive. The SCOPE trial (Lithell et al., 2003) included a much older (70–89 years) patient group and excluded those with stroke or myocardial infarction in previous 6 months. Candesartan (angiotensin II type 1 [AT1] receptor blocker) was not found to have any positive effect on progression of cognitive impairment over 3.7 years. However, antihypertensives were used in 84 per cent of the controls and the mean blood pressure difference achieved between active and placebo groups was very small.

The statistical power of these studies is limited by the low incident risk of dementia in these studies because of the young age and modest study durations. In all RCTs, incident dementia has been a secondary outcome, heart disease or stroke being the primary outcomes, and generally brief assessment instruments lacking sensitivity to subtle changes have been employed. Also, epidemiological evidence suggests that the time lapse between diagnosis of hypertension and

Table 41.1 *Effect of antihypertensive treatment on cognitive function and dementia*

Randomized controlled trials	Sample size	Participants (characteristics, age in years)	Duration	Treatment	Impact on dementia or cognition
Forette et al., 1998 (Syst-Eur)	2418	>60 systolic hypertension	2 years	Nitrendipine	50% reduction in the incidence of dementia (7.7 to 3.8 cases per 1000 patient-years, $P = 0.05$)
Forette et al., 2002 (Extended follow-up of Syst-Eur)	2902	>60 systolic hypertension	3.9 years	Nitrendipine, enalapril maleate, hydrochlorothiazide	55% reduction in the risk of dementia (7.4 to 3.3 cases per 1000 patient-years, $P < 0.001$)
Applegate et al., 1994 (Systolic Hypertension in the Elderly)	2034	>60 systolic hypertension	5 years	Chlorthalidone	No significant impact of cognition or incident dementia
Prince et al., 1996 (MRC Older people with HT)	2584	65–74 systolic BP: 160–209 mmHg	4.5 years	Atenolol, hydrochlorothiazide amiloride	No significant impact on cognition or incident dementia
Bosch et al., 2002 (HOPE)	9297	>55 left ventricular dysfunction	4.5 years	Ramipril, vitamin E	Significantly better outcome with respect to cognition and function
The PROGRESS Collaborative Group (Tzourio et al., 2003)	6105	mean age 64; stroke or TIA with and without hypertension	4 years	Perindopril, indapamide	Significant reduction in cognitive decline and incident dementia associated with recurrent stroke
Lithell et al., 2003 (SCOPE)	4964	70–89 systolic and or diastolic hypertension	3.7 years	Candesartan (antihypertensive used in 84% of controls)	No difference on progression of cognitive impairment

onset of dementia can be over 15 years, and it is not known whether the protective effect of starting antihypertensives on incident dementia extends throughout this period.

The treatment issues may be slightly different in established VaD. One study has indicated that maintaining systolic blood pressure (BP) within upper limits of normal (135–150 mmHg) was more beneficial in preserving cognitive functions than reducing systolic BP below this level (Meyer et al., 1986). Another issue which needs further clarification is whether the risk reduction is related to actual reduction in the BP and/or some other neuroprotective action of the individual hypertensive, such as calcium channel antagonists, ACE inhibitors or AT1 receptor blockers. In animal studies, angiotensin II has been shown to inhibit acetylcholine release while AT1 receptor blockers improve cognitive performance (Barnes et al., 1989; Fogari et al., 2003).

41.1.2 Hypercholesterolaemia

41.1.2.1 BIOLOGICAL BASIS FOR IMPORTANCE IN PREVENTION OF AD

Hypercholesterolaemia, especially increased low density lipoproteins, is a known risk factor for coronary heart disease, atherosclerosis and stroke, which are all associated with increased risk of dementia. The ApoE ε4 allele affects stabilization of membrane lipoproteins and is a risk factor for hypercholesterolaemia, as well as AD. Lowering of cholesterol promotes the non-amyloidogenic α-secretase pathway (Kojro et al., 2001). Statins reduce cholesterol levels by inhibiting the enzyme 3-hydroxy-3-methylglutaryl coenzyme A (HMG-CoA). In addition, statins have an antioxidant action, they decrease pro-inflammatory process and improve cerebral blood flow. Lovastatin was shown to reduce amyloid beta protein 42 ($A\beta_{42}$) in cultured hippocampal neurones (Simons et al., 1998) and simvastatin had a similar effect in cerebrospinal fluid (CSF) and brain tissue of guineapigs (Fassbender et al., 2001).

41.1.2.2 CLINICAL EVIDENCE

A number of case–control and epidemiological studies have reported hypercholesterolaemia as a risk factor for dementia, including AD. For example, Moroney et al. (1999) followed over 2000 older people in New York City over 2 years and found those with cholesterol levels in the highest quartile to be at increased risk of dementia, especially VaD (OR = 3–4) compared with those in the lowest quartile. A similar sized study but with much longer follow up (21 years), from eastern Finland, reported that raised cholesterol in mid life

(>6.5 mmol/L) to more than double the risk of dementia, including AD, independently of other risk factors such as hypertension and ApoE ε4 (Kivipelto et al., 2002).

There are some important inconsistencies in the epidemiological evidence. For example, some studies have found risk reduction with lipid lowering agents (LLAs) in general, while others suggest the risk reduction to be more specifically associated with use of statins. A recent meta-analysis of seven observational studies indicated risk reduction in cognitive impairment to be significant for only statins (OR = 0.43) and not other LLAs (Etminan et al., 2003). Other inconsistencies may relate to differential effect in certain age groups (statins and lower risk of AD in those <80 years, Rockwood et al., 2002) and specific actions of individual statins. For example, simvastatin acts directly on processing of amyloid precursor protein (APP) by inhibiting both α- and β-secretase (Sjogren et al., 2003).

The results of intervention trials, with cognition as one of the many secondary outcomes, have been disappointing. MRC/BHF Heart Protection Study (Heart Protection Study Collaborative Group, 2002), comparing simvastatin versus placebo, found simvastatin to reduce the risk of major vascular events by one-third. The study examined a potential effect on cognition using a modification of the Telephone Interview for Cognitive Status (TICS). There was no difference between two groups in either proportion of patients scoring below the cut-off of 22 out of 39 or in the mean TICS score. The PROSPER study (Shepherd et al., 2002), an RCT of pravastatin (n = 2891) versus placebo (n = 2913) over 3 years, found pravastatin to significantly reduce mortality from coronary disease but to have no effect on cognition. The statistical power of both studies was limited by the low incident dementia in study subjects (0.3 per cent in active or placebo group in the Heart Protection Study).

41.1.3 Elevated homocysteine

Plasma or serum homocysteine, or total homocysteine (tHcy), refers to the sum of the sulfhydryl amino acid homocysteine and the homocysteinyl moieties of the disulfides homocysteine and homocystein-cysteine, whether free or bound to plasma proteins. A number of factors such as age, diet, vitamin B_{12} and folate, plasma albumin, use of diuretics and renal function influence homocysteine levels in the blood. Elevated tHcy may lead to an excessive production of homocysteic acid and cysteine sulfinic acid, which act as endogenous agonists of NMDA receptors. In addition to this excitotoxic effect, homocysteine is also known to cause damage to vascular endothelium.

41.1.3.1 PREVALENCE AND IMPORTANCE IN CVD

Elevated tHcy is found in 61 per cent of hospitalized older patients (Ventura et al., 2001). Gottfries et al. (2001) identified elevated tHcy in 31 per cent of patients with mild cognitive impairment (MCI), 45 per cent of patients with AD, and 62 per cent of patients with VaD. Elevated tHcy is known to increase the risk of coronary artery disease, peripheral vascular

disease, and cerebrovascular disease. Elevated tHcy is also associated with increased risk of silent brain infarcts and white matter lesions (Vermeer et al., 2002). A case–control study from Northern Ireland, reported moderately high tHcy levels to be associated with stroke, VaD and AD, independent of vascular risk factors and nutritional status (McIlroy et al., 2002). A meta-analysis from Homocysteine Studies Collaboration group (2002), which included individual participant data from 30 prospective or retrospective studies, indicated that after adjusting for known cardiovascular risk factors low tHcy levels (3.0 ± 0.41 μmol/L) were associated with 11 per cent lower risk of ischaemic heart disease and 19 per cent lower risk of stroke.

41.1.3.2 ROLE IN COGNITION AND AD

In older people without dementia, elevated tHcy is associated with more subtle cognitive impairment. Dufouil et al. (2003) followed up 1241 subjects aged 61–73 years over 4 years and found higher concentrations of tHcy to be associated with poor performance on all neuropsychological tests with the odds of cognitive decline 2.8-fold ($P < 0.05$) higher in subjects with tHcy levels above 15 μmol/L compared with those with levels below 10 μmol/L. Fasting tHcy levels were shown to predict cognitive decline in a follow-up study of 32 healthy elderly people over 5 years ($P < 0.001$), especially word recall, orientation and special copying skills (McCaddon et al., 2001). Case–control studies have shown elevated tHcy to be associated with AD after adjusting for age, sex, nutritional status and ApoE ε4 allele (Clarke et al., 1998). A large epidemiological study in Framingham, USA, involving 1092 older residents in the community (mean age 76 years, median follow up 8 years) reported that the risk of AD nearly doubled (relative risk, RR 1.8; confidence intervals, CI 1.3–2.5) with one standard deviation increase in tHcy levels at baseline (Seshadri et al., 2002).

41.1.3.3 CAN LOWERING HOMOCYSTEINE PREVENT COGNITIVE DECLINE?

Although elevated tHcy has been shown to be associated with cognitive impairment in AD, the effect of reducing homocysteine levels on cognition and global functioning has not been adequately investigated. In a small prospective study involving 33 patients, Nilsson et al. (2001) reported an improvement in cognitive function after 2 months of cobalamine (B_{12}) and folate treatment in individuals with mild to moderate dementia who had elevated tHcy. Patients with severe dementia and those who had normal tHcy did not, however, show clinical improvement.

Intervention trials to lower homocysteine levels need to consider three things:

- first, whether to target people with tHcy levels in the highest quartile of local population or use an arbitrary cut-off of such as >15 μmol/L;
- second, the best treatment combination to lower tHcy from various forms of B_{12} and folate needs to be

determined, also considering merits of additional nutrients such as n-acetyl cysteine;

- third, a better understanding is required of factors affecting tHcy levels and their response to vitamin supplementation. Age, plasma albumin, use of diuretics and renal function are just some of them (Ventura et al., 2001).

C677T mutation of methylenetetrahydrofolate reductase (MTHFR) gene, present in about one-fifth of people with AD, may be yet another important factor that affecting treatment response. MTHFR acts as a methyl donor for homocysteine methylation and hence reduces homocysteine levels. C677T mutation is common in the Caucasian population (30 per cent), which results in lower MTHFR activity and elevated tHcy (Bottiglieri et al., 2001; Frosst et al., 1995).

41.1.4 Other cardiovascular risk factors

Diabetes, carotid atherosclerosis, heart disease and smoking are risk factors for stroke, VaD and AD. Their control reduces the occurrence of cerebrovascular disease and one would expect a similar risk reduction in AD, but so far there is no RCT. Nonetheless, understanding underlying pathophysiological mechanisms may open new avenues for prevention. For example, mutations in insulin degrading enzyme (IDE) that induce diabetes, also impair degradation of β-amyloid (Farris et al., 2004). Similarly, spontaneous cerebral microemboli (SCE), common in carotid disease but thought to be asymptomatic, have been associated with cognitive impairment following carotid and heart bypass surgery. We examined the frequency of SCE in AD and VaD by transcranial Doppler monitoring of middle cerebral arteries over 1 hour. Among 85 AD–control and 85 VaD–control pairs, we found SCE in 37–38 per cent of patients with AD or VaD compared with 13–14 per cent of their controls ($P < 0.001$; Purandare et al., 2003). SCE are potentially treatable and if they are found to be predictive of cognitive decline then they could be a target in prevention of dementia, both AD and VaD.

Yet another example would be smoking. Whilst smoking overall appears to be associated with a doubling of the risk of AD (presumably because of cardiovascular factors), nicotine itself may have neuroprotective properties and possibly reduce amyloid burden (Nordberg et al., 2002).

41.2 CONTROL OF SUBCLINICAL INFLAMMATORY PROCESSES

41.2.1 Biological basis

The importance of inflammatory processes in causation of dementia is established with evidence from biochemical, neuropathological and epidemiological studies. Primary inflammatory cytokines such as interleukins 1β (IL-1β), IL-6, and α2-macroglobulin are increased in brains of patients with AD. The neuropathological features of AD include accumulation of microglia and astrocytes around senile plaques. Both express HLA antigens and are involved in activation of the complement cascade. These inflammatory changes are thought to lead to further amyloid deposition and neuronal damage.

Non-steroidal anti-inflammatory drugs (NSAIDs) differ in their mechanisms of action and as yet we do not know the mechanism that is most important in offering neuroprotection in AD. Traditional NSAIDs such as ibuprofen, indomethacin affect both cyclo-oxygenases (Cox-1 and Cox-2). Newer NSAID such as celecoxib and rofecoxib specifically inhibit Cox-2 and hence have less propensity to cause gastrointestinal side effects. Cox-1 is prominent in CA-1 of hippocampus and is involved in microglial activation surrounding senile plaques. Cox-2 is prominent in dendrites of pyramidal neurones and is increased in many areas of brains in AD. Cox-2 levels correlate with Aβ-amyloid levels in the AD brains. Cox-2 is required in neurones with NMDA receptors responsible for glutamate-induced excitotoxicity in AD. NSAIDs also exhibit actions other than suppression of inflammation. NSAIDs inhibit Cox in platelets (resulting in reduced platelet aggregation and reduced Aβ-amyloid in blood) and in vascular endothelium (protecting the endothelium from free radicals). The importance of non-inflammatory actions of NSAIDs is highlighted by observations that both 'low' and 'high' doses offer neuroprotection. It is also possible that some NSAIDs influence amyloid deposition by inhibiting γ-secretase, independent of cyclo-oxygenase activity (Weggen et al., 2001).

41.2.2 Clinical evidence

A number of epidemiological studies have shown long-term use of NSAIDs to be associated with 2–4-fold reduced risk of AD, but some have been inconclusive (McGeer et al., 1996). A more recent systematic review and meta-analysis of nine observational studies concluded that NSAIDs do offer some protection against AD (Etminan et al., 2003). In't Veld et al. (2001) suggest that the conflicting evidence may be related to inaccurate recording and reliance on patients'/relatives' memory or incomplete medical records. They examined computerized pharmacy records in the follow-up study of almost 7000 residents of Rotterdam over 7 years. NSAIDs were associated with reduced risk of AD depending on the duration of the use (<1 month: RR 0.95; 1–24 months: RR 0.83; >24 months: RR 0.20). Zandi and Breitner (2001) suggest that to be protective in AD, NSAIDs would need to be taken several years before the disease onset, and secondary or tertiary prevention trials were unlikely to show a positive effect. This is in keeping with a very modest effect observed in RCTs of low-dose prednisone and NSAIDs in AD, including a recent trial of rofecoxib (Cox-2 inhibitor) or naproxen versus placebo with negative results (Aisen et al., 2000, 2003). The results of the Alzheimer's Disease Anti-inflammatory

Prevention Trial (ADAPT) should be interesting as it is examining efficacy of celecoxib and naproxen in older people (over 70s with family history of AD), and is attempting to exclude people with prodromal AD.

41.3 CONTROL OF OXIDATIVE STRESS AND FREE RADICALS

41.3.1 Biological basis

Oxidative stress can cause lipoprotein oxidation, Aβ polymerization and generation of excessive free radicals. *In vitro* studies suggest that ApoE ε4 reduces anti-oxidant capacity of neurones. Vitamins E and C along with alcohol (in moderation) scavenge these free radicals.

41.3.2 Clinical evidence

A number of epidemiological studies have found higher dietary intake of vitamins E and C, and moderate alcohol consumption to lower risk of dementia. In the Rotterdam study (Ruitenberg *et al.*, 2002), which followed over 5000 people for an average 6 years, a moderate alcohol consumption (1–3 drinks per day) was associated with reduced risk of dementia including both AD and VaD (hazards ratio, HR 0.58). Orgogozo *et al.* (1997) found 250–500 mL daily consumption of wine to reduce risk of dementia even further (OR 0.19). Additional studies are needed to examine the effect of type of alcohol on risk reduction, as micronutrients in red wine, especially resveratrol, may offer specific protection against β-amyloid toxicity, an effect also observed with green tea extracts and curry spice, curcumin.

There are no specific clinical trials examining the prevention of dementia with anti-oxidants. The key RCT, in which 341 patients with moderate to severe AD were randomized to receive selegiline (monoamine oxidase inhibitor) and vitamin E (either alone or in combination) or placebo found all active treatments, including vitamin E alone, to slow progression of AD over 2 years, as measured by time to occurrence of death, institutionalization, loss of ability to perform basic activities of daily living or severe dementia, but with no effect specifically on cognition (Sano *et al.*, 1997).

41.4 IMPROVING FUNCTIONAL NEURONAL CAPACITY

41.4.1 Role of cognitive, physical and social activities

A number of cross-sectional and retrospective studies have found an inverse relationship between activities (cognitive, physical or leisure) in mid-life and latter risk of dementia.

The repetition of cognitive skills may improve processing skills such as working memory and perceptual speed by possibly increasing dendritic plasticity. Physical exercise can increase insulin-like growth factor (IGF-1) and somatostatin levels, which are decreased in AD. IGF-1 has been shown to reduce tau phosphorylation and have an anti-apoptotic effect. In experiments on rats, environmental enrichment has been shown to inhibit spontaneous apoptosis, increase neurogenesis in dentate gyrus and improve spatial memory (Nilsson *et al.*, 1999; Young *et al.*, 1999). This may suggest a possible link between environment/social stimulation and regenerative brain processes.

41.4.2 Clinical evidence

There are no RCTs, but four large observational studies have shown reduced activities as an independent risk factor for AD. Wilson *et al.* (2002) followed 801 older clergy over 4 years and found 111 developed AD. They recorded seven common activities involving information processing as a core component (e.g. reading, watching TV, doing crosswords, etc.). The frequency of each activity was rated on a 5-point scale (1 = once a year, 5 = everyday) and responses to each item averaged to calculate a composite score (range: 1–5). The authors in their previous work had shown this to be a reliable method compared with differential weighing of each item depending on the perceived cognitive demand. After controlling for age, sex and education, a 1-point increase in cognitive activity was associated with 33 per cent reduction in risk of AD (HR 0.67). The epidemiological evidence for physical activity in prevention of dementia is mixed. Wilson *et al.* (2002) and Verghese *et al.* (2003) suggested that risk reduction was specifically due to cognitively stimulating activities. Friedland *et al.* (2001) found that reduced activity (intellectual, passive or physical) in mid-life increased the risk of developing AD by 250 per cent. The mixed results could be partly explained by how each study divided activities into physical, cognitive or social. For example, 'dancing' (Verghese *et al.*, 2003) or 'going to museum' (Wilson *et al.*, 2002) often included as cognitive activities include a strong physical component. Activities, either cognitive or physical, often include social aspects and are done as leisure activities. The social aspect of the activities or rich social network itself may be beneficial in reducing risk of dementia. Wang *et al.* (2002) in their analysis of the Kungsholmen project found that engagement in stimulating activities (mental, social or productive) reduced the risk of developing dementia over 6 years by 50 per cent (RR 0.54–0.58).

However, care has to be taken with interpretation of these studies as activities may be a proxy to some other factors such as education, socioeconomic status and generally healthy lifestyle. Although reduced activities have been shown to exist many years prior to onset of dementia, one cannot completely rule out the possibility of a prolonged prodrome.

41.5 TARGET POPULATIONS

Many of the risk factors for AD and the beginning of losses in key neuronal receptor systems (Perry *et al.*, 2001) come into play in mid-life, 15 to 20 years prior to onset of AD. This would suggest targeting prevention strategies at people with risk factors in their mid-life, who may not have any identifiable cognitive impairment. The economics of such trials make them impractical, due to low incident dementia and prolonged follow up over two decades. Identification of surrogate markers of subclinical disease progression is crucial for their viability.

Another approach would be to target older people who have developed some cognitive impairment but which is not severe enough to cause functional impairment and warrant diagnosis of dementia. A somewhat loose and controversial term 'mild cognitive impairment' (MCI) is most widely used to describe this population, which has community prevalence of 17–34 per cent with annual 'conversion' to dementia of between 3 and 15 per cent depending upon the population (Burns and Zaudig, 2002). Mild 'vascular cognitive impairment' (mVCI), which describes people with early cognitive impairment related to cerebrovascular disease, may be a more specific target owing to importance of vascular risk factors in causation of AD.

41.6 CONCLUSION

The epidemiological evidence suggests that it is possible to delay, if not prevent, the onset of dementia, both AD and VaD. The RCT evidence is building up for antihypertensives but remains sparse for other strategies. Most of the ongoing RCTs focus on one or two vascular risk factors and assess dementia only as a secondary outcome. There is a need for RCTs that will target multiple risk factors in at risk people with MCI or mVCI with incident dementia as a primary outcome. The design of such RCTs should be guided by the up-to-date basic research on pathophysiological mechanisms involved in causation of common dementias.

REFERENCES

Aisen PS, Davis KL, Berg JD *et al.* (2000) A randomized controlled trial of prednisone in Alzheimer's disease. Alzheimer's Disease Cooperative Study. *Neurology* **54**: 588–593

Aisen PS, Schafer KA, Grundman M *et al.* (2003) Alzheimer's Disease Cooperative Study. Effects of rofecoxib or naproxen versus placebo on Alzheimer disease progression: a randomised controlled trial. *JAMA* **289**: 2819–2826

Applegate WB, Pressel S, Wittes J. (1994) Impact of the treatment of isolated systolic hypertension on behavioral variables. Results from the systolic hypertension in the elderly program. *Archives of Internal Medicine* **154**: 2154–2160

Barnes JM, Barnes NM, Costall B, Horovitz ZP, Naylor RJ. (1989) Angiotensin II inhibits the release of [3H]acetylcholine from rat entorhinal cortex *in vitro*. *Brain Research* **491**: 136–143

Bosch J, Yusuf S, Pogue J *et al.* (2002) HOPE Investigators. Heart outcomes prevention evaluation. Use of ramipril in preventing stroke: double blind randomized trial. *BMJ* **324**: 699–702

Bottiglieri T, Parnetti L, Arning E *et al.* (2001) Plasma total homocysteine levels and the C677T mutation in the methylenetetrahydrofolate reductase (MTHFR) gene: a study in an Italian population with dementia. *Mechanics of Ageing Development* **122**: 2013–2023

Burns A and Zaudig M. (2002) Mild cognitive impairment in older people. *Lancet* **360**: 1963–1965

Clarke R, Smith AD, Jobst KA *et al.* (1998) Folate, vitamin B12, and serum total homocysteine levels in confirmed Alzheimer disease. *Archives of Neurology* **55**: 1407–1408

Dufouil C, Alperovitch A, Ducros V *et al.* (2003) Homocysteine, white matter hyperintensities, and cognition in healthy elderly people. *Annals of Neurology* **53**: 214–221

Etminan M, Gill S, Samii A. (2003) The role of lipid-lowering drugs in cognitive function: a meta-analysis of observational studies. *Pharmacotherapy* **23**: 726–730

Farris W, Mansourian S, Leissring MA *et al.* (2004) Partial loss-of-function mutations in insulin-degrading enzyme that induce diabetes also impair degradation of amyloid beta-protein. *American Journal of Pathology* **164**: 1424–1434

Fassbender K, Simons M, Bergmann C *et al.* (2001) Simvastatin strongly reduces levels of Alzheimer's disease beta-amyloid peptides Abeta 42 and Abeta 40 *in vitro* and in vivo. *Proceedings of the National Academy of Sciences of the United States of America* **98**: 5856–5861

Fogari R, Mugellini A, Zoppi A *et al.* (2003) Influence of losartan and atenolol on memory function in very elderly hypertensive patients. *Journal of Human Hypertension* **17**: 781–785

Forette F, Seux ML, Staessen JA *et al.* (1998) Prevention of dementia in randomised double-blind placebo-controlled systolic hypertension in Europe (Syst-Eur) trial. *Lancet* **352**: 1347–1351

Forette F, Seux ML, Staessen JA *et al.* (2002) The prevention of dementia with antihypertensive treatment: new evidence from the Systolic Hypertension in Europe (Syst-Eur) study. *Archives of Internal Medicine* **162**: 2046–2052

Friedland RP, Fritsch T, Smyth KA *et al.* (2001) Patients with Alzheimer's disease have reduced activities in midlife compared with healthy control-group members. *Proceedings of the National Academy of Sciences of the United States of America* **98**: 3440–3445

Frosst P, Blom HJ, Milos R *et al.* (1995) A candidate genetic risk factor for vascular disease: a common mutation in methylenetetrahydrofolate reductase. *Nature Genetics* **10**: 111–113

Gottfries J, Blennow K, Lehmann MW *et al.* (2001) One-carbon metabolism and other biochemical correlates of cognitive impairment as visualized by principal component analysis. *Journal of Geriatric Psychiatry and Neurology* **14**: 109–114

Guo Z, Qiu C, Viitanen M *et al.* (2001) Blood pressure and dementia in persons 75+ years old: 3-year follow-up results from the Kungsholmen Project. *Journal of Alzheimer's Disease* **3**: 585–591

Heart Protection Study Collaborative Group. (2002) MRC/BHF Heart Protection Study of cholesterol lowering with simvastatin in 20 536 high-risk individuals: a randomised placebo-controlled trial. *Lancet* **360**: 7–22

Homocysteine Studies Collaboration. (2002) Homocysteine and risk of ischemic heart disease and stroke: a meta-analysis. *JAMA* **288**: 2015–2022

In't Veld BA, Ruitenberg A, Hofman A et al. (2001) Nonsteroidal antiinflammatory drugs and the risk of Alzheimer's disease. New England of Medicine 345: 1515–1521

Jorm AF, Korten AE, Henderson AS. (1987) The prevalence of dementia: a quantitative integration of the literature. Acta Psychiatrica Scandinavica 76: 465–479

Kivipelto M, Helkala EL, Laakso MP et al. (2002) Apolipoprotein E epsilon4 allele, elevated midlife total cholesterol level, and high midlife systolic blood pressure are independent risk factors for late-life Alzheimer disease. Annals of Internal Medicine 137: 149–155

Kojro E, Gimpl G, Lammich S, Marz W, Fahrenholz F. (2001) Low cholesterol stimulates the nonamyloidogenic pathway by its effect on the alpha -secretase ADAM 10. Proceedings of the National Academy of Sciences of the United States of America 98: 5815–520

Lithell H, Hansson L, Skoog I et al. (2003) SCOPE Study Group. The Study on Cognition and Prognosis in the Elderly (SCOPE): principal results of a randomized double-blind intervention trial. Journal of Hypertension 21: 875–886

McCaddon A, Hudson P, Davies G et al. (2001) Homocysteine and cognitive decline in healthy elderly. Dementia and Geriatric Cognitive Disorders 12: 309–313

McGeer PL, Schulzer M, McGeer EG. (1996) Arthritis and anti-inflammatory agents as possible protective factors for Alzheimer's disease: a review of 17 epidemiologic studies. Neurology 47: 425–432

McIlroy SP, Dynan B, Lawson JT et al. (2002) Moderately elevated plasma homocysteine, methylenetetrahydrofolate reductase genotype, and risk for stroke, vascular dementia, and Alzheimer's disease in Northern Ireland. Stroke 33: 2351–2356

Meyer JS, Judd BW, Tawaklna T et al. (1986) Improved cognition after control of risk factors for multi-infarct dementia. JAMA 256: 2203–2209

Moroney JT, Tang MX, Berglund L et al. (1999) Low-density lipoprotein cholesterol and the risk of dementia with stroke. JAMA 282: 254–260

Murray MD, Lane KA, Gao S et al. (2002) Preservation of cognitive function with antihypertensive medications: a longitudinal analysis of a community-based sample of African Americans. Archives of Internal Medicine:162: 2090–2096

Nilsson M, Perfilieva E, Johansson U et al. (1999) Enriched environment increases neurogenesis in the adult rat dentate gyrus and improves spatial memory. Journal of Neurobiology 39: 569–578

Nilsson K, Gustafson L, Hultberg B. (2001) Improvement of cognitive functions after cabolmin/folate supplementation in elderly patients with dementia and elevated plasma homocysteine. International Journal of Geriatric Psychiatry 16: 609–614

Nordberg A, Hellstrom-Lindahl E, Lee M et al. (2002) Chronic nicotine treatment reduces beta-amyloidosis in the brain of a mouse model of Alzheimer's disease (APPsw). Journal of Neurochemistry 81: 655–658

Orgogozo JM, Dartigues JF, Lafont S et al. (1997) Wine consumption and dementia in the elderly: a prospective community study in the Bordeaux area. Revista de Neurologia (Paris) 153: 185–192

Peila R, White LR, Petrovich H et al. (2001) Joint effect of the APoE gene and midlife systolic blood pressure on late-life cognitive impairment: the Honolulu-Asia aging study. Stroke 32: 2882–2889

Perry EK, Martin-Ruiz CM, Court JA. (2001) Nicotinic receptor subtypes in human brain related to aging and dementia. Alcohol 24: 63–68

Prince MJ, Bird AS, Blizard RA et al. (1996) Is the cognitive function of older patients affected by antihypertensive treatment? Results from 54 months of the Medical Research Council's trial of hypertension in older adults. BMJ 312: 801–805

Purandare N, Welsh S, Hutchinson S et al. (2003) Cerebral emboli and venous to arterial circulation shunt (v-aCS) in dementia [abstract]. International Psychogeriatrics 15 (Suppl. 2): 115

Rockwood K, Kirkland S, Hogan DB et al. (2002) Use of lipid-lowering agents, indication bias, and the risk of dementia in community-dwelling elderly people. Archives of Neurology 59: 223–227

Ruitenberg A, van Swieten JC, Witteman JC et al. (2002). Alcohol consumption and risk of dementia: The Rotterdam study. Lancet 359: 281–286

Sano M, Ernesto C, Thomas RG et al. (1997) A controlled trial of selegiline, alpha-tocopherol, or both as treatment for Alzheimer's disease. The Alzheimer's Disease Cooperative Study. New England of Medicine 336: 1216–1222

Seshadri S, Beiser A, Selhub J et al. (2002) Plasma homocysteine as a risk factor for dementia and Alzheimer's disease. New England of Medicine 346: 466–468

Shepherd J, Blauw GJ, Murphy MB et al. (2002) Pravastatin in elderly individuals at risk of vascular disease (PROSPER): a randomised controlled trial. Lancet 360: 1623–1630

Simons M, Keller P, De Strooper B et al. (1998) Cholesterol depletion inhibits the generation of beta-amyloid in hippocampal neurons. Proceedings of the National Academy of Sciences of the United States of America 26: 6460–6464

Sjogren M, Gustafsson K, Syversen S et al. (2003) Treatment with simvastatin in patients with Alzheimer's disease lowers both alpha- and beta-cleaved amyloid precursor protein. Dementia and Geriatric Cognitive Disorders 16: 25–30

Tzourio C, Anderson C, Chapman N et al. (2003) PROGRESS Collaborative Group. Effects of blood pressure lowering with perindopril and indapamide therapy on dementia and cognitive decline in patients with cerebrovascular disease. Archives of Internal medicine 163: 1069–1075

Ventura P, Panini R, Verlato C et al. (2001) Hyperhomocysteinemia and related factors in 600 hospitalized elderly subjects. Metabolism 50: 1466–1471

Verghese J, Lipton RB, Katz MJ et al. (2003) Leisure activities and the risk of dementia in the elderly. New England of Medicine 348: 2508–2516

Vermeer SE, van Dijk EJ, Koudstaal PJ et al. (2002) Homocysteine, silent brain infarcts, and white matter lesions: The Rotterdam Scan Study. Annals of Neurology 51: 285–289

Wang H-X, Karp A, Winblad B et al. (2002) Late-life engagement in social and leisure activities is associated with a decreased risk of dementia: a longitudinal study from the Kungsholmen project. American Journal of Epidemiology 155: 1081–1087

Weggen S, Eriksen JL, Das P et al. (2001) A subset of NSAIDs lower amyloidogenic Abeta42 independently of cyclooxygenase activity. Nature 8: 212–216

Wilson RS, Mendes De Leon CF, Barnes LL et al. (2002) Participation in cognitively stimulating activities and risk of incident Alzheimer disease. JAMA 287: 742–748

Young D, Lawlor PA, Leone P et al. (1999) Environmental enrichment inhibits spontaneous apoptosis, prevents seizures and is neuroprotective. Nature Medicine 5: 448–453

Zandi PP and Breitner JC. (2001) Do NSAIDs prevent Alzheimer's disease? And, if so, why? The epidemiological evidence. Neurobiology of Aging 22: 811–817

42

Trial design

SERGE GAUTHIER

Any therapy, whether pharmacological or not, requires proof of safety and efficacy. This chapter will outline the various trial design issues that have been encountered in the modern pharmacological treatment of Alzheimer's disease (AD). The experience gained so far has been predominantly in the symptomatic treatment of AD, using parallel group designs over 3–12 months. A number of randomized clinical studies attempting to modify progression of AD are under way, using parallel groups or survival designs over 1 year or longer.

The natural history of AD will be described first, introducing the concepts of disease stages, disease milestones and symptomatic domains that fluctuate in intensity as the disease runs through its course. Lessons from the symptomatic studies using cholinesterase inhibitors and memantine will be summarized. Current disease modification study designs will be outlined.

42.1 NATURAL HISTORY OF ALZHEIMER'S DISEASE

The natural history of AD can be broadly considered as a presymptomatic stage, during which a number of pathological events take place (see Chapters 28–30), an early symptomatic or prodromal stage with affective and/or cognitive manifestations, and symptomatic mild, moderate and severe stages. Each of these stages could be targeted for specific treatments, requiring different trial designs and outcomes (Table 42.1).

Disease milestones can also be defined in AD (Box 42.1). Some of these can be a target for treatment, with considerable face validity and impact on care (Galasko *et al.*, 1995). For example, studies in mild cognitive impairment (MCI) of the amnestic type may demonstrate that the diagnosis of dementia (predominantly AD) is delayed by 6 months or

Table 42.1 *Examples of trial design and outcomes for each stage of Alzheimer's disease*

Stage	Target population	Trial design	Primary outcome
Presymptomatic	Healthy elderly	Survival over 5 years	Incident dementia
Prodromal	Mild cognitive impairment; amnestic subtype	Survival over 3 years	Conversion to dementia
Mild to moderate	AD in the community	Six months parallel groups	Cognition and global impression of change
Moderate to severe	AD in the community or in assisted-living	Six months parallel groups	Global impression of change
Severe	AD in institution	Six months parallel groups	Behaviour

Box 42.1 *Clinical milestones in Alzheimer's disease*

- Emergence of cognitive symptoms
- Progression from amnestic mild cognitive impairement to diagnosable dementia
- Loss of instrumental activities of daily living (ADL)
- Emergence of behavioural and psychological symptoms of dementia
- Nursing home placement
- Loss of self-care ADL
- Death

longer. Delaying loss of autonomy for self-care and even death in moderate to severe stages of AD using α-tocopherol in only one study by the Alzheimer Disease Cooperative Study group (Sano *et al.*, 1997) has influenced clinical practice to use vitamin E in all stages of AD, at least in the USA. Delaying the loss of autonomy for instrumental activities of daily living (ADL) or the need for nursing home care would reduce the need for supportive care. Delaying emergence of some of the behavioural and psychological symptoms of dementia (BPSD) would reduce caregiver burden and later need for nursing home placement.

Symptomatic domains in dementia include cognition, ADL and behaviour. One can even add a domain of changes in motricity, since patients with AD will manifest some features of parkinsonism late in the disease. In many patients early changes in mood and anxiety precede the formal diagnosis of AD, sometimes with spontaneous improvement as insight into the disease is lost. Cognitive and functional ADL decline are relatively linear over time, whereas BPSD peak midway into the disease course and resolve spontaneously through the severe stage as motricity becomes impaired (Gauthier *et al.*, 2001). These natural fluctuations in the intensity of individual symptomatic domains through the stages of AD have an impact into trial design and outcomes (Table 42.2). It should be noted that studies can be of shorter duration and/or of smaller numbers of subjects in moderate compared with mild

stages of AD because of the faster rate of decline in the moderate stage, which may be related to the sensitivity of measurement scales, or to the progression of AD.

42.2 SYMPTOMATIC CLINICAL TRIALS USING CHOLINESTERASE INHIBITORS AND MEMANTINE

The modern treatment for AD was initiated by the report that tacrine improved some aspects of cognition and daily life. The follow-up confirmatory studies used cross-over and parallel group designs. The FDA published 'guidelines' (Leber, 1990), which greatly influenced the choice of outcomes for proof of efficacy of drugs improving symptoms in AD: a cognitive performance-based scale such as the ADAS-cog and an interview-based impression of change became the primary outcomes in mild to moderate AD, usually defined operationally as scores between 10 and 26 on the Mini-Mental State Examination (MMSE; Folstein *et al.*, 1975). Unfortunately, as these FDA guidelines cautioned against the 'pseudospecificity' of measurable benefits on neuropsychiatric manifestations in AD, they delayed research in this symptomatic domain. More recent discussions and publications from the FDA and other regulatory agencies have been more accepting of ADL and behaviour as important outcomes.

The following study designs have been used in the proof of efficacy for cholinesterase inhibitors (ChEIs): parallel groups over 3–12 months, and survival to a predefined clinical end point over 1 year or longer.

The parallel groups offer the possibility of short-term (minimum of 3 months) studies comparing the efficacy of different doses of the drug versus placebo. The primary analysis is done on outcomes at the end of the study using the last observation carried forward (LOCF) or intent to treat (ITT) analyses, which compensate for missing values in case of dropouts. Although LOCF/ITT has been favoured by the FDA, investigators and other regulatory agencies are now suggesting that for studies of 12 months or longer duration,

Table 42.2 *Examples of impact of symptoms through stages of AD on trial design and outcomes*

Stage	Prominent features	Types of outcomes	Examples
Mild	Depression may be present; few BPSD; cognitive decline slow but predominant feature; some instrumental ADL losses	Cognition; instrumental ADL	ADAS-cog, ADCS-ADL, DAD
Moderate	Cognitive decline more rapid; functional decline more rapid; BPSD emerge	Cognition; instrumental and basic ADL; behaviour	ADAS-cog, DAD, ADCS-ADL, NPI, BEHAVE-AD
Severe	Cognitive losses harder to measure (floor effect); few self-care ADL remaining; BPSD abating; parkinsonism emerging	Cognition; self-care ADL; behaviour; parkinsonism	SIB, ADCS-ADL, NPI, UPDRS

ADAS-cog, Alzheimer Disease Assessment Scale – cognitive subscale (Rosen *et al.*, 1984); ADCS-ADL, Alzheimer Disease Cooperative Study ADL scale (Galasko *et al.*, 1997); BEHAVE-AD, Behavioral symptoms in Alzheimer's disease (Reisberg *et al.*, 1987); DAD, Disability Assessment in Dementia (Gélinas *et al.*, 1999); NPI, Neuropsychiatric Inventory (Cummings *et al.*, 1994); SIB, Severe Impairment Battery (Panisset *et al.*, 1994); UPDRS, United Parkinson Disease Rating Scale (Fahn and Elton, 1987) the primary analysis should be done on observed cases (OC), i.e. completers. For practical purpose both types of analysis will usually be performed. Although 'cognitive enhancement' was the main hope for ChEIs as a therapeutic class, the reality that has emerged from 6 months studies with open-label extensions and the one-year placebo-controlled Nordic study (Winblad et al., 2001) is that, although there is a small but statistically significant improvement in cognition peaking at 3 months with the ChEIs, the most clinically relevant finding has been the stabilization of cognitive decline with 'return to baseline' at 9–12 months for the actively treated groups at the higher therapeutic doses, compared with placebo treated groups who decline steadily. It should be noted that this natural decline varies greatly between studies in AD, and is even less evident in AD with cerebrovascular disease or in vascular dementia (VaD), where control of vascular risk factors appear to modify progression, at least in studies of 6 months' duration (Schneider, 2003).

Survival studies have primarily targeted loss of ADL, and have successfully demonstrated a delay in the loss of autonomy for patients on ChEIs compared with placebo. Parallel group studies of 6 months' duration in patients ranging from mild to moderately severe AD (MMSE 5–26) have also established that ADL are stable on treatment, but show no benefit on instrumental ADL (so called 'tutoring effect').

The most difficult domain to study, although very significant clinically, has been behaviour. The availability of general BPSD scales such as the NPI and BEHAVE-AD, as well as specific scales such as Cohen-Mansfield Agitation Inventory (Cohen-Mansfield et al., 1989), has not yet allowed unequivocal demonstration of benefit in severe stages of AD. New methods of analysis of behaviour have been proposed (Gauthier et al., 2002), and will likely be more successful in defining categories of BPSD symptoms most responsive to ChEIs (anxiety, hallucinations), memantine (agitation) and other drugs.

Memantine as a new therapeutic class has been found to be effective in a range of studies using parallel groups, in moderate to severe AD (Doody et al., 2004). Scales appropriate for this stage of disease, such as the SIB, the ADCS-ADL and the NPI have been used and accepted by the FDA and other regulatory agencies. Of great importance is the novel design of adding memantine or placebo to a stable dose of a ChEI used successfully, paving the way to a number of studies where novel drugs or placebo are added to 'standard treatment'.

42.3 DISEASE MODIFICATION STRATEGIES

Although no trial design has yet led to a successful treatment for disease modification, many attempts have been made using parallel groups >1 year. Recent refinements of this design include adding the novel drug or a placebo to standard treatment over 1 year, selection of outcomes that demonstrate relatively linear changes over time such as the Clinical Dementia Rating sum of boxes (Hughes et al. 1982),

---

Box 42.2 *Add-on design for disease modification*

- One year is the minimum period for meaningful clinical observations in mild to moderate AD considering natural decline (may need to be longer in mild AD)
- Ethically long duration studies without 'standard treatment' are not possible
- There are scales with relatively linear changes over 1 year, such as the CDR sum of boxes, the ADAS-cog, the DAD and the ADCS-ADL, allowing analysis for slopes of decline
- A randomized wash-out from active treatment at the end of the study could demonstrate a lack of return to placebo
- A demonstrable reduction in rate of brain atrophy associated with differences in clinical decline would offer great face validity

---

randomized wash-out at the end of the year, and volumetric brain measurements using magnetic resonance imaging at beginning and end of year (Mohr et al., 2004). The reasoning behind this 'add-on design' is summarized in Box 42.2.

Although this design appears promising, there are uncertainties and limitations. For instance the difference in rate of brain atrophy may be absent or opposite to expectations, with accelerated atrophy in the actively treated group. Wash-out from an active treatment will not be acceptable to all institutional review boards, and a previous attempt in using this design with patients treated with propentofylline failed to convince regulatory agencies (Whitehouse et al., 1998).

One of the most difficult issues in disease modification strategies is the decision of the stage of disease where the proposed drug is most likely to work. On this 'proof-of-concept' phase II/III efficacy and safety study hinges the entire future of the drug. For example, numerous attempts at treating patients with AD in mild to moderate stages using non-steroidal anti-inflammatory drugs have failed, despite the weight of evidence from epidemiological research and the biological plausibility of an inflammatory response to β-amyloid deposition. It may be that treatment in the late presymptomatic or in the prodromal stages would be the most appropriate time. On the other hand studies in these stages of AD would require 3–5 years, a very long time for a 'proof-of-concept'. Alternative patients groups could be considered, such as presenilin mutation carriers or amnestic MCI, perhaps with additional risk factors for rapid conversion to AD such as apolipoprotein E.

A survival design is currently being tested extensively in order to delay progression from amnestic MCI to diagnosable dementia, predominantly AD (Geda and Petersen, 2001). These studies are unlikely to be considered as 'disease modifying', but rather as early symptomatic treatment in the prodromal stage of AD.

42.4 FUTURE STRATEGIES TO DELAY EMERGENCE OF ALZHEIMER'S DISEASE

As hypotheses on the pathophysiology of AD emerge from epidemiological research in human populations, post-mortem and biomarkers studies in patients, and animal models, we will need to establish whether new therapies can delay the onset of symptoms in asymptomatic people at varying degrees of risk of AD. The prototype of trial design to establish the safety and efficacy of such therapies is an ongoing 5-year survival study comparing *Ginkgo biloba* to placebo in elderly subjects, with incident dementia as primary end point. Variations of this design may be possible, by enriching the study population with different levels of risk, such as a positive family history of AD and/or selected gene markers, although it should be remembered that any enrichment of a study population may limit the applicability of findings to the population as a whole.

REFERENCES

Cohen-Mansfield J, Marx MS, Rosenthal AS. (1989) A description of agitation in a nursing home. *Journal of Gerontology* **44**: M77–M84

Cummings JL, Mega M, Gray K *et al.* (1994) The Neuropsychiatric Inventory: comprehensive assessment of psychopathology in dementia. *Neurology* **44**: 2308–2314

Doody RS, Winblad B, Jelic V. (2004) Memantine: a glutamate antagonist for treatment of Alzheimer's disease. In: S Gauthier, P Scheltens, JL Cummings (eds), *Alzheimer's Disease and Related Disorders Annual 2004*. London, Martin Dunitz, pp. 137–144

Fahn S and Elton R. (1987) United Parkinson's Disease Rating Scale. In: S Fahn, C Marsden, M Golstein *et al.* (eds), *Recent Development in Parkinson's Disease*. Florham Park, Macmillan Healthcare, pp. 153–163

Folstein MF, Folstein SE, McHugh PR. (1975) Mini-mental State: a practical method for grading the cognitive state of patients for the clinician. *Journal of Psychiatric Research* **12**: 189–198

Galasko D, Edland SD, Morris JC *et al.* (1995) The Consortium to Establish a Registry for Alzheimer's Disease (CERAD). Part IX. Clinical milestones in patients with Alzheimer's disease followed over 3 years. *Neurology* **45**: 1451–1455

Galasko D, Bennett D, Sano M *et al.* (1997) An inventory to assess activities of daily living for clinical trials in Alzheimer's disease. *Alzheimer Disease and Associated Disorders* **11** (Suppl. 2): S33–S39

Gauthier S, Thal LJ, Rossor MN. (2001) The future diagnosis and management of Alzheimer's disease. In: S Gauthier (ed.), *Clinical Diagnosis and Management of Alzheimer's Disease*. London, Martin Dunitz, pp. 369–378

Gauthier S, Feldman H, Hecker J *et al.* (2003) Efficacy of donepezil on behavioral symptoms in patients with moderate to severe Alzheimer's disease. *International Psychogeriatrics* **14**: 389–404

Geda YE and Petersen RC. (2001) Clinical trials in mild cognitive impairment. In: S Gauthier, JL Cummings (eds), *Alzheimer's Disease and Related Disorders Annual (2001)*. London, Martin Dunitz, pp. 69–83

Gélinas I, Gauthier L, McIntyre M, Gauthier S. (1999) Development of a functional measure for persons with Alzheimer's disease: the Disability Assessment for Dementia. *American Journal of Occupational Therapy* **53**: 471–481

Hughes CP, Berg L, Danziger WL, Coben LA, Martin RL. (1982) A new clinical scale for the staging of dementia. *British Journal of Psychiatry* **140**: 566–572

Leber P. (1990) *Guidelines for Clinical Evaluation of Antidementia Drugs*. Washington, DC, US Food and Drug Administration

Mohr E, Barclay CL, Anderson R, Constant J. (2004) Clinical trial design in the age of dementia treatments: challenges and opportunities. In: S Gauthier, P Scheltens, JL Cummings (eds), *Alzheimer's Disease and Related Disorders Annual 2004*. London, Martin Dunitz, pp. 97–122

Panisset M, Roudier M, Saxton J *et al.* (1994) Severe Impairment Battery: a neuropsychological test for severely demented patients. *Archives of Neurology* **51**: 41–45

Reisberg B, Borenstein J, Salob SP *et al.* (1987) Behavioral symptoms in Alzheimer's disease: phenomenology and treatment. *Journal of Clinical Psychiatry* **48** (Suppl.): 9–15

Rosen WG, Mohs RC, Davis KL. (1984) A new rating scale for Alzheimer's disease. *American Journal of Psychiatry* **141**: 1356–1364

Sano M, Ernesto C, Thomas RG *et al.* (1997) A controlled trial of selegiline, alpha-tocopherol, or both as treatment for Alzheimer's disease. *New England Journal of Medicine* **336**: 1216–1222

Schneider LS. (2003) Cholinesterase inhibitors for vascular dementia? *Lancet Neurology* **2**: 658–659

Whitehouse PJ, Kittner B, Roessner M *et al.* (1998) Clinical trial designs for demonstrating disease-course-altering effects in dementia. *Alzheimer Disease and Associated Disorders* **12**: 281–294

Winblad B, Engedal K, Soininen H *et al.* (2001) Donepezil Nordic Study Group: a 1-year, randomized, placebo-controlled study of donepezil in patients with mild to moderate AD. *Neurology* **57**: 489–495

PART 4

Cerebrovascular disease and cognitive impairment

43

Vascular cognitive impairment

TIMO ERKINJUNTTI

43.1 HISTORICAL BACKGROUND

As early as 1896 'arteriosclerotic dementia' (referring to vascular dementia – VaD) was separated from 'senile dementia' (referring to Alzheimer's disease – AD) (Berchtold and Cotman, 1998). Alzheimer together with Binswanger recognized the heterogeneity of VaD by describing four clinico-pathological variants of VaD (Román, 2001), as well as vascular lesions in the Alzheimer brain. Nevertheless, until the 1960s and 1970s, cerebral atherosclerosis by causing chronic strangulation of blood supply to the brain was thought to be the commonest cause of dementia, and AD was regarded as a rare cause affecting only younger patients. Tomlinson et al. (1970) reinvented AD as the more frequent cause of dementia than that of arteriosclerotic dementia. In 1979 Hachinski and colleagues used the term multi-infarct dementia (MID) to describe the mechanism by which they considered VaD was produced (Hachinski et al., 1974). As the pendulum swung in the direction of AD, vascular forms of dementia became relegated to a position of relative obscurity (Brust, 1988).

Despite until 1990s the concept of VaD has been that it is a dementia caused by small or large brain infarcts, that of MID (Hachinski et al., 1974; Erkinjuntti and Hachinski, 1993), VaD has come full circle with the resurgence of interest of the whole spectrum of vascular causes of cognitive impairment and dementia (Hachinski, 1990). The new term is vascular cognitive impairment (VCI), which reflects the reinvention of the importance of vascular burden of brain and cognition (Bowler and Hachinski, 1995; O'Brien et al., 2003a, b). The

original findings of Alois Alzheimer have been 'reinvented'. Important are new data highlighting complex interactions between vascular aetiologies, changes in the brain, host factors and cognition (Chui, 1989; Tatemichi, 1990; Desmond, 1996; Pasquier and Leys, 1997; Skoog, 1998). Also reinvention of the heterogeneity of VaDs has fuelled the discussion, and subcortical vascular disease and dementia is seen the cardinal subtype (Erkinjuntti et al., 2000; Erkinjuntti and Pantoni, 2000; Román et al., 2002). Further the facts that vascular factors relate and coexist with AD have strengthened interest in the vascular burden of cognition (Kalaria and Ballard, 1999; Skoog et al., 1999).

43.2 VASCULAR BURDEN OF THE BRAIN AND COGNITION

The VaDs are the second most common single causes of dementia (Rocca et al., 1991; Hebert and Brayne, 1995; Lobo et al., 2000; Rockwood et al., 2000; Doody et al., 2001). Cerebrovascular disease (CVD) relates to a high risk of cognitive impairment and dementia (Tatemichi et al., 1992; Tatemichi et al., 1994a). In addition, vascular factors such as coexisting stroke and white matter lesions (WMLs) relate also to AD (Snowdon et al., 1997). Thus vascular causes are an important cause of cognitive impairment worldwide (Hachinski, 1992; O'Brien et al., 2003b).

CVD and ischaemic brain injury have been seen as the primary cause of clinical deficits in VCI and the VaDs (Erkinjuntti, 1999). The multiplicity of vascular causes, associated risk factors and clinical manifestations of dementia related to CVD makes VCI and VaD a complex area of research (Wallin and Blennow, 1993; Erkinjuntti, 1999; Pohjasvaara et al., 2000). Even though a number of sets of diagnostic criteria have been produced for epidemiological studies of VaD, opinions are divided over the definition of VaD subtypes. How wide should the definition of the cognitive syndrome and the vascular cause be, and which patients should be excluded from a diagnosis of VCI and VaD?

Also, debate centres on difficulties in distinguishing between dementia owing to AD and that arising from CVD, as there are large overlaps in clinical signs and symptoms. Both result in cognitive, functional and behavioural impairment. There are also similarities in pathophysiological mechanisms (e.g. WMLs, delayed neuronal death and apoptosis) (Pantoni and Garcia, 1997; Snowdon et al., 1997; Skoog et al., 1999), associated risk factors (e.g. age, education, arterial hypertension; Skoog, 1994; Skoog et al., 1999) and neurochemical deficits (e.g. cholinergic dysfunction) (Togi et al., 2002; Wallin et al., 2002) shared with these two dementia causes.

More important, however, is the fact that AD and VaD coexist in a large proportion of patients (Kalaria and Ballard, 1999; Rockwood, 1997; Rockwood et al., 2000). AD with CVD (referred also to as mixed dementia) could present clinically either as AD with evidence of cerebrovascular lesions in brain imaging, or with features of both AD and VaD (Rockwood et al., 1999). Based on the findings from the Nun Study, it has been suggested that CVD may play an important role in determining the presence and severity of clinical symptoms of AD (Snowdon et al., 1997). Either way, the prevalence of AD with CVD has previously been underestimated (Kalaria and Ballard, 1999).

43.3 VASCULAR COGNITIVE IMPAIRMENT

The recognition of AD as the commonest cause of dementia resulted in criteria of dementia based on the clinical picture of AD (Bowler and Hachinski, 1995; Erkinjuntti et al., 1997). Features of dementia included early and prominent memory loss, progression, irreversibility and a level of cognitive impairment sufficient to affect normal activities of daily living (ADL). Unexplained different definitions of dementia required different combinations of impairment in different domains of cognition (Erkinjuntti et al., 1997).

In AD involvement of the medial temporal lobe results with dense episodic memory impairment. By contrast, patients with vascular lesions have no such predilection (Rockwood et al., 1999, 2000). The emphasis on dementia underestimates the vascular burden of cognition, as well as distracts focus on prevention and treatment. Accordingly, it has been suggested to abandon the 'alzheimerized' dementia concept in the setting of CVD, and substitute it with a broader category of VCI (Hachinski, 1992; Bowler and Hachinski, 1995; Bowler et al., 1999; O'Brien et al., 2003a, b).

In VCI, vascular refers to all causes of ischaemic CVD, and cognitive impairment encompasses all levels of cognitive decline, from the earliest step to a more severe and broad dementia-like cognitive syndrome (Bowler et al., 1999; O'Brien et al., 2003a, b). VCIs that do not meet the criteria of dementia have been labelled also as vascular cognitive impairment with no dementia, vascular CIND (Rockwood et al., 1999, 2000). VCI is expected to include cases with cognitive impairment related to CVD (transient ischaemic attack [TIA], stroke), multiple cortico-subcortical infarcts, silent infarcts, strategic infarcts, small vessel disease with WMLs and lacunae, as well as AD pathology with coexisting CVD lesions. The concept and definition of VCI or CIND is still in evolution. The two main factors to be defined include the level of severity of cognitive impairment and the pattern of cognitive impairment (O'Brien et al., 2003a, b); in particular identification of a cognitive syndrome signalling a high risk of further cognitive decline, vascular mild cognitive decline (VMCI), a group of patients similar to that of amnestic MCI as a risk state for AD (Petersen et al., 2002), is a challenge.

43.4 EPIDEMIOLOGY

Our understanding of the population distribution of VCI and its outcomes are subject to the variety of definitions used to identify it (Rocca et al., 1991; Lobo et al., 2000). For example, if mixed AD/VaD is included, then VCI may even be the most common cause of chronic progressive cognitive impairment in elderly people (Rockwood et al., 2000).

The prevalence of VCI has been estimated at 5 per cent of people over age 65 in a Canadian Study (Rockwood et al., 2000). This included patients with CIND. The prevalence of vascular CIND was 2.4 per cent; that of AD with CVD 0.9 per cent and that of VaD 1.5 per cent. By contrast, in the same study, the prevalence of AD without a vascular component was 5.1 per cent, and at all ages up to age 85 was less common than VCI.

As traditionally conceived, VaD is the second most common single cause of dementia accounting for 10 and even up to 50 per cent of the cases, depending on the geographic location, patient population and clinical methods used (Rocca et al., 1991; Hebert and Brayne, 1995; Lobo et al., 2000). The prevalence of VaD has been higher in earlier studies in China and Japan, compared with Europe and United States. The prevalence of VaD has ranged from 1.2 to 4.2 per cent in persons aged 65 years and older (Hebert and Brayne, 1995). In a European collaborative study using population-based studies of people aged 65 years and older conducted in the 1990s the age-standardized prevalence of dementia was 6.4 per cent (all causes), 4.4 per cent for AD and 1.6 per cent for VaD (Lobo et al., 2000). In this study 15.8 per cent of the cases had VaD and 53.7 per cent AD.

The incidence of VaD has varied between 6 and 12 cases per year in 1000 persons aged 70 years and older (Hebert and Brayne, 1995). The incidence of VaD increases with increasing age, without any substantial difference between men and women in a European collaborative study (Fratiglioni *et al.*, 2000).

In the Canadian study, the mean duration of survival in VCI was 41 months (Rockwood *et al.*, 2000). The highest impact on mortality arose from VaD in women (Ostbye *et al.*, 2002). In general, survival from VaD is around 5 years (Hebert and Brayne, 1995), less than that for the general population or those with AD (Mölsä *et al.*, 1995; Skoog *et al.*, 1993). Also post-stroke dementia is an independent predictor of mortality (Tatemichi *et al.*, 1994b).

The cognitive outcome of patients with VaD may be as severe as in AD but their morbidity and mortality are usually worse. Chui and Gonthier (1999) reviewed studies showing shorter survival in VaD than in AD; also, those who survived VaD had a more variable course. Survival variability may produce a length bias whereby patients whose disease progresses too rapidly are usually excluded in prevalence surveys (Wolfson *et al.*, 2001).

Although natural history studies have found poor cognitive outcome in patients with VaD, this has not been seen in clinical trials in VaD. In such trials, patients in the placebo groups have had little progression of impairment – the so-called 'stable placebo response' (Kittner *et al.*, 1997; Kittner for the European/Canadian Propentofyllinen Study Group, 1999). The most likely explanation is the degree of exclusion of cases with mixed AD plus CVD, since these mixed patients usually have a progression mid-way between AD and VaD cases (Erkinjuntti *et al.*, 2002). Other explanations have been proposed, including selection bias since patients enrolled in trials are generally more fit than patients studied in natural history settings, expectation bias, placebo effect and co-intervention, resulting in better control of vascular risk factors, that might also explain both less disease progression and lower mortality rates. Finally, outcome measures used in these trials and adopted from AD trials may be relatively less unresponsive to decline.

43.5 DISEASE MECHANISMS

VCI and VaDs as a general entity include many syndromes, which themselves reflect a variety of vascular mechanisms and changes in the brain, with different causes and clinical manifestations. The pathophysiology incorporates interactions between vascular aetiologies (CVD and vascular risk factors), changes in the brain (infarcts, WMLs, atrophy), and host factors (age, education) (Chui, 1989; Tatemichi, 1990; Desmond, 1996; Pasquier and Leys, 1997; Skoog, 1998).

43.5.1 Aetiologies

Aetiologies of VCI include both CVDs and risk factors (Box 43.1). The main CVDs include large artery disease, cardiac embolic events, small vessel disease and haemodynamic

---

Box 43.1 *Aetiologies of vascular dementia*

Cerebrovascular disorders
- Large artery disease
  - artery-to-artery embolism
  - occlusion of an extra- or intracranial artery
- Cardiac embolic events
- Small vessel disease
  - lacunar infarcts
  - ischaemic white matter lesions
- Haemodynamic mechanisms
- Specific arteriopathies
- Haemorrhages
  - intracranial haemorrhage
  - subarachnoidal haemorrhage
- Haematological factors
- Venous diseases
- Hereditary entities

Risk factors
- Vascular
  - arterial hypertension
  - atrial fibrillation
  - myocardial infarction
  - coronary heart disease
  - diabetes
  - generalized atherosclerosis
  - lipid abnormalities
  - smoking
- Demographic factors
  - high age
  - low education
- Genetic factors
  - family history
  - specific genetic factors
- Stroke-related farctors
  - type of CVD
  - site and size of infarcts

---

mechanisms (Brun, 1994; Wallin and Blennow, 1994; Pantoni and Garcia, 1995; Amar and Wilcock, 1996; Erkinjuntti, 1996).

Risk factors related to VCI (Box 43.1) include risk factors for CVD, stroke, WMLs, but, at the same time, also those of any cognitive decline and AD (Skoog, 1998). They can be divided into vascular factors (e.g. arterial hypertension, atrial fibrillation, myocardial infarction, coronary heart disease, diabetes, generalized atherosclerosis, lipid abnormalities, smoking), demographic factors (e.g. age, education), genetic factors (e.g. family history and specific genetic features), and stroke-related factors (e.g. type of CVD, site and size of stroke) (Skoog, 1998; Gorelick, 1997). Hypoxic ischaemic events (cardiac arrhythmias, congestive heart failure, myocardial infarction, seizures, pneumonia) may be an important risk factor for incident dementia in patients with stroke (Moroney *et al.*, 1996).

43.5.2 Brain changes

The changes in the brain related to VaD include both ischaemic and non-ischaemic factors (Chui, 1989; Tatemichi, 1990; Brun, 1994; Erkinjuntti, 1996) (Box 43.2). The static ischaemic lesions include arterial territorial infarct, distal field (watershed) infarct, lacunar infarct, ischaemic WMLs and incomplete ischaemic injury. Incomplete ischaemic injury include, for example, focal gliosis and incomplete white matter infarctions in areas of selective vulnerability (Englund et al., 1988; Pantoni and Garcia, 1997). The functional ischaemic changes include both focal (around the ischaemic lesion) and remote (disconnection, diaschisis) effects. The volume of functionally inactive tissue exceeds that of static ischaemic lesions in VaD (Mielke et al., 1992). Current technologies in clinical work-up have limitations in detection of incomplete ischaemic injury and functional ischaemic changes. Also distinction between ischaemic and degenerative origin of atrophic changes awaits discovery (Vinters et al., 2000).

43.5.3 Brain mechanisms

Pathophysiological mechanisms related to VaD include: volume of brain infarcts (size reaching a critical threshold), number of infarcts (additive, synergistic), site of infarcts (bilateral, strategic cortical or subcortical sites), WMLs (extent, site, type, density), other ischaemic factors (incomplete ischaemic injury, delayed neuronal death, functional changes), atrophy (location, extent), and additive effects of other pathologies (AD, Lewy body dementia) (Chui, 1989; Tatemichi, 1990; Desmond, 1996; Erkinjuntti, 1996). Relationship between vascular factors and cognition is essential: whether the identified vascular factors cause, compound or only coexist with the VaD syndrome (Box 43.3) (Tatemichi et al., 1994a; Erkinjuntti et al., 1988). Another important question is, whether they contribute to the risk and clinical picture of AD (Pasquier and Leys, 1997; Snowdon et al., 1997). Questions of type, extent, side, site and tempo of vascular lesions in the brain relating to different types of VaD have no firm answers (Chui, 1989; Tatemichi, 1990; Desmond, 1996; Erkinjuntti, 1996).

43.5.4 Anatomical brain imaging

Computed tomography (CT) and magnetic resonance imaging (MRI) studies on VaD indicate that bilateral ischaemic lesions are of importance (Erkinjuntti and Hachinski, 1993; DeCarli and Scheltens, 2002). Regarding locations some emphasize deep infarcts in the frontal and limbic areas, other cortical ones, especially in the temporal and parietal areas. There are also controversies in regard to the number and volume of the infarcts, as well as the extent and location of atrophy. The diffuse WMLs have been offered as an important factor leading to functional disconnection of cortical brain areas.

Generalizations and summary in regard to lesion and cognition interaction in VaD can be made (Erkinjuntti et al., 1999; Román et al., 2002; O'Brien et al., 2003a, b):

- Not a single feature, but a combination of infarct features, extent and type of WMLs, degree and site of atrophy, and host factors characterizations are correlates of VCI/VaD.
- Infarct features favouring VaD include: bilaterality, multiplicity (>2), location in the dominant hemisphere and location in the fronto-subcortical and limbic structures.
- WML features favouring VaD are extensive WMLs (extending periventricular WMLs and confluent to extending WMLs in the deep white matter).
- It is doubtful that only a single small lesion could support an imaging evidence for a diagnosis of VaD. However, exceptions are rare cases with strategic infarcts.
- Absence of CVD lesions on CT or MRI are against a diagnosis of VaD.

Box 43.2   *Brain changes in vascular dementia*

Static lesions
- Arterial territorial infarct
- Distal field (watershed) infarct
- Lacunar infarct
- Ischaemic white matter lesions
- Incomplete ischaemic injury
- Atrophy

Functional ischaemic changes
- Focal (around the ischaemic lesion)
- Remote (disconnection, diaschisis)

Box 43.3   *Relation between ischaemic brain changes and dementia*

Causal
- Vascular dementia
- Post-stroke dementia

Contributory
- Post-stroke dementia
- Degenerative dementias
  - Alzheimer's disease
  - Lewy body dementia
  - Frontal lobe dementia

Coincidental
- All causes

43.6 MAIN SUBTYPES OF VASCULAR DEMENTIAS

The subtypes of VaD included in current classifications are the cortical VaD or MID also referred to as post-stroke VaD, the subcortical ischaemic vascular disease and dementia (SIVD) or the small vessel dementia, and the strategic infarct dementia (Box 43.4) (Erkinjuntti, 1987b; Román *et al.*, 1993; Brun, 1994; Cummings, 1994; Wallin and Blennow, 1994; Loeb and Meyer, 1996; Konno *et al.*, 1997; Wallin *et al.*, 2003) and many include also the hypoperfusion dementia (Sulkava and Erkinjuntti, 1987; Román *et al.*, 1993; Brun, 1994; Cummings, 1994). Further subtypes suggested include haemorrhagic dementia, hereditary vascular dementia, and AD with CVD (also labelled as combined or mixed dementia).

43.6.1 Cortical VaD

Cortical VaD, post-stroke VaD (MID) relates to large vessel disease, cardiac embolic events and also hypoperfusion. It shows predominantly cortical and cortico-subcortical arterial territorial and distal field (watershed) infarcts. Typical clinical features are lateralized sensorimotor changes and abrupt onset of cognitive impairment and aphasia (Erkinjuntti, 1987b; Erkinjuntti *et al.*, 1988). In addition, some combination of different cortical neuropsychological syndromes are present in cortical VaD (Mahler and Cummings, 1991).

43.6.2 Strategic infarct dementia

In strategic infarct dementia focal, often small, ischaemic lesions involving specific sites critical for higher cortical functions have been classified separately. Of the cortical sites, the hippocampal formation, angular gyrus and gyrus cinguli are examples. The subcortical sites include thalamus, fornix, basal forebrain, caudate, globus pallidus and the genu or anterior limb of the internal capsule (Tatemichi, 1990; Erkinjuntti and Hachinski, 1993; Erkinjuntti, 1996). Depending on the strategic location in question, the time-course and clinical features vary greatly.

Box 43.4 *Subtypes of vascular dementia*

- Cortical VaD, multi-infarct dementia (MID), post-stroke VaD
- Subcortical VaD, subcortical vascular disease and dementia (SIVD), small vessel dementia
- Strategic infarct dementia
- Hypoperfusion dementia
- Haemorrhagic dementia
- Hereditary vascular dementias
- Other vascular dementias
- Alzheimer's disease with CVD ('combined or mixed dementia')

43.6.3 Subcortical VaD

Subcortical ischaemic vascular dementia (SIVD), the small vessel dementia, incorporates two entities 'the lacunar state' and 'Binswanger disease' (Román *et al.*, 2002). It relates to small vessel disease and is characterized by lacunar infarcts, focal and diffuse ischaemic WMLs, and incomplete ischaemic injury (Erkinjuntti, 1987b; Román, 1987; Mahler and Cummings, 1991; Wallin *et al.*, 2003). The ischaemic lesions in SIVD affect the prefrontal subcortical circuit and the subcortical syndrome is the cardinal clinical manifestation (Cummings, 1993; Erkinjuntti *et al.*, 2000). Clinically, small vessel dementia is characterized by pure motor hemiparesis, bulbar signs and dysarthria, gait disorder, depression and emotional lability, and, especially, deficits in executive functioning (Ishii *et al.*, 1986; Babikian and Ropper, 1987; Román, 1987; Mahler and Cummings, 1991; Wallin *et al.*, 1991).

The patients with the SIVD having multiple lacunes and extensive WMLs on neuroimaging often give only a clinical history of 'prolonged TIA' or 'multiple TIAs' (which mostly are minor strokes) without residual symptoms and only mild focal findings (e.g. drift, reflex asymmetry, gait disturbance), which supports the importance of neuroimaging requirements in the criteria (Erkinjuntti *et al.*, 2000).

43.7 CLINICAL FEATURES

Early cognitive syndrome of SIVD is characterized by dysexecutive syndrome including slowed information processing, memory deficit (may be mild), and behavioural and psychological symptoms (Román *et al.*, 2002). The dysexecutive syndrome in SIVD includes impairment in goal formulation, initiation, planning, organizing, sequencing, executing, set-sifting and set-maintenance, as well as in abstracting (Mahler and Cummings, 1991; Cummings, 1994; Desmond *et al.*, 1999). The memory deficit in SIVD may be milder than, for example, in AD, and is specified by impaired recall, relative intact recognition, less severe forgetting, and better benefit from cues (Desmond *et al.*, 1999). Behavioural and psychological symptoms in SIVD include depression, personality change, emotional lability and incontinence, as well as inertia, emotional bluntness and psychomotor retardation (Mahler and Cummings, 1991; Román *et al.*, 1993; Cummings, 1994).

The early cognitive syndrome of cortical VaD includes some memory impairment (by definition), which may be mild, some heteromodal cortical symptom(s) such as aphasia, apraxia, agnosia, visuospatial or constructional difficulty. In addition most patients have some degree of dysexecutive syndrome.

Clinical neurological findings (Box 43.5) especially early in the course of SIVD include episodes of mild upper motor neurone signs (drift, reflex asymmetry, incoordination), gait disorder (apractic-atactic or small-stepped), imbalance and falls, urinary frequency and incontinence, dysarthria, dysphagia, as well as extrapyramidal signs (hypokinesia, rigidity)

Box 43.5   *Clinical features of vascular dementia*

Course
- Frequently an insidious onset and progressive deterioration
- Often stepwise deterioration (some recovery after worsening) and fluctuating course (e.g. difference between days) of cognitive symptoms
- May be relatively abrupt onset (days to weeks) of cognitive impairment

Symptoms and signs
- Clinical neurological findings indicating focal brain lesion early in the course:
  - mild motor or sensory deficits, decreased coordination, brisk tendon reflexes, Babinski's sign, field cut
- Bulbar signs including dysarthria and dysphagia
- Gait disorder: hemiplegic, apractic-atactic, small-stepped
- Unsteadiness and unprovoked falls
- Urinary frequency and urgency
- Psychomotor slowing, abnormal executive functioning
- Depression, anxiety, emotional lability
- Relatively preserved personality and insight in mild and moderate cases

Comorbid findings
- History of cardiovascular diseases (not always present), e.g. arterial hypertension, coronary heart disease, atrial fibrillation

CT or MRI
- Focal infarcts (70–90%). Diffuse or patchy white matter lesions (70–100%), often more extensive

SPECT or PET
- Often patchy reduction of regional blood flow and decreased white matter flow

EEG
- Compared to Alzheimer's disease, more often normal. If abnormal, more focal findings. Overall, abnormality increases with more severe intellectual decline

Laboratory
- No known specific tests. Often findings related to concomitant diseases, e.g. hyperlipidaemia, diabetes, cardiac abnormality

(Ishii *et al.*, 1986; Babikian and Ropper, 1987; Erkinjuntti, 1987a; Román, 1987; Román *et al.*, 1993, 2002). However, often these focal neurological signs are subtle only (Fischer *et al.*, 1990; Skoog, 1997).

Patients with cortical VaD, having multiple cortico-subcortical infarcts often show field cut, lower facial weakness, lateralized sensorimotor changes and gait impairment (hemiplegic, apractic-atactic) (Erkinjuntti, 1987a).

In SIVD the onset is variable. For example in the series of Babikian and Ropper (Babikian and Ropper, 1987), 60 per cent of the patients had a slow, less abrupt onset, and only 30 per cent an acute onset of cognitive symptoms. The course was gradual without (40 per cent) and with (40 per cent) acute deficits (Babikian and Ropper, 1987).

Traditionally cortical VaD (MID, post-stroke VaD) has been characterized by a relative abrupt onset (days to weeks), a step-wise deterioration (some recovery after worsening), and fluctuating course (e.g. difference between days) of cognitive functions (Román, 1987; Erkinjuntti, 1987b; Fischer *et al.*, 1990; Chui *et al.*, 1992; Román *et al.*, 1993; Skoog, 1997).

43.8   CLINICAL CRITERIA

Since the 1970s several clinical criteria for VaD have been used (Erkinjuntti, 1994; Rockwood *et al.*, 1994; Wetterling *et al.*, 1996). The most widely used criteria for VaD include the DSM-IV (American Psychiatric Association, 1994), the ICD-10 (World Health Organization, 1993), the ADDTC criteria (Chui *et al.*, 1992), and the NINDS-AIREN criteria (Román *et al.*, 1993).

The two cardinal elements implemented in the clinical criteria for VaD are the definition of the cognitive syndrome of dementia (Erkinjuntti *et al.*, 1997), and the definition of the vascular cause of the dementia (Erkinjuntti, 1994; Wetterling *et al.*, 1994, 1996). Variation in defining these two critical elements has created different definitions giving different point prevalence estimates, identifying different groups of subjects, and consequently also identifying different types and distribution of brain lesions (Skoog *et al.*, 1993; Wetterling *et al.*, 1996; Erkinjuntti *et al.*, 1997, 1999; Pohjasvaara *et al.*, 1997). Further, this heterogeneity may have been a factor for negative results in prior clinical trials on VaD (Inzitari *et al.*, 2000). All the clinical criteria used are consensus criteria, which are neither derived from prospective community-based studies on vascular factors affecting the cognition, nor based on detailed natural histories (Chui *et al.*, 1992; Román *et al.*, 1993; Erkinjuntti, 1994, 1997; Rockwood *et al.*, 1994). All the cited criteria are mainly based on the ischaemic infarct concept and designed to have high specificity, although they have been poorly implemented and validated (Rockwood *et al.*, 1994; Erkinjuntti, 1997).

The NINDS-AIREN criteria:

- emphasize heterogeneity of VaD syndromes and pathologic subtypes including not only ischaemic stroke but also other causes of CVD including cerebral hypoxic-ischaemic events, WMLs, and haemorrhagic strokes;
- recognize the variability in clinical course, which may be static, remitting, or progressive;
- highlight the question of the location of ischaemic lesions and the need to establish a causal relationship between vascular brain lesions and cognition;

- recognize the need to establish a temporal relationship between stroke and dementia onset;
- include specific findings early in the course that support a vascular rather than a degenerative cause;
- emphasize the importance of brain imaging to support clinical findings; and
- give value of neuropsychological testing to document impairments in multiple cognitive domains.

The NINDS-AIREN criteria handle VaD as a syndrome with different aetiologies and different clinical manifestations and not as a single entity, and they list possible subtypes to be used in research studies. The focus is on consequences of CVD, but the criteria takes also into account different aetiologies. These criteria incorporate also different levels of certainty of the clinical diagnosis (probable, possible, definite).

In a neuropathological series, sensitivity of the NINDS-AIREN criteria for probable and possible VaD was 58 per cent and specificity 80 per cent (Gold et al., 1997). The criteria successfully excluded AD in 91 per cent of cases, and the proportion of combined cases misclassified as probable VaD was 29 per cent. Compared with the other modern criteria, the ADDTC criteria (Chui et al., 1992), the NINDS-AIREN criteria are more specific and they better exclude combined cases (54 per cent versus 29 per cent). In a more recent series the sensitivity of NINDS-AIREN criteria for probable VaD was 20 per cent and specificity 93 per cent; the corresponding figures for probable ADDTC were 25 and 91 per cent (Gold et al., 2002). The interrater reliability of the NINDS-AIREN criteria is moderate to substantial (kappa 0.46 to 0.72) (Lopez et al., 1994).

43.9 DIFFERENTIAL DIAGNOSIS

Differential diagnosis of VaD include besides differentiation between VaD and AD a number of other conditions (Box 43.6). We focus here on AD and AD + CVD.

Box 43.6 *Differential diagnosis of vascular dementia*

- Alzheimer's disease
- Alzheimer's disease with cerebrovascular disease (CVD)
- Normal pressure hydrocephalus (NPH)
- Non-ischaemic white matter lesions and dementia
- Frontal lobe tumour
- Intracranial mass
- Vascular dementia and Alzheimer's disease (mixed)
- Lewy body dementia
- Frontotemporal dementia
- Parkinson's disease and dementia
- Progressive supranuclear palsy
- Multisystem atrophy

43.9.1 Alzheimer's disease

AD has typical neuropathological stages (transentorhinal, limbic and neocortical) corresponding to clinical stages (preclinical, early and mild dementia) (Braak and Braak, 1991). Accordingly, AD is a typical stage concurrent disorder, progressing from mild cognitive impairment (MCI), to early predementia AD and then to stages of AD dementia (Petersen, 1995), and is not a diagnosis of exclusion. Taken the clinical series on differential diagnosis between AD and VaD, the main limitations have included definition of the cognitive syndrome, the dementia syndrome, definition of the cause/aetiology of the dementia syndrome, and heterogeneity of patient populations, especially that of VaDs. The traditional concept of dementia has been based on the typical clinical features of AD (McKhann et al., 1984; Erkinjuntti et al., 1997). The definition has been the prison of AD, as the focus has been early episodic memory impairment, more or less global cognitive syndrome, with progressive course, and major restrictions of ADL. These are features different from that in early cases of VaD, and these criteria merely detect an endstage of VaD.

The most widely used definition of the cause of these cognitive syndromes includes the NINDS-AIREN for probable VaD (Román et al., 1993) and the NINCDS-ADRDA for probable AD (McKhann et al., 1984). These criteria define a stereotyped set of patient groups: probable VaD characterized by abrupt onset, or fluctuating and stepwise course with clinical signs of CVD and relevant CVD on brain imaging. On the contrary AD is characterized by insidious onset, progressive course, without clinical signs of CVD and without signs of CVD in brain imaging. Accordingly, in typical cases the differentiation between probable VaD and AD using common clinical tools is direct (Erkinjuntti et al., 1988).

Hachinski Ischaemic Score has been widely used to differentiate patients with VaD and AD (Hachinski et al., 1975) (Table 43.1). In most clinical series the majority of the items differentiate VaD from probable AD – as a matter of fact this is based on the clinical definitions used. However, in a large

Table 43.1 *Hachinski Ischaemic Score*

Item	Score value
Abrupt onset	2
Stepwise deterioration	1
Fluctuating course	2
Nocturnal confusion	1
Relative preservation of personality	1
Depression	1
Somatic complaints	1
Emotional incontinence	1
History of hypertension	1
History of strokes	2
Evidence of associated atherosclerosis	1
Focal neurological symptoms	2
Focal neurological signs	2

neuropathologically confirmed series by Moroney *et al.* (1997), the independent correlates of VaD were stepwise deterioration (OR 6.1), fluctuating course (OR 7.6), history of hypertension (OR 4.3), history of stroke (OR 4.3) and history of focal neurological symptoms (OR 4.4).

43.9.2 Alzheimer's disease with CVD

AD and CVD (mixed dementia) is a challenge. Increasing evidence shows that different vascular factors are related to AD, and frequently CVD coexist with AD (Kalaria and Ballard, 1999; Skoog *et al.*, 1999). This overlap is increasingly important in older populations. Clinical recognition of patients with mixed dementia or AD with CVD, however, is a problem. As detailed in the neuropathological series of Moroney *et al.* (1997) these patients have a clinical history and signs of CVD, being clinically more close to VaD. In fact, in this series fluctuating course (OR 0.2) and history of strokes (OR 0.1) were the only items differentiating AD from the mixed cases.

Problematic clinical examples include stroke unmasking AD in patients with post-stroke dementia, insidious onset and/or slow progressive course in VaD patients, and cases where difficulty exists in assessing the role of less extensive WMLs or of distinct infarcts on neuroimaging. AD with CVD (referred also as mixed dementia) could present clinically either as AD with evidence of cerebrovascular lesions in brain imaging, or with features of both AD and VaD (Rockwood *et al.*, 1999). In a Canadian study, typical AD presentations with one or more features pointing to 'vascular aspects', derived from the Hachinski Ischaemia Scale score, were used successfully to diagnose AD + CVD in combination with neuroimaging of ischaemic lesions (Rockwood *et al.*, 2000). Vascular risk factors, and focal neurological signs and symptoms were present more often in AD with CVD than in 'pure' AD. Other visible clinical clues for a diagnosis of AD with CVD were gained from analyses of disease course characteristics, and presentations of patchy cognitive deficits, early onset of seizures or gait disorder.

A solution to recognize patients with AD + CVD could be to find reliable biological markers of clinical AD. Potential markers include, for example, early prominent episodic memory impairment, early and significant medial temporal lobe atrophy on magnetic resonance imaging (MRI), bilateral parietal hypoperfusion on single photon emission computed tomography (SPECT), change in cerebrospinal fluid (CSF) β-amyloid and tau-protein, or presence of ApoE ε4 allele.

43.10 CLINICAL EXAMINATION

Clinical evaluation of patients with memory impairment has two diagnostic approaches: first, the symptomatic diagnosis,

i.e. evaluation of the type and extent of cognitive impairment; and second, the aetiological diagnosis, i.e. evaluation of vascular cause(s) and related factors. The prevalent symptomatic categories besides dementia include delirium, circumscribed neuropsychological syndromes, e.g. aphasia, and functional psychiatric disorders, e.g. depression (Erkinjuntti, 1997). Steps in the aetiological diagnosis include diagnosis of the specific causes, especially the potentially treatable conditions, evaluation of secondary factors able to affect the cognitive functioning and more detailed differentiation between specific causes, especially that between VaD and AD.

Elements in the clinical examination of the patients with suspected vascular dementia have been detailed in Box 43.7. The cornerstone in the evaluation are traditional clinical skills to perform detailed clinical and neurological history and examination, including interview of a close informant. These patients are challenging and we should allocate enough time for the consultation, often 40–60 minutes.

Bedside mental status examination include the Mini-Mental State Examination (Folstein *et al.*, 1975); it has limitations as it emphasizes language, does not include timed elements and recognition portion of the memory tests, is insensitive to mild deficits, and is influenced by education and age. Other proposed screening instruments for VaD include a 4–10 word memory test with delayed recall, cube

---

Box 43.7 *Clinical examinations of patients with suspected vascular dementia*

Symptomatic diagnosis (type and extent of cognitive impairment)

- Interview of the patient and caregiver
- Bedside mental status examination
- Neuropsychological examination
- Assessment of social functions and activities of daily life
- Assessment of psychiatric and behavioural symptoms

Aetiological diagnosis (vascular cause[s] and related factors)

- Clinical and neurological history and examination
- Ischaemic scores
- Brain imaging: computed tomography (CT) or preferably magnetic resonance imaging (MRI) of the brain
- Routine laboratory investigations
- Chest X-ray
- Electrocardiography (ECG)
- Single photon emission computed tomography (SPECT)
- Electroencephalography (EEG)
- Extended laboratory investigations including coagulation studies
- Doppler ultrasonography/magnetic angiography of the carotid arteries
- Echocardiography
- 24-hour ECG and blood pressure monitoring

drawing test for copy, verbal fluency test (number of animals named in 1 minute), and Luria's alternating hang sequence or finger rings and letter cancellation test (neglect) (Román et al., 1993). This has given rise to proposals to incorporate such testing in future clinical trials, and to the development of the vascular equivalent of the ADAS-cog, the VaDAS-cog (Ferris and Gauthier, 2002).

Often more detailed neuropsychological tests and test batteries are needed. The test battery should cover the main cognitive domains including memory functions (short- and long-term memory), abstract thinking, judgement, aphasia, apraxia, agnosia, orientation, attention, executive functions, and speed of information processing (Erkinjuntti et al., 1997; Pohjasvaara et al., 1998; Hietanen et al., 2003; Tingus et al., 2003). Assessment of a person's social and emotional functioning is also part of basic evaluation.

Clinical evaluations to define the aetiological diagnosis include clinical and neurological history and examination (Box 43.7).

Brain imaging should be performed at least once during the initial diagnostic workout; because of its higher sensitivity and ability to demonstrate medial temporal lobe and basal forebrain areas MRI is preferred. Chest X-ray, electrocardiography and screening laboratory tests are part of the basic evaluation (Erkinjuntti and Sulkava, 1991; Amar and Wilcock, 1996; Orrell and Wade, 1996; DeCarli and Scheltens, 2002). In selected cases extended laboratory investigations, analysis of the CSF, electroencephalography (EEG), quantitative EEG and SPECT are done, as well as examinations of the extra- and intracranial arteries and detailed cardiological investigations.

43.11 PREVENTION

Primary prevention aims to reduce incident disease by eliminating its cause or the main risk factors (Last, 1988) (Table 43.2). In primary prevention, the target is the person with a 'brain at risk' of CVD before cognitive impairment or stroke occur. The intent is to treat putative risk factors and to promote protection. In this contexts the effect of primary prevention in populations free of cognitive impairment still remains less well known. Most cardiovascular and cerebrovascular studies on primary prevention have missed the opportunity to study cognition as an end point. The Medical Research Council's treatment trial of hypertension in older adults did not show an effect on subsequent cognitive function (Prince et al., 1996). In contrast, the SYST-EUR Study demonstrated that the treatment of isolated systolic hypertension in the elderly with a calcium-channel agent decreased significantly the incidence of dementia (Forette et al., 1998, 2002). Other inferences about the positive effects of primary prevention are based on cumulative experience with the treatment of vascular risk factors in the primary prevention of stroke.

Table 43.2 *Prevention and treatment of vascular dementia*

Type of therapy	Main target	Degree of cognitive impairment	Action
Prevention			
Primary	Brain at risk of CVD and any cognitive impairment	Normal	Treatment of and action on risk factors; promotion of protective factors
Secondary	CVD brain at risk of VCI and VaD	Normal; mild diffuse in several; significant in one domain	Diagnosis of the type of CVD; acute intervention on ischemic brain changes; treatment according to CVD type; untensifying treatment of risk factors
Treatment			
Slowing progression	Risk of progression of VCI and VaD	Significant in several domains; dementia	Intensifying primary and secondary prevention
Symptomatic			Targeted medications to: increase cerebral blood flow; support neuronal metabolism; modify neurotransmission; neuroprotection
Secondary factors	Risk of intensifying VCI and VaD		Treatment of secondary factors affecting the cognition
AD strategies			AD treatments to prevent, slow progression and treat symptoms of impairment of cognition and behaviour

AD, Alzheimer's disease; CVD, cerebrovascular disease; VaD, vascular dementia; VCI, vascular cognitive impairment

Secondary prevention aims to prevent disease progression by means of early detection and appropriate treatment. In secondary prevention, the target is CVD in the brain at risk of VCI and VaD. The basis of secondary prevention therefore includes diagnosis and treatment of acute stroke in order to limit the extent of ischaemic brain changes and to promote recovery, prevention of recurrence of stroke, according to the type of CVD, slowing the progression of brain changes associated with VaD (e.g. ischaemic white matter lesions, management of risk factors of incident dementia), as well as intensifying treatment of risk factors. There have been significant advances in acute stroke therapy, particularly in regard to antiplatelet agents, thrombolysis and acute stroke care (Wardlaw, 2001), although neuroprotection has been disappointing (Gorelick, 2000). Treatments for recurrent stroke prevention are also well defined (Gorelick, 2002). Selection of treatment is guided by the aetiology of CVD such as large artery disease (e.g. antiplatelet agents, carotid endarterectomy), cardiac embolic events (e.g. anticoagulation), small-vessel disease (e.g. aspirin), and haemodynamic mechanisms (e.g. control of hypotension and cardiac arrhythmias) (Gorelick, 2002). Hypoxic ischaemic events (cardiac arrhythmias, congestive heart failure, myocardial infarction, seizures, pneumonia) are important risk factors for incident dementia in patients with stroke (Moroney et al., 1996). There is a dearth of knowledge on the effects of secondary prevention of VaD. Most trials on acute stroke and secondary prevention of stroke have missed the opportunity to study cognition as an end point.

Perindopril, an angiotensin-converting enzyme inhibitor used in a trial of secondary prevention of stroke (PROGRESS Collaborative Group, 2003), showed a beneficial effect (usually coupled with the diuretic indapamide) in patients who had a previous stroke. Lowering of blood pressure was associated with a reduction in the risk of dementia and severe cognitive impairment among patients who experienced recurrent stroke.

Given that HMG Co-A reductase inhibitors (statins) are import in the secondary prevention of stroke (Callahan, 2001), there are incentives to undertake trials in patients with mild VaD.

In general, drugs initiated for the treatment of CVD and prevention of its adverse outcomes should be continued even as cognitive impairment manifests itself. Often, the drugs that modify vascular risk factors are used less frequently as the dementia becomes more severe. As dementia progresses lower blood pressure is often seen with severe disease. In small series, patients with VaD benefited from blood pressure control and cessation of smoking (Meyer et al., 1986). Routine use of acetylsalicylic acid in VaD is controversial (Molnar et al., 1999). Effects of vitamins to reduce plasma homocysteine levels await randomized controlled trials (Welch and Loscalzo, 1998). Further, the absence of progressive cognitive decline in patients receiving placebo in symptomatic treatment trials of VaD may also reflect an effect of intensified risk factor control (Rother et al., 1998).

43.12 TREATMENT

A vascular aetiology underlay the use of several compounds purported to be useful in the symptomatic treatment of VaD. These included antithrombotics, ergot alkaloids, nootropics, TRH-analogue, *Ginkgo biloba* extract, plasma viscosity drugs, hyperbaric oxygen, antioxidants, serotonin and histamine receptor antagonists, vasoactive agents, xanthine derivates and calcium antagonists (Erkinjuntti, 1999; Doody et al., 2001; Erkinjuntti and Rockwood, 2001; Rockwood et al., 2002; Inzitari et al., 2003). These studies have mostly had negative results, were based on small numbers, short treatment periods, variations in diagnostic criteria and tools, often included mixed populations, and have had variations in the application of clinical end points. Currently there is not a widely accepted standard symptomatic treatment of VaD (Doody et al., 2001). Two drugs which were carefully studied are propentofylline (Rother et al., 1998) and nimodipine (Pantoni et al., 1996; Lopez-Arieta 2001).

Propentofylline, a glial modulator, is no longer under study despite observed beneficial effect on learning and memory (Mielke et al., 1998). Unpublished results of several European and Canadian double-blind, placebo-controlled, randomized, parallel group trials on the efficacy and safety of long-term treatment with propentofylline, compared with placebo, in patients with mild to moderate VaD according to NINDS-AIREN criteria (Román et al., 1993) have been shown as a poster (Pischel, 1998). This 24-week study showed a significant symptomatic improvement and long-term efficacy in ADAS-Cog and CIBIC-plus up to 48 weeks. In addition, sustained treatment effects for at least 12 weeks after withdrawal were present suggesting an effect on disease progression.

Nimodipine, a dihydropyridine calcium antagonist was used in subcortical VaD. Nimodipine is held to effect vasodilatation, without a steal effect, so as to reduce the influx of calcium ions into depolarized neurones. In consequence, it is held to have a neuroprotective effect that is not directly related to changes in cerebral blood flow. In addition the drug has a specific effect on small vessels. Encouraging results from an open-label trial (Pantoni et al., 1996) led to a subgroup analysis of a larger double-blind, placebo-controlled study known as the Scandinavian Multi-Infarct Dementia Trial. Patients were divided between MID and subcortical VaD groups, according to CT findings and were blindly assessed. Nimodipine had a beneficial effect on attention and psychomotor performances in the subcortical group, although no clear advantage was seen in the combined sample (Pantoni et al., 2000a, b). These preliminary results are currently being tested in an international, multicentre, randomized, double-blind trial enrolling patients with subcortical VaD, defined on a clinical-radiological basis (Erkinjuntti et al., 2000). For the moment, the Cochrane Collaboration review concluded that there is no convincing evidence that nimodipine is a useful treatment for the symptoms of vascular dementia (Lopez-Arieta, 2001).

43.12.1 Current treatment of VaD

At present, there is evidence-based data that two types of drugs modulating neurotransmission abnormalities appear to be useful in VaD; these neurotransmitter abnormalities are acetylcholine deficit (acetylcholinesterase inhibitors, AChEIs) and glutamate excess (memantine).

Memantine is a moderate-affinity, voltage-dependent, uncompetitive NMDA receptor antagonist with fast receptor kinetics (Görtelmeyer and Erbler, 1992). Initial data from a double-blind, placebo-controlled nursing home trial in severe dementia of mixed aetiology (51 per cent of patients had VaD), showed that memantine (10 mg/day) was well tolerated, improved function, and reduced care dependency in treated patients with severe dementia, compared with patients on placebo (Winblad and Poritis, 1998). Based on the hypothesis of glutamate-induced neurotoxicity in cerebral ischaemia, two randomized, placebo-controlled 6-month trials have studied memantine (20 mg/day) in patients with mild to moderate probable NINDS-AIREN VaD (Orgogozo et al., 2002; Wilcock et al., 2002).

The study MMM 300 randomized 147 patients on memantine and 141 on placebo (Orgogozo et al., 2002). After 28 weeks, the mean ADAS-cog scores were significantly improved relative to placebo: the memantine group mean score had gained an average of 0.4 points, whereas the placebo group mean score declined by 1.6, i.e. a difference of 2.0 points ($P = 0.0016$). The response rate for CIBIC-plus, defined as improved or stable, was 60 per cent with memantine compared with 52 per cent with placebo ($P = 0.227$). The Gottfries-Bråne-Steen (GBS) Scale and the Nurses' Observation Scale for Geriatric Patients (NOSGER) total scores at week 28 did not differ significantly between the two groups. However, the GBS Scale intellectual function subscore and the NOSGER disturbing behaviour dimension also showed a difference in favour of memantine ($P = 0.04$ and $P = 0.07$, respectively).

The study MMM 500 randomized 277 patients on memantine and 271 on placebo (Wilcock et al., 2002). At 28 weeks the active group had gained 0.53 and placebo declined by 2.28 points in ADAS-cog, a significant difference of 1.75 ADAS-cog points between the groups ($P < 0.05$). The global assessment CGIC, the MMSE, GBS or NOSGER did not reveal differences between the groups. Memantine was well tolerated in the two studies. In a *post hoc* pooled subgroup analysis of these two studies by baseline severity as assessed by MMSE, the more advanced patients obtained a larger cognitive benefit than the mildly affected patients did. The subgroup with an MMSE score <15 at baseline showed an ADAS-cog improvement of 3.2 points over placebo (Möbius and Stöffler, 2003). Subgroup analyses by radiological findings at baseline showed that the cognitive treatment effect for memantine was more pronounced in the small vessel type group of patients who had no signs of cortical infarctions in their brain scans (CT or MRI). In addition, the placebo decline in this group was clearly more pronounced than in

patients with (cortical) large-vessel type VaD (Möbius and Stöffler, 2002).

43.12.2 Cholinergic dysfunction in VaD

Cholinergic deficit in VaD, independently of any concomitant AD pathology, has been documented. Cholinergic structures are vulnerable to ischaemic damage. Indeed, hippocampal CA1 neurones are particularly susceptible to experimental ischaemia, and hippocampal atrophy is common in patients with VaD in the absence of AD (Vinters et al., 2000). Selden et al. (1998) described two highly organized and discrete bundles of cholinergic fibres in human brains that extend from the nucleus basalis to the cerebral cortex and amygdala. Both pathways travel in the white matter, and together carry widespread cholinergic input to the neocortex. Localized ischaemic focal lesions or white matter lesions may interrupt these cholinergic bundles. Mesulam et al. (2003) demonstrated cholinergic denervation from pathway lesions, in the absence of AD, in a young patient with CADASIL, a pure genetic form of VaD.

In experimental rodent models, such as the spontaneously hypertensive stroke-prone rat, there is a significant reduction in cholinergic markers including acetylcholine (ACh) in the neocortex, hippocampus and CSF (Togashi et al., 1994). White matter infarction in rodent models results in substantial decreases in cholinergic markers, presumably through an impact on cholinergic projection fibres (Freidle, 1967). In human disease there is a reported loss of cholinergic neurones in 70 per cent of AD cases and in 40 per cent of VaD patients examined neuropathologically, and reduced ACh activity in the cortex, hippocampus, striatum and CSF (Court et al., 2002).

43.12.3 Cholinesterase inhibitors in VaD

Four cholinesterase inhibitors (ChEIs) have been approved for use in AD: tacrine, donepezil, rivastigmine and galantamine. In controlled trials, secondary outcomes have varied, but often included ADL and behavioural scales. Studies have shown a modest improvement of cognition peaking at 3 months and decline below the baseline or starting point at 9–12 months. There is good evidence for stabilization of ADL decline for at least 6 months, and improvement of some behaviours associated with AD (predominantly apathy and hallucinations). A description of reasonable therapeutic expectations was published by Winblad et al. (2001).

By 2004 pivotal randomized clinical trials with ChEIs had been conducted in patients with probable and possible VaD (donepezil) and in probable VaD or AD + CVD (galantamine). A smaller series on SIVD with rivastigmine has been published. Large clinical trials on VaD are ongoing with galantamine (GAL-INT-26) and rivastigmine (Vantage).

Donepezil's safety and efficacy has been studied in the largest clinical trial of pure VaD to date (Pratt et al., 2002). A total of 1219 subjects were recruited for a 24-week, randomized, placebo-controlled, multicentre, multinational study divided in two identical trials, 307 and 308 (Black *et al.*, 2003; Wilkinson *et al.*, 2003). The patients were randomized to one of three groups: placebo, donepezil at a dosage of 5 mg/day or donepezil 10 mg/day. The group receiving 10 mg/day initially received 5 mg/day for 4 weeks; the dosage was then titrated up to 10 mg/day. Patients with a diagnosis of either possible or probable VaD according to the NINDS-AIREN criteria were eligible for inclusion in the study (Román *et al.*, 1993). All patients had brain imaging prior to the study (CT or MRI) with demonstration of relevant cerebrovascular lesions. Patients with pre-existing AD were excluded, as were patients with the so-called 'mixed dementia', better defined as AD + CVD. Although patients with concomitant AD may not be totally excluded, the NINDS-AIREN criteria are able to classify patients into probable or possible VaD categories (Erkinjuntti *et al.*, 1988; Gold *et al.*, 2002).

Probable VaD was present in 73 per cent of the patients in the two studies. Probable VaD was diagnosed by the presence of mild to moderate dementia, clinical and brain imaging evidence of relevant CVD, and a clear temporal relationship between stroke and cognitive decline, with onset of dementia within 3 months of a clinically eloquent stroke or a stepwise course. Possible VaD was diagnosed in cases with indolent onset of the cognitive decline, and accounted for 27 per cent of the cases. Possible VaD included patients with silent stroke, extensive white matter disease or an atypical clinical course. There were no differences in trial results between these two subgroups.

The end points included cognition measured with the ADAS-cog, MMSE, global function as measured with the Clinicians' Interview-Based Impression of Change – Plus (CIBIC-plus), the Sum of Boxes of the Clinical Dementia Rating (CDR-SB) and ADL as measured with Alzheimer's Disease Functional Assessment and Change Scale (ADFACS).

In the study 307 (Black *et al.*, 2003), the donepezil treatment group showed statistically significant improvement in cognitive functioning measured by ADAS-cog; the mean changes from baseline score was: donepezil 5 mg/day, -1.90 ($P = 0.001$); donepezil 10 mg/day, -2.33 ($P < 0.001$). The MMSE also showed statistically significant improvement versus placebo. The treated group showed as well significant improvement in global function on the CIBIC-plus in the 5 mg/day group ($P = 0.014$), which did not reach significance in the 10 mg/day group ($P = 0.27$). CDR-SB showed non significant benefit in the 5 mg/day group, but was significant in the 10 mg/day group ($P = 0.022$). The ADL showed significant benefits in donepezil-treated patients over placebo using the ADFACS in both treatment groups ($P < 0.05$).

In the study 308 (Wilkinson *et al.*, 2003), the donepezil treatment group showed statistically significant improvement in cognitive functioning measured with the ADAS-cog; the mean changes from baseline score was: donepezil 5 mg/day, -1.65 ($P = 0.003$); donepezil 10 mg/day, -2.09

($P = 0.0002$). The MMSE also showed statistically significant improvement versus placebo. The treated group showed as well significant improvement in global function of the CIBIC-plus in the 5 mg/day day group ($P = 0.004$), which did not reach significance in the 10 mg/day group ($P = 0.047$). CDR-SB showed non-significant benefit in the 5 mg/day group, but was significant in the 10 mg/day group ($P = 0.03$). The ADL showed superiority in the donepezil-treated patients over placebo using the ADFACS in both treatment groups, which, however, did not reach significance at the end of the study compared with placebo.

Of interest, cognitive decline in untreated patients with VaD in this trial was less severe than in placebo-treated patients with AD during 24 weeks of study, using similar instruments. These differences were also noted for global effects, measured by the CIBIC-plus version; and, in contrast with AD, patients with VaD showed actual improvements in global function. In contrast with AD trials, these VaD studies enrolled more men than women (58 per cent versus 38 per cent), their mean age was older (74.5 ± 0.2 versus 72 ± 0.2 years), their HIS score more elevated (6.6 ± 0.2 versus < 4), with higher percentages of subjects with hypertension, cardiovascular disease, diabetes, smoking, hypercholesterolaemia, previous stroke and TIAs, suggesting that the two populations are clearly different (Pratt *et al.*, 2002).

Donepezil was generally well tolerated, although more adverse effects were reported in the 10 mg group than in the 5 mg or placebo groups. The adverse effects were assessed as mild to moderate and transient, and were typically diarrhoea, nausea, arthralgia, leg cramps, anorexia and headache. The incidence of bradycardia and syncope was not significantly different from the placebo group. The discontinuation rates for the groups were 15 per cent for placebo, 18 per cent for the 5 mg group, and 28 per cent for the 10 mg group. There was no significant interaction with the numerous cardiovascular medications and antithrombotic agents used by this population. Donepezil was demonstrated to be effective and well tolerated in the treatment of patients with VaD.

Galantamine is a cholinesterase inhibitor that also modulates central nicotinic receptors to increase cholinergic neurotransmission. In a multicentre, double-blind, 6-month randomized controlled trial patients diagnosed with probable VaD, or with AD combined with CVD, received galantamine 24 mg/day (n = 396) or placebo (n = 196) (Erkinjuntti *et al.*, 2002). Eligible patients met the clinical criteria of probable VaD of the NINDS-AIREN (Román *et al.*, 1993), or possible AD according to the NINCDS-ADRDA (McKhann *et al.*, 1984). They also showed significant radiological evidence of CVD on CT or MR (i.e. they had AD and CVD). Evidence of CVD on a recent (within 12 months) scan included multiple large-vessel infarcts or a single, strategically placed infarct (angular gyrus, thalamus, basal forebrain, territory of the posterior or anterior cerebral artery), or at least two basal ganglia and white matter lacunae, or white matter changes involving at least 25 per cent of the total white matter. They had to score 10–25 on the MMSE and 12 or more in the ADAS-cog/11, and had to be between ages of 40 and 90 years.

Primary end points were cognition, as measured using the ADAS-cog/11, and global functioning, as measured using the CIBIC-plus. Secondary end points included assessments of activities of daily living, using the Disability Assessment in Dementia (DAD), and behavioural symptoms, using the Neuropsychiatric Inventory (NPI) (Erkinjuntti et al., 2002).

Analysing both groups as a whole, galantamine demonstrated efficacy on all outcome measures. Galantamine showed greater efficacy than placebo on ADAS-cog (2.7 points, $P \le 0.001$) and CIBIC-plus (74 per cent versus 59 per cent of patients remained stable or improved, $P \le 0.001$). Activities of daily living and behavioural symptoms were also significantly improved compared with placebo (both $P < 0.05$). Galantamine was well tolerated (Erkinjuntti et al., 2002).

In an open label extension the original galantamine group of patients with probable VaD or AD + CVD showed similar sustained benefits in terms of maintenance of or improvement in cognition (ADAS-cog), functional ability (DAD) and behaviour (NPI) after 12 months (Erkinjuntti et al., 2003).

Although the study was not designed to detect differences between subgroups, the subgroup of patients with AD + CVD on galantamine (n = 188; 48 per cent) showed greater efficacy than placebo (n = 97; 50 per cent) at 6 months on ADAS-cog ($P \le 0.001$) and CIBIC-plus ($P = 0.019$) (Erkinjuntti et al., 2002). In the open-label extension patients with AD + CVD continuously treated with galantamine maintained cognitive abilities at baseline for 12 months (Small et al., 2003).

Probable VaD was diagnosed in 81 (41 per cent) of the placebo patients and in 171 (43 per cent) of the patients on galantamine. In the probable VAD group, ADAS-cog scores improved significantly (mean change from baseline, 2.4 points, $P < 0.0001$) in patients treated with galantamine for 6 months, but not in the patients treated with placebo (mean change from baseline, 0.4; treatment difference versus galantamine 1.9, $P = 0.06$) (Erkinjuntti, 2002; Erkinjuntti et al., 2002). More patients treated with galantamine than with placebo-maintained or improved global function (CIBIC-plus, 31 per cent versus 23 per cent); however, it was not statistically significant. In these patients, the cognitive benefits of galantamine were maintained at least up to 12 months, demonstrating a mean change of -2.1 in the ADAS-cog score compared with baseline (Small et al., 2003) and the active group was still close to baseline at 24 months (Kurz et al., 2003).

Rivastigmine is an acetylcholinesterase and butyrylcholinesterase inhibitor. The effects of rivastigmine in the treatment of cognitive impairment associated with general VaD remain to be established. It has been shown in a small study of patients with subcortical VaD that rivastigmine improved cognition (clock drawing test), reduced caregiver stress and improved behaviour (Moretti et al., 2001). AD patients with vascular risk factors showed relatively larger effect size in cognitive response (ADAS-cog) than those without vascular risk factors (Kumar et al., 2000; Erkinjuntti et al., 2002).

REFERENCES

Amar K and Wilcock G. (1996) Vascular dementia. BMJ 312: 227–231

American Psychiatric Association. (1994) Diagnostic and Statistical Manual of Mental Disorders, 4th edition. Washington DC, American Psychiatric Association

Babikian V and Ropper AH. (1987) Binswanger's disease: a review. Stroke 18: 2–12

Berchtold NC and Cotman CW. (1998) Evolution in the conceptualization of dementia and Alzheimer's disease: Greco Roman period to the 1960s. Neurobiological Aging 19: 173–189

Black S, Román GC, Geldmacher DS et al. (2003) Efficacy and tolerability of donepezil in vascular dementia. Positive results of a 24-week, multicenter, international, randomized, placebo-controlled clinical trial. Stroke 34: 2323–2332

Bowler JV and Hachinski V. (1995) Vascular cognitive impairment: a new approach to vascular dementia. Baillière's Clinical Neurology 1995; 4: 357–376

Bowler JV, Steenhuis R, Hachinski V. (1999) Conceptual background of vascular cognitive impairment. Alzheimer Disease and Associated Disorders 13: S30–S37

Braak H and Braak E. (1991) Neuropathological staging of Alzheimer-related changes. Acta Neuropathologica (Berlin) 82: 239–259

Brun A. (1994) Pathology and pathophysiology of cerebrovascular dementia: pure subgroups of obstructive and hypoperfusive etiology. Dementia 5: 145–147

Brust JC. (1988) Vascular dementia is overdiagnosed. Archives of Neurology 45: 799–801

Callahan A. (2001) Cerebrovascular disease and statins: a potential addition to the therapeutic armamentarium for stroke prevention. American Journal of Cardiology 88: 33J–37J.

Chui HC. (1989) Dementia: a review emphasizing clinicopathologic correlation and brain-behaviour relationships. Archives of Neurology 46: 806–814

Chui HC and Gonthier R. (1999) Natural history of vascular dementia. Alzheimer Disease and Associated Disorders 13 (Suppl. 3): S124–S130

Chui HC, Victoroff JI, Margolin D, Jagust W, Shankle R, Katzman R. (1992) Criteria for the diagnosis of ischemic vascular dementia proposed by the State of California Alzheimer's Disease Diagnostic and Treatment Centers. Neurology 42: 473–480

Court JA, Perry EK, Kalaria RN. (2002) Neurotransmitter control of the cerebral vasculature and abnormalities in vascular dementia. In: T Erkinjuntti and S Gauthier (eds), Vascular Cognitive Impairment. London, Martin Dunitz Ltd, pp. 167–185

Cummings JL. (1993) Fronto-subcortical circuits and human behavior. Archives of Neurology 50: 873–880

Cummings JL. (1994) Vascular subcortical dementias: clinical aspects. Dementia 5: 177–180

DeCarli C and Scheltens P. (2002) Structural brain imaging. In: T Erkinjuntti and S Gauthier (eds), Vascular Cognitive Impairment. London, Martin Dunitz Ltd, pp. 433–457

Desmond DW. (1996) Vascular dementia: a construct in evolution. Cerebrovascular and Brain Metabolism Reviews 8: 296–325

Desmond DW, Erkinjuntti T, Sano M *et al.* (1999) The cognitive syndrome of vascular dementia: implications clinical trials. *Alzheimer Disease and Associated Disorders* **13** (Suppl. 3): S21–S29

Doody RS, Stevens JC, Beck C *et al.* (2001) Practice parameter: Management of dementia (an evidence-based review). Report of the Quality Standards Subcommittee of the American Academy of Neurology. *Neurology* **56**: 1154–1166

Englund E, Brun A, Alling C. (1988) White matter changes in dementia of Alzheimer's type. Biochemical and neuropathological correlates. *Brain* **111**: 1425–1439

Erkinjuntti T. (1987a) Differential diagnosis between Alzheimer's disease and vascular dementia: evaluation of common clinical methods. *Acta Neurologica Scandinavica* **76**: 433–442

Erkinjuntti T. (1987b) Types of multi-infarct dementia. *Acta Neurologica Scandinavica* **75**: 391–399

Erkinjuntti T. (1994) Clinical criteria for vascular dementia: The NINDS-AIREN criteria. *Dementia* **5**: 189–192

Erkinjuntti T. (1996) Clinicopathological study of vascular dementia. In: I Prohovnik, J Wade, S Knezevic TK Tatemichi T Erkinjuntti T (eds), *Vascular Dementia. Current Concepts.* Chichester, John Wiley and Sons, pp. 73–112

Erkinjuntti T. (1997) Vascular dementia: challenge of clinical diagnosis. *International Psychogeriatrics* **9** (Suppl. 1): 51–58

Erkinjuntti T. (1999) Cerebrovascular dementia. Pathophysiology, diagnosis and treatment. *CNS Drugs* 1999; **12**: 35–48

Erkinjuntti T. (2002) Cognitive decline and treatment options for patients with vascular dementia. *Acta Neurologica Scandinavica* **106** (Suppl. 178): 15–18

Erkinjuntti T and Sulkava R. (1991) Diagnosis of multi-infarct dementia. *Alzheimer Disease and Associated Disorders* **5**: 112–121

Erkinjuntti T and Hachinski VC. (1993) Rethinking vascular dementia. *Cerebrovascular Disease* **3**: 3–23

Erkinjuntti T and Pantoni L. (2000) Subcortical vascular dementia. In: S Gauthier and JL Cummings (eds), *Alzheimer's Disease and Related Disorders Annual.* London, Martin Dunitz Ltd, pp. 101–133

Erkinjuntti T and Rockwood K. (2001) Vascular cognitive impairment. *Psychogeriatrics* **1**: 27–38

Erkinjuntti T, Haltia M, Palo J, Sulkava R, Paetau A. (1988) Accuracy of the clinical diagnosis of vascular dementia: a retrospective clinical and post-mortem neuropathological study. *Journal of Neurology, Neurosurgery, and Psychiatry* **51**: 1037–1044

Erkinjuntti T, Ostbye T, Steenhuis R, Hachinski V. (1997) The effect of different diagnostic criteria on the prevalence of dementia. *New England Journal of Medicine* **337**: 1667–1674

Erkinjuntti T, Bowler JV, DeCarli C *et al.* (1999) Imaging of static brain lesions in vascular dementia: implications for clinical trials. *Alzheimer Disease and Associated Disorders* **13** (Suppl. 3): S81–S90

Erkinjuntti T, Inzitari D, Pantoni L *et al.* (2000) Research criteria for subcortical vascular dementia in clinical trials. *Journal of Neural Transmission* **59** (Suppl. 2): 23–30

Erkinjuntti T, Kurz A, Gauthier S, Bullock R, Lilienfeld S, Chandrasekhar Rao VD. (2002) Efficacy of galantamine in probable vascular dementia and Alzheimer's disease combined with cerebrovascular disease: a randomized trial. *Journal of the American Geriatrics Society* **359**: 1283–1290

Erkinjuntti T, Skoog I, Lane R, Andrews C. (2002) Rivastigmine in patients with Alzheimer's disease and concurrent hypertension. *International Journal of Clinical Practice* **56**: 791–796

Erkinjuntti T, Kurz A, Small GW, Bullock R, Lilienfeld S, Damaraju CV. (2003) An open-label extension trial of galantamine in patients with probable vascular dementia and mixed dementia. *Clinical Therapeutics* **25**: 1765–1782

Ferris S and Gauthier S. (2002) Cognitive outcome measures in vascular dementia. In: T Erkinjuntti and S Gauthier (eds), *Vascular Cognitive Impairment.* London, Martin Dunitz Ltd, pp. 395–400

Fischer P, Gatterer G, Marterer A, Simanyi M, Danielczyk W. (1990) Course characteristics in the differentiation of dementia of the Alzheimer type and multi-infarct dementia. *Acta Psychiatrica Scandinavica* **81**: 551–553

Folstein MF, Folstein SE, McHugh PR. (1975) 'Mini-mental State': A practical method for grading the cognitive state of patients for the clinician. *Journal of Psychiatric Research* **12**: 189–198

Forette F, Seux ML, Staessen JA *et al.* (1998) Prevention of dementia in randomized double-blind placebo-controlled Systolic Hypertension in Europe (Syst-Eur) trial. *Journal of the American Geriatrics Society* **352**: 1347–1351

Forette F, Seux ML, Staessen JA *et al.* (2002) The prevention of dementia with antihypertensive treatment. New evidence from the systolic hypertension in Europe (Sys-Eur) study. *Archives of Internal Medicine* **162**: 2046–2052

Fratiglioni L, Launer LJ, Andersen K *et al.* (2000) Incidence of dementia and major subtypes in Europe: A collaborative study of population-based cohorts. *Neurology* **54** (Suppl. 5): S10–S15

Freidle RL. (1967) A comparative histochemical mapping of the distribution of butyrylcholinesterase in the brains of four species of animals, including man. *Acta Anatomica (Basel)* **66**: 161–177

Gold G, Giannakopoulos P, Montes-Paixao JC *et al.* (1997) Sensitivity and specificity of newly proposed clinical criteria for possible vascular dementia. *Neurology* **49**: 690–694

Gold G, Bouras C, Canuto A *et al.* (2002) Clinicopathological validation study of four sets of clinical criteria for vascular dementia. *American Journal of Psychiatry* **159**: 82–87

Gorelick PB. (1997) Status of risk factors for dementia associated with stroke. *Stroke* **28**: 459–463

Gorelick PB. (2000) Neuroprotection in acute ischemic stroke: a tale of for whom the bell tolls? *Journal of the American Geriatrics Society* **355**: 1925–1926

Gorelick PB. (2002) Stroke prevention therapy beyond antithrombotics: unifying mechanisms in ischaemic stroke pathogenesis and implications for therapy. *Stroke* **33**: 862–875

Görtelmeyer R and Erbler H. (1992) Memantine in treatment of mild to moderate dementia syndrome. *Drug Research* **42**: 904–912

Hachinski VC. (1990) The decline and resurgence of vascular dementia. *Canadian Medical Association Journal* **142**: 107–111

Hachinski V. (1992) Preventable senility: a call for action against the vascular dementias. *Journal of the American Geriatrics Society* **340**: 645–648

Hachinski VC, Lassen NA, Marshall J. (1974) Multi-infarct dementia. A cause of mental deterioration in the elderly. *Journal of the American Geriatrics Society* **ii**: 207–210

Hachinski VC, Iliff LD, Zilhka E *et al.* (1975) Cerebral blood flow in dementia. *Archives of Neurology* **32**: 632–637

Hebert R and Brayne C. (1995) Epidemiology of vascular dementia. *Neuroepidemiology* **14**: 240–257

Hietanen M, Hänninen T, Almkvist O. (2003) Neuropsychological examination of memory. In: T Erkinjuntti and S Gauthier (eds), *Vascular Cognitive Impairment.* London, Martin Dunitz Ltd, pp. 365–382

Inzitari D, Erkinjuntti T, Wallin A, del Ser T, Romanelli M, Pantoni L. (2000) Subcortical vascular dementia as a specific target for clinical trials. *Annals of the New York Academy of Sciences* **903**: 510–521

Inzitari D, Lamassa M, Pantoni L. (2003) Treatment of vascular dementias. In: JV Bowler and V Hachinski (eds), *Vascular Cognitive Impairment Preventable Dementia*. Oxford, Oxford University Press, pp. 277–292

Ishii N, Nishihara Y, Imamura T. (1986) Why do frontal lobe symptoms predominate in vascular dementia with lacunes? *Neurology* **36**: 340–345

Kalaria RN and Ballard C. (1999) Overlap between pathology of Alzheimer disease and vascular dementia. *Alzheimer Disease and Associated Disorders* **13** (Suppl. 3): S115–S123

Kittner B, Rossner M, Rother M. (1997) Clinical trials in dementia with propentofylline. *Annals of the New York Academy of Sciences* **826**: 307–316

Kittner B for the European/Canadian Propentofyllinen Study Group. (1999) Clinical trials of Propentofylline in vascular dementia. *Alzheimer Disease and Associated Disorders* **13** (Suppl. 3): S166–S171

Konno S, Meyer JS, Terayama Y, Margishvili GM, Mortel KF. (1997) Classification, diagnosis and treatment of vascular dementia. *Drugs and Aging* **11**: 361–373

Kumar V, Anand R, Messian J. (2000) An efficacy and safety analysis of Exelon in Alzheimer's disease with concurrent vascular risk factors. *European Journal of Neurology* **7**: 159–169

Kurz AF, Erkinjuntti T, Small GW, Lilienfeld S, Venkata Damarju CR. (2003) Long-term safety and cognitive effects of galantamine in the treatment of probable vascular dementia or Alzheimer's disease with cerebrovascular disease. *European Journal of Neurology* **10**: 663–640

Last JM. (1988) *A Dictionary of Epidemiology*, 2nd edition. New York, Oxford University Press

Lobo A, Launer LJ, Fratiglioni L *et al.* (2000) Prevalence of dementia and major subtypes in Europe: a collaborative study of population-based cohorts. *Neurology* **54** (Suppl. 5): S4–S9

Loeb C and Meyer JS. (1996) Vascular dementia: still a debatable entity? *Journal of the Neurological Sciences* **143**: 31–40

Lopez-Arieta BJ. (2001) Nimodipine for primary degenerative, mixed and vascular dementia. *Cochrane Database of Systematic Reviews* **1**: CD000147

Lopez OL, Larumbe MR, Becker JT *et al.* (1994) Reliability of NINDS-AIREN clinical criteria for the diagnosis of vascular dementia. *Neurology* **44**: 1240–1245

Mahler ME and Cummings JL. (1991) The behavioural neurology of multi-infarct dementia. *Alzheimer Disease and Associated Disorders* **5**: 122–130

McKhann G, Drachman D, Folstein M, Katzman R, Price D, Stadlan EM. (1984) Clinical diagnosis of Alzheimer's disease: report of the NINCDS-ADRDA Work Group under the auspices of Department of Health and Human Services Task Force on Alzheimer's Disease. *Neurology* **34**: 939–944

Mesulam M, Siddique T, Cohen B. (2003) Cholinergic denervation in a pure multi-infarct state: observations on CADACIL. *Neurology* **60**: 1183–1185

Meyer JS, Judd BW, Tawaklna T, Rogers RL, Mortel KF. (1986) Improved cognition after control of risk factors for multi-infarct dementia. *JAMA* **256**: 2203–2209

Mielke R, Herholz K, Grond M, Kessler J, Heiss WD. (1992) Severity of vascular dementia is related to volume of metabolically impaired tissue. *Archives of Neurology* **49**: 909–913

Mielke R, Möller H-J, Erkinjuntti T, Rosenkranz B, Rother M, Kittner B. (1998) Propentofylline in the treatment of vascular dementia and Alzheimer-type dementia: overview of phase I and phase II clinical trials. *Alzheimer Disease and Associated Disorders* **12** (Suppl. 2): 29–35

Möbius HJ and Stöffler A. (2002) New approaches to clinical trials in vascular dementia: memantine in small vessel disease. *Cerebrovascular Disease* **13** (Suppl. 2): 61–66

Möbius HJ and Stöffler A. (2003) Memantine in vascular dementia. *International Psychogeriatrics* **15** (Suppl. 1): 207–213

Molnar F, Hing M, St John P, Brymer C, Rockwood K, Hachinski V. (1999) National survey on the treatment of and future research into subcortical vascular dementia. *Canadian Journal of Neurological Sciences* **25**: 320–324

Mölsä PK, Marttila RJ, Rinne UK. (1995) Long-term survival and predictors of mortality in Alzheimer's disease and multi-infarct dementia. *Acta Neurologica Scandinavica* **91**: 159–164

Moretti R, Torre P, Antonello RM, Cazzato G. (2001) Rivastigmine in subcortical vascular dementia: a comparison trial on efficacy and tolerability for 12 months follow-up. *European Journal of Neurology* **8**: 361–362

Moretti R, Torre P, Antonello RM, Cazzato G, Bava A. (2002) Rivastigmine in subcortical vascular dementia: an open 22-month study. *Journal of the Neurological Sciences* **203**: 141–146

Moroney JT, Bagiella E, Desmond DW, Paik MC, Stern Y, Tatemichi TK. (1996) Risk factors for incident dementia after stroke. Role of hypoxic and ischemic disorders. *Stroke* **27**: 1283–1289

Moroney JT, Bagiella E, Desmond DW *et al.* (1997) Meta-analysis of the Hachinski Ischemic Score in pathologically verified dementias. *Neurology* **49**: 1096–1105

O'Brien J, Reisberg B, Erkinjuntti T. (2003a) Vascular burden of the brain. *International Psychogeriatrics* **15** (Suppl. 1): 11–13

O'Brien JT, Erkinjuntti T, Reisberg B *et al.* (2003b) Vascular cognitive impairment. *Lancet Neurology* **2**: 89–98

Orgogozo J.-M, Rigaud A.-S, Stöffler A, Möbius H-J, Forette F. (2002) Efficacy and safety of memantine in patients with mild to moderate vascular dementia. A randomized, placebo-controlled trial (MMM 300). *Stroke* **33**: 1834–1839

Orrell RW and Wade JPH. (1996) Clinical diagnosis: How good is it and how should it be done. In: I Prohovnik, J Wade, S Knezevic, TK Tatemichi, T Erkinjuntti (eds), *Vascular Dementia. Current Concepts*. Chichester, John Wiley and Sons, pp. 143–163

Ostbye T, Hill G, Steenhuis R. (2002) Mortality in elderly Canadians with and without dementia. *Neurology* **53**: 521–526

Pantoni L and Garcia JH. (1995) The significance of cerebral white matter abnormalities 100 years after Binswanger's report. A review. *Stroke* **26**: 1293–1301

Pantoni L and Garcia JH. (1997) Pathogenesis of leukoaraiosis: a review. *Stroke* **28**: 652–659

Pantoni L, Carosi M, Amigoni S, Mascalchi M, Inzitari D. (1996) A preliminary open trial with nimodipine in patients with cognitive impairment and leukoaraiosis. *Clinical Neuropharmacology* **19**: 497–506

Pantoni L, Bianchi C, Beneke M, Inzitari D, Wallin A, Erkinjuntti T. (2000a) The Scandinavian multi-infarct dementia trial: a double-blind, placebo-controlled trial on nimodipine in multi-infarct dementia. *Journal of the Neurological Sciences* **175**: 116–123

Pantoni L, Rossi R, Inzitari D *et al.* (2000b) Efficacy and safety of nimodipine in subcortical vascular dementia: a subgroup analysis of the Scandinavian multi-infarct dementia trial. *Journal of the Neurological Sciences* **175**: 124–134

Pasquier F and Leys D. (1997) Why are stroke patients prone to develop dementia? *Journal of Neurology* **244**: 135–142

Petersen RC. (1995) Normal aging, mild cognitive impairment, and early Alzheimer's disease. *The Neurologist* 1: 326–344

Petersen RC, Doody R, Kurz A *et al.* (2002) Current concepts in mild cognitive impairment. *Archives of Neurology* 58: 1985–1992

Pischel T. (1998) Long-term-efficacy and safety of propentofylline in patients with vascular dementia. Results of a 12 months placebo-controlled trial. *Neurobiological Aging* 19(4S): S182

Pohjasvaara T, Erkinjuntti T, Vataja R, Kaste M. (1997) Dementia three months after stroke. Baseline frequency and effect of different definitions of dementia in the Helsinki Stroke Aging Memory Study (SAM) cohort. *Stroke* 28: 785–792

Pohjasvaara T, Erkinjuntti T, Ylikoski R, Hietanen M, Vataja R, Kaste M. Clinical determinants of poststroke dementia. *Stroke* 1998; 29: 75–81

Pohjasvaara T, Mäntylä R, Salonen O *et al.* (2000) How complex interactions of ischemic brain infarcts, white matter lesions and atrophy relate to poststroke dementia. *Archives of Neurology* 57: 1295–1300

Pratt RD, Perdomo CA, the Donepezil VaD 307 and 308 Study Groups. (2002) Donepezil-treated patients with probable vascular dementia demonstrate cognitive benefits. *Annals of the New York Academy of Science* 977: 513–522

Prince MJ, Bird AS, Blizard RA, Mann AH. (1996) Is the cognitive function of older patients affected by antihypertensive treatment? Results from 54 months of the Medical Research Council's trial of hypertension in older adults. *BMJ* 312: 801–805

PROGRESS Collaborative Group. (2003) Effects of blood pressure lowering with perindopril and indapimine therapy on dementia and cognitive decline in patients with cerebrovascular disease. *Archives of Internal Medicine* 163: 1069–1075

Rocca WA, Hofman A, Brayne C *et al.* (1991) The prevalence of vascular dementia in Europe: facts and fragments from 1980–1990 studies. EURODEM-Prevalence Research Group. *Annals of Neurology* 30: 817–824

Rockwood K. (1997) Lesions from mixed dementia. *International Psychogeriatrics* 9: 245–249

Rockwood K, Parhad I, Hachinski V *et al.* (1994) Diagnosis of vascular dementia: Consortium of Canadian Centres for Clinical Cognitive Research consensus statement. *Canadian Journal of Neurological Sciences* 21: 358–364

Rockwood K, Howard K, MacKnight C, Darvesh S. (1999) Spectrum of disease in vascular cognitive impairment. *Neuroepidemiology* 18: 248–254

Rockwood K, Wenzel C, Hachinski V, Hogan DB, MacKnight C, McDowell I. (2000) Prevalence and outcomes of vascular cognitive impairment. *Neurology* 54: 447–451

Rockwood K, Gauthier S, Erkinjuntti T. (2002) Prevention and treatment of vascular dementia. In: T Erkinjuntti and S Gauthier (eds), *Vascular Cognitive Impairment*. London, Martin Dunitz Ltd, pp. 587–595

Román GC. (1987) Senile dementia of the Binswanger type. A vascular form of dementia in the elderly. *JAMA* 258: 1782–1788

Román GC. (2001) Historic evolution of the concept of dementia: a systematic review from 2000 BC to 2000 AD. In: N Qizilbash, L Schneider, H Chui, P Tariot, H Brodaty, J Kaye *et al.* (eds), *Evidence-Based Dementia: A Practical Guide to Diagnosis and Management*. Oxford, Blackwell *Science*

Román GC, Tatemichi TK, Erkinjuntti T *et al.* (1993) Vascular Dementia: Diagnostic Criteria for Research Studies. Report of the NINDS-AIREN International Work Group. *Neurology* 43: 250–260

Román GC, Erkinjuntti T, Pantoni L, Wallin A, Chui HC. (2002) Subcortical ischaemic vascular dementia. *Lancet Neurology* 1: 426–436

Rother M, Erkinjuntti T, Roessner M, Kittner B, Marcusson J, Karlsson I. (1998) Propentofylline in the treatment of Alzheimer's disease and vascular dementia. *Dementia and Geriatric Cognitive Disorders* 9 (Suppl. 1): 36–43

Selden NR, Gitelman DR, Salamon-Murayama N, Parrsh TB, Mesulam MM. (1998) Trajectories of cholinergic pathways within the cerebral hemispheres of the human brain. *Brain* 121: 2249–2257

Skoog I. (1994) Risk factors for vascular dementia: a review. *Dementia* 5: 137–144

Skoog I. (1997) Blood pressure and dementia. In: L Hansson and WH Birkenhäger (eds), *Handbook of Hypertension. Vol 18. Assessment of Hypertensive Organ Damage*. Amsterdam, Elsevier Science BV, pp. 303–331

Skoog I. (1998) Status of risk factors for vascular dementia. *Neuroepidemiology* 17: 2–9

Skoog I, Nilsson L, Palmertz B, Andreasson L.-A, Svanborg A. (1993) A population-based study on dementia in 85-year-olds. *New England Journal of Medicine* 328: 153–158

Skoog I, Kalaria RN, Breteler MMB. (1999) Vascular factors and Alzheimer's disease. *Alzheimer Disease and Associated Disorders* 13 (Suppl. 3): S106–S114

Small G, Erkinjuntti T, Kurz A, Lilienfeld S. (2003) Galantamine in the treatment of cognitive decline in patients with vascular dementia or Alzheimer's disease with cerebrovascular disease. *CNS Drugs* 17: 905–914

Snowdon DA, Greiner LH, Mortimer JA, Riley KP, Greiner PA, Markesbery WR. (1997) Brain infarction and the clinical expression of Alzheimer disease. The Nun Study. *JAMA* 277: 813–817

Sulkava R and Erkinjuntti T. (1987) Vascular dementia due to cardiac arrhythmias and systemic hypotension. *Acta Neurologica Scandinavica* 76: 123–128

Tatemichi TK. (1990) How acute brain failure becomes chronic. A view of the mechanisms and syndromes of dementia related to stroke. *Neurology* 40: 1652–1659

Tatemichi TK, Desmond DW, Mayeux R *et al.* (1992) Dementia after stroke: baseline frequency, risks, and clinical features in a hospitalized cohort. *Neurology* 42: 1185–1193

Tatemichi TK, Paik M, Bagiella E, Desmond DW, Pirro M, Hanzawa LK. (1994a) Dementia after stroke is a predictor of long-term survival. *Stroke* 25: 1915–1919

Tatemichi TK, Paik M, Bagiella E *et al.* (1994b) Risk of dementia after stroke in a hospitalized cohort: results of a longitudinal study. *Neurology* 44: 1885–1891

Tingus K, McPherson S, Cummings JL. (2003) Neuropsychological examination of executive functions. In: T Erkinjuntti and S Gauthier (eds), *Vascular Cognitive Impairment*. London, Martin Dunitz Ltd, pp. 339–363

Togashi H, Matsumoto K, Yoshida M. (1994) Neurochemical profiles in cerebrospinal fluid of stroke-prone spontaneously hypertensive rat. *Neuroscience Letters* 166: 117–120

Togi H, Abe T, Kimura M, Saheki M, Takahashi S. (2002) Cerebrospinal fluid acetylcholine and choline in vascular dementia of Binswanger and multiple small infarct types as compared with Alzheimer-type dementia. *Journal of Neural Transmission* 103: 1211–1220

Tomlinson BE, Blessed G, Roth M. (1970) Observations on the brains of demented old people. *Journal of the Neurological Sciences* 11: 205–242

Vinters HV, Ellis WG, Zarow C *et al.* (2000) Neuropathologic substrates of ischemic vascular dementia. *Journal of Neuropathology and Experimental Neurology* **60**: 658–659

Wallin A and Blennow K. (1993) Heterogeneity of vascular dementia: mechanisms and subgroups. *Journal of Geriatric Psychiatry and Neurology* **6**: 177–188

Wallin A and Blennow K. (1994) The clinical diagnosis of vascular dementia. *Dementia* **5**: 181–184

Wallin A, Blennow K, Gottfries CG. (1991) Subcortical symptoms predominate in vascular dementia. *International Journal of Geriatric Psychiatry* **6**: 137–146

Wallin A, Blennow K, Gottfries CG. (2002) Neurochemical abnormalities in vascular dementia. *Dementia* **1**: 120–130

Wallin A, Milos V, Sjögren M, Pantoni L, Erkinjuntti T. (2003) Classification and subtypes of vascular dementia. *International Psychogeriatrics* **15** (Suppl. 1): 27

Wardlaw J. (2001) Overview of Cochrane thrombolysis meta-analysis. *Neurology* **57**:S69–S76

Welch GN and Loscalzo J. (1998) Mechanisms of disease: homocysteine and atherothrombosis. *New England Journal of Medicine* **338**: 1042–1050

Wetterling T, Kanitz RD, Borgis KJ. (1994) The ICD-10 criteria for vascular dementia. *Dementia* **5**: 185–188

Wetterling T, Kanitz RD, Borgis KJ. (1996) Comparison of different diagnostic criteria for vascular dementia (ADDTC, DSM-IV, ICD-10, NINDS-AIREN). *Stroke* **27**: 30–36

Wilcock G, Möbius HJ, Stöffler A, on behalf of the MMM 500 group. (2002) A double-blind, placebo-controlled multicentre study of memantine in mild to moderate vascular dementia (MMM500). *International Journal of Clinical Psychopharmacology* **17**: 297–305

Wilkinson D, Doody R, Helme R *et al.* (2003) Donepezil in vascular dementia. A randomized, placebo-controlled study. *Neurology* **61**: 479–486

Winblad B, Brodaty H, Gauthier S *et al.* (2001) Pharmacotherapy of Alzheimer's disease: is there a need to redefine treatment success? *International Journal of Geriatric Psychiatry* **16**: 388–390

Winblad B and Poritis N. (1998) Clinical improvement in a placebo-controlled trial with memantine in care-dependent patients with severe dementia. *Neurobiology of Aging* **19**: S303

Wolfson C, Wolfson DB, Asgharian M *et al.* (2001) A re-evaluation of the duration of survival after the onset of dementia. *New England Journal of Medicine* **344**: 1111–1116

World Health Organization. (1993) *ICD-10 Classification of Mental and Behavioural Disorders: Diagnostic Criteria for Research.* Geneva, WHO

Leukoaraiosis and cognitive impairment

LEONARDO PANTONI AND DOMENICO INZITARI

44.1 LEUKOARAIOSIS: HISTORICAL NOTES, DEFINITION AND RADIOLOGICAL–PATHOLOGICAL CORRELATES

44.1.1 Historical notes

A possible relation between cerebral white matter changes and impairment in cognitive functions was first suggested by Binswanger. In 1894, in a lengthy manuscript dealing with the differential diagnosis of general paresis of the insane, Binswanger described the case of a syphilitic man in his mid-50s, who had developed a progressive decline in mental functions characterized by speech and memory disorders, depression and personality changes (Binswanger, 1894; Blass et al., 1991). At autopsy, the dura mater at the base of the skull showed granular deposits; there was minimal intracranial atherosclerosis, considerable enlargement of the lateral ventricles, marked atrophy of the cerebral white matter, and multiple ependymal thickenings (Binswanger, 1894; Blass et al., 1991). Binswanger neither provided microscopic descriptions nor illustrated any findings of this single case, which remained the sole publication in which he dealt with the topic of white matter disease (Schneider and Wieczorek, 1991). In 1902, Alzheimer referred to the case described by his mentor Otto Binswanger, added a short histological description of what he considered was an analogous case and, intuitively, attributed the white matter changes to arteriosclerosis of the long penetrating vessels (Alzheimer, 1902; Schorer, 1992).

In 1962, Olszewski was the first to doubt that Binswanger's original report contained sufficient data to define a new disease, and suggested that the lesions in the dura mater and in

the ependyma, together with the history of syphilis, made Binswanger's a likely case of neurosyphilis. Accordingly, Olszewski proposed the term subcortical arteriosclerotic encephalopathy to describe 'a form of cerebral arteriosclerosis in which vessels of the white matter and subcortical grey matter are affected predominantly' (Olszewski, 1962). In subsequent years, the diagnosis of 'Binswanger's disease' remained restricted to rare descriptions, and careful revision of previous cases shows that many of them were ascribable to heterogeneous pathological processes (Pantoni et al., 1996b; Pantoni and Garcia, 1996).

The diagnosis of 'Binswanger's disease' acquired new popularity after the introduction of computed tomography (CT) and the first reports based exclusively on clinical-radiological findings (Rosenberg et al., 1979) that led many to assume that 'Binswanger's disease' could be diagnosed premortem (Loizou et al., 1981; Tomonaga et al., 1982; Young et al., 1983; Bradley et al., 1984a; Kinkel et al., 1985, 1986; Gerard and Weisberg, 1986). However, it soon became apparent that alterations of the hemispheric white matter, detected by either CT or magnetic resonance imaging (MRI), were common both in symptomatic and asymptomatic subjects.

Careful discussion about the historical appropriateness and usefulness of the eponym 'Binswanger's disease' is beyond the scope of this chapter and has been already dealt with in a collection of papers (Bogousslavsky et al., 1996). Nowadays, many authors still use the eponym to describe a form of vascular dementia with prevalent damage of subcortical structures. Bennett et al. (1990) have proposed clinical criteria for 'Binswanger's disease' which, unfortunately, were validated against pathological criteria on which no consensus exists. In the NINDS-AIREN criteria for vascular dementia

'Binswanger's disease' somehow overlaps with the more general definition of 'small-vessel disease with dementia' (Román *et al.*, 1993). Therefore what is by some still considered as a well-defined disease entity ('Binswanger's disease') probably represents only the most severe expression of a pathological process-radiological picture encompassing normal and pathological states without a clear cut-off.

44.1.2 Definition of leukoaraiosis

The term leukoaraiosis (originally leuko-araiosis) (LA) is a neologism coined in the 1980s to describe the radiological alterations detected by CT in the brains of elderly neurologically normal subjects and, more frequently, in demented patients (Hachinski *et al.*, 1986, 1987). The term derives from the Greek *leuko* (white) and *araiosis* (rarefaction), and was intentionally meant to be descriptive in an attempt to overcome the diffuse tendency to identify these neuroimaging abnormalities of uncertain origin and unclear clinical significance with a disease. LA designates areas of hypodensity on CT in the periventricular or subcortical white matter. The lesions can be focal, initially confluent, or diffuse according to the severity; are usually symmetric in the two hemispheres; and can be differentiated from other cerebrovascular processes such as territorial infarcts. In the original group of papers that reported on the new term and on the clinical correlates of LA, only CT-detected lesions were considered (Hachinski *et al.*, 1987; Inzitari *et al.*, 1987; Steingart *et al.*, 1987a, b). However, in the following years the term leukoaraiosis was also used to describe the MRI white matter lesions of analogue significance. On MRI these lesions appear as areas of hyperintensity on T2-weighted images and, given the better spatial resolution of this technique, can be differentiated into those in the periventricular region and those in the deep white matter of the corona radiata or centrum semiovale. A number of studies then pointed out differences, similarities and correlations between the lesions detected by CT and MRI (Brant-Zawadzki *et al.*, 1983; Bradley *et al.*, 1984b; Salgado *et al.*, 1986; Zimmerman *et al.*, 1986; Erkinjuntti *et al.*, 1987a; Johnson *et al.*, 1987; Lechner *et al.*, 1988). Recently, a systematic approach to the harmonization of CT and MRI LA rating has also been proposed (Pantoni *et al.*, 2002).

Over the following years, a large number of visual scales have been developed to rate and classify LA mainly in order to detect a cut-off score to define a pathological status. These scales are described in detailed in a review paper (Scheltens *et al.*, 1998). Being based on visual evaluation, many scales are prone to high interrater variability. The complexity of different scales is very variable. The scales based on MRI evaluation are usually more complex than those based on CT. Based on the above mentioned collaborative work by the European Task Force on Age-Related White Matter Changes, harmonization of the scales has been proposed. The main results of this collaboration are the creation of a new visual rating that can be used for both CT and MRI (Wahlund *et al.*, 2001), the development of methods to convert the score of one visual rating scale into that of another (Pantoni *et al.*, 2002), and definition of the agreement between visual and volumetric assessment of white matter changes (Kapeller *et al.*, 2003).

In recent years, computer-assisted volumetric evaluation of LA as detected by MRI has been used and proposed as a more valuable tool to assess the impact of these changes on clinical functions (Schmidt *et al.*, 1993). Volumetric assessment techniques are time consuming but likely more reliable than visual rating for the assessment of the progression of LA that is to be considered a rather slow but measurable process (Kapeller *et al.*, 2003). One of the most relevant advances in the field is the recent demonstration of the progression of white matter changes in a group of patients with severe degrees of LA (Schmidt *et al.*, 2003). Also based on the experience gathered in other neurological diseases such as multiple sclerosis, the volumetric assessment of LA has thus been proposed as an outcome measure for clinical trials focused on small vessel-related diseases that are characterized by prominent LA, such as subcortical vascular dementia (Schmidt *et al.*, 2004).

44.1.3 Radiological–pathological correlates of leukoaraiosis

The pathological correlates of LA are not definitely established. At the histological level, heterogeneous changes may all result in radiological pictures of white matter hypodensity on CT and hyperintensity on MRI. A number of studies have investigated the radiological-pathological correlates of LA, performing either neuroimaging and pathological studies after a short interval or post-mortem MRI examination.

LA in the periventricular white matter correlates with decreased myelin content (Sze *et al.*, 1986; Leifer *et al.*, 1990; Fazekas *et al.*, 1991; Grafton *et al.*, 1991; van Swieten *et al.*, 1991a; Chimowitz *et al.*, 1992; Scarpelli *et al.*, 1994; Moody *et al.*, 1995), loss of ependymal cell layer, reactive gliosis (the combination of the two above is also called granular ependymitis) at the tip of the frontal horns (Sze *et al.*, 1986; Jungreis *et al.*, 1988; Fazekas *et al.*, 1991; Grafton *et al.*, 1991; Chimowitz *et al.*, 1992; Scarpelli *et al.*, 1994), as well as with increased content of periependymal extracellular fluid, and with smaller and fewer number of axons per unit area (Sze *et al.*, 1986). Some authors also have described enlarged perivascular spaces at these periventricular locations (Grafton *et al.*, 1991) but, because small lesions in the periventricular white matter exist in all age groups (Sze *et al.*, 1986; Moody *et al.*, 1995), many authors do not consider these as indicative of true pathology.

The histological correlates of subcortical white matter changes, detectable by MRI, are less consistent than those reported for periventricular white matter changes. In these MRI studies, tiny focal abnormalities correspond to enlarged perivascular spaces (Chimowitz *et al.*, 1992; Scarpelli *et al.*,

1994), small cavitary infarcts (or lacunes) (Braffman *et al.*, 1988a; Marshall *et al.*, 1988; Muñoz *et al.*, 1993), demyelinating plaques, brain cysts and congenital diverticuli of the lateral ventricles (Braffman *et al.*, 1988b). MRI methods seem adequate to distinguish between enlarged perivascular Virchow–Robin spaces and lacunar infarcts (Braffman *et al.*, 1988b; Jungreis *et al.*, 1988). The more typical diffuse lesions in the centrum semiovale have been related to myelin rarefaction that in most instances spares the U fibres (Révész *et al.*, 1989; Chimowitz *et al.*, 1992). Sometimes these diffuse lesions are accompanied by astrogliosis (Fazekas *et al.*, 1991, 1993) and diffuse vacuolization of the white matter (Muñoz *et al.*, 1993). The white matter rarefaction corresponds to loss of myelinated axons, decreased number of oligodendrocytes, and vacuolation without clear aspects of necrosis (Awad *et al.*, 1986b; Lotz *et al.*, 1986; Janota *et al.*, 1989; Révész *et al.*, 1989). Thickening of the wall of the small vessels (arteriolosclerosis) is commonly found in areas of white matter rarefaction (Lotz *et al.*, 1986; Marshall *et al.*, 1988; Révész *et al.*, 1989; Leifer *et al.*, 1990; Fazekas *et al.*, 1991; van Swieten *et al.*, 1991b).

44.2 LEUKOARAIOSIS: PATHOGENIC ASPECTS

The pathogenesis of LA is still under investigation although the most recent data all point to a possible vascular (i.e. related to vessel disease) origin of these changes. Which vascular mechanism is involved cannot be considered, however, as definitively clarified.

Since the original, although largely incomplete and anecdotal, reports by Binswanger (Binswanger, 1894; Blass *et al.*, 1991) and Alzheimer (Alzheimer, 1902; Schorer, 1992), the white matter changes seen in demented patients were intuitively linked with vessel abnormalities. More recently, a number of clues suggest that vascular, and more specifically ischaemic, mechanisms are responsible for these alterations (Pantoni and Garcia, 1997). Among these are:

- The higher frequency of LA in patients with cerebrovascular diseases and in subjects with vascular risk factors (arterial hypertension, heart disease, diabetes mellitus, etc.) (Liao *et al.*, 1996; Longstreth *et al.*, 1996);
- The higher frequency of cardiovascular events at follow up in patients with LA (Inzitari *et al.*, 1995, 1997; Longstreth *et al.*, 2002; Wong *et al.*, 2002; Yamauchi *et al.*, 2002; Henon *et al.*, 2003; Vermeer *et al.*, 2003a);
- Some preliminary observations by positron emission tomography showing an ischaemic state of areas of LA (Yao *et al.*, 1992);
- The recent demonstration of the high susceptibility of white matter components to ischaemia (Pantoni *et al.*, 1996a; Petito *et al.*, 1998; Pantoni, 2000).

Central to the vascular theory is the role played by deep small vessel alterations. Changes of the arteriolosclerotic type

in the small vessels (loss of smooth muscle cells, fibrohyalinization of the tunica media, thickening of the wall) are commonly seen in areas of white matter alterations and have been associated particularly with ageing, arterial hypertension and diabetes mellitus (Alex *et al.*, 1962; Furuta *et al.*, 1991; Ostrow and Miller 1993). These changes may result in stenosis or occlusion of the vessels with consequent sudden or more chronic oligoaemia of the parenchyma. Moreover, the arteriolosclerotic changes lead the small arteries and arterioles located in the deep white matter and basal ganglia to lose their physiologic capacity to dilate and constrict in response to variations of systemic blood pressure (autoregulation). Accordingly, the areas supplied by these vessels may suffer from cerebral blood flow fluctuations (either drops or increases) in response to changes of systemic blood pressure.

Both these types of mechanism may be particularly harmful to the brain parenchyma since the blood supply of the deep cerebral structures is of the terminal type with scarce, if any, anastomoses (Rowbotham and Little, 1965; Van den Bergh and van der Eecken, 1968). This vascular damage to the white matter would not be sufficient to provoke complete necrosis of the tissue (with the exception of some areas where true lacunar infarcts are recognizable) but could cause selective damage to some histological components. Brun and Englund were among the first to propose that the diffuse changes of the white matter seen in demented patients were to be considered a form of incomplete infarction (Brun and Englund, 1986). Although this remains a hypothesis, there are now experimental data showing that white matter components are extremely vulnerable to ischaemia and can be damaged in the absence of neuronal injury (Pantoni *et al.*, 1996a; Petito *et al.*, 1998).

As far as the pathogenesis of LA in Alzheimer's disease (AD) is concerned, there are a few hypotheses that have been put forward. The majority of AD patients show cerebral amyloid angiopathy, another type of small vessel disease. Cerebral amyloid angiopathy is histologically characterized by thickening of the wall of small- and medium-size subarachnoid and cortical arteries and arterioles caused by the deposition in the media and adventitia of an amorphous, eosinophilic material that shows typical yellow-green birefringence when stained with Congo Red and viewed under polarized light (Vinters, 1987). The hypothesis that amyloid angiopathy in AD patients may be causally linked to white matter alterations is supported by the observation that subcortical leukoencephalopathy was demonstrated in patients with cerebral amyloid angiopathy who lacked changes characteristic of AD (Gray *et al.*, 1985; Tabaton *et al.*, 1991).

The hypothesis that white matter damage in patients with AD might simply reflect Wallerian changes secondary to cortical loss of neurones (Leys *et al.*, 1991) seems less likely. The histological markers of Wallerian changes, such as abundant lipid-laden macrophages, are in fact missing in most areas of leukoencephalopathy. Moreover, it is difficult to understand why many AD patients with severe cortical atrophy and loss of neurones lack demonstrable white matter changes at autopsy (Brun and Englund, 1986). Magnetic resonance spectroscopy data confirm that decreases in myelin phospholipids exist in areas of LA, in the absence of changes in the concentration of N-acetyl-aspartate, a marker for neuronal perikarya (Constans et al., 1995). This reinforces the hypothesis that the changes in the white matter can occur independent of the alterations involving the grey matter. A second possible cause of white matter damage in AD patients are changes affecting the tunica media and tunica adventitia of the white matter vessels, the extent and frequency of which is higher than in age-matched controls (Brun and Englund, 1986; Scheltens et al., 1995). A third possible cause could be changes in the permeability of the blood–brain barrier to proteins and the accumulation of fluid in the extracellular space. This leakiness might be the result of structural alterations, such as thickening of the basal lamina and pericapillary gliosis affecting the precapillary arterioles (Buée et al., 1994).

As alternatives to the possible ischaemic origin of LA, other hypotheses have been raised. In our view, these mechanisms are not mutually exclusive and may concur to the development of the final pathological picture. The small vessel alterations also could lead to damage of the blood–brain barrier and chronic leakage of fluid and macromolecules in the white matter. White matter changes characterized by pallor sparing the U fibres, accompanied by reactive astrogliosis and small vessel thickening have been described in conditions with antecedent brain oedema (Feigin and Popoff, 1963). This suggests that transient cerebral oedema might be an additional cause of white matter changes. The increased interstitial fluid concentration in abnormal white matter may be also a consequence of arterial hypertension. The blood–brain barrier may be leaky, and the capillary permeability to proteins may be increased in patients with systemic hypertension (Nag, 1984). Abnormalities in the blood–brain barrier, in the form of increased concentration of cerebrospinal fluid proteins, have been described in a group of patients with LA (Pantoni et al., 1993) and in a pathological series of patients with subcortical vascular encephalopathy (Akiguchi et al., 1998). In addition to the effects of sustained hypertension, hypertensive bouts of short duration could cause fluid transudation and protein leakage.

In addition to acquired vascular risk factors and conditions, genetically determined factors also could play an important role in the development of white matter alterations in the elderly. At least one form of vascular leukoencephalopathy exists that is genetically determined. It is called CADASIL (cerebral autosomal dominant arteriopathy with subcortical infarcts and leukoencephalopathy) and has been recently recognized and genetically characterized (Joutel et al., 1996). It is caused by a point mutation in the Notch3 gene located on chromosome 19p13.1. The clinical features of CADASIL are similar to those encountered in patients with sporadic age-related LA (cognitive deterioration, mood and gait disorders, recurrent subcortical strokes), but the age of onset of these disturbances is classically in the fourth and fifth decades and the course is usually very severe (Chabriat

et al., 1995; Dichgans et al., 1998; Desmond et al., 1999; Sarti and Pantoni, 2000). Moreover, migraine in young ages is another hallmark of the disease. From the radiological point of view, CADASIL patients present with diffuse cerebral white matter alterations associated with small focal lesions of the lacunar type. Histological studies have shown a degeneration of small vessel smooth muscle cells with deposition of granular osmiophilic material in the vessel wall (Ruchoux and Maurage, 1997; Sarti and Pantoni, 2000). The epidemiological relevance of CADASIL is under evaluation. Once reputed a rare disease, the number of described patients is now continuously increasing with cases reported at older ages and with more benign course raising the possibility of different patterns of transmission or penetrance (Pantoni et al., 2004).

Genetic factors may also contribute, by interaction with conventional risk factors, to the development of white matter injury in non-familiar cases. The heritability of LA has been shown by two studies in a consistent extent of about 65–70 per cent (Carmelli et al., 1998; Turner et al., 2004). Among possible genetic factors, angiotensinogen gene promoter haplotype (Schmidt et al., 2001) and paraoxonase specific polymorphisms (Schmidt et al., 2000) already have been found to be associated with LA. Another genetic factor with possible influence on the presence an extension of LA could be apolipoprotein (ApoE). The ApoE $\varepsilon4$ allele (Skoog et al., 1998) has been associated with damage of cerebral subcortical structures in one CT-based community survey, while the $\varepsilon2$-$\varepsilon3$ ApoE genotype has been found to be associated with white matter changes among population subjects free of neuropsychiatric disease (Schmidt et al., 1997). While the possible specific role of these genetic factors in the origin of LA remains to be explored, their influence could explain why not all the patients with vascular risk factors, for example hypertension, develop white matter alterations at follow up.

44.3 LEUKOARAIOSIS: EPIDEMIOLOGICAL ASPECTS

LA is frequently detected by CT and MRI both in asymptomatic people older than 60 years and in cognitively impaired individuals, especially those who have evidence of either cerebrovascular disease or risk factors associated with stroke (Pantoni and Garcia, 1995). Among series of patients with dementia of presumed vascular origin, LA is detected by CT with a frequency ranging from 41 to 100 per cent (London et al., 1986; Inzitari et al., 1987; Erkinjuntti et al., 1987a, b; Aharon-Peretz et al., 1988; Jayakumar et al., 1989; Wallin et al., 1989; Kobari et al., 1990a, b; Parnetti et al., 1990; Räihä et al., 1993), and by MRI in 64 to 100 per cent of the cases (Erkinjuntti et al., 1987a; Fazekas et al., 1987; Hershey et al., 1987; Kertesz et al., 1990; Kobari et al., 1990b; Mirsen et al., 1991; Almkvist et al., 1992; Liu et al., 1992; Schmidt, 1992; Wahlund et al., 1994). Although the frequency of LA is the highest in patients with cerebrovascular diseases, with or without dementia, a large proportion of AD patients, ranging from 19 to 78 per cent in CT-based studies have LA (George *et al.*, 1986a; London *et al.*, 1986; Erkinjuntti *et al.*, 1987a; Inzitari *et al.*, 1987; Rezek *et al.*, 1987; Steingart *et al.*, 1987b; Aharon-Peretz *et al.*, 1988; Erkinjuntti *et al.*, 1989; Fazekas *et al.*, 1989; Wallin *et al.*, 1989; Kobari *et al.*, 1990a, b; Blennow *et al.*, 1991; Diaz *et al.*, 1991; Lopez *et al.*, 1992; Räihä *et al.*, 1993), and from 7.5 to 100 per cent in MRI studies (George *et al.*, 1986b; Erkinjuntti *et al.*, 1987a; Fazekas *et al.*, 1987; Bondareff *et al.*, 1988; Wilson *et al.*, 1988; Fazekas *et al.*, 1989; Kertesz *et al.*, 1990; Kobari *et al.*, 1990b; Kozachuk *et al.*, 1990; McDonald *et al.*, 1991; Mirsen *et al.*, 1991; Almkvist *et al.*, 1992; Schmidt, 1992; Wahlund *et al.*, 1994; Waldemar *et al.*, 1994). However, the changes in white matter density are usually less severe in AD patients than in those with cerebrovascular disorders (Fazekas *et al.*, 1987; Steingart *et al.*, 1987b; Bowen *et al.*, 1990; Kertesz *et al.*, 1990; Almkvist *et al.*, 1992; Wahlund *et al.*, 1994).

LA in normal controls is usually less severe than in demented patients (Harrell *et al.*, 1991; Schmidt, 1992; Waldemar *et al.*, 1994), but is, however, frequent, occurring in up to 21 per cent of asymptomatic subjects evaluated with CT (London *et al.*, 1986; Inzitari *et al.*, 1987; Steingart *et al.*, 1987a; Kobari *et al.*, 1990b; Räihä *et al.*, 1993; George *et al.*, 1986a; Rezek *et al.*, 1987; Fazekas *et al.*, 1989) and up to 100 per cent among those evaluated with MRI (George *et al.*, 1986b; Fazekas *et al.*, 1987, 1988; Fazekas, 1989; Hendrie *et al.*, 1989; Hunt *et al.*, 1989; Rao *et al.*, 1989; Bowen *et al.*, 1990; Kertesz *et al.*, 1990; Kobari *et al.*, 1990b; Kozachuk *et al.*, 1990; Zubenko *et al.*, 1990; McDonald *et al.*, 1991; Mirsen *et al.*, 1991; Schmidt *et al.*, 1991, 1993; Almkvist *et al.*, 1992; Boone *et al.*, 1992; Schmidt, 1992; Tupler *et al.*, 1992; Waldemar *et al.*, 1994). The prevalence of MRI-detected LA in the general population has been evaluated in some recent community-based studies (Breteler *et al.*, 1994b; Lindgren *et al.*, 1994; Schmidt *et al.*, 1995; Ylikoski *et al.*, 1995; Liao *et al.*, 1996; Longstreth *et al.*, 1996). The figures are shown in Table 44.1.

Although figures are variable, the frequency of LA in these studies generally is very high. When any degree of white matter alterations was considered, almost all the subjects in the sample proved to have LA (Liao *et al.*, 1996; Longstreth *et al.*, 1996). In all these studies the severity and the extent of hyperintense images in the white matter increased with age.

One of these studies (Liao *et al.*, 1996) evaluated the possible difference in frequency of white matter alterations and risk factors between white and African American subjects. The higher prevalence of LA among African Americans was explained by the higher prevalence of hypertension in this racial group. No data exist so far on the prevalence of white matter changes among Asians among whom hypertension is highly prevalent.

Only one study has used CT to estimate the prevalence of white matter changes in the population. The study performed in Sweden in a cohort of very old (85-year-old) subjects reported an over-30 per cent prevalence of moderate to

Table 44.1 *Frequency of MRI-detected white matter changes in population based studies*

Author	Age	Number of subjects evaluated by MRI	Prevalence of white matter changes
Lindgren *et al.*, 1994	>35	77	62.3%*
Breteler *et al.*, 1994b	65–84	111	27%*
Ylikoski *et al.*, 1995	55–85	128	PVH: 39%
			DWH: 22%
Schmidt *et al.*, 1996	45–75	355	44.8%*
Longstreth *et al.*, 1996	>65	3301	95.6%*
Liao *et al.*, 1996	55–72	1920	85%*

*Considering any degree of white matter changes
DWH, deep white matter hyperintensities; PVH, periventricular hyperintensities

severe LA among non-demented subjects of this age group (Skoog *et al.*, 1994). In the same Swedish community an ongoing survey has recently reported the presence of LA of any degree to be present in about 55 per cent of the subjects with a mean age of 74 years (Simoni *et al.*, 2003).

Discrepant data on the frequency of LA across studies can be attributed to the inclusion of subjects of different ages or with different frequency of associated vascular risk factors. In addition, in MRI studies, the diverse strengths of magnetic field and variations in pulse sequence may lead to different results. Other possible reasons are the different criteria used for defining LA, including whether minimal periventricular lesions are considered or not.

44.4 RELEVANCE OF LEUKOARAIOSIS TO COGNITIVE IMPAIRMENT

44.4.1 Specificity of the association between leukoaraiosis, dementia and dementia type

The first reports of radiologically detected white matter changes regarded anecdotal cases of patients with dementia and other neurological deficits consistent with the diagnosis of 'Binswanger's disease'. In ensuing studies of series of patients collected for presenting with white matter abnormalities on CT, dementia or intellectual impairment was not invariably present (Valentine *et al.*, 1980; Goto *et al.*, 1981; Loizou *et al.*, 1981). The prevalence of demented patients varied across these series according to the different study settings and selection. The frequency of mental deterioration appeared to increase with the extension of white matter disease in a study performed in two Japanese geriatric hospitals (Goto *et al.*, 1981). All 15 patients in the series of Loizou *et al.* selected for fulfilling diagnostic criteria for a diagnosis of subcortical arteriosclerotic encephalopathy were mildly to moderately demented (Loizou *et al.*, 1981). Mental abnormalities included mostly impaired visual-motor skills and executive functions, mood and other frontal lobe disturbances related to white matter disease predominantly located in the frontal lobes. In the same study, a second small series of clinically unselected patients with white matter changes comprised subjects who were not demented, and, who, according to the authors, could exemplify early stages of subcortical arteriosclerotic encephalopathy (Loizou *et al.*, 1981).

LA was then examined in series of demented patients compared with non-demented controls. These studies provided conclusive evidence that the mere presence of LA was not synonymous with dementia. George *et al.* (1986a) were the first to indicate that what they called 'brain lucencies' were observable in demented patients as well as in normal aged individuals and a strict correlation with age was observed. They also suggested that in their AD patients the presence of lucencies seemed to worsen the dementing disorder. MRI soon proved to be more sensitive than CT in revealing changes in white matter. Awad *et al.* (1986a) investigated 'incidental subcortical lesions' on MRI scans of elderly individuals. Prevalence of these lesions was definitely correlated with increasing age, history of hypertension and ischaemic cerebrovascular disease, but was independent of any particular clinical entity, including dementia. However, George *et al.* (1986b) found that in demented patients the extent of white matter involvement on MRI was greater than in normal controls.

A similar finding was reported by others (Rezek *et al.*, 1987). In a study of demented patients compared with age-matched controls, Inzitari *et al.* (1987) addressed the question to what extent LA was linked with dementia, adjusting for factors associated with both conditions. Prevalence of LA was 35 per cent among 140 demented patients and about 11 per cent among 110 aged controls, a difference that was statistically highly significant. However, the strong association between dementia and LA disappeared in a multivariate statistical model including vascular risk factors and history of stroke as possible confounding factors, and the association between dementia and LA turned out mainly to be explained by the effect of stroke. In this study, history of stroke proved to be the major independent predictor of LA and deep lacunar infarct was the stroke type most frequent among demented patient with stroke history. Regarding dementia types, 100 per cent of patients classified as having multi-infarct dementia had LA. However, 33 per cent of the patients classified in the AD subgroup also showed LA.

This last finding, while confirming previous observations, was in contrast with the very low prevalence (1.5 per cent) of LA in AD patients found by Erkinjuntti *et al.* (1987b) in a study of the same period. The difference appeared less marked, but still significant, when MRI was used to replicate the study (Erkinjuntti *et al.*, 1987a); all the 29 vascular dementia patients had white matter changes in this second study, as opposed to 8 of 22 (36 per cent) in the AD group. These findings induced the authors to indicate imaging techniques as a tool for discriminating between different dementia types.

Schmidt (1992) made similar observations comparing MRI scans of 31 patients with vascular dementia with those of 27 patients with AD type dementia and those of 18 normal controls. Almost all the vascular dementia patients had white matter changes; these consisted in irregular periventricular halos in 94 per cent of patients, whereas large confluent subcortical lesions were observable in only half of these patients. AD patients showed almost exclusively punctate lesions which, however, were present in the large majority (78 per cent) of the patients. These findings suggest that between the two types of dementia, besides difference in the absolute prevalence of white matter lesions, there are quantitative differences and different morphological patterns, possibly expressing different pathological substrates.

The study by Hershey *et al.* (1987) found no statistically significant difference in the prevalence of white matter lesions between cerebrovascular patients with and without dementia, confirming that cerebral vascular disease is more important than dementia in relation to these lesions. Ventricular enlargement was the only abnormality discriminating between demented and non-demented patients in this study. Tanaka *et al.* (1989) performed a similar study in the setting of lacunar infarction. Demented patients had more severe white matter disease, but also a greater degree of brain atrophy.

From the evaluation of these first cross-sectional and observational data all the difficulties and uncertainties linked with the interpretation of the pathophysiological role of LA in relation to dementia emerge, even in relation to the vascular dementia setting where LA is most frequently observable, and where the current view considers white matter changes an important factor to be taken into account. Regarding LA associated with AD, we have seen that, after the first observations, this rather surprising finding has been reported repeatedly, although with a wide variation in the observed prevalence.

44.4.2 Effect of leukoaraiosis on severity of dementia and on pattern of cognitive impairment

Several early studies attempted to evaluate the impact of white matter abnormality on the severity of dementia or on pattern of cognitive impairment (Table 44.2). Patients included in these studies were for the large majority AD patients. Concerning neuropsychological measurements, there were studies that employed screening tools for dementia or dementia scales, and studies that used comprehensive test batteries or tests of selective cognitive functions.

From the evaluation of the results reported in Table 44.2, the following conclusions may be made. First, CT studies are not numerous and their results seem to be much influenced by the effect of age. In one population-based study examining a fairly wide patient sample in the oldest age group, demented patients compared with and without LA, proved

Table 44.2 *Studies examining the impact of leukoaraiosis on severity of dementia, or type of cognitive impairment in demented patients*

Authors	No. of patients with LA/total sample	Mean age of patients with LA/patients without LA or of total sample	Association (±) of cognitive impairment with LA and type of impairment
CT studies			
Steingart *et al.*, 1987b	39/113	75.2/70.0	Lower score of Extended Scale for Dementia among AD patients with LA accounted for by age. Significantly lower score among less advanced AD cases with LA
Johnson *et al.*, 1987	36	69.8	Correlation with dementia severity on the Blessed Scale
Diaz *et al.*, 1991	34/85	75.1/68.0	Correlation with dementia severity on Extend Scale for Dementia
Lopez *et al.*, 1992	22	72.5	No correlation with MMSE and Blessed Scale scores
Skoog *et al.*, 1996	67/98	85	Demented subjects with LA scoring lower in tests of spatial ability and secondary memory
Amar *et al.*, 1996	37/68	75.2/71.6	AD patients with LA performing worse on test of visuospatial function and cognitive speed
MRI studies			
Fazekas *et al.*, 1987	13/16	nr	No correlation with dementia severity
Kertesz *et al.*, 1990	19/38	74.0/72.1	Attention and comprehension deficit among demented patient with LA
Kozachuk *et al.*, 1990	4/22	66.7	No correlation with dementia severity (MMSE)
Bondareff *et al.*, 1990	18/19	78.6	Correlation with Blessed and MMSE scores, deficit of verbal memory, naming, and attention
Libon *et al.*, 1990	8/40	72.6/75.1	No correlation with scores of any selective function test in a comprehensive test battery
Leys *et al.*, 1990	17	64.5	No correlation with MMSE score
Bowen *et al.*, 1990	113	73.0	No correlation with MMSE score
Harrell *et al.*, 1991	45	68.8	Patients with severe periventricular hyperintensities worse in total MDRS and MDRS memory subscale
Mirsen *et al.*, 1991	38/41	nr	No association with Extended Scale for Dementia score
McDonald *et al.*, 1991	12/22	64.1	No correlation with MMSE score
Almkvist *et al.*, 1992	48/105	78.7/72.3	Patients with LA more impaired in attention, visuoconstruction, and finger motor speed
Bennett *et al.*, 1992	29/106	73.4/70.7	No correlation with MMSE score
Marder *et al.*, 1995	55	70.5	No correlation between number of lesions or periventricular caps and MMSE or Blessed scale score
O'Brien *et al.*, 1996b	61	71.2	No correlation with CAMCOG score
Stout *et al.*, 1996	52	71.7	Correlation between abnormal white matter volume and MDRS or MMSE score
Starkstein *et al.*, 1997	15/38	73.9/70.3	No difference between AD patients with and without LA in any test score of a comprehensive battery

AD, Alzheimer's disease; CAMCOG, Cambridge Cognitive Examination for the Elderly; LA, leukoaraiosis; MDRS, Mattis Dementia Rating Scale; MMSE, Mini-Mental State Examination; nr, not reported.

more impaired in both global and selective cognitive functions (Skoog *et al.*, 1996). It is noteworthy that subcortical functions were the ones found to be selectively affected. Second, in MRI studies, discrepant results are apparent. Data may be influenced by small sample sizes, different age groups, patient selection, and use of different tools for measuring cognition. In this last connection, abnormalities of global cognitive function seem less prone to be associated with the presence of LA, in comparison with those of selective functions.

However, in one study, measuring quantitatively abnormal white matter volume, Stout *et al.* (1996) were able to find a correlation between this volume and scores of tests of global cognition such as the Mini-Mental State Examination (MMSE) and the Mattis Dementia Rating Scale. MRI study results may be influenced by different lesion patterns of white matter abnormalities (i.e. differently located and shaped lesions, periventricular halos, punctate or confluent focal deep or subcortical lesions).

Fazekas *et al.* (1996), confirming a finding previously reported by others (Mirsen *et al.*, 1991), have shown that computer-measured, rather than visually rated, periventricular hyperintensity was significantly greater in AD patients than in controls matched for risk factors. They also observed a significant association between periventricular hyperintensity thickness and lateral ventricular enlargement. Based on these observations, it has been suggested that the more likely explanation for the discrepancy of reports on the association between MRI assessed LA and dementia may be due to difference in brain atrophy across the various groups of patients investigated (Fazekas *et al.*, 1998). This may explain the lack of difference in brain hyperintensities between early AD and control subjects reported by Erkinjuntti *et al.* (1994).

A positive association between ventricular dilatation and cognitive impairment has been observed in numerous, both cross-sectional and longitudinal, studies on LA and cognitive decline, and in the setting of either vascular or AD dementia. Studies using detailed and comprehensive tests batteries tended to discover more abnormalities linked with presence and severity of LA than those using global screening tools for dementia assessment. Again, functions found consistently to be impaired in many studies were those linked to subcortical-frontal connections. For example, attention and visual construction proved to be selectively impaired in some studies (Bondareff *et al.*, 1988; Kertesz *et al.*, 1990; Almkvist *et al.*, 1992).

44.4.3 Leukoaraiosis as a predictor of dementia progression

Longitudinal studies examining the prognostic significance of LA in relation to dementia development or progression are very scanty. Morris *et al.* (1990) followed up 12 AD patients with and 26 AD patients without LA over a period of 66 months (Morris *et al.*, 1990). At the end of the follow up, AD patients with LA had not experienced greater dementia progression or mortality. No progression of LA was observed during the study period, but in patients with LA ventricular size tended to increase. The rate of disease progression was examined by Lopez *et al.* (1992) in 22 patients with probable AD and LA compared with 22 AD patients without LA. Executive/attention, lexical/semantic, memory/learning, and visuospatial functions did not differ between the two groups at baseline or at the 1-year follow-up examination. However, patients with AD and LA were more likely to develop cerebrovascular disease during follow up than AD controls without LA.

Bracco *et al.* (1993) examined MRI features as possible predictors of cognitive decline in 24 patients with cerebrovascular disease and LA. All the patients underwent an extensive clinical and neuropsychological assessment on admission, and 19 patients were followed with repeated cognitive examinations for an average of 48 months. Neither extent nor location of LA predicted the development or the progression of mental deterioration in patients who were mentally healthy or already cognitively impaired at entry.

44.4.4 Leukoaraiosis and dementia onset after acute stroke

In the last few years a number of studies have focused on the frequency, characteristics and determinants of dementia occurring in patients with an acute stroke. In this sense, efforts have been made in order to characterize the structural correlates of this frequent condition from the radiological point of view (Erkinjuntti *et al.*, 1999; Pantoni *et al.*, 1999), and LA has been hypothesized to be one potential radiological substrate of post-stroke dementia. This hypothesis is based on the evaluation of some studies.

Liu *et al.* (1992) compared clinical and MRI features in 24 patients who became demented after having a stroke and 29 patients who did not. The total area of LA was 10 times larger among patients who developed dementia. LA was the factor that best discriminated between the two groups of patients among several others, including age, total area of infarction and location in the dominant hemisphere. Out of 146 patients with a first-ever stroke, examined for dementia 3 months after the event by Censori *et al.* (1996) 15 were found to have become demented. LA was present in one-third of patients with post-stroke dementia as opposed to one-sixth of those without dementia, a difference that was not statistically significant owing to low statistical power. Patients who developed post-stroke dementia more frequently had diabetes mellitus, atrial fibrillation, aphasia, large middle cerebral artery infarction and more severe neurological deficits at entry and at 3 months than did non-demented patients, underlining the fact that the onset of post-stroke dementia is likely to be a multifactorial process.

The most comprehensive data about LA as predictor of dementia in stroke patients come from studies that have followed up patients with lacunar stroke: 95 of 215 Japanese patients with a first-ever lacunar stroke had LA on admission CT scan (Miyao *et al.*, 1992). One month after stroke, 15.1 per cent of patients with LA were found to be demented compared with 1.7 per cent of patients without LA, rates that, at the end of the 25-month follow up, had increased to 22.1 per cent and 2.5 per cent, respectively (Miyao *et al.*, 1992). The new onset dementia was attributed to stroke recurrence (mostly recurrent lacunar stroke) in all but one patient with LA.

In another study performed in Italy and aimed at investigating the risk and determinants of dementia among patients with lacunar stroke, 25 of 108 patients (23.1 per cent) developed dementia over a period of 4 years (Loeb *et al.*, 1992). The frequency of LA did not differ between patients who became demented and those who did not, while the recurrence of stroke was by far the most important determinant of subsequent dementia.

The discrepancy on the role of LA in predicting dementia between these two studies (Loeb *et al.*, 1992; Miyao *et al.*, 1992) may be due to the different case-mix. In fact, in the Italian study, patients had more severe disease at baseline, all presenting multiple lacunar infarcts on entry CT scan.

A parallel progression of LA and lacunar infarct was clearly demonstrated by Van Zagten *et al.* (1996) who examined by CT scanning repeated over 3 years the evolution of LA and associated vascular lesions in 63 patients with a first-ever symptomatic lacunar stroke, and in 44 patients with cortical territorial stroke. Progression of LA occurred in 27 patients (26 per cent) and was strongly associated with symptomatic or silent lacunar stroke at entry. Although no evaluation of evolution of functional, including cognitive, deficits was performed in this study, the results indirectly support the hypothesis that in patients with stroke, even if LA progresses over time, this is accompanied by progression of lacunar lesions, which may be the primary determinant of cognitive decline in these patients.

In a smaller study, Tarvonen-Schröder *et al.* (1995) did not find any association between progression of LA and a selective infarct type: 11 (29 per cent) of the 38 patients with either pure LA or LA combined with radiological evidence of infarction proved to have significant and rapid progression of LA during a 3-year follow-up period, irrespective of whether the infarct was small, deep, or cortical on baseline CT scan. No difference in the occurrence or type of dementia was detected at the end of the follow-up period between patients with progressive and non-progressive LA, but progressive LA was paralleled by the increase in cortical atrophy.

More recently, the presence of LA in stroke patients has been related to the occurrence of executive dysfunction reinforcing the idea that the type of cognitive change associated with LA is likely to be of the frontal type (Vataja *et al.*, 2003).

44.4.5 The role of leukoaraiosis in criteria for vascular dementia

Despite the controversies existing about the effect of the presence or the severity of white matter changes on cognition, current consensus criteria for vascular dementia and vascular dementia subtypes list LA as one of the radiological correlates of the disease. The ICD-10 criteria require the presence of dementia, hypertension, and LA to reach a diagnosis of subcortical vascular dementia (Wetterling *et al.*, 1994). According to the NINDS-AIREN criteria, LA involving at least one-fourth of the cerebral white matter is one of the radiological correlates supporting the clinical diagnosis of vascular dementia (Román *et al.*, 1993). These latter radiological criteria have been more recently operationalized (van Straaten *et al.*, 2003). The presence of extensive LA finally has been taken as one of the two radiological hallmarks of subcortical vascular dementia (the other one is the presence of multiple lacunar infarcts) in the set of clinicoradiological criteria specifically developed to define this subtype of cerebrovascular dementia in research settings (Erkinjuntti *et al.*, 2000).

44.4.6 Leukoaraiosis and cognitive functions in non-demented subjects

The possibility that LA, frequently observed in elderly subjects, produces subtle or selective cognitive deficits not sufficient for a clinical definition of dementia was first suggested by Steingart *et al.* (1987a). They observed that elderly volunteers participating in a dementia study as non-demented controls and showing LA on CT scan scored lower on a extended scale for dementia than control subjects without LA, and had difficulties in selective tasks involving time orientation, construction of sentences and memory. This finding put forward important questions about the role of LA in contributing to cognitive decline in the elderly to a level not severe enough to imply a diagnosis of dementia but still able to produce difficulties in everyday life. Neuropsychological tools to be used in this case have of course to be much more sensitive and selective than those commonly used to screen out patients with dementia. Studies in this setting have been numerous, but the results, as for the dementia setting, are discrepant. Table 44.3 lists such studies.

From the evaluation of Table 44.3 there are difficulties in drawing unequivocal conclusions. Conflicting results were obtained even by studies using similar instruments to measure cognitive functions and examining subjects comparable in age (the lack of effect was not surprising when the mean age of the sample was low, as in the study of Schmidt *et al.* [1991]). Studies exploring selective functions in a more or less detailed fashion tended to achieve more positive results compared with studies evaluating global cognitive functions. The reasons for discrepancy are again, besides age, size and mode of selection of investigational cohorts, different MRI equipment (varying from 0.02 to 1.5 Tesla), and different lesion patterns considered for their correlation with cognitive test scores. Moreover, the effect of age and other vascular risk factors was not taken into account in all the studies. The fact that two out of the three CT studies found an effect of LA on cognitive performance may be explained by the greater severity of white matter lesions as expressed by CT-evidenced LA. This may suggest that, if only confluent large changes were considered in MRI-assessed LA, an association with cognitive impairment could have been demonstrated.

Only some of the studies reported in Table 44.3 took into account concomitant structural lesions such as brain atrophy or silent infarcts. For example, a more strict association was found between cognitive deficits and ventricular enlargement than with white matter lesions in the one study, which considered cognitive impairment as possibly related to either structural abnormality (Breteler *et al.*, 1994a). Regarding the cognitive domains affected, results are rather consistent in indicating a predominant involvement of functions linked with fronto-subcortical circuits. Impairments of attention,

Table 44.3   *Effect of leukoaraiosis on cognitive functions in non-demented subjects*

Author, Year	Number of patients with LA/total sample	Mean age of patients with LA/patients without LA or of total sample	Association (±) of cognitive impairment with LA and type of impairment
CT studies			
Steingart *et al.*, 1987	9/105	75.3/70.8	Lower score on extended scale for dementia, especially items 12 (sentences construction and memory) and 13 (orientation to time)
Masdeu *et al.*, 1989	40	83.3	No effect on Blessed and Mattis dementia scales
Skoog *et al.*, 1996	46/134	85	Subjects with LA scoring lower in MMSE and in tests of verbal ability, spatial ability, perceptual speed, secondary memory, and basic arithmetics
MRI studies			
Rao *et al.*, 1989	10/50	47.1/42.8	Lack of association with any test of a comprehensive battery
Hendrie *et al.*, 1989	16/27	76.4/67.5	No variation of MMSE, CAMCOG and WAIS digit symbol
Hunt *et al.*, 1989	34/46	78.2	Lack of association with any test of a comprehensive battery after controlling for age
Mirsen *et al.*, 1991	39	73.2	No association between any pattern of LA and performance on Extended Scale for Dementia
Harrell *et al.*, 1991	25	65.6	No correlation between severity of either periventricular or deep hyperintensities and MMSE and MDRS
Schmidt *et al.*, 1991	12/32	43.3/35.8	No difference between subjects with and without white matter lesions on a computerized test of vigilance and reaction time, a test of visual attention and a test of learning and memory
Tupler *et al.*, 1992	48/66	69.9/64.3	No difference between subjects with and without subcortical white matter hyperintensities in Benton Facial Recognition Test and WAIS digit symbol after controlling for age and education
Boone *et al.*, 1992	54/100	62.8	Subjects with extensive ($>10\,cm^2$) white matter lesions more impaired in basic attention and selected frontal lobe skills
Matsubayashi *et al.*, 1992	60/73	70	Correlation with MMSE and Hasegawa score, and visuospatial cognitive performance test
Schmidt *et al.*, 1993	74/150	61.3/58.5	Difference between subjects with and without white matter hyperintensities in form B of Trail Making Test, a complex reaction time task, and the assembly procedures of the Purdue Pegboard test
Ylikoski *et al.*, 1993	48/120	Range 55–85	Significant association of total LA and results of Trail Making Test A, Stroop test (words/time and difference/time) and compound score of speed and attention
Fukui *et al.*, 1994	38/43	66.1/55.3	No direct correlation between white matter hyperintensities score and any cognitive test. Periventricular hyperintensity associated with reduced performance in the Stroop test
Breteler *et al.*, 1994b	29/111	Range 65–84	Borderline correlation between degree of white matter lesions and CAMCOG score. White matter lesions significantly associated with subjective mental decline
Breteler *et al.*, 1994a	23/96	73.6	White matter lesions associated with word fluence (letter B), Trail Making Test A and B, Word List Learning (delayed recall)
Baum *et al.*, 1995	16/41	50.8	White matter foci related to performance on immediate visual memory/visuoperceptual skills, visuomotor tracking/psychomotor speed and, to a lesser degree, learning capacity and abstract and conceptual reasoning skills
Longstreth *et al.*, 1996	3301	75	Association of white matter lesions and modified MMSE, and Digit Symbol Substitution Test

CAMCOG, Cambridge Cognitive Examination for the Elderly; LA, leukoaraiosis; MDRS, Mattis Dementia Rating Scale; MMSE, Mini-Mental State Examination visuospatial memory, visuospatial skills and frontal skills were the abnormalities most frequently reported.

That specific rather than general cognitive tasks are affected by the severity rather than by the mere presence of LA has been shown by other more recent surveys (de Groot et al., 2000; Leaper et al., 2001). Moreover, even in subjects who score high on neuropsychological tests, the severity of LA can be reflected by subjective cognitive dysfunction and reporting of progression of these dysfunctions (de Groot et al., 2001).

Studies examining only subjects with vascular risk factors were not included in Table 44.3 since they cannot be considered strictly normal. Three studies have investigated hypertensive subjects compared with non-hypertensive controls (Schmidt et al., 1991, 1995; van Swieten et al., 1991a). In the study of van Swieten et al. (1991a), 10 of 42 hypertensive elderly subjects had confluent white matter lesions on MRI versus only one from an equal number of controls. The performances on MMSE, Stroop colour-word test, Trail Making test, and the visual subtest of the Wechsler Memory Scale were worse among hypertensive patients with confluent lesions. In the 1991 study of Schmidt et al., 35 hypertensive subjects performed worse than non-hypertensive controls on verbal memory, total learning and memory capacity, although there was no difference in cognitive performance between hypertensives with and without punctate white matter lesions on MRI (Schmidt et al., 1991). In a second study by Schmidt et al. (1995), 89 hypertensives tended to perform worse than 89 non-hypertensive controls when assessed for attentional and visuopractic skills. Twenty-seven out of 43 non-demented patients with history of stroke, different vascular risk factors and periventricular white matter CT hypodensity were studied with a detailed neuropsychological examination by Gupta et al. (1988). Even in patients with the lowest degree of white matter abnormalities there was a defect in sustained mental concentration and attention. Slowness in acquisition, difficulty in organizing material to be learned, lack of consistency in recall, and difficulties in spontaneous recall were also reported in the investigated patients.

Similar patients were studied by Junquè et al. (1990). Among functions explored by a comprehensive test battery, the main cognitive abnormality was a reduced speed of information processing, especially complex processes, an abnormality that was independent of age. The authors concluded that slowness of thought was the main characteristics of cognitive functioning in patients with LA (Junquè et al., 1990). This slowness could affect encoding and retrieval processes in memory, although the overall results of the study tended to exclude the presence of an encoding deficit.

In none of the reported studies of the effect of LA in non-demented subjects have behavioural aspects been taken into account. Mood disorders, including depression and irritability, possibly concurring with cognitive deficits in affecting behaviour, can be substantiated by several observations in either non-demented or demented subjects with LA (O'Brien et al., 1996a, b, 1998).

44.4.7 Leukoaraiosis as predictor of dementia in normal subjects and in subjects with mild cognitive impairment

Because subtle cognitive deficits are found frequently in non-demented patients with LA, the question arises whether these subjects are particularly prone to develop a more severe cognitive impairment or even overt dementia over time. Until very recently, the answer was not available and only very preliminary observations were accessible (Fein et al., 1990; Guerriero Austrom et al., 1990; Wohl et al., 1994). Data from a large cohort of community-dwelling normal subjects, sequentially studied with MRI and detailed neuropsychological testing, have been more recently reported (Schmidt et al., 1999). After 3 years, progression of LA was noted in 22 (8.1 per cent) of the 273 subjects but was not associated with cognitive decline. However, the recently published results from a large population-based study enrolling more than 700 subjects demonstrated that the presence of LA (together with that of silent lacunar infarcts) significantly predicts dementia onset (Vermeer et al., 2003b). The relative risk of becoming demented over a 3.6-year follow up was about 1.6 for subjects with periventricular LA at baseline MRI.

In the National Heart, Lung and Blood Institute Twin Study, higher LA volume together with increasing age, ApoE ε4 genotype, elevated mid-life blood pressure, and lower alcohol consumption, significantly increased the risk of mild cognitive impairment (DeCarli et al., 2001).

Many open questions in relation to the role of LA in the development of cognitive impairment or dementia may find an answer only from the results of longitudinal studies. The LADIS (Leukoaraiosis And DISability) study is an international collaborative study that aims to assess the predictive values of different severity degrees of LA on the transition to disability in a group of 639 normally functioning subjects enrolled in 12 European centres (www.ladis.unifi.it). While disability is the main outcome of the 3-year follow up, relevant information will be also collected as far as cognition is concerned, and dementia and mild cognitive impairment will be relevant secondary outcome measures (Pantoni et al., 2005). The preliminary cross-sectional data show that subjects with more severe degrees of LA have poorer cognitive performance and are subjected to a higher risk of transition to a disabled functional status (Inzitari et al., 2003) than subjects with mild LA. If confirmed at the end of the follow up, these data will provide a clear answer on the independent effect of LA on cognition.

Linked with the above mentioned question there is another one that concerns the possible role of LA in the transition from mild cognitive impairment to dementia. A preliminary study aimed at testing possible radiological markers of this transition found that CT-detected LA and temporal lobe atrophy were significant predictors of AD in a small group of 27 patients with mild cognitive impairment (Wolf et al., 2000). These findings have been corroborated by the results of another study performed in a Japanese sample of 46 patients with mild cognitive impairment defined on the basis of a MMSE score <24 and the lack of fulfilment of DSM-IV criteria for dementia (Koga *et al.*, 2002); in this study, larger quantities of LA were found to be one of the factors predicting cognitive impairment together with cerebral atrophy and lower education level (Koga *et al.*, 2002).

44.4.8 Comments on the role of leukoaraiosis in predicting cognitive impairment

In the previous edition of this book, we concluded that 'The reported evidence does not support LA as an independent prognostic factor for future development of dementia in healthy subjects …'. Four years later, the scenario appears changed and the last reported studies advocate modification of that statement. Not only the presence (and the severity) of LA is associated with dysfunction of specific cognitive tasks that depend on the frontal lobes, but it also predicts the development of cognitive impairment and dementia. The effect of LA in specific disease conditions requires some comments.

In patients with stroke, particularly in those with the lacunar type, the presence of LA at stroke onset seems to predict an evolution towards dementia. However, in this setting, the effect of LA seems to be strictly interrelated with that of other lesions with common underlying pathological substrates such as deep lacunar infarcts. In patients with established vascular dementia the net contribution of LA to dementia progression remains to be determined, as it does in relation to other commonly associated lesions (i.e. infarcts, atrophy and ventricular enlargement). However, it appears inappropriate to make a general conclusion on the role of LA in vascular dementia considering that the latter cannot any longer be considered as a homogeneous entity. In fact, the role of LA is likely more prominent in contributing to the clinical picture of patients with the subcortical type of vascular dementia (Erkinjuntti *et al.*, 2000; Román *et al.*, 2002) while its role is probably less prominent in forms characterized by large cortical infarcts. The clinical significance of LA in patients with AD remains instead less clear and the presence of LA does not appear to determine a greater cognitive decline (Hirono *et al.*, 2000). However, the inference from follow-up studies performed with cognitively healthy subjects or AD patients is limited by the small sample sizes, and by observation periods that always are too short.

Another major limitation appears to be the type of cognitive assessment used to define the mental status and the requirement of current criteria for diagnosis of dementia. As LA is unlikely to cause prominent memory problems, being instead more related to frontal lobe executive dysfunctions, it will be difficult to find it associated with forms of dementia such as AD, the essential requirement of which are memory dysfunctions.

44.4.9 Possible mechanisms by which leukoaraiosis may cause or contribute to cognitive impairment

Pathophysiological mechanisms by which LA may cause or contribute to cognitive impairment remain predominantly hypothetical. The hypotheses may be grouped into two main categories discussed below.

44.4.9.1 DIRECT EFFECT

The main question is whether LA is able to produce cognitive impairment *per se*, in other terms what is its exclusive or net contribution, considering risk factors including age, associated with both dementia and LA, or concomitant structural lesions, such as focal (lacunar) infarcts or neurodegenerative changes, that frequently are associated with LA. In the case of a direct effect of LA on cognition, the alteration of myelinated fibres and accompanying tissue abnormalities (e.g. gliosis) known to underlie LA could disconnect functionally-related cortical and subcortical structures (Cummings, 1993). Unfortunately, according to Fazekas *et al.* (1998) 'such estimate is complicated by our ignorance about the actual severity of damage to connecting fiber tracts based on CT or routine MRI findings'. Hints may proceed from studies of dementia and white matter changes in diseases, such as multiple sclerosis, in which lesions are almost exclusively limited to white matter (Fazekas *et al.*, 1998). For a long time it has been recognized that cognitive dysfunctions frequently occur in multiple sclerosis, but only recently has the use of extensive neuropsychological testing provided accurate information about prevalence and type of cognitive attaint (Rao *et al.*, 1991). Deficits involve predominantly attention, visuospatial functions, memory retrieval and abstraction. The same functions proved to be affected in many of the above reported studies on LA.

Concerning the clinical expression of LA on cognitive grounds, several factors have to be taken into account:

- *Lesion pattern.* What is seen as LA on CT is usually resolved by MRI into differently seated and shaped lesions including periventricular caps, rims, or haloes; deep focal punctate lesions; large confluent or diffuse subcortical lesions. Different pathological processes are now thought to underlie each type of lesion. While focal punctate lesions, a very frequent finding in normal ageing and present even at younger ages, are generally considered of small importance in relation to cognitive impairment, there is evidence that large confluent areas of LA are involved more directly in cognitive decline. Unfortunately, in patients presenting with this type of lesion, the number of lacunar infarcts is also elevated, making it difficult to evaluate the respective role of each. Regarding periventricular abnormalities, we have reported data showing a role in relation to dementia in AD patients, but the effect of this abnormality can be hardly considered independent since it is also associated with brain atrophy.

- *Location and volume.* Scattered evidence exists as to whether the location of LA is important in relation to the expression of cognitive impairment. Intuitively, lesions predominantly seated in the frontal white matter may sustain the typical pattern of cognitive dysfunction reported in subjects with LA. There are also clues suggesting that location in the posterior white matter is associated with selective dysfunction of areas and tracts involved in visuospatial cognitive performance (Fukui *et al.*, 1994). Although not invariably, changes affecting the entire subcortical white matter, are likely to produce global cognitive dysfunction that are more easily measurable, even with unrefined instruments such as dementia rating scales. Regarding volume of LA (area on CT or MRI scan), there are theories and some evidence that suggest a possible threshold volume above which dementia becomes evident. In one study of healthy elderly patients, the threshold area for cognitive dysfunction was $10 \, cm^2$ (Boone *et al.*, 1992), consistent with the findings of Erkinjuntti *et al.* (1987b) who observed that a white matter lesion area exceeding one-fourth of the total white matter area discriminates between multi-infarct and AD patients, and that of Liu *et al.* (1992) who found that the mean white matter lesion area in demented stroke patients was $26.7 \, cm^2$, as compared with $2.5 \, cm^2$ in non-demented patients.

- *Metabolic status of the tissue.* One positron emission tomography (PET) study (Yao *et al.*, 1992) has demonstrated low flow and increased oxygen extraction in the areas of white matter changes in non-demented subjects, while in patients who were demented the blood flow was decreased and oxygen extraction was normal, indicating a low metabolic rate. The possibility that the threshold for dementia associated with LA is metabolic or functional has been scarcely explored as yet. Some more information in this regard may derive from recently developed MR techniques. Diffusion MRI allows the determination of the directionality of free water in brain tissues. In normal cerebral white matter, diffusion is highly related to the direction of the myelinated axonal bundles (this directionality is called 'anisotropy'). If damage to the white matter occurs, diffusion is increased but to a lesser extent than in the centre of cavitated large infarcts, and anisotropy is lost. Diffusion MRI might detect signal changes (i.e. loss of anisotropy) in the case of disruption of the white matter architecture at very early stages when conventional MRI does not show any signal change (O'Sullivan *et al.*, 2001). These diffusion alterations in the normal-appearing white matter were found to correlate with a test of executive dysfunctions in a small group of patients (O'Sullivan *et al.*, 2001) and with the degree of LA in other white matter areas (Helenius *et al.*, 2002).

44.4.9.2 INTERACTION WITH OTHER PROCESSES INVOLVED IN COGNITIVE IMPAIRMENT

Subcortical infarcts, especially lacunar infarcts, and atrophy, either cortical or subcortical (of which ventricular dilatation may be an expression), are commonly seen in association with LA in aged patients and in those with vascular risk factors. From the reviewed evidence, lacunar infarcts remain the main confounder for the association between LA and cognitive impairment in patients with vascular risk factors, in particular arterial hypertension. However, at least two other morphologic aspects are to be taken into account, corpus callosum atrophy (Yamauchi *et al.*, 2000) and hippocampal atrophy (Mungas *et al.*, 2001; Wu *et al.*, 2002) as they may interact with LA in determining cognitive impairment. It should be noted that what is seen on MRI as hippocampal atrophy may also be the results of ischaemic, not necessarily degenerative, insults. The pathological nature of LA in AD is not well understood. Wallerian degeneration (Leys *et al.*, 1991), incomplete infarction linked with systemic hypoperfusion (Brun and Englund, 1986), and amyloid angiopathy (Gray *et al.*, 1985) are among the advocated causes. Recent MRI studies have shown that LA in AD patients is due mainly to periventricular changes and that these are associated with the degree of brain atrophy. This evidence further supports a marginal role of LA in relation to dementia in pure AD dementia cases. In patients with a mixed type of dementia, particularly frequent at older ages, the role of subcortical lesions of ischaemic origin may be substantial. The Nun Study has convincingly demonstrated that at old ages, in the presence of AD changes, vascular lesions play a crucial role in the manifestation of dementia (Snowdon *et al.*, 1997). In post-stroke dementia the role of LA has to be seen as synergistic with that of other vascular lesions such as volume and site of infarction (Pohjasvaara *et al.*, 2000).

44.5 CONCLUSIONS

Although not synonymous with dementia, LA is potentially involved in cognitive impairment in elderly individuals. Given the pathogenesis, very likely predominantly ischaemic, linked with small vessel disease, the setting in which LA is more closely associated with dementia is that of vascular dementia, particularly of the subcortical type. LA has been described in a noticeable proportion of patients with AD, although, from either retrospective or prospective studies, besides the pathophysiology, the contribution to cognitive deterioration is still unclear. In non-demented elderly individuals it is very likely that LA is associated with subtle cognitive changes, involving predominantly subcortical functions, like attention and speed of mental processes. Its presence is moreover associated with an increased risk of developing cognitive impairment or dementia at follow up.

Regarding mechanisms by which LA causes dementia, they are for large part conjectural, although disconnection among areas involved in cognition appears the most probable one. Damage to the white matter pathways connecting subcortical structures to the frontal lobes is one of the most likely causes. However, since LA is almost invariably associated with concomitant lesions such as brain atrophy, ventricular dilatation and multiple focal ischaemic lesions, all known possibly to have a role in cognitive impairment, the net contribution of LA is difficult to establish. Future studies, including volumetric MRI techniques, functional imaging (spectroscopy, diffusion-weighted and perfusion images), and other cerebral blood studies, may help to clarify several issues on the relationship between LA and cognitive impairment.

REFERENCES

Aharon-Peretz J, Cummings JL, Hill MA. (1988) Vascular dementia and dementia of the Alzheimer type. Cognition, ventricular size, and leuko-araiosis. *Archives of Neurology* **45**: 719–721

Akiguchi I, Tomimoto H, Suenaga T *et al.* (1998) Blood–brain barrier dysfunction in Binswanger's disease; an immunohistochemical study. *Acta Neuropathologica (Berlin)* **95**: 78–84

Alex M, Baron EK, Goldenberg S, Blumenthal HT. (1962) An autopsy study of cerebrovascular accident in diabetes mellitus. *Circulation* **25**: 663–673

Almkvist O, Wahlund L-O, Andersson-Lundman G *et al.* (1992) White-matter hyperintensity and neuropsychological functions in dementia and healthy aging. *Archives of Neurology* **49**: 626–632

Alzheimer A. (1902) Die Seelenstörungen auf arteriosklerotischer Grundlage. Allgemeine *Zeitschrift für Psychiatrie* **59**: 695–701

Amar K, Bucks RS, Lewis T *et al.* (1996) The effect of white matter low attenuation on cognitive performance in dementia of the Alzheimer type. *Age and Ageing* **25**: 443–448

Awad IA, Spetzler RF, Hodak JA *et al.* (1986a) Incidental subcortical lesions identified on magnetic resonance imaging in the elderly. I. Correlation with age and cerebrovascular risk factors. *Stroke* **17**: 1084–1089

Awad IA, Johnson PC, Spetzler RF, Hodak JA. (1986b) Incidental subcortical lesions identified on magnetic resonance imaging in the elderly. II. Postmortem pathological correlations. *Stroke* **17**: 1090–1097

Baum KA, Schulte C, Girke W *et al.* (1996) Incidental white-matter foci on MRI in 'healthy' subjects: evidence of subtle cognitive dysfunction. *Neuroradiology* **38**: 755–760

Bennett DA, Wilson RS, Gilley DW, Fox JH. (1990) Clinical diagnosis of Binswanger's disease. *Journal of Neurology, Neurosurgery, and Psychiatry* **53**: 961–965

Bennett DA, Gilley DW, Wilson RS *et al.* (1992) Clinical correlates of high signal lesions on magnetic resonance imaging in Alzheimer's disease. *Journal of Neurology* **239**: 186–190

Binswanger O. (1894) Die Abgrenzung der allgemeinen progressiven paralyse. *Berliner Klinische Wochenschrift* **31**: 1102–1105, 1137–1139, 1180–1186

Blass JP, Hoyer S, Nitsch R. (1991) A translation of Otto Binswanger article, 'The delineation of the generalized progressive paralyses.' *Archives of Neurology* **48**: 961–972

Blennow K, Wallin A, Uhlemann C, Gottfries CG. (1991) White-matter lesions on CT in Alzheimer patients: relation to clinical symptomatology and vascular factors. *Acta Neurologica Scandinavica* **83**: 187–193

Bogousslavsky J, Mast H, Mohr JP *et al.* (1996) Binswanger's disease: does it exist? *Cerebrovascular Diseases* **6**: 255–263

Bondareff W, Raval J, Colletti PM, Hauser DL. (1988) Quantitative magnetic resonance imaging and the severity of dementia in Alzheimer's disease. *American Journal of Psychiatry* **145**: 853–856

Bondareff W, Raval J, Woo B *et al.* (1990) Magnetic resonance imaging and the severity of dementia in older adults. *Archives of General Psychiatry* **47**: 47–51

Boone KB, Miller BL, Lesser IM *et al.* (1992) Neuropsychological correlates of white-matter lesions in healthy elderly subjects. A threshold effect. *Archives of Neurology* **49**: 549–554

Bowen BC, Barker WW, Loewenstein DA *et al.* (1990) MR signal abnormalities in memory disorders and dementia. *American Journal of Neuroradiology* **11**: 283–290

Bracco L, Campani D, Baratti E *et al.* (1993) Relation between MRI features and dementia in cerebrovascular disease patients with leucoaraiosis: a longitudinal study. *Journal of the Neurological Sciences* **120**: 131–136

Bradley WG Jr, Waluch V, Brandt-Zawadzki M *et al.* (1984a) Patchy, periventricular white matter lesions in the elderly: a common observation during NMR imaging. *Noninvasive Medical Imaging* **1**: 35–41

Bradley WG Jr, Waluch V, Yadley RA, Wycoff RR. (1984b) Comparison of CT and MR in 400 patients with suspected disease of the brain and cervical spinal cord. *Radiology* **152**: 695–702

Braffman BH, Zimmerman RA, Trojanowski JQ *et al.* (1988a) Brain MR. Pathologic correlation with gross and histopathology. 1. Lacunar infarction and Virchow-Robin spaces. *American Journal of Neuroradiology* **9**: 621–628

Braffman BH, Zimmerman RA, Trojanowski JQ *et al.* (1988b) Brain MR. Pathologic correlation with gross and histopathology. Hyperintense white-matter foci in the elderly. *American Journal of Neuroradiology* **9**: 629–636

Brant-Zawadzki M, David PL, Crooks LE *et al.* (1983) NMR demonstration of cerebral abnormalities: comparison with CT. *American Journal of Roentgenology* **140**: 847–854

Breteler MMB, van Amerongen NM, van Swieten JC *et al.* (1994a) Cognitive correlates of ventricular enlargement and cerebral white matter lesions on magnetic resonance imaging: the Rotterdam Study. *Stroke* **25**: 1109–1115

Breteler MMB, van Swieten JC, Bots ML *et al.* (1994b) Cerebral white matter lesions, vascular risk factors, and cognitive function in a population-based study: the Rotterdam Study. *Neurology* **44**: 1246–1252

Brun A and Englund E. (1986) A white matter disorder in dementia of the Alzheimer type: a pathoanatomical study. *Annals of Neurology* **19**: 253–262

Buée L, Hof PR, Bouras C *et al.* (1994) Pathological alterations of the cerebral microvasculature in Alzheimer's disease and related dementing disorders. *Acta Neuropathologica (Berlin)* **87**: 469–480

Carmelli D, DeCarli C, Swan GE *et al.* (1998) Evidence for genetic variance in white matter hyperintensity volume in normal elderly male twins. *Stroke* **29**: 1177–1181

Censori B, Manara O, Agostinis C *et al.* (1996) Dementia after first stroke. *Stroke* **27**: 1205–1210

Chabriat H, Vahedi K, Iba-Zizen MT *et al.* (1995) Clinical spectrum of CADASIL; a study of 17 families. Cerebral autosomal dominant arteriopathy with subcortical infarcts and leukoencephalopathy. *Lancet* **346**: 934–939

Chimowitz MI, Estes ML, Furlan AJ, Awad IA. (1992) Further observations on the pathology of subcortical lesions identified

on magnetic resonance imaging. *Archives of Neurology*
49: 747–752

Constans JM, Meyerhoff DJ, Norman D *et al.* (1995) 1H and 31P magnetic resonance spectroscopic imaging of white matter signal hyperintensities areas in elderly subjects. *Neuroradiology* **37**: 615–623

Cummings JL. (1993) Frontal-subcortical circuits and human behavior. *Archives of Neurology* **50**: 873–880

DeCarli C, Miller BL, Swan GE *et al.* (2001) Cerebrovascular and brain morphologic correlates of mild cognitive impairment in the National Heart, Lung, and Blood Institute Twin Study. *Archives of Neurology* **58**: 643–647

de Groot JC, de Leeuw F-E, Oudkerk M *et al.* (2000) Cerebral white matter lesions and cognitive function: the Rotterdam Scan Study. *Annals of Neurology* **47**: 145–151

de Groot JC, de Leeuw F-E, Oudkerk M *et al.* (2001) Cerebral white matter lesions and subjective cognitive dysfunction. The Rotterdam Scan Study. *Neurology* **56**: 1539–1545

Desmond DW, Moroney JT, Lynch T *et al.* (1999) The natural history of CADASIL: a pooled analysis of previously published cases. *Stroke* **30**: 1230–1233

Diaz JF, Merskey H, Hachinski VC *et al.* (1991) Improved recognition of leukoaraiosis and cognitive impairment in Alzheimer's disease. *Archives of Neurology* **48**: 1022–1025

Dichgans M, Mayer M, Uttner I *et al.* (1998) The phenotypic spectrum of CADASIL: clinical findings in 102 cases. *Annals of Neurology* **44**: 731–739

Erkinjuntti T, Ketonen L, Sulkava R *et al.* (1987a) Do white matter changes on MRI and CT differentiate vascular dementia from Alzheimer's disease? *Journal of Neurology, Neurosurgery, and Psychiatry* **50**: 37–42

Erkinjuntti T, Ketonen L, Sulkava R *et al.* (1987b) CT in the differential diagnosis between Alzheimer's disease and vascular dementia. *Acta Neurologica Scandinavica* **75**: 262–270

Erkinjuntti T, Sulkava R, Palo J, Ketonen L. (1989) White matter low attenuation on CT in Alzheimer's disease. *Archives of Gerontology and Geriatrics* **8**: 95–104

Erkinjuntti T, Gao F, Lee DH *et al.* (1994) Lack of difference in brain hyperintensities between patients with early Alzheimer's disease and control subjects. *Archives of Neurology* **51**: 260–268

Erkinjuntti T, Bowler JV, DeCarli CS *et al.* (1999) Imaging of static brain lesions in vascular dementia: implications for clinical trials. *Alzheimer Disease and Associated Disorders* **13** (Suppl. 3): S81–S90

Erkinjuntti T, Inzitari D, Pantoni L *et al.* (2000) Research criteria for subcortical vascular dementia in clinical trials. *Journal of Neural Transmission* **59** (Suppl.): 23–30

Fazekas F. (1989) Magnetic resonance signal abnormalities in asymptomatic individuals: their incidence and functional correlates. *European Neurology* **29**: 164–168

Fazekas F, Chawluk JB, Alavi A *et al.* (1987) MR signal abnormalities at 1.5 T in Alzheimer's dementia and normal aging. *American Journal of Neuroradiology* **8**: 421–426

Fazekas F, Niederkorn K, Schmidt R *et al.* (1988) White matter signal abnormalities in normal individuals: correlation with carotid ultrasonography, cerebral blood flow measurements, and cerebrovascular risk factors. *Stroke* **19**: 1285–1288

Fazekas F, Alavi A, Chawluk JB *et al.* (1989) Comparison of CT, MR, and PET in Alzheimer's dementia and normal aging. *Journal of Nuclear Medicine* **30**: 1607–1615

Fazekas F, Kleinert R, Offenbacher H *et al.* (1991) The morphologic correlate of incidental punctate white matter hyperintensities on MR images. *American Journal of Neuroradiology* **12**: 915–921

Fazekas F, Kleinert R, Offenbacher H *et al.* (1993) Pathologic correlates of incidental MRI white matter signal hyperintensities. *Neurology* **43**: 1683–1689

Fazekas F, Kapeller P, Schmidt R *et al.* (1996) The relation of cerebral magnetic resonance signal hyperintensities to Alzheimer's disease. *Journal of the Neurological Sciences* **142**: 121–125

Fazekas F, Schmidt R, Roob G, Kapeller P. (1998) White matter changes in dementia. In: D Leys, F Pasquier, P Scheltens (eds), *Stroke and Alzheimer's Disease*. The Hague, Holland Academic Graphics, pp.183–195

Feigin I and Popoff N. (1963) Neuropathological changes late in cerebral oedema: the relationship to trauma, hypertensive disease and Binswanger's encephalopathy. *Journal of Neuropathology and Experimental Neurology* **22**: 500–511

Fein G, Van Dyke C, Davenport L *et al.* (1990) Preservation of normal cognitive functioning in elderly subjects with extensive white-matter lesions of long duration. *Archives of General Psychiatry* **47**: 220–223

Fukui T, Sugita K, Sato Y *et al.* (1994) Cognitive functions in subjects with incidental cerebral hyperintensities. *European Neurology* **34**: 272–276

Furuta A, Ishii N, Nishihara Y, Horie A. (1991) Medullary arteries in aging and dementia. *Stroke* **22**: 442–446

George AE, de Leon MJ, Gentes CI *et al.* (1986a) Leukoencephalopathy in normal and pathologic aging: 1. CT of brain lucencies. *American Journal of Neuroradiology* **7**: 561–566

George AE, de Leon MJ, Kalnin A *et al.* (1986b) Leukoencephalopathy in normal and pathologic aging: 2. MRI of brain lucencies. *American Journal of Neuroradiology* **7**: 567–570

Gerard G and Weisberg LA. (1986) MRI periventricular lesions in adults. *Neurology* **36**: 998–1001

Goto K, Ishii N, Fukasawa H. (1981) Diffuse white-matter disease in the geriatric population. *Radiology* **141**: 687–695

Grafton ST, Sumi SM, Stimac GK *et al.* (1991) Comparison of postmortem magnetic resonance imaging and neuropathologic findings in the cerebral white matter. *Archives of Neurology* **48**: 293–298

Gray F, Dubas F, Rouller E, Escourolle R. (1985) Leukoencephalopathy in diffuse hemorrhagic cerebral amyloid angiopathy. *Annals of Neurology* **18**: 54–59

Guerriero Austrom M, Thompson RF, Hendrie HC *et al.* (1990) Foci of increased T$_2$ signal intensity in MR images of healthy elderly subjects. A follow-up study. *Journal of the American Geriatrics Society* **38**: 1133–1138

Gupta SR, Naheedy MH, Young JC *et al.* (1988) Periventricular white matter changes and dementia: clinical, neuropsychological, radiological, and pathological correlation. *Archives of Neurology* **45**: 637–641

Hachinski VC, Potter P, Merskey H. (1986) Leuko-araiosis: an ancient term for a new problem. *Canadian Journal of Neurological Sciences* **13**: 533–534

Hachinski VC, Potter P, Merskey H. (1987) Leuko-araiosis. *Archives of Neurology* **44**: 21–23

Harrell LE, Duvall E, Folks DG *et al.* (1991) The relationship of high-intensity signals on magnetic resonance images to cognitive and psychiatric state in Alzheimer's disease. *Archives of Neurology* **48**: 1136–1140

Helenius J, Soinne L, Salonen O *et al.* (2002) Leukoaraiosis, ischemic stroke, and normal white matter on diffusion-weighted MRI. *Stroke* **33**: 45–50

Hendrie HC, Farlow MR, Austrom Guerriero M *et al.* (1989) Foci of increased T2 signal intensity on brain MR scans of healthy elderly subjects. *American Journal of Neuroradiology* **10**: 703–707

Henon H, Vroylandt P, Durieu I et al. (2003) Leukoaraiosis more than dementia is a predictor of stroke recurrence. Stroke 34: 2935–2940

Hershey LA, Modic MT, Greenough PG, Jaffe DF. (1987) Magnetic resonance imaging in vascular dementia. Neurology 37: 29–36

Hirono N, Kitagaki H, Kazui H. (2000) Impact of white matter changes on clinical manifestation of Alzheimer's disease. A quantitative study. Stroke 31: 2182–2188

Hunt AL, Orrison WW, Yeo RA et al. (1989) Clinical significance of MRI white matter lesions in the elderly. Neurology 39: 1470–1474

Inzitari D, Diaz F, Fox A et al. (1987) Vascular risk factors and leuko-araiosis. Archives of Neurology 44: 42–47

Inzitari D, Di Carlo A, Mascalchi M et al. (1995) The cardiovascular outcome of patients with motor impairment and extensive leukoaraiosis. Archives of Neurology 52: 687–691

Inzitari D, Cadelo M, Marranci ML et al. (1997) Vascular deaths in elderly neurological patients with leukoaraiosis. Journal of Neurology, Neurosurgery, and Psychiatry 62: 177–181

Inzitari D, Pantoni L, Basile AM et al. (2003) Age-related white matter changes as predictor of disability in the elderly: the LADIS (Leukoaraiosis And DISsability) project. European Journal of Neurology 10 (Suppl. 1): 231

Janota J, Mirsen TR, Hachinski VC et al. (1989) Neuropathological correlates of leuko-araiosis. Archives of Neurology 46: 1124–1128

Jayakumar PN, Taly AB, Shanmugam V et al. (1989) Multi-infarct dementia: a computed tomographic study. Acta Neurologica Scandinavica 73: 292–295

Johnson KA, Davis KR, Buonanno FS et al. (1987) Comparison of magnetic resonance and roentgen ray computed tomography in dementia. Archives of Neurology 44: 1075–1080

Joutel A, Corpechot C, Ducros A et al. (1996) Notch 3 mutations in CADASIL, a hereditary adult-onset condition causing stroke and dementia. Nature 383: 707–710

Jungreis CA, Kanal E, Hirsch WL et al. (1988) Normal perivascular spaces mimicking lacunar infarction: MR imaging. Radiology 169: 101–104

Junqué C, Pujol J, Vendrell P et al. (1990) Leuko-araiosis on magnetic resonance imaging and speed of mental processing. Archives of Neurology 47: 151–156

Kapeller P, Barber R, Vermeulen RJ et al. (2003) Visual rating of age-related white matter changes on magnetic resonance imaging: scale comparison, interrater agreement, and correlations with quantitative measurements. Stroke 34: 441–445

Kertesz A, Polk M, Carr T. (1990) Cognition and white matter changes on magnetic resonance imaging in dementia. Archives of Neurology 47: 387–391

Kinkel WR, Jacobs L, Polachini I et al. (1985) Subcortical arteriosclerotic encephalopathy (Binswanger's disease). Computed tomographic, nuclear magnetic resonance, and clinical correlations. Archives of Neurology 42: 951–959

Kinkel WR, Jacobs L, Polachini I et al. (1986) Binswanger's disease. Archives of Neurology 43: 641–642

Kobari M, Meyer JS, Ichijo M. (1990a) Leuko-araiosis, cerebral atrophy, and cerebral perfusion in normal aging. Archives of Neurology 47: 161–165

Kobari M, Meyer JS, Ichijo M, Oravez WT. (1990b) Leukoaraiosis: correlation of MR and CT findings with blood flow, atrophy, and cognition. American Journal of Neuroradiology 11: 273–281

Koga H, Yuzuriha T, Yao H et al. (2002) Quantitative MRI findings and cognitive impairment among community dwelling elderly subjects. Journal of Neurology, Neurosurgery, and Psychiatry 72: 737–741

Kozachuk WE, DeCarli C, Schapiro MB et al. (1990) White matter hyperintensities in dementia of Alzheimer's type and in healthy

subjects without cerebrovascular risk factors. A magnetic resonance imaging study. Archives of Neurology 47: 1306–1310

Leaper SA, Murray AD, Lemmon HA et al. (2001) Neuropsychologic correlates of brain white matter lesions depicted on MR images: 1921 Aberdeen Birth Cohort. Radiology 221: 51–55

Lechner H, Schmidt R, Bertha G et al. (1988) Nuclear magnetic resonance image white matter lesions and risk factors for stroke in normal individuals. Stroke 19: 263–265

Leifer D, Buonanno FS, Richardson EP. Jr. (1990) Clinicopathologic correlations of cranial magnetic resonance imaging of periventricular white matter. Neurology 40: 911–918

Leys D, Soetaert G, Petit H et al. (1990) Periventricular and white matter magnetic resonance imaging hyperintensities do not differ between Alzheimer's disease and normal aging. Archives of Neurology 47: 524–527

Leys D, Pruvo JP, Parent M et al. (1991) Could Wallerian degeneration contribute to 'leuko-araiosis' in subjects free of any vascular disorder? Journal of Neurology, Neurosurgery, and Psychiatry 54: 46–50

Liao D, Cooper L, Cai J et al. (1996) Presence and severity of cerebral white matter lesions and hypertension, its treatment, and its control. The ARIC Study. Atherosclerosis Risk in Communities Study. Stroke 27: 2262–2270

Libon DJ, Scanlon M, Swenson R, Coslet HB. (1990) Binswanger's disease: some neuropsychological considerations. Journal of Geriatric Psychiatry and Neurology 3: 31–40

Lindgren A, Roijer A, Rudling O et al. (1994) Cerebral lesions on magnetic resonance imaging, heart disease, and vascular risk factors in subjects without stroke. Stroke 25: 929–934

Liu CK, Miller BL, Cummings JL et al. (1992) A quantitative MRI study of vascular dementia. Neurology 42: 138–143

Loeb C, Gandolfo C, Croce R, Conti M. (1992) Dementia associated with lacunar infarction. Stroke 23: 1225–1229

Loizou LA, Kendall BE, Marshall J. (1981) Subcortical arteriosclerotic encephalopathy: a clinical and radiological investigation. Journal of Neurology, Neurosurgery, and Psychiatry 44: 294

London E, de Leon MJ, George AE et al. (1986) Periventricular lucencies in the CT scans of aged and demented patients. Biological Psychiatry 21: 960–962

Longstreth WT, Manolio TA, Arnold A et al. (1996) Clinical correlates of white matter findings on cranial magnetic resonance imaging of 3301 elderly people. The Cardiovascular Health Study. Stroke 27: 1274–1282

Longstreth WT Jr, Dulberg C, Manolio TA et al. (2002) Incidence, manifestations, and predictors of brain infarcts defined by serial cranial magnetic resonance imaging in the elderly: the Cardiovascular Health Study. Stroke 33: 2376–2382

Lopez OL, Becker JT, Rezek D et al. (1992) Neuropsychiatric correlates of cerebral white-matter radiolucencies in probable Alzheimer's disease. Archives of Neurology 49: 828–834

Lotz PR, Ballinger WE Jr, Quisling RG. (1986) Subcortical arteriosclerotic encephalopathy: CT spectrum and pathologic correlation. American Journal of Neuroradiology 7: 817–822

McDonald WM, Krishnan KRR, Doraiswamy PM et al. (1991) Magnetic resonance findings in patients with early-onset Alzheimer's disease. Biological Psychiatry 29: 799–810

Marder K, Richards M, Bello J et al. (1995) Clinical correlates of Alzheimer's disease with and without silent radiographic abnormalities. Archives of Neurology 52: 146–151

Marshall VG, Bradley WG Jr, Marshall CE et al. (1988) Deep white matter infarction: correlation of MR imaging and histopathologic findings. Radiology 167: 517–522

Masdeu JC, Wolfson L, Lantos G *et al.* (1989) Brain white-matter changes in the elderly prone to falling. *Archives of Neurology* **46**: 1292–1296

Matsubayashi K, Shimada K, Kawamoto A, Ozawa T. (1992) Incidental brain lesions on magnetic resonance imaging and neurobehavioral functions in the apparently healthy elderly. *Stroke* **23**: 175–180

Mirsen TR, Lee DH, Wong CJ *et al.* (1991) Clinical correlates of white-matter changes on magnetic resonance imaging scans of the brain. *Archives of Neurology* **48**: 1015–1021

Miyao S, Takano A, Teramoto J, Takahashi A. (1992) Leukoaraiosis in relation to prognosis for patients with lacunar infarction. *Stroke* **23**: 1434–1438

Moody DM, Brown WR, Challa VR, Anderson RL. (1995) Periventricular venous collagenosis: association with leukoaraiosis. *Radiology* **194**: 469–476

Morris JC, Gado M, Torack RM, McKeel DW. (1990) Binswanger's disease or artifact: a clinical, neuroimaging, and pathological study of periventricular white matter changes in Alzheimer's disease. *Advances in Neurology* **51**: 47–52

Mungas D, Jagust WJ, Reed BR *et al.* (2001) MRI predictors of cognition in subcortical ischemic vascular disease and Alzheimer's disease. *Neurology* **57**: 2229–2235

Muñoz DG, Hastak SM, Harper B *et al.* (1993) Pathologic correlates of increased signals of the centrum ovale on magnetic resonance imaging. *Archives of Neurology* **50**: 492–497

Nag S. (1984) Cerebral changes in chronic hypertension: combined permeability and immunohistochemical studies. *Acta Neuropathologica (Berlin)* **62**: 178–184

O'Brien JT, Ames D, Schweitzer I. (1996a) White matter changes in depression and Alzheimer's disease: a review of magnetic resonance imaging studies. *International Journal of Geriatric Psychiatry* **11**: 681–694

O'Brien J, Desmond P, Ames D *et al.* (1996b) A magnetic resonance imaging study of white matter lesions in depression and Alzheimer's disease. *British Journal of Psychiatry* **168**: 477–485

O'Brien J, Ames D, Chiu E *et al.* (1998) Severe deep white matter lesions and outcome in elderly patients with major depressive disorder: follow-up study. *BMJ* **317**: 982–984

Olszewski J. (1962) Subcortical arteriosclerotic encephalopathy. *World Neurology* **3**: 359–375

Ostrow PT and Miller LL. (1993) Pathology of small artery disease. *Advances in Neurology* **62**: 93–123

O'Sullivan M, Summers PE, Jones DK *et al.* (2001) Normal-appearing white matter in ischemic leukoaraiosis: a diffusion tensor MRI study. *Neurology* **57**: 2307–2310

Pantoni L. (2000) Cerebral white matter ischemia and anoxia: data from experimental models. In: L Pantoni, D Inzitari, A Wallin (eds), *The Matter of White Matter. Clinical and Pathophysiological Aspects of White Matter Disease Related to Cognitive Decline and Vascular Dementia.* Utrecht, Academic Pharmaceutical Productions, pp. 377–388

Pantoni L and Garcia JH. (1995) The significance of cerebral white matter abnormalities 100 years after Binswanger's report. A review. *Stroke* **26**: 1293–1301

Pantoni L and Garcia JH. (1996) Binswanger's disease: what's in a name? *Cerebrovascular Diseases* **6**: 255–263

Pantoni L and Garcia JH. (1997) Pathogenesis of leukoaraiosis: a review. *Stroke* **28**: 652–659

Pantoni L, Inzitari D, Pracucci G *et al.* (1993) Cerebrospinal fluid proteins in patients with leucoaraiosis: possible abnormalities in blood–brain barrier function. *Journal of the Neurological Sciences* **115**: 125–131

Pantoni L, Garcia JH, Gutierrez JA. (1996a) Cerebral white matter is highly vulnerable to ischemia. *Stroke* **27**: 1641–1646

Pantoni L, Moretti M, Inzitari D. (1996b) The first Italian report on 'Binswanger's disease'. *Italian Journal of Neurological Sciences* **17**: 367–370

Pantoni L, Leys D, Fazekas F *et al.* (1999) The role of white matter lesions in cognitive impairment of vascular origin. *Alzheimer Disease and Associated Disorders* **13** (Suppl. 3): S49–S54

Pantoni L, Simoni M, Pracucci G *et al.* (2002) Visual rating scales for age-related white matter changes (leukoaraiosis): can the heterogeneity be reduced? *Stroke* **33**: 2827–2833

Pantoni L, Basile AM, Pracucci G *et al.* (2005) Impact of age-related cerebral white matter changes on the transition to disability – The LADIS Study: rationale, design, and methodology. *Neuroepidemiology* **24**: 51–62

Pantoni L, Sarti C, Pescini F *et al.* (2004) Thrombophilic risk factors and unusual clinical features in three Italian CADASIL patients. *European Journal of Neurology* **11**: 782–787

Parnetti L, Mecocci P, Santucci C *et al.* (1990) Is multi-infarct dementia representative of vascular dementia? A retrospective study. *Acta Neurologica Scandinavica* **81**: 484–487

Petito CK, Olarte J-P, Roberts B *et al.* (1998) Selective glial vulnerability following transient global ischemia in rat brain. *Journal of Neuropathology and Experimental Neurology* **57**: 231–238

Pohjasvaara T, Mäntyla R, Salonen O *et al.* (2002) How complex interactions of ischemic brain infarcts, white matter lesions, and atrophy relate to poststroke dementia. *Archives of Neurology* **57**: 1295–1300

Räihä I, Tarvonen S, Kurki T *et al.* (1993) Relationship between vascular factors and white matter low attenuation of the brain. *Acta Neurologica Scandinavica* **87**: 286–289

Rao SM, Mittenberg W, Bernardin L *et al.* (1989) Neuropsychological test findings in subjects with leucoaraiosis. *Archives of Neurology* **46**: 40–44

Rao SM, Leo GJ, Bernardin L, Unverzagt F. (1991) Cognitive dysfunction in multiple sclerosis. I. Frequency, patterns, and prediction. *Neurology* **41**: 685–691

Révész T, Hawkins CP, du Boulay EPGH *et al.* (1989) Pathological findings correlated with magnetic resonance imaging in subcortical arteriosclerotic encephalopathy (Binswanger's disease). *Journal of Neurology, Neurosurgery, and Psychiatry* **52**: 1337–1344

Rezek DL, Morris JC, Fulling KH, Gado MH. (1987) Periventricular white matter lucencies in senile dementia of the Alzheimer type and in normal aging. *Neurology* **37**: 1365–1368

Román GC, Tatemichi TK, Erkinjuntti T *et al.* (1993) Vascular dementia: diagnostic criteria for research studies. Report of the NINDS-AIREN International Workshop. *Neurology* **43**: 250–260

Román GC, Erkinjuntti T, Wallin A *et al.* (2002) Subcortical ischaemic vascular dementia. *Lancet Neurology* **1**: 426–436

Rosenberg GA, Kornfeld M, Stovring J, Bicknell JM. (1979) Subcortical arteriosclerotic encephalopathy (Binswanger): computerized tomography. *Neurology* **29**: 1102–1106

Rowbotham GF and Little E. (1965) Circulation of the cerebral hemispheres. *British Journal of Surgery* **52**: 8–21

Ruchoux MM and Maurage CA. (1997) CADASIL: cerebral autosomal dominant arteriopathy with subcortical infarcts and leukoencephalopathy. *Journal of Neuropathology and Experimental Neurology* **56**: 947–964

Salgado ED, Weistein M, Furlan AJ *et al.* (1986) Proton magnetic imaging in ischemic cerebrovascular disease. *Annals of Neurology* **20**: 502–507

Sarti C and Pantoni L. (2000) CADASIL and other hereditary forms of vascular leukoencephalopathy. In: L Pantoni, D Inzitari, A Wallin (eds), *The Matter of White Matter. Clinical and Pathophysiological Aspects of White Matter Disease Related to Cognitive Decline and Vascular Dementia.* Utrecht, Academic Pharmaceutical Productions, pp. 335–345

Scarpelli M, Salvolini U, Diamanti L *et al.* (1994) MRI and pathological examination of post-mortem brains: the problem of white matter high signal areas. *Neuroradiology* **36**: 393–398

Scheltens P, Barkhof F, Leys D *et al.* (1995) Histopathological correlates of white matter changes on MRI in Alzheimer's disease and normal aging. *Neurology* **45**: 883–888

Scheltens P, Erkinjuntti T, Leys D *et al.* (1998) White matter changes on CT and MRI: an overview of visual rating scales. European Task Force on Age-Related White Matter Changes. *European Neurology* **39**: 80–89

Schmidt R. (1992) Comparison of magnetic resonance imaging in Alzheimer's disease, vascular dementia and normal aging. *European Neurology* **32**: 164–169

Schmidt R, Fazekas F, Offenbacher H *et al.* (1991) Magnetic resonance imaging white matter lesions and cognitive impairment in hypertensive individuals. *Archives of Neurology* **48**: 417–420

Schmidt R, Fazekas F, Offenbacher H *et al.* (1993) Neuropsychological correlates of MRI white matter hyperintensities: a study of 150 normal volunteers. *Neurology* **43**: 2490–2494

Schmidt R, Fazekas F, Koch M *et al.* (1995) Magnetic resonance imaging cerebral abnormalities and neuropsychologic test performance in elderly hypertensive subjects. A case–control study. *Archives of Neurology* **52**: 905–910

Schmidt R, Hayn M, Fazekas F, Kapeller P, Esterbauer H. (1996) Magnetic resonance imaging white matter hyperintensities in clinically normal elderly individuals. Correlations with plasma concentrations of naturally occurring antioxidants. *Stroke* **27**: 2043–2047

Schmidt R, Schmidt H, Fazekas F *et al.* (1997) Apolipoprotein E polymorphism and silent microangiopathy-related cerebral damage. Results of the Austrian Stroke Prevention Study. *Stroke* **28**: 951–956

Schmidt R, Fazekas F, Kapeller P *et al.* (1999) A 3-year follow-up study on MRI white-matter hyperintensities in normal persons: rate, predictors, and neuropsychologic consequences of progression. *Neurology* **53**: 132–139

Schmidt R, Schmidt H, Fazekas F *et al.* (2000) MRI cerebral white matter lesions and paraoxonase PON1 polymorphisms. Three-year follow-up of the Austrian Stroke Prevention Study. *Arteriosclerosis Thrombosis and Vascular Biology* **20**: 1811–1816

Schmidt H, Fazekas F, Kostner GM *et al.* (2001) Angiotensinogen gene promoter haplotype and microangiopathy-related cerebral damage: results of the Austrian Stroke Prevention Study. *Stroke* **32**: 405–412

Schmidt R, Enzinger C, Ropele S *et al.* (2003) Progression of cerebral white matter lesions: 6-year results of the Austrian Stroke Prevention Study. *Lancet* **361**: 2046–2048

Schmidt R, Scheltens P, Erkinjuntti T *et al.* (2004) White matter lesion progression: a surrogate endpoint for trials in cerebral small-vessel disease. *Neurology* **63**: 139–144

Schneider R and Wieczorek V. (1991) Otto Binswanger (1852–1929). *Journal of the Neurological Sciences* **103**: 61–64

Schorer CE. (1992) Alzheimer and Kraepelin describe Binswanger's disease. *Journal of Neuropsychiatry and Clinical Neuroscience* **4**: 55–58

Skoog I, Berg S, Johansson B *et al.* (1996) The influence of white matter lesions on neuropsychological functioning in demented and non-demented 85-year-olds. *Acta Neurologica Scandinavica* **93**: 142–148

Skoog I, Palmertz B, Andreasson L-A. (1994) The prevalence of white-matter lesions on computed tomography of the brain in demented and non-demented 85-year olds. *Journal of Geriatric Psychiatry and Neurology* **7**: 169–175

Skoog I, Hesse C, Aevarsson O *et al.* (1998) A population study of ApoE genotype at the age of 85: relation to dementia, cerebrovascular disease, and mortality. *Journal of Neurology, Neurosurgery, and Psychiatry* **64**: 37–43

Simoni M, Pantoni L, Pracucci G *et al.* (2003) Prevalence of different cerebral computed tomography-detected lesions in an elderly population sample living in Göteborg, Sweden. In: *Abstract Book of the First Congress of the International Society for Vascular Behavioural and Cognitive Disorders*, Göteborg, Sweden, August 28–30, 2003, pp. 32–33

Snowdon DA, Greiner LH, Mortimer JA *et al.* (1997) Brain infarction and the clinical expression of Alzheimer disease. The Nun Study. *JAMA* **277**: 813–817

Starkstein SE, Sabe L, Vazquez S *et al.* (1997) Neuropsychological, psychiatric, and cerebral perfusion correlates of leukoaraiosis in Alzheimer's disease. *Journal of Neurology, Neurosurgery, and Psychiatry* **63**: 66–73

Steingart A, Hachinski VC, Lau C *et al.* (1987a) Cognitive and neurologic findings in subjects with diffuse white matter lucencies on computed tomographic scan (Leuko-araiosis). *Archives of Neurology* **44**: 32–35

Steingart A, Hachinski VC, Lau C *et al.* (1987b) Cognitive and neurologic findings in demented patients with diffuse white matter lucencies on computed tomographic scan (Leuko-araiosis). *Archives of Neurology* **44**: 36–39

Stout JC, Jernigan TL, Archibald SL, Salmon DP. (1996) Association of dementia severity with cortical gray matter and abnormal white matter volumes in dementia of the Alzheimer type. *Archives of Neurology* **53**: 742–749

Sze G, De Armond SJ, Brant-Zawadzki M *et al.* (1986) Foci of MRI signal (pseudolesions) anterior to the frontal horns: histologic correlations of a normal finding. *American Journal of Neuroradiology* **7**: 381–387

Tabaton M, Caponnetto C, Mancardi G, Loeb C. (1991) Amyloid beta protein deposition in brains from elderly subjects with leukoaraiosis. *Journal of the Neurological Sciences* **106**: 123–127

Tanaka Y, Tanaka O, Mizuno Y, Yoshida M. (1989) A radiological study of dynamic processes in lacunar dementia. *Stroke* **20**: 1488–1493

Tarvonen-Schröder S, Räihä I, Kurki T *et al.* (1995) Clinical characteristics of rapidly progressive leukoaraiosis. *Acta Neurologica Scandinavica* **91**: 399–404

Tomonaga M, Yamanouchi H, Tohgi H, Kameyama M. (1982) Clinicopathologic study of progressive subcortical vascular encephalopathy (Binswanger type) in the elderly. *Journal of the American Geriatrics Society* **30**: 524–529

Tupler LA, Coffey CE, Logue PE *et al.* (1992) Neuropsychological importance of subcortical white matter hyperintensity. *Archives of Neurology* **49**: 1248–1252

Turner ST, Jack CR, Fornage M *et al.* (2004) Heritability of leukoaraiosis in hypertensive sibships. *Hypertension* **43**: 483–487

Valentine AR, Moseley IF, Kendall BE. (1980) White matter abnormality in cerebral atrophy: clinicoradiological correlations. *Journal of Neurology, Neurosurgery, and Psychiatry* **43**: 139–142

Van den Bergh R and van der Eecken H. (1968) Anatomy and embryology of cerebral circulation. *Progress in Brain Research* **30**: 1–26 van Straaten EC, Scheltens P, Knol DL *et al.* (2003) Operational definitions for the NINDS-AIREN criteria for vascular dementia: an interobserver study. *Stroke* **34**: 1907–1912

van Swieten JC, Geyskes GG, Derix MMA *et al.* (1991a) Hypertension in the elderly is associated with white matter lesions and cognitive decline. *Annals of Neurology* **30**: 825–830

van Swieten JC, van Den Hout JHW, van Ketel BA *et al.* (1991b) Periventricular lesions in the white matter on magnetic resonance imaging in the elderly. A morphometric correlation with arteriolosclerosis and dilated perivascular spaces. *Brain* **114**: 761–774

Van Zagten M, Boiten J, Kessels F, Lodder J. (1996) Significant progression of white matter lesions and small deep (lacunar) infarcts in patients with stroke. *Archives of Neurology* **53**: 650–655

Vataja R, Pohjasvaara T, Mäntyla R *et al.* (2003) MRI correlates of executive dysfunction in patients with ischaemic stroke. *European Journal of Neurology* **10**: 625–631

Vermeer SE, Hollander M, van Dijk EJ *et al.* (2003a) Silent brain infarcts and white matter lesions increase stroke risk in the general population: the Rotterdam Scan Study. *Stroke* **34**: 1126–1129

Vermeer SE, Prins ND, den Heijer T *et al.* (2003b) Silent brain infarcts and the risk of dementia and cognitive decline. *New England Journal Medicine* **348**: 1215–1222

Vinters HV. (1987) Cerebral amyloid angiopathy. A critical review. *Stroke* **18**: 311–324

Wahlund L-O, Basun H, Almkvist O *et al.* (1994) White matter hyperintensities in dementia: does it matter? *Magnetic Resonance Imaging* **12**: 387–394

Wahlund L-O, Barkhof F, Fazekas F *et al.* (2001) A new rating scale for age-related white matter changes applicable to MRI and CT. *Stroke* **32**: 1318–1322

Waldemar G, Christiansen P, Larsson HBW *et al.* (1994) White matter magnetic resonance hyperintensities in dementia of the Alzheimer type: morphological and regional cerebral blood flow correlates. *Journal of Neurology, Neurosurgery, and Psychiatry* **57**: 1458–1465

Wallin A, Blennow K, Uhlemann C *et al.* (1989) White matter low attenuation on computed tomography in Alzheimer's disease and vascular dementia – diagnostic and pathogenetic aspects. *Acta Neurologica Scandinavica* **80**: 518–523

Wetterling T, Kanitz RD, Borgis KJ. (1994) The ICD-10 criteria for vascular dementia. *Dementia* **5**: 185–188

Wilson RS, Bennett D, Fox JH *et al.* (1988) Alzheimer's disease: prevalence and clinical significance of white-matter lesions on magnetic resonance imaging. *Annals of Neurology* **24**: 160–161

Wohl MA, Mehringer CM, Lesser IM *et al.* (1994) White matter hyperintensities in healthy older adults: a longitudinal study. *International Journal of Geriatric Psychiatry* **9**: 273–277

Wolf H, Ecke GM, Bettin S *et al.* (2000) Do white matter changes contribute to the subsequent development of dementia in patients with mild cognitive impairment? A longitudinal study. *International Journal of Geriatric Psychiatry* **15**: 803–812

Wong TY, Klein R, Sharrett AR *et al.* (2002) Atherosclerosis Risk in Communities Study. Cerebral white matter lesions, retinopathy, and incident clinical stroke. *JAMA* **288**: 67–74

Wu CC, Mungas D, Petkov CI *et al.* (2002) Brain structure and cognition in a community sample of elderly Latinos. *Neurology* **59**: 383–391

Yamauchi H, Fukuyama H, Shio H. (2000) Corpus callosum atrophy in patients with leukoaraiosis may indicate global cognitive impairment. *Stroke* **31**: 1515–1520

Yamauchi H, Fukuda H, Oyanagi C. (2002) Significance of white matter high intensity lesions as a predictor of stroke from arteriolosclerosis. *Journal of Neurology, Neurosurgery, and Psychiatry* **72**: 576–582

Yao H, Sadoshima S, Ibayashi S *et al.* (1992) Leukoaraiosis and dementia in hypertensive patients. *Stroke* **23**: 1673–1677

Ylikoski R, Ylikoski A, Erkinjuntti T *et al.* (1993) White matter changes in healthy elderly persons correlate with attention and speed of mental processing. *Archives of Neurology* **50**: 818–824

Ylikoski A, Erkinjuntti T, Raininko R *et al.* (1995) White matter hyperintensities on MRI in the neurologically non-diseased elderly. Analysis of cohorts of consecutive subjects aged 55 to 85 years living at home. *Stroke* **26**: 1171–1177

Young IR, Randell CP, Kaplan PW *et al.* (1983) Nuclear magnetic resonance (NMR) imaging in white matter disease of the brain using spin-echo sequences. *Journal of Computer Assisted Tomography* **7**: 290–294

Zimmerman RD, Fleming CA, Lee BCP *et al.* (1986) Periventricular hyperintensity as seen by magnetic resonance: prevalence and significance. *American Journal of Neuroradiology* **7**: 13–20

Zubenko GS, Sullivan P, Nelson JP *et al.* (1990) Brain imaging abnormalities in mental disorders of late life. *Archives of Neurology* **47**: 1107–1111

SUGGESTED READING

Ferro JM and Madureira S. (2002) Age-related white matter changes and cognitive impairment. *Journal of the Neurological Sciences* **203–204**: 221–225

Gunning-Dixon FM and Raf N. (2000) The cognitive correlates of white matter abnormalities in normal aging: a quantitative review. *Neuropsychology* **14**: 224–232

45

Vascular dementia: neuropathological features

RAJ N KALARIA

Cerebrovascular disease is distinctly heterogeneous but may lead to vascular cognitive impairment or vascular dementia (VaD). Previous autopsy series of dementia cases have reported frequencies of VaD to vary widely (0.03–58 per cent) but use of current clinical diagnostic criteria suggests worldwide prevalence to be 10–15 per cent. Atherothromboembolism and intracranial small vessel disease are the main causes of brain infarction. Consistent with the subclassification of VaD lacunar infarcts or multiple microinfarcts in the basal ganglia, thalamus, brain stem and white matter are associated with more than 50 per cent of the cases. White matter changes including regions of incomplete infarction are usually widespread in VaD but their contribution to impairment is not explicit. Other pathologies including remote hippocampal injury, neocortical neuronal demise and Alzheimer type of lesions may modify the course of dementia. While most of VaD occurs sporadically, only a small proportion of cases bear apparent familial traits. CADASIL is likely the most common form of hereditary VaD, which arises from small vessel disease. Relative to other common dementias, the neuropathological substrates of VaD need unambiguous definition to impact on preventative and treatment strategies, and are critical for selective recruitment to clinical trials.

45.1 INTRODUCTION

Thomas Willis (1672) deserves the credit for advancing the obvious link between the cerebral circulation and dementia before the twentieth century. However, Alois Alzheimer and Emil Kraeplin among other neuropsychiatrists had specifically ascribed arteriosclerotic dementia resulting from gradual strangulation of the blood supply to the brain as the main cause of dementia (Berrios and Freeman, 1991). The clear concept of subclasses of VaD was introduced by Otto Binswanger when he described subcortical arteriosclerotic encephalopathy upon pathological verification of cerebral white matter disorder in a group of eight patients (Berrios and Freeman, 1991). Today we accept that cerebrovascular disease causes the second most common form of age-related dementia. VaD may, however, result from all forms of cerebrovascular lesions that sometimes includes post-stroke syndromes (O'Brien et al., 2003). The challenge of defining the pathological substrates of VaD is complicated by the heterogeneous nature of cerebrovascular disease and coexistence of other pathologies including Alzheimer type of lesions. Blood vessel size, origin of vascular occlusion and genetic factors are critical factors in defining subtypes of VaD (Box 45.1). Multi-infarct dementia is caused by large vessel disease whereas Binswanger type of VaD involving subcortical regions including the white matter results from small vessel changes. Subcortical ischaemic VaD appears the most significant subtype of VaD (Román et al., 2002). Other factors that may define the subtype and degree of impairment include multiplicity, size, anatomical location, laterality and age of the lesion (Box 45.1). Several brain regions including the territories of the anterior, posterior and middle cerebral arteries, the angular gyrus, caudate and medial thalamus in the dominant hemisphere, the amygdala and hippocampus as well as the hippocampus have been implicated in VaD (Markesbery, 1998). For purposes of prevention and treatment it is imperative to recognize subtypes of VaD yet not devise numerous categories to make the task overly complicated (Román et al., 1993).

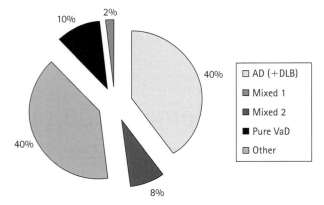

Figure 45.1   *Pathological outcome of clinically diagnosed Vascular dementia (VaD). Mixed type 1 revealed large infarcts whereas mixed type 2 predominantly exhibited small vessel disease with microinfarction. 'Other' includes dementia with mild Parkinson's disease and depression. AD, Alzheimer's disease; DLB, dementia with Lewy bodies.*

45.2 CEREBROVASCULAR DISEASE, VASCULAR DEMENTIA AND MIXED DEMENTIA

There is now a general consensus that the clinical diagnosis of VaD in demented patients with evidence of cerebrovascular lesions applies only when other causes of dementia are ruled out (Erkinjuntti, 1994; see Chapter 43 in this volume). As with diagnosis of other causes of dementia, criteria may be derived from a range of investigations including a detailed clinical history, timing of event, neuropsychometric tests, neuroimaging and neuropathological reports in accord with the DSM criteria. Perhaps inevitably like in the Alzheimer's disease (AD) model, diagnostic criteria based on the pathological findings should be quantified and related to the progression of cognitive impairment (Mirra, 1997). The frequencies of VaD in autopsy series range from as low as 0.03 per cent to as high as 58 per cent with an overall mean rate of 17 per cent (Markesbery, 1998; Jellinger, 2002). In cases where currently accepted criteria have been applied, the frequencies are even lower with a mean of 7 per cent. Perhaps not surprisingly in Japanese studies the incidence of VaD cases was found to be 35 per cent (Seno *et al.*, 1999) and 22 per cent (Akatsu *et al.*, 2001). Taking this into account the worldwide frequency of VaD in autopsy verified cases might be estimated to be between 10 and 15 per cent.

In addition to VaD the diagnosis of mixed dementia (AD and VaD or less frequently dementia with Lewy bodies and VaD) particularly among the oldest old (>85 years of age) is a challenge. Clinical and pathological evidence indicates that combined neurodegenerative and vascular pathologies worsen presentation and outcome of dementia (Snowdon *et al.*, 1997;

Esiri *et al.*, 1999; Rossi *et al.*, 2004). A high proportion of individuals fulfilling the neuropathological diagnosis of AD have significant cerebrovascular lesions including silent infarcts upon imaging and extensive white matter disease (Premkumar *et al.*, 1996; Heyman *et al.*, 1998; Nagy *et al.*, 1998; Kalaria and Ballard, 1999). Conversely, clinically diagnosed VaD patients frequently show extensive AD-type neuropathological changes (Hulette *et al.*, 1997; Erkinjuntti *et al.*, 1988; Kalaria and Ballard, 1999). Nolan *et al.* (1998) reported that 87 per cent of the patients enrolled in a prospective series to examine VaD in a dementia clinic were found to have AD either alone (58 per cent) or in combination with cerebrovascular disease (42 per cent) at post mortem. All of the patients with signs of cerebrovascular disease were also found to have some concomitant neurodegenerative disease (Figure 45.1). Similarly, another study indicated that large numbers of VaD cases without coexisting neuropathological evidence of AD suggests that 'pure' VaD is very uncommon (Hulette *et al.*, 1997). Thus current clinical diagnostic criteria serve to detect pathology but not 'pure' pathology. Early validation studies indicated that while mixed dementia could be distinguished from AD, it could not be separated from VaD (Rosen *et al.*, 1980). Recent studies suggest that 30–50 per cent of mixed AD and VaD cases are misclassified as VaD (Gold *et al.*, 1997, 2002) and the neuroimaging component of the NINDS AIREN criteria does not distinguish between people with and without dementia in the context of cerebrovascular disease (Ballard *et al.*, 2003). The potential overlap of pathologies is therefore complex, with different types of cerebrovascular lesions including cortical and subcortical infarction and small vessel disease (Esiri *et al.*, 1997; Ballard *et al.*, 2000), and different types and severity of neurodegenerative changes involving tau, amyloid and α-synuclein pathology. While evidence-based pathological criteria for the diagnosis of mixed dementia remains to be perfected, the diagnosis should be made when a primary neurodegenerative disease known to cause dementia exists with one or more of the pathological lesions

Box 45.2 *Key variables to define pathology of VaD*

- Identify as ischaemic or haemorrhagic infarct(s)
- Presence of lacunes and lacunar infarcts: *état lacunaire* (grey) and *état crible* (WM)
- Location of infarcts: cortex, WM, basal ganglia, brain stem (pontine), cerebellum
- Circulation involved: arterial territories – anterior, middle or posterior
- Laterality: right or left anterior and posterior
- Sizes and number of infarcts = dimension: 0–4 mm, 5–15 mm, 16–30 mm, 31–50 mm and >50 mm; if size < 5 mm determine as small or microinfarcts
- Presence and location of small vessel disease: lipohyalinosis; fibroid necrosis; CAA
- Presence of white matter disease: rarefaction or incomplete infarction
- Degree of gliosis: mild, moderate or severe
- Presence of Alzheimer pathology (incl. NFT and neuritic plaque staging). If degree > stage III, the case is mixed AD and VaD
- Presence of hippocampal sclerosis

For reporting purposes each of above features can be scored numerically to provide a summary. For example, 0 is absent and 1 means present. Less frequent lesions including watershed infarcts and laminar necrosis. Increasing numerical value may also be assigned to the infarcts

CAA, cerebral amyloid angiopathy; NFT, neurofibrillary tangles; WM, white matter

Table 45.1 *Dementia associated with different cerebrovascular pathologies*

VaD subtypes related to:	Subtype
Large infarct or several infarcts (≥50 mL loss of tissue); MID	I
Multiple small or microinfarcts (>3 with minimum diameter 5 mm); Small vessel disease* (involving ≥3 coronal levels; hyalinization, CAA, lacunar infarcts, perivascular changes)	II
Strategic infarcts (e.g. thalamus, hippocampus)	III
Cerebral hypoperfusion (hippocampal sclerosis, ischaemic-anoxic damage, cortical laminar necrosis, borderzone infarcts involving 3 different coronal levels)	IV
Cerebral haemorrhages (lobar, ICH or SAH)	V
Cerebrovascular changes with AD pathology (above Braak III); mixed dementia	VI

In all of above, the age of the vascular lesion(s) should correspond with the time when disease began. The proposed Newcastle categorization includes six subtypes (Polvikoski T and Kalaria RN, unpublished observations). The post-stroke cases are usually included in subtypes I–III. While these may not be much different from other published subtypes (Román *et al.*, 1993; Jellinger 2002), they are practical and simple to use. Cases with extensive white matter disease in the absence of significant other features are included under small vessel disease
*Subtype I may result from large vessel occlusion (atherothromboembolism), artery to artery embolism or cardioembolism. Subtype II usually involves descriptions of arteriosclerosis, lipohyalinosis, hypertensive, arteriosclerotic, amyloid or collagen angiopathy. Subtypes I–II and V may result from aneurysms, arterial dissections, arteriovenous malformations and various forms of arteritis (vasculitis)
AD, Alzheimer's disease; CAA, cerebral amyloid angiopathy; ICH, intracerebral haemorrhage; SAH, subarachnoid haemorrhage; VaD, vascular dementia

defining the VaD subtypes (Box 45.2). Therefore a combination of the nominal three or more infarctions and Alzheimer pathology above stage III may warrant such a diagnosis.

From the essential information derived at autopsy (Box 45.1), we have proposed the neuropathological diagnosis of probable VaD or less popular 'pure VaD' be based on the exclusion of a primary neurodegenerative disease known to cause dementia and the presence of cerebrovascular pathology that defines one or more of the VaD subtypes (Box 45.2). These would include dementia among post-stroke survivors who fulfil the NINDS-AIREN (Román *et al.*, 1993) criteria for probable VaD. Those stroke survivors with mild cognitive impairment could be classed as exhibiting vascular cognitive impairment but the criteria for this extension are not widely accepted (O'Brien *et al.*, 2003). The diagnosis of possible VaD may be used when the brain contains vascular pathology, which does not fulfil the criteria for one of the subtypes but where no other explanation for dementia is found.

45.3 BRAIN VASCULAR LESIONS AND VASCULAR DEMENTIA

The majority of arterial territory infarctions, which may be admixed in cortical and subcortical regions, result from atherothromboembolism. This may be responsible for up to 50 per cent of all ischaemic strokes whereas intracranial small vessel disease causes 25 per cent of the infarcts (Kalimo *et al.*, 2002a). Small vessel alternations involve arteriosclerosis and hyalinosis and associated with lacunar infarcts and lacunes predominantly occurring in the subcortical structures. White matter disease or subcortical leukoencephalopathy with incomplete infarction and small vessel disease are common pathological changes in cerebrovascular disease. Others features include border zone (watershed) infarctions, laminar necrosis and amyloid angiopathy (Box 45.2). Complicated angiopathies such as fibromuscular dysplasia, arterial dissections, granulomatous angiitis, collagen vascular disease and giant cell arteritis are rarer causes of cerebrovascular disease (Kalimo *et al.*, 2002a) and VaD.

Previous studies have recorded ischaemic, oedematous and haemorrhagic lesions affecting the brain circulation or perfusion to be associated with VaD (Table 45.1). In four studies where VaD was diagnosed 75 per cent of the cases revealed cortical and subcortical infarcts suggesting other vascular pathologies involving incomplete infarction or border zone infarcts could be important factors. Among other lesions

25 per cent of the cases had cystic infarcts whereas 50 per cent of the cases had lacunar infarcts or microinfarcts. Lacunar infarcts, however, appear to be a common category of infarcts, and currently recognized as the most frequent cause of stroke (dissections, granulomatous angiitis, collagen vascular disease and giant-cell arteritis are rarer causes of cerebrovascular disease (Kalimo *et al.*, 2002a). Severe amyloid angiopathy was present in 10 per cent of the cases. Most interestingly, 55 per cent of the cases revealed hippocampal atrophy in one study (Vinters *et al.*, 2000). One of the studies concluded that ischaemic vascular disease appears to correlate with widespread small ischaemic lesions distributed throughout the central nervous system (CNS) (Vinters *et al.*, 2000).

45.3.1 Large infarction and large vessel pathology

Large infarction or macroinfarction is usually defined as that visible upon gross examination of the brain at autopsy. Stenosis arising from atherosclerosis within large vessels is considered to be the main cause of large infarction, which may sometimes extend beyond the arterial territories. The stages of atherosclerosis may vary from accumulation of foam cells causing fatty streaks to complicated atheromas involving extracellular matrix components and even viral or bacterial infections. Occlusion of the extracranial arteries such as the internal carotid artery and the main intracranial arteries of the circle of Willis including the middle cerebral artery can lead to multi-infarct dementia, which forms approximately 15 per cent of VaD (Brun, 1994). In severe cases medium-sized arteries in the leptomeninges and proximal perforating arteries could be involved. The damage could be worse depending upon the presence of hypertension. Artery-to-artery embolism involves breaking of thrombi from the often ulcerated lesions in the extracranial arteries, e.g. at the bifurcation of common carotid artery or the heart. The thrombi may contain, in addition to coagulated blood and platelets, cholesterol and calcified deposits from the underlying atheromatous plaque. Various types of cardiogenic emboli may also find their way to the anterior or particularly the posterior cerebral circulation, to cause infarcts in the territory of the posterior cerebral artery or superior cerebellar artery.

Arterial territorial infarctions involve four principal areas particularly those supplied by the major arteries: anterior, middle cerebral artery, posterior artery and the territory between the anterior and middle cerebral artery (Kalimo *et al.*, 2002a). The size of these infarctions is determined by assessing the two largest diameters of each lesion (Box 45.2). The typical infarct comprises the central core with complete infarction surrounded by a narrow perifocal hypoperfused (or penumbra) zone of incomplete infarction, which may be oedematous, and leads into normal appearing tissue. The core may involve both the cortex and underlying white matter that is devoid of functional components such as neurones, axons and oligodendrocytes and may in time form cavitated lesions or scars devoid of cells or haemosiderin. Prior to scar formation

between 3 and 14 days, infarct cores attract neutrophils, lipid-laden macrophages or microglia and astrocytes in the lesion, which is easily assessed upon routine staining. The intensity of gliosis, both astrocytic and microgliosis, is an important consideration in judging the degree and age of infarction. Degrees of gliosis or glial scars may be noted in brains subjected to global ischaemia, i.e. after transient cardiac arrest where responses may be observed in vulnerable neuronal groups within the hippocampus or neocortical laminae (Box 45.2).

45.3.2 Microinfarction, lacunar infarcts and lacunes

Microinfarcts have been variably described but widely thought to be small ischaemic lesions visible only upon light microscopy (see Plate 15a, b). These lesions of up to 5 mm diameter may or may not involve a small vessel at its centre but are foci with pallor, neuronal loss, axonal damage (white matter) and gliosis. Sometimes these may include regions of incomplete infarction or rarefied (subacute) change. Microinfarcts have also been described as attenuated lesions of indistinct nature occurring in both cortical or subcortical regions. Such lesions or combination of these should be reported when there are multiple or at least more than three present in any region (Table 45.2). Microinfarcts and lacunar infarcts appear central to the most common cause of VaD and predict poor outcome in the elderly (Esiri *et al.*, 1997; Ballard *et al.*, 2000; Vinters *et al.*, 2000; White *et al.*, 2002). Interestingly, in the autopsied older Japanese-American men the importance of microvascular lesions as a likely explanation for dementia was nearly equal to that of Alzheimer lesions (White *et al.*, 2002). Microinfarction in the subcortical structures has been emphasized as substrate of cognitive impairment, and correlated with increased Alzheimer type of pathology, but cortical microinfarcts also appear to contribute significantly to the progression of cognitive deficits in brain ageing (Kovari *et al.*, 2004). Furthermore microinfarcts even in border zone (watershed) regions may aggravate the degenerative process as indicated by worsening

Table 45.2 *Types of vascular and hippocampal lesions reported in VaD*

Pathological feature	% Cases
Complete infarctions (cortical and subcortical)	75
Lacunar infarcts (mostly WM and BG)	50
Small or microinfarcts	50
Cystic infarcts	25
Cerebral amyloid angiopathy	10
Intracerebral haemorrhages	2
Hippocampal atrophy and sclerosis	55

Data compiled from 70 cases reported in previous studies (Esiri *et al.*, 1997; Hulette *et al.*, 1997; Vinters *et al.*, 2000; Kalaria *et al.*, unpublished observations). Per cent cases are averaged from two or more reported studies. Cystic infarcts (possibly also lacunar) with typically ragged edges were admixed in both cortical and subcortical structures
BG, basal ganglia; WM, white matter

impairment in AD (Suter *et al.*, 2002). Thus multiple micro-infarction appears strongly correlated with dementia indicated by several studies (Jellinger, 2002).

Lacunes are complete or cavitating infarcts as defined above, measuring up to 15 mm in diameter seen radiologically and upon gross examination at autopsy (Box 45.2; Figure 45.2). These lesions are largely confined to the cerebral white matter and subcortical structures including the thalamus, basic ganglia and brain stem. Most lacunes, remnants of small infarcts, are detected in the cystic or chronic stage with no viable central tissue, but could have perifocal regions with incomplete infarction, particularly in the white matter. A few lacunes may represent healed or reabsorbed minute or petechial haemorrhages. Microlacunes have also been described, which essentially should be thought of as large cystic microinfarcts. To distinguish perivascular cavities, it has been suggested that lacunes be classed into three subtypes: lacunar infarcts, lacunar haemorrhages and dilated perivascular spaces (Poirier *et al.*, 1985). Lacunar infarcts usually result from progressive small vessel disease manifested as hypertensive angiopathy that may involve stenosis caused by hyalinosis. Small vessel disease in a perforating artery, for example, may also reveal regions of incomplete infarction, attenuation or rarefaction usually recognized by pallor upon microscopic examination. However, lacunar lesions can also be caused by infections and neoplasms. Lacunes are associated with small perivascular cavities up to 2 mm in diameter often found in the basal ganglia and the white matter. Perivascular cavities or empty spaces resulting from distortion or elongation of small arteries collectively referred to as *état lacunaire* in the grey matter and *état crible* in the white matter may be numerous in older subjects.

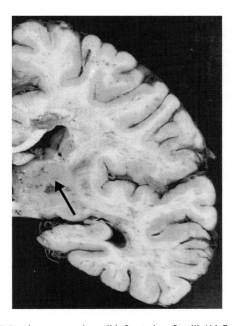

Figure 45.2 *Lacunes and small infarcts in a familial VaD. Typical lacunar lesion (arrow) in the thalamus of a 60 year-old-man diagnosed with CADASIL bearing a single missense mutation in the Notch3 gene. Lacunes in sporadic VaD cases are qualitatively similar.*

45.3.3 Small vessel disease

Small vessels including intracerebral end-arteries and arterioles undergo progressive age-related changes (Lammie, 2000), which may result in lacunar or microinfarcts. These range from wall thickening by hyalinosis, reduction or increment of the intima to severe arteriosclerosis and fibroid necrosis (Plate 15b). Uncomplicated hyalinosis is characterized by almost complete degeneration of vascular smooth muscle cells (becomes acellular) with concentric accumulation of extracellular matrix components like the collagens and fibroblasts (Lammie, 2000). These changes are most common in the small vasculature of the white matter (Plate 15b). Small vessel changes likely promote occlusion or progressive stenosis with consequent acute or chronic ischaemia of the tissue behind it. Alternatively, arteriosclerotic changes located in small vessels in the deep white matter and basal ganglia may lose their elasticity to dilate and constrict in response to variations of systemic blood pressure or loss of autoregulation. This in turn causes fluctuations in blood flow response and changes in cerebral perfusion. The deep cerebral structures would be rendered most vulnerable because the vessels are end-arteries almost devoid of anastomoses. Small vessel pathology could lead also oedema and damage of the blood–brain barrier (BBB) with chronic leakage of fluid and macromolecules in the white matter (Ho and Garcia, 1999).

45.3.4 Cerebral amyloid angiopathy (CAA)

While CAA is most common in AD and consistently present in Down's syndrome (Premkumar *et al.*, 1996; Kalaria, 2001) it also occurs in elderly subjects with cerebrovascular disease in the general absence of Alzheimer lesions (Cohen *et al.*, 1997). Amyloid β protein accumulation within or juxtaposed to the vasculature may lead to degeneration of vascular cells in both larger perforating arterial vessels as well as cerebral capillaries that represent the BBB. These likely result in microinfarctions and perivascular cavities similar to those seen in hyalinized vessels in subcortical structures. CAA is an important cause of intracerebral and lobar haemorrhages leading to profound ischaemic damage (Vonsattel *et al.*, 1991). CAA also appears to be causally related to white matter changes described by subcortical leukoencephalopathy in patients with CAA, who lacked changes characteristic of AD (Lammie, 2000). Genetic factors such as the apolipoprotien E (ApoE) ε4 allele associated with severity of CAA may modify or attenuate the perfusion of the white matter (Kalaria, 2001).

45.3.5 Alzheimer–type pathology

Alzheimer lesions including amyloid β plaques and neurofibrillary pathology occur more often in cases of cerebrovascular disease than in normal ageing elderly (Kalaria and Ballard, 1999). We reported that amyloid deposits and tangles were three times greater in VaD cases with small (<15 mL) compared with larger volume of infarction. However, the burden of Alzheimer lesions was just barely associated with dementia scores (Ballard *et al.*, 2000). While these findings corroborated the importance of microvascular disease rather than macroscopic infarction as the critical substrate in VaD and in AD (Kalaria, 1996), the burden of Alzheimer lesions was just barely associated with dementia scores in VaD (Ballard *et al.*, 2000).

Cerebral amyloid angiopathy is also frequent in VaD even where the amyloid deposits may be rare in the parenchyma. Although conventional histopathological staining methods may not reveal classical amyloid and neurofibrillary pathology the accumulation of amyloid β and tau peptides may be revealed by immunochemical methods. Our preliminary findings suggest that accumulation of soluble amyloid β_{42} in the temporal lobe of VaD patients is almost similar as that in AD subjects by the eighth decade (Kalaria *et al.*, 1999). These observations implied that total amyloid β peptides increase in brains of patients who succumb to cerebral ischaemia and that brains of the very elderly who suffer from stroke produce large amounts of soluble amyloidogenic peptides almost like AD patients.

Amyloid precursor protein accumulation along white matter tracts has also been previously demonstrated in cerebral ischaemia even in middle-aged subjects (Cochran *et al.*, 1991). It may be hypothesized that, concomitant with ageing, small vessel disease along with white matter lesions in the brain causes vascular injury and may induce tissue pH changes, oxidative damage, amyloid precursor protein expression and subsequent aggregation of soluble amyloid β.

A similar argument may be made for parallel changes that induce tau-like pathology and other neuronal changes. This is supported by the demonstration that increases in cerebrospinal fluid (CSF) tau are not restricted to AD but also evident in various forms of VaD (Blennow *et al.*, 1995; Munroe *et al.*, 1995; Skoog *et al.*, 1995). Concentrations of tau in lumbar CSF in patients diagnosed with probable VaD were reported to be comparable to those in AD and were significantly increased compared with those in non-demented elderly controls (Skoog *et al.*, 1995). Similarly, the concentrations of soluble synaptophysin were found to be decreased in VaD as well as in AD (Zhan *et al.*, 1994). These findings not only suggest that axonal degeneration occurs in VaD as evident in AD but support the notion that ischaemic or oligaemic events in the elderly are early events leading to increases in known markers of Alzheimer pathology. Other biological markers for AD such as decreased ApoE levels in CSF have also been reported in VaD (Skoog *et al.*, 1997).

VaD cases may also bear other AD type lesions including cholinergic and monoamine neuronal deficits (Kalaria and Ballard, 1999). Two different groups had previously shown that compared with AD patients choline acetyltransferase activity was also reduced, albeit to a lesser degree, in the temporal cortex and hippocampus in patients diagnosed with multi-infarct dementia or VaD (Perry *et al.*, 1977; Gottfries *et al.*, 1994). However, despite these deficits there do not appear to be pronounced effects in the cholinergic cell bodies of the basal forebrain in VaD (Mann *et al.*, 1986; Keverne *et al.*, 2003).

Subsequent studies had reported deficits in other neuro-transmitters particularly 5-hydroxytryptamine (5HT) in the basal ganglia and neocortex of VaD subjects (Gottfries *et al.*, 1994). These findings indicate that a variety of Alzheimer-type of changes are also associated with VaD. The pathological diagnosis of VaD in such cases may be dictated by the degree and location of Alzheimer pathology. If it is restricted to the hippocampus and the density of neuritic plaques or tangles does not exceed stage III of the criteria defined by Thal *et al.* (2002) and Braak and Braak (1995), they could be diagnosed as VaD. This is similar to the notion where dementia cases meeting CERAD criteria for probable AD may exhibit infarctions or white matter changes. However, cases of cerebrovascular disease fulfilling the criteria for VaD (Box 45.2, p. 567) with concomitant Alzheimer pathology above stage III for plaques and tangles may be designated as mixed dementia.

45.3.6 White matter disease

White matter lesions (or subcortical leukoencephalopathy) incorporating myelin loss are considered a consequence of vascular disease. The frequency of white matter changes is increased in patients with cerebrovascular disease and those at risk for vascular disease including arterial hypertension, cardiovascular disease and diabetes mellitus (O'Brien *et al.*, 2003). White matter lesions occur in ≈30 per cent of AD and dementia with Lewy body (DLB) cases and may be present irrespective of the focal lesions in VaD (Englund, 1998). It is often argued that white matter damage in patients with AD might simply reflect Wallerian changes secondary to cortical loss of neurones. However, this is unlikely since histological changes characteristic of Wallerian degeneration are not evident as white matter pallor. Conversely, in AD patients with severe loss of cortical neurones similar white matter lesions are not apparent (Englund, 1998).

Lesions in the deep white matter (0.5–1 cm away from ventricle in coronal plane) have been correlated with dementia including VaD (Kalaria and Ballard, 1999; O'Brien *et al.*, 2003). Conflicting data with respect to periventricular lesions may depend on definition of the boundaries between the periventricular and deep white matter if the coursing of the fibres are used as markers. Lacunar infarcts are produced when the ischaemic damage is focal and of sufficient severity to result in a small area of necrosis, whereas diffuse white matter change is considered a form of rarefaction or incomplete infarction where there may be selective damage to some cellular components (Plate 16). While the U-fibres are usually spared, white matter disease comprises several patterns of alterations including pallor or swelling of myelin, loss of oligodendrocytes, axons and myelin fibres, cavitations with or without presence of macrophages and areas of reactive astrogliosis, where the astrocytic cytoplasm and cell processes may be visible with standard stains. Lesions in the white matter also include spongiosis, i.e. vacuolization of the white matter structures and widening of the perivascular spaces.

45.3.7 Hippocampal sclerosis and atrophy

Hippocampal neurones in the Sommer's sector are highly vulnerable to disturbances in the cerebral circulation or hypoxia caused by systemic or cardiovascular disease. Severe loss of hippocampal neurones within the CA fields and infarctions along Ammon's horn are evident in a proportion (10–20 per cent) of usually older (>80 years) VaD cases. The loss of cells should be graded when this is evident, together with any microinfarctions within the hippocampal formation (Dickson *et al.*, 1994). Hippocampal sclerosis is a likely major contributing factor in the hippocampal atrophy described at gross examination. Hippocampal changes remote to ischaemic injury have also been emphasized in subcortical ischaemic vascular dementia (Vinters *et al.*, 2000).

45.3.8 Border zone (watershed) infarcts

Border zone or watershed infarctions mostly occur from haemodynamic events, usually in patients with severe internal carotid artery stenosis. They could occur bilaterally or unilaterally, and disposed to regions between two main arterial territories, deep and superficial vessel systems. Typical border zone infarctions may be 5 mm or more wide as wedge shaped regions of pallor and rarefaction extending into the white matter. Larger areas of incomplete infarction may extend into the white matter (Brun, 1994; Kalimo *et al.*, 2002a). These are characterized by mild to moderate loss of oligodendrocytes, myelin and axons in areas where there may be hyalinized vessels (Brun, 1994). These features may be accompanied by astrogliosis, some microgliosis and macrophage infiltration.

45.3.9 Laminar necrosis

Laminar necrosis is characterized by neuronal ischaemic changes leading to neuronal loss and gliosis in the cortical ribbon. This is particularly apparent in cases where global ischaemia or hypoperfusion has occurred as in cardiac arrest. Typical topographic distribution of spongy form change can be readily apparent with standard stains. They appear more commonly at the arterial border zones (Brun, 1994; Kalimo *et al.*, 2002a) that may fall into the subtype IV of VaD pathology (Box 45.2, p. 567).

45.4 FAMILIAL VASCULAR DEMENTIA AND GENETIC FACTORS

Cerebral autosomal dominant arteriopathy with subcortical infarcts and leukoencephalopathy (CADASIL) is a small vessel disease that emerges as the most common hereditary form of stroke leading to progressive dementia (Kalaria, 2001; Kalimo *et al.*, 2002b). Several other hereditary conditions presenting with ischaemic strokes or focal infarcts unrelated to the amyloid angiopathies have been described. These include hereditary multi-infarct dementia (Sourander and Walinder, 1977; Zhang *et al.*, 1994) rare occlusive conditions such as hereditary endotheliopathy retinopathy nephropathy with stroke or HERNS (Jen *et al.*, 1997) and chronic familial vascular encephalopathy (Stevens *et al.*, 1977), which actually proved to be *Notch 3* type CADASIL. In view of the striking pathology (Plate 15, Figure 45.2) including multiple subcortical infarcts, small vessel disease, severe arteriosclerosis, profound white matter rarefaction CADASIL has also been considered a familial form of Binswanger's disease.

Several genes have also been considered to be associated with cerebrovascular disease or stroke risk factors (Kalaria, 2001). The precise functions of the products of these genes, however, in light of the pathogenetic processes remain unclear. The ApoE gene is accepted to be unequivocally linked to late-onset AD but its role in cerebrovascular disease not associated with Alzheimer pathology (i.e. VaD) is not clear. In accord with the implications that ApoE might promote pathological alterations in the vascular wall, the ApoE ε4 allele is a strong factor in the development of CAA but not an independent risk factor in CAA-related intracerebral haemorrhages (Greenberg *et al.*, 1995; Nicoll *et al.*, 1997; Olichney *et al.*, 1996; Premkumar *et al.*, 1996; Zarow *et al.*, 1999). Surprisingly, the ApoE ε2 allele is considered a strong factor for intracerebral haemorrhage in amyloid-laden vessels that may cause rupture of the vessel walls by inducing specific cellular changes (Greenberg *et al.*, 1998; McCarron and Nicoll, 1999). However, a meta-analysis revealed significantly higher ApoE ε4 allele frequencies in patients diagnosed with ischaemic cerebrovascular disease (Kalmijn *et al.*, 1996; McCarron *et al.*, 1999); Frisoni *et al.* (1994) had previously implicated comparably high ε4 allele frequencies in cerebrovascular disease-associated dementia but these observations remain unconfirmed. On the other hand, Traykov *et al.* (1999) showed that the frequency of ApoE ε4 allele in over 70-year-olds with clinically diagnosed VaD or vascular cognitive impairment did not differ from controls. Similarly, pathologically verified studies showed that ε4 allele frequencies did not differ between Binswanger's disease and other forms of VaD (Higuchi *et al.*, 1996).

45.5 CONCLUSIONS

The heterogeneous nature of cerebrovascular disease compels better understanding of the neuropathological substrates of VaD for wide application. Small vessel disease leading to multiple microinfarcts or lacunes in the subcortical structures appear most involved in VaD. White matter pathology is frequent in VaD but it needs evaluation to enable correlation with cognitive decline. Whether hippocampal changes remote from sites of ischaemic injury or Alzheimer pathology contribute to the disease progression is unclear. The systematic classification of VaD pathological subtypes should be applied universally. The clear definition of the neuropathological correlates of VaD would be useful for preventative and treatment strategies.

REFERENCES

Akatsu H, Takahashi M, Matsukawa N *et al.* (2001) Subtype analysis of neuropathologically diagnosed patients in a Japanese geriatric hospital. *Journal of the Neurological Sciences* **196**: 63–70

Ballard C, McKeith I, O'Brien J *et al.* (2000) Neuropathological substrates of dementia and depression in vascular dementia, with a particular focus on cases with small infarct volumes. *Dementia and Geriatric Cognitive Disorders* **11**: 59–55

Ballard C, Stephens S, Kenny R *et al.* (2003) Profile of neuro-psychological deficits in older stroke survivors without dementia. *Dementia and Geriatric Cognitive Disorders* **16**: 52–56

Berrios GE and Freeman HL. (1991) *Alzheimer and the Dementias. Eponymists in Medicine Series.* London, Royal Society of Medicine Services, pp. 69–76

Blennow K, Wallin A, Agren H *et al.* (1995) Tau protein in cerebrospinal fluid: a biochemical marker for axonal degeneration in Alzheimer disease? *Molecular Chemistry and Neuropathology* **26**: 231–245

Braak H and Braak E. (1995) Staging of Alzheimer's disease-related neurofibrillary changes. *Neurobiological Aging* **16**: 271–278

Brun A. (1994) Pathology and pathophysiology of cerebrovascular dementia: pure subgroups and hypoperfusive etiology. *Dementia* **5**: 145–147

Cochran E, Bacci B, Chen Y *et al.* (1991) Amyloid precursor protein and ubiquitin immunoreactivity in dystrophic axons is not unique to Alzheimer's disease. *American Journal of Pathology* **139**: 485–489

Cohen DL, Hedera P, Premkumar DRD *et al.* (1997) Amyloid-β angiopathies masquerading as Alzheimer's disease. *Annals of the New York Academy of Science* **826**: 390–395

Dickson DW, Davies P, Bevona C *et al.* (1994) Hippocampal sclerosis: a common pathological feature of dementia in very old (> or = 80 years of age) humans. *Acta Neuropathologica* **88**: 212–221

Englund E. (1998) Neuropathology of white matter changes in Alzheimer's disease and vascular dementia. *Dementia and Geriatric Cognitive Disorders* **1**: 6–12

Erkinjuntti T. (1994) Clinical criteria for vascular dementia: The NINDS-AIREN criteria. *Dementia* **5**: 189–192

Erkinjuntti T, Haltia M, Palo J *et al.* (1988) Accuracy of the clinical diagnosis of vascular dementia: a prospective clinical and post-mortem neuropathological study. *Journal of Neurology, Neurosurgery, and Psychiatry* **51**: 1037–1044

Esiri MM, Wilcock GK, Morris, JH. (1997) Neuropathological assessment of the lesions of significance in vascular dementia. *Journal of Neurology, Neurosurgery, and Psychiatry* **63**: 749–753

Esiri MM, Nagy Z, Smith MZ *et al.* (1999) Cerebrovascular disease and threshold for dementia in the early stages of Alzheimer's disease. *Lancet* **354**: 919–920

Frisoni GB, Calabresi L, Geroldi C *et al.* (1994) Apolipoprotein E ε4 allele in Alzheimer's disease and vascular dementia. *Dementia* **5**: 240–242

Gold G, Giannakopoulos P, Montes-Paixao JC *et al.* (1997) Sensitivity and specificity of newly proposed clinical criteria for possible vascular dementia. *Neurology* **49**: 690–694

Gold G, Bouras C, Canuto A *et al.* (2002) Clinicopathological validation study of four sets of clinical criteria for vascular dementia. *American Journal of Psychiatry* **159**: 82–87

Gottfries CG, Blennow K, Karlsson I, Wallin A. (1994) The neurochemistry of vascular dementia. *Dementia* **5**: 163–167

Greenberg SM, Vonsattelm JP, Rebeck GW *et al.* (1995) Apolipoprotein E ε 4 and cerebral hemorrhage associated with amyloid angiopathy. *Annals of Neurology* **38**: 254–259

Greenberg SM, Vonsattel P, Segal AZ *et al.* (1998) Association of apolipoprotein E ε 2 and vasculopathy in cerebral amyloid angiopathy. *Neurology* **50**: 961–965

Heyman A, Fillenbaum GG, Welsh-Bohmer KA *et al.* (1998) Cerebral infarcts in patients with autopsy-proven Alzheimer's disease. CERAD Part XVIII. *Neurology* **51**: 159–162

Higuchi S *et al.* (1996) The apolipoprotein E gene in Binswanger's disease and vascular dementia. *Clinical Genetics* **5**: 459–461

Ho K-L and Garcia JH. (2000) Neuropathology of the small blood vessels in selected disease of the cerebral white matter. In: L Pantoni, D Inzitaria, A Wallin (eds), *The Matter of White Matter. Current Issues in Neurodegenerative Diseases*, Vol. 10. Utrecht, Academic Pharmaceutical Productions, pp. 247–73

Hulette C, Nochlin D, McKeel D *et al.* (1997) Clinical-neuropathologic findings in multi-infarct dementia: a report of six autopsied cases. *Neurology* **48**: 668–672

Jellinger KA. (2002) Vascular-ischemic dementia: an update. *Journal of Neural Transmission* **62** (Suppl.): 1–23

Jen J, Cohen AH, Yuem Q *et al.* (1997) Hereditary endotheliopathy with retinopathy, nephropathy, and stroke (HERNS). *Neurology* **49**: 1322–1330

Kalaria RN. (1996) Cerebral vessels in ageing and Alzheimer's disease. *Pharmaceutical Therapy* **72**: 193–214

Kalaria RN. (2001) Advances in molecular genetics and pathology of cerebrovascular disorders. *Trends in Neuroscience* **24**: 392–400

Kalaria RN and Ballard CG. (1999) Overlap between pathology of Alzheimer disease and vascular dementia. *Alzheimer Disease and Associated Disorders* **13**: S115–S123

Kalaria RN, Lewis HD, Thomas NJ, Shearman MS. (1999) Brain Aβ42 and Aβ40 concentrations in multi-infarct dementia and Alzheimer's disease. *Society of Neuroscience Abstracts* **23**: 1114

Kalimo H, Kaste M and Haltia, M. (2002a) Vascular diseases. In: D Graham and P Lantos (eds), *Greenfield's Neuropathology*. London, Arnold Press, pp. 281–255

Kalimo H, Ruchoux MM, Viitanen M, Kalaria RN. (2002b) CADASIL: a common form of hereditary arteriopathy causing brain infarcts and dementia. *Brain Pathology* **12**: 317–384

Kalmijn S, Feskens EJM, Launer LJ *et al.* (1996) Cerebrovascular disease, the apolipoprotein ε4 allele and cognitive decline in a community based study of elderly men. *Stroke* **27**: 2230–2235

Keverne J, Court J, Piggott M *et al.* (2003) Cholinergic neurones and microvascular pathology in dementia. *British Neuroscience Association Abstracts* **17**: 78

Kovari E, Gold G, Hermann FR *et al.* (2004) Cortical microinfarcts and demyelination significantly affect cognition in brain aging. *Stroke* **35**: 410–414

Lammie GA. (2000) Pathology of small vessel stroke. *British Medical Bulletin* **56**: 296–206

McCarron MO and Nicoll JR. (1999) The apolipoprotein E epsilon 2 allele and the pathological features in cerebral amyloid angiopathy-related haemorrhage. *Journal of Neuropathology and Experimental Neurology* **158**: 711–718

McCarron MO et al. (1999) APoE genotype as a risk factor for ischemic cerebrovascular disease: a meta-analysis. Neurology 53: 1308–1311

Mann DMA, Yates PO, Marcyniuk B. (1986) The nucleus basalis of Myenert in multi-infarct (vascular) dementia. Acta Neuropathologica 71: 332–337

Markesbery W. (1998) Vascular dementia. In: WR Markesbery (ed.), Neuropathology of Dementing Disorders. London, Arnold, pp. 293–311

Mirra SS. (1997) The CERAD neuropathology protocol and consensus recommendations for the postmortem diagnosis of Alzheimer's disease: a commentary. Neurobiological Aging 18: S91–S94

Munroe WA, Southwick PC, Chang L et al. (1995) Tau protein in cerebrospinal fluid as an aid in the diagnosis of Alzheimer's disease. Annals of Clinical Laboratory Science 25: 207–217

Natte R, Maat-Schieman ML, Haan J et al. (2001) Dementia in hereditary cerebral hemorrhage with amyloidosis-Dutch type is associated with cerebral amyloid angiopathy but is independent of plaques and neurofibrillary tangles. Annals of Neurology 50: 765–772

Nagy Z, Esiri MM, Joachim C et al. (1998) Comparison of pathological diagnostic criteria for Alzheimer disease. Alzheimer Disease and Associated Disorders 12: 182–189

Nicoll JA, Burnett C, Love S et al. (1997) High frequency of apolipoprotein ε 2 allele in hemorrhage due to cerebral amyloid angiopathy. Annals of Neurology 41: 716–721

Nolan KA, Lino MM, Seligmann AW et al. (1998) Absence of vascular dementia in an autopsy series from a dementia clinic. Journal of the American Geriatrics Society 46: 597–604

O'Brien JT, Erkinjuntti T, Reisberg B et al. (2003) Vascular cognitive impairment. Lancet Neurology 2: 89–88

Olichney JM, Hansen LA, Hofstetter CR et al. (1996) Apolipoprotein ε 4 allele is associated with increased neuritic plaques and CAA in Alzheimer's disease and Lewy body variant. Neurology 47: 190–196

Perry EK, Gibson PH, Blessed G et al. (1977) Neurotransmitter enzyme abnormalities in senile dementia, Journal of the Neurological Sciences 34: 247–265

Poirier J, Gray F, Gherardi R et al. (1985) Cerebral lacunae: a new neuropathological classification. Journal of Neuropathology and Experimental Neurology 44: 312–320

Premkumar DRD, Cohen DL, Hedera P et al. (1996) Apolipoprotein E ε4 alleles in cerebral amyloid angiopathy and cerebrovascular pathology associated with Alzheimer's disease. American Journal of Pathology 148: 2083–2095

Román GC, Tatemichi TK, Erkinjuntti T et al. (1993) Vascular Dementia: Diagnostic Criteria for Research Studies. Report of the NINDS-AIREN International Work Group. Neurology 43: 250–260

Román GC, Erkinjuntti T, Wallin A et al. (2002) Subcortical ischaemic vascular dementia. Lancet Neurology 1: 426–436

Rosen WG, Terry RD, Fuld PA et al. (1980) Pathological verification of ischemic score in differentiation of dementias. Annals of Neurology 7: 486–488

Rossi R, Joachim C, Geroldi C et al. (2004) Association between subcortical vascular disease on CT and neuropathological findings. International Journal of Geriatric Psychiatry 19: 690–695

Seno H, Ishino H, Inagaki T et al. (1999) A neuropathological study of dementia in nursing homes over a 17-year period in Shimane Prefecture, Japan. Gerontology 45: 44–48

Skoog I, Vanmechelen E, Andreasson LA et al. (1995) A population-based study of tau protein and ubiquitin in cerebrospinal fluid in 85-year-olds: relation to severity of dementia and cerebral atrophy, but not to the apolipoprotein ε4 allele. Neurodegeneration 4: 433–442

Skoog I, Hesse C, Fredman P et al. (1997) Apolipoprotein E in cerebrospinal fluid in 85-year-olds. Relation to dementia, apolipoprotein E polymorphism, cerebral atrophy, and white-matter lesions. Archives of Neurology 54: 267–272

Snowdon DA, Greiner LH, Mortimer JA et al. (1997) Brain infarction and the clinical expression of Alzheimer disease. The Nun Study. JAMA 277: 813–817

Sourander P and Walinder J (1977) Hereditary multi-infarct dementia. Acta Neuropathica 39: 247–254

Stevens DL, Hewlett RH, Brownell B. (1977) Chronic familial vascular encephalopathy. Lancet I: 1364–1365

Suter OC, Sunthorn T, Kraftsik R et al. (2002) Cerebral hypoperfusion generates cortical watershed microinfarcts in Alzheimer disease. Stroke 33: 1986–1992

Thal DR, Rub U, Orantes M et al. (2002) Phases of Abeta-deposition in the human brain and its relevance for the development of AD. Neurology 58: 1791–1700

Traykov L, Rigaud AS, Caputo L et al. (1999) Apolipoprotein E phenotypes in demented and cognitively impaired patients with and without cerebrovascular disease. European Journal of Neurology 6: 415–421

Vinters HV, Ellis WG, Zarow C et al. (2000) Neuropathologic substrates of ischemic vascular dementia. Journal of Neuropathology and Experimental Neurology 59: 931–945

Vonsattel JP, Myers RH, Hedley-Whyte ET et al. (1991) Cerebral amyloid angiopathy without and with cerebral hemorrhages: a comparative histological study. Annals of Neurology 30: 637–649

White L, Petrovitch H, Hardman J et al. (2002) Cerebrovascular pathology and dementia in autopsied Honolulu-Asia aging study participants. Annals of the New York Academy of Science 977: 9–23

Willis T. (1672) Two Discourses concerning The Soul of Brutes, Which is that of the Vital and Sensitive of Man. Oxford. [Two editions, quarto and octavo]. [English translation by Samuel Pordage, London, 1683]

Yanagawa S, Ito N, Arima K, Ikeda S. (2002) Cerebral autosomal recessive arteriopathy with subcortical infarcts and leukoencephalopathy. Neurology 58: 817–820

Zarow C, Zaias B, Lyness SA, Chui H. (1999) Cerebral amyloid angiopathy in Alzheimer's disease is associated with apolipoprotein α4 and cortical neuron loss. Alzheimer Disease and Associated Disorders 13: 1–8

Zhan SS, Beyreuther K, Schmitt HP. (1994) Synaptophysin immunoreactivity of the cortical neuropil in vascular dementia of Binswanger type compared with the dementia of the Alzheimer type and nondemented controls. Dementia 5: 79–87

Zhang H, Sourander P, Olsson Y. (1994) The microvascular changes in cases of hereditary multi-infarct disease of the brain. Acta Neuropathica 87: 317–324

46

Therapeutic strategies for vascular dementia

GUSTAVO ROMÁN

The few years elapsed since the publication of this chapter in the Second Edition of *Dementia* (2000) have seen the completion of a number of promising treatment trials in patients with vascular dementia (VaD). Moreover, successful enrolment for these studies demonstrated that by using strict criteria it is feasible to diagnose and identify patients with clinically unmixed VaD, and that the subjects recruited for these trials disclose clinical features and progression patterns that are clearly different from those observed in patient populations selected for clinical trials of Alzheimer disease (AD).

The therapeutic management of VaD is particularly challenging because of the multiple types of cerebrovascular injuries and circulatory events that may lead to vascular cognitive decline and eventual dementia. This multiplicity of pathogenetic mechanisms results in a variety of clinical presentations that hampered in the past the formulation of diagnostic criteria and the ascertainment of cases for controlled clinical trials. In addition, VaD is often complicated with neuropsychiatric symptoms, in particular depression, apathy, aggressiveness and other behavioural changes that require careful management.

In addition to the symptomatic therapeutic trials, a limited number of studies have also shown promise for the prevention of VaD, giving support to the concept that vigorous treatment of vascular risk factors in patients with cognitive decline short of dementia (the so-called vascular cognitive impairment – VCI) could spare the progression to dementia.

46.1 DEFINITIONS

46.1.1 Vascular cognitive disorder (VCD)

VCD is the global category of cognitive decline resulting from cerebrovascular disease (CVD), ranging from VCI to VaD (Román *et al.*, 2004).

46.1.2 Vascular cognitive impairment

VCI was initially coined as an umbrella term to include all forms of vascular cognitive decline (Bowler and Hachinski, 1995; Erkinjuntti and Gauthier, 2002; O'Brien *et al.*, 2003). However, by analogy to mild cognitive impairment (MCI), considered the earliest manifestation of AD (Petersen *et al.*, 1999), the definition of VCI is restricted here to vascular forms of cognitive impairment without dementia.

46.1.3 Vascular dementia

Román (2002b, 2003a) defined VaD as an aetiological category of dementia characterized by acquired intellectual impairment, severe enough to interfere with social and personal independence, resulting from ischaemic or haemorrhagic stroke, as well as from ischaemic hypoperfusive brain injuries, affecting brain regions important for memory, cognition and behaviour. The most common neuropathological lesions capable of producing VaD are hypoperfusive and ischaemic (occlusive) vascular brain injuries (Brun, 1994; Parnetti, 1999; Mikol and Vallat-Decouvelaere, 2000; Vinters *et al.*, 2000). These include:

- *Hypoperfusion dementia* (Román, 2004): global anoxia, selective vulnerability, border-zone infarcts, and periventricular incomplete white matter ischaemia;
- *ischaemic lesions* involving large vessels: strategic single strokes, multi-infarct dementia (MID); small vessel disease (cortical, subcortical and cortico-subcortical ischaemia), as well as venous occlusions.

46.2 RISK FACTORS FOR VASCULAR DEMENTIA

A number of case–control studies of post-stroke dementia have provided a useful quantification of risk factors for VaD (Tatemichi *et al.*, 1990; Pohjasvaara *et al.*, 1997; Barba *et al.*, 2000). In patients with ischaemic stroke, the most important risk factors for development of post-stroke VaD are older age, lower educational level, recurrent stroke, as well as presence of dysphagia, gait limitations and urinary impairment. The left-sided predominance of lesions in demented patients with large vessel stroke in the territories of the anterior and posterior cerebral arteries has been repeatedly demonstrated (Leys and Pasquier, 2000). Recently, Johnston and colleagues (2004) observed progressive decline in cognitive function among Cardiovascular Health Study participants with stenosis of the left internal carotid artery (ICA), but not in those with stenosis of the right ICA, in the absence of stroke. Possible explanations include the fact that the left hemisphere has larger cholinergic innervation than the right one does; and tests such as the Mini-Mental State Examination (MMSE) (Folstein *et al.*, 1975), and the CAMCOG, the cognitive portion of the CAMDEX (Cambridge Mental Disorders of the Elderly Examination) (Huppert *et al.*, 1995), rely heavily on language functions.

Other risk factors in patients with post-stroke VaD include current smoking, lower blood pressure, orthostatic hypotension, and larger periventricular white matter ischaemic lesions on brain computed tomography (CT) or magnetic resonance imaging (MRI) (Liu *et al.*, 1991; Gorelick *et al.*, 1992). Orthostatic hypotension is a strong predictor of periventricular white matter ischaemic lesions (Longstreth *et al.*, 1996). Hypoxic and ischaemic complications of acute stroke (e.g. seizures, cardiac arrhythmias, aspiration pneumonia, etc.) are independent risk factors for post-stroke dementia (Moroney *et al.*, 1996); these complications increase more than 4-fold the risk of developing post-stroke dementia (OR 4.3; 95 per cent CI 1.9–9.6, after adjustment for demographic factors, recurrent stroke, and baseline cognitive function). Post-stroke VaD is also a strong predictor of poor outcome (Desmond *et al.*, 1998; Barba *et al.*, 2000; Linden *et al.*, 2004). In Rochester (Minnesota), 10 per cent of 482 incident cases of dementia had onset or worsening of the dementia within 3 months of a stroke (Knopman *et al.*, 2003). Overall, patients with vascular dementia had worse mortality than matched subjects (relative risk [RR] 2.7), particularly among cases of post-stroke VaD (RR 4.5).

46.3 DIAGNOSTIC CRITERIA AND METHODOLOGY OF CLINICAL TRIALS IN VASCULAR DEMENTIA

46.3.1 Vascular cognitive impairment

There are currently no widely accepted diagnostic criteria for VCI. The Canadian Study on Health and Aging (2000) used the following criteria (Rockwood *et al.*, 2000; Ingles *et al.*, 2002) to classify subjects with VCI without dementia (VCIND):

- The subjects' cognitive impairment did not meet the DSM-IIIR criteria for dementia (American Psychiatric Association, 1987); these criteria require impairment of memory and other cognitive domain causing functional deficits.
- Cognitive impairment was judged to have a vascular cause as based on presence of signs of ischaemia/ infarction; e.g. sudden onset, stepwise progression, patchy cortical deficits on cognitive testing, other evidence of atherosclerosis, and a high Hachinski Ischaemic Score (HIS) (Hachinski *et al.*, 1975). Presence of vascular risk factors alone was insufficient for a VCIND diagnosis. Global functional impairment was defined as having difficulty in any two of the following domains:
  - performing household chores
  - managing money
  - feeding self
  - dressing and
  - incontinence.

Using these criteria in the Canadian cohort of 10 263 randomly selected persons aged ⩾65 years, a total of 149 were diagnosed with VCIND (Ingles *et al.*, 2002). Follow-up cognitive diagnoses were available for 102 individuals and after 5 years, 45 patients (44 per cent) developed dementia; the rates of institutionalization and mortality were equivalent to those of AD (Wentzel *et al.*, 2001, 2002). In this study, the progression to dementia was similar to that seen in MCI suggesting that, in all likelihood, the population identified by these criteria was actually a mixture of AD with CVD. Moreover, a number of patients improved their cognitive scores (Wentzel *et al.*, 2002) indicating that VCIND, in contrast with VCI, does not follow a unidirectional progression towards dementia. In summary, valid criteria for VCI are needed at present.

46.3.2 Vascular dementia

The existence of multiple diagnostic criteria for the diagnosis of VaD – and their lack of agreement on patient selection – has been the main argument brandished to deny the existence of VaD as an independent form of dementia, clinically and pathologically separate from AD. In fact, the criteria differ among themselves since they were designed for different purposes (hospital discharges, research studies, epidemiological surveys, etc.); in addition, they lack sensitivity (particularly when strict imaging criteria are mandatory) since it is virtually impossible to include all forms of VaD within a single set of criteria. Finally, given the importance of CVD in the clinical expression of dementia in patients with lesions of AD, the inclusion of mixed dementia (AD + CVD) is a common occurrence with most criteria.

Román *et al.* (2004) have recently proposed a definition of dementia of vascular origin as characterized by abnormal executive control function, severe enough to interfere with social or occupational functioning. This definition corrects the problem of definitions of dementia that require memory loss as the *sine qua non* for dementia diagnosis. Obligate memory loss in patients with VaD may result in over-sampling of subjects with AD worsened by stroke (AD + CVD).

Existing criteria include the Hachinski Ischaemic Score or HIS (Hachinski *et al.*, 1975); the criteria from the 4th revision of the American Psychiatric Association's *Diagnostic and Statistical Manual of Mental Disorders*, better known as DSM-IV (American Psychiatric Association, 1994); the 10th revision of the International Classification of Diseases or ICD-10 (World Health Organization, 1992); the California Criteria for Ischaemic VaD or ADDTC (Chui *et al.*, 1992), and the consensus criteria proposed by Román and colleagues (1993) or NINDS-AIREN criteria. Although all of them are useful in selecting VaD patients with varying degrees of sensitivity and specificity, they are not interchangeable (Verhey *et al.*, 1996; Wetterling *et al.*, 1996; Chui *et al.*, 2000; Pohjasvaara *et al.*, 2000).

The NINDS-AIREN criteria (Román *et al.*, 1993) were developed specifically for research studies in VaD and include a number of vascular aetiologies and clinical manifestations. These criteria have the highest specificity and have been used in most modern controlled clinical trials in VaD (López-Pousa *et al.*, 1997; Kittner, 1999; Erkinjuntti *et al.*, 2002a; Orgogozo *et al.*, 2002; Wilcock *et al.*, 2002; Black *et al.*, 2003; Wilkinson *et al.*, 2003). These criteria recognize patients with multiple forms of stroke and CVD (i.e. ischaemic, haemorrhagic, hypoperfusive) but establish strict requirements to classify patients appropriately. Two cardinal elements of the clinical syndrome of VaD must be identified, namely the cognitive syndrome of dementia and the definition of the vascular cause of the dementia. Cerebrovascular disease is defined by the presence of focal neurological signs and detailed brain imaging showing evidence of stroke or ischaemic changes in the brain. A defining element of the criteria is the need for a temporal relationship between dementia and the cerebrovascular disorder whereby dementia onset should occur within 3 months following a recognized stroke. The temporal relationship may prove to be difficult to fulfil, particularly in patients with silent strokes and in the subcortical form of VaD. These elements are summarized in Box 46.1.

46.3.3 Mixed dementia (AD + CVD)

Specific brain pathological lesions define the two most common forms of senile dementia, AD and VaD. Stroke and cerebrovascular disease are the hallmarks of VaD, while senile plaques and neurofibrillary tangles typify AD. When these two pathologies are combined, the neuropathological diagnosis of AD + CVD or 'mixed dementia' is invoked (Zekry *et al.*, 2002a). Coexistent lesions occur in up to one-third of unselected elderly demented patients (Kalaria and Ballard, 1999; Zekry *et al.*, 2002b, c), or in 10–15 per cent of cases of post-stroke dementia (Hénon *et al.*, 1997, 2001; Barba *et al.*, 2001), but mixed lesions also occur in patients without dementia (Román and Royall, 2004).

Separating AD from VaD may be a frequent problem in patients with pre-existing and progressive memory loss worsened by an acute vascular episode. The NINDS-AIREN criteria (Román *et al.*, 1993) accurately separate VaD from AD or from AD associated to cerebrovascular lesions (AD + CVD) as demonstrated in validation neuropathological studies comparing various sets of diagnostic criteria. The NINDS-AIREN criteria (Román *et al.*, 1993) consistently obtained the highest specificity values, ranging from 0.80 (Gold *et al.*, 1997), 0.86 (Zekry *et al.*, 2002b), 0.93 (Gold *et al.*, 2002) to 0.95 (Holmes *et al.*, 1999). Specificity defines the capacity to identify true negative cases. Therefore, with neuropathology as the gold standard, several studies confirmed that the NINDS-AIREN criteria (Román *et al.*, 1993) successfully exclude AD cases, and have the lowest proportion of mixed cases misclassified. The NINDS-AIREN criteria for VaD (Román *et al.*, 1993) have slightly better specificity than the NINCDS-ADRDA criteria for AD (McKhann *et al.*, 1984; Holmes *et al.*, 1999).

The accuracy of the NINDS-AIREN criteria increases by excluding subjects with pre-existing diagnosis of AD, those with isolated memory impairment (MCI), as well as those with history of obvious progressive cognitive decline prior to a stroke (Hénon *et al.*, 1997, 2001). VaD dementia typically occurs in patients with stroke and multiple vascular risk factors. The HIS quantifies this profile with high interrater reliability (kappa = 0.61). A score >4 in the HIS usually excludes AD.

Using the NINDS-AIREN criteria (Román *et al.*, 1993) along the guidelines described above, two international trials of donepezil in VaD (Black *et al.*, 2003; Wilkinson *et al.*, 2003) were able to recruit more than 1200 patients with relatively pure or unmixed VaD. The VaD population selected was older and had a male preponderance, in agreement with population-based epidemiological data on VaD and in contrast with the female preponderance in AD trials. Furthermore, the 6-month progression of the placebo groups selected in the donepezil VaD studies was different from placebo groups in AD (Román and Rogers, 2004) as well as in mixed AD plus CVD trials (Erkinjuntti *et al.*, 2002a), further indicating the separate identity of the VaD cases selected (Pratt, 2002).

In summary, VaD is a well-defined form of dementia that can be clinically diagnosed with reasonable accuracy. Of all available criteria, the NINDS-AIREN criteria (Román *et al.*,

---

Box 46.1 *NINDS-AIREN diagnostic criteria for vascular dementia**

I. The criteria for the diagnosis of *probable* VaD include *all* of the following:

  1 **Dementia**: Impairment of memory and two or more cognitive domains (including executive function), interfering with ADL and not due to physical effects of stroke alone.

  Exclusion criteria: Alterations of consciousness, delirium, psychoses, severe aphasia or deficits precluding testing, systemic disorders, Alzheimer's disease or other forms of dementia.

  2 **Cerebrovascular disease**: Focal signs on neurological examination (hemiparesis, lower facial weakness, Babinski sign, sensory deficit, hemianopsia, dysarthria) consistent with stroke (with or without history of stroke, *and* evidence of relevant CVD by brain CT or MRI including *multiple large vessel infarcts* or a *single strategically placed infarct* (angular gyrus, thalamus, basal forebrain, or PCA or ACA territories), as well as *multiple basal ganglia* and *white matter lacunes* or *extensive periventricular white matter lesions,* or combinations thereof.

  Exclusion criteria: Absence of cerebrovascular lesions on CT or MRI.

  3 **A Relationship between the above two disorders**: Manifested or inferred by the presence of one or more of the following:

    a. onset of dementia within 3 months following a recognized stroke

    b. abrupt deterioration in cognitive functions; or fluctuating, stepwise progression of cognitive deficits.

II. Clinical features *consistent* with the diagnosis of *probable* VaD include the following:

    a. early presence of gait disturbances (small step gait or *marche à petits pas*, or magnetic, apraxic-ataxic or parkinsonian gait)

    b. history of unsteadiness and frequent, unprovoked falls

    c. early urinary frequency, urgency, and other urinary symptoms not explained by urological disease

    d. pseudobulbar palsy

    e. personality and mood changes, abulia, depression, emotional incontinence, or other deficits including psychomotor retardation and abnormal executive function.

III. Features that make the diagnosis of VaD uncertain or unlikely include:

    a. Early onset of memory deficit and progressive worsening of memory and other cognitive functions such as language (transcortical sensory aphasia), motor skills (apraxia), and perception (agnosia), in the absence of corresponding focal lesions on brain imaging

    b. Absence of focal neurological signs, other than cognitive disturbances

    c. Absence of CVD on CT or MRI.

ACA, anterior cerebral artery; ADL, activities of daily living; CT, computed tomography; CVD, cerebrovascular disease; MRI, magnetic resonance imaging; PCA, posterior cerebral artery; VaD, vascular dementia.
*Adapted from Román *et al.* (1993)

1993) have the highest specificity in neuropathology-confirmed cases, effectively ruling out cases of mixed dementia. The population thus selected is different from that of AD and mixed dementia trials. Several controlled clinical trials on VaD have successfully used the NINDS-AIREN criteria, effectively making these criteria the most suitable current choice for VaD studies. In addition, careful interview of relatives and caregivers allows a successful diagnosis of prestroke dementia. In most instances, probable AD is a likely aetiology for the progressive memory loss or MCI occurring prior to the ictus (Jagust, 2001).

46.3.4 Methodological aspects of clinical trials in VaD

The methodological requirements for controlled clinical trials in patients with dementia have been reviewed by the International Working Group on Harmonization of Dementia Drug Guidelines at the Sixth International Congress on AD and Related Disorders in Amsterdam (Whitehouse *et al.*, 1998),

and at the 1998 Osaka Conference on VaD (Erkinjuntti and Sawada, 1999; Erkinjuntti *et al.*, 1999); for more recent reviews see Mills and Chow (2003), Mani (2004), and Erkinjuntti *et al.* (2004). The first and foremost requirement for a valid trial in dementia, and VaD in particular, is the use of appropriate inclusion and exclusion criteria. This requirement is crucial for the selection of a homogeneous population that would allow the generalized application of the trial results. Given the clinical variety of VaD, some authors have suggested limiting the trials to patients with subcortical VaD using various sets of criteria (Pantoni *et al.*, 1996, 2000; Erkinjuntti *et al.*, 2000; Moretti *et al.*, 2001, 2002), or to cases of mixed dementia, including AD + CVD (Erkinjuntti *et al.*, 2002a, b) or AD plus arterial hypertension (Kumar *et al.*, 2000). However, as discussed above, the criteria proposed by Román *et al.* (1993) are appropriate for VaD trials. Several instruments (MMSE, CAMCOG, Clinical Dementia Rating [CDR]) are used to ensure that dementia severity is comparable across the trial.

The next requirement is an appropriate number of participants (sample size). The sample size is a function not only of the effectiveness of the drug, but also of the degree of responsiveness – or lack thereof – of the measuring instruments, as well as of the accuracy of the end points selected for the trial. Instruments that are relatively insensitive to change, require larger sample sizes in order to demonstrate a statistically significant difference from the placebo or untreated group.

Other requirements include randomization with appropriate group allocation concealment, placebo-controlled, double-blinded design with parallel group, and specific outcome measures, adequate instruments, and well-defined end points. Potential targets for the symptomatic treatment of VaD include:

- symptomatic improvement of the core symptoms (cognition, function and behaviour);
- slowing of progression; and
- treatment of neuropsychiatric symptoms (e.g. depression, anxiety, agitation).

All the current VaD trials have used the same primary outcome measures used in AD trials, as recommended by the United States Food and Drug Administration (FDA). These instruments include the cognitive portion of the Alzheimer's Disease Assessment Scale (ADAS-cog) (Rosen et al., 1984), the Clinician's Interview-Based Impression of change plus caregiver input (CIBIC-plus) (Schneider et al., 1997), or the Clinical Global Impression of Change (CGIC) (Berg, 1988). The European Commission for Medicinal and Pharmaceutical Compounds (CPMC) also requires positive impact on activities of daily living (ADL), using a scale similar to the Alzheimer's Disease Functional Assessment and Change Scale (ADFACS) that provides a measure of instrumental and basic ADL (Mohs et al., 2001). The CPMC also requires a responder analysis; another useful measure is the Disability Assessment for Dementia scale (Gélinas et al., 1999). To the extent that ADAS-cog and CIBIC-plus assess the multiple cognitive domains affected in all forms of dementia, including VaD, it is not unreasonable to use the same measures in both AD and VaD patient populations. However, Quinn and colleagues (2000) showed difficulties with CIBIC-plus ratings in instances of clinical improvement. Physicians fail to recognize successful disease treatment beyond reversal of progression.

Furthermore, current tests are relatively insensitive to frontal/subcortical dysfunction, a key cognitive domain in VaD (Román and Royall, 1999; Pohjasvaara et al., 2002). Future clinical trials should incorporate tests such as the vascular equivalent of the ADAS-cog, the VaDAS-cog (Ferris and Gauthier, 2002), as well as others tests that include formal measurement of executive function. Of interest, ADL are considered a proxy evaluation of executive function. Pohjasvaara et al. (2002) confirmed that executive dysfunction was the main determinant of abnormalities in both basic ADL and instrumental ADLs (IADLs) in patients with post-stroke VaD. Executive function tests, including IADLs, may be sensitive tools for the diagnosis of VaD and could accurately measure the effects of potential therapies.

46.4 CLINICAL FORMS OF VASCULAR DEMENTIA

Despite the anatomical and pathophysiological complexity of VaD, Román (1999a, 2002b) has simplified the clinical forms into two groups, acute and subacute, according to the temporal profile of presentation.

46.4.1 Acute forms of VaD

Acute VaD is defined by new onset of dementia after a demonstrated stroke, either a single 'strategic stroke' resulting from occlusion (or rupture) of a large-size vessel, after a symptomatic lacunar stroke caused by ischaemic small vessel disease, or from recurrent strokes (MID). VaD can result from a single stroke located in one of the following three possible areas (Delay and Brion, 1962):

- posterior cerebral artery (PCA) territory, involving ventral-medial temporal lobe, hippocampus, occipital structures and thalamus;
- anterior cerebral artery (ACA) territory and medial frontal lobe lesions, often from an anterior communicating artery aneurysm rupture; and
- basal ganglia and thalamus, usually from small vessel disease; this is the so-called 'thalamic dementia of vascular origin' caused by butterfly-shaped bilateral paramedian thalamic polar infarcts. Some cases of caudate stroke may also result in VaD.

Numerous reports have confirmed the occurrence of true 'lacunar dementia', i.e. acute VaD resulting from a single lacunar stroke involving the inferior genu of the internal capsule and causing ipsilateral blood flow reduction to the inferomedial frontal cortex by a mechanism of diaschisis (Tatemichi et al., 1992, 1995; Chukwudelunzu et al., 2001). This thalamocortical disconnection syndrome is manifested by sudden change in cognitive function, often associated with fluctuating attention, memory loss, confusion, abulia, striking psychomotor retardation, inattention, and other features of frontal lobe dysfunction but with mild focal findings such as hemiparesis or dysarthria.

46.4.2 Subacute-subcortical forms of VaD

Subacute VaD is defined clinically by insidious onset of subcortical dementia with frontal lobe deficits, depressive mood changes – the so-called 'vascular depression' (Alexopoulos et al., 2002), along with psychomotor slowing, parkinsonian features, urinary disturbances and pseudobulbar palsy, usually resulting from small vessel disease (Román et al., 2002f). Symptoms are due to interruption by ischaemic lesions of prefrontal-subcortical circuits for executive control of working memory, organization, language, mood, regulation of attention, constructional skills, motivation, and socially responsive behaviours (Cummings, 1993). Prefrontal-subcortical loops may be severed by lacunes in the striatum, globus pallidus or thalamus, or by white matter lesions that disconnect prefrontal or anterior cingulate cortexes from their basal ganglia or thalamocortical connections (Swartz et al., 2003; Vataja et al., 2003).

Loss of executive function is a major component of VaD (Román and Royall, 1999), leading to cognitive disability and clinically significant loss of planning capacity, working memory, attention, concentration, discrimination, abstraction, conceptual flexibility, and self-control (Román and Royall, 1999; Vataja et al., 2003). Some patients are unable to initiate the required behaviour, others fail to inhibit irrelevant behaviours, and most can perform individual steps of a complex problem but are unable to provide a correct strategy to solve it. These symptoms often lead to post-stroke depression and functional disability (Pohjasvaara et al., 1998, 2002).

The main clinical forms of subacute VaD are Binswanger's disease (état lacunaire), cerebral autosomal dominant arteriopathy with subcortical infarcts and leukoencephalopathy (CADASIL), and rare instances of cerebral amyloid angiopathy, including those that present with leukoencephalopathy (Gray et al., 1985; Sarazin et al., 2002). The temporal profile of presentation of these conditions is typically subacute, with a chronic course marked by fluctuations and progressive worsening.

46.4.2.1   BINSWANGER'S DISEASE

Binswanger's disease is characterized by the presence of ischaemic periventricular leukoencephalopathy typically sparing the arcuate subcortical U-fibres (Román, 1987). Brain imaging (CT and MRI) usually correlates well with the pathological features that include diffuse myelin pallor, loss of oligodendrocytes and astrocytic gliosis. Under the microscope, there is loss of myelin and axons resulting in rarefaction, spongiosis and vacuolization without definite necrosis (incomplete white matter infarction); in addition, lesions of arteriolosclerosis and other hypertensive lesions (Lammie, 2002), and état criblé or widening of perivascular spaces are present. Advanced white matter lesions include focal necrosis and cavitations (lacunes); there are also lacunar infarcts in the basal ganglia and the pons. Román (1985a) suggested the identity of Binswanger's disease and a remarkably similar clinical condition, état lacunaire (Marie, 1901), characterized by multiple lacunes, ventricular dilatation and lesions of the white matter with a moth-eaten appearance. The syndrome included mild residual hemiparesis, a peculiar gait with short steps (marche à petits pas), dysarthria, pseudobulbar palsy, and extrapyramidal features such as inexpressive facies, slowness of movement, axial rigidity, loss of postural reflexes and frequent falls.

Dementia is not a salient feature of état lacunaire (Marie, 1901), but some intellectual deficit is constantly present. However, Fisher (1965) remarked that lacunar strokes typically do not cause disturbances in higher cerebral functions, and when present 'always exclude a lacunar diagnosis'. Among 114 patients with lacunes he examined at necropsy, dementia

was uncommon or mild. Population-based studies of elderly subjects indicate that in the vast majority of cases, lacunes are silent (Longstreth et al., 1998); however, silent lacunes particularly in the thalamus more than double the risk of dementia (hazard ratio 2.26; 95 per cent CI 1.09–4.70) (Vermeer et al., 2003). Hospital-based series of lacunar infarctions show that about 30 per cent of these patients develop dementia (Babikian et al., 1990; Tatemichi et al., 1993). In a clinico-pathological review of 100 consecutive autopsies of patients with lacunar strokes at the Hôpital de la Salpêtrière (Román, 1985b), 72 cases with multiple lacunes were found, but only 36 per cent were clinically demented (état lacunaire). In six cases, Alzheimer disease and lacunes coexisted and six had Binswanger's disease (Mikol, 1968). In the demented patients, dilatation of the lateral ventricles was the only morphological feature that separated état lacunaire patients from cases with multiple lacunes but without dementia, suggesting that either white matter disease or normal pressure hydrocephalus could have contributed to the dementia.

Neuropathological data indicates that up to 60 per cent of patients with AD have Binswanger-type white matter lesions (Brun and Englund, 1986; Englund et al., 1988). These lesions have been postulated as being caused by cerebral hypoperfusion resulting from cardiac disease or orthostatic hypotension; this form could be called AD type B (with Binswanger-type lesions), in contrast with AD type A, with exclusive cortical involvement. Moreover, Snowdon and colleagues (1997) in the Nun Study reported that in very old subjects lacunes are an important factor in the clinical expression of AD. Likewise, according to Jellinger and Mitter-Ferstl (2003) the presence of cerebrovascular pathology in patients with AD is significantly higher at autopsy than in controls (48 versus 7.4 per cent). Zekry and co-workers (2002b, c) demonstrated at postmortem examination the synergistic effect of vascular lesions in patients with dementia of AD. The presence of vascular lesions had a direct correlation with the severity of the dementia. Furthermore, the density of AD lesions (neuritic plaques, focal amyloid β deposits, and neurofibrillary tangles) was significantly lower when vascular lesions were present.

46.4.2.2   CADASIL

CADASIL was described in France in the early 1990s (Bousser and Tournier-Lasserve, 1994); it was originally called 'familial Binswanger' (van Bogaert, 1955) and 'hereditary multi-infarct dementia' (Sourander and Walinder, 1977; Sonninen and Savontaus, 1987). Currently, CADASIL appears to be the most common genetic form of VaD. Recently, Chabriat and Bousser (2003), Dichgans (2002) and Kalimo et al. (2002) have provided excellent reviews. This autosomal dominant disorder of cerebral small vessels maps to chromosome 19 and is caused by Notch3 gene mutations. The underlying vascular lesion is a unique non-amyloid non-atherosclerotic microangiopathy involving arterioles (100–400 μm in diameter) and capillaries, primarily in the brain but also in other organs. The diagnosis may be established by skin biopsy with confirmation by immunostaining with a Notch3 monoclonal antibody. CADASIL offers a natural model for the study of subcortical-subacute forms of VaD, in particular Binswanger's disease. Numerous pedigrees have been described in Europe and North America. Clinical manifestations include transient ischaemic attacks (TIAs) and strokes (80 per cent), cognitive deficits and VaD (50 per cent), migraine with focal deficits (40 per cent), mood disorders (30 per cent) and epilepsy (10 per cent). Onset is usually in early adulthood (mean age: 46 years) in the absence of risk factors for vascular disease, culminating in dementia and death usually about 20 years after onset of symptoms. The dementia is slow in onset, subcortical, frontal in type, accompanied by gait and urinary disturbances, and pseudobulbar palsy clinically identical to that of sporadic Binswanger's disease. MRI reveals a combination of small lacunar lesions and diffuse white matter abnormalities, including, typically, lesions of the corpus callosum; MRI lesions are often present in asymptomatic relatives. Also, cerebral blood flow (CBF) reactivity to inhaled carbon dioxide is impaired. Widespread smooth-muscle cell loss results in decreased regional CBF; these values correlate inversely with cognitive performance. The disease is caused by highly stereotyped mutations in the Notch3 gene that encodes a phyllogenetically old transmembrane cell-surface receptor that regulates cell fate during embryonic development. The large extracellular domain of Notch3 contains 34 tandem epidermal growth factor (EGF)-like repeats where the mutations result in gain or loss of a cysteine residue.

46.4.2.3 CEREBRAL AMYLOID ANGIOPATHY

Cerebral amyloid angiopathy or CAA is a heterogeneous group of disorders characterized by deposition of amyloid in the walls of leptomeningeal and cerebral cortical blood vessels, manifested clinically by recurrent or multiple lobar haemorrhages, cognitive deterioration, and ischaemic strokes. Cerebral MRI displays diffuse white matter abnormalities along with ischaemic or haemorrhagic focal brain lesions. On histology, the vessels show amyloid deposition, micro-aneurysms and fibrinoid necrosis.

There are several autosomal dominant forms of CAA with differences in their clinical, genetic, biochemical and pathologic findings. $A\beta$, the major amyloid component in the Dutch, Flemish, and Iowa-type of familial CAA, is also the major amyloid component in sporadic CAA and in AD. Familial British dementia (FBD) with amyloid angiopathy is an autosomal dominant condition characterized by VaD, progressive spastic paraparesis and cerebellar ataxia with onset in the sixth decade (Mead et al., 2000). A point mutation in the BRI gene has been shown to be the genetic abnormality. On brain MRI, Binswanger-type deep white matter hyperintensities and lacunar infarcts are seen, but without intracerebral haemorrhages. The corpus callosum is severely affected and atrophic. Plaques and tangles are present but the amyloid subunit (ABri) found in FBD brains is entirely different and unrelated to other amyloid proteins. FBD combines neurodegeneration and dementia with systemic amyloid deposition.

46.5 PHARMACOLOGICAL THERAPY OF VASCULAR DEMENTIA

A review of the history of VaD (Román, 2002c, d) suggests that the prevailing concepts of pathogenesis at a given time influence not only the elaboration of clinical criteria, but also the approach to therapy. Until the 1970s, VaD was believed to be caused by progressive strangulation of blood flow to the brain resulting in chronic cerebral hypoperfusion. Therefore, beginning with nicotinic acid, a number of vasodilating agents were recommended for years for the treatment of non-specific senile symptoms, cognitive decline and dementia. Following the same logic, Walsh (Walsh, 1968; Walsh et al., 1978) claimed significant improvement of symptoms of presenile and senile dementia with a combination of warfarin anticoagulation and psychotherapy. A vascular pathogenesis also underlay the use of antithrombotics, ergot alkaloids, nootropics, thyrotropin-releasing hormone (TRH)-analogue, Ginkgo biloba extract, plasma viscosity drugs, hyperbaric oxygen, antioxidants, serotonin and histamine receptor antagonists, vasoactive agents, xanthine derivatives and calcium antagonists (Román, 2000). With increasing recognition of AD and new knowledge of neurotransmitters, neuronal metabolism and biochemical tissue reactions to ischaemia–hypoxia and oxidative stress, more specific medications were developed leading to the current of neuroprotection (Mondadori, 1993). The most recent advance in the treatment of VaD has been the development of medications to enhance specific neurotransmitters, such as acetylcholine. Furthermore, these products have been studied following closely the standard recommendations for controlled clinical trials. The cholinesterase inhibitors will be discussed first, followed by the NMDA-receptor antagonist of glutamatergic neurotransmission, memantine, the calcium channel blockers, the nootropic agents, the xanthines, the ergot derivatives, the vasodilators, and then other various treatments for VaD.

46.5.1 Cholinergic dysfunction in VaD

Cholinergic dysfunction is well documented in VaD, independently of any concomitant AD pathology; these deficits consist of decreased levels of acetylcholine (ACh) in the cerebrospinal fluid (CSF), and reduced cholinergic markers such as choline acetyltransferase (ChAT) in the brain (Szilagyi et al., 1987; Wallin et al., 1989; Wallin and Gottfries, 1990; Gottfries et al., 1994; Tohgi et al., 1996). Hippocampal ChAT deficits of up to 60 per cent have been reported in the brains of both AD and VaD patients (Perry et al., 1977; Sakurada et al., 1990; Kalaria et al. 2001). The cholinergic basal forebrain nuclei are irrigated by penetrating arterioles and are therefore susceptible to the effects of arterial hypertension. Moreover, ischaemic lesions in the white matter and the basal ganglia can interrupt the cholinergi projections (Swartz et al., 2003). Selden and co-workers (1998) described in the human brain two highly organized and discrete bundles of cholinergic fibres extending from the nucleus basalis of Meynert (nbM) to the cerebral cortex and amygdala. Mesulam *et al.* (2003) demonstrated cholinergic denervation from ischaemic pathway lesions in CADASIL, a pure genetic form of VaD, entirely unmixed with AD lesions.

Cholinergic mechanisms play a role in the modulation of regional CBF (Sato *et al.*, 2001). Stimulation of the nbM results in increased blood flow in the cerebral cortex (Biesold *et al.*, 1989). This cholinergic vasodilatory system relies upon activation of both muscarinic and nicotinic cholinergic receptors and the response declines with age (Lacombe *et al.*, 1997; Uchida *et al.*, 2000). Therefore, there is loss of cholinergic function in patients with VaD, and this is associated with reductions in CBF (Court *et al.*, 2002).

The above observations provide reasonable arguments to justify the use of cholinesterase inhibitors in VaD (Román, 2005), both unmixed with AD, as well as in patients with AD + CVD. Three of the acetylcholinesterase inhibitors (AChEIs) approved for use in AD – donepezil, galantamine and rivastigmine – have also been studied in VaD and will be reviewed below.

46.5.1.1 DONEPEZIL

Donepezil hydrochloride (E2020, Aricept) is a piperidine-based, reversible, non-competitive AChEI with highly selective central action, approved for treatment of mild to moderate AD (Román and Rogers, 2004). Donepezil is unrelated to other cholinesterase inhibitors, and has greater selectivity for cerebral AChE than for butyrylcholinesterse (BuChE). It reaches peak plasma concentrations 3–4 hours after oral administration. Oral absorption is excellent and is unaffected by food or by time of administration; a single bedtime dose is recommended because of its long half-life. Therapeutic levels are obtained with a dose of 5 mg/day, reaching steady state plasma levels after 15 days. Donepezil is 96 per cent bound to plasma proteins (75 per cent to albumin and 21 per cent to $\alpha 1$ acid glycoprotein). Donepezil is metabolized primarily by the cytochrome P450 system (CYP 450 isoenzymes 2D6 and 3A4) with extensive first-pass metabolism; it also undergoes glucuronidation (Román and Rogers, 2004).

The safety and efficacy of donepezil has been studied in the largest clinical trial of pure VaD to date (Goldsmith and Scott, 2003). A total of 1219 subjects were recruited for a 24-week, randomized, placebo-controlled, multicentre, multinational study divided in two identical trials, 307 (Black *et al.*, 2003) and 308 (Wilkinson *et al.*, 2003). The patients were randomized to one of three groups: placebo, donepezil at a dosage of 5 mg/day or donepezil, 10 mg/day. The group receiving 10 mg/day initially received 5 mg/day for four weeks; the dosage was then titrated up to 10 mg/day. Most patients (73 per cent) fulfilled diagnosis of probable VaD according to the NINDS-AIREN criteria (Román *et al.*, 1993). All had brain imaging prior to enrolment (CT or MRI) with demonstration of cerebrovascular lesions. Patients with pre-existing AD and those with 'mixed dementia,' (AD + CVD) were excluded.

Exclusion criteria also included other neurodegenerative or psychiatric disorders such as schizophrenia or major depression, a MMSE (Folstein *et al.*, 1975) score >26 or <10, the occurrence of new strokes within the 28 days prior to baseline, or myocardial infarction within 3 months of enrolment. These two VaD studies enrolled more men than women (58 versus 38 per cent) and their mean age was older than in AD (74.5 ± 0.2 versus 72 ± 0.2 years). The more severe vascular pathology of VaD was reflected in the high HIS score (6.6 ± 0.2 versus <4 in AD); most subjects had hypertension, hypercholesterolaemia, cardiovascular disease, diabetes, smoking, previous stroke and TIAs.

There were three main end points:

- cognition, measured with the ADAS-cog (Rosen *et al.*, 1984) and the MMSE (Folstein *et al.*, 1975);
- global function, evaluated with the CIBIC-plus (Schneider *et al.*, 1997) and with the Sum of Boxes of the Clinical Dementia Rating (CDR-SB) scale (Berg, 1988); and
- ADL, measured with the Alzheimer's Disease Functional Assessment and Change Scale (ADFACS) (Mohs *et al.*, 2001).

In study 307 (Black *et al.*, 2003), both donepezil treatment group showed statistically significant cognitive improvement measured with the MMSE and the ADAS-cog; the mean changes from baseline ADAS-cog scores were: donepezil 5 mg/day, −1.90 ($P = 0.001$); donepezil 10 mg/day, −2.33 ($P < 0.001$). The donepezil 5 mg/day group also showed significant improvement in global function on the CIBIC-plus but this did not reach significance in the 10 mg/day group ($P = 0.27$). The CDR-SB showed non-significant benefit in the 5 mg/day group and statistical significance in the 10 mg/day group ($P = 0.022$). Compared with placebo, there was significant benefit in ADL ($P < 0.05$) in both donepezil groups using the ADFACS.

Similar results were observed in study 308 (Wilkinson *et al.*, 2003); donepezil treatment resulted in significant improvement in cognition measured with the MMSE and the ADAS-cog. For the latter, the mean changes from baseline score were: donepezil 5 mg/day, −1.65 ($P = 0.003$); donepezil 10 mg/day, −2.09 ($P = 0.0002$). Global function on the CIBIC-plus was significantly better in the 5 mg/day group ($P = 0.004$), and was barely below signficance in the 10 mg/day group ($P = 0.047$). The CDR-SB showed benefits with 5 mg/day (non-significant), and it reached significance with 10 mg/day ($P = 0.03$). The ADL were improved in patients treated with donepezil when compared with placebo using the ADFACS, but did not reach significance at the end of the study. Comparison of cortical versus subcortical forms of VaD showed no differences in the overall results of the trial (Salloway *et al.*, 2003).

In comparison with AD patients, cognitive decline in untreated patients with VaD during 24 weeks of study in these trials was less severe, using similar instruments. These differences were also noted for global effects, measured by the CIBIC-plus version. Substantial decline of instrumental ADL was noted in untreated VaD patients. A combined analysis of the total population confirmed the effects on cognition and global function. Of interest, donepezil-treated patients demonstrated statistically significant improvements in instrumental IADLs compared with decline in the placebo group (least squares [LS] mean change from baseline at end point: placebo, 0.60; 5 mg/day -0.09, $P < 0.05$; 10 mg/day -0.18, $P < 0.01$). These results suggest that donepezil treatment may improve or maintain the patients' abilities to perform ADL. Executive dysfunction is a major component of disability in patients with VaD and the beneficial effect of donepezil on IADLs may be related to improvement or stabilization of executive function.

Donepezil was generally well tolerated, although more adverse effects were reported in the 10 mg/day group than in the 5 mg/day or placebo groups. The adverse effects were assessed as mild to moderate and transient, and were typically diarrhoea, nausea, arthralgia, leg cramps, anorexia and headache. The incidence of bradycardia and syncope was not significantly different from the placebo group. The discontinuation rates for the groups were 15 per cent for placebo, 18 per cent for 5 mg, and 28 per cent for the 10 mg group. There was no significant interaction with cardiovascular medications or antithrombotic agents. These two large trials offer evidence that donepezil is effective and well tolerated in patients with VaD (Malouf and Birks, 2004).

46.5.1.2 GALANTAMINE

Galantamine (galanthamine, Remynil, Proneurax, Prometax) is a tertiary alkaloid currently approved for the treatment of mild to moderate AD. Galantamine is a reversible specific inhibitor of AChE, and in addition it modulates central nicotinic receptors to increase cholinergic neurotransmission. Galantamine was initially isolated from the bulbs of the snowdrop plant, *Galanthus woronowii*, and from several Amaryllidaceae plants; commercially, galantamine is extracted from *Leucojum aestivum*, the common snowflake (Harvey, 1995; Pearson, 2001). Galantamine has high bioavailability from the oral route; maximum plasma levels are obtained about 1–2 hours after oral administration, with 18 per cent protein binding. Galantamine is metabolized by the CYP2D6 system into three inactive metabolites, O-demethyl-galantamine, N-demethyl-galantamine, and epi-galantamine; elimination half-life is 5–7 hours. Cytochrome CYP2D6 inhibitors will increase the serum concentration of galantamine. The starting daily dose of galantamine is 8 mg/day (4 mg twice daily), but therapeutic levels are reached with 8 mg/day and doses up to 24–32 mg/day are used in AD. The safety and efficacy of galantamine in AD has been studied in randomized, controlled trials recruiting more than 2600 patients. Improvement or stabilization of cognition, function, behaviour and caregiver burden were demonstrated over 6 months; a few 12-month trials confirmed slowing of decline or maintained baseline performance (Corey-Bloom, 2003; Raskind, 2003; Dengiz and

Kershaw, 2004). Galantamine is safe and well tolerated when the dosage is escalated gradually. Galantamine HBr is available in 4 mg, 8 mg and 12 mg tablets.

Galantamine has been studied in VaD in a large phase III, randomized, multicentre, double-blind, placebo-controlled clinical trial in patients with probable VaD, or with AD combined with CVD (Erkinjuntti *et al.*, 2002a). Patients received galantamine 24 mg/day (n = 396) or placebo (n = 196) for 6 months; the age of the patients ranged from 40 to 90 years. Eligible subjects met either the clinical criteria of probable VaD by NINDS-AIREN criteria (Román *et al.*, 1993), or of possible AD according to the NINCDS-ADRDA criteria (McKhann *et al.*, 1984). Radiological evidence of CVD on brain CT or MR was required (i.e. AD + CVD), including multiple large-vessel infarcts or a single, strategically placed infarct (angular gyrus, thalamus, basal forebrain, territory of the posterior or anterior cerebral artery), or at least two basal ganglia and white matter lacunes, or white matter changes involving at least 25 per cent of the total white matter. Mild to moderate dementia was defined by a score of $\geqslant 12$ in the ADAS-cog/11 (Rosen *et al.*, 1984) and 10–25 on the MMSE (Folstein *et al.*, 1975).

Primary end points were cognition, as measured using the ADAS-cog/11 (Rosen *et al.*, 1984), and global functioning as measured using the CIBIC-plus (Schneider *et al.*, 1997). Secondary end points included assessments of activities of daily living, using the Disability Assessment in Dementia (DAD) (Gélinas *et al.*, 1999), and behavioural symptoms, using the Neuropsychiatric Inventory (NPI) (Cummings *et al.*, 1994). Galantamine demonstrated greater efficacy than placebo on all outcome measures in analyses of both groups of patients as a whole: ADAS-cog (2.7 points, $P \leqslant 0.001$), on the CIBIC-plus (74 versus 59 per cent of patients remained stable or improved, $P \leqslant 0.001$). ADL and behavioural symptoms in the NPI were also significantly improved compared with placebo (both $P < 0.05$). Galantamine was safe and well tolerated; however, nausea was reported six times as often by VaD patients on galantamine than those on placebo. In comparison nausea was twice as common in patients with AD treated with galantamine compared with placebo-treated patients (Erkinjuntti *et al.*, 2002a), suggesting lesser tolerability in patients with VaD.

In an open label extension (Erkinjuntti *et al.*, 2003a), the original galantamine group of patients with probable VaD or AD + CVD showed similar sustained benefits in terms of maintenance of or improvement in cognition (ADS-cog), functional ability (DAD), and behaviour (NPI) after 12 months. Although not designed to detect differences between subgroups, the subgroup of patients with AD + CVD on galantamine (n = 188, 48 per cent) showed greater efficacy than placebo (n = 97, 50 per cent) at 6 months on the ADAS-cog ($P \leqslant 0.001$) and the CIBIC-plus ($P = 0.019$) (Erkinjuntti *et al.*, 2002a). In the open-label extension, patients with AD + CVD on galantamine maintained cognition at baseline for 12 months (Erkinjuntti *et al.*, 2003a). The subgroup of patients with probable VaD, compared those on placebo (n = 81, 41 per cent) with 171 subjects (43 per cent) on galantamine. In the subgroup of patients with VaD treated with galantamine for 6 months, the ADAS-cog scores improved significantly (mean change from baseline, 2.4 points, $P < 0.0001$), compared with no response in placebo group (mean change from baseline, 0.4; treatment difference versus galantamine 1.9, $P = 0.06$) (Erkinjuntti et al., 2003a). More patients treated with galantamine than with placebo maintained or improved global function (CIBIC-plus, 31 per cent versus 23 per cent; not statistically significant). In these patients, the cognitive benefits of galantamine were maintained at least up to 12 months, demonstrating a mean change of -2.1 in the ADAS-cog score compared with baseline, and the active group was still close to baseline at 24 months (Erkinjuntti et al., 2003a). During the 12-month trial, the most frequently reported adverse events were depression (13 per cent), agitation (12 per cent) and insomnia (11 per cent).

46.5.1.3 RIVASTIGMINE

Rivastigmine (Exelon) is a second-generation carbamate slowly reversible AChEI and butyryl-cholinesterase (BuChE) inhibitor currently approved for use in mild to moderate AD (Farlow, 2003). Rivastigmine binds to the AChE molecule in a pseudo-irreversible manner; the acetyl moiety of ACh is dissociated rapidly but the carbamyl moiety remains longer. Rivastigmine is therefore metabolized at the synapse rather than by hepatic cytochrome enzymes; hence, there are no drug–drug interactions (Polinsky, 1998). Rivastigmine has a half-life at the synapse of 9 hours and should be given twice daily. Initial dosage is 3 mg/day and should be slowly escalated to 6 mg/day, 9 mg/day and 12 mg/day. The role of BuChE inhibition in glial cells in AD remains unclear. After treatment of AD with rivastigmine for 12 months, CSF and plasma AChE activity decreased by 46 per cent and BuChE by 65 per cent from baseline (Darreh-Shori et al., 2002). There was a significant correlation between plasma ChE inhibition and cognition, particularly in relation to attention (Almkvist et al., 2004).

The effects of rivastigmine in VaD remain to be determined in phase III, randomized, double-blind, placebo-controlled clinical trials (Moretti et al., 2004). Rivastigmine was used in small open-label studies of patients with subcortical VaD followed for 12 months (Moretti et al., 2001) and 22 months (Moretti et al., 2002); rivastigmine resulted in stabilization of cognition and ADL, with slight improvement of executive function and planning, less caregiver stress and improved behaviour.

Regarding the use of rivastigmine in patients with AD + CVD, Kumar and colleagues (2000) compared the outcomes of AD patients with or without concurrent vascular risk factors; cognitive effects were seen in both groups but patients with AD and vascular risk had greater clinical benefit. These findings were confirmed by Erkinjuntti and colleagues (2002b) in an open-label extension study of 104 weeks. Compared with non-hypertensive patients with AD,

significant treatment differences were observed in the hypertensive subgroup on the Progressive and Global Deterioration Scales (PDS and GDS). Furthermore, Erkinjuntti et al. (2003b) stratified 725 patients with AD treated with rivastigmine, according to the presence or absence of arterial hypertension at baseline. Rivastigmine 6–12 mg/day provided better outcomes than placebo on the PDS in the hypertensive ($P = 0.031$) and non-hypertensive ($P = 0.035$) subgroups. All patients receiving rivastigmine 6–12 mg/day had superior CIBIC-plus scores than those receiving placebo. The additional apparent benefits on disease progression detected in patients with AD and hypertension may be linked to drug effects on cerebrovascular risk factors, or to a larger underlying cholinergic deficit in patients with AD and hypertension.

46.5.2 Memantine

Memantine (Namenda, Ebixa, Axura) is a moderate-affinity, voltage-dependent, uncompetitive, potent antagonist of the N-methyl-d-aspartate (NMDA) receptor (Farlow, 2004). Experimentally, memantine inhibits and reverses the abnormal activity of protein phosphatase (PP-2A) that leads to tau hyperphosphorylation and to neurofibrillary degeneration in AD (Li et al., 2004). Memantine has been shown to be effective and well tolerated in patients with severe AD (Reisberg et al., 2003), and was recently approved by the FDA for the treatment of moderate to severe AD (Möbius, 2003). Furthermore, Tariot and colleagues (2004) showed that, in patients with moderate to severe AD receiving stable doses of donepezil, memantine resulted in significantly better outcomes than placebo in cognition, ADL, global outcome and behaviour. These findings suggest that this dual therapy could be useful.

Memantine has been used also in patients with VaD based on its experimental efficacy in animal models of ischaemia. Memantine acts on potentially contributing factors such as neuronal depolarization, mitochondrial dysfunction, magnesium effects on NMDA receptors and chronic glutamatergic overstimulation; it also has shown positive effects on long-term potentiation and cognitive tests in standard animal models of impaired synaptic plasticity (Möbius, 1999).

Orgogozo and colleagues (2002) and Wilcock and co-workers (2002), recently completed two randomized, placebo-controlled 6-month trials of memantine (20 mg/day) in mild to moderate probable VaD, diagnosed according to the NINDS-AIREN criteria (Román et al., 1993). In study MMM 300 Orgogozo et al. (2002) randomized 147 patients to memantine and 141 to placebo. After 28 weeks, the mean ADAS-cog scores were significantly improved relative to placebo: the memantine group gained an average of 0.4 points, versus a decline of 1.6 in the placebo group, a difference of 2.0 points ($P = 0.0016$). The CIBIC-plus improved or stable response, reached 60 per cent with memantine compared with 52 per cent with placebo ($P = 0.227$). The Gottfries-Bråne-Steen (GBS) Scale (Gottfries et al., 1982) and the Nurses' Observation Scale for Geriatric

Patients (NOSGER) (Spiegel *et al.*, 1991) total scores at week 28 did not differ significantly between the two groups. However, the GBS Scale intellectual function subscore and the NOSGER disturbing behaviour dimension also showed a difference favouring memantine ($P = 0.04$ and $P = 0.07$, respectively).

In study MMM 500 Wilcock *et al.* (2002) randomized 277 patients to memantine and 271 to placebo. At 28 weeks the active group had gained 0.53 points and the placebo declined by 2.28 points in ADAS-cog, a significant difference of 1.75 ADAS-cog points between the groups ($P < 0.05$). There were no differences in CGIC, MMSE, GBS or NOSGER between groups. Memantine was well tolerated in both studies. Möbius and Stoffler (2002) performed a *post hoc* pooled analysis of the above two placebo-controlled trials of memantine in VaD. Baseline severity, as assessed by MMSE, showed larger cognitive benefit in patients with more advanced disease. Also, the cognitive treatment effect for memantine was more pronounced in the small-vessel type group without cortical infarctions by CT or MRI. Finally, the placebo subgroup of patients with large vessel disease showed less cognitive decline than the other subgroup.

46.5.3 Calcium channel blockers

The main calcium channels blockers used for the treatment of VaD include nimodipine, lacidipine and fasudil.

46.5.3.1 NIMODIPINE

Nimodipine (Nimotop) is a dihydropyridinic calcium channel blocker used as an antihypertensive agent. Due to its highly lipophilic properties it readily crosses the blood–brain barrier (BBB), affects autoregulation of cerebral blood flow and produces vasodilatation of small cerebral blood vessels (Jansen *et al.*, 1991). Nimodipine has been shown to reduce the severity of neurological outcome in patients after subarachnoid haemorrhage secondary to ruptured aneurysms, probably by decreasing cerebral vasospasm, although this effect has not been demonstrated by angiography or transcranial Doppler (Ohman *et al.*, 1991). In addition to its vascular effects, nimodipine appears to have nootropic properties. There is a high density of nimodipine binding sites in hippocampus, caudate nucleus and cerebral cortex (Traber and Gibsen, 1989). Nimodipine binds to slow L-type calcium receptors, preventing influx of calcium into vascular smooth muscle cells and into ischaemic neurones (Greenberg *et al.*, 1990); experimentally, it provides protection against age-associated microvascular abnormalities in the rat brain (De Jong *et al.*, 1990). Although a neuroprotective effect has been postulated in stroke patients, nimodipine showed only a trend for better outcome when used within the first 12 hours of stroke onset (Gelmers and Hennerici, 1990).

A Cochrane review on nimodipine by Lopez-Arrieta and Birks (2002) concluded that, owing to limitations in the available data, there was no convincing evidence for the efficacy of nimodipine in AD, VaD or mixed forms of dementia.

However, a re-analysis of the Scandinavian Trial of Nimodipine in MID (Pantoni *et al.*, 2000) showed a beneficial effect in tests of attention and psychomotor performance in the subgroup of patients with subcortical small vessel VaD, but not in patients with post-stroke dementia of the MID type.

A pilot open label trial of nimodipine in patients with small vessel VaD was positive (Pantoni *et al.*, 1996). In this study, subcortical VaD was defined according to ICD-10 criteria (World Health Organization, 1992), and inclusion criteria required the patients to have mild to moderate dementia (MMSE, 12–24; Global Deterioration Scale, 3–5), as well as CT evidence of extensive leukoaraiosis and at least one lacunar infarct. The primary measure of efficacy was the Sandoz Clinical Assessment – Geriatric (SCAG) scale (Shader *et al.*, 1974). Using similar criteria and outcome measures, a large multicentre, randomized, double-blind, placebo-controlled trial of nimodipine in subcortical VaD is being conducted in Italy and Spain.

46.5.3.2 LACIDIPINE AND LERCANIDIPINE

Lacidipine and lercanidipine are third-generation dihydropyridine calcium antagonists that cause systemic vasodilatation by blocking calcium entry through L-type calcium channels in cell membranes; these agents also improve carotid atherosclerosis (Zanchetti *et al.*, 2004), small vessel disease (Frishman, 2002) and cerebral flow (Semplicini *et al.*, 2000) in hypertensive patients and offer some promise for the treatment of vascular dementia.

46.5.3.3 FASUDIL

Fasudil hydrochloride is a novel intracellular calcium antagonist, with Rho-kinase inhibitory activity on arterial walls affecting vessel remodelling (Pearce *et al.*, 2004). Kamei and colleagues (1996) reported the use of fasudil in the treatment of two patients with Binswanger's disease using ^{31}P-magnetic resonance spectroscopy and Xenon-computed tomography. Treatment with fasudil at 30 or 60 mg/day orally for 8 weeks controlled the fluctuating symptoms of Binswanger's disease in both patients. Mental tests and imaging also improved during the treatment.

46.5.4 Nootropic agents

The name nootropic (Greek *nous*, mind; *trophikos*, nourishing) describes a category of agents with neuroprotective capacity against anoxic or oxidative injuries. Piracetam, oxiracetam and citicoline will be reviewed here.

46.5.4.1 PIRACETAM

Piracetam (2-oxo-1-pyrrolidine acetamide), the first of the nootropic agents, is a cyclic derivative of γ-aminobutyric acid (GABA) which can cross the blood–brain barrier (Hitzenberger *et al.*, 1998) to concentrate selectively in the brain cortex (Vernon and Sorkin, 1991). At low doses, piracetam increases both oxygen and glucose utilization via ATP pathways and the release of some neurotransmitters – in particular dopamine metabolites – whilst at higher dosages, it is associated with platelet anti-aggregation and rheological effects with antithrombotic properties (Moriau *et al.*, 1993). It enhances the microcirculation by promoting erythrocyte deformability and by reducing adherence to endothelial cells. However, studies of piracetam in acute stroke have been inconclusive, although improvement of aphasia in patients treated within 7 hours of stroke onset was seen (Hitzenberger *et al.*, 1998). Several animal studies showed effects of piracetam on memory and facilitation of retention over 24 hours. A Cochrane review (Flicker and Grimley Evans, 2001) concluded that the usefulness of piracetam in patients with AD and VaD in small clinical trials has been unclear, based mainly on subjective Global Impression of Change. A recent review of 19 trials in patients with several forms of dementia (Waegemans *et al.*, 2002) and a protective effect in patients undergoing coronary artery bypass surgery (Uebelhack *et al.*, 2003) appear to provide some support for a moderate effect of piracetam on cognitive impairment.

46.5.4.2 OXIRACETAM

Oxiracetam is a structural analogue of the nootropic agent piracetam. This compound has enhancing effects on vigilance and memory. In comparison with piracetam, oxiracetam exhibits greater improvement in memory (Itil *et al.*, 1986) and has been used extensively for the treatment of dementia, including AD, VaD, MID (Dysken *et al.*, 1989; Baumel *et al.*, 1989) and mixed forms. Green and colleagues (1992) failed to demonstrate a difference with placebo in AD patients. In contrast, Maina and co-workers (1989) studied 289 patients with MID in a double-blind placebo-controlled trial and after 12 weeks of treatment found that oxiracetam reduced behavioural symptoms.

46.5.4.3 CITICOLINE

Citicoline (Somazina), also known as CDP-choline or cytidine-5′-diphosphate choline, is a naturally occurring endogenous nucleoside that functions as an intermediate in three major metabolic pathways (Conant and Schauss, 2004):

- *Synthesis of phosphatidylcholine* (lecithin), one of the major cell membrane phospholipids with an important role in the formation of lipoproteins. Citicoline formation is the rate-limiting step in the synthesis of phosphatidylcholine.
- *Synthesis of acetylcholine*: citicoline by providing choline for this neurotransmitter could limit choline availability for membrane synthesis. This 'auto-cannibalism' of choline-containing membrane phospholipids as a source of acetylcholine has been postulated in AD (Ulus *et al.*, 1989).
- *Oxidation to betaine*, a methyl donor. The main components of citicoline, choline and cytidine, are readily absorbed in the gastrointestinal tract and cross the blood–brain barrier. As a dietary supplement, choline is grouped with the B vitamins.

In animal studies, citicoline is biologically active, enhancing repair of ischaemic neuronal injury and increasing levels of acetylcholine and dopamine (Secades and Frontera, 1995). In aged animals, citicoline increased dopamine release, improving learning and memory tasks (Cacabelos *et al.*, 1993). In a pooled analysis of clinical trials on acute ischaemic stroke, citicoline was shown to enhance the possibility of recovery (Davalos *et al.*, 2002). Citicoline has been used in a number of trials in patients with AD showing modest results in improvement of memory and behaviour (Cacabelos *et al.*, 1993). In a Cochrane review (Fioravanti and Yanagi, 2000) of four studies in VaD with a total of 217 patients (citicoline = 115, placebo = 102), evaluation with the Global Impression of Change showed a significant improvement in contrast with the placebo group. The effect size was very large (8.89 CI = 5.19–15.22) indicating a strong drug effect (Fioravanti and Yanagi, 2000). However, a more recent, placebo-controlled trial, on 30 patients showed no evidence of cognitive improvement (Cohen *et al.*, 2003).

46.5.5 Xanthine derivatives

The main xanthine derivatives used in the treatment of VaD are pentoxifylline or oxpentifylline (Trental), denbufylline – a phosphodiesterase 4 (PDE4) inhibitor, and propentofylline (PPF). Pentoxifylline, derived from theobromine, has haemorheological effects both on the microcirculation and on peripheral vascular disease (in particular for the treatment of intermittent claudication). Pentoxifylline has immunomodulatory properties, increasing the rate of neutrophil migration, suppressing monocyte production of tumour necrosis factor (TNF)-α, and inhibiting leukocyte stimulation by TNF-α and interleukin-1 (IL-1). These properties are strong contributors to its haemorheological effects (Samlaska and Winfield, 1994). PPF exhibits adenosine-mediated nootropic properties against post-anoxic neuronal cell damage, and glial-modulation effects with inhibition of microglial activation.

46.5.5.1 PENTOXIFYLLINE

Haemorheological changes are found in patients with AD and in some forms of VaD, such as Binswanger's disease, in comparison with age-matched controls (Solerte *et al.*, 2000). Abnormalities included hyperviscosity, increased sedimentation rate, hyperfibrinogenaemia and increased acute-phase reactants; these changes correlate with increased levels of TNF-α and interferon(IFN)-γ. Pentoxifylline (Trental) treatment lowers fibrinogen and TNF-α levels. Black and colleagues (1992) demonstrated beneficial effects of pentoxifylline in patients with MID. These preliminary findings were confirmed in the larger, multicentre European Pentoxifylline Multi-Infarct Dementia Study (1996) that demonstrated significant cognitive improvement in the MID form of VaD in comparison with placebo.

46.5.5.2 PROPENTOFYLLINE

Beneficial effects on learning and memory were observed in several European and Canadian double-blind, placebo-controlled, randomized, parallel group trials of PPF in AD and VaD (Kittner et al., 1997; Mielke et al., 1998; Kittner, 1999; Pischel, 1998). Most studies included patients with mild to moderate VaD according to NINDS-AIREN criteria (McKhann et al., 1984). Significant symptomatic improvement and long-term efficacy in ADAS-cog and CIBIC-plus were noted up to 48 weeks of treatment compared with placebo. In addition, sustained treatment effects for at least 12 weeks after withdrawal suggested an effect on disease progression (Pischel, 1998; Rother et al., 1998). Despite these positive results in controlled clinical trials in AD and VaD, the clinical development of PPF was halted in 2000.

46.5.5.3 DENBUFYLLINE

Denbufylline, a xanthine derivative and PDE4 inhibitor, has interesting effects such as vasodilatation of cerebral vessels (Willette et al., 1997) and potent activation of the hypothalamo-pituitary–adrenal axis. PDE4 is one of the cyclic AMP (cAMP) specific phosphodiesterases whose tissue distribution is important in pathologies related to the central nervous and immune systems. In the experimental animal, denbufylline increases adrenocortico tropic hormone, circulating corticosterone, luteinizing hormone, corticotrophin releasing hormone, and cAMP content of the hypothalamic tissue, but is without effect on arginine vasopressin (Kumari et al., 1997). It also stimulates inhibition of bone loss suggesting therapeutic potential for the treatment of osteoporosis (Miyamoto et al., 1997). Treves and Korczyn (1999) studied a group of patients with AD, mixed dementia, and VaD treated with denbufylline. No significant differences were found in comparison with placebo for the treatment of AD or VaD, although patients who received denbufylline tended to improve in their cognitive scores.

46.5.6 Vasodilators

Yesavage and colleagues (1979) reviewed 102 studies from the literature on the use of vasodilating agents in senile dementias; the postulated effect of these agents was to counteract the 'hardening of the arteries'. Recommendations for most of these agents were based in trials invalidated by the small number of participants, short open treatment periods, and variations in diagnostic criteria and clinical end points. Cochrane himself (1979) strongly criticized the poor quality of the evidence thus obtained.

The principal pharmacological agents with primary effect on smooth muscle resulting in vasodilatation include cyclandelate (Cyclospasmol), papaverine (Pavabid), isoxsuprine (Vasodilan), cinnarizine (Stugeron), and nafronyl (Pralixene). No significant effects have been demonstrated with the use of vasodilating agents in VaD (Cook and James, 1981).

Nicotinic acid (niacin), used for many years for its vasodilating properties, has received renewed attention due to its effects in the treatment of primary hypercholesterolaemia and mixed dyslipidaemia. Nicotinic acid is the only drug that primarily lowers concentrations of non-esterified fatty acids and thereby lowers VLDL triglycerides. Nicotinic acid also seems to improve insulin resistance and to stimulate cholesterol mobilization from macrophages, offering an avenue for regression of the vascular lesions of atherosclerosis (Karpe and Frayn, 2004).

46.5.7 Ergot derivatives

The main ergot derivatives used for the treatment of VaD are nicergoline (Sermion) and codergocrine or ergoloid mesylates (Hydergine) – a mixture of the mesylated form of four dehydrogenated ergot peptide derivatives (in a 3:3:2:1 ratio), dihydroergocornine, dihydroergocristine, dihydro-α-ergocryptine, and dihydro-β-ergocryptine (Wadworth and Chrisp, 1992).

46.5.7.1 ERGOLOID MESYLATES

The metabolic effects of ergoloid mesylates (Hydergine) are incompletely understood; however, enhancement of noradrenergic, dopaminergic and serotinergic functions (Weil, 1988) and reduction of free radical formation (Favit et al., 1995) have been proposed. Schneider and Olin (1994) reviewed 151 reports on the use of ergoloid mesylates (Hydergine) in senile dementia, but only 47 of these trials (31 per cent) met strict criteria for meta-analysis. The review by Schneider and Olin (1994) and a subsequent Cochrane report (Olin et al., 2001) confirmed that patients with VaD appeared to benefit more from Hydergine than patients with AD in terms of cognition, clinical global ratings, and combined measures. However, compared with placebo, efficacy was very modest, at best, and there are at present no grounds to recommend its use.

46.5.7.2 NICERGOLINE

Nicergoline (Sermion) is an ergot derivative used for the treatment of cognitive, affective and behavioural disorders of the elderly. Although initially considered a vasoactive drug indicated for cerebrovascular disorders, nicergoline appears to have protective effects against degeneration of cholinergic neurones (Giardino et al., 2002) and has been used for the treatment of various forms of dementia, including AD and VaD (Fioravanti and Flicker, 2001). The therapeutic effects of nicergoline were evident by 2 months of treatment and were maintained for 6 months. Cognitive assessment with the MMSE was performed in 261 patients. The difference between treatment and control groups on the MMSE favoured nicergoline; at 12 months the effect size was 2.86 (0.98, 4.74). Herrmann and colleagues (1997) conducted a randomized double-blind placebo-controlled trial involving 136 patients with MID. After 6 months of treatment, nicergoline was significantly better than placebo. Another placebo-controlled pilot study by Bes and colleagues (1999), recruited 72 elderly hypertensive patients with VCI and evidence of leukoaraiosis, randomly assigned to either nicergoline (n = 36) or placebo (n = 36) for 24 months. Nicergoline (30 mg b.i.d. for 24 months) was well tolerated and attenuated the cognitive decline of elderly hypertensive patients with VCI.

46.5.8 Posatirelin

Posatirelin is a TRH analogue (L-6-ketopiperidine-2-carbonyl-L-leucyl-proline amide). In an experimental model of brain cholinergic deficit in the rat by lesion of the nucleus basalis magnocellularis, posatirelin treatment was shown to rescue cholinergic neurones of the nbM and their cholinergic projections to the cerebral cortex (Sabbatini et al., 1998). Posatirelin has been used in patients with AD and VaD (Parnetti et al., 1995, 1996). VaD patients treated with posatirelin showed a significant improvement in intellectual performance, orientation, motivation and memory as compared with controls. The drug was well tolerated.

46.5.9 Antithrombotic agents

Antiplatelet drugs have been shown to effectively prevent TIAs and ischaemic stroke (Easton, 2003). Aspirin provides a relative reduction of 19 per cent in the rate of major vascular events in patients with arterial disease in general, and 13 per cent in patients with ischaemic CVD (van Gijn and Algra, 2003). Other antiplatelet agents, such as sulfinpyrazone, ticlopidine, clopidogrel, dipyridamole and orally administered IIb/IIIa inhibitors have similar effects, although the combination of aspirin and dipyridamole may be more efficacious than aspirin alone. The Antithrombotic Trialists' Collaboration (Easton, 2003) assessed the effect of antiplatelet therapy in 135 000 patients. Antiplatelet therapy reduces the combined odds of stroke, myocardial infarction or vascular death by 22 per cent, and antiplatelet agents reduce the odds of a non-fatal stroke by 25 per cent in patients with or without a history of stroke. Likewise, among patients with non-valvular atrial fibrillation, anticoagulation (INR $\geq$ 2.0) reduces not only the frequency and severity, but also the mortality of ischaemic stroke (Hart, 2003; Hylek et al., 2003). The few trials of antiplatelet agents conducted in patients with VaD will be mentioned below.

46.5.9.1 ASPIRIN

A population-based study by Sturmer and colleagues (1996) showed that aspirin (ASA) users have a slight protection against cognitive decline with an odds ratio ranging from 0.97 to 0.87. A single randomized trial used ASA (325 mg/day) in patients with mild MID type of VaD (Meyer et al., 1989). Cognitive tests and CBF studies were performed at onset and 1 year later. Stabilization or mild improvement was seen in the active group compared with untreated controls. However, a recent Cochrane review (Williams et al. 2000) concluded that there is no evidence that aspirin is effective in treating patients with VaD.

46.5.9.2 TRIFLUSAL

Triflusal (Disgren) is an antiplatelet agent structurally related to the salicylates, but it is not derived from ASA. Triflusal and its active metabolite (3-hydroxy-4-trifluoro-methylbenzoic acid or HTB) produce specific inhibition of platelet arachidonic acid metabolism (McNeely and Goa, 1998). A single open-label trial of triflusal in 73 patients with VaD (López-Pousa et al., 1997) showed, after 12 months of therapy, less decline in MMSE scores in the active group compared with the untreated subjects.

46.5.9.3 *GINKGO BILOBA*

Ginkgo, extract EGb 761 from the *Ginkgo biloba* tree (the maidenhair tree), has been widely used in several European countries and more recently in North America, for the treatment of 'chronic cerebral circulatory insufficiency' (Kleijnen and Knipschild, 1992; Gertz and Kiefer, 2004). *Ginkgo biloba* extracts are considered to have vasodilating and antioxidant properties, as well as haemorheological and nootropic effects, and to decrease platelet aggregability and blood viscosity, but the mechanism of action remains poorly understood (Zimmermann et al., 2002; Gertz and Kiefer, 2004). Several trials have used ginkgo in patients with MID or with AD + CVD, with modest positive results (Le Bars et al., 1997; Kanowski and Hoerr, 2003; van Dongen et al., 2003). Using Cochrane data, Kurz and Van Baelen (2004) showed significant benefit versus placebo with ginkgo treatment only when all doses were pooled, although the effects appeared to be minimal. Ginkgo treatment in the elderly, has been associated with subarachnoid haemorrhage and other haemorrhagic complications such as subdural haematoma, intracranial and intraocular bleeding (Vale, 1998; Fong and Kinnear, 2003; Meisel et al., 2003).

46.5.10 Choto-san

Choto-san (Gouteng-san) is a traditional Japanese (Kampo) herbal medicine with apparent neuroprotective effect against glutamate-induced neuronal death (Itoh et al., 1999; Watanabe et al., 2003). Choto-san was administered for 12 weeks to 10 patients with post-stroke VCI; P3 event-related brain potentials, MMSE, and verbal fluency tests significantly improved with treatment (Yamaguchi et al., 2004). In a larger trial, Choto-san resulted in improvement of ADL, global rating, and subjective and psychiatric symptoms (Itoh et al., 1999).

46.5.11 Jiannao yizhi

Zhang and colleagues (2002) evaluated the safety and efficiency of Jiannao yizhi, a Chinese herbal medicine, in the treatment of VaD. A multicentre, double-blind, randomized, placebo-controlled method was used to study 242 patients with mild to moderate VaD; 89 cases were randomized to the active group (Jiannao Yizhi Granules), 106 cases to the Western medicine group and 47 to the placebo group. MMSE and Blessed Dementia Scale were used to evaluate the therapeutic effect after 60 days of therapy. Treatment with Jiannao Yizhi was superior to Western medicine and to placebo.

46.5.12 Vinpocetine

Vinpocetine is a synthetic ethyl ester of apovincamine, a vinca alkaloid obtained from the leaves of the lesser periwinkle (*Vinca minor*). For many years, vinpocetine has been used for the treatment of cognitive impairment but the mechanism of action remains unclear (Szatmari and Whitehouse, 2003). A recent Cochrane review of three short-term studies involving 583 patients with dementia (AD, VaD, mixed) treated with vinpocetine or placebo, concluded that patients treated with vinpocetine (30–60 mg/day) showed modest benefit compared with placebo (Szatmari and Whitehouse, 2003).

46.5.13 Dehydroepiandrosterone

Dehydroepiandrosterone (DHEA) is a weakly androgenic adrenal steroid and an intermediary in the biosynthesis of androgens and oestrogens. It is considered a neurohormone, since small quantities of DHEA are produced in the brain (Knopman and Henderson, 2003). DHEA or its sulphate ester metabolite (dehydroepiandrosterone sulphate, DHEAS) is the most abundant circulating steroid and declines in serum and CSF with aging. Bicikova and colleagues (2004) have suggested that variations in levels of these neurohormones could discriminate between AD and VaD. However, Kim *et al.* (2003) observed that DHEAS levels in the CSF were significantly decreased in both AD and VaD.

DHEA is classified as a dietary supplement; its effect on dementia could result from a direct action, or through testosterone, oestradiol, and other metabolites. However, there is no association between DHEAS levels and duration or severity of symptoms in AD. Wolkowitz and co-workers (2003) conducted a 6-month, randomized double-blind study of DHEA for AD. A modest improvement was seen with DHEA but increasing confusion, agitation and paranoid reactions were seen among DHEA-treated participants. A high dropout may have compromised the study. DHEA alone seems unlikely to be superior to currently available anticholinesterases for AD. A single open-label trial of DHEA in the MID type of VaD (Azuma *et al.*, 1999) used intravenous DHES (200 mg/day) for 4 weeks; the treatment markedly increased serum and CSF levels of DHEAS in seven MID patients; however, improvement of ADL and emotional disturbances was seen in only three patients.

46.5.14 Cerebrolysin

Cerebrolysin is a peptidergic drug produced from purified brain proteins, with postulated neurotrophic activity (Windisch *et al.*, 1998; Windisch, 2000) and probable neuroprotective effects (Rockenstein *et al.*, 2003). A small open-label trial in patients with AD and VaD (Rainer *et al.*, 1997) showed minimal improvement in cognitive tests and clinical global impression.

46.5.15 Sulodexide

Sulodexide is a medium molecular weight glycosaminoglycan with effects on plasma viscosity by lowering plasma fibrinogen concentrations (Lunetta and Salanitri, 1992). Sulodexide is effective and well tolerated in peripheral occlusive arterial disease with claudication (Shustov, 1997). In Italy, Parnetti and colleagues (1997) conducted a trial of sulodexide in patients that fulfilled NINDS-AIREN criteria for probable VaD; 46 patients were included in the active treatment group, compared with 40 in the pentoxifylline group. Larger reductions of plasma fibrinogen levels were seen with sulodexide, and both groups showed a slight reduction in activated factor VII levels. Dementia scores improved more in the sulodexide group.

46.5.16 Thrombin inhibitors

There is evidence indicating that hypercoagulable states could result in increased risk of dementia (Mari *et al.*, 1996). Bots and colleagues (1998) from the Dutch Vascular Factors in Dementia Study in Rotterdam, found that dementia, particularly post-stroke VaD, was associated with increased thrombin generation. In this population, increased levels of thrombin-antithrombin complex (TAT), cross-linked D-dimer and tissue-type plasminogen activator (tPA) activity were associated with increased risk of dementia. In addition, coagulation abnormalities have been described in patients with Binswanger's disease. Schneider and colleagues (1987) found increased fibrinogen levels and hyperviscosity in patients with Binswanger's disease. Iwamoto and co-workers (1995) demonstrated increased platelet activation in Binswanger's disease that was manifested by increased plasma β-thromboglobulin levels. Tomimoto and colleagues (1999, 2001) found coagulation activation leading to hypercoagulable state in Japanese patients with Binswanger's disease; levels of fibrinogen, TAT complex, prothrombin fragment 1 + 2, and D-dimer were found to be significantly increased, particularly in patients with recent aggravation of their deficits.

There are no controlled clinical trials of Binswanger's disease, but the above results point toward several potential therapeutic options (Román, 1999b). Iwamoto and co-workers (1995) reported that the use of ticlopidine hydrochloride in eight patients with Binswanger's disease resulted in lower levels of platelet activation, without major clinical change. There is a need for controlled trials of ticlopidine and other antiplatelet agents, such as aspirin, dipyridamole, and clopidogrel, alone or in combination, in Binswanger's disease.

Hyperfibrinogenaemia has deleterious effects on haemorheological conditions in the cerebral microcirculation that result in hyperviscosity and slowing of blood flow in deep border-zone territories in Binswanger's disease.

Therefore, the use of medications such as pentoxifylline (Trental), ancrod (Sherman, 2002) or bezafibrate (Tanne *et al.*, 2001) to lower fibrinogen levels could be indicated.

46.5.16.1 ANCROD

Ancrod, a defibrinating enzyme obtained from the venom of a Malayan pit viper (Sherman, 2002), was used by Ringelstein and colleagues (1988) in 10 patients with Binswanger's disease. Mean plasma levels of fibrinogen decreased from 3.26 g/L (SD 1.3) prior to treatment (normal 2.5–4.0 g/L), to 1.52 g/L (SD 0.53) after 1 month of treatment with subcutaneous ancrod. Treatment resulted in significant improvement of the timed retinal arteriovenous circulation (abnormally slow prior to treatment), and increase of CO_2-induced cerebral vasomotor response measured by transcranial Doppler. However, clinical condition and neuropsychological tests were unchanged, and there was no decrease in stroke recurrences during a 6-month observation period.

46.5.16.2 ARGATROBAN

As mentioned earlier, Walsh (1968, 1978) claimed significant improvement of dementia symptoms with a treatment based on warfarin anticoagulation. Currently, this treatment is reserved for patients with non-valvular atrial fibrillation (Hart, 2003), heart valve replacement, or with the anticardiolipin antibody syndrome. Direct thrombin inhibitors are equally effective; they inhibit fibrin-bound thrombin, produce a predictable anticoagulant response that is unaffected by platelet factor 4 and require no long-term monitoring and no dose adjustment (Weitz and Crowther, 2002; Donnan *et al.*, 2003). There are three parenteral direct thrombin inhibitors (hirudin, bivalirudin and argatroban), and one oral agent, ximelagatran (Francis *et al.*, 2003; Schulman *et al.*, 2003).

Argatroban, a selective competitive inhibitor of thrombin, was successfully used by Akiguchi and colleagues (1999) for the treatment of a Japanese patient with Binswanger's disease with antiphospholipid antibody syndrome, and a hypercoagulable state with abnormally high levels of TAT and fibrinogen. A long-term therapeutic regimen with argatroban (20 mg/day i.v. for 28 days), improved gait disturbances and mental dysfunction. Argatroban reduced TAT and improved levels of fibrinogen and other coagulation markers to normal limits. Kario and colleagues (1999) also reported similar positive effects with the use of argatroban in reducing silent ischaemic strokes in a patient with VaD.

46.5.16.3 HEPARIN–MEDIATED EXTRACORPOREAL LDL/FIBRINOGEN PRECIPITATION (HELP)

Since 1993, Walzl (1993, 2000) in Austria has developed an haemorheological treatment that he called HELP (**H**eparin-mediated **E**xtracorporeal **L**DL/fibrinogen **P**recipitation) to reduce elevated fibrinogen levels and increased lipid fractions and to control thereby the high viscosity of plasma and whole blood, as well as to reduce the aggregability or sludging of red blood cells. HELP was used in 141 patients with the MID type of VaD. Laboratory and clinical evaluations were performed before and after treatment. Each HELP treatment reduced whole blood and plasma viscosity and red cell transit time. Total cholesterol, low density lipoproteins and triglycerides were reduced significantly. Neurological improvement was documented by improved scores in MMSE, Mathew Scale and ADL.

46.5.17 Hyperbaric oxygen treatment

Vila and colleagues (1999), from Buenos Aires, reported on the use of hyperbaric oxygen treatment (HOT) in four patients with Binswanger's disease. Patients received daily sessions of HOT at 2.5 atmospheres absolute (ATA) for 45 minutes, for a total of 10 days. Controls received room air at 1.1 ATA. The procedure was well tolerated. After active treatment, noticeable improvements in gait, urinary and cognitive tests was observed in all subjects, with increase in independence. This improvement persisted for up to 5 months, after which the previous deficits reappeared but responded again to repeated HOT treatment. Despite the promise of the method, there has been no independent confirmation of the benefits of HOT in Binswanger's disease (Román, 1999c).

46.6 GENERAL MEDICAL MANAGEMENT OF THE PATIENT WITH VASCULAR DEMENTIA

Epidemiological studies have confirmed the increased risk of dementia associated with vascular risk factors, in particular hypertension (Launer *et al.*, 1995, 2000; Skoog *et al.*, 1996, 1998; Kilander *et al.*, 1998; Tzourio *et al.*, 1999). In a population-based study in France, Tzourio and colleagues (1999) found that in 4 years, untreated hypertensive persons (59–71 years of age) multiplied by four the risk of cognitive decline (OR 4.3, 95 per cent CI 2.1–8.8) compared with 1.9 (95 per cent CI 0.8–4.4) in those being treated.

Other important risk factors, include diabetes mellitus (Ott *et al.*, 1999; Stewart and Liolitsa, 1999), raised homocysteine (Seshadri *et al.*, 2002), and smoking (Ott *et al.*, 1998). These vascular risk factors increase the risk of both VaD and AD. Other than apolipoprotein (ApoE), genetic and racial factors are probably important. In Alabama, southern USA, Zamrini and colleagues (2004a) showed that Black Americans had higher rates of hypertension than White Americans, whereas the latter had a higher incidence of atrial fibrillation, coronary artery disease, and higher cholesterol. Therefore, primary and secondary prevention of stroke and CVD appears to be mandatory for the prevention of dementia (Lechner, 1998; Erkinjuntti and Gauthier, 2002; O'Brien *et al.*, 2003). There are clear guidelines for the use of anticoagulants (Hart, 2003) and antiplatelet medication in the prevention of stroke (Elkind, 2004).

46.6.1 Treatment of hypertension

Treatment of hypertension protects against cognitive decline even in the absence of stroke (Forette *et al.*, 1998, 2002; Clarke, 1999). No deleterious effects on cognition, mood and quality of life have been demonstrated with the treatment of hypertension in the elderly (Applegate *et al.*, 1994; Starr *et al.*, 1996; Prince *et al.*, 1996; Prince, 1997). On the contrary, Forette and collaborators (2002) confirmed that treatment of systolic hypertension with nitrendipine, a long-acting dihydropyridine calcium channel blocker, protects against dementia in older patients. Compared with placebo, long-term antihypertensive therapy reduced the risk of dementia by 55 per cent, from 7.4 to 3.3 cases per 1000 patient-years. After adjustment for sex, age, education and entry blood pressure, the relative hazard rate associated with the use of nitrendipine was 0.38 (95 per cent CI 0.23–0.64; $P < 0.001$). Treatment of 1000 patients for 5 years can prevent 20 cases of dementia (95 per cent CI 7–33) (Forette *et al.*, 1998, 2002). The most appropriate levels of blood pressure control remain undecided. The results of the ongoing SPS3 study should help solve this issue (Benavente, 2003).

Recently, the Study on Cognition and Prognosis in the Elderly (SCOPE) confirmed that treatment of mild to moderate hypertension in the elderly prevents stroke and dementia (Lithell *et al.*, 2003). SCOPE enrolled 4964 patients aged 70–89 years, with systolic blood pressure of 160–179 mmHg, and/or diastolic blood pressure of 90–99 mmHg, and a MMSE test score ≥24; patients were treated with candesartan, an angiotensin-receptor blocker, or with placebo, plus open-label active antihypertensive therapy added as needed. Blood pressure reduction was slightly better with candesartan therapy, compared with control therapy; this was associated with a modest, statistically non-significant, reduction in major cardiovascular events and with a marked reduction in non-fatal stroke. Cognitive function was well maintained in both treatment groups in the presence of substantial blood pressure reductions.

Finally, control of hypertension in patients with stroke (secondary prevention) is also helpful in preventing dementia. The PROGRESS trial (2001), a randomized clinical trial of perindopril, an angiotensin-converting enzyme (ACE) inhibitor, and a diuretic (indapamide) used in 6105 individuals with previous stroke or TIA, showed that after a follow up of 3.9 years, blood pressure was reduced, lowering the risks of stroke and other major vascular events. Dementia was also decreased, with a relative risk reduction of 12 per cent (Tzourio *et al.*, 2003). Cognitive decline occurred in 9.1 per cent of the actively treated group and 11.0 per cent of the placebo group (risk reduction, 19 per cent). In summary, active treatment resulted in reduced risks of dementia and of the cognitive decline associated with recurrent stroke (Tzourio *et al.*, 2003).

46.6.2 Treatment of hyperlipidaemia with statins

The most recent recommendations for the management of hyperlipidaemia suggest a reduction of low density lipoprotein (LDL) cholesterols to below 100 mg/dL, and drug therapy for high-risk patients whose LDL ranges from 100 to 129 mg/dL (Grundy *et al.*, 2004). High-risk patients have coronary heart disease or disease of the blood vessels to the brain or extremities, or diabetes, or multiple (two or more) risk factors (e.g. smoking, hypertension) that give them >20 per cent chance of having a heart attack within 10 years. Very high-risk patients are those who have cardiovascular disease together with either multiple risk factors (especially diabetes), or severe and poorly controlled risk factors (e.g. continued smoking), or metabolic syndrome (a constellation of risk factors associated with obesity including high triglycerides and low high density lipoproteins – HDL). Patients hospitalized for acute coronary syndromes or stroke are also at very high risk (Grundy *et al.*, 2004).

There are indications suggesting that the use of statins (3-hydroxy-3-methylglutaryl-coenzyme A [HMG-CoA] reductase inhibitors) can reduce the risk of dementia (Jick *et al.*, 2000; Rockwood *et al.*, 2002; Zamrini *et al.*, 2004b). In Boston, Jick and colleagues (2000) studied 284 patients with dementia and 1080 controls older than 50 years of age; the adjusted relative risk for those prescribed statins was 0.29 (95 per cent CI 0.13–0.63; $P = 0.002$) indicating a substantially lowered risk of developing dementia, independent of the presence or absence of untreated hyperlipidaemia. Furthermore, Zamrini and co-workers (2004b) conducted between 1997 and 2001 a study of veterans in Birmingham, Alabama, USA; patients with a new diagnosis of AD (n = 309) were compared with age-matched non-AD controls (n = 3088). In this group, statins users had a 39 per cent lower risk of AD relative to non-statin users (odds ratio 0.61, 95 per cent CI 0.42–0.87). These results indicate a possible antidementia effect of statins, perhaps related to the anti-inflammatory effects. However, the use of statins in non-demented, non-hyperlipidaemic patients cannot be recommended at this time (Miller and Chacko, 2004).

46.6.3 Control of diabetes

The abnormalities in carbohydrate, lipid and protein metabolism resulting from diabetes mellitus produce injury of blood vessels, nerves and other tissues. Diabetes increases up to 4-fold the relative risk for cardiovascular disease and CVD due to the microvascular (retinopathy, nephropathy, neuropathy, lacunes), and macrovascular (coronary heart disease, stroke, peripheral arterial disease) complications. Diabetes produces cognitive decline with doubling of the overall risk of dementia (Ott *et al.*, 1999; Stewart and Liolitsa, 1999).

Diabetes results in increased blood viscosity from hyperglycaemia, endothelial oxidative damage, loss of nitric oxide (NO)-mediated endothelial functions, and alterations of the blood–brain barrier (Mooradian *et al.*, 1997), as a result of excessive glycation as well as from glycoxidized LDLs. The end result is the impairment of perfusion through the cerebral and retinal microcirculation. In addition, stress-activated pathways such as the Jun-kinases play a major role in diabetic microangiopathy (Evans *et al.*, 2002). The most current guidelines for treatment are the 2004 American Diabetes Association Clinical Practice Recommendations and those of the US Veterans Hospitals (Pogach *et al.*, 2004).

46.6.4 Cessation of smoking

Smokers double the risk of coronary artery disease, congestive heart failure, and peripheral vascular disease, and increase 1.5 times the risk of stroke and dementia (Ott *et al.*, 1998). Smoke, in addition to nicotine and carbon monoxide, contains a complex mixture of free radicals including quinone/hydroquinone, NO and nitrogen dioxide (NO_2) that cause morphological irregularities of the endothelium, formation of blebs, leakage of macromolecules and increased endothelial cell death (Pittilo, 2000). Smoke reduces prostacyclin release, enhances endothelium-derived vasodilatation, and decreases NO concentrations and cGMP production, increasing aggregation of platelets and leukocytes. Smoking worsens atheromatous plaque formation in carotid arteries, increases hypertension, blood coagulability, serum viscosity and fibrinogen. Smokers have worse cognitive performances than non-smokers including reduced psychomotor speed and reduced cognitive flexibility. This effect is observed in subjects as young as 45 years of age (Kalmijn *et al.*, 2002).

46.6.5 Diet

It is clear that dietary change with reduced sodium intake, is a crucial component of the treatment of arterial hypertension. The Dietary Approaches to Stop Hypertension (DASH) diet (Sacks *et al.*, 2001), is currently recommended by the US Department of Health and Human Services. This diet is rich in magnesium, potassium, calcium, protein and fibre and is low in saturated fat, cholesterol and total fat. There is emphasis in fruits, vegetables, and low fat dairy foods, whole grain products, fish, poultry and nuts. A recent clinical trial (McGuire *et al.*, 2004) randomized hypertensive patients to advice-only group; to a group treated with weight loss, increased physical activity and reduced sodium and alcohol intake; and to a third group that included the latter plus the DASH diet. At 6 months, compared with the advice-only group, the other groups had a decline of mean systolic blood pressure of 3.7 mmHg ($P < 0.001$) and 4.3 mmHg for the DASH diet group ($P < 0.001$) respectively. The study confirmed that hypertension control requires multiple lifestyle changes including an appropriate eating plan.

Epidemiological data suggested an association between dietary factors, in particular antioxidants, and cognition (Deschamps *et al.*, 2001). Similarities in the diets of patients with AD and VaD have been reported in Japan (Otsuka *et al.*, 2002), with higher energy intake from fats, in particular polyunsaturated fatty acids and decrease in antioxidant vitamins B, C and carotene. However, in the Honolulu-Asia Aging Study, mid-life intakes of antioxidants, such as beta-carotene, flavonoids, and vitamins E and C, did not modify the risk for late life dementia, including AD and VaD (Laurin *et al.*, 2004). Likewise, no effect of fat intake in the development of dementia was found in the Rotterdam study (Engelhart *et al.*, 2002).

Wald and colleagues (2002) concluded, based on evidence from genetic and prospective studies, that the association between increased homocysteine and cardiovascular disease is causal. On this basis, lowering homocysteine concentrations by 3 μmol/L from current levels (achievable by increasing folic acid intake) would reduce the risk of ischaemic heart disease (IHD) by 16 per cent (11–20 per cent), deep vein thrombosis by 25 per cent (8–38 per cent) and stroke by 24 per cent (15–33 per cent). However, meta-analysis of observational studies suggests that elevated homocysteine is at most a modest independent predictor of ischaemic heart disease and stroke risk in healthy populations (Homocysteine Studies Collaboration, 2002).

Moreover, folic acid/vitamin B_{12} is not an effective treatment of dementia; a Cochrane review (Malouf *et al.*, 2003) concluded that in older patients with mild to moderate cognitive decline, supplementation with 750 μg/day of folic acid, with or without B_{12}, had no beneficial effects on measures of cognition or mood, although folic acid plus vitamin B_{12} effectively reduced serum homocysteine concentrations. Along the same lines, a trial on the use of vitamins to prevent recurrent stroke gave negative results (Toole *et al.*, 2004).

Nonetheless, a diet rich in antioxidant phytophenols, such as those found in olive oil and red wine, appears to effectively inhibit endothelial adhesion molecule expression, explaining in part the protection from atherosclerosis afforded by Mediterranean diets (Carluccio *et al.*, 2003).

46.6.6 Chronic inflammation

Recent evidence indicates that markers of inflammation such as C-reactive protein (CRP) are important predictors of atherosclerotic disease, particularly in patients with diabetes (Rader, 2000). Chronic infections, including periodontal disease and persistent intracellular infection with *Chlamydia pneumoniae* have been associated with increased risk of vascular events (Kalayoglu *et al.*, 2002).

46.7 PUBLIC HEALTH ASPECTS OF VASCULAR DEMENTIA

Based on current population trends, the ageing of the population will lead to increasing incidence of stroke and heart disease in the near future. It is predicted that VaD will become the most common cause of senile dementia, both by itself and as a contributor to other degenerative dementias (Román, 2002e).

There is growing evidence that preventive measures to decrease the vascular burden on the brain may also decrease vascular dementia in the elderly. VaD and AD share with stroke a number of vascular risk factors, as demonstrated in large epidemiological studies. The most important of the modifiable factors is hypertension, a treatable risk factor that explains at least half of the attributable risk of stroke. As mentioned above, three large controlled trials (Forette *et al.*, 1998, 2002; Lithell *et al.*, 2003; Tzourio *et al.*, 2003) have demonstrated that blood pressure lowering has a significant effect in decreasing the risk of dementia, including VaD and AD. Overall, these data suggest that interventions aiming at reducing the level of vascular risk factors might prevent dementia. The expected benefit of these interventions could be estimated from data provided by epidemiological studies; however, there is a dearth of large population-based controlled studies to demonstrate the efficacy of preventive interventions at public health level (Román, 2003b; Alperovitch *et al.*, 2004; Williams, 2004). Prevention appears to be the most promising avenue for decreasing the incidence of the two most common forms of senile dementia, AD and VaD.

REFERENCES

Akiguchi I, Tomimoto H, Kinoshita M *et al.* (1999) Effects of antithrombin on Binswanger's disease with antiphospholipid antibody syndrome. *Neurology* **52**: 398–401

Alexopoulos GS, Kiosses DN, Klimstra S *et al.* (2002) Clinical presentation of the 'depression-executive dysfunction syndrome' of late life. *American Journal of Geriatric Psychiatry* **10**: 98–106

Almkvist O, Darreh-Shori T, Stefanova E *et al.* (2004) Preserved cognitive function after 12 months of treatment with rivastigmine in mild Alzheimer's disease in comparison with untreated AD and MCI patients. *European Journal of Neurology* **11**: 253–261

Alperovitch A, Schwarzinger M, Dufouil C *et al.* (2004) Towards a prevention of dementia. *Revue Neurologique (Paris)* **160**: 256–60.

American Psychiatric Association. (1987) *Diagnostic and Statistical Manual of Mental Disorders*, revised 3rd edition (DSM-IIIR). Washington, DC, American Psychiatric Association

American Psychiatric Association. (1994) *Diagnostic and Statistical Manual of Mental Disorders*, 4th edition (DSM-IV). Washington, DC, American Psychiatric Association

Applegate WB, Pressel S, Wittes J *et al.* (1994) Impact of the treatment of isolated systolic hypertension on behavioural variables. Results from the systolic hypertension in the elderly program. *Archives of Internal Medicine* **154**: 2154–2160

Azuma T, Nagai Y, Saito T *et al.* (1999) The effect of dehydroepiandrosterone sulfate administration to patients with multi-infarct dementia. *Journal of the Neurological Sciences* **162**: 69–73

Babikian VL, Wolfe N, Linn R *et al.* (1990) Cognitive changes in patients with multiple cerebral infarcts. *Stroke* **21**: 1013–1018

Barba R, Martinez-Espinosa S, Rodriguez-Garcia E *et al.* (2000) Poststroke dementia: clinical features and risk factors. *Stroke* **31**: 1494–1501

Barba R, Castro MD, del Mar Morin M *et al.* (2001) Prestroke dementia. *Cerebrovascular Diseases* **11**: 216–224

Baumel B, Eisner L, Karukin M *et al.* (1989) Oxiracetam in the treatment of multi-infarct dementia. *Progress in Neuropsychopharmacology and Biological Psychiatry* **13**: 673–682

Benavente O. (2003) Antithrombotic therapy in small subcortical strokes (lacunar infarcts). *Advances in Neurology* **92**: 275–280

Berg L. (1988) Clinical Dementia Rating (CDR). *Psychopharmacology Bulletin* **24**: 637–639

Bes A, Orgogozo JM, Poncet M *et al.* (1999) A 24-month, double-blind, placebo-controlled multicentre pilot study of the efficacy and safety of nicergoline 60 mg per day in elderly hypertensive patients with leukoaraiosis. *European Journal of Neurology* **6**: 313–322

Bicikova M, Ripova D, Hill M *et al.* (2004) Plasma levels of 7-hydroxylated dehydroepiandrosterone (DHEA) metabolites and selected amino-thiols as discriminatory tools of Alzheimer's disease and vascular dementia. *Clinical Chemistry Laboratory Medicine* **42**: 518–524

Biesold D, Inanami O, Sato A, Sato Y. (1989) Stimulation of the nucleus basalis of Meynert increases cerebral cortical blood flow in rats. *Neuroscience Letters* **98**: 39–44

Black RS, Barclay LL, Nolan KA *et al.* (1992) Pentoxifylline in cerebrovascular dementia. *Journal of the American Geriatrics Society* **40**: 237–244

Black S, Román GC, Geldmacher DS *et al.* for the Donepezil 307 Vascular Dementia Study Group. (2003) Efficacy and tolerability of donepezil in vascular dementia. Positive results of a 24-week, multicenter, international, randomized, placebo-controlled clinical trial. *Stroke* **34**: 2323–2330

Bots ML, Breteler MM, van Kooten F *et al.* (1998) Coagulation and fibrinolysis markers and risk of dementia. The Dutch Vascular Factors in Dementia Study. *Haemostasis* **28**: 216–222

Bousser MG and Tournier-Lasserve E. (1994) Summary of the proceedings of the First International Workshop on CADASIL. Paris, 19–21 May 1993. *Stroke* **25**: 704–707

Bowler JV and Hachinski V. (1995) Vascular cognitive impairment: a new approach to vascular dementia. *Baillière's Clinical Neurology* **4**: 357–376

Brun A. (1994) Pathology and pathophysiology of cerebrovascular dementia: pure subgroups of obstructive and hypoperfusive etiology. *Dementia* **5**: 145–147

Brun A and Englund E. (1988) A white matter dementia of the Alzheimer type: a pathoanatomical study. *Annals of Neurology* **19**: 253–262

Cacabelos R, Alvarez XA, Franco-Maside A *et al.* (1993) Effect of CDP-choline on cognition and immune function in Alzheimer's disease and multi-infarct dementia. *Annals of the New York Academy of Sciences* **695**: 321–323

Canadian Study of Health and Aging Working Group (2000) The incidence of dementia in Canada. *Neurology* **55**: 66–73

Carluccio MA, Siculella L, Ancora MA *et al.* (2003) Olive oil and red wine antioxidant polyphenols inhibit endothelial activation: antiatherogenic properties of Mediterranean diet phytochemicals. *Arteriosclerosis, Thrombosis, and Vascular Biology* **23**: 622–629

Chabriat H and Bousser MG. (2003) CADASIL. Cerebral autosomal dominant arteriopathy with subcortical infarcts and leukoencephalopathy. *Advances in Neurology* **92**: 147–150

Chui HC, Victoroff JI, Margolin D *et al.* (1992) Criteria for the diagnosis of ischaemic vascular dementia proposed by the State of California Alzheimer's Disease Diagnostic and Treatment Centers. *Neurology* **42**: 473–480

Chui HC, Mack W, Jackson JE *et al.* (2000) Clinical criteria for the diagnosis of vascular dementia: a multicenter study of comparability and interrater reliability. *Archives of Neurology* **57**: 191–196

Chukwudelunzu FE, Meschia JF, Graff-Radford NR, Lucas JA. (2001) Extensive metabolic and neuropsychological abnormalities associated with discrete infarction of the genu of the internal capsule. *Journal of Neurology, Neurosurgery, and Psychiatry* **71**: 658–662

Clarke CE. (1999) Does the treatment of isolated hypertension prevent dementia? *Journal of Human Hypertension* 13: 357–358

Cochrane AL. (1979) Concluding remarks. In: G Tognoni and S Garattini (eds), *Treatment and Prevention in Cerebrovascular Disorders*. Amsterdam, Elsevier, pp. 453–455

Cohen RA, Browndyke JN, Moser DJ et al. (2003) Long-term citicoline (cytidine diphosphate choline) use in patients with vascular dementia: neuroimaging and neuropsychological outcomes. *Cerebrovascular Diseases* 16: 199–204

Conant R and Schauss AG. (2004) Therapeutic applications of citicoline for stroke and cognitive dysfunction in the elderly: a review of the literature. *Alternative Medicine Review* 9: 17–31

Cook P and James I. (1981) Drug therapy: cerebral vasodilators. *New England Journal of Medicine* 305: 1508–1513; 1560–1564

Corey-Bloom J. (2003) Galantamine: a review of its use in Alzheimer's disease and vascular dementia. *International Journal of Clinical Practice* 57: 219–223

Court JA, Perry EK, Kalaria RN. (2002) Neurotransmitter control of the cerebral vasculature and abnormalities in vascular dementia. In: T Erkinjuntti and S Gauthier (eds), *Vascular Cognitive Impairment*. London, Martin Dunitz Ltd, pp. 167–185

Cummings JL. (1993) Frontal-subcortical circuits and human behavior. *Archives of Neurology* 50: 873–880

Cummings JL, Mega M, Gray K et al. (1994) The Neuropsychiatric Inventory. Comprehensive assessment of psychopathology in dementia. *Neurology* 44: 2308–2314

Darreh-Shori T, Almkvist O, Guan ZZ et al. (2002) Sustained cholinesterase inhibition in AD patients receiving rivastigmine for 12 months. *Neurology* 59: 563–572

Davalos A, Castillo J, Alvarez-Sabin J et al. (2002) Oral citicoline in acute ischaemic stroke: an individual patient data pooling analysis of clinical trials. *Stroke* 33: 2850–2857

De Jong GI, de Weerd H, Schuurman T et al. (1990) Microvascular changes in aged rat forebrain. Effects of chronic nimodipine treatment. *Neurobiology of Aging* 11: 381–389

Delay J and Brion S. (1962) *Les Démences Tardives*. Paris, Masson et Cie

Dengiz AN and Kershaw P. (2004) The clinical efficacy and safety of galantamine in the treatment of Alzheimer's disease. *CNS Spectrums* 9: 377–392

Deschamps V, Barberger-Gateau P, Peuchant E, Orgogozo JM. (2001) Nutritional factors in cerebral aging and dementia: epidemiological arguments for a role of oxidative stress. *Neuroepidemiology* 20: 7–15

Desmond DW, Moroney JT, Bagiella E et al. (1998) Dementia as a predictor of adverse outcomes following stroke. An evaluation of diagnostic methods. *Stroke* 29: 69–74

Dichgans M. (2002) Cerebral autosomal dominant arteriopathy with subcortical infarcts and leukoencephalopathy: phenotypic and mutational spectrum. *Journal of the Neurological Sciences* 203–204: 77–80

Donnan GA, Dewey HM, Chambers BR. (2004) Warfarin for atrial fibrillation: the end of an era? *Lancet Neurology* 3: 305–308

Dysken MW, Katz R, Stallone F, Kuskowski M. (1989) Oxiracetam in the treatment of multi-infarct dementia and primary degenerative dementia. *Journal of Neuropsychiatry and Clinical Neurosciences* 1: 249–252

Easton D. (2003) Evidence with antiplatelet therapy and ADP-receptor antagonists. *Cerebrovascular Diseases* 16 (Suppl. 1): 20–26

Elkind MS. (2004) Secondary stroke prevention: review of clinical trials. *Clinical Cardiology* 27 (5 Suppl. 2): II 25–II 35

Engelhart MJ, Geerlings MI, Ruitenberg A et al. (2002) Diet and risk of dementia: Does fat matter?: the Rotterdam Study. *Neurology* 59: 1915–1921

Englund E, Brun A, Alling C. (1988) White matter changes in dementia of the Alzheimer's type. Biochemical and neuropathological correlates. *Brain* 111: 1425–1439

Erkinjuntti T and Gauthier S (eds). (2002) *Vascular Cognitive Impairment*. London, Martin Dunitz Ltd

Erkinjuntti T and Sawada T (eds) (1999) Summary of the 1st International Conference on Development of Drug Treatment for Vascular Dementia, by the International Working Group on Harmonization of Dementia Drug Guidelines, 7–9 October 1998, Osaka, Japan. *Alzheimer Disease and Associated Disorders* 13 (Suppl. 3): S1–S212

Erkinjuntti T, Sawada T, Whitehouse PJ. (1999) The Osaka Conference on Vascular Dementia 1998. *Alzheimer Disease and Associated Disorders* 13 (Suppl. 3): S1–S3

Erkinjuntti T, Inzitari D, Pantoni L et al. (2000) Research criteria for subcortical vascular dementia in clinical trials. *Journal of Neural Transmission* 59 (Suppl. 1): 23–30

Erkinjuntti T, Kurz A, Gauthier S et al. (2002a) Efficacy of galantamine in probable vascular dementia and Alzheimer's disease combined with cerebrovascular disease: a randomized trial. *Lancet* 359: 1283–1289

Erkinjuntti T, Skoog I, Lane R, Andrews C. (2002b) Rivastigmine in patients with Alzheimer's disease and concurrent hypertension. *International Journal of Clinical Practice* 56: 791–796

Erkinjuntti T, Kurz A, Small GW et al. (2003a) An open-label extension trial of galantamine in patients with probable vascular dementia and mixed dementia. *Clinical Therapeutics* 25: 1765–1782

Erkinjuntti T, Skoog I, Lane R, Andrews C. (2003b) Potential long-term effects of rivastigmine on disease progression may be linked to drug effects on vascular changes in Alzheimer brains. *International Journal of Clinical Practice* 57: 756–760

Erkinjuntti T, Román G, Gauthier S et al. (2004) Emerging therapies for vascular dementia and vascular cognitive impairment. *Stroke* 35: 1010–1017

European Pentoxifylline Multi-Infarct Dementia Study. (1996) *European Neurology* 36: 315–321

Evans JLK, Goldfine ID, Maddux BA, Grodsky GM. (2002) Oxidative stress and stress-activated signaling pathways: a unifying hypothesis of type 2 diabetes. *Endocrine Reviews* 23: 599–622

Farlow MR. (2003) Update on rivastigmine. *The Neurologist* 9: 230–234

Farlow MR. (2004) NMDA receptor antagonists. A new therapeutic approach for Alzheimer's disease. *Geriatrics* 59: 22–27

Favit A, Sortino MA, Aleppo G et al. (1995) The inhibition of peroxide formation as a possible substrate for the neuroprotective action of dehydroergocryptine. *Journal of Neural Transmission* 45 (Suppl.): 297–305

Ferris S and Gauthier S. (2002) Cognitive outcome measures in vascular dementia. In: T Erkinjuntti and S Gauthier (eds), *Vascular Cognitive Impairment*. London, Martin Dunitz Ltd, pp. 395–400

Fioravanti M and Flicker L. (2001) Efficacy of nicergoline in dementia and other age associated forms of cognitive impairment. *Cochrane Database of Systematic Reviews* 4: CD00315

Fioravanti M and Yanagi M. (2000) Cytidinediphosphocholine (CDP choline) for cognitive and behavioural disturbances associated with chronic cerebral disorders in the elderly. *Cochrane Database of Systematic Reviews* 4: CD000269

Fisher CM. (1965) Lacunes: small deep cerebral infarcts. *Neurology* 15: 774–784

Flicker L and Grimley Evans G. (2001) Piracetam for dementia or cognitive impairment. *Cochrane Database of Systematic Reviews* 2: CD001011

Folstein MF, Folstein SE, McHugh PH. (1975) 'Mini-mental state'. A practical method for grading the cognitive state of patients for the clinician. *Journal of Psychiatric Research* 12:189–198

Fong KC and Kinnear PE. (2003) Retrobulbar haemorrhage associated with chronic *Ginkgo biloba* ingestion. *Postgraduate Medical Journal* 79: 531–532

Forette F, Seux ML, Staessen JA *et al.* for the Syst-Eur investigators. (1998) Prevention of dementia in randomised double-blind placebo-controlled Systolic Hypertension in Europe (Syst-Eur) trial. *Lancet* 352: 1347–1351

Forette F, Seux ML, Staessen JA *et al.* for the Syst-Eur investigators. (2002) The prevention of dementia with antihypertensive treatment: new evidence from the Systolic Hypertension in Europe (Syst-Eur) study. *Archives of Internal Medicine* 162: 2046–2052

Francis CW, Berkowitz SD, Comp PC *et al.* for the EXULT A Study Group. (2003) Comparison of ximelagatran with warfarin for the prevention of venous thromboembolism after total knee replacement. *New England Journal of Medicine* 349: 1703–1712

Frishman WH. (2002) Are antihypertensive agents protective against dementia? A review of clinical and preclinical data. *Heart Diseases* 4: 380–386

Gélinas I, Gauthier L, McIntyre M, Gauthier S. (1999) Development of a functional measure for persons with Alzheimer's disease: the Disability Assessment for Dementia. *American Journal of Occupational Therapy* 53: 471–481

Gelmers HJ and Hennerici M. (1990) Effect of nimodipine on acute ischemic stroke. Pooled results from five randomized trials. *Stroke* 21 (Suppl. 12): IV 81–84

Gertz HJ and Kiefer M. (2004) Review about *Ginkgo biloba* special extract EGb 761 (Ginkgo). *Current Pharmaceutical Design* 10: 261–264

Giardino L, Giuliani A, Battaglia A *et al.* (2002) Neuroprotection and aging of the cholinergic system: a role for the ergoline derivative nicergoline (Sermion). *Neuroscience* 109:487–497

Gold G, Giannakopoulos P, Montes-Paixao Junior C *et al.* (1997) Sensitivity and specificity of newly proposed clinical criteria for possible vascular dementia. *Neurology* 49: 690–694

Gold G, Bouras C, Canuto A *et al.* (2002) Clinicopathological validation study of four sets of clinical criteria for vascular dementia. *American Journal of Psychiatry* 159: 82–87

Goldsmith DR and Scott LJ. (2003) Donepezil in vascular dementia. *Drugs and Aging* 20: 1127–1136

Gorelick PB, Chatterjee A, Patel D *et al.* (1992) Cranial computed tomographic observations in multi-infarct dementia: a controlled study. *Stroke* 23: 804–811

Gottfries CG, Bråne G, Steen G. (1982) A new rating scale for dementia syndromes. *Gerontology* 28 (Suppl. 2): 20–31

Gottfries CG, Blennow K, Karlsson I, Wallin A. (1994) The neurochemistry of vascular dementia. *Dementia* 5: 163–167

Gray F, Dubas F, Roullet E, Escourolle R. (1985) Leukoencephalopathy in diffuse hemorrhagic cerebral amyloid angiopathy. *Annals of Neurology* 18: 54–59

Green RC, Goldstein FC, Auchus AP *et al.* (1992) Treatment trial of oxiracetam in Alzheimer's disease. *Archives of Neurology* 49: 1135–1136

Greenberg JH, Uematsu D, Araki N *et al.* (1990) Cytosolic free calcium during focal cerebral ischemia and the effects of nimodipine on calcium and histological damage. *Stroke* 21 (Suppl. 2): IV 72–77

Grundy SM, Cleeman JI, Bairey Merz CN *et al.* for the Coordinating Committee of the National Cholesterol Education Program. (2004) Implications of Recent Clinical Trials for the National Cholesterol Education Program Adult Treatment Panel III Guidelines. *Circulation* 110: 227–239

Hachinski VC, Iliff LD, Zilhka E *et al.* (1975) Cerebral blood flow in dementia. *Archives of Neurology* 32: 632–637

Hart RG. (2003) Atrial fibrillation and stroke prevention. *New England Journal of Medicine* 349: 1015–1016

Harvey AL. (1995) The pharmacology of galanthamine and its analogues. *Pharmacology and Therapeutics* 68: 113–128

Hénon H, Pasquier F, Durieu I *et al.* (1997) Preexisting dementia in stroke patients. Baseline frequency, associated factors, and outcome. *Stroke* 28: 2429–2436

Hénon H, Durieu I, Guerouaou D *et al.* (2001) Poststroke dementia: incidence and relationship to prestroke cognitive decline. *Neurology* 57: 1216–1222

Herrmann WM, Stephan K, Gaede K, Apeceche M. (1997) A multicenter randomized double-blind study on the efficacy and safety of nicergoline in patients with multi-infarct dementia. *Dementia and Geriatric Cognitive Disorders* 8: 9–17

Hitzenberger G, Rameis H, Manigley C. (1998) Pharmacological properties of piracetam. *CNS Drugs* 9 (Suppl. 1): 19–27

Holmes C, Cairns N, Lantos P, Mann A. (1999) Validity of current clinical criteria for Alzheimer's disease, vascular dementia and dementia with Lewy bodies. *British Journal of Psychiatry* 174: 45–50

Homocysteine Studies Collaboration. (2002) Homocysteine and risk of ischemic heart disease and stroke: a meta-analysis. *JAMA* 288: 2015–2022

Huppert FA, Brayne C, Gill C *et al.* (1995) CAMCOG – a concise neuropsychological test to assist dementia diagnosis: sociodemographic characteristics in an elderly population sample. *British Journal of Clinical Psychology* 34: 529–541

Hylek EM, Go AS, Chang Y *et al.* (2003) Effect of intensity of oral anticoagulation on stroke severity and mortality in atrial fibrillation. *New England Journal of Medicine* 349: 1019–1026

Ingles JL, Wentzel C, Fisk JD, Rockwood K. (2002) Neuropsychological predictors of incident dementia in patients with vascular cognitive impairment, without dementia. *Stroke* 33: 1999–2002

Itil TM, Menon GN, Songar A, Itil KZ. (1986) CNS pharmacology and clinical therapeutic effects of oxiracetam. *Clinical Neuropharmacology* 9 (Suppl. 3): S70–S72

Itoh T, Shimada Y, Terasawa K. (1999) Efficacy of Choto-san on vascular dementia and the protective effect of the hooks and stems of *Uncaria sinensis* on glutamate-induced neuronal death. *Mechanisms of Ageing and Development* 111: 155–173

Iwamoto T, Kubo H, Takasaki M. (1995) Platelet activation in the cerebral circulation in different subtypes of ischemic stroke and Binswanger's disease. *Stroke* 26: 52–56

Jagust W. (2001) Untangling vascular dementia. *Lancet* 358: 2097–2098

Jansen I, Tfelt-Hansen P, Edvinsson L. (1991) Comparison of the calcium entry blockers nimodipine and flunarizine on human cerebral and temporal arteries: role in cerebral disorders. *European Journal of Clinical Pharmacology* 40: 7–15

Jellinger KA and Mitter-Ferstl E. (2003) The impact of cerebrovascular lesions in Alzheimer disease – a comparative autopsy study. *Journal of Neurology* 250: 1050–1055

Jick H, Zornberg GL, Jick SS *et al.* (2000) Statins and the risk of dementia. *Lancet* 356: 1627–1631

Johnston SC, O'Meara ES, Manolio TA et al. (2004) Cognitive impairment and decline are associated with carotid artery disease in patients without clinically evident cerebrovascular disease. Annals of Internal Medicine 140: 237–247

Kalaria RN and Ballard C. (1999) Overlap between pathology of Alzheimer disease and vascular dementia. Alzheimer Disease and Associated Disorders 13 (Suppl. 3): S115–S123

Kalaria RN, Ballard CG, Ince PG et al. (2001) Multiple substrates of late-onset dementia: implications for brain protection. Novartis Foundation Symposium 235: 49–60

Kalayoglu MV, Libby P, Byrne GI. (2002) Chlamydia pneumoniae as an emerging risk factor in cardiovascular disease. JAMA 288: 2724–2731

Kalimo H, Ruchoux M-M, Viitanen M, Kalaria RN. (2002) CADASIL: a common form of hereditary arteriopathy causing brain infarcts and dementia. Brain Pathology 12: 371–384

Kalmijn S, van Boxtel MP, Verschuren MW et al. (2002) Cigarette smoking and alcohol consumption in relation to cognitive performance in middle age. American Journal of Epidemiology 156: 936–944

Kamei S, Oishi M, Takasu T. (1996) Evaluation of fasudil hydrochloride treatment for wandering symptoms in cerebrovascular dementia with 31P-magnetic resonance spectroscopy and Xe-computed tomography. Clinical Neuropharmacology 19: 428–438

Kanowski S and Hoerr R. (2003) Ginkgo biloba extract EGb 761 in dementia: intent-to-treat analyses of a 24-week, multi-center, double-blind, placebo-controlled, randomized trial. Pharmacopsychiatry 36: 297–303

Kario K, Matsuo T, Hoshide S et al. (1999) Effect of thrombin inhibition in vascular dementia and silent cerebrovascular disease. An MR spectroscopy study. Stroke 30: 1033–1037

Karpe F and Frayn KN. (2004) The nicotinic acid receptor – a new mechanism for an old drug. Lancet 363: 1892–1894

Kilander L, Nyman H, Boberg M et al. (1998) Hypertension is related to cognitive impairment: a 20-year follow-up of 999 men. Hypertension 31: 780–786

Kim SB, Hill M, Kwak YT et al. (2003) Neurosteroids: cerebrospinal fluid levels for Alzheimer's disease and vascular dementia diagnostics. Journal of Clinical Endocrinology and Metabolism 88: 5199–5206

Kittner B. (1999) Clinical trials of propentofylline in vascular dementia. The European/Canadian Propentofylline Study Group. Alzheimer Disease and Associated Disorders 13 (Suppl. 3): S166–S171

Kittner B, Rossner M, Rother M. (1997) Clinical trials in dementia with propentofylline. Annals of the New York Academy of Sciences 826: 307–316

Kleijnen J and Knipschild P. (1992) Ginkgo biloba. Lancet 340: 1136–1139

Knopman D and Henderson VW. (2003) DHEA for Alzheimer's disease: a modest showing by a superhormone. Neurology 60: 1060–1061

Knopman DS, Rocca WA, Cha RH et al. (2003) Survival study of vascular dementia in Rochester, Minnesota. Archives of Neurology 60: 85–90

Kumar V, Anand R, Messina J et al. (2000) An efficacy and safety analysis of Exelon in Alzheimer's disease patients with concurrent vascular risk factors. European Journal of Neurology 7: 159–169

Kumari M, Cover PO, Poyser RH, Buckingham JC. (1997) Stimulation of the hypothalamo-pituitary-adrenal axis in the rat by three selective type-4 phosphodiesterase inhibitors: in vitro and in vivo studies. British Journal of Pharmacology 121: 459–468

Kurz A and Van Baelen B. (2004) Ginkgo biloba compared with cholinesterase inhibitors in the treatment of dementia: a review

based on meta-analyses by the Cochrane Collaboration. Dementia and Geriatric Cognitive Disorders 18: 217–26

Lacombe P, Sercombe R, Vaucher E, Seylaz J. (1997) Reduced cortical vasodilatory response to stimulation of the nucleus basalis of Meynert in the aged rat and evidence for a control of the cerebral circulation. Annals of the New York Academy of Sciences 826: 410–415

Lammie A. (2002) Hypertensive cerebral small vessel disease and stroke. Brain Pathology 12: 358–370

Launer LJ, Masaki K, Petrovitch H et al. (1995) The association between midlife blood pressure levels and late-life cognitive function. The Honolulu-Asia Aging Study. JAMA 274: 1846–1851

Launer LJ, Ross GW, Petrovik H et al. (2000) Midlife blood pressure and dementia: the Honolulu-Asia aging study. Neurobiology of Aging 21: 49–55

Laurin D, Masaki KH, Foley DJ et al. (2004) Midlife dietary intake of antioxidants and risk of late-life incident dementia: the Honolulu-Asia Aging Study. American Journal of Epidemiology 159: 959–967

Le Bars PL, Katz MM, Berman N et al. for the North American EGb Study Group. (1997) A placebo-controlled, double-blind, randomized trial of an extract of Ginkgo biloba for dementia. JAMA 278: 1327–1332

Lechner H. (1998) Status of treatment of vascular dementia. Neuroepidemiology 17: 10–13

Leys D and Pasquier F. (2000) How can cerebral infarcts and hemorrhages lead to dementia? Journal of Neural Transmission 59 (Suppl.): 31–36

Li L, Sengupta A, Haque N et al. (2004) Memantine inhibits and reverses the Alzheimer type abnormal hyperphosphorylation of tau and associated neurodegeneration. FEBS Letters 566: 261–269

Linden T, Skoog I, Fagerberg B, Steen B, Blomstrand C. (2004) Cognitive impairment and dementia 20 months after stroke. Neuroepidemiology 23: 45–52

Lithell H, Hansson L, Skoog I et al. for the SCOPE Study Group. (2003) The Study on Cognition and Prognosis in the Elderly (SCOPE): principal results of a randomized double-blind intervention trial. Journal of Hypertension 21: 875–886

Liu CK, Miller BL, Cummings JL et al. (1991) A quantitative MRI study of vascular dementia. Neurology 42: 138–143

Longstreth WT Jr, Manolio TA, Arnold A et al. for the Cardiovascular Health Study. (1996) Clinical correlates of white matter findings on cranial magnetic resonance imaging of 3301 elderly people. Stroke 27: 1274–1282

Longstreth WT Jr, Bernick C, Manolio T et al. (1998) Lacunar infarcts defined by magnetic resonance imaging of 3660 elderly people. Archives of Neurology 55: 1217–1225

Lopez-Arrieta JM and Birks J. (2002) Nimodipine for primary degenerative, mixed and vascular dementia. Cochrane Database of Systematic Reviews 3: CD000147

López-Pousa S, Mercadal-Dalmau J, Marti-Cuadros AM et al. (1997) Triflusal in the prevention of vascular dementia. Revista de Neurología (Barcelona) 25: 1525–1528

Lunetta M and Salanitri T. (1992) Lowering of plasma viscosity by the oral administration of the glycosaminoglycan sulodexide in patients with peripheral vascular disease. Journal of International Medical Research 20: 45–53

McGuire HL, Svetkey LP, Harsha DW et al. (2004) Comprehensive lifestyle modification and blood pressure control: a review of the PREMIER trial. Journal of Clinical Hypertension (Greenwich) 6, 383–390

McKhann G, Drachman D, Folstein M et al. (1984) Clinical diagnosis of AD: report of the NINCDS-ADRDA Work Group under the auspices of

Department of Health and Human Services Task Force on AD. *Neurology* **34**: 939–944

McNeely W and Goa KL. (1998) Triflusal. *Drugs* **55**: 823–833

Maina G, Fiori L, Torta R *et al.* (1989) Oxiracetam in the treatment of primary degenerative and multi-infarct dementia: a double-blind, placebo-controlled study. *Neuropsychobiology* **21**: 141–145

Malouf R and Birks J. (2004) Donepezil for vascular cognitive impairment. *Cochrane Database of Systematic Reviews* **1**: CD004395.

Malouf M, Grimley EJ, Areosa SA. (2003) Folic acid with or without vitamin B_{12} for cognition and dementia. *Cochrane Database of Systematic Reviews* **4**: CD004514

Mani RB. (2004) The evaluation of disease modifying therapies in Alzheimer's disease: a regulatory viewpoint. *Statistics in Medicine* **23**: 305–314

Mari D, Parnetti L, Coppola R *et al.* (1996) Hemostasis abnormalities in patients with vascular dementia and Alzheimer's disease. *Thrombosis and Haemostasis* **75**: 216–218

Marie P. (1901) Des foyers lacunaires de désintégration et de différents autres états cavitaires du cerveau. *Revue de Médecine (Paris)* **21**: 281–298

Mead S, James-Galton M, Revesz T *et al.* (2000) Familial British dementia with amyloid angiopathy: early clinical, neuropsychological and imaging findings. *Brain* **123**: 975–991

Meisel C, Johne A, Roots I. (2003) Fatal intracerebral mass bleeding associated with *Ginkgo biloba* and ibuprofen. *Atherosclerosis* **167**: 367

Mesulam M, Siddique T, Cohen B. (2003) Cholinergic denervation in a pure multi-infarct state: observations on CADASIL. *Neurology* **60**: 1183–1185

Meyer JS, Rogers RL, McClintic K *et al.* (1989) Randomized clinical trial of daily aspirin therapy in multi-infarct dementia. A pilot study. *Journal of the American Geriatrics Society* **37**: 549–555

Mielke R, Möller H-J, Erkinjuntti T *et al.* (1998) Propentofylline in the treatment of vascular dementia and Alzheimer-type dementia: overview of phase I and phase II clinical trials. *Alzheimer Disease and Associated Disorders* **12** (Suppl. 2): 29–35

Mikol J. (1968) Binswanger's disease and related forms. Contribution to the study of arteriosclerotic leukoencephalopathies. *Revue Neurologique (Paris)* **118**: 111–132

Mikol J and Vallat-Decouvelaere AV. (2000) Vascular dementia. *Annales de Pathologie* **20**: 470–478

Miller LJ and Chacko R. (2004). The role of cholesterol and statins in Alzheimer's disease. *Annals of Pharmacotherapy* **38**: 91–98

Mills EJ and Chow TW. (2003) Randomized controlled trials in long-term care residents with dementia: a systematic review. *Journal of the American Medical Directors Association* **4**: 302–307

Miyamoto K, Waki Y, Horita T *et al.* (1997) Reduction of bone loss by denbufylline, an inhibitor of phosphodiesterase 4. *Biochemical Pharmacology* **54**: 613–617

Möbius HJ. (1999). Pharmacologic rationale for memantine in chronic cerebral hypoperfusion, especially vascular dementia. *Alzheimer Disease and Associated Disorders* **13** (Suppl. 3): S172–S178

Möbius HJ. (2003) Memantine: update on the current evidence. *International Journal of Geriatric Psychiatry* **18** (Suppl. 1): S47–S54

Möbius HJ and Stoffler A. (2002) New approaches to clinical trials in vascular dementia: memantine in small vessel disease. *Cerebrovascular Diseases* **13** (Suppl. 2): 61–66

Mohs RC, Doody RS, Morris JC *et al.* (2001) A 1-year placebo-controlled preservation of function survival study of donepezil in AD patients. *Neurology* **57**: 481–488

Mondadori C. (1993) The pharmacology of the nootropics: new insights and new questions. *Behavioural Brain Research* **59**: 1–9

Mooradian AD. (1997) Central nervous system complications of diabetes mellitus-a perspective from the blood-brain barrier. *Brain Research and Brain Research Reviews* **23**: 210–218

Moretti R, Torre P, Antonello RM, Cazzato G. (2001) Rivastigmine in subcortical vascular dementia: a comparison trial on efficacy and tolerability for 12 months follow-up. *European Journal of Neurology* **8**: 361–362

Moretti R, Torre P, Antonello RM *et al.* (2002) Rivastigmine in subcortical vascular dementia: an open 22-month study. *Journal of the Neurological Sciences* **203**: 141–146

Moretti R, Torre P, Antonello RM *et al.* (2004) Rivastigmine in vascular dementia. Expert *Opinion in Pharmacotherapy* **5**: 1399–1410

Moriau M, Crasborn L, Lavenne-Pardonge E *et al.* (1993) Platelet antiaggregant and rheological properties of piracetam. A pharmacodynamic study in normal subjects. *Arzneimittel-Forschung/Drug Research* **43**: 110–118

Moroney JT, Bagiella E, Desmond DW *et al.* (1996) Risk factors for incident dementia after stroke. Role of hypoxic ischemic disorders. *Stroke* **27**: 1283–1289

O'Brien JT, Erkinjuntti T, Reisberg B, Román G *et al.* (2003) Vascular cognitive impairment. *Lancet Neurology* **2**: 89–98

Ohman J, Servo A, Heiskanen O. (1991) Long-term effects of nimodipine on cerebral infarcts and outcome after aneurysmal subarachnoid hemorrhage and surgery. *Journal of Neurosurgery* **74**: 8–13

Olin J, Schneider I, Novit A, Luczak S. (2001) Hydergine for dementia. *Cochrane Database of Systematic Reviews* **2**: CD000359

Orgogozo J-M, Rigaud AS, Stoffler A *et al.* (2002) Efficacy and safety of memantine in patients with mild to moderate vascular dementia: a randomized, placebo-controlled trial (MMM 300). *Stroke* **33**: 1834–1839

Otsuka M, Yamaguchi K, Ueki A. (2002) Similarities and differences between Alzheimer's disease and vascular dementia from the viewpoint of nutrition. *Annals of the New York Academy of Sciences* **977**: 155–161

Ott A, Slooter AJ, Hofman A *et al.* (1998) Smoking and risk of dementia and Alzheimer's disease in a population-based cohort study: the Rotterdam Study. *Lancet* **351**: 1840–1843

Ott A, Stolk RP, van Harskamp F *et al.* (1999) Diabetes mellitus and the risk of dementia: the Rotterdam Study. *Neurology* **53**: 1937–1942

Pantoni L, Carosi M, Amigoni S *et al.* (1996) A preliminary open trial with nimodipine in patients with cognitive impairment and leukoaraiosis. *Clinical Neuropharmacology* **19**: 497–506

Pantoni L, Rossi R, Inzitari D *et al.* (2000) Efficacy and safety of nimodipine in subcortical vascular dementia: a subgroup analysis of the Scandinavian Multi-Infarct Dementia Trial. *Journal of the Neurological Sciences* **175**: 124–134

Parnetti L. (1999) Pathophysiology of vascular dementia and white matter changes. *Revue Neurologique (Paris)* **155**, 754–758

Parnetti L, Ambrosoli L, Abate G *et al.* (1995) Posatirelin for the treatment of late-onset Alzheimer's disease: a double-blind multicentre study vs citicoline and ascorbic acid. *Acta Neurologica Scandinavica* **92**: 135–140

Parnetti L, Ambrosoli L, Agliati G *et al.* (1996) Posatirelin in the treatment of vascular dementia: a double-blind multicentre study vs placebo. *Acta Neurologica Scandinavica* **93**: 456–463

Parnetti L, Mari D, Abate G *et al.* (1997) Vascular dementia Italian sulodexide study (VAD.IS.S.). Clinical and biological results. *Thrombosis Research* **87**: 225–233

Pearce JD, Li J, Edwards MS *et al.* (2004) Differential effects of Rho-kinase inhibition on artery wall mass and remodeling. *Journal of Vascular Surgery* **39**: 223–228

Pearson VE. (2001) Galantamine: a new Alzheimer drug with a past life. *Annals of Pharmacotherapy* **35**: 1406–1413

Perry EK, Gibson PH, Blessed G *et al.* (1977) Neurotransmitter enzyme abnormalities in senile dementia. Choline acetyltransferase and glutamic acid decarboxylase activities in necropsy brain tissue. *Journal of the Neurological Sciences* **34**: 247–265

Petersen RC, Smith GE, Waring SC *et al.* (1999) Mild cognitive impairment: clinical characterization and outcome. *Archives of Neurology* **56**: 303–308

Pischel T. (1998) Long-term-efficacy and safety of propentofylline in patients with vascular dementia. Results of a 12 months placebo-controlled trial. *Neurobiology of Aging* **19** (Suppl. 4): S182

Pittilo RM. (2000) Cigarette smoking, endothelial injury and cardiovascular disease. *International Journal of Experimental Pathology* **81**: 219–230

Pogach LM, Brietzke SA, Cowan CL. Jr *et al.* for the VA/DoD Diabetes Guideline Development Group. (2004) Development of evidence-based clinical practice guidelines for diabetes: the Department of Veterans Affairs/Department of Defense guidelines initiative. *Diabetes Care* **27** (Suppl. 2): B82–B89

Pohjasvaara T, Erkinjuntti T, Vataja R, Kaste M. (1997) Dementia three months after stroke. Baseline frequency and effect of different definitions of dementia in the Helsinki Stroke Aging Memory Study (SAM) cohort. *Stroke* **28**: 785–792

Pohjasvaara T, Leppavouri A, Siira I *et al.* (1998) Frequency and clinical determinants of post-stroke depression. *Stroke* **29**: 2311–2317

Pohjasvaara T, Mantyla R, Ylikoski R *et al.* (2000) Comparison of different clinical criteria (DSMIII, ADDTC, ICD-10, NINDS-AIREN, DSM-IV) for the diagnosis of vascular dementia. *Stroke* **31**: 2952–2957

Pohjasvaara T, Leskela M, Vataja R *et al.* (2002) Post-stroke depression, executive dysfunction and functional outcome. *European Journal of Neurology* **9**: 269–275

Polinsky RJ. (1998) Clinical pharmacology of rivastigmine: a new generation acetylcholinesterase inhibitor for the treatment of Alzheimer's disease. *Clinical Therapeutics* **20**: 634–647

Pratt RD. (2002) Patient populations in clinical trials of the efficacy and tolerability of donepezil in patients with vascular dementia. *Journal of the Neurological Sciences* **203-204**: 57–65

Prince MJ. (1997) The treatment of hypertension in older people and its effect on cognitive function. *Biomedicine and Pharmacotherapy* **51**: 208–212

Prince MJ, Bird AS, Blizard RA, Mann AH. (1996) Is the cognitive function of older patients affected by antihypertensive treatment? Results from 54 months of the Medical Research Council's trial of hypertension in older adults. *BMJ* **312**: 801–805

PROGRESS Collaborative Group. (2001) Randomised trial of a perindopril-based blood-pressure-lowering regimen among 6:105 individuals with previous stroke or transient ischaemic attack. *Lancet* **358**: 1033–1041

Quinn J, Moore M, Benson DF *et al.* (2000) A videotaped CIBIC for dementia patients: validity and reliability in a simulated clinical trial. *Neurology* **58**: 433–437

Rader DJ. (2000) Inflammatory markers of coronary risk. *New England Journal of Medicine* **343**: 1179–1182

Rainer M, Brunnbauer M, Dunky A *et al.* (1997) Therapeutic results with Cerebrolysin in the treatment of dementia. *Wiener Medizinische Wochenschrift* **147**: 426–431

Raskind MA. (2003) Update on Alzheimer drugs (galantamine). *The Neurologist* **9**: 235–240

Reisberg B, Doody R, Stoffler A *et al.* for the Memantine Study Group. (2003) Memantine in moderate-to-severe Alzheimer's disease. *New England Journal of Medicine* **348**: 1333–1341

Ringelstein EB, Mauckner A, Schneider R *et al.* (1988) Effects of enzymatic blood defibrination in subcortical arteriosclerotic encephalopathy. *Journal of Neurology, Neurosurgery, and Psychiatry* **51**: 1051–1057

Rockenstein E, Adame A, Mante M *et al.* (2003) The neuroprotective effects of Cerebrolysin in a transgenic model of Alzheimer's disease are associated with improved behavioral performance. *Journal of Neural Transmission* **110**: 1313–1327

Rockwood K, Wentzel C, Hachinski V *et al.* (2000) Prevalence and outcomes of vascular cognitive impairment. Vascular Cognitive Impairment Investigators of the Canadian Study on Health and Aging. *Neurology* **54**: 447–451

Rockwood K, Kirkland S, Hogan DB. (2002) Use of lipid-lowering agents, indication bias, and the risk of dementia in community-dwelling elderly people. *Archives of Neurology* **59**: 223–237

Román GC. (1985a) The identity of lacunar dementia and Binswanger disease. *Medical Hypotheses* **16**: 389–391

Román GC. (1985b) Lacunar dementia. In: JT Hutton and AD Kenny (eds), *Senile Dementia of the Alzheimer Type*. New York, Alan R Liss Inc, pp. 131–151

Román GC. (1987) Senile dementia of the Binswanger type: a vascular form of dementia in the elderly. *JAMA* **258**: 1782–1788

Román GC. (1999a) Vascular dementia today. *Revue Neurologique (Paris)* **155** (Suppl. 4): S64–S72

Román GC. (1999b) Editorial: new insight into Binswanger disease. *Archives of Neurology* **56**: 1061–1062

Román GC. (1999c) [Hyperbaric oxygenation: a promising treatment for Binswanger's disease]. *Revista de Neurología (Barcelona)* **28**: 707

Román GC. (2000) Perspectives in the treatment of vascular dementia. *Drugs of Today* **36**: 641–653

Román GC. (2002a) Vascular dementia revisited: diagnosis, pathogenesis, treatment, and prevention. *Medical Clinics of North America* **86**: 477–499

Román GC. (2002b) Defining dementia: clinical criteria for the diagnosis of vascular dementia. *Acta Neurologica Scandinavica* **178** (Suppl.): 6–9

Román GC. (2002c) On the history of lacunes, état criblé, and the white matter lesions of vascular dementia. *Cerebrovascular Diseases* **13** (Suppl. 2): 1–6

Román GC. (2002d) Historical evolution of the concept of dementia: a systematic review from 2000 BC to AD (2000) In: N Qizilbash, LS Schneider, H Chui *et al.* (eds), *Evidence-based Dementia Practice*. Oxford, Blackwell Science, pp. 199–227

Román GC. (2002e) Vascular dementia may be the most common form of dementia in the elderly. *Journal of the Neurological Sciences* **203-204**: 7–10

Román GC. (2003a) Vascular dementia: distinguishing characteristics, treatment, and prevention. *Journal of the American Geriatrics Society* **51** (Suppl. 5): S296–S304

Román GC. (2003b) Stroke, cognitive decline and vascular dementia: the silent epidemic of the 21st century. *Neuroepidemiology* **22**: 161–164

Román GC. (2004) Brain hypoperfusion: a critical factor in vascular dementia. *Neurological Research* **26**: 454–458

Román GC. (2005) Cholinergic dysfunction in vascular dementia. *Current Psychiatric Reports* **7**: 18–26

Román GC and Royall DR. (1999) Executive control function: a rational basis for the diagnosis of vascular dementia. *Alzheimer Disease and Associated Disorders* **13** (Suppl. 3): S69–S80

Román GC and Rogers SJ. (2004) Donepezil: a clinical review of current and emerging indications. *Expert Opinion in Pharmacotherapy* **5**: 161–180

Román GC and Royall DR. (2004) A diagnostic dilemma: is 'Alzheimer's dementia' Alzheimer's disease. vascular dementia, or both? *Lancet Neurology* **3**:141

Román GC, Tatemichi TK, Erkinjuntti T *et al.* (1993) Vascular dementia: diagnostic criteria for research studies. Report of the NINDS-AIREN International Workshop. *Neurology* **43**: 250–260

Román GC, Erkinjuntti T, Wallin A *et al.* (2002) Subcortical ischaemic vascular dementia. *Lancet Neurology* **1**: 426–436

Román GC, Sachdev P, Royall DR *et al.* (2004) Vascular cognitive disorder: a new diagnostic category updating vascular cognitive impairment and vascular dementia. *Journal of the Neurological Sciences* **226**: 81–87

Rosen WG, Mohs RC, Davis KL. (1984) A new rating scale for Alzheimer's Disease. *American Journal of Psychiatry* **14**: 1356–1364

Rother M, Erkinjuntti T, Roessner M *et al.* (1998) Propentofylline in the treatment of Alzheimer's disease and vascular dementia: a review of phase III trials. *Dementia and Geriatric Cognitive Disorders* **9** (Suppl. 1): 36–43

Sabbatini M, Coppi G, Maggioni A *et al.* (1998) Effect of lesions of the nucleus basalis magnocellularis and of treatment with posatirelin on cholinergic neurotransmission enzymes in the rat cerebral cortex. *Mechanisms of Ageing and Development* **104**: 183–194

Sacks FM, Svetkey LP, Vollmer WM *et al.* for the DASH-Sodium Collaborative Research Group. (2001) Effects on blood pressure of reduced dietary sodium and the Dietary Approaches to Stop Hypertension (DASH) diet. *New England Journal of Medicine* **344**: 3–10

Sakurada T, Alufuzoff I, Winblad B, Nordberg A. (1990) Substance P-like immunoreactivity, choline acetyltransferase activity and cholinergic muscarinic receptors in Alzheimer's disease and multi-infarct dementia. *Brain Research* **521**: 329–332

Salloway S, Pratt RD, Perdomo CA, for the Donepezil 307 and 308 Study Groups. (2003) A comparison of the cognitive benefits of donepezil in patients with cortical versus subcortical vascular dementia: a subanalysis of two 24-week, randomized, double-blind, placebo-controlled trials. *Neurology* **60** (Suppl. 1): A141–A142

Samlaska CP and Winfield EA. (1994) Clinical review: pentoxifylline. *Journal of the American Academy of Dermatology* **30**: 603–621

Sarazin M, Amarenco P, Mikol J *et al.* (2002) Reversible leukoencephalopathy in cerebral amyloid angiopathy presenting as subacute dementia. *European Journal of Neurology* **9**: 353–358

Sato A, Sato Y, Uchida S. (2001) Regulation of regional cerebral blood flow by cholinergic fibers originating in the basal forebrain. *International Journal of Developmental Neuroscience* **19**: 327–337

Schneider LS and Olin JT. (1994) Overview of clinical trials of Hydergine in dementia. *Archives of Neurology* **51**: 787–798

Schneider R, Ringelstein EB, Kiesewetter H, Jung F. (1987) The role of plasma hyperviscosity in subcortical arteriosclerotic encephalopathy (Binswanger's disease). *Journal of Neurology* **234**: 67–73

Schneider LS, Olin JT, Doody RS *et al.* (1997) Validity and reliability of the Alzheimer's Disease Cooperative Study – Clinical Global Impression of Change. *Alzheimer Disease and Associated Disorders* **11**: S22–S32

Schulman S, Wahlander K, Lundstrom T *et al.* for the THRIVE III Investigators. (2003) Secondary prevention of venous thromboembolism with the oral direct thrombin inhibitor ximelagatran. *New England Journal of Medicine* **349**: 1713–1721

Secades JJ and Frontera G. (1995) CDP-choline: pharmacological and clinical review. *Methods and Findings in Experimental and Clinical Pharmacology* **17** (Suppl. B): 1–54

Selden NR, Gitelman DR, Salamon-Murayama N *et al.* (1998) Trajectories of cholinergic pathways within the cerebral hemispheres of the human brain. *Brain* **121**: 2249–22457

Semplicini A, Maresca A, Simonella C *et al.* (2000) Cerebral perfusion in hypertensives with carotid artery stenosis: a comparative study of lacidipine and hydrochlorothiazide. *Blood Pressure* **9**: 34–9

Seshadri S, Beiser A, Selhub J *et al.* (2002) Plasma homocysteine as a risk factor for dementia and Alzheimer's disease. *New England Journal of Medicine* **346**: 476–483

Shader RI, Harmatz JS, Salzman C. (1974) A new scale for clinical assessment in geriatric populations: Sandoz Clinical Assessment – Geriatric (SCAG). *Journal of the American Geriatrics Society* **22**: 107–113

Sherman DG. (2002) Ancrod. *Current Medical Research and Opinion* **18** (Suppl. 2): S48–S52

Shustov SB. (1997) Controlled clinical trial on the efficacy and safety of oral sulodexide in patients with peripheral occlusive arterial disease. *Current Medical Research and Opinion* **13**: 573–582

Skoog I, Lernfelt B, Landahl S. (1996) 15-year longitudinal study of blood pressure and dementia. *Lancet* **347**: 1141–1145

Skoog I, Marcusson J, Blennow K. (1998) Dementia: it's getting better all the time. *Lancet* **352** (Suppl. 4): S1–S4

Snowdon D, Greiner LH, Mortimer JA *et al.* (1997) Brain infarction and the clinical expression of Alzheimer disease. The Nun Study. *JAMA* **277**: 813–817

Solerte SB, Ceresini G, Ferrari E, Fioravanti M. (2000) Hemorheological changes and overproduction of cytokines from immune cells in mild to moderate dementia of the Alzheimer's type: adverse effects on cerebromicrovascular system. *Neurobiology of Aging* **21**: 271–281

Sonninen V and Savontaus ML. (1987) Hereditary multi-infarct dementia. *European Neurology* **27**: 209–215

Sourander P and Walinder J. (1977) Hereditary multi-infarct dementia. Morphological and clinical studies of a new disease. *Acta Neuropathologica (Berlin)* **39**: 247–254

Spiegel R, Brunner C, Ermini-Funfschilling D *et al.* (1991) A new behavioral assessment scale for geriatric out- and in-patients: the NOSGER (Nurses' Observation Scale for Geriatric Patients). *Journal of the American Geriatrics Society* **39**: 339–347

Starr JM, Whalley LJ, Deary IJ (1996) The effects of antihypertensive treatment on cognitive function: results from the HOPE study. *Journal of the American Geriatrics Society* **44**: 411–415

Stewart R and Liolitsa D. (1999) Type 2 diabetes mellitus, cognitive impairment and dementia. *Diabetic Medicine* **16**: 93–112

Sturmer T, Glynn RJ, Field TS *et al.* (1996) Aspirin use and cognitive function in the elderly. *American Journal of Epidemiology* **143**: 683–691

Swartz RH, Sahlas DJ, Black SE *et al.* (2003) Strategic involvement of cholinergic pathways and executive dysfunction: does location of white matter signal hyperintensity matter? *Journal of Stroke and Cerebrovascular Diseases* **12**: 29–36

Szatmari SZ and Whitehouse PJ. (2003) Vinpocetine for cognitive impairment and dementia. *Cochrane Database of Systematic Reviews* **1**: CD003119

Szilagyi AK, Nemeth A, Martini E *et al.* (1987) Serum and CSF cholinesterase activity in various kinds of dementia. *European Archives of Psychiatry and Neurological Sciences* **236**: 309–311

Tanne D, Benderly M, Goldbourt U et al. for the Bezafibrate Infarction Prevention Study Group. (2001) A prospective study of plasma fibrinogen levels and the risk of stroke among participants in the bezafibrate infarction prevention study. American Journal of Medicine 111: 457–463

Tariot PN, Farlow MR, Grossberg GT et al. for the Memantine Study Group. (2004). Memantine treatment in patients with moderate to severe Alzheimer disease already receiving donepezil: a randomized controlled trial. JAMA 291: 317–324

Tatemichi TK, Foulkes MA, Mohr JP et al. (1990) Dementia in stroke survivors in the Stroke Data Bank cohort: prevalence, incidence, risk factors, and computed tomographic findings. Stroke 21: 858–866

Tatemichi TK, Desmont DW, Prohovnik I et al. (1992) Confusion and memory loss from capsular genu infarction: a thalamocortical disconnection syndrome? Neurology 42: 1966–1979

Tatemichi TK, Desmont DW, Paik M et al. (1993) Clinical determinants of dementia related to stroke. Annals of Neurology 33: 568–575

Tatemichi TK, Desmont DW, Prohovnik I et al. (1995) Strategic infarcts in vascular dementia. A clinical and imaging experience. Arzneimittel-Forschung/Drug Research 45: 371–385

Tohgi H, Abe T, Kimura M et al. (1996) Cerebrospinal fluid acetylcholine and choline in vascular dementia of Binswanger and multiple small infarct types as compared with Alzheimer-type dementia. Journal of Neural Transmission 103: 1211–1220

Tomimoto H, Akiguchi I, Wakita H et al. (1999) Coagulation activation in patients with Binswanger disease. Archives of Neurology 56: 1104–1108

Tomimoto H, Akiguchi I, Ohtani R et al. (2001) The coagulation-fibrinolysis system in patients with leukoaraiosis and Binswanger disease. Archives of Neurology 58: 1620–1625

Toole JF, Malinow MR, Chambless LE et al. (2004) Lowering homocysteine in patients with ischemic stroke to prevent recurrent stroke, myocardial infarction, and death: the Vitamin Intervention for Stroke Prevention (VISP) randomized controlled trial. JAMA 291: 565–575

Traber WH and Gibsen J. (1989) Nimodipine and Central Nervous System Function: New Vistas. Stuttgart, Schattauaer-Verlag

Treves TA and Korczyn AD. (1999) Denbufylline in dementia: a double-blind controlled study. Dementia and Geriatric Cognitive Disorders 10: 505–510

Tzourio C, Dufouil C, Ducimetiere P, Alperovitch A. (1999) Cognitive decline in individuals with high blood pressure: a longitudinal study in the elderly. EVA Study Group. Epidemiology of Vascular Aging. Neurobiology 53: 1948–1952

Tzourio C, Anderson C, Chapman N et al. for the PROGRESS Collaborative Group. (2003). Effects of blood pressure lowering with perindopril and indapamide therapy on dementia and cognitive decline in patients with cerebrovascular disease. Archives of Internal Medicine 163: 1069–1075

Uchida S, Suzuki A, Kagitani F, Hotta H. (2000) Effects of age on cholinergic vasodilatation of cortical cerebral blood vessels in rats. Neuroscience Letters 294: 109–112

Uebelhack R, Vohs K, Zytowski M et al. (2003) Effect of piracetam on cognitive performance in patients undergoing bypass surgery. Pharmacopsychiatry 36: 89–93

Ulus IH, Wurtman RJ, Mauron C, Blusztajn JK. (1989) Choline increases acetylcholine release and protects against the stimulation-induced decrease in phosphatide levels within membranes of rat corpus striatum. Brain Research 484: 217–127

Vale S. (1998) Subarachnoid haemorrhage associated with Ginkgo biloba. Lancet 352: 36

van Bogaert L. (1955) Encéphalopathie sous-corticale progressive (Binswanger) à evolution rapide chez deux soeurs. Médecine Hellénique 24: 961–972

van Dongen M, van Rossum E, Kessels A et al. (2003) Ginkgo for elderly people with dementia and age-associated memory impairment: a randomized clinical trial. Journal of Clinical Epidemiology 56: 367–376

van Gijn J and Algra A. (2003) Aspirin and stroke prevention. Thrombosis Research 110: 349–353

Vataja R, Pohjasvaara T, Matyla R et al. (2003) MRI correlates of executive dysfunction in patients with ischaemic stroke. European Journal of Neurology 10: 625–631

Verhey FR, Lodder J, Rosendaal N, Jolles J. (1996) Comparison of seven sets of criteria used for the diagnosis of vascular dementia. Neuroepidemiology 15: 166–172

Vermeer SE, Den Heijer T, Koudstaal PJ et al. (2003) Silent brain infarcts and the risk of dementia and cognitive decline. New England Journal of Medicine 348: 1215–1222

Vernon MW and Sorkin EM. (1991) Piracetam: an overview of its pharmacological properties and a review of its therapeutic use in senile cognitive disorders. Drugs and Aging 1: 17–35

Vila JF, Balcarce PE, Abiusi GR et al. (1999) [Hyperbaric oxygenation in subcortical frontal syndrome due to small artery disorders with leukoaraiosis]. Revista de Neurología (Barcelona) 28, 655–660

Vinters HV, Ellis WG, Zarow C et al. (2000) Neuropathological substrate of ischemic vascular dementia. Journal of Neuropathology and Experimental Neurology 59: 931–945

Wadworth AN and Chrisp P. (1992) Co-dergocrine mesylate. A review of its pharmacodynamic and pharmacokinetic properties and therapeutic use in age-related cognitive decline. Drugs and Aging 2: 153–173

Waegemans T, Wilsher CR, Danniau A et al. (2002) Clinical efficacy of piracetam in cognitive impairment: a meta-analysis. Dementia and Geriatric Cognitive Disorders 13: 217–224

Wald DS, Law M, Morris JK. (2002) Homocysteine and cardiovascular disease: evidence on causality from a meta-analysis. BMJ 325: 1202

Wallin A and Gottfries CG. (1990) Biochemical substrates in normal aging and Alzheimer's disease. Pharmacopsychiatry 23: 37–43

Wallin A, Blennow K, Gottfries CG. (1989) Neurochemical abnormalities in vascular dementia. Dementia 1: 120–130

Walsh AC. (1968) Anticoagulant therapy as potentially effective method for the prevention of presenile dementia: two case reports. Journal of the American Geriatrics Society 16: 472–481

Walsh AC, Walsh BH, Melaney C. (1978) Senile-presenile dementia: follow-up data on an effective psychotherapy-anticoagulant regimen. Journal of the American Geriatrics Society 26: 467–470

Walzl M. (1993) Effect of heparin-induced extracorporeal low-density lipoprotein precipitation and bezafibrate on hemorheology and clinical symptoms in cerebral multiinfarct disease. Haemostasis 23: 192–202

Walzl M. (2000) A promising approach to the treatment of multi-infarct dementia. Neurobiology of Aging 21: 283–287

Watanabe H, Zhao Q, Matsumoto K et al. (2003) Pharmacological evidence for antidementia effect of Choto-san (Gouteng-san), a traditional Kampo medicine. Pharmacology Biochemistry and Behavior 75: 635–643

Weil C. (1988) Hydergine: Pharmacologic and Clinical Facts. Berlin, Springer-Verlag

Weitz JI and Crowther M. (2002) Direct thrombin inhibitors. Thrombosis Research 106: V275–V284

Wentzel C, Rockwood K, MacKnight C et al. (2001) Progression of impairment in patients with vascular cognitive impairment without dementia. Neurology 57: 714–716

Wentzel C, Fisk JD, Rockwood K. (2002) Neuropsychological predictors of incident dementia in patients with vascular cognitive impairment, without dementia. Stroke 33: 1999–2002

Wetterling T, Kanitz RD, Borgis KJ. (1996) Comparison of different diagnostic criteria for vascular dementia (ADDTC, DSM-IV, ICD-10, NINDS-AIREN). Stroke 27: 30–36

Whitehouse PJ, Kittner B, Roessner M et al. (1998) Clinical trial designs for demonstrating disease-course-altering effects in dementia. Alzheimer Disease and Associated Disorders 12: 281–294

Wilcock G, Möbius HJ, Stoffler A, the MMM 500 group. (2002) A double-blind, placebo-controlled multicentre study of memantine in mild to moderate vascular dementia (MMM 500). International Clinical Psychopharmacology 17: 297–305

Wilkinson D, Doody R, Helme R et al. (2003) Donepezil in vascular dementia. A randomized, placebo-controlled study. Neurology 61: 479–486

Willette RN, Shiloh AO, Sauermelch CF et al. (1997) Identification, characterization, and functional role of phosphodiesterase type IV in cerebral vessels: effects of selective phosphodiesterase inhibitors. Journal of Cerebral Blood Flow and Metabolism 17: 210–219

Williams B. (2004) Protection against stroke and dementia: an update on the latest clinical trial evidence. Current Hypertension Reports 6: 307–313

Williams PS, Rands G, Orrel M, Spector A. (2000) Aspirin for vascular dementia. Cochrane Database of Systematic Reviews 4: CD001296

Windisch M. (2000) Approach towards an integrative drug treatment of Alzheimer's disease. Journal of Neural Transmission 59: 301–313

Windisch M, Gschanes A, Hutter-Paier B. (1998) Neurotrophic activities and therapeutic experience with a brain derived peptide preparation. Journal of Neural Transmission 53 (Suppl.): 289–298

Wolkowitz OM, Kramer JH, Reus VI et al. for the DHEA-Alzheimer's Disease Collaborative Research. (2003) DHEA treatment of Alzheimer's disease: a randomized, double-blind, placebo-controlled study. Neurology 60: 1071–1076

World Health Organization. (1992) International Statistical Classification of Diseases and Related Health Problems, 10th Revision. Geneva, World Health Organization

Yamaguchi S, Matsubara M, Kobayashi S. (2004) Event-related brain potential changes after Choto-san administration in stroke patients with mild cognitive impairments. Psychopharmacology (Berlin) 171: 241–249

Yesavage JA, Tinkleberg JR, Hollister LE, Berger PA. (1979) Vasodilators in senile dementia: a review of the literature. Archives of General Psychiatry 36: 220–223

Zamrini E, Parrish JA, Parsons D, Harrell LE. (2004a) Medical comorbidity in black and white patients with Alzheimer's disease. Southern Medical Journal 97: 2–6

Zamrini E, McGwin G, Roseman JM. (2004b) Association between statin use and Alzheimer's disease. Neuroepidemiology 23: 94–98

Zanchetti A, Bond MG, Hennig M et al. for the ELSA Investigators. (2004) Absolute and relative changes in carotid intima-media thickness and atherosclerotic plaques during long-term antihypertensive treatment: further results of the European Lacidipine Study on Atherosclerosis (ELSA). Journal of Hypertension 22: 1201–1212

Zekry D, Hauw J-J, Gold G. (2002a) Mixed dementia: epidemiology, diagnosis, and treatment. Journal of the American Geriatrics Society 50: 1431–1438

Zekry D, Duyckaerts C, Belmin J et al. (2002b) Alzheimer's disease and brain infarcts in the elderly. Agreement with neuropathology. Journal of Neurology 249: 1529–1534

Zekry D, Duyckaerts C, Moulias R et al. (2002c) Degenerative and vascular lesions of the brain have synergistic effects in dementia of the elderly. Acta Neuropathologica (Berlin) 103: 481–487

Zhang BL, Wang YY, Chen RX. (2002) Clinical randomized double-blinded study on treatment of vascular dementia by jiannao yizhi granule. [Article in Chinese] Zhongguo Zhong Xi Yi Jie He Za Zhi [Chinese Journal of Integrated Traditional and Western Medicine] 22: 577–580

Zimmermann M, Colciaghi F, Cattabeni F, Di Luca M. (2002) Ginkgo biloba extract: from molecular mechanisms to the treatment of Alzheimer's disease. Cellular and Molecular Biology (Noisy-le-grand, France) 48: 613–623

PART 5

Dementia with Lewy bodies and Parkinson's disease

Dementia with Lewy bodies: a clinical overview

IAN G McKEITH

47.1 TERMINOLOGY, SPECTRUM AND EPIDEMIOLOGY

47.1.1 Dementia with Lewy bodies: what's in a name?

Dementia with Lewy bodies (DLB) is now the preferred term (McKeith *et al.*, 1996a) for a variety of clinical diagnoses including diffuse LB disease (DLBD) (Kosaka *et al.*, 1984; Dickson *et al.*, 1987; Lennox *et al.*, 1989), dementia associated with cortical Lewy bodies (DCLB) (Byrne *et al.*, 1991), the LB variant of Alzheimer's disease (LBVAD) (Hansen *et al.*, 1990; Förstl *et al.*, 1993), senile dementia of LB type (SDLT) (Perry *et al.*, 1989a, b; 1990) and LB dementia (LBD) (Gibb *et al.*, 1987). Initially thought to be uncommon, DLB is now thought to account for up to 20 per cent of all elderly cases of dementia reaching autopsy (Perry *et al.*, 1989a; Jellinger, 1996). This chapter reviews the evolution of clinical knowledge about the disorder. The term DLB is used throughout except when reference is made to specific reports in which authors have used alternative terminology. Pathology, neuropsychological changes and therapeutic aspects of DLB are considered in subsequent chapters.

47.1.2 The spectrum of Lewy body disease

Current thinking about Lewy body (LB) related disorders suggests that there is a spectrum of disease, the clinical presentation varying according to the site of LB formation and associated neuronal loss (Jackson *et al.*, 1995; Lowe *et al.*, 1996). Three broad patterns of disease can be identified:

- nigrostriatal involvement producing motor features of parkinsonism;

- cortical involvement producing cognitive impairment and neuropsychiatric symptoms;
- sympathetic nervous system involvement producing autonomic failure.

This may prove to be an oversimplified view since there are generally poor correlations between LB density and severity of clinical symptoms (Gómez-Tortosa *et al.*, 1999; Colosimo *et al.*, 2003). The majority of cases seen in clinical practice, particularly elderly patients, have a combination of these clinical features, reflecting multisite (diffuse) pathology. DLB is important in clinical practice because:

- it usually has a clinical presentation and course that differs from Alzheimer's disease (AD) and other non-AD dementias;
- the management of psychosis and behavioural disturbances, which are common in DLB, is complicated by sensitivity to neuroleptic medication;
- accumulating evidence (Chapter 50) suggests that DLB may be particularly amenable to treatment with cholinergic enhancers.

47.1.3 Epidemiology

Several studies in a range of settings have suggested that DLB accounts for just under 20 per cent of all cases of dementia referred for neuropathological autopsy (Perry *et al.*, 1989a, 1990; Jellinger, 1996). The male to female ratio in these autopsy series is 1.5:1, but it is unclear to what extent this represents increased male susceptibility to disease or reduced survival in men with DLB. A Finnish community study of people aged 85 and over found 5.0 per cent to meet Consensus Criteria for DLB (3.3 per cent probable, 1.7 per cent possible) representing 22 per cent of all demented cases (Rahkonen *et al.*, 2003), higher than that in a London-based community sample of people aged 65 and over, in which 10.9 per cent of demented cases had DLB, which is consistent with estimates of LB prevalence in a dementia case register followed to autopsy (Holmes *et al.*, 1999). Twenty-six per cent of clinical referrals to an old age psychiatry service with dementia (Shergill *et al.*, 1994; Stevens *et al.*, 2002) and 24 per cent of demented day hospital attenders met clinical criteria for DLB (Ballard *et al.*, 1993).

Age at onset in reported series ranges from 50–83 years to 68–92 years at death (Papka *et al.*, 1998). Survival in DLB was initially reported as being significantly reduced compared with AD, but more recent series have not confirmed a general tendency to reduced survival or more rapid cognitive decline. It is possible that mean values could conceal disease heterogeneity, and survival times in DLB may be skewed to the left (McKeith, 1998) with very rapid progression in a few individuals (Armstrong *et al.*, 1991). Classical epidemiological studies to determine age and sex variation and potential risk factors for DLB have not yet been reported.

47.2 HISTORICAL DEVELOPMENTS AND DIAGNOSTIC CRITERIA FOR DEMENTIA WITH LEWY BODIES

47.2.1 Early case reports

When Friedrich Lewy first described the eosinophilic, neuronal inclusions that we now call Lewy bodies, in the brain stem of patients with paralysis agitans (Parkinson's disease – PD), he did not associate the inclusions with cognitive impairment and psychiatric disorder (Forster and Lewy, 1912). This was despite half of his sample being clinically demented and a quarter having mood disorders, hallucinations and paranoid delusions (Förstl and Levy, 1991). Although Woodard (1962) cites Hassler (1938) as reporting cortical Lewy bodies in association with dementia, the first case reports specifically describing patients with DLB did not appear until 1961 when Okazaki *et al.* (1961) published two cases, both elderly men, presenting with cognitive decline and subsequently developing severe dementia. Over the next 20 years, 34 similar cases were reported, all by Japanese workers. Kosaka *et al.* (1984) noted a 3:1 male predominance, with memory disturbance as the presenting feature in 67 per cent, psychotic states (*sic*) in 17 per cent and dizziness due to orthostatic hypotension in 17 per cent. Progressive dementia with muscular rigidity occurred eventually in 80 per cent although only 25 per cent of cases were diagnosed as parkinsonian. The first substantial listing of these Japanese cases in the Western literature was in 1987 by Gibb *et al.* (1987) who added four new UK cases.

47.2.2 Early diagnostic criteria

The following year, Burkhardt *et al.* (1988) listed 34 cases and carried out a simple meta-analysis. The most common

presentation was a 'neurobehavioural syndrome'; memory impairment and other cognitive deficits were typical, all but one patient eventually becoming demented. Psychotic features such as depression, hallucinations and paranoia were seen in 10 patients (29 per cent), two being psychotic for many years before developing other symptoms. Parkinsonian features, the most common of which was rigidity, were usually overshadowed by dementia; in only five cases (15 per cent) were no extrapyramidal features present. Duration of illness was very variable (1–20 years) with an end state of severe dementia, rigidity, akinetic mutism, quadriparesis in flexion and emaciation. The most common reported cause of death was aspiration pneumonia. Based upon these observations, Burkhardt *et al.* (1988) were the first to attempt a general description of the clinical syndrome associated with diffuse Lewy body disease, distinguishing it as separate from PD with dementia. They concluded that 'DLBD should be suspected in any elderly patient who presents with a rapidly progressive dementia, followed in short order by rigidity and other parkinsonian features. Myoclonus may be present.'

Crystal *et al.* (1990) in a paper entitled 'Antemortem diagnosis of diffuse Lewy body disease', criticized this approach on the grounds that 'extrapyramidal features occur in many patients with severe AD and since dementia occurs in many subjects with PD, the clinical criteria for the diagnosis of DLBD remain unclear'. The authors proposed alternative criteria of 'progressive dementia with gait disorder, psychiatric symptoms and a burst pattern on EEG at the time of moderate dementia'. No particular characteristics of the pattern of cognitive impairment were noted.

Although these early clinical definitions were important in drawing attention to the existence of DLB and describing some of its salient characteristics, neither could be regarded as satisfactory for clinical diagnostic purposes, since they lacked detail and were not operationalized in a way which would allow acceptable interrater reliability (Hansen and Galasko, 1992).

47.2.3 The Nottingham Group for the Study of Neurodegenerative Disorders

In 1989, Byrne *et al.* (1989) reviewed the situation, citing 51 pathologically confirmed cases and remarking upon the brevity of clinical details in most of these. Gibb *et al.* (1987) were among the first to describe fluctuating levels of consciousness and episodic confusion, now recognized as key features of DLB.

The Nottingham group reported the clinical characteristics of 15 new UK cases in considerable detail, the largest individual series published at that time (Byrne *et al.*, 1989). Seven were men, the mean age at onset was 72 years and the mean duration of illness, 5.5 years. Forty per cent presented with symptoms and signs of idiopathic PD, with cognitive impairment occurring 1–4 years later. A further 20 per cent had parkinsonism and mild cognitive impairment at presentation and the remaining 40 per cent showed motor features later in their illnesses, gait disturbance and postural abnormalities being most common. These latter cases presented with neuropsychiatric features only, in various combinations of cognitive impairment, paranoid delusions and visual or auditory hallucinations; 14 of the 15 were demented before death, the exception presenting with classic PD and later becoming depressed, irritable and mildly forgetful with frequent falls. Fluctuating cognition with episodic confusion for which no adequate underlying cause could be found, was observed in 80 per cent of the Nottingham cases. Byrne *et al.* (1989) also drew attention to the frequent occurrence of depression (20 per cent) and psychosis (33 per cent). This led to the first formal proposal of operational criteria for dementia associated with cortical Lewy bodies (DCLB) (Byrne *et al.*, 1991) – see Box 47.1.

The presence of extrapyramidal features was mandatory although these could be mild and occur late in the course of the illness. Since at least 25 per cent of DLB cases reported in the whole literature (McKeith, 1997; Kosaka and Iseki, 1998; Papka *et al.*, 1998) never have motor parkinsonism, the sensitivity of

the Nottingham criteria was inevitably restricted by this requirement, which may have been influenced by the inclusion in their sample of five cases who had motor only PD diagnosed for at least 12 months before neuropsychiatric features developed. These cases would according to current criteria (McKeith *et al.* 1996a) be regarded as having PD + dementia and not a primary diagnosis of DLB (see section below on patients previously diagnosed with PD for further discussion of this).

47.2.4 The Newcastle criteria

At around the same time, Perry *et al.* identified 14 cases with the neuropathological features of 'senile dementia of Lewy body type' (SDLT) (Perry *et al.*, 1989a, b, 1990) accounting for 15 per cent of a series of dementia autopsies. These SDLT cases had been regarded as clinically atypical 'causing much diagnostic perplexity'. Acute onset, fluctuating course, more rapid deterioration, early and prominent hallucinatory and behavioural disturbances, and associated mild parkinsonian

---

Box 47.1 *Nottingham criteria for dementia associated with cortical Lewy bodies (Byrne* et al., *1991, reproduced by kind permission of S. Karger AG, Basel)*

A, B, C and D should be present for a diagnosis to be made of *probable* dementia associated with cortical Lewy bodies

A Either 1, 2 or 3
1. Gradual onset of dementia syndrome (which fulfils DSM-IIIR criteria) with prominent attentional deficits
or
The appearance early in the course of apparent acute confusional states for which no underlying toxic, metabolic, infective or other cause is identified
or
2. 'Classical' Parkinson's disease (defined as levodopa responsive parkinsonism) at onset with the later emergence of dementia syndrome (as described in 1)
or
3. The simultaneous occurrence at onset of dementia (as described in 1) and parkinsonism

B Both 1 and 2 should be fulfilled
1. The absence of any unequivocal history of stroke
2. No focal signs other than parkinsonism

C Three of more of the following should be present
1. Tremor
2. Rigidity
3. Postural change
4. Bradykinesia
5. Gait abnormality
These symptoms may be mild and may develop late in the course of the illness, and abnormal involuntary movements resulting from levodopa treatment are unusual in parkinsonism with cortical Lewy bodies

D Other causes of dementia syndrome or parkinsonism have been excluded (eg boxer's encephalopathy, chronic phenothiazine poisoning), after thorough clinical and laboratory investigation

A, B, C and D should be present to make a diagnosis of *possible* dementia associated with cortical Lewy bodies

A Either 1 or 2
1. Dementia (as described above) with acute onset and rapid course, sometimes associated with plateaux (periods where the symptoms do not progress) and frequently associated with psychiatric symptoms (depression or delusional states)
or
Dementia (as described above) with late presentation of parkinsonian symptoms which fulfil B

B One or two of the following
1. Tremor
2. Rigidity
3. Bradykinesia
4. Postural change
5. Gait abnormality

C Both 1 and 2 should be fulfilled
1. The absence of any unequivocal history of stroke
2. No focal signs other than parkinsonism

D Other causes of dementia syndrome and parkinsonism have been excluded, after thorough clinical and laboratory investigation

Source: Nottingham Group for the Study of Neurodegenerative Disorders

Table 47.1a   *Mental state symptoms in Newcastle upon Tyne autopsy confirmed cases of senile dementia of Lewy body type (SDLT, n = 21) and dementia of Alzheimer type (DAT, n = 20). (From McKeith et al., 1992a – figures are percentages of patients)*

Symptom	Symptoms at presentation		Symptoms occurring after presentation		Symptoms occurring at any stage	
	SDLT	DAT	SDLT	DAT	SDLT	DAT
Fluctuating cognitive impairment	81.0	10.8¶	4.8	8.1	86.0	18.9¶
Clouding of consciousness	38.1	8.1†	43.0	8.1†	81.0	13.5¶
Visual hallucinations	33.3	8.1*	14.0	8.1	47.6	16.2†
Auditory hallucinations	14.3	2.7	4.8	0	19.0	2.7*
Paranoid delusions	47.6	8.1†	9.5	2.7	57.1	10.8†
Depression (total)	38.1	16.2*	0	5.4	38.1	21.6*
Depression (major)	14.3	0*	0	5.4	14.3	5.4
Depression (minor)	23.8	16.2	0	0	23.8	16.2

Comparisons made using Fisher's exact test
* $P < 0.05$
† $P < 0.01$
‡ $P < 0.001$
¶ $P < 0.0001$

Table 47.1b   *Physical symptoms in Newcastle upon Tyne autopsy confirmed cases of senile dementia of Lewy body type (SDLT, n = 21) and dementia of Alzheimer type (DAT, n = 20). (From McKeith et al., 1992a – figures are percentages of patients)*

Symptom	Symptoms at presentation		Symptoms occurring after presentation		Symptoms occurring at any stage	
	SDLT	DAT	SDLT	DAT	SDLT	DAT
Unexplained falls	38.1	5.4†	4.8	5.4	43.0	10.8*
Observed disturbances of consciousness	4.8	0	38.1	5.4†	43.0	5.4†
Parkinsonian features:	9.5	8.1	62.0	21.6†	71.0	29.7*
1) rigidity	0	5.4	52.4	24.3	52.4	29.7
2) tremor	4.8	5.4	28.6	10.8	33.3	16.2
3) hypokinesia	9.5	5.4	52.4	13.5†	62.0	18.9†
4) hypersalivation	4.8	0	4.8	0	9.5	0
5) drug-induced parkinsonism	0	0	57.1	16.2†	57.1	16.2†
pyramidal signs	4.8	2.7	14.3	18.9	19.0	21.6

Comparisons made using Fisher's exact test
* $P < 0.05$
† $P < 0.01$
‡ $P < 0.001$
¶ $P < 0.0001$
Both tables reproduced by kind permission of Cambridge University Press

features were present. In 1992, McKeith and colleagues published further clinical details of two separate SDLT cohorts (21 and 20 cases respectively) and compared these with autopsy-confirmed AD (n = 57) cases (McKeith *et al.*, 1992a, b). SDLT patients were predominantly male (25:16) with mean survival reduced by about 50 per cent compared with AD. Tables 47.1a and 47.1b show clinical details of the first series of cases.

Depressive symptoms, unexplained falls, observed disturbances of consciousness and excessive sensitivity to side effects of neuroleptic medication were added to the list of clinical characteristics with potential to distinguish DLB pathology cases from AD.

Based upon these observations, an attempt was made to describe the typical course of illness (McKeith *et al.*, 1992a) and new clinical diagnostic criteria proposed with an emphasis upon cognitive dysfunction and neuropsychiatric features that could occur in the absence of extrapyramidal motor signs (Box 47.2).

The first stage is often recognized only in retrospect and may extend back 1–3 years prepresentation with occasional minor episodes of forgetfulness, sometimes described as lapses of concentration or 'switching off'. A brief period of delirium is sometimes noted for the first time, often associated with genuine physical illness and/or surgical procedures.

Box 47.2 *Operational criteria for senile dementia of Lewy body type (SDLT)*

A Fluctuating cognitive impairment affecting both memory and higher cortical functions (such as language, visuospatial ability, praxis or reasoning skills). The fluctuation is marked with the occurrence of both episodic confusion and lucid intervals, as in delirium, and is evident either on cognitive testing or by variable performance in daily living skills

B At least one of the following:
1. Visual and/or auditory hallucinations which are usually accompanied by secondary paranoid delusions
2. Mild spontaneous extrapyramidal features or neuroleptic sensitivity syndrome, i.e. exaggerated adverse responses to standard doses of neuroleptic medication
3. Repeated unexplained falls and/or transient clouding or loss of consciousness

C Despite the fluctuating pattern, the clinical features persist over a long period of time (weeks or months) unlike delirium which rarely persists as long. The illness progresses, often rapidly, to an end stage of severe dementia

D Exclusion of any underlying physical illness adequate to account for the fluctuating cognitive state, by appropriate examination and investigation

E Exclusion of past history of confirmed stroke and/or evidence of cerebral ischaemic damage on physical examination or brain imaging

Disturbed sleep, nightmares and daytime drowsiness often persist after recovery.

Progression to the second stage frequently prompts psychiatric or medical referral. A more sustained cognitive impairment is established, albeit with marked fluctuations in severity. Recurrent confusional episodes are accompanied by vivid hallucinatory experiences, visual misidentification syndromes and topographical disorientation. Extensive medical screening is usually negative. Attentional deficits are apparent as apathy, and daytime somnolence and sleep behaviour disorder may be severe. Gait disorder and bradykinesia are often overlooked, particularly in elderly subjects. Frequent falls occur owing to either postural instability or syncope.

The third and final stage often begins with a sudden increase in behavioural disturbance leading to requests for sedation or hospital admission by perplexed and exhausted carers. The natural course from this point is variable and obscured by the high incidence of adverse reactions to neuroleptic medication. For patients not receiving, or tolerating, neuroleptics, a progressive decline into severe dementia with dysphasia and dyspraxia occurs over months or years, with death usually due to cardiac or pulmonary disease. During this terminal phase patients show continuing behavioural disturbance including vocal and motor responses to hallucinatory phenomena. Lucid intervals with some retention of recent memory function and insight may still be apparent. Neurological disability is often profound with fixed flexion deformities of the neck and trunk and severe gait impairment.

Applied retrospectively to the original sample of autopsy-confirmed cases, these criteria identified 71 per cent of SDLT cases on initial presentation and 86 per cent between presentation and death (McKeith *et al.*, 1992a). Although some of the SDLT cases also met clinical criteria for AD, no AD cases met the proposed criteria for SDLT. Mega *et al.* (1996) reported a sensitivity of 50 per cent and a specificity of 71 per cent for the Newcastle criteria in a similar case note study.

Applied to another independent sample of DLB, AD and vascular dementia (VaD) patients, the Newcastle criteria yielded a 74 per cent sensitivity rate, averaged across four raters, and a specificity of 95 per cent. Interrater agreement was highest and diagnosis most accurate (90 per cent versus 55 per cent sensitivity) among more experienced clinicians. The most common errors among less experienced clinicians were failure to recognize cognitive fluctuations unique to DLB patients, and a tendency to overvalue comorbid disease as responsible for the clinical presentation (McKeith *et al.*, 1994a).

47.2.5 The Consensus criteria

By the early 1990s it was becoming apparent that DLB was a relatively common cause of dementia in old age and that the several research groups investigating it were adopting different terminologies for what were essentially the same patients. The Consortium on DLB therefore met in October 1995 to agree common clinical and pathological methods and nomenclature. The Consensus clinical criteria (McKeith *et al.*, 1996a) (Box 47.3) are largely based on the previous Newcastle scheme, but do differ in some important aspects.

The particular characteristics of the cognitive impairments of DLB are described in some detail as differing from the dementia syndrome of AD, in which memory deficits predominate. In DLB, attentional deficits and prominent visuospatial dysfunction are the main features (Sahgal *et al.*, 1992, 1995; Salmon and Galasko, 1996). Symptoms of persistent or prominent memory impairment are not always present early in the course of illness, although with disease progression they are likely to develop in most patients. DLB patients therefore perform better than AD patients on tests of verbal recall, but relatively worse on tests of copying and drawing (Gnanalingham *et al.*, 1997). With the progression of dementia, this selective pattern of cognitive deficits may be lost, making differential diagnosis based on neuropsychological examination difficult during the later stages. Probable DLB can be diagnosed if any two of the three key symptoms in Box 47.3 are present, namely fluctuation, visual hallucinations, or spontaneous motor features of parkinsonism and possible DLB if only one is present.

Box 47.3 *Consensus criteria for the clinical diagnosis of probable and possible dementia with Lewy bodies (DLB). Reproduced by kind permission of Lippincott, Williams & Wilkins. From McKeith IG, Galasko D, Kosaka K et al. (1996a) Consensus guidelines for the clinical and pathological diagnosis of dementia with Lewy bodies (DLB): report of the consortium on DLB international workshop.* Neurology **47**: 1113–1124

1 The central feature required for a diagnosis of DLB is progressive cognitive decline of sufficient magnitude to interfere with normal social or occupational function. Prominent or persistent memory impairment may not necessarily occur in the early stages but is usually evident with progression. Deficits on tests of attention and of fronto-subcortical skills and visuospatial ability may be especially prominent

2 Two of the following core features are essential for a diagnosis of *probable* DLB, one is essential for *possible* DLB:
   a) Fluctuating cognition with pronounced variations in attention and alertness
   b) Recurrent visual hallucinations which are typically well formed and detailed
   c) Spontaneous motor features of parkinsonism

3 Features supportive of the diagnosis are:
   a) Repeated falls
   b) Syncope
   c) Transient loss of consciousness
   d) Neuroleptic sensitivity
   e) Systematized delusions
   f) Hallucinations in other modalities

4 A diagnosis of DLB is less likely in the presence of:
   a) Stroke disease, evident as focal neurological signs or on brain imaging
   b) Evidence on physical examination and investigation of any physical illness, or other brain disorder, sufficient to account for the clinical picture

Several retrospective and two prospective studies have examined the predictive accuracy of Consensus clinical criteria for probable DLB (Litvan *et al.*, 2003) (Table 47.2). These show that sensitivity of case detection is variable and although high in one prospective study (McKeith *et al.*, 2000) was unacceptably low in several others. In contrast, specificity is generally found to be high, suggesting that the clinical criteria for probable DLB are best used for confirmation of diagnosis (few false positives) whereas those for possible DLB may be of more value in screening but have a relatively high false negative rate. Improved methods of identifying the core feature 'fluctuation' have potential to increase diagnostic accuracy (Walker *et al.*, 2000a; Ferman *et al.*, 2004; Bradshaw *et al.*, 2004) as do biological markers such as FP-CIT SPECT neuroimaging (O'Brien *et al.*, 2004).

47.2.5.1 REPORT OF THE SECOND INTERNATIONAL WORKSHOP OF THE CONSORTIUM ON DLB

The Second International DLB Workshop met in July 1998 (McKeith *et al.*, 1999). The objectives were to review developments since publication of the Consensus guidelines and to determine whether these yet require to be modified. It was recommended that the clinical Consensus criteria should continue to be used in their current format although two additional features, supportive of a diagnosis of DLB, were identified.

47.2.5.2 RECENT DEVELOPMENTS

In an effort to further review and clarify current knowledge, concepts and methods for further enquiry, a specialist meeting was held in November 2002 by the International Psychogeriatric Association (IPA) with input from the European Movement Disorder Society (MDS). The product of this

Table 47.2 *Diagnostic accuracy of dementia with Lewy bodies. Consensus criteria validated against autopsy. (Adapted from Litvan et al., 2003)*

Reference	Numbers of cases and pathological diagnosis	Probable/possible category	Sensitivity	Specificity	PPV	NPV
Mega *et al.*, 1996	4 DLB/24 AD	Prob.	75	79	100	93
		Poss.	NA	NA	NA	NA
Litvan *et al.*, 1998	14 DLB/105 PD, PSP, MSA, CBD, AD		18	99	75	89
Holmes *et al.*, 1999	9 DLB/80 AD and VaD	Prob.	22	100	100	91
		Poss.	NA	NA	NA	NA
Luis *et al.*, 1999	35 DLB/56 AD	Prob.	57	90	91	56
		Poss.	NA	NA	NA	NA
Verghese *et al.*, 1999	18 DLB/94 AD	Prob.	61	84	48	90
		Poss.	89	28	23	91
Lopez *et al.*, 1999	8 DLB/40 AD		0	100	0	80
Hohl *et al.*, 2000	5 DLB/10 AD	Prob.	100	8	83	100
		Poss.	100	0	NA	NA
McKeith *et al.*, 2000	29 DLB/50 AD and VaD	Prob.	83	95	96	80
		Poss.	NA	NA	NA	NA
Lopez *et al.*, 2002	13 DLB/26 AD	Prob.	23	100	100	43
		Poss.	NA	NA	NA	NA

AD, Alzheimer's disease; CBD, corticobasal degeneration; DLB, dementia with Lewy bodies; MSA, multisystem atrophy; NA, not available; NPV, negative predictive value; PD, Parkinson's disease; PPV, positive predictive value; PSP, progressive supranuclear palsy; VaD, vascular dementia international meeting was a systematic review of the current state of scientific knowledge about DLB that identified key issues requiring clarification and research necessary to advance knowledge in this area (McKeith *et al.*, 2004a). The Third Meeting of the International Consortium on DLB in September 2003 suggested revisions to the clinical and pathological diagnostic criteria and devised the first treatment algorithm. The Consortium also incorporated discussions about Parkinson's disease with dementia (PDD) in view of emerging clinical and pathological evidence that DLB and PDD share more similarities than was previously supposed (Emre, 2003). A report of this meeting will be published in 2005 and the new recommendations about assessment and diagnosis of DLB will be accompanied by guidelines for patient management (McKeith *et al.*, submitted for publication).

47.3 DIFFERENTIAL DIAGNOSIS OF DEMENTIA WITH LEWY BODIES IN CLINICAL PRACTICE

47.3.1 Clinical presentations of DLB

DLB patients may present to psychiatric services (cognitive impairment, psychosis or behavioural disturbance), internal medicine (acute confusional state or syncope) or neurology (movement disorder or disturbed consciousness). The details of clinical assessment and differential diagnoses will to a large extent be shaped by these symptom and specialty biases (McKeith *et al.*, 1995; Barber *et al.*, 2001). In all cases a detailed history from patient and reliable informants should document the time of onset of relevant key symptoms, the nature of their progression, and their effects on social, occupational and personal function.

47.3.1.1 COGNITIVE IMPAIRMENT

Although brief bedside tests of mental status may confirm the presence of cognitive impairment, more detailed psychometric examination is usually required to reveal a profile of deficits that helps to distinguish DLB from AD or other dementias. Prominent deficits on tests of executive function and problem solving, such as the Trail Making Test and verbal fluency for categories and letters, may be useful clinical discriminators (Salmon and Galasko, 1996), as may disproportional impairment on tests of visuospatial performance (Sahgal *et al.*, 1995; Gnanalingham *et al.*, 1997). Walker *et al.* (1996) tested DLB and AD patients with the CAMCOG battery, which is widely used in clinical practice. Although the mean, total CAMCOG scores were identical, significant differences were found in mean scores for the delayed recall subtest (DLB performing better) and the visuospatial praxis subtest (DLB performing worse). Disproportionately severe impairment on computer-based tasks of attentional function are characteristic of DLB (Ayre *et al.*, 1996) and wide test–retest variation in performance of such tasks (Walker *et al.*, 2000b) may ultimately provide a

reliable and widely applicable quantified measure well correlated with clinical expert estimates of fluctuating performance.

47.3.1.2 CORE FEATURES

A review of nine studies, which reported clinical details on 190 autopsy-confirmed DLB cases and compared them with 261 AD cases, provided a useful source of prevalence and incidence of the core features of DLB (Byrne *et al.*, 1989; McKeith *et al.*, 1992a, b; Förstl *et al.*, 1993; Galasko *et al.*, 1996; Klatka *et al.*, 1996; Hely *et al.*, 1996; Weiner *et al.*, 1996; Ala *et al.*, 1997; McKeith, 1998). The wide frequency ranges reported most likely reflect sampling biases and different methods of symptom ascertainment.

Fluctuation. Fluctuations in cognitive function, which may vary over minutes, hours or days, occur in 58 per cent of DLB cases at the time of presentation (range 8–85 per cent) and are observed at some point during the course of the illness in 75 per cent (45–90 per cent). Substantial changes in mental state and behaviour may be seen within the duration of a single interview or between consecutive examinations. Fluctuation includes, and indeed may be based on, pronounced variations in attention and alertness. Excessive daytime drowsiness with transient confusion on waking commonly occurs. Such episodes may last from a few seconds to several hours leading to misdiagnosis of transient ischaemic attack, with obvious implications for misdiagnosis of dementia subtype. These can be assessed by caregiver report, observer rating (Walker *et al.*, 2000a) or using computer-based measures of variation in attentional performance (Walker *et al.*, 2000b). Questions such as, 'Are there episodes when his/her thinking seems quite clear and then becomes muddled?' may be useful probes (Ballard *et al.*, 1993, Bradshaw *et al.*, 2004), although Ferman *et al.* (2004) found carers reports of fluctuation to be less reliable predictors of DLB diagnosis than more objective questions about daytime sleepiness, episodes of staring blankly or incoherent speech.

Visual hallucinations. Visual hallucinations are present in 33 per cent of DLB cases at the time of presentation (range 11–64 per cent) and occur at some point during the course of the illness in 46 per cent (13–80 per cent). Well-formed, detailed and animate figures are experienced, provoking emotional responses varying through fear, amusement or indifference, usually with some insight into the unreality of the episode once it is over. It is the persistence of visual hallucinations in DLB (McShane *et al.*, 1995) that helps distinguish them from the episodic perceptual disturbances that occur transiently in dementias of other aetiology or during a delirium provoked by an external cause (McKeith *et al.*, 1996a). It has been suggested that they arise from a combination of faulty perceptual processing of environmental stimuli, and less detailed recollection of experience, combined with intact image generation (Barnes *et al.*, 2003; Collerton *et al.*, in press) Visual hallucinations in DLB are associated with greater deficits in cortical acetylcholine (Perry *et al.*, 1991) and predict better response to cholinesterase inhibitors (McKeith *et al.*, 2004b).

Motor parkinsonism. Extrapyramidal signs (EPS) are reported in 25–50 per cent of DLB cases at diagnosis and the majority develop some EPS during the natural course. Up to 25 per cent of autopsy-confirmed cases may, however, have no record of EPS indicating that parkinsonism is not necessary for clinical diagnosis of DLB and indeed the principal cause for 'missing' DLB clinically in a prospective clinico-pathological study was the absence of EPS (McKeith *et al.*, 2000). Initial suggestions that parkinsonism in DLB is mild have not been supported by studies finding equal severity with non-demented PD patients (Aarsland *et al.*, 2001) with similar annual progression rates in United Parkinson's Disease Rating Scale (UPDRS) motor scores (Ballard *et al.*, 2000). The pattern of EPS in DLB shows an axial bias, e.g. greater postural instability and facial impassivity, with a tendency towards less tremor and consistent with greater 'non-dopaminergic' motor involvement (Burn *et al.*, 2003).

47.3.1.3 SUPPORTIVE FEATURES

Repeated falls, syncope, and transient losses of consciousness. Dementia of any aetiology is probably a risk factor for all three of these clinical features and it can be difficult clearly to distinguish between them. Repeated falls may be due to posture, gait and balance difficulties, particularly in patients with parkinsonism. Reported fall rates are 28 per cent at the time of presentation (range 10–38 per cent) and 37 per cent (22–50 per cent) at some point during the illness. Syncopal attacks in DLB with complete loss of consciousness and muscle tone may represent the extension of LB associated pathology to involve the brain stem and autonomic nervous system (as described in Section 47.1.2, p. 603). The associated phenomenon of transient episodes of unresponsiveness without loss of muscle tone may represent one extreme of fluctuating attention and cognition. Episodes of this type were recorded in 15 per cent of DLB cases at presentation and in 46 per cent during the whole course of illness (McKeith *et al.*, 1992a, b).

Neuroleptic sensitivity. The hypothesis made by the Newcastle group, of an abnormal sensitivity to adverse effects of neuroleptic medication was based upon two sets of independent observations. In the first (McKeith *et al.*, 1992a) 67 per cent (14/21) DLB patients received neuroleptics and 57 per cent (8/14) deteriorated rapidly after either receiving them for the first time, or following a dose increase. Mean survival time for these eight patients was reduced to 7.4 months (95 per cent CI 3.5–11.3) significantly less than for the six patients who had only mild to no adverse reaction, 28.5 months (12.9–44.1), and the seven never receiving neuroleptics, 17.8 months (−7.4–43.0). In the second study 54 per cent (7/16) neuroleptic treated DLB patients had neuroleptic sensitivity reactions and their mortality risk, estimated by survival analysis was increased by a factor of 2.7 (McKeith *et al.*, 1992b). Although this phenomenon had not previously been reported, literature review reveals that a small number of case reports of rapid deterioration following neuroleptic use were published from 1988 onwards (McKeith *et al.*, 1996b). A severe adverse reaction to neuroleptic medication may be an important indicator of underlying LB disorder but is of more importance in management than in the diagnostic process, especially if neuroleptic prescribing is routinely and desirably avoided in patients suspected of having DLB (Committee on Safety of Medicines, 1994). Newer atypical antipsychotics used at low dose may be safer in this regard but sensitivity reactions have been documented with most and they should be used with great caution (McKeith *et al.*, 2004a).

Systematized delusions and hallucinations in other modalities. Delusions are common in DLB, in 56 per cent at the time of presentation and 65 per cent at some point during the illness (McKeith *et al.*, 1992a, b). They are usually based on recollections of hallucinations and perceptual disturbances and consequently often have a fixed, complex and bizarre content that contrasts with the mundane and often poorly formed persecutory ideas encountered in AD patients, which are based on forgetfulness and confabulation.

Auditory hallucinations occur in 19 per cent (13–30 per cent) at presentation and 19 per cent (13–45 per cent) at any point. Together with olfactory and tactile hallucinations, these may be important features in some DLB cases and can lead to initial diagnoses of late onset psychosis (Birkett *et al.*, 1992) and temporal lobe epilepsy (McKeith *et al.*, 1992a).

Sleep disorder. Rapid eye movement (REM) sleep behaviour disorder (SBD) is a parasomnia manifested by vivid and often frightening dreams associated with simple or complex motor behaviour during REM sleep. It is frequently associated with DLB, PD and multisystem atrophy (MSA) but rarely occurs in AD (Boeve *et al.*, 2001). REM sleep-wakefulness dissociations (SBD, daytime hypersomnolence, hallucinations, cataplexy), characteristic of narcolepsy may explain several features of DLB. Sleep disorders may contribute to fluctuations typical of DLB and their treatment may improve fluctuations and quality of life (Ferman *et al.*, 2001).

Depression. Depressive symptoms are reported in 33–50 per cent of DLB cases, a rate higher than in AD and similar to that in PD. In the first Newcastle clinical study (McKeith *et al.*, 1992a), depression was diagnosed at presentation in 38 per cent (AD = 16 per cent, $P < 0.05$, χ^2), and was the primary reason for referral in five of the eight patients in whom it was present. Klatka *et al.* (1996) found depression in 14/28 (50 per cent) DLB, 8/58 (14 per cent) AD and 15/26 (58 per cent) PD cases with autopsy diagnosis, and Papka *et al.* (1998) suggest that depression is sufficiently more common in DLB than AD to be a significant diagnostic predictor.

47.3.2 Differential diagnosis

There are four main categories of disorder that should be considered in the differential diagnosis of DLB. These are:

- other dementia syndromes
- other causes of delirium
- other neurological syndromes
- other psychiatric disorders.

47.3.2.1 OTHER DEMENTIA SYNDROMES

Sixty five per cent of autopsy-confirmed DLB cases meet the NINCDS-ADRDA clinical criteria for probable or possible AD (McKeith *et al.*, 1994b) and this is the most frequent clinical misdiagnosis of DLB patients who present with a primary dementia syndrome. Between 12 and 36 per cent of cases meeting NINCDS criteria for a clinical diagnosis of AD are unexpectedly found to have LB pathology at autopsy (Burns *et al.*, 1990; Hansen *et al.*, 1990). This suggests that DLB routinely should be excluded before the diagnosis of AD is made. Up to a third of DLB cases are additionally misclassified as VaD by the Hachinski Ischaemic Index by virtue of items such as fluctuating nature and course of illness. Pyramidal and focal neurological signs are, however, usually absent. When a false positive diagnosis of vascular dementia is made in a patient with DLB pathology, it is often associated at autopsy with concomitant microvascular abnormalities and a mixed pathology.

47.3.2.2 OTHER CAUSES OF DELIRIUM

In patients with intermittent delirium, appropriate examination and laboratory tests should be performed during the acute phase to maximize the chances of detecting infective, metabolic, inflammatory or other aetiological factors. Pharmacological causes are particularly common in elderly patients. Although the presence of any of these features makes a diagnosis of DLB less likely, comorbidity is not unusual in elderly patients and the diagnosis should not be excluded simply on this basis.

47.3.2.3 OTHER NEUROLOGICAL SYNDROMES

In patients with a prior diagnosis of PD, the onset of visual hallucinations and fluctuating cognitive impairment may be attributed to side effects of antiparkinsonian medications, and this must be tested by dose reduction or withdrawal (Harrison and McKeith, 1995; Goetz *et al.*, 1998). Other atypical parkinsonian syndromes associated with poor levodopa response, cognitive impairment and postural instability include progressive supranuclear palsy (Fearnley *et al.*, 1991), MSA and corticobasal degeneration. The development of myoclonus in patients with a rapidly progressive form of DLB may lead the clinician to suspect Creutzfeldt–Jakob disease. Syncopal episodes in DLB are often incorrectly attributed to transient ischaemic attacks, despite an absence of focal neurological signs. Recurrent disturbances in consciousness accompanied by complex visual hallucinations may suggest complex partial seizures (temporal lobe epilepsy) and vivid dreaming with violent movements during sleep may meet criteria for REM sleep behaviour disorder (Boeve *et al.*, 2001).

Patients with a previous diagnosis of Parkinson's disease. Patients who initially present with motor symptoms of PD, and who only develop the typical features of DLB after many years of severe motor disability, present some problems of classification. Antiparkinsonian medications are usually held

responsible for hallucinations and confusion in PD, but research findings do not fully support this clinical impression. Factors associated with the development of visual hallucinosis are: later age of onset of PD, total duration of illness and the presence of cognitive impairment. Hallucinators and non-hallucinators are distinguished neither by severity of motor disability nor dosage of antiparkinsonian medication. Patients with early onset of hallucinations are particularly likely to subsequently develop DLB (Goetz *et al.*, 1998). The DLB Consensus statement recommends that, if a syndrome meeting diagnostic criteria for DLB develops in a patient who has had motor PD for at least 12 months prior to the onset of neuropsychiatric features, a diagnosis of PD + DLB, should be made. This arbitrary 12-month rule is helpful in the diagnosis of individual cases and in selecting samples for clinical research studies, but is increasingly difficult to justify from a neurobiological point of view.

47.3.2.4 OTHER PSYCHIATRIC DISORDERS

If a patient spontaneously develops parkinsonian features or cognitive decline, or shows excessive sensitivity to neuroleptic medication, in the course of late onset delusional disorder, depressive psychosis or mania (Birkett *et al.*, 1992; Mullan *et al.*, 1996), DLB should be considered.

47.4 CLINICAL INVESTIGATION

Detailed psychometric testing (see Chapter 49) and expert neurological examination are likely to be informative and should be carried out whenever DLB is suspected (McKeith *et al.*, 1996a). No specific biomarkers for DLB have yet been identified but there have been sufficient studies to allow the conclusion that neuroimaging investigations can be helpful in supporting the clinical diagnosis.

47.4.1 Neuroimaging – structural and functional

Prominent atrophy of the medial temporal lobes on CT or MRI is indicative of AD rather than DLB (Barber *et al.*, 1999). Periventricular lesions and white matter hyperintensities are often present in (Barber *et al.*, 2000a) but, similar to measures of generalized atrophy and rates of progression of whole brain tissue loss (O'Brien *et al.*, 2001), are not helpful in differential diagnosis. Dopamine transporter loss in the caudate and putamen, a marker of nigrostriatal degeneration can be detected in DLB but not AD by dopaminergic SPECT. Abnormal scans in DLB were reported as more accurate in predicting neuropathological diagnosis than the application of clinical Consensus criteria (Walker *et al.*, 2002). A sensitivity of 88 per cent for detecting probable DLB with a specificity of 85 per cent for AD and 95 per cent for controls has been reported (O'Brien *et al.*, 2004), a flatter rostrocaudal gradient of loss along the striatum indicating relatively greater loss in the caudate and lesser loss in the putamen compared with PD.

47.4.2 EEG

The electroencephalogram (EEG) is diffusely abnormal in over 90 per cent of DLB patients. Early slowing of the dominant rhythm, with 4–7 Hz transient activity over the temporal lobe area, is characteristic and correlates with a clinical history of loss of consciousness (Briel *et al.*, 1999). It is not possible reliably to differentiate DLB and AD subjects on the basis of the EEG, however (Barber *et al.*, 2000b). The diagnostic significance of bursts of bilateral frontal rhythmic delta activity, reported to be more common in DLB than AD, has yet to be established (Calzetti *et al.*, 2002).

47.4.3 Genotyping

No specific genetic markers for DLB have been identified and genetic testing cannot be recommended as part of the diagnostic process at present. DLB patients have an elevated apolipoprotein ε4 allele frequency (Benjamin *et al.*, 1994; Pickering-Brown *et al.*, 1994) similar to that reported in AD so a positive ε4 test does not provide additional information in the differential diagnosis of AD and DLB. Most DLB cases are sporadic, although there are a few reports of autosomal dominant Lewy body disease families.

REFERENCES

Aarsland D, Ballard C, McKeith I *et al.* (2001) Comparison of extrapyramidal signs in dementia with Lewy bodies and Parkinson's disease. *Journal of Neuropsychiatry and Clinical Neurosciences* **13**: 374–379

Ala TA, Yang K-H, Sung JH, Frey WHI. (1997) Hallucinations and signs of parkinsonism help distinguish patients with dementia and cortical Lewy bodies from patients with Alzheimer's disease. *Journal of Neurology, Neurosurgery, and Psychiatry* **62**: 16–21

Armstrong TP, Hansen LA, Salmon DP *et al.* (1991) Rapidly progressive dementia in a patient with the Lewy body variant of Alzheimer's disease. *Neurology* **41**: 1178–1180

Ayre GA, Sahgal A, Wesnes K, McKeith IG. (1996) Psychological function in dementia with Lewy bodies and senile dementia of Alzheimer's type. *Neurobiology of Aging* **17**: 205

Ballard CG, Mohan RNC, Patel A, Bannister C. (1993) Idiopathic clouding of consciousness – do the patients have cortical Lewy body disease? *International Journal of Geriatric Psychiatry* **8**: 571–576

Ballard C, O'Brien J, Swann A *et al.* (2000) One year follow-up of parkinsonism in dementia with Lewy bodies. *Dementia and Geriatric Cognitive Disorders* **11**: 219–222

Barber R, Gholkar A, Scheltens P *et al.* (1999) Medial temporal lobe atrophy on MRI in dementia with Lewy bodies. *Neurology* **52**: 1153–1158

Barber R, Ballard C, McKeith IG *et al.* (2000a) MRI volumetric study of dementia with Lewy bodies. A comparison with AD and vascular dementia. *Neurology* **54**: 1304–1309

Barber PA, Varma AR, Lloyd JJ *et al.* (2000b) The electroencephalogram in dementia with Lewy bodies. *Acta Neurologica Scandinavica* **101**: 53–56

Barber R, Panikkar A, McKeith IG. (2001) Dementia with Lewy bodies: diagnosis and management. *International Journal of Geriatric Psychiatry* **16**: S12–S18

Barnes J, Boubert L, Harris J *et al.* (2003) Reality monitoring and visual hallucinations in Parkinson's disease. *Neuropsychologia* **41**: 565–574

Benjamin R, Leake A, Edwardson JA *et al.* (1994) Apolipoprotein E genes in Lewy body and Parkinson's disease. *Lancet* **343**: 1565

Birkett DP, Desouky A, Han L, Kaufman M. (1992) Lewy bodies in psychiatric patients. *International Journal of Geriatric Psychiatry* **7**: 235–240

Boeve B, Silber M, Ferman T *et al.* (2001) Association of REM sleep behavior disorder and neurodegenerative disease may reflect an underlying synucleinopathy. *Movement Disorders* **16**: 622–630

Bradshaw J, Saling M, Hopwood M *et al.* (2004) Fluctuating cognition in dementia with Lewy bodies and Alzheimer's disease is qualitatively distinct. *Journal of Neurology, Neurosurgery, and Psychiatry* **75**: 382–387

Briel RCG, McKeith IG, Barker WA *et al.* (1999) EEG findings in dementia with Lewy bodies and Alzheimer's disease. *Journal of Neurology, Neurosurgery, and Psychiatry* **66**: 401–440

Burkhardt CR, Filley CM, Kleinschmidt-DeMasters BK *et al.* (1988) Diffuse Lewy body disease and progressive dementia. *Neurology* **38**: 1520–1528

Burn DJ, Rowan EN, Minett T *et al.* (2003) Extrapyramidal features in Parkinson's disease with and without dementia and dementia with Lewy bodies: a cross-sectional comparative study. *Movement Disorders* **18**: 884–889

Burns A, Luthert P, Levy R *et al.* (1990) Accuracy of clinical diagnosis of Alzheimer's disease. *BMJ* **301**: 1026

Byrne EJ, Lennox G, Lowe J, Godwin-Austen RB. (1989) Diffuse Lewy body disease: clinical features in 15 cases. *Journal of Neurology, Neurosurgery, and Psychiatry* **52**: 709–717

Byrne EJ, Lennox G, Godwin-Austen RB *et al.* (1991) Dementia associated with cortical Lewy bodies. Proposed diagnostic criteria. *Dementia* **2**: 283–284

Calzetti S, Bortone E, Negrotti A *et al.* (2002) Frontal intermittent rhythmic delta activity (FIRDA) in patients with dementia with Lewy bodies: a diagnostic tool? *Neurological Sciences* **23**: S65–S66

Colosimo C, Hughes AJ, Kilford L, Lees AJ. (2003) Lewy body cortical involvement may not always predict dementia in Parkinson's disease. *Journal of Neurology, Neurosurgery, and Psychiatry* **74**: 852–856

Collerton D, Perry E, McKeith I. (in press) Why do people see things that are not there? *Behavioral and Brain Sciences*

Committee on Safety of Medicines. (1994) Neuroleptic sensitivity in patients with dementia. *Current Problems in Pharmacovigilance* **20**: 6

Crystal HA, Dickson DW, Lizardi JE *et al.* (1990) Antemortem diagnosis of diffuse Lewy body disease. *Neurology* **40**: 1523–1518

Dickson DW, Davies P, Mayeux R *et al.* (1987) Diffuse Lewy body disease. Neuropathological and biochemical studies of six patients. *Acta Neuropathologica* **75**: 8–15

Emre M. (2003) Dementia associated with Parkinson's disease. *Lancet Neurology* **2**: 229–237

Fearnley JM, Revesz T, Brooks DJ *et al.* (1991) Diffuse Lewy body disease presenting with a supranuclear gaze palsy. *Journal of Neurology, Neurosurgery, and Psychiatry* **54**: 159–161

Ferman T, Boeve B, Silber M et al. (2001) Is fluctuating cognition in dementia with Lewy bodies attributable to an underlying sleep disorder? *Sleep* **24**: A374

Ferman T, Smith GE, Boeve BF et al. (2004) DLB fluctuations: specific features that reliably differentiate from AD and normal aging. *Neurology* **62**: 181–187

Forster E and Lewy FH. (1912) Paralysis agitans. I. Pathologische Anatomie. In M Lewandowsky (ed.), *Handbuch der Neurologie*. Berlin, Springer, pp. 920–933

Förstl H and Levy R. (1991) FH. Lewy on Lewy bodies, parkinsonism and dementia. *International Journal of Geriatric Psychiatry* **6**: 757–766

Förstl H, Burns A, Luthert P et al. (1993) The Lewy-body variant of Alzheimer's disease. Clinical and pathological findings. *British Journal of Psychiatry* **162**: 385–392

Galasko D, Katzman R, Salmon DP, Thal LJ, Hansen L. (1996) Clinical and neuropathological findings in Lewy body dementias. *Brian and Cognition* **31**: 166–175

Gibb WRG, Esiri MM, Lees AJ. (1987) Clinical and pathological features of diffuse cortical Lewy body disease (Lewy body dementia). *Brain* **110**: 1131–1153

Gnanalingham KK, Byrne EJ, Thornton A et al. (1997) Motor and cognitive function in Lewy body dementia: comparison with Alzheimer's and Parkinson's diseases. *Journal of Neurology, Neurosurgery, and Psychiatry* **62**: 243–252

Goetz CG, Vogel C, Tanner CM, Stebbins GT. (1998) Early dopaminergic drug-induced hallucinations in parkinsonian patients. *Neurology* **51**: 811–814

Gómez-Tortosa E, Newell K, Irizarry MC et al. (1999) Clinical and quantitative pathological correlates of dementia with Lewy bodies. *Neurology* **53**: 1284–1291

Hansen L, Salmon D, Galasko D et al. (1990) The Lewy body variant of Alzheimer's disease: a clinical and pathologic entity. *Neurology* **40**: 1–8

Hansen LA and Galasko D. (1992) Lewy body disease. *Current Opinion in Neurology and Neurosurgery* **5**: 889–894

Harrison RH and McKeith IG. (1995) Senile dementia of Lewy body type – a review of clinical and pathological features: implications for treatment. *Journal of Geriatric Psychiatry* **10**: 919–926

Hassler R. (1938) Zur pathologie der paralysis agitans und des postenzephalitischen parkinsonismus. *Journal Psychologie und Neurologie* **48**: 387–476

Hely MA, Reid WGJ, Halliday GM et al. (1996) Diffuse Lewy body disease: clinical features in nine cases without coexistent Alzheimer's disease. *Journal of Neurology, Neurosurgery, and Psychiatry* **60**: 531–538

Hohl U, Tiraboschi P, Hansen LA et al. (2000) Diagnostic accuracy of dementia with Lewy bodies. *Archives of Neurology* **57**: 347–351

Holmes C, Cairns N, Lantos P, Mann A. (1999) Validity of current clinical criteria for Alzheimer's disease, vascular dementia and dementia with Lewy bodies. *British Journal of Psychiatry* **174**: 45–50

Jackson M, Lennox G, Balsitis M, Lowe J. (1995) Lewy body dysphagia. *Journal of Neurology, Neurosurgery, and Psychiatry* **58**: 756–757

Jellinger KA. (1996) Structural basis of dementia in neurodegenerative disorders. *Journal of Neural Transmission* **47**: 1–29

Klatka LA, Louis ED, Schiffer RB. (1996) Psychiatric features in diffuse Lewy body disease: findings in 28 pathologically diagnosed cases. *Neurology* **47**: 1148–1152

Kosaka K and Iseki E. (1998) Recent advances in dementia research in Japan: non-Alzheimer type degenerative dementias. *Psychiatry and Clinical Neurosciences* **52**: 367–373

Kosaka K, Yoshimura M, Ikeda K, Budka H. (1984) Diffuse type of Lewy body disease: progressive dementia with abundant cortical Lewy bodies and senile changes of varying degree – a new disease? *Clinical Neuropathology* **3**: 185–192

Lennox G, Lowe J, Byrne EJ et al. (1989) Diffuse Lewy body disease. *Lancet* **1**: 323–324

Litvan I, MacIntyre A, Goetz CG et al. (1998) Accuracy of the clinical diagnoses of Lewy body disease, Parkinson's disease, and dementia with Lewy bodies. *Archives of Neurology* **55**: 969–978

Litvan I, Bhatia KP, Burn DJ et al. (2003) SIC Task Force Appraisal of clinical diagnostic criteria for parkinsonian disorders. *Movement Disorders* **18**: 467–486

Lopez OL, Litvan I, Catt KE et al. (1999) Accuracy of four clinical diagnostic criteria for the diagnosis of neurodegenerative dementias. *Neurology* **53**: 1292–1299

Lopez OL, Becher JT, Kaufer DI et al. (2002) Research evaluation and prospective diagnosis of dementia with Lewy bodies. *Archives of Neurology* **59**: 43–46

Louis E, Klatka L, Lui Y et al. (1997) Comparison of extrapyramidal features in 31 pathologically confirmed cases of diffuse Lewy body disease and 34 pathologically confirmed cases of Parkinson's disease. *Neurology* **48**: 376–380

Lowe JS, Mayer RJ, Landon M. (1996) Pathological significance of Lewy bodies in dementia. In: R Perry, I McKeith, E Perry (eds.), *Dementia with Lewy Bodies*. New York, Cambridge University Press, pp. 195–203

Luis CA, Barker WW, Gajaraj K et al. (1999) Sensitivity and specificity of three clinical criteria for dementia with Lewy bodies in an autopsy-verified sample. *International Journal of Geriatric Psychiatry* **14**: 526–533

McKeith IG. (1997) Dementia with Lewy bodies. In: C Holmes and R Howard (eds), *Advances in Old Age Psychiatry: Chromosomes to Community Care*. Petersfield, Wrightson Biomedical Publishing Ltd, pp. 52–63

McKeith IG. (1998) Dementia with Lewy bodies: clinical and pathological diagnosis. *Alzheimer's Reports* **1**: 83–87

McKeith IG. (2002) Dementia with Lewy bodies. *British Journal of Psychiatry* **180**: 144–147

McKeith IG, Perry RH, Fairbairn AF et al. (1992a) Operational criteria for senile dementia of Lewy body type (SDLT). *Psychological Medicine* **22**: 911–922

McKeith I, Fairbairn A, Perry R et al. (1992b) Neuroleptic sensitivity in patients with senile dementia of Lewy body type. *BMJ* **305**: 673–678

McKeith IG, Fairbairn AF, Bothwell RA et al. (1994a) An evaluation of the predictive validity and inter-rater reliability of clinical diagnostic criteria for senile dementia of Lewy body type. *Neurology* **44**: 872–827

McKeith IG, Fairbairn AF, Perry RH, Thompson P. (1994b) The clinical diagnosis and misdiagnosis of senile dementia of Lewy body type (SDLT) *British Journal of Psychiatry* **165**: 324–332

McKeith IG, Galasko D, Wilcock GK, Byrne EJ. (1995) Lewy body dementia – diagnosis and treatment. *British Journal of Psychiatry* **167**: 709–717

McKeith IG, Galasko D, Kosaka K et al. (1996a) Consensus guidelines for the clinical and pathologic diagnosis of dementia with Lewy bodies (DLB): report of the consortium on DLB international workshop. *Neurology* **47**: 1113–1124

McKeith IG, Fairbairn AF, Harrison R. (1996b) Management of the noncognitive symptoms of Lewy body dementia. In: R Perry, I McKeith, E Perry (eds), *Dementia with Lewy Bodies*. New York, Cambridge University Press, pp. 381–396

McKeith IG, Perry EK, Perry RH. (1999) Report of the second dementia with Lewy body international workshop. Diagnosis and treatment. *Neurology* **53**: 902–905

McKeith IG, Ballard CG, Perry RH *et al.* (2000) Prospective validation of Consensus criteria for the diagnosis of dementia with Lewy bodies. *Neurology* **54**: 1050–1058

McKeith I, Mintzer J, Aarsland D *et al.* (2004a) Dementia with Lewy bodies. *Lancet Neurology* **3**: 19–28

McKeith IG, Wesnes K, Perry E, Ferrara R. (2004b) Greater attentional deficits and responses to rivastigmine in dementia with Lewy body patients with visual hallucinations. *Dementia and Geriatric Cognitive Disorders* **18**: 94–100

McKeith IG, Dickson D, Emre M *et al.* (submitted for publication) Dementia with Lewy bodies: diagnosis and management: Third report of the DLB Consortium.

McShane R, Gedling K, Reading M *et al.* (1995) Prospective study of relations between cortical Lewy bodies, poor eyesight, and hallucinations in Alzheimer's disease. *Journal of Neurology, Neurosurgery, and Psychiatry* **59**: 185–188

Mega MS, Masterman DL, Benson F *et al.* (1996) Dementia with Lewy bodies: reliability and validity of clinical and pathologic criteria. *Neurology* **47**: 1403–1409

Mullan E, Cooney C, Jones E. (1996) Mania and cortical Lewy body dementia. *International Journal of Geriatric Psychiatry* **11**: 837–839

O'Brien JT, Paling S, Barber R *et al.* (2001) Progressive brain atrophy on serial MRI in dementia with Lewy bodies, AD, and vascular dementia. *Neurology* **56**: 1386–1388

O'Brien JT, Colloby SJ, Fenwick J *et al.* (2004) Dopamine transporter loss visualised with FP-CIT SPECT in Dementia with Lewy bodies. *Archives of Neurology* **61**: 919–925

Okazaki H, Lipton LS, Aronson SM. (1961) Diffuse intracytoplasmic ganglionic inclusions (Lewy type) associated with progressive dementia and quadraparesis in flexion. *Journal of Neurology, Neurosurgery, and Psychiatry* **20**: 237–244

Papka M, Rubio A, Schiffer RB. (1998) A review of Lewy body disease, an emerging concept of cortical dementia. *Journal of Neuropsychiatry and Clinical Neuroscience* **10**: 267–279

Perry RH, Irving D, Blessed G *et al.* (1989a) Clinically and neuropathologically distinct form of dementia in the elderly. *Lancet* **1**: 166

Perry RH, Irving D, Blessed G *et al.* (1989b) Senile dementia of Lewy body type and spectrum of Lewy body disease. *Lancet* **i**: 1088

Perry RH, Irving D, Blessed G *et al.* (1990) Senile dementia of Lewy body type. A clinically and neuropathologically distinct form of Lewy body dementia in the elderly. *Journal of the Neurological Sciences* **95**: 119–139

Perry EK, McKeith I, Thompson P *et al.* (1991) Topography, extent, and clinical relevance of neurochemical deficits in dementia of Lewy body type, Parkinson's disease and Alzheimer's disease. *Annals of the New York Academy of Sciences* **640**: 197–202

Pickering-Brown SM, Mann DMA, Bourke JP *et al.* (1994) Apolipoprotein E4 and Alzheimer's disease pathology in Lewy body disease and in other beta-amyloid-forming diseases. *Lancet* **343**: 1155

Rahkonen T, Eloniemi-Sulkava U, Rissanen S *et al.* (2003) Dementia with Lewy bodies according to the consensus criteria in a general population aged 75 years or older. *Journal of Neurology, Neurosurgery, and Psychiatry* **74**: 720–724

Sahgal A, Galloway PH, McKeith IG *et al.* (1992) A comparative study of attentional deficits in senile dementias of Alzheimer and Lewy body types. *Dementia* **3**: 350–354

Sahgal A, McKeith IG, Galloway PH *et al.* (1995) Do differences in visuospatial ability between senile dementias of the Alzheimer and Lewy body types reflect differences solely in mnemonic function. *Journal of Clinical and Experimental Neuropsychology* **17**: 35–43

Salmon D and Galasko D. (1996) Neuropsychological aspects of Lewy body dementia. In: R Perry, I McKeith, E Perry (eds.), *Dementia with Lewy Bodies*. New York, Cambridge University Press, pp. 99–114

Shergill S, Mullan E, D'ath P, Katona C. (1994) What is the clinical prevalence of Lewy body dementia? *International Journal of Geriatric Psychiatry* **9**: 907–912

Stevens T, Livingston G, Kitchen G *et al.* (2002) Islington study of dementia subtypes in the community. *British Journal of Psychiatry* **180**: 270–276

Verghese J, Crystal HA, Dickson DW, Lipton RB. (1999) Validity of clinical criteria for the diagnosis of dementia with Lewy bodies. *Neurology* **53**: 1974–1982

Walker Z, Allen RL, Shergill S, Katona C. (1996) Neuropsychological performance in Lewy body dementia and Alzheimer's disease. *British Journal of Psychiatry* **170**: 156–158

Walker MP, Ayre GA, Cummings JL *et al.* (2000a) The Clinician Assessment of Fluctuation and the One Day Fluctuation Assessment Scale. Two methods to assess fluctuating confusion in dementia. *British Journal of Psychiatry* **177**: 252–256

Walker MP, Ayre GA, Cummings JL *et al.* (2000b) Quantifying fluctuation in dementia with Lewy bodies, Alzheimer's disease, and vascular dementia. *Neurology* **54**: 1616–1624

Walker Z, Costa DC, Walker RW *et al.* (2002) Differentiation of dementia with Lewy bodies from Alzheimer's disease using a dopaminergic presynaptic ligand. *Journal of Neurology, Neurosurgery, and Psychiatry* **73**: 134–140

Weiner MF, Risser RC, Cullum CM *et al.* (1996) Alzheimer's disease and its Lewy body variant: a clinical analysis of post-mortem verified cases. *American Journal of Psychiatry* **153**: 1269–1273

Woodard JS. (1962) Concentric hyaline inclusion body formation in mental disease: analysis of twenty-seven cases. *Journal of Neuropathology and Experimental Neurology* **21**: 442–449

48

Pathology of dementia with Lewy bodies

PAUL G INCE AND ELAINE K PERRY

The pathology of dementia with Lewy bodies (DLB) is that of a primary degenerative dementia with pathological features shared with both Alzheimer's (AD) and Parkinson's diseases (PD). There is a variable burden of Alzheimer-type pathology, together with Lewy bodies (LB) in both cortical and subcortical regions. Often the neocortical senile plaque formation is at densities equivalent to that found in AD, but neocortical neurofibrillary tangles are infrequent (Kosaka et al., 1984; Dickson et al., 1987; Hansen et al., 1989, 1990; Perry et al., 1990d). A group of DLB patients have only minimal plaque pathology, and a virtual absence of paired helical filament (PHF)-tau pathology including neurofibrillary tangles.

Controversies surrounding DLB and its relationship to AD remain unresolved and comparison of pathology data in the literature must be viewed from the perspective of the varied clinical provenance of case series from neurology and old age psychiatry. Problems also remain in defining the relationship between DLB and dementia occurring as part of PD. Lewy bodies are found as coincidental pathology in a wide range of conditions (Table 48.1) but are characteristically associated with idiopathic PD (Gibb and Lees, 1989; Lewy, 1912). Dementia is recognized to be a clinical component of PD (Mayeux et al., 1990), especially in older patients. It is apparent that the range of clinical syndromes in which Lewy bodies form a characteristic part of the pathological substrate includes extrapyramidal movement disorders, cognitive impairment, autonomic dysfunction and gut motility disorders (Table 48.2). The concept of a spectrum of Lewy body disorders, among which PD is the most familiar (Yoshimura, 1983; Kosaka, 1993; Ince et al., 1998), best accounts for this phenotypic diversity. The clinical manifestation of Lewy body

Table 48.1 *Disorders in which 'incidental' Lewy bodies have been described*

Disorder	References
Ataxia telangiectasia	DeLeon et al., 1976; Monaco et al., 1988
Corticobasal degeneration	Paulus and Selim, 1990; Horoupian and Chu, 1994; Wakabayashi et al., 1994b
Down's syndrome	Raghavan et al., 1993; Bodhireddy et al., 1994
Familial early-onset Alzheimer's disease	Lantos et al., 1994
Hallervorden–Spatz disease	Helfand, 1935; Defendini et al., 1973; Dooling et al., 1974; Kalyanasundaram et al., 1980; Gaytan-Garcia et al., 1990; Wakabayashi et al., 1994b
Motor neurone disease	Hedera et al., 1995; Williams et al., 1995
Multiple system atrophy	Morin et al., 1980; Gibb, 1986; Sima et al., 1987
Neuraxonal dystrophy	Vuia, 1977; Williamson et al., 1982; Sugiyama et al., 1993
Progressive supranuclear palsy	Gibb, 1986; Mori et al., 1986
Subacute sclerosing panencephalitis	Gibb et al., 1990
Diffuse neurofibrillary tangles with calcification	Yokota et al., 2002

Table 48.2   *Spectrum of 'Lewy body diseases'*

Syndrome	Neocortex	Limbic cortex	Substantia nigra	Dorsal vagus nucleus	Lateral grey horn/ sympathetic ganglia	Myenteric ganglia
Dementia with Lewy bodies	++/+++	++/+++	+++	+/++	+/+++	??
Parkinson's disease	+/++	++/+++	+++	+/+++	+/++	+/++
Pure autonomic failure	0	0	0/+	+/++	++/+++	?
LB dysphagia	0	0	0/+	0	?	++/+++

0, no LB; +, mild LB formation/neuronal loss; ++ , moderate LB and neuronal loss; +++, severe LB and neuronal loss; ?, not yet reported

pathology depends on the severity and anatomical distribution of Lewy body involvement in the central and peripheral nervous system (Kosaka *et al.*, 1989; Kosaka, 1993; Kosaka and Iseki, 1996).

A major advance in the understanding of pathogenetic relationships among these Lewy body disorders arose from the finding that familial PD is caused by a mutation of the gene encoding α-synuclein (αS) in a few families (Polymeropoulos, 1997) and subsequently that all sporadic Lewy body pathology has αS as the major underlying filamentous inclusion body protein (Spillantini *et al.*, 1997, 1998). These disorders are now classified as 'α-synucleinopathies'.

The pathogenesis of the different syndromes within this spectrum is not yet worked out. The biochemical basis for inclusion body formation related to αS is emerging in relation to the ubiquitin/proteasome system and aberrant phosphorylation of αS. The availability of αS immunocytochemistry has revealed extensive neuritic accumulation of fibrillated αS and a 'neuritic dystrophy hypothesis' of Lewy degeneration has been proposed (Duda, 2004). The balance of genetic and environmental factors that give rise to this disease process are unknown and may vary among individuals (De Palma *et al.*, 1998). Similarly, it is not known why individuals have different anatomical patterns of selective vulnerability to αS, although it seems that the population comprises major groups in terms of the disease phenotype that develop. Studies in this area currently focus heavily on genetic determinants, despite an earlier consensus that genetic influences in PD were of little significance.

Many pathological studies draw attention to the overlap, and common concurrence of the pathologies of PD and AD in the same patient (Forno *et al.*, 1978; Hakim and Mathieson, 1979; Boller *et al.*, 1980; Gaspar and Gray, 1984; Ditter and Mirra, 1987; Burkhardt *et al.*, 1988; Joachim *et al.*, 1988). The pathology of DLB therefore raises two areas of controversy, i.e.:

- What are the clinical, pathological and aetiological relationships among the 'α-synucleinopathies'?
- How does DLB relate to AD?

These issues have been reflected in the difficulty of classifying such patients, and the confusing nomenclature in the earlier literature (Box 48.1). Consensus guidelines on clinical diagnosis and pathological evaluation have been

Box 48.1   *Nomenclature previously used to classify DLB cases*

- Alzheimer's disease with incidental Lewy bodies
- Cortical Lewy body disease
- Diffuse Lewy body disease
- Lewy body dementia
- Lewy body variant of Alzheimer's disease
- Parkinson's disease plus Alzheimer's disease
- Parkinson's disease with dementia
- Senile dementia of the Lewy body type

adopted so that clinical work and research can be compared between centres (McKeith *et al.*, 1996). The outcome of this consensus, and subsequent revisions, is a compromise that leaves important issues unresolved. Two are of particular importance.

First, the term 'dementia with Lewy bodies' was adopted because it does not prejudge the significance of Lewy bodies as a pathological substrate for dementia. This approach creates the difficulty that any demented patient in whom a Lewy body can be demonstrated at autopsy could be regarded as a 'dementia with Lewy bodies'. What the clinical diagnostic guidelines for DLB seek to achieve is to define a particular neuropsychological syndrome in the elderly. Thus there is still a place in routine clinical practice for a more specific diagnostic label. The International DLB Consortium explicitly left open the possibility of using favoured terminology (Box 48.1) in routine clinical practice. Currently the most frequently used of these terms are 'diffuse Lewy body disease (DLBD)', the 'Lewy body variant of Alzheimer's disease (LBVAD)' and 'senile dementia of Lewy body type (SDLT)'. For many practical purposes these terms are interchangeable.

Second, the Consensus pathological guidelines were designed only to allow uniform semiquantification of the pathological features. This allows any case with Lewy bodies to be put into one of three categories: 'neocortical', 'limbic (transitional)', and 'brain stem predominant'. There is no explicit assumption or requirement that patients must be in any of these categories to be classified as DLB. Evidence for the evolution of αS pathology along a definable anatomical hierarchy, beginning in medullary centres has been proposed (Braak *et al.*, 2003) analogous to that proposed in 'Braak staging' of AD (Braak and Braak, 1991). However, data from a large sample of older brains undermines the absolute validity of this concept (Parkkinen *et al.*, 2003). While there is an expectation that dementia will be most frequent in cases in the neocortical or limbic categories, it is not necessary for them to be in a particular pathological category to be regarded as 'dementia with Lewy bodies', and a diagnosis of DLB should be made only on the basis of a clinical picture which fulfils the clinical diagnostic criteria. Finally, the diagnosis of DLB (or one of the more specific terms) does not preclude other diagnoses. Alzheimer-type pathology especially should be assessed, according to established diagnostic criteria for AD, e.g. CERAD (Mirra *et al.*, 1991, 1993), NIA-Reagan Institute (National Institute for Aging [NIA], 1997), or Braak stage (Braak and Braak, 1991) and an opinion given as to whether there is sufficient pathology to warrant that diagnosis.

48.1 VALIDATION OF CONSENSUS CLINICAL DIAGNOSTIC CRITERIA

Studies of the sensitivity and specificity of clinical diagnostic criteria for DLB show values similar to comparable studies of AD. Early studies were retrospective and the patients were diagnosed by using one of two protocols which preceded the DLB Consensus guidelines (Byrne *et al.*, 1989; McKeith *et al.*, 1992b). On average the sensitivity and specificity of the diagnostic criteria reported in these studies is around 80 per cent (McKeith *et al.*, 1994a, b; Mega *et al.*, 1996). Prospective evaluation of the performance of the Consensus Guidelines shows sensitivity of 83 per cent and specificity of 92 per cent compared with comparable values of 78 per cent and 87 per cent for a diagnosis of 'probable AD' (NINCDS-ARDRA criteria) in the same study (McKeith *et al.*, 2000a). There are a minority of patients reported in these series in which the pathological subtype is 'brain stem predominant', indicating that the clinical phenotype is not exclusively dependent on a pathologically demonstrable substrate (i.e. density of cortical Lewy bodies) based on quantifying Lewy bodies.

48.2 PREVALENCE OF DEMENTIA WITH LEWY BODIES AND α-SYNUCLEINOPATHY IN AGEING POPULATIONS

The true prevalence of α-synucleinopathy can only be established on the basis of pathology studies because none of the associated clinical phenotypes (e.g. PD, DLB) predict for the underlying pathologic substrate in better than four of five cases. Population-based data are limited. The UK Cognitive Function and Ageing cohort showed Lewy bodies in 11 per cent of 209 autopsies (Neuropathology Group MRC, 2001). This study is limited in that the sample is not truly representative of the population as a whole, being weighted to individuals with cognitive decline and to the more physically frail. The frequency

of Lewy bodies was no different between demented and non-demented people (12 per cent versus 10 per cent) and only a minority of demented individuals with Lewy bodies had clinical features suggestive of DLB. A recent Japanese study showed α-synucleinopathy in 19.5 per cent of a cohort of 1241 aged but only 4 per cent of the sample showed significant cortical αS pathology (Saito *et al.*, 2004). In the Hisayama study the prevalence of α-synucleinopathy at autopsy was 22.5 per cent of the sample, comprising 41 per cent of demented people. Only one other very large autopsy sample has been reported (Parkkinen *et al.*, 2001). In this Finnish sample the overall prevalence of Lewy body pathology was 14 per cent. Whether these differences between European and Asian populations reflect true differences in genetic factors and exposures, or different sampling strategies, remains to be confirmed.

48.3 PATHOLOGICAL PHENOTYPES

48.3.1 Spectrum of Lewy body disorders

The neuropathology of DLB is part of a spectrum in which α-synucleinopathy is regarded as a primary component of the disorder. These conditions can be interpreted in part on the basis of the anatomical distribution and severity of the degenerative process (see Table 48.2). The motor features of Lewy body disorders usually manifest as an extrapyramidal syndrome (e.g. PD with a 'paucity of movement'), but in some rare cases may be associated with dystonia (e.g. Meig's syndrome with an 'excess of movement'; Mark *et al.*, 1994) and such differences in clinical phenotype are not a specific consequence of Lewy body degeneration.

Rare cases of atypical dementia, with parkinsonism and cortical Lewy bodies, were first described by Okazaki *et al.* (1961) and the concept of a spectrum of Lewy body diseases was originally proposed by Kosaka and colleagues (Kosaka *et al.*, 1980; Kosaka and Iseki, 1996). The peripheral and central nervous system involvement by Lewy bodies in PD includes hypothalamic nuclei, nucleus basalis of Meynert, dorsal raphé, locus caeruleus, substantia nigra, dorsal vagus nucleus and intermediolateral nucleus (Den Hartog Jager and Bethlem, 1960). In addition, a 'neuritic' form of αS degeneration has been described, and is especially common in the dorsal vagus nucleus, sympathetic ganglia and myenteric autonomic ganglia. Kosaka and colleagues later demonstrated cases with extensive cortical and basal ganglia involvement (Kosaka, 1978; Kosaka and Mehraein, 1979). A spectrum of Lewy body diseases was proposed, categorized into three types (brain stem, transitional and diffuse), and this concept is now the basis for the categories defined by the Consensus Guidelines on the evaluation of DLB (McKeith *et al.*, 1996).

More recently, Kosaka proposed a 'cerebral' subtype of Lewy body disease in a patient with progressive dementia, no detectable parkinsonian features (Kosaka *et al.*, 1996) and widespread neocortical and limbic Lewy body involvement.

The pigmented brain stem nuclei only showed a few Lewy bodies with no neuronal loss, and the patient had no significant Alzheimer-type pathology. The significance of these observations relates especially to the evolution and spread of Lewy body pathology. In AD there is evidence that 'tangle' pathology follows a hierarchic evolution from medial temporal lobe regions to other 'limbic' areas and then to temporal, parietal, frontal and occipital neocortex (Arnold et al., 1991; Braak and Braak, 1991). Within the spectrum of Lewy body diseases evidence for such hierarchic spread has been proposed (Braak et al., 2003) but remains controversial (see above): cases present with brain stem Lewy bodies, clinically manifesting as PD, who do not dement and show few cortical Lewy bodies at autopsy. By contrast, DLB patients (including the 'cerebral Lewy body disease' patient described above) may get severe cortical involvement as an early feature with minimal brain stem disease. In addition, patients may develop predominant involvement of the peripheral nervous system, e.g. Lewy body dysphagia (Jackson et al., 1995) and primary autonomic failure, with minimal central involvement. Isolated involvement of the amygdala is well documented (Parkkinen et al., 2003).

The role of pathology in the evaluation of a case with an appropriate clinical history, is to address two questions:

- Is this disorder associated with αS/Lewy body pathology?
- What is the anatomical distribution of Lewy bodies and what is the regional severity of involvement?

In relation to the second question, the pathology section of the Consensus Guidelines for the evaluation of cortical Lewy bodies were offered as a means of standardizing assessment of Lewy body pathology in cortical regions (McKeith et al., 1996). They were designed to be equally applicable to a survey of cortical Lewy body pathology in cases with or without dementia. With the advent of immunocytochemistry for αS this protocol needs to be re-assessed and reformulated taking account of neuritic changes.

48.3.2 Alzheimer and vascular pathologies

Both Alzheimer changes and cerebrovascular pathology are found in the brain of DLB patients at autopsy. The relationship between DLB and AD is not resolved. From studies of AD pathology in DLB there is an emerging consensus that cases can usually be assigned to one of two broad groups. In the first of these, and numerically the more numerous, there is sufficient AD pathology either to satisfy published pathological criteria for AD (Mirra et al., 1991), or such that it is likely that AD pathology contributes significantly as a substrate for the neuropsychiatric phenotype. This 'common form' of DLB has been called 'Lewy body variant of AD' (Hansen et al., 1989, 1990, 1997). The second group comprises cases in which the extent of AD pathology is within a spectrum from mild to negligible, and therefore is not a plausible substrate for cognitive impairment. This 'pure form' of DLB has been called 'diffuse

Lewy body disease' (Hansen, 1997). The SDLT cases (Perry et al., 1990d) include both forms of DLB. A number of studies have recently reported on the clinical phenotype of DLB patients with and without significant AD pathology. They conclude that patients with more severe AD pathology are likely to resemble AD clinically (Merdes et al., 2003; Ballard et al., 2004). Other authors have suggested that 'common form' DLB patients may have more intense cortical Lewy body formation than 'pure' BLB and may show a more severe dementia than in pure AD or DLB (Serby et al., 2003).

The Consensus clinical diagnostic criteria for DLB exclude cases where vascular disease is a demonstrable component of the clinical picture, either as infarcts on neuroimaging or as focal neurological deficits. Despite this it is the authors' experience that, in common with AD cases, microvascular pathology is a frequent finding in DLB at autopsy (Ince et al., 1998). Other studies have emphasized this aspect of CLB pathology (Londos et al., 2002) so that exclusion of cases with vascular features may be of value in selecting the 'pure' disease for research studies but has no value in a routine clinical diagnostic setting. Thus the pathological diagnosis of DLB needs to be qualified by explicit confirmation of the extent of AD and vascular pathology.

48.4 PATHOLOGY OF DEMENTIA WITH LEWY BODIES

The pathological lesions encountered in DLB are listed in Box 48.2. None of these is exclusive to the disorder.

48.4.1 Lewy bodies – conventional and molecular pathology

Lewy bodies are encountered in both subcortical nuclei (e.g. substantia nigra as in PD) and also in cerebral cortical regions. In the pigmented brain stem nuclei Lewy bodies show a

---

Box 48.2 *Pathological features associated with DLB*

Essential for the diagnosis of DLB
- Lewy bodies

Associated with DLB but not essential
- Lewy neurites
- Alzheimer-type pathology
- Senile plaques
- Neurofibrillary tangles
- Regional neuronal loss, especially affecting substantia nigra, locus caeruleus, and nucleus basalis of Meynert
- Microvacuolation
- Synapse loss
- Neurochemical abnormalities/neurotransmitter deficits

Source: McKeith et al., 1996, reprinted with permission

classical morphology comprising an eosinophilic core and peripheral halo (Plate 17a). In the cortex they are much less distinct in conventional stains, appearing as diffusely granular, eosinophilic spheroids with no halo (Plate 17b). In routine practice most laboratories now use αS rather than ubiquitin immunocytochemistry (ICC) to demonstrate cortical Lewy bodies (Plate 17c), although haematoxylin and eosin (H&E) remains of value for brain stem lesions. It has been reported that ubiquitin ICC is more than twice as sensitive in the detection of cortical Lewy bodies compared with H&E (Lennox et al., 1989), but others have shown either no difference between these methods or higher counts with H&E. Formal evaluation of αS ICC against other methods has not been published but experience suggests this method will detect rather more lesions, first because of variable ubiquitination of αS (Sampathu et al., 2003) and second because the method reveals far more extensive pathology than ubiquitin ICC (Duda et al., 2002). The only silver staining method that can reliably demonstrate cortical Lewy bodies is Campbell–Switzer (Braak et al., 1995). The most important practical problem in the evaluation of cortical Lewy bodies is the distinction from small globular tangles in those cases with combined Alzheimer-type and Lewy body pathologies (Plate 17d). Since Lewy bodies are usually unstained by antibodies to PHF-tau it has been suggested that Lewy bodies should only be confirmed, in cases with cortical neurofibrillary tangles, if they are negative for a reliable anti-PHF tau antibody.

Since the discovery that a small minority of cases of familial autosomal dominant PD are associated with mutations in the gene encoding αS (Polymeropoulos et al., 1997; Higuchi et al., 1998; Vaughan et al., 1998; Aarsland et al., 2001) and that antibodies to αS are very consistent markers of Lewy bodies (Baba et al., 1998; Spillantini et al., 1997, 1998; Wakabayashi et al., 1997b; Takeda et al., 1998) (Plate 18a, b), this problem is largely historical. αS immunocytochemistry has therefore confirmed that:

- the different appearances of cortical and subcortical Lewy bodies are likely to be due to factors related to the cell types affected, not molecular pathogenesis;
- PD and DLB share a common molecular pathology suggesting close pathogenetic links.

48.4.2 Lewy bodies – anatomical pathology

In the substantia nigra, the frequency of Lewy bodies may be low in DLB, and there is often not a severe loss of neurones as compared with that in PD patients. DLB patients show substantia nigra neurone counts that are intermediate between PD and AD (Perry et al., 1990d; Ince et al., 1995), although individual cases vary and there may be substantia nigra neurone loss in the PD range associated with variable expression of parkinsonian symptoms. Another brain stem nucleus regularly affected in PD, the cholinergic pedunculopontine tegmental nucleus, may also be preferentially affected in DLB. Individual patients also vary in the involvement of serotonergic

raphé nucleus subdivisions, although no quantitative studies are published. The locus caeruleus is often severely affected by neuronal loss and Lewy bodies in both PD and DLB patients (Perry et al., 1990d; Zweig et al., 1993).

Between 75 and 95 per cent of PD cases have some degree of cortical Lewy body involvement whether or not the patient has dementia (Hughes et al., 1993; Mattila et al., 1998), with a tendency for dementia to be associated with neocortical Lewy bodies (Sugiyama et al., 1994), although this is not an invariable correlate of cognitive decline (Colosimo et al., 2003). Thus the difference between PD and DLB in terms of cortical Lewy body pathology is quantitative, not qualitative. In both DLB and PD the distribution of Lewy bodies in the cortex is most frequent in limbic areas. Quantitative studies have shown that cingulate cortex involvement is more marked in Brodmann area 23 compared with 24 (Perry et al., 1990d). The amygdaloid complex, insula, entorhinal and transentorhinal cortices have been shown to be sites of predilection for Lewy body formation (Kosaka et al., 1984; Braak et al., 1994; Iseki et al., 1995; Rezaie et al., 1996; Schmidt et al., 1996). They were rarely described in the hippocampal formation prior to αS ICC but this region is now considered to fall within the spectrum of selective vulnerability (Harding et al., 2002b). Neocortical involvement is usually most severe in the temporal lobe and follows the gradient: temporal > parietal = frontal > occipital (Kosaka et al., 1984; Perry et al., 1990d). The Consensus Guidelines do not include the occipital region where Lewy bodies are infrequent, even in the most severely involved cases of DLB, and where their presence does not contribute to a significant distinction between clinical phenotypes or pathological subgroups (Perry et al., 1990d).

Cortical Lewy bodies are found in deeper cortical layers (especially cortical layers 4, 5 and 6) in all affected regions (Kosaka et al., 1984), although the population of affected neurones has yet to be fully characterized. On morphological grounds they are small and medium-sized neurones (Kosaka et al., 1984; Dickson et al., 1987), which includes pyramidal neurones on the basis of expression of neurofilament (NF) medium and heavy subunits, and the absence of parvalbumin, a marker of GABAergic interneurones (Smith et al., 1995; Wakabayashi et al., 1995). The total number of SMI32 positive neurones was reported to be reduced by 70 per cent in DLB, suggesting that Lewy body formation is associated with severe neuronal dysfunction or death (Wakabayashi et al., 1995). However, a recent study based on optical dissector stereometry found the opposite (Shepherd et al., 2002). There was also 40 per cent reduction in parvalbumin-immunoreactive neurones, suggesting that any selective vulnerability of pyramidal neurones is only relative. Cortical Lewy body frequency may be positively correlated with the intensity of dementia (Samuel et al., 1996), although this finding remains controversial. Thus the extent to which Lewy bodies are themselves the substrate for dementia in DLB or PD is in doubt. Even in the most severely affected cases of DLB the frequency of cortical Lewy bodies (demonstrated by

H&E, ubiquitin ICC or αS ICC) is at least 10^{-3} times less than would be the case for neurofibrillary tangles in AD patients with a similar level of cognitive deficit (Perry *et al.*, 1990d). It is likely that the substrate of cognitive deficits in 'pure' DLB cases will eventually be explained on the basis of a complex interaction of pathological lesions (cortical and subcortical), diffuse molecular pathological changes, and neurochemical alterations in both cortical and subcortical neurotransmission. Recent work using αS ICC suggests that the more extensive pathological changes revealed by this method significantly contribute to the pathological substrate of DLB (Duda *et al.*, 2002).

48.4.3 Lewy neurites (Lewy–related neurites)

Ubiquitin-immunoreactive neuritic processes were first described in the CA2 sector of the hippocampus in DLB (Dickson *et al.*, 1991, 1994) and were proposed as a means of distinguishing hippocampal pathology in AD and cases of DLB where Alzheimer-type pathology can be significant (Plate 19a, b). Whilst this concept remains valid, further reports have shown that LB neurites are also a consistent feature of PD and do not predict dementia (de Vos *et al.*, 1995) simply by virtue of their presence. Neurites are immunoreactive for αS (Plate 19b, c), ubiquitin and (variably) neurofilament epitopes (especially phosphorylated epitopes). Immunoreactivity to Alz50 and Tau-2 have also been reported (Plate 19d), but not to neurofibrillary tangle-specific tau isoforms (Dickson *et al.*, 1994). Electron microscopy confirms a major component of αS filaments within these structures. They are also described in the amygdala (Braak *et al.*, 1994), basal forebrain, substantia nigra (Plate 19f), pedunculopontine nucleus, raphé nuclei, dorsal vagal nucleus and neocortex (Plate 19e) (Gai *et al.*, 1995; Pellise *et al.*, 1996). In all these sites neurites can be present in very high density but they are not co-localized with immunoreactivity to tyrosine hydroxylase, suggesting that they do not arise in distal projections of the substantia nigra. Lewy bodies and neurites coexist (Kim *et al.*, 1995) and in one study the intensity of CA2 neurites and cortical Lewy body formation were shown to be correlated (Pollanen *et al.*, 1993b).

The significance of Lewy neurites in DLB is uncertain both in terms of their pathogenesis and their role in neuronal dysfunction or clinical phenotype. Recent work using αS ICC in Lewy body disorders shows more extensive neuritic pathology than was previously appreciated with methods such as ubiquitin ICC (Baba *et al.*, 1998; Duda *et al.*, 2002). The appreciation that neuritic changes are frequently extensive and more prominent than Lewy bodies, and work in animal models of α-synucleinopathy (Giasson *et al.*, 2002) underpins the 'neuritic dystrophy hypothesis' of Lewy neurodegeneration (Duda, 2004).

48.4.4 Alzheimer–type pathology

Many cases of DLB have Alzheimer-type pathology which has led to concepts of the disorder being a variant of AD (Hansen *et al.*, 1990), or that the diseases represent phenotypic clustering along a continuous 'spectrum of neurodegeneration' (Perl *et al.*, 1998). However, there are pathological observations that support the distinction of DLB from AD:

- There are cases with no significant Alzheimer-type pathology (DLB 'pure form').
- Quantitative and qualitative analysis of the Alzheimer-type pathology shows differences between DLB and AD.
- The similarity is predominantly at the level of β-amyloid deposition, so that the neuronal inclusion pathology remains distinct.

Most cases of DLB have αS accumulation with low or minimal PHF-tau accumulation. The picture is reversed in AD where PHF-tau predominates and αS deposition is less prominent or absent.

The published series of autopsy cases which drew attention to DLB as a distinct dementing syndrome in the elderly included a minority of cases with virtually no Alzheimer-type pathology (Kosaka *et al.*, 1984; Dickson *et al.*, 1987; Perry *et al.*, 1990d), including cases with absence of senile plaques of any type. They were clinically indistinguishable from other DLB cases, and the burden of Alzheimer-type pathology was less than in many cognitively intact, age-matched individuals (Lippa *et al.*, 1994). These cases correspond to the category of 'pure diffuse Lewy body disease' described by Kosaka (1993) or the diffuse Lewy body disease of Hansen (1997) to distinguish them from those cases with Alzheimer-type pathology who comprise the 'common form of DLBD' of Kosaka (1993), or 'Lewy body variant of Alzheimer disease' of Hansen (1997).

Nevertheless, this relationship between AD and Lewy body diseases remains problematic. Various observations predating the emergence of DLB as a distinct entity are difficult to apply to the current debate because it is not clear to which disease categories the cases would now be assigned on clinical and pathological grounds. Such observations include:

- more frequent Alzheimer-type pathology in PD cases than in age-matched control (Forno *et al.*, 1978; Hakim and Mathieson, 1979; Boller *et al.*, 1980; Gibb, 1986; Hughes *et al.*, 1993);
- the frequency of Lewy bodies in familial AD (Ditter and Mirra, 1987; Joachim *et al.*, 1988; Lantos *et al.*, 1994; Halliday *et al.*, 1997).

Since these studies also predate a widespread awareness of the frequency of cortical Lewy bodies and neurites, and the use of sensitive methods to detect them, they are difficult to interpret in the context of more recent concepts. It is likely that DLB represents an undiagnosed group within many of the older reported cohorts, and account for much of the clinicopathological overlap described between AD and PD. Review of cases in the Newcastle centre prior to 1982 include a proportion of demented cases that correspond to the entity 'senile dementia of the Lewy body type'. This is certainly the case with respect to the category 'plaque-only AD', where re-examination of the original cohort from whom this diagnostic category was formulated showed that most patients could be rediagnos as DLB (Hansen *et al.*, 1993).

In the neocortex, quantitative studies show that the burden of senile plaques is similar in many DLB cases and age-matched AD patients, even in cohorts among whom the DLB patients died more rapidly after onset of dementia (Plate 20a, b) (Hansen *et al.*, 1990; Perry *et al.*, 1990d). In image analysis studies of DLB and AD cohorts, matched for age and degree of dementia, the area occupied by βA4 immunoreactive deposits was reported to be equal, and there was no difference in the ratio of different morphological categories of plaque type (Gentleman *et al.*, 1992; McKenzie *et al.*, 1996). Qualitatively this reflects the burden of βA4 amyloidosis, and not the cytoskeletal pathology of AD. The major difference between the senile plaques of AD and those in DLB is the paucity of a neuritic component that is immunoreactive for PHF-tau (Plate 20c, d). This is not to say that DLB plaques of 'classical' appearance with neuritic involvement are not frequent, but rather that these neurites do not contain Alzheimer disease-related tau (Dickson *et al.*, 1989; Samuel *et al.*, 1997b). Reports indicate that these plaque neurites in DLB are reactive for αS (Takeda *et al.*, 1998). It is also reported that neuritic plaques in DLB have a higher expression of GAP-43 (Masliah *et al.*, 1993), interpreted as increased neuronal sprouting, compared with downregulation of GAP-43 expression in AD (de la Monte *et al.*, 1995). The extent to which clinical DLB cases have neocortical neurofibrillary tangles is very variable. In most cases tangles are infrequent and largely confined to the medial temporal lobe (Hansen *et al.*, 1990; Ince *et al.*, 1991). Some cases undoubtedly do have a burden of neocortical neurofibrillary tangles comparable with AD cases but they are a minority (Hansen *et al.*, 1990; Ince *et al.*, 1995), and recent work suggests this burden of tangle pathology is likely to be associated with clinical features more like AD (Merdes *et al.*, 2003; Ballard *et al.*, 2004). This distinction is one of the key features that discriminate AD from DLB. The possibility that AD-related PHF-tau changes occur in DLB without the formation of neurofibrillary tangles has been studied using ELISA of extracted cortical proteins and shows no evidence for a global alteration in tau isoforms towards insoluble PHF-related species (Harrington *et al.*, 1994; Strong *et al.*, 1995). It is now clear that the cortical dysfunction associated with DLB is not explicable on the basis of neurofibrillary pathology, and the more likely culprit is abnormal αS metabolism.

DLB cases have an excess of hippocampal Alzheimer-type pathology when compared with age-matched controls and with both demented and non-demented PD patients (Ince *et al.*, 1991; Harding *et al.*, 2002b). The burden of amyloidosis in the entorhinal cortex may be equal to AD in those DLB cases corresponding to the 'common form', but cases of 'pure form' DLB have much lower densities of senile plaques in this region (Armstrong *et al.*, 1997). Neurofibrillary tangles show intermediate densities with considerable intercase variation (Ince *et al.*, 1991). Morphological markers of the integrity of the perforant pathway also show intermediate changes in

DLB of lesser severity than in AD (Lippa *et al.*, 1997; Wakabayashi *et al.*, 1997a). Whilst these changes may contribute to neuropsychological features such as defective short-term memory, they do not account for much of the clinical picture of DLB.

The above discussion encapsulates the problem of defining the relationship between AD and DLB, and the confusion of nomenclature in the older literature. The issue centres around the criteria used to define AD. In the American literature these criteria have evolved from a scheme in which only the numerical burden of neocortical senile plaques was evaluated (Khachaturian, 1985), through the CERAD criteria (Mirra *et al.*, 1991, 1993) and its revisions, which rely on neuritic plaques, to the latest NIA-Reagan Institute guidelines, which include evaluation of both plaques and neocortical tangles (NIA and RI Working Group, 1997). Many authors would now also include a high score using the 'Braak stage' method as an additional part of the pathological diagnosis of AD (Braak and Braak, 1991). This represents a convergence towards the view that requires both neocortical plaques and tangles (Tomlinson *et al.*, 1970). Thus the extent to which DLB cases represent a variant of AD is entirely dependent on the diagnostic criteria used (Hansen and Samuel, 1997). If a plaque-based method is used, then many DLB patients can be interpreted to have AD, depending on the qualification of plaque molecular pathology. If a requirement for neocortical tangles, or PHF-tau plaque neurites, is adopted, then most DLB patients fall short of AD. If it is mistakenly assumed that cortical Lewy pathology, in the absence of consensus clinical features of DLB, is a basis for diagnosis then many AD patients would fall into the DLB spectrum.

48.4.5 Regional neuronal loss

A characteristic of the core clinical syndrome of DLB is the presence of parkinsonian signs which may be of a spectrum of severity ranging from fully developed PD to very subtle extrapyramidal features. In contrast to the cognitive features of DLB, the pathological and neurochemical substrate for this motor component is well characterized. DLB patients on average have substantia nigra degeneration intermediate between that seen in PD and normal control individuals of the same age (Perry *et al.*, 1990d; Agid, 1991). The degree of depigmentation of the substantia nigra is often only moderate, and microscopic evidence of neurone loss and incontinence of pigment is usually less than in PD. The mechanism of neuronal loss associated with Lewy body diseases is not known, although evidence supports the possibility of apoptosis (Tompkins *et al.*, 1997). The cellular pathology in the substantia nigra is identical in PD and DLB and includes both classical Lewy bodies and pale bodies, together with a variable background of neuritic changes best demonstrated by αS ICC. Pale bodies contain ubiquitin and αS, are regarded as a precursor lesion to Lewy bodies, and may be more numerous than Lewy bodies (Dale *et al.*, 1992). By contrast,

AD patients do not usually have significant nigral degeneration, although some cases have substantia nigra neurofibrillary tangles, and a small proportion may develop frank parkinsonism (Alvord et al., 1974) sufficient to warrant a clinical diagnosis of PD arising on the basis of tangle pathology. Atypical AD patients may attract an erroneous clinical diagnosis of DLB due to the prominence of parkinsonian signs (Ince et al., 1998). Erroneous diagnoses of DLB may also arise in the context of other atypical variants of tau-related neurodegenerative disorders including progressive supranuclear palsy and corticobasal degeneration (Chin and Goldman, 1996; Feany et al., 1996).

Some cases of DLB have fully developed PD and in these cases the nigral cell loss will exceed the commonly cited threshold for the development of PD (<70 per cent of substantia nigra counts in age-matched controls). Occasional cases are encountered where there is marked substantia nigra neurone loss but no overt parkinsonism. In these cases it is postulated that additional pathology in the striatum produces a compensatory effect with no overall loss in the balance of neurotransmitter activity. The locus caeruleus is routinely more severely affected than the substantia nigra and is often totally depigmented to the naked eye. Lewy bodies are usually frequent in the surviving neurones. Some cases with additional significant Alzheimer-type pathology may show tangle formation in substantia nigra neurones in addition to Lewy bodies.

Other brain stem and mid-brain nuclei that project into the cerebrum contain Lewy bodies, including the serotinergic raphé subdivisions and the pedunculopontine nucleus. No quantitative studies have compared these nuclei in DLB, AD, PD and controls, but neuronal loss would be expected to occur. Neuronal loss in the cholinergic nucleus basalis of Meynert has been reported (Jellinger and Bancher, 1996). In PD, DLB and AD, the degree of cell loss is approximately 70 per cent of age-matched controls. In DLB cases with significant AD pathology this neuronal population may contain both Lewy bodies and neurofibrillary tangles.

48.4.6 Microvacuolation

Early reports of DLB emphasized the presence of cortical spongiform changes in the temporal cortex (Plate 21) (Hansen et al., 1989). The appearance of this pathology was said to closely resemble prion disease, although the anatomical distribution was distinctive. The possible involvement of prion disease has been excluded on the basis of failed animal transmission experiments and lack of immunocytochemical staining for prion protein (Mancardi et al., 1982; Smith et al., 1987). There is no clear relationship between spongiosis and the distribution or severity of cortical Lewy body pathology in individual cases. However, affected areas have been shown to be related to the presence of 'ubiquitin-positive granular structures' (UPGS) (Iseki et al., 1997). Spongiform degeneration is also encountered in otherwise typical cases of AD but there is a reduction in the frequency of UPGS (Iseki et al.,

1996). The frequency of αS reactive neurites in relation to spongiform changes has not been reported.

48.4.7 Synaptic loss

Reduced synaptic densities of up to 50 per cent have been reported in AD patients (Masliah et al., 1991; Clinton et al., 1994) and it is claimed that this abnormality is a major substrate for the reduced cognitive performance of Alzheimer patients compared with controls. Similar data have been reported for other diseases including vascular dementia (VaD) (Zhan et al., 1994) and AIDS (Masliah et al., 1991). Data relating to DLB are less easy to interpret. Reported synaptic loss in the neocortex and entorhinal cortex of DLB patients were equivalent to those of patients with AD (Masliah et al., 1993; Wakabayashi et al., 1994a). However, these patients were all from the 'common form' subgroup in whom there was significant concomitant Alzheimer-type pathology, especially in the entorhinal region. Thus the synaptic loss demonstrated may be due to Alzheimer-type and not Lewy body pathology. In a more recent study, a dot-blot assay for cortical synaptophysin was used to compare LBVAD patients with 'pure DLBD', and concluded that a significant synaptic loss of 20 per cent was present in LBVAD patients whereas the pure DLBD group showed only a non-significant decrease of 10 per cent (Samuel et al., 1997a). A second study has confirmed this difference between the 'pure' and 'common' forms of DLB (Hansen et al., 1998).

48.5 NEUROTRANSMITTERS AND NEUROCHEMISTRY IN DEMENTIA WITH LEWY BODIES

The neurochemical profile of the brain in DLB in comparison to AD and PD has been studied from three perspectives:

- correlation with the clinical features;
- correlation with the severity and distribution of pathological lesions;
- the identification of rational therapeutic targets.

Drugs currently used to treat psychotic features, depression, anxiety and cognitive impairment act on specific neurotransmitter systems (dopamine, 5-hydroxytryptamine (5HT), gamma-aminobytyric acid (GABA) and acetylcholine). In degenerative conditions such as AD, such therapies are considered to be symptomatic or palliative at best but evidence of neurotrophic consequences of neurotransmitter signalling, mediated at the level of alterations in gene transcription, indicate that chronic manipulation of neurotransmitter function can have either neurotoxic or neuroprotective effects. In DLB the major clinical features, particularly psychotic features, can occur in the absence of cortical Alzheimer-type pathology or synaptic loss and may be at least partly functional. The fluctuating course of the disease also supports this idea. Such observations raise the possibility that neurotransmitter-targeted therapies may be of particular benefit in DLB compared with AD.

Neuronal loss occurs in specific subcortical nuclei in DLB as it does in AD and PD (see above). The systems that have received the most neurochemical attention in DLB, because of consistently observed abnormalities and likely clinical correlates, are the cholinergic (relating to cognitive and psychotic symptoms) and the dopaminergic (relating to parkinsonism). The role of noradrenergic or 5HT systems in depression or delusions, as has been suggested in AD, has not yet been explored in DLB, nor the significance of neuropeptide changes, e.g. somatostatin or corticotropin-releasing factor (CRF) which are evident in DLB (Dickson *et al.*, 1987; Leake *et al.*, 1990).

48.5.1 Cholinergic systems

Cortical cholinergic abnormalities and degeneration of basal forebrain nuclei are considered to contribute to cognitive impairments including memory loss in AD. In PD, cortical cholinergic activities and nucleus basalis neurone counts are lower in demented compared with non-demented individuals. In DLB, neocortical choline acetyltransferase (ChAT) is lower than in AD and similar to that in demented PD (Dickson *et al.*, 1987; Langlais *et al.*, 1993; Perry *et al.*, 1994). In comparison with AD the cortical loss of ChAT is a relatively 'early' and severe phenomenon in DLB (Tiraboschi *et al.*, 2002). Cognitive impairment is generally less severe in DLB than AD, and the clinical correlate of this neocortical cholinergic deficit may not be cognitive but neuropsychiatric, specifically visual hallucinations. Cholinergic activity is lower in hallucinating compared with non-hallucinating DLB cases whereas 5HT activity is relatively preserved (Perry *et al.*, 1990a). This observation may be linked to the tendency of antimuscarinic agents such as atropine and hyoscine (scopolamine) to induce visual hallucinations of a type similar to those experienced by patients with DLB (Perry and Perry, 1995). Such drugs interact with muscarinic M1, M3 and M4 receptor subtypes, which predominate in the cortex, thalamus and striatum.

Loss of striatal ChAT in DLB (Langlais *et al.*, 1993), which reflects pathology of intrinsic local circuit neurones, may account for the reduced severity of extrapyramidal clinical symptoms in some DLB patients who have equivalent loss of dopaminergic substantia nigra neurones as PD patients (Perry *et al.*, 1998). The reticular nucleus receives joint innervation from basal forebrain and brain stem pedunculopontine cholinergic nuclei. Disturbances in its function may lead to disruption of sensory processing and affect attentional or perceptive processes, possibly contributing to visual hallucinations.

In DLB, the muscarinic M1 subtype is elevated in the cortex, as it is in PD (Perry *et al.*, 1990c), reflecting upregulation of postsynaptic receptors in response to cholinergic denervation. Together with a normal extent of receptor coupling via G proteins, this suggests that cholinoceptive neurones are intact in DLB (Perry *et al.*, 1998). By contrast, there is no upregulation of the M1 subtype in AD, at least in advanced

cases, and receptor uncoupling is widely reported. These differences reflect the more 'destructive' cortical pathology, including neurofibrillary tangle formation, in AD. In contrast striatal M1 receptor density is lower in DLB, and parallels low D2 receptor density, which may relate to the relatively mild movement disorder (Piggott *et al.*, 2003).

The nicotinic receptor, which binds nicotine with high affinity (considered to consist primarily of α4β2 subunits), is equally reduced in the cortex in DLB compared with AD and PD (Perry *et al.*, 1990c). In the substantia nigra, where nicotine binding is concentrated in the pars compacta in association with the pigmented dopaminergic neurones, receptor binding is as depleted in DLB as in PD, despite the greater loss of neurones in PD (Perry and Perry, 1995). This suggests that loss or down-regulation of the receptor may precede neurodegeneration. However, expression of various receptor subunits (α2, α7, β2, β3 nAChR) is unchanged in DLB suggesting a problem at the level of receptor assembly (Martin-Ruiz *et al.*, 2002). Nicotinic agonists upregulate the receptor and possible protective effects of nicotine may involve reversal of age- or disease-related loss of the receptor. Another nicotinic receptor subtype, comprising α7 subunits, binds α-bungarotoxin and is not affected in the cortex in DLB or AD. In the thalamus this receptor is concentrated in the reticular nucleus and is reduced in both disorders (Perry *et al.*, 1998), although a clinical correlate of this additional thalamic cholinergic abnormality is not established.

The therapeutic implications of the cholinergic neurochemical pathology so far identified in DLB can be summarized as follows:

- Since cortical cholinergic abnormalities exist in most cases in the absence of typical Alzheimer pathology (especially tangles), and muscarinic receptors are functionally intact, cholinergic replacement therapy (anticholinesterases, muscarinic or nicotinic agonists) is likely to be more effective than in AD.
- Since the cortical cholinergic deficits in DLB relate more to psychiatric than cognitive symptoms, therapy may be more effective in alleviating the former.

There is already some support for the second of these propositions. In AD patients the anticholinesterase tacrine has been reported to be more effective in alleviating psychotic features such as hallucinations and delusions than in improving cognition (Cummings, 1997). In a small series of patients with PD and dementia, hallucinations have been reported to be reduced or abolished in all cases treated with tacrine (Hutchinson and Fazzini, 1996). Paradoxically, given that extrapyramidal movement disorder is relieved by muscarinic antagonists, parkinsonian features were not exacerbated but actually alleviated. One explanation of this effect of tacrine may be that elevating acetylcholine in the striatum leads to nicotinic as well as muscarinic stimulation, resulting in greater release of nigral dopamine. Stimulation of nicotinic receptors as a therapeutic strategy in DLB may be of particular relevance because both mental and motor symptoms should be relieved. The possibility that nicotinic stimulation may also be neuroprotective has been raised by epidemiological studies of smoking in PD and AD (Court and Perry, 1994). Recent interest in the correlation between butyrylcholinesterase activity in DLB and cognitive decline suggests that inhibitors of this enzyme might also have therapeutic potential (Perry et al., 2003).

48.5.2 Dopaminergic systems

The loss of pigmented substantia nigra neurones and clinical evidence of parkinsonian symptoms in DLB indicate disruption of the dopaminergic input to the striatum. Reduced dopamine or the metabolite (homovanillic acid):dopamine ratio have been reported in autopsy tissue in DLB (Perry et al., 1990b; Langlais et al., 1993). Whilst a correlation between nigral neurone loss and striatal dopamine loss has been reported (Perry et al., 1993), interpretation is complicated by selection of patients (e.g. via neurology or old age psychiatry, with less emphasis on extrapyramidal symptoms in the latter), and by treatment with neuroleptic drugs (which block D2 receptors and also reduce dopamine metabolism).

The dopamine transporter molecule is affected in both PD and DLB. Single photon emission computed tomography (SPECT) imaging shows that the striatal/cerebellar ratio is significantly lower in DLB compared with AD (2.1 versus 5.5) (Donnemiller et al., 1997). Loss of mazindol binding, which also marks the transporter, also distinguishes DLB from AD (Perry et al., 1990b). Compared with the striatum, there is much less dopamine in the cortex and, in autopsy tissue, no marked changes have been observed in those cortical areas that have been examined (Perry et al., 1993). Although L-dopa may induce hallucinations in PD, no dopaminergic parameters distinguish between patients with and without hallucinations.

The status of dopaminergic receptors in DLB is less clear. Autopsy findings suggest no alteration in D1, D2 or D3 subtypes in unmedicated patients (Perry et al., 1990b; Piggott et al., 1999). The absence of any D2 upregulation, such as occurs in the course of PD in response to diminishing dopaminergic input, is surprising and suggests that basal ganglia pathology may be distinct between the two diseases. There is also clinical evidence to support this possibility. In a retrospective survey of cases, rest tremor and response to L-dopa were significantly less prevalent and myoclonus significantly more prevalent in DLB compared with PD (Louis et al., 1997) and DLB patients are unusually sensitive to typical neuroleptic D2 antagonists (McKeith et al., 1992a). This neuroleptic sensitivity may be related to a dysregulation in D2 receptors: receptor numbers were upregulated in patients tolerant of the drugs but not in the drug-sensitive group (Piggott et al., 1994). In vivo SPECT or PET imaging shows a reduced caudate:putamen ratio in DLB compared with AD and has diagnostic value (Walker et al., 1997; O'Brien et al., 2004; Gilman et al., 2004).

The limited neurochemical studies so far conducted in DLB show some features similar to those in PD (cortical cholinergic and striatal dopaminergic deficits), and others to those in AD (striatal cholinergic deficits). D2-receptor dysregulation and changes in cortical 5HT and turnover levels may differ in DLB compared with both AD or PD (Perry et al., 1993). The Consensus Guidelines for clinical diagnosis of DLB (McKeith et al., 1996) raise the possibility that DLB patients will be distinguished by their therapeutic response to cholinergic and dopaminergic therapies. Initial clinical evidence from trials supports this hypothesis (McKeith et al., 2000b).

48.6 MOLECULAR AND ANATOMICAL PATHOLOGY CORRELATES OF CLINICAL FEATURES IN DEMENTIA WITH LEWY BODIES

48.6.1 Structural brain imaging

Data on regional atrophy in DLB when compared with related disorders, including AD and PD with no cognitive decline, and with elderly controls have largely come from in vivo brain imaging using voxel-based morphometry to analyse structural MRI studies. In DLB there is grey matter volume loss in frontal, temporal and insular cortices compared with controls (Burton et al., 2002). However, the medial temporal lobe (including hippocampus and amygdala) are relatively preserved in comparison with AD patients but there is also increased thalamic atrophy in AD. The caudate nucleus is atrophic in AD, commensurate with overall global brain volume loss (Almeida et al., 2003). Caudate volume is also reported to be reduced in DLB (Barber et al., 2002) but not in PD (Almeida et al., 2003).

48.6.2 Cognitive decline in DLB

Neurochemical pathology (see Section 48.4.5, pp. 621–622) already establishes a number of neurotransmitter-related changes that correlate with cognition in DLB. Establishing the possible role of molecular pathological changes as a basis for the substrate of cognitive decline in DLB is complicated by the frequent co-existence of significant ATP (i.e. in 'common form' DLB). The possibility that α-synucleinopathy and ATP may interact synergistically on cognition is raised by the finding of more severe cognitive disability in 'common form' DLB compared with AD or 'pure' DLB (Serby et al., 2003). Whether the anatomical distribution of α-synucleinopathy, and the quantitative expression of pathology, influence cognitive decline is not fully resolved. Many authors have interpreted the consensus guidelines for documenting Lewy body pathology (McKeith et al., 1996) as diagnostic guidelines. implying that dementia is associated with at least 'limbic' pathological stage. However, it is quite clear that patients with only 'brain stem' LB pathology can have the full clinical expression of DLB (McKeith et al., 2000a). In general there is a strong body of evidence that increased neocortical Lewy body pathology is associated with cognitive decline in DLB and PD (Samuel *et al.*, 1996; Hurtig *et al.*, 2000; Maffila *et al.*, 2000; Kovari *et al.*, 2003).

48.6.3 Visual hallucinations

The obvious candidate regions studied as correlates of visual hallucinations in DLB are the components of the visual pathways and related higher processing brain areas. Neurochemical studies have indicated that cortical cholinergic activity is lower in patients with hallucinations whilst serotonergic neurotransmission is relatively preserved (Perry *et al.*, 1990a). No studies have reported on the relative burden of pathology in serotonergic projection pathways or in the raphé nuclei in DLB in relation to this observation. It has long been appreciated that the occipital neocortex is relatively spared from α-synucleinopathy in terms of Lewy body formation (Perry *et al.*, 1990d) but occipital hypometabolism has been consistently demonstrated in DLB compared with AD (Imamura *et al.*, 2001; Lobotesis *et al.*, 2001). In one study visual hallucination was more frequent in DLB patients with a lower Braak score (Merdes *et al.*, 2003). It is also suggested that an increased burden of medial temporal lobe (parahippocampus, amygdala) Lewy body pathology is an important correlate of visual hallucination (Harding *et al.*, 2002a). Finally it has been proposed that an intrinsic α-synucleinopathy of the retina may characterize hallucinations in DLB (Maurage *et al.*, 2003).

48.6.4 Parkinsonism

The pathological and neurochemical basis of mild parkinsonian features of DLB are probably the most satisfactorily characterized aspect of DLB pathology. The presence of nigral dopamine neurone loss with reduced presynaptic dopamine transporter activity in the striatum now form the basis for a clinical diagnostic strategy (Walker *et al.*, 1997; Gilman *et al.*, 2004; O'Brien *et al.*, 2004) to distinguish DLB from other dementia syndromes. Rather less well resolved is the whole debate about the relationship between DLB and PD, especially in those cases of PD who go on to develop dementia. This topic is beyond the scope of the present chapter and has not been resolved through pathological studies to date. The opportunity to extend studies of α-synucleinopathy from quantification of Lewy bodies to include the neuritic component of the disorder, which can be abundant within the basal ganglia, may well illuminate this question in the future (Duda *et al.*, 2002).

49.6.5 Fluctuation in conscious level

The neuroanatomical structures that are key to regulation of consciousness are not well characterized so that clear candidate brain regions have not been established for the changes found in DLB. One potential candidate brain region is the thalamic intralaminar nuclei (Henderson *et al.*, 2000), which have been shown to be affected in PD.

48.6.6 Supportive features of DLB

Pathological correlates for some of the supportive features of DLB are beginning to emerge or have been hypothesized:

- *Repeated falls.* Orthostatic hypotension is a very frequent correlate of PD and is thought to reflect α-synucleinopathy affecting central (dorsal vagus, medullary reticular formation) and peripheral (autonomic, cardiac) nervous tissues involved in cardiovascular regulation. It is likely that similar changes occur in DLB and contribute to the increased risk of falls in this disorder compared with AD (Imamura *et al.*, 2000; Kaufmann *et al.*, 2001; Londos *et al.*, 2002).
- *REM sleep disorder.* REM-sleep behaviour disorder (RBD) is now regarded as a supportive feature of the diagnosis of DLB following revision of the Consensus diagnostic criteria (McKeith *et al.*, 2004). There is now an impressive body of evidence indicating that RBD is frequently a correlate of α-synucleinopathy and is associated with DLB (Turner *et al.*, 2000; Ferman *et al.*, 2002; Boeve *et al.*, 2003).

48.7 PATHOGENESIS OF DEMENTIA WITH LEWY BODIES

48.7.1 Molecular pathology of Lewy bodies

The biogenesis of Lewy bodies remains incompletely understood. There is a group of disorders in which the formation of αS inclusion bodies is a characteristic, invariable, and apparently primary component of the pathogenetic cascade (Table 48.2, p. 616). In addition, there is a large group of conditions in which Lewy bodies, as defined by modern immunocytochemical concepts, are sometimes associated (Table 48.1, p. 615). The development of animal models of αS aggregation is rapidly increasing understanding of the pathogenesis of α-synucleinopathy (Giasson *et al.*, 2002).

48.7.2 α-Synuclein

The finding that point mutations of the gene encoding αS are associated with the development of autosomal dominant familial PD has had a major impact on studies of the pathology and pathogenesis of Lewy body disorders (Polymeropoulos *et al.*, 1997). It is now apparent that all the major features of the cellular pathology of Lewy body disorders (Lewy bodies, pale bodies, neurites) are intensely immunoreactive for this protein (Spillantini *et al.*, 1997, 1998; Takeda *et al.*, 1998).

The function of the synuclein family is not yet defined. αS is concentrated within synaptic fractions of brain extracts but is not a component of the synaptic vesicle mechanism. A proportion of αS is transported via the rapid vesicle-moving component of axonal transport (Jensen *et al.*, 1998). This vesicle-binding property is abolished by one of the mutations found in familial PD patients. αS is homologous with the β-, γ-synucleins and Persyn, as a family of small, soluble, heat-stable and abundant brain proteins (Buchman *et al.*, 1998; Clayton and George, 1998). αS exists as two alternatively spliced isoforms in man and three in rat (Maroteaux and Scheller, 1991; Hashimoto *et al.*, 1997). The avian homologue of αS is synelfin, which is implicated in synaptic remodelling during song learning (George *et al.*, 1995). Persyn is particularly interesting because it has been shown to promote the disassembly of neurofilament heavy chain subunits when overexpressed in neural cells (Buchman *et al.*, 1998). The possibility is therefore raised that abnormal neurofilament metabolism in Lewy body degeneration results from an abnormal interaction with αS.

An alternative hypothesis has been proposed on the basis of the tendency of αS to self-aggregate. Experiments *in vitro* with human recombinant αS show that certain conditions (e.g. low pH, high temperature) favour the development of thioflavin-S-positive aggregates, which resemble amyloid fibrils (Hashimoto *et al.*, 1998). This is pertinent for two reasons:

- αS was first recognized to be relevant to neurodegeneration when it was unexpectedly isolated from plaque amyloid in AD (Iwai *et al.*, 1995a, b).
- Filamentous proteins can be isolated from Lewy body cases (including both PD and DLB) using a method for isolating paired helical filaments from AD brain. The extracted filaments are either straight or twisted and appear to be composed of regularly orientated αS molecules (Spillantini *et al.*, 1998).

These data therefore suggest that self-aggregation of αS may be a primary mechanism for Lewy body formation. Subsequent enzymatic modifications are reported including phosphorylation (Fujiwara *et al.*, 2002) and proteolytic truncation (Tofaris *et al.*, 2003). It has been argued that ubiquitination of αS in PD and DLB is predominantly by mono-, di- or tri-ubiquitin chains and may represent a proteasome-independent and disease-specific sequence of biochemical changes (Tofaris *et al.*, 2003). Other work suggests that ubiquitination of αS (see below) is not required for inclusion body formation (Sampathu *et al.*, 2003).

48.7.3 Neurofilaments

By analogy with other conditions (e.g. hepatic Mallory body formation), the Lewy body was originally regarded as an intermediate filament inclusion, a view which was supported by immunoelectron microscopic studies, which indicated that the core filamentous component contains neurofilaments (Pollanen *et al.*, 1993a). Since the formation of another intermediate filament inclusion, the Mallory body, can be studied in murine models of hepatocellular toxicity (Denk *et al.*, 1976), this approach has been used to gain insight into Lewy body formation (Pollanen *et al.*, 1994). There is no evidence for an underlying alteration in neurofilament expression in

Lewy body formation (Bergeron *et al.*, 1996), although the mechanism may involve primary damage to neurofilaments. However, the primary pathogenetic insult may be directed at intracellular targets that are crucial to the regulation and maintenance of neurofilament assembly, transport or disassembly. The currently favoured candidate is αS (see Section 48.4.4, pp. 620–621). In this alternative model, the subsequent phosphorylation and truncation of aggregated neurofilaments occurs as a secondary process (Lowe *et al.*, 1996).

Candidate enzymes involved in the phosphorylation of neurofilaments incorporated into Lewy bodies have been sought. Cyclin-dependent kinase 5 has been proposed as a likely candidate on the basis of immunolocalization, in both cortical and subcortical Lewy bodies (Brion and Couck, 1995), together with its regulatory subunit p35nck5a (Nakamura *et al.*, 1997). Such studies do not overcome the problem of whether phosphorylation of neurofilaments precedes or follows Lewy body formation.

48.7.4 Ubiquitin

Much interest has focused on the role of the ubiquitin pathway in Lewy body formation and the concept has developed of Lewy bodies as a cellular protective mechanism (Lowe *et al.*, 1996). Cortical Lewy bodies purified from DLB brains react predominantly to an antibody recognizing polyubiquitin chains rather than free ubiquitin or monoubiquitinated forms (Iwatsubo *et al.*, 1996). The possibility was raised that incomplete activation of ubiquitin-mediated proteolytic pathways may contribute to the pathogenesis of Lewy body degeneration. The dynamic nature of Lewy body formation in comparison to some other inclusion bodies in neurodegenerative diseases has been suggested (Lowe *et al.*, 1990, 1992; Iwatsubo *et al.*, 1996). Differences in the expression of both ubiquitin and the 26S proteasome in Lewy bodies compared with neurofibrillary tangles have been described (Ii *et al.*, 1997).

48.7.5 Other proteins

A large diversity of other peptide constituents have been detected in Lewy bodies by immunocytochemical methods (Table 48.3), but the significance of many of these should be interpreted with caution because of their normal widespread cytosolic distribution.

48.6 SUMMARY

The relationship between DLB, PD and AD is complex and incompletely understood. Within the spectrum of Lewy body disorders there is a neuropsychiatric syndrome, with associated parkinsonism, in the elderly, which is sufficiently distinct in terms of its clinical, pathological and neurochemical profile to warrant recognition as a distinct condition. The

Table 48.3 *Cellular constituents found in Lewy bodies*

Constituent	References
Proteins regarded as major constituents related to formation of Lewy bodies	
α-Synuclein	Spillantini *et al.*, 1997
Neurofilaments (NF)	
• Light, medium and heavy chains	Goldman *et al.*, 1983; Forno *et al.*, 1986; Galloway *et al.*, 1988; Pollanen *et al.*, 1992; Pollanen *et al.*, 1993a
• NF phosphorylation and truncation	Bancher *et al.*, 1989; Hill *et al.*, 1991; Schmidt *et al.*, 1991
• NF cross-linking	Pollanen *et al.*, 1993a, b
Ubiquitin and cell stress or ubiquitination-related proteins	
Ubiquitin	Lowe *et al.*, 1988
Ubiquitin C-terminal hydrolase	Lowe *et al.*, 1990
Polyubiquitin chains	Iwatsubo *et al.*, 1996
26S proteasome	Fergusson *et al.*, 1996; Ii *et al.*, 1997
α-B crystallin	Lowe *et al.*, 1992
Multicatalytic protease	Kwak *et al.*, 1991; Masaki *et al.*, 1994
Cu/Zn superoxide dismutase	Nishiyama *et al.*, 1995
Parkin (E3 ligase)	Schlossmacher *et al.*, 2002
Dorfin (E3 ligase)	Hishikawa *et al.*, 2003
Amyloid precursor protein	Arai *et al.*, 1992
Ca²⁺/calmodulin-dependent protein kinase II	Iwatsubo *et al.*, 1991
Synaptophysin	Nishimura *et al.*, 1994
Chromogranin A	Nishimura *et al.*, 1994
MAP 5	Gai *et al.*, 1996
Cyclin-dependent kinase 5	Brion and Couck, 1995
p35nck5a	Nakamura *et al.*, 1997
Chondroitin sulphate proteoglycan	DeWitt *et al.*, 1994
Sept 4/H5	Ihara *et al.*, 2003
Clusterin	Sasaki *et al.*, 2002

syndrome can be reliably diagnosed by the Consensus Guidelines and has particular therapeutic and other management implications compared with PD or AD. The pathology and neurochemistry of the disorder should be considered from two perspectives:

- α-Synucleinopathy is central to DLB and PD but with a different anatomical distribution of the major burden of lesions.
- The Alzheimer-type pathology, which frequently, but not invariably, complicates the pathological picture, may change the clinical and neurochemical features so that they more closely resemble AD. Genetic studies indicate that DLB cases tend to share many risk factors for AD.

Most elderly demented patients whose clinical course fulfils the Consensus diagnostic criteria for DLB and who have

Lewy body pathology will be compatible with a diagnosis of DLB. Others may more comfortably be interpreted as 'AD with incidental Lewy bodies' or 'dementia in PD'. Clarification of the relationship between patients within these and other diagnostic categories is emerging based on pathological, genetic and neurochemical data in order to understand pathogenesis.

REFERENCES

Aarsland D, Ballard C, Larsen J, McKeith I. (2001) A comparative study of psychiatric symptoms in dementia with Lewy bodies and Parkinson's disease with and without dementia. *International Journal of Geriatric Psychiatry* **16**: 528–536

Agid Y. (1991) Parkinson's disease: pathophysiology. *Lancet* **337**: 1321–1324

Almeida O, Burton E, McKeith I, Gholkar A, Burn D, O'Brien J. (2003) MRI study of caudate nucleus volume in Parkinson's disease with and without dementia with Lewy bodies and Alzheimer's disease. *Dementia and Geriatric Cognitive Disorders* **16**: 57–63

Alvord EC, Forno LS, Kusske JA, Kauffman RJ, Rhodes JS, Goetowski CR. (1974) The pathology of parkinsonism: a comparison of degenerations in cerebral cortex and brain stem. *Advances in Neurology* **5**: 175–193

Arai H, Lee VM-Y, Hill WD, Greenberg BD, Trojanowski JQ. (1992) Lewy bodies contain beta-amyloid precursor proteins of Alzheimer's disease. *Brain Research* **585**: 386–390

Armstrong RA, Cairns NJ, Lantos PL. (1997) Beta-Amyloid (A beta) deposition in the medial temporal lobe of patients with dementia with Lewy bodies. *Neuroscience Letters* **227**: 193–196

Arnold SE, Hyman BT, Flory J, Damasio AR, Van Hoesen GW. (1991) The topographical and neuroanatomical distribution of neurofibrillary tangles and neuritic plaques in cerebral cortex of patients with Alzheimer's disease. *Cerebral Cortex* **1**: 103–116

Baba M, Nakajo S, Tu P-H *et al.* (1998) Aggregation of α-synuclein in Lewy bodies of sporadic Parkinson's disease and Dementia with Lewy bodies. *American Journal of Pathology* **152**: 879–884

Ballard C, Jacoby R, Del Ser T *et al.* (2004) Neuropathological substrates of psychiatric symptoms in prospectively studied patients with autopsy-confirmed dementia with Lewy bodies. *American Journal of Psychiatry* **161**: 843–849

Bancher C, Lassmann H, Budka H *et al.* (1989) An antigenic profile of Lewy bodies: immunocytochemical indication for protein phosphorylation and ubiquitination. *Journal of Neuropathology and Experimental Neurology* **48**: 81–93

Barber R, McKeith I, Balland C, O'Brien JT. (2002) Volumetric MRI study of the caudate nucleus in patients with dementia with Lewy bodies, Alzheimer's disease, and vascular dementia. *Journal of Neurology, Neurosurgery, and Psychiatry* **72**: 406–407

Bergeron C, Petrunka C, Weyer L, Pollanen MS. (1996) Altered neurofilament expression does not contribute to Lewy body formation. *American Journal of Pathology* **148**: 1267–1272

Bodhireddy S, Dickson DW, Mattiace L, Weidenheim KM. (1994) A case of Down's syndrome with diffuse Lewy body disease and Alzheimer's disease. *Neurology* **44**: 159–161

Boeve B, Silber M, Parisi J *et al.* (2003) Synucleinopathy pathology and REM sleep behavior disorder plus dementia or parkinsonism. *Neurology* **61**: 40–45

Boller E, Mizutani T, Roessmann U, Gambetti P. (1980) Parkinson's disease, dementia and Alzheimer's disease: clinicopathological correlations. *Annals of Neurology* **7**: 329–335

Braak H and Braak E. (1991) Neuropathological staging of Alzheimer-related changes. *Acta Neuropathologica (Berlin)* **82**: 239–259

Braak H, Braak E, Yilmazer D *et al.* (1994) Amygdala pathology in Parkinson's disease. *Acta Neuropathologica (Berlin)* **88**: 493–500

Braak H, Braak E, Yilmazer D, de Vos R, Jansen EN, Bohl J. (1995) Nigral and extranigral pathology in Parkinson's disease. *Journal of Neural Transmission* **46** (Suppl.): 15–31

Braak H, Del Tredici K, Rub U, Jansen-Steur E, Braak E. (2003) Staging of brain pathology related to sporadic Parkinson's disease. *Neurobiology of Aging* **24**: 197–211

Brion JP and Couck AM. (1995) Cortical and brain stem-type Lewy bodies are immunoreactive for the cyclin-dependent kinase 5. *American Journal of Pathology* **147**: 1465–1476

Buchman VL, Adu J, Pinon LGP, NinKina NN, Davies AM. (1998) Persyn, a member of the synuclein family, influences neurofilament network integrity. *Nature Neuroscience* **1**: 101–103

Burkhardt CR, Filet CM, Kleinschmidt-DeMasters BK, de la Monte S, Norenberg MD, Schneck SA. (1988) Diffuse Lewy body disease and progressive dementia. *Neurology* **38**: 1520–1528

Burton E, Karas G, Paling S *et al.* (2002) Patterns of cerebral atrophy in dementia with Lewy bodies using voxel-based morphometry. *Neuroimage* **17**: 618–630

Byrne EJ, Lennox G, Lowe J, Godwin-Austen RB. (1989) Diffuse Lewy body disease: clinical features in 15 cases. *Journal of Neurology, Neurosurgery, and Psychiatry* **52**: 709–717

Chin SS-M and Goldman JE. (1996) Glial inclusions in CNS degenerative diseases. *Journal of Neuropathology and Experimental Neurobiology* **55**: 499–508

Clayton DF and George JM. (1998) The synucleins: a family of proteins involved in synaptic function, plasticity, neurodegeneration and disease. *Trends in Neuroscience* **21**: 249–254

Clinton J, Blackman SE-A, Royston MC, Roberts GW. (1994) Differential synaptic loss in the cortex in Alzheimer's disease: a study using archival material. *NeuroReport* **5**: 497–500

Colosimo C, Hughes A, Kilford L, Lees A. (2003) Lewy body cortical involvement may not always predict dementia in Parkinson's disease. *Journal of Neurology, Neurosurgery, and Psychiatry* **74**: 852–856

Court JA and Perry EK. (1994) CNS nicotinic receptors: the therapeutic target in neurodegeneration. *CNS Drugs* **2**: 216–233

Cummings J. (1997) Changes in neuropsychiatric symptoms as outcome measures in clinical trials with cholinergic therapies for Alzheimer's disease. *Alzheimer Disease and Associated Disorders* **11**: 51–59

Dale GE, Probst A, Luthert P, Martin J, Anderton BH, Leigh PN. (1992) Relationship between Lewy bodies and pale bodies in Parkinson's disease. *Acta Neuropathologica (Berlin)* **83**: 525–529

de la Monte SM, Ng SC, Hsu DW. (1995) Aberrant GAP-43 gene expression in Alzheimer's disease. *American Journal of Pathology* **147**: 934–946

De Palma G, Mozzoni P, Mutti A, Calzetti S, Negrotti A. (1998) Case-control study of interactions between genetic and environmental factors in Parkinson's disease. *Lancet* **352**: 1986–1987

de Vos RA, Jansen EN, Stam FC, Ravid R, Swaab DF. (1995) 'Lewy Body Disease': clinicopathological correlations in 18 consecutive cases of Parkinson's disease with and without dementia. *Clinical Neurology and Neurosurgery* **97**: 13–22

Defendini R, Markesbury W, Mastri A, Duffy P. (1973) Hallervorden-Spatz disease and infantile neuraxonal dystrophy. *Journal of the Neurological Sciences* **20**: 7–23

DeLeon G, Grover W, Huff D. (1976) Neuropathological changes in ataxia telangiectasia. *Neurology* **26**: 947–951

Den Hartog Jager WA, Bethlem J. (1960) The distribution of Lewy bodies in the central and autonomic nervous system in idiopathic paralysis agitans. *Journal of Neurology, Neurosurgery, and Psychiatry* **23**: 283–290

Denk H, Eckerstorfer R, Gschnait F, Konrad K, Wolff K. (1976) Experimental induction of hepatocellular hyaline (Mallory bodies) in mice by griseofulvin treatment: 1. Light microscopic observations. *Laboratory Investigation* **35**: 377–382

DeWitt DA, Richey PL, Silver J, Perry G. (1994) Chondroitin sulphate proteoglycans are a common component of neuronal inclusions and astrocytic reaction in neurodegenerative diseases. *Brain Research* **656**: 205–209

Dickson DW, Davies P, Mayeux R *et al.* (1987) Diffuse Lewy body disease: Neuropathological and biochemical studies of six patients. *Acta Neuropathologica (Berlin)* **75**: 8–15

Dickson DW, Crystal H, Mattiace LA *et al.* (1989) Diffuse Lewy body disease: light and electron microscopic immunocytochemistry of senile plaques. *Acta Neuropathologica (Berlin)* **78**: 572–584

Dickson DW, Ruan D, Crystal H *et al.* (1991) Hippocampal degeneration differentiates diffuse Lewy body disease (DLBD) from Alzheimer's disease. *Neurology* **41**: 1402–1409

Dickson DW, Schmidt ML, Lee VM, Zhao ML, Yen SH, Trojanowski JC. (1994) Immunoreactivity profile of hippocampal CA2/3 neurites in diffuse Lewy body disease. *Acta Neuropathologica (Berlin)* **87**: 269–276

Ditter SM and Mirra SS. (1987) Neuropathological and clinical features of Parkinson's disease patients. *Neurology* **37**: 754–760

Donnemiller E, Heilmann J, Wenning GK *et al.* (1997) Brain perfusion scintigraphy with 99mTc-HMPAO or 99mTc-ECD and 123I-beta-CIT single-photon emission tomography in dementia of the Alzheimer-type and diffuse Lewy body disease. *European Journal of Nuclear Medicine* **24**: 320–325

Dooling E, Schoene W, Richardson E. (1974) Hallervorden-Spatz syndrome. *Archives of Neurology* **30**: 70–83

Duda J. (2004) Pathology and neurotransmitter abnormalities of dementia with Lewy Bodies. *Dementia and Geriatric Cognitive Disorders* **17** (Suppl. 1): 3–14

Duda J, Giasson B, Mabon M, Lee V, Trojanowski J. (2002) Novel antibodies to synuclein show abundant striatal pathology in Lewy body diseases. *Annals of Neurology* **52**: 205–210

Feany MB, Mattiace LA, Dickson DW. (1996) Neuropathologic overlap of progressive supranuclear palsy, Pick's disease and corticobasal degeneration. *Journal of Neuropathology and Experimental Neurology* **55**: 53–67

Fergusson J, Landon M, Lowe J *et al.* (1996) Pathological lesions of Alzheimer's disease and dementia with Lewy bodies brains exhibit immunoreactivity to an ATPase that is a regulatory subunit of the 26S proteasome. *Neuroscience Letters* **219**: 167–170

Ferman T, Boeve B, Smith G *et al.* (2002) Dementia with Lewy bodies may present as dementia and REM sleep behavior disorder without parkinsonism or hallucinations. *Journal of International Neuropsychology* **8**: 907–914

Forno LS, Barbour PJ, Norville RL. (1978) Presenile dementia with Lewy bodies and neurofibrillary tangles. *Archives of Neurology* **35**: 818–822

Forno LS, Sternberger L, Sternberger N, Strefling A, Swanson K, Eng L. (1986) Reaction of Lewy bodies with antibodies to phosphorylated and non-phosphorylated neurofilaments. *Neuroscience Letters* **64**: 253–258

Fujiwara H, Hasegawa M, Dohmae N *et al.* (2002) a-Synuclein is phosphorylated in synucleinopathy lesions. *Nature Cell Biology* **4**: 160–164

Gai WP, Blessing WW, Blumbergs PC. (1995) Ubiquitin-positive degenerating neurites in the brain stem in Parkinson's disease. *Brain* **118**: 1447–1459

Gai WP, Blumbergs PC, Blessing WW. (1996) Microtubule-associated protein 5 is a component of Lewy bodies and Lewy neurites in the brainstem and forebrain regions affected in Parkinson's disease. *Acta Neuropathologica (Berlin)* **91**: 78–81

Galloway P, Grunde-Iqbal I, Iqbal K, Perry G. (1988) Lewy bodies contain epitopes both shared and distinct from Alzheimer's neurofibrillary tangles. *Journal of Neuropathology and Experimental Neurology* **47**: 654–663

Gaspar P and Gray F. (1984) Dementia in idiopathic Parkinson's disease. A neuropathological study of 32 cases. *Acta Neuropathologica (Berlin)* **64**: 43–52

Gaytan-Garcia S, Kaufmann JC, Young G. (1990) Adult onset Hallervorden-Spatz syndrome or Seitelberger's disease with late onset: variants of the same entity? a clinicopathological study. *Clinical Neuropathology* **9**: 136–142

Gentleman SM, Williams B, Royston MC *et al.* (1992) Quantification of βA4 protein deposition in the medial temporal lobe: a comparison of Alzheimer's disease and senile dementia of Lewy body type. *Neuroscience Letters* **142**: 9–12

George JM, Jin H, Woods WS, Clayton DF. (1995) Characterization of a novel protein regulated during the critical period for song learning in the zebra finch. *Neuron* **15**: 361–372

Giasson B, Duda J, Quinn S, Zhang B, Trojanowski J, Lee V. (2002) Neuronal α-synucleinopathy with severe movement disorder in mice expressing A53T human α-synuclein. *Neuron* **34**: 521–533

Gibb WRG. (1986) Idiopathic Parkinson's disease and the Lewy body disorders. *Neuropathology and Applied Neurobiology* **12**: 223–234

Gibb WRG and Lees AJ. (1989) The significance of the Lewy body in the diagnosis of idiopathic Parkinson's disease. *Neuropathology and Applied Neurobiology* **15**: 27–44

Gibb WRG, Scaravilli F, Michaud J. (1990) Lewy bodies and subacute sclerosing panencephalitis. *Journal of Neurology, Neurosurgery, and Psychiatry* **53**: 710–711

Gilman S, Koeppe R, Little R *et al.* (2004) Striatal monoamine terminals in Lewy body dementia and Alzheimer's disease. *Annals of Neurology* **556**: 774–780

Goldman J, Yne S-H, Chiu F, Peress N. (1983) Lewy bodies of Parkinson's disease contain neurofilament antigens. *Science* **221**: 1082–1084

Hakim AM and Mathieson G. (1979) Dementia in Parkinson's disease: a neuropathologic study. *Neurology* **29**: 1209–1214

Halliday G, Brooks W, Arthur H, Creasey H, Broe GA. (1997) Further evidence for an association between a mutation in the APP gene and Lewy body formation. *Neuroscience Letters* **227**: 49–52

Hansen LA. (1997) The Lewy body variant of Alzheimer disease. *Journal of Neural Transmission* **51** (Suppl.): 83–93

Hansen LA and Samuel W. (1997) Criteria for Alzheimer's disease and the nosology of dementia with Lewy bodies. *Neurology* **48**: 126–132

Hansen LA, Masliah E, Terry RD, Mirra SS. (1989) A neuropathological subset of Alzheimer's disease with concomitant Lewy body disease and spongiform change. *Acta Neuropathologica (Berlin)* **78**: 194–201

Hansen L, Salmon D, Galasko D *et al.* (1990) The Lewy body variant of Alzheimer's disease: a clinical and pathological entity. *Neurology* **40**: 1–8

Hansen LA, Masliah E, Galasko D, Terry RD. (1993) Plaque-only Alzheimer's disease is usually the Lewy body variant and vice versa. *Journal of Neuropathology and Experimental Neurology* **52**: 648–654

Hansen LA, Daniel SE, Wilcock GK, Love S. (1998) Frontal cortical synaptophysin in Lewy body diseases: relation to Alzheimer's disease and dementia. *Journal of Neurology, Neurosurgery, and Psychiatry* **64**: 653–656

Harding A, Broe G, Halliday G. (2002a) Visual hallucinations in Lewy body disease related to Lewy bodies in the temporal lobe. *Brain* **125**: 391–403

Harding A, Lakay B, Halliday G. (2002b) Selective hippocampal neuron loss in dementia with Lewy bodies. *Annals of Neurology* **51**: 125–128

Harrington CR, Perry RH, Perry EK *et al.* (1994) Senile dementia of Lewy body type and Alzheimer type are biochemically distinct in terms of paired helical filaments and hyperphosphorylated tau protein. *Dementia and Geriatric Cognitive Disorders* **5**: 216–228

Hashimoto M, Yoshimoto M, Sisk A *et al.* (1997) NACP, a synaptic protein involved in Alzheimer's disease, is differentially regulated during megakaryocyte differentiation. *Biochemical and Biophysical Research Communications* **237**: 611–616

Hashimoto M, Hsu LJ, Sisk A, Xia Y, Takeda A, Sundsmo M, Masliah E. (1998) Human recombinant NACP/α-synuclein is aggregated and fibrillated in vitro: relevance for Lewy body disease. *Brain Research* **799**: 301–306

Hedera P, Lerner AJ, Castellani R, Freiland RP. (1995) Concurrence of Alzheimer's disease, Parkinson's disease, diffuse Lewy body disease and amyotrophic lateral sclerosis. *Journal of the Neurological Sciences* **128**: 219–224

Helfand M. (1935) Status pigmentatus: its pathology and relation to Hallervorden-Spatz disease. *Journal of Nervous and Mental Disorders* **81**: 662–675

Henderson JM, Carpenter K, Cartwright H, Halliday GM. (2000) Loss of thalamic intralaminar nuclei in progressive supranuclear palsy and Parkinson's disease: clinical and therapeutic implications. *Brain* **123**: 1410–1421

Higuchi S, Arai H, Matsushita S *et al.* (1998) Mutation in the α-synuclein gene and sporadic Parkinson's disease, Alzheimer's disease and Dementia with Lewy bodies. *Experimental Neurology* **153**: 164–166

Hill WD, Lee VM-Y, Hurtig HI, Murrat JM, Trojanowski JQ. (1991) Epitopes located in spatially separated domains of each neurofilament subunit are present in Parkinson's disease Lewy bodies. *Journal of Comparative Neurology* **309**: 150–160

Hishikawa N, Hashizume Y, Yoshida M, Sobue G. (2003) Clinical and neuropathological correlates of Lewy body disease. *Acta Neuropathologica (Berlin)* **105**: 341–350

Horoupian D and Chu P. (1994) Unusual case of corticobasal degeneration with tau/Gallyas-positive neuronal and glial tangles. *Acta Neuropathologica (Berlin)* **82**: 592–598

Hughes AJ, Daniel SE, Blankson S, Lees AJ. (1993) A clinicopathological study of 100 cases of Parkinson's disease. *Archives of Neurology* **50**: 140–148

Hurtig H, Trojanowski J, Galvin J *et al.* (2000) Alpha-synuclein cortical Lewy bodies correlate with dementia in Parkinson's disease. *Neurology* **54**: 1916–1921

Hutchinson M and Fazzini E. (1996) Cholinesterase inhibition in Parkinson's disease. *Journal of Neurology, Neurosurgery, and Psychiatry* **61**: 324–325

Ihara M, Tomimoto H, Kitayama H *et al.* (2003) Association of the cytoskeletal GTP-binding protein Sept4/H5 with cytoplasmic inclusions found in Parkinson's disease and other synucleinopathies. *Journal of Biological Chemistry* **278**: 24095–24102

Ii K, Ito H, Tanaka K, Hirano A. (1997) Immunocytochemical co-localisation of the proteasome in ubiquitinated structures in neurodegenerative disease and the elderly. *Journal of Neuropathology and Experimental Neurology* **56**: 125–131

Imamura T, Hirono N, Hashimoto *et al.* (2000) Fall-related injuries in dementia with Lewy bodies (DLB) and Alzheimer's disease. *European Journal of Neurology* **7**: 77–79

Imamura T, Ishii K, Hirono N *et al.* (2001) Occipital glucose metabolism in dementia with Lewy bodies with and without parkinsonism: a study using positron emission tomography. *Dementia and Geriatric Cognitive Disorders* **12**: 194–197

Ince P, Irving D, MacArthur F, Perry RH. (1991) Quantitative neuropathology in the hippocampus: comparison of senile dementia of Alzheimer type, senile dementia of Lewy body type, Parkinson's disease and non-demented elderly control patients. *Journal of the Neurological Sciences* **106**: 142–152

Ince PG, McArthur FK, Bjertness E, Torvik A, Candy JM, Edwardson JA. (1995) Neuropathological diagnoses in elderly patients in Oslo: Alzheimer's disease, Lewy body disease and vascular lesions. *Dementia and Geriatric Cognitive Disorders* **6**: 162–168

Ince P, Morris C, Perry E. (1998) Dementia with Lewy bodies: a distinct non-Alzheimer dementia? *Brain Pathology* **8**: 299–324

Iseki E, Odawara T, Kosaka, K. (1995) A quantitative study of Lewy bodies and senile changes in the amygdala in diffuse Lewy body disease. *Neuropathology and Applied Neurobiology* **15**: 112–116

Iseki E, Odawara T, Li F, Kosaka K, Nishimura T, Akiyama H, Ikeda K. (1996) Age-related ubiquitin-positive granular structures in non-demented subjects and neurodegenerative disorders. *Journal of the Neurological Sciences* **142**: 25–29

Iseki E, Li F, Kosaka K. (1997) Close relationship between spongiform change and ubiquitin-positive granular structures in diffuse Lewy body disease. *Journal of the Neurological Sciences* **146**: 53–57

Iwai A, Masliah E, Yoshimoto M *et al.* (1995a) The precursor protein of non-A beta component of Alzheimer's disease is a presynaptic protein of the central nervous system. *Neuron* **14**: 467–475

Iwai A, Yoshimoto M, Masliah E, Saitoh T. (1995b) Non-Aβ component of Alzheimer's disease amyloid (NAC) is amyloidogenic. *Biochemistry* **34**: 10139–10145

Iwatsubo T, Nakano I, Fukunaga K, Miyamoto E. (1991) Ca2+/calmodulin-dependent protein kinase II immunoreactivity in Lewy bodies. *Acta Neuropathologica (Berlin)* **82**: 159–163

Iwatsubo T, Yamaguchi H, Fujimoro M *et al.* (1996) Purification and characterisation of Lewy bodies from the brains of patients with diffuse Lewy body disease. *American Journal of Pathology* **148**: 1517–1529

Jackson M, Lennox G, Balsitis M, Lowe J. (1995) The cortical neuritic pathology of Huntington's disease. *Journal of Neurology, Neurosurgery, and Psychiatry* **58**: 756–758

Jellinger KA and Bancher C. (1996) Dementia with Lewy bodies: relationships to Parkinson's and Alzheimer's diseases. In: R Perry, I McKeith, E Perry (eds), *Dementia with Lewy Bodies*. New York, Cambridge University Press

Jensen PH, Nielsen MS, Jakes R, Dotti CG, Goedert M. (1998) Binding of α-synuclein to brain vesicles is abolished by familial Parkinson's disease mutation. *Journal of Biological Chemistry* **273**: 26292–26294

Joachim CL, Morris JH, Selkoe DJ. (1988) Clinically diagnosed Alzheimer's disease: autopsy results in 150 cases. *Annals of Neurology* **24**: 50–56

Kalyanasundaram S, Srivinas HV, Deshpande DH. (1980) An adult with Hallervorden-Spatz disease: clinical and pathological study. *Clinical Neurology and Neurosurgery* **82**: 245–249

Kaufmann H, Hague K, Perl D. (2001) Accumulation of alpha-synuclein in autonomic nerves in pure autonomic failure. *Neurology* **56**: 980–981

Khachaturian ZS. (1985) The diagnosis of Alzheimer's disease. *Archives of Neurology* **42**: 1097–1105

Kim H, Gearing M, Mirra SS. (1995) Ubiquitin-positive CA2/3 neurites in hippocampus coexist with cortical Lewy bodies. *Neurology* **45**: 1768–1770

Kosaka K. (1978) Lewy bodies in the cerebral cortex. Report of three cases. *Acta Neuropathologica (Berlin)* **42**: 127–134

Kosaka K. (1993) Dementia and neuropathology in Lewy body disease. *Advances in Neurology* **60**: 456–463

Kosaka K and Iseki E. (1996) Diffuse Lewy body disease within the spectrum of Lewy body disease. In: R Perry, I McKeith, E Perry (eds), *Dementia with Lewy Bodies*. New York, Cambridge University Press

Kosaka K and Mehraein P. (1979) Dementia-parkinsonism with numerous Lewy bodies and senile plaques in cerebral cortex. *Archiv für Psychiatrie und Nervenkrankheiten* **226**: 241–250

Kosaka K, Matsushita M, Oyanagi S, Mehraein P. (1980) A clinicopathological study of the 'Lewy Body Disease'. *Psychiatria et Neurologia* **82**: 292–311

Kosaka K, Yoshimura M, Ikeda K, Budka H. (1984) Diffuse type of Lewy body disease: progressive dementia with abundant cortical Lewy bodies and senile changes of varying degree – a new disease? *Clinical Neuropathology* **3**: 185–192

Kosaka K, Tsuchiya K, Yoshimura M. (1989) Lewy body disease with and without dementia: a clinicopathological study of 35 cases. *Clinical Neuropathology* **7**: 299–305

Kosaka K, Iseki E, Odawara T. (1996) Cerebral type of Lewy body disease. *Neuropathology* **16**: 32–35

Kovari E, Gold G, Herrmann F *et al.* (2003) Lewy body densities in the entorhinal and anterior cingulate cortex predict cognitive deficits in Parkinson's disease. *Acta Neuropathologica (Berlin)* **106**: 83–88

Kwak S, Masaki T, Ishiura S, Sugita H. (1991) Multicatalytic proteinase is present in Lewy bodies and neurofibrillary tangles in diffuse Lewy body disease brains. *Neuroscience Letters* **128**: 21–24

Langlais PJ, Thal L, Hansen L, Galasko D, Alford M, Masliah E. (1993) Neurotransmitters in basal ganglia and cortex of Alzheimer's disease with and without Lewy bodies. *Neurology* **43**: 1927–1934

Lantos PL, Ovenstone IM, Johnson J, Clelland CA, Roques P, Rossor MN. (1994) Lewy bodies in the brains of two members of a family with the 717 (Val to Ile) mutation of the amyloid precursor protein gene. *Neuroscience Letters* **172**: 77–79

Leake A, Perry EK, Perry RH, Fairbairn AF, Ferrier IN. (1990) Cortical concentrations of corticotropin-releasing factor and its receptor in Alzheimer type dementia and major depression. *Biological Psychiatry* **28**: 603–608

Lennox G, Lowe J, Morrell K, Landon M, Mayer RJ. (1989) Anti-ubiquitin immunocytochemistry is more sensitive than conventional techniques in the detection of diffuse Lewy body disease. *Journal of Neurology, Neurosurgery, and Psychiatry* **52**: 67–71

Lewy FH. (1912) Paralysis agitans. I. Pathologische anatomie. In: M Lewandowsky (ed.), *Handbuch der Neurologie*. Berlin, Springer

Lippa CF, Smith TW, Swearer JM. (1994) Alzheimer's disease and Lewy body disease: a comparative clinicopathological study. *Annals of Neurology* **35**: 81–88

Lippa CF, Pulaski-Salo D, Dickson DW, Smith TW. (1997) Alzheimer's disease, Lewy body disease and aging: a comparative study of the perforant pathway. *Journal of the Neurological Sciences* **147**: 161–166

Lobotesis K, Fenwick J, Phipps A et al. (2001) Occipital hypoperfusion on SPECT in dementia with Lewy bodies but not AD. Neurology 56: 643-649

Londos E, Passant U, Risberg J, Gustafson L, Brun A. (2002) Contributions of other brain pathologies in dementia with Lewy bodies. Dementia and Geriatric Cognitive Disorders 13: 130-148

Louis ED, Klatka LA, Lui Y, Fahn S. (1997) Comparison of extrapyramidal features in 31 pathologically confirmed cases of diffuse Lewy body disease and 34 pathologically confirmed cases of Parkinson's disease. Neurology 48: 376-380

Lowe J, Blanchard A, Morrell K et al. (1988) Ubiquitin is a common factor in intermediate filament inclusion bodies of diverse type in man, including those of Parkinson's disease, Pick's disease and Alzheimer's disease as well as Rosenthal fibres in cerebellar astrocytomas, cytoplasmic bodies in muscle and Mallory bodies in alcoholic liver disease. Journal of Pathology 155: 9-15

Lowe J, McDermott H, Landon M, Mayer RJ, Wilkinson K. (1990) Ubiquitin carboxyl-terminal hydrolase (PGP9.5) is selectively present in ubiquitinated inclusion bodies characteristic of human neurodegenerative diseases. Journal of Pathology 161: 153-160

Lowe J, McDermott H, Pike I, Spendlove I, Landon M, Mayer RJ. (1992) Alpha B crystallin expression in non-lenticular tissues and selective presence in ubiquitinated inclusion bodies in human disease. Journal of Pathology 166: 61-68

Lowe JS, Mayer RJ, Landon M. (1996) Pathological significance of Lewy bodies in dementia. In: R Perry, I McKeith, E Perry (eds), Dementia with Lewy Bodies. New York, Cambridge University Press

McKeith IG, Fairbairn A, Perry RH, Thompson P, Perry EK. (1992a) Neuroleptic sensitivity in patients with senile dementia of Lewy body type. BMJ 305: 673-678

McKeith IG, Perry RH, Fairbairn AF, Jabeen S, Perry EK. (1992b) Operational criteria for senile dementia of Lewy body type. Psychological Medicine 22: 911-922

McKeith IG, Fairbairn AF, Bothwell RA et al. (1994a) An evaluation of the predictive value and interrater reliability of clinical diagnostic criteria for senile dementia of Lewy body type. Neurology 44: 872-877

McKeith IG, Fairbairn AF, Perry RH, Thompson P. (1994b) The clinical diagnosis and misdiagnosis of senile dementia of Lewy body type. British Journal of Psychiatry 165: 324-332

McKeith IG, Galasko D, Kosaka K et al. (1996) Consensus guidelines for the clinical and pathological diagnosis of dementia with Lewy bodies (DLB): report of the consortium on DLB International Workshop. Neurology 47: 1113-1124

McKeith IG, Ballard CG, Perry RH et al. (2000a) Prospective validation of consensus criteria for the diagnosis of dementia with Lewy bodies. Neurology 54: 1050-1058

McKeith I, Del Ser T, Spano P et al. (2000b) Efficacy of rivastigmine in dementia with Lewy bodies: a randomized, double-blind, placebo-controlled, international study. Lancet 356: 2031-2036

McKeith I, Mintzer J, Aarsland D et al. (2004) International Psychogeriatric Association Expert Meeting on DLB. Dementia with Lewy bodies. Lancet Neurology 3: 19-28

McKenzie JE, Edwards RJ, Gentleman SM, Ince PG, Perry RH, Royston MC. (1996) A quantitative comparison of plaque types in Alzheimer's disease and senile dementia of the Lewy body type. Acta Neuropathologica 91: 526-529

Maffila P, Rinne J, Helenius H, Dickson D, Roytta M. (2000) Alpha-synuclein-immunoreactive cortical Lewy bodies are associated with cognitive impairment in Parkinson's disease. Acta Neuropathologica (Berlin) 100: 285-290

Mancardi GI, Mandybur TI, Liwnicz BH. (1982) Spongiform-like changes in Alzheimer's disease. Acta Neuropathologica (Berlin) 56: 146-150

Mark MH, Sage JI, Dickson DW et al. (1994) Meige syndrome in the spectrum of Lewy body disease. Neurology 44: 1432-1436

Maroteaux L and Scheller RH. (1991) The rat brain synucleins: family of proteins transiently associated with neuronal membrane. Molecular Brain Research 11: 335-343

Martin-Ruiz C, Lawrence S, Piggott M et al. (2002) Nicotinic receptors in the putamen of patients with dementia with Lewy bodies and Parkinson's disease: relation to changes in α-synuclein expression. Neuroscience Letters 335: 134-138

Masaki T, Ishiura S, Sugita H, Kwak S. (1994) Multicatalytic proteinase is associated with characteristic oval structures in cortical Lewy bodies. Journal of the Neurological Sciences 122: 127-134

Masliah E, Terry RD, Alford M, De Teresa R, Hansen LA. (1991) Cortical and subcortical patterns of synaptophysin-like immunoreactivity in Alzheimer's disease. American Journal of Pathology 138: 235-246

Masliah E, Mallory M, deTeresa R, Alford M, Hansen LA. (1993) Differing patterns of aberrant neuronal sprouting in Alzheimer's disease with and without Lewy bodies. Brain Research 617: 258-266

Mattila PM, Röttyä M, Torikka H, Dickson DW, Rinne JO. (1998) Cortical Lewy bodies and Alzheimer-type changes in patients with Parkinson's disease. Acta Neuropathologica (Berlin) 95: 576-582

Maurage C, Ruchoux M, de Vos R, Surguchov A, Destee A. (2003) Retinal involvement in dementia with Lewy bodies: a clue to hallucinations? Annals of Neurology 54: 542-547

Mayeux R, Chen J, Mirabello E et al. (1990) An estimate of the incidence of dementia in patients with idiopathic Parkinson's disease. Neurology 40: 1513-1517

Mega MS, Masterman DL, Benson et al. (1996) Dementia with Lewy bodies: reliability and validity of clinical and pathological criteria. Neurology 47: 1403-1409

Merdes A, Hansen L, Jeste D et al. (2003) Influence of Alzheimer pathology on clinical diagnostic accuracy in dementia with Lewy bodies. Neurology 60: 1586-1590

Mirra SS, Heyman A, McKeel D et al. (1991) The consortium to establish a registry of Alzheimer's disease (CERAD) Part II. Standardization of the neuropathologic assessment of Alzheimer's disease. Neurology 41: 479-486

Mirra SS, Hart M, Terry RD. (1993) Making a diagnosis of Alzheimer's disease: a primer for the practicing pathologist. Archives of Pathology and Laboratory Medicine 117: 132-144

Monaco S, Nardelli E, Moretto G, Cavallaro T, Rizzuto N. (1988) Cytoskeletal pathology in ataxia telangiectasia. Clinical Neuropathology 7: 44-45

Mori H, Yoshimura M, Tomonaga M, Yamanouchi H. (1986) Progressive supranuclear palsy with Lewy bodies. Acta Neuropathologica (Berlin) 71: 344-346

Morin P, Lechavelier B, Bianco C. (1980) Cerebellar atrophy associated with lesions of the pallidum and Luys' body and the presence of Lewy bodies. Relationships with degenerative disorders of the pallidum, substantia nigra and Luys' body. Revue Neurologique 136: 381-390

Nakamura S, Kawamoto Y, Nakano S, Akiguchi I, Kimura J. (1997) p35nck5a and cyclin-dependent kinase 5 colocalise in Lewy bodies in brains with Parkinson's disease. Acta Neuropathologica (Berlin) 94: 153-157

NIA and Reagan Institute. (1997) Consensus recommendations for the postmortem diagnosis of Alzheimer's disease. Neurobiology of Aging 18: S1-S2

Neuropathology Group of MRCCFAS. (2001) Pathological correlates of late-onset dementia in a multicentre, community-based population in England Wales. *Lancet* **357**: 169–175

Nishimura M, Tomimoto H, Suenaga T *et al.* (1994) Synaptophysin and chromogranin A immunoreactivities of Lewy bodies in Parkinson's disease. *Brain Research* **634**: 339–344

Nishiyama K, Murayama S, Shimizu J *et al.* (1995) Cu/Zn superoxide dismutase-like immunoreactivity is present in Lewy bodies from Parkinson's disease: a light and electron microscopic immunocytochemical study. *Acta Neuropathologica (Berlin)* **89**: 471–474

O'Brien JT, Colloby S, Fenwick J *et al.* (2004) Dopamine transporter loss visualized with FP-CIT SPECT in the differential diagnosis of dementia with Lewy bodies. *Archives of Neurology* **61**: 919–925

Okazaki H, Lipkin LS, Aronson SM. (1961) Diffuse intracytoplasmic ganglionic inclusions (Lewy type) associated with progressive dementia and quadriparesis in flexion. *Journal of Neuropathology and Experimental Neurology* **20**: 237–244

Parkkinen L, Soininen H, Laakso M, Alafuzoff I. (2001) α-Synuclein pathology is highly dependent on the case selection. *Neuropathology and Applied Neurobiology* **27**: 314–325

Parkkinen L, Soininen H, Alfuzoff I. (2003) Regional distribution of alpha-synuclein pathology in unimpaired aging and Alzheimer's disease. *Journal of Neuropathology and Experimental Neurology* **62**: 363–367

Paulus W and Selim M. (1990) Corticonigral degeneration with neuronal achromasia and basal neurofibrillary tangles. *Acta Neuropathologica (Berlin)* **81**: 89–94

Pellise A, Roig C, Barraquer-Bordas LI, Ferrer I. (1996) Abnormal ubiquitinated cortical neurites in patients with diffuse Lewy body disease. *Neuroscience Letters* **206**: 85–88

Perl DP, Olanow CW, Calne D. (1998) Alzheimer's disease and Parkinson's disease: distinct entities or extremes of a spectrum of neurodegeneration. *Annals of Neurology* **44** (Suppl. 1): S19–S31

Perry EK and Perry RH. (1995) Acetylcholine and hallucinations: disease-related compared with drug-induced alterations in human consciousness. *Brain and Cognition* **28**: 240–258

Perry EK, Marshall E, Kerwin J *et al.* (1990a) Evidence of a monoaminergic:cholinergic imbalance related to visual hallucinations in Lewy body dementia. *Journal of Neurochemistry* **55**: 1544–1546

Perry EK, Marshall E, Perry RH *et al.* (1990b) Cholinergic and dopaminergic activities in senile dementia of Lewy body type. *Alzheimer Disease and Associated Disorders* **4**: 87–95

Perry EK, Smith CJ, Court JA, Perry RH. (1990c) Cholinergic nicotinic and muscarinic receptors in dementia of Alzheimer, Parkinson and Lewy body types. *Journal of Neural Transmission* **2**: 149–158

Perry RH, Irving D, Blessed G, Fairbairn A, Perry EK. (1990d) Senile dementia of Lewy body type: a clinically and neuropathologically distinct form of Lewy body dementia in the elderly. *Journal of the Neurological Sciences* **95**: 119–139

Perry EK, Marshall E, Thompson P *et al.* (1993) Monoaminergic activities in Lewy body dementia: relation to hallucinosis and extrapyramidal features. *Journal of Neural Transmission* **6**: 167–177

Perry EK, Haroutunian V, Davis KL *et al.* (1994) Neocortical cholinergic activities differentiate Lewy body dementia from classical Alzheimer's disease. *NeuroReport* **5**: 747–749

Perry EK, Court JA, Goodchild R *et al.* (1998) Clinical neurochemistry: developments in dementia research based on brain bank material. *Journal of Neural Transmission* **105**: 915–933

Perry E, McKeith I, Ballard C. (2003) Butyryl-cholinesterase and progression of cognitive deficits in dementia with Lewy bodies. *Neurology* **60**: 1852–1853

Piggott MA, Perry RH, McKeith IG, Marshall E, Perry EK. (1994) Dopamine D2 receptors in demented patients with severe neuroleptic sensitivity. *Lancet* **343**: 1044–1045

Piggott MA, Marshall EF, Thomas N. (1999) Dopaminergic activities in the human striatum: rostrocaudal gradients of uptake sites and of D1 and D2 but not of D3 receptor binding or dopamine. *Neuroscience* **90**: 433–445

Piggott M, Owens J, O'Brien J *et al.* (2003) Muscarinic receptors in basal ganglia in dementia with Lewy bodies, Parkinson's disease and Alzheimer's disease. *Journal of Chemical Neuroanatomy* **25**: 161–173

Pollanen MS, Bergeron C, Weyer L. (1993a) Deposition of detergent-resistant neurofilaments into Lewy body fibrils. *Brain Research* **603**: 121–124

Pollanen MS, Dickson DW, Bergeron C. (1993b) Pathology and biology of the Lewy body. *Journal of Neuropathology and Experimental Neurology* **52**: 183–191

Pollanen MS, Markiewicz P, Weyer L, Goh MC, Bergeron C. (1994) Mallory body filaments become insoluble after normal assembly into intermediate filaments. *American Journal of Pathology* **145**: 140–147

Polymeropoulos MH, Lavedan C, Leroy E *et al.* (1997) Mutation in the α-synuclein gene identified in families with Parkinson's disease. *Science*: **276**: 2045–2047

Raghavan R, Khin-Nu C, Brown A *et al.* (1993) Detection of Lewy bodies in trisomy 21 (Down's syndrome). *Canadian Journal of Neurological Science* **20**: 48–51

Rezaie P, Cairns NJ, Chadwick A, Lantos PL. (1996) Lewy bodies are located preferentially in limbic areas in diffuse Lewy body disease. *Neuroscience Letters* **212**: 111–114

Saito Y, Ruberu N, Sawabe M *et al.* (2004) Lewy body-related α-synucleinopathy in aging. *Journal of Neuropathology and Experimental Neurology* **63**: 742–749

Sampathu D, Giasson B, Pawlyk A, Trojanowski J, Lee V. (2003) Ubiquitination of α-synuclein is not required for formation of pathological inclusions in α-synucleinopathies. *American Journal of Pathology* **163**: 91–100

Samuel W, Galasko D, Masliah E, Hansen LA. (1996) Neocortical Lewy body counts correlate with dementia in the Lewy body variant of Alzheimer's disease. *Journal of Neuropathology and Experimental Neurology* **55**: 44–52

Samuel W, Alford M, Hofstetter CR, Hansen L. (1997a) Dementia with Lewy bodies versus pure Alzheimer's disease: differences in cognition, neuropathology, cholinergic dysfunction, and synaptic density. *Journal of Neuropathology and Experimental Neurology* **56**: 499–508

Samuel W, Crowder R, Hofstetter CR, Hansen L. (1997b) Neuritic plaques in the Lewy body variant of Alzheimer's disease lack paired helical filaments. *Neuroscience Letters* **223**: 73–76

Sasaki K, Doh-ura K, Wakisaka Y, Iwaki T. (2002) Clusterin/apolipoprotein J is associated with cortical Lewy bodies: immunohistochemical study in cases with α-synucleinopathies. *Acta Neuropathologica (Berlin)* **104**: 225–230

Schlossmacher M, Frosch M, Gai W *et al.* (2002) Parkin localizes to the Lewy bodies of Parkinson's disease and dementia with Lewy bodies. *American Journal of Pathology* **160**: 1655–1667

Schmidt ML, Murray JM, Lee VM-Y Hill, WD Wertkin A, Trojanowski JQ. (1991) Epitope map of neurofilament protein domains in cortical and peripheral nervous system Lewy bodies. *American Journal of Pathology* **139**: 53–65

Schmidt ML, Martin JA, Lee VM-Y, Trojanowski JQ. (1996) Convergence of Lewy bodies and neurofibrillary tangles in amygdala neurons of Alzheimer's disease and Lewy body disorders. *Acta Neuropathologica (Berlin)* **91**: 475–481

Serby M, Brickman A, Haroutunian V *et al.* (2003) Cognitive burden and excess Lewy-body pathology in the Lewy-body variant of Alzheimer's disease. *American Journal of Geriatric Psychiatry* **11**: 371–374

Shepherd C, McCann H, Thiel E, Halliday G. (2002) Neurofilament-immunoreactive neurons in Alzheimer's disease and dementia with Lewy bodies. *Neurobiology of Disease* **9**: 249–57

Sima AA, Hoag G, Rozdilsky B. (1987) Shy-Drager syndrome: the transitional variant. *Clinical Neuropathology* **6**: 49–54

Smith TW, Anwer U, De Girolami U, Drachman DA. (1987) Vacuolar change in Alzheimer's disease. *Archives of Neurology* **44**: 1225–1228

Smith MC, Mallory M, Hansen LA, Ge N, Masiah E. (1995) Fragmentation of the neuronal cytoskeleton in the Lewy body variant of Alzheimer's disease. *NeuroReport* **6**: 673–679

Spillantini MG, Schmidt ML, Lee VM-Y, Trojanowski JQ, Jakes R, Goedert M. (1997) α-Synuclein in Lewy bodies. *Nature* **388**: 839–840

Spillantini MG, Crowther RA, Jakes R, Hasegawa M. (1998) α-synuclein in filamentous inclusions of Lewy bodies from Parkinson's disease and Dementia with Lewy bodies. *Proceedings of the National Academy of Sciences of the United States of America* **95**: 6469–6473

Strong C, Anderton BH, Perry RH, Perry EK, Ince PG, Lovestone S. (1995) Abnormally phosphorylated tau protein in senile dementia of Lewy body type and Alzheimer's disease: evidence that the disorders are distinct. *Alzheimer Disease and Associated Disorders* **9**: 21–222

Sugiyama H, Hainfeller JA, Schmid SB, Budka H. (1993) Neuraxonal dystrophy combined with diffuse Lewy body disease in a young adult. *Clinical Neuropathology* **12**: 147–152

Sugiyama H, Hainfellner JA, Yoshimura M, Budka H. (1994) Neocortical changes in Parkinson's disease, revisited. *Clinical Neuropathology* **13**: 55–59

Takeda A, Mallory M, Sundsmo M, Hansen L, Masliah E. (1998) Abnormal accumulation of α-synuclein in neurodegenerative disorders. *American Journal of Pathology* **152**: 367–372

Tiraboschi P, Hansen L, Alford M *et al.* (2002) Early and widespread cholinergic losses differentiate dementia with Lewy bodies from Alzheimer disease. *Archives of General Psychiatry* **59**: 947–951

Tofaris C, Razzaq A, Ghetti B, Lilley K, Spillantini M. (2003) Ubiquitination of α-synuclein in Lewy bodies in a pathological event not associated with impairment of proteasome function. *Journal of Biological Chemistry* **278**: 44405–44411

Tomlinson BE, Blessed G, Roth M. (1970) Observations on the brains of demented old people. *Journal of the Neurological Sciences* **11**: 205–242

Tompkins MM, Basgall EJ, Zamrini E, Hill WD. (1997) Apoptotic-like changes in Lewy-body-associated disorders and normal aging in substantia nigral neurons. *American Journal of Pathology* **150**: 119–131

Turner R, D'Amata C, Chervin R, Blaivas M. (2000) The pathology of REM sleep behaviour disorder with comorbid Lewy body dementia. *Neurology* **55**: 1730–1732

Vaughan JR, Farrer MJ, Wszolek *et al.* (1998) For the European Consortium on Genetic Susceptibility in Parkinson's Disease. Sequencing of the α-synuclein gene in a large series of cases of familial Parkinson's disease fails to reveal any further mutations. *Human Molecular Genetics* **7**: 751–753

Vuia O. (1977) Neuraxonal dystrophy: a juvenile adult form. *Clinical Neurology and Neurosurgery* **79**: 305–315

Wakabayashi K, Honer WG, Masliah E. (1994a) Synapse alterations in the hippocampal-entorhinal formation in Alzheimer's disease with and without Lewy bodies. *Brain Research* **667**: 24–32

Wakabayashi K, Oyanagi K, Makifuchi T *et al.* (1994b) Corticobasal degeneration: etiopathological significance of the cytoskeletal alterations. *Acta Neuropathologica (Berlin)* **87**: 545–553

Wakabayashi K, Hansen LA, Masliah E. (1995) Cortical Lewy body-containing neurons are pyramidal cells: laser scanning confocal imaging of double-immunolabelled sections with anti-ubiquitin. *Acta Neuropathologica (Berlin)* **89**: 404–408

Wakabayashi K, Hansen LA, Vincent I, Mallory M, Masliah E. (1997a) Neurofibrillary tangles in the dentate granule cells of patients with Alzheimer's disease, Lewy body disease and progressive supranuclear palsy. *Acta Neuropathologica (Berlin)* **93**: 7–12

Wakabayashi K, Matsumoto K, Takayama K, Yoshimoto M, Takahashi H. (1997b) NACP, a presynaptic protein, immunoreactivity in Lewy bodies in Parkinson's disease. *Neuroscience Letters* **239**: 45–48

Walker Z, Costa DC, Janssen AG, Walker RW, Livingstone G, Katona CL. (1997) Dementia with Lewy bodies: a study of post-synaptic dopaminergic receptors with iodine-123 iodobenzamide single photon emission tomography. *European Journal of Nuclear Medicine* **24**: 609–614

Williams T, Shaw PJ, Lowe J, Bates D, Ince PG. (1995) Parkinsonism in motor neuron disease: case report and literature review. *Acta Neuropathologica (Berlin)* **89**: 275–283

Williamson K, Sima A, Curry B, Ludwin S. (1982) Neuraxonal dystrophy in young adults: a clinicopathological study of two unrelated cases. *Annals of Neurology* **11**: 335–343

Yokota O, Terada S, Ishizu H *et al.* (2002) NACP/α-synuclein immunoreactivity in diffuse neurofibrillary tangles with calcification (DNTC). *Acta Neuropathologica (Berlin)* **104**: 333–341

Yoshimura M. (1983) Cortical changes in the parkinsonian brain: a contribution to the delineation of 'diffuse Lewy body disease'. *Journal of Neurology* **229**: 17–32

Zhan S-S, Beyreuther K, Schmitt HP. (1994) Synaptophysin immunoreactivity of the cortical neuropil in vascular dementia of Binswanger type compared with the dementia of Alzheimer type and non-demented controls. *Dementia and Geriatric Cognitive Disorders* **5**: 79–87

Zweig RM, Cardillo JE, Cohen M, Giere S, Hedreen JC. (1993) The locus ceruleus and dementia in Parkinson's disease. *Neurology* **43**: 986–991

Neuropsychological changes in dementia with Lewy bodies

DAVID P SALMON AND JOANNE M HAMILTON

Dementia with Lewy bodies (DLB; [McKeith *et al.*, 1996b]) refers to a clinicopathologic condition in which the brains of patients who exhibited insidious and progressive cognitive decline during life are found to have a diffuse distribution of Lewy bodies and cell loss in subcortical structures and in widespread regions of the neocortex (Kosaka *et al.*, 1984; Gibb *et al.*, 1985; Dickson *et al.*, 1987; Gibb *et al.*, 1989; Lennox *et al.*, 1989; Hansen *et al.*, 1990; Kosaka, 1990; Perry *et al.*, 1990). The subcortical pathology that occurs in DLB is similar to that of Parkinson's disease (PD), but the number of Lewy bodies and the degree of cell loss in the substantia nigra and in other pigmented brain stem nuclei (e.g. locus caeruleus and dorsal vagal nucleus) is usually intermediate between that of patients with PD and age-matched normal individuals (for reviews, see Perry *et al.*, 1990; Hansen and Galasko, 1992; Ince *et al.*, 1998). The cortical Lewy body pathology of DLB occurs primarily in the cingulate, insula, amygdaloid complex, entorhinal cortex, and transentorhinal cortex, and in the neocortex (usually in deeper layers such as 4, 5, and 6) of the temporal, parietal, and frontal lobes (Double *et al.*, 1996; Kosaka and Iseki, 1996; Ince *et al.*, 1998; Gómez-Tortosa *et al.*, 1999; Gómez-Tortosa *et al.*, 2000; Harding *et al.*, 2002). Some Lewy body pathology also occurs in the occipital cortex (Kosaka and Iseki, 1996; Pellise *et al.*, 1996; Rezaie *et al.*, 1996; Gómez-Tortosa *et al.*, 1999; Harding *et al.*, 2002), but white matter spongiform change with coexisting gliosis appears to be the most prominent feature of occipital lobe pathology associated with DLB (Higuchi *et al.*, 2000). This occipital pathology is accompanied by hypometabolism and decreased blood flow in primary visual and visual association cortex that is evident with positron emission tomography (PET) or single photon emission computed tomography (SPECT) scanning (Albin, *et al.*, 1996; Ishii *et al.*, 1998; Imamura *et al.*, 1999; Higuchi *et al.*, 2000; Imamura *et al.*, 2001; Lobotesis *et al.*, 2001; Minoshima *et al.*, 2001).

The majority of patients with DLB have concomitant Alzheimer's disease (AD) pathology (i.e. neuritic plaques, neurofibrillary tangles) that is sufficient to meet standard criteria for AD (e.g. Khachaturian, 1985; Mirra *et al.*, 1993). This AD pathology occurs in the same general distribution throughout the brain as in patients with 'pure' AD (Armstrong *et al.*, 1998; Gómez-Tortosa *et al.*, 2000), although the severity of AD pathology is usually less than in pure AD (Samuel *et al.*, 1996; Brown *et al.*, 1998; Gearing *et al.*, 1999; Heyman *et al.*, 1999). Neuropathological (Lippa *et al.*, 1994, 1998) and neuroimaging studies (Hashimoto *et al.*, 1998; Barber *et al.*, 2000, 2001) also indicate that medial temporal lobe structures, and the hippocampus in particular, are somewhat less atrophic in DLB patients than in patients with AD. Patients with DLB have abnormal ubiquitinated neurites in the CA 2/3 region of the hippocampus that are not present in AD (Dickson *et al.*, 1991, 1994; Lippa *et al.*, 1994).

A number of neurochemical abnormalities have been identified in patients with DLB (for review, see Ince *et al.*, 1998). As in PD, one of the primary neurochemical changes is a disruption of dopaminergic input to the striatum due to the loss of pigmented substantia nigra neurones (Perry *et al.*, 1990). This loss may be as severe as that in PD (Langlais *et al.*, 1993) and most likely mediates the extrapyramidal motor dysfunction that usually accompanies DLB (see below). Cortical dopamine, in contrast, has been reported to not markedly decrease in DLB (Perry *et al.*, 1993). DLB is also characterized by a widespread depletion of striatal and neo-cortical choline acetyltransferase (ChAT) that is greater than that observed in pure AD (Reid et al., 2000; Tiraboschi et al., 2000, 2002). Loss of ChAT activity occurs in the striatum due to pathology of intrinsic local circuit neurones and, as suggested by Perry et al. (1990) and Langlais et al. (1993), this loss may attenuate the manifestation of the severe motor dysfunction that usually occurs with the loss of striatal dopamine in PD. The severe loss of neocortical ChAT activity in DLB is thought to contribute to the cognitive and neuropsychiatric features (e.g. visual hallucinations) of the disorder (Aarsland et al., 2001; Perry et al., 2003). There is also some evidence that the grey matter level of a particular cholinesterase involved in the breakdown of acetylcholine, butyryl-cholinesterase, is correlated with rate of cognitive decline in patients with DLB (Perry et al., 2003).

49.1 CLINICAL MANIFESTATIONS OF DEMENTIA WITH LEWY BODIES

The initial clinical manifestation of DLB is usually the insidious onset of cognitive decline with no other prominent neurological abnormalities (Hansen et al., 1990; McKeith et al., 1996b). Memory impairment is often the earliest feature of DLB but, with time, cognitive deficits become widespread and patients inexorably progress to severe dementia. These aspects of DLB are similar to the dementia syndrome associated with AD, and patients with DLB are often clinically diagnosed as having probable or possible AD during life (e.g. Hansen et al., 1990; Merdes et al., 2003). Because of the extensive pathological, clinical, and genetic overlap that DLB often shares with AD (Galasko et al., 1994; Hansen et al., 1994; Katzman, et al., 1995; Olichney et al., 1996), Hansen and colleagues (1990) distinguish between what they refer to as the Lewy body variant (LBVAD) of AD and diffuse Lewy body disease (DLBD) without concomitant AD.

Despite the general similarities in the two disorders, numerous retrospective studies that have compared the clinical features present in autopsy-confirmed DLB and AD patients have identified a number of distinguishing characteristics (Hansen et al., 1990; McKeith et al.,1992; Beck, 1995; McShane et al., 1995; Galasko et al., 1996; Hely et al., 1996; Weiner et al., 1996; Ala et al., 1997; Graham et al., 1997; for reviews, see Perry et al., 1996; Cercy and Bylsma, 1997). These studies have demonstrated that patients with DLB are more likely than those with pure AD to manifest extrapyramidal motor features (e.g. bradykinesia, rigidity, masked facies; but without a resting tremor) at some point during the course of the disease (Hansen et al., 1990; McKeith et al., 1992; Galasko et al., 1996). In addition, it is estimated that 40–45 per cent of patients with DLB experience well-formed visual hallucinations (Galasko et al., 1996; McKeith et al., 1996b; Verghese et al., 1999; Harding et al., 2002; Merdes et al., 2003) in comparison to approximately 25 per cent of patients with pure AD

(Ballard et al., 1999) or PD (Aarsland and Karlsen, 1999; Fenelon et al., 2000). Patients with DLB are more likely than those with AD to exhibit fluctuations in cognition and consciousness and to have unexplained falls (McKeith et al., 1992; Ballard et al., 2001).

Patients with DLB may develop urinary incontinence earlier in the course of the disease than do AD patients (Del-Ser et al., 1996); they appear to be quite susceptible to REM sleep disorder (Turner et al., 1997; Boeve et al., 1998; Ferman et al., 2002); they respond poorly to neuroleptic treatment for their psychotic symptoms (for review, see McKeith et al., 1996a), and they may show a better clinical response than AD patients to acetylcholinesterase (AChE) inhibitor treatment of their cognitive deficits (Levy et al., 1994). Patients with DLB have also been shown to decline more rapidly than patients with AD (Olichney et al., 1998; McKeith et al., 2000), although some investigators have found similar rates of progression and survival in DLB and AD (Heyman et al., 1999; Stern et al., 2001).

There is some evidence that the clinical manifestation of DLB is directly related to the distribution and severity of Lewy body pathology. In a study of 46 patients with autopsy-confirmed DLB (25 with LBVAD, 10 with DLBD, and 11 with PD or PD + AD), Haroutunian and colleagues (2000) found a significant correlation ($r = 0.34$) between the total number of Lewy bodies in the entire brain and scores achieved 6 months before death on the Clinical Dementia Rating (CDR) scale. When the analysis was limited to neocortical Lewy bodies only, the relationship with CDR scores was even stronger ($r = 0.52$). This relationship remained significant after the severity of AD pathology was accounted for by means of partial correlation analysis ($r = 0.32$), indicating that the extent of Lewy body pathology in DLB contributes to level of dementia severity independent of AD pathology. In another study, Gómez-Tortosa and colleagues (1999) compared clinical features in 13 patients with autopsy-confirmed DLBD and 12 patients with autopsy-confirmed LBVAD in order to determine if Lewy body pathology alone could produce the typical clinical presentation associated with DLB. The results of the study showed no differences in initial clinical symptoms, including age at onset, age at death, or disease duration. In addition, comparison of pathological changes showed no difference in the distribution of Lewy bodies within the brains of the two groups, and there were no significant differences in regional Lewy body counts for patients with and without initial parkinsonism, hallucinations, recurrent falls, fluctuations, or delusions. Although the relationship between Lewy body pathology and clinical symptoms is complex, these results indicate that this pathology makes a distinct contribution to the clinical manifestation of DLB.

Many of the clinical features of DLB that are described above have been incorporated into the primary clinical criteria for the disorder that were adopted by the International Consortium on DLB (McKeith et al., 1996b). These criteria include, in addition to dementia, spontaneous motor features of parkinsonism, recurrent and well-formed visual hallucinations, and fluctuating cognition with pronounced variations in attention or alertness. Probable DLB is diagnosed if two of these three features are present; possible DLB if only one is present. An examination of the performance of these consensus guidelines against autopsy verification of DLB demonstrated 83 per cent sensitivity and 91 per cent specificity (McKeith et al., 2000). This was comparable to the 87 per cent sensitivity and 83 per cent specificity for AD (using NINCDS-ADRDA criteria) that was obtained in the same study. Despite these reports of relatively high sensitivity and specificity for the DLB clinical criteria, other studies have reported less success in using these criteria to distinguish between DLB and AD during life (e.g. Lopez et al., 2000; Hohl et al., 2002; Merdes et al., 2003). Furthermore, at least two studies have shown that some autopsy-confirmed DLB patients displayed none of the core features of the disorder, other than dementia, during life (Stern et al., 2001; Merdes et al., 2003). The results of these studies indicate that additional ways to clinically identify patients with DLB are needed. As reviewed in the ensuing sections, neuropsychological studies of the disease indicate that DLB may be associated with a distinct pattern of cognitive changes that might aid in differentiating DLB from AD.

49.2 NEUROPSYCHOLOGICAL FEATURES OF DEMENTIA WITH LEWY BODIES

The specific neuropsychological deficits associated with DLB have been largely identified through the retrospective examination of prospectively collected data from patients in whom the disease was neuropathologically confirmed. Early studies of cognitive changes in DLB clearly demonstrated that the disorder is characterized by global cognitive dysfunction and a pattern of deficits that is very similar to the one associated with AD, including memory impairment, dysphasia, constructional dyspraxia, executive dysfunction and attention deficits (Gibb et al., 1985; Byrne et al., 1989). Several studies have directly compared the nature and severity of the neuropsychological deficits associated with the relatively early stages of DLB and pure AD. Förstl and colleagues (1993), for example, found similar degrees of language, praxis, and memory impairment on the cognitive portion of the Cambridge Mental Disorders of the Elderly Examination (CAMCOG) in eight autopsy-confirmed DLB patients and eight patients with AD. In another study, McKeith and colleagues (1992) found that 21 patients with autopsy-verified DLB performed significantly better than 37 patients with pure AD on the standardized Mental Test Score of Blessed. The superior performance of the DLB patients was most evident on the recall component of the test, and occurred despite similar degrees of impairment on measures of temporal and parietal lobe function.

A more detailed comparison of the neuropsychological deficits associated with DLB and AD was carried out by Hansen and colleagues (1990) who retrospectively examined the cognitive performance of nine patients with autopsy-proven

DLB (all with LBVAD) and nine patients with pure AD. As part of a prospective study of cognitive deficits associated with dementia, all patients had been evaluated with a comprehensive neuropsychological test battery that included measures of memory, language, executive functions, attention and visuospatial abilities. The DLB and AD patients included in the study were matched one-to-one on the basis of age, education, overall level of global dementia as assessed by the Information-Memory-Concentration test of Blessed, and the interval between cognitive testing and death. The results of this study showed that the DLB and AD patients were equally impaired (relative to elderly normal control subjects) on tests of episodic memory, confrontation naming (e.g. Boston Naming Test), and arithmetic (Wechsler Adult Intelligence Scale – Revised [WAIS-R] Arithmetic subtest), but the patients with DLB performed significantly worse than those with AD on a test of attention (WAIS-R Digit Span subtest) and on tests of visuospatial and constructional ability (Wechsler Intelligence Scale for Children – Revised [WISC-R] Block Design subtest and Copy-a-Cross test). In addition, the DLB and AD patients produced different patterns of impairment on tests of verbal fluency: the DLB group scored significantly lower than the AD group on the phonemically based letter fluency task (i.e. generating words that begin with a particular letter) but the two groups performed similarly on the semantically based category fluency task (i.e. producing words that belong to a particular category such as 'animals').

Subsequent studies have generally replicated these findings in much larger cohorts of autopsy-confirmed DLB and AD patients (Yeatman et al., 1994; Gnanalingham et al., 1996; Wagner et al., 1996; Connor et al., 1998; Galasko et al., 1998; Hamilton et al., 2004). Hamilton and colleagues (2004), for example, found that 24 patients with autopsy-confirmed DLB (all with LBVAD) performed significantly worse than 24 patients with autopsy-confirmed AD on several tests of visuospatial ability (e.g. the WISC-R Block Design Test, copying figures from the Visual Reproduction Test) but significantly better than the AD patients on verbal tests of episodic memory (see Figure 49.1). These differences in the cognitive changes associated with the two disorders occurred despite similar levels of impairment on a test of language production (Boston Naming Test) and equivalent levels of overall dementia as measured by the Mini-Mental State Examination (MMSE). The apparent double dissociation between the severity of visuospatial and episodic memory deficits in the two groups suggests that the distinct patterns of performance cannot be easily attributed to differences in dementia severity or difficulty of the various cognitive tasks, but instead reflects a true difference in the brain–behaviour relationships underlying DLB and AD.

In a related study of 66 patients with autopsy-verified DLB and 132 patients with autopsy-verified AD, Salmon et al. (2002) found that a derived measure of the difference between memory test and visuoconstructive test standardized scores revealed the same dissociation observed by Hamilton and colleagues (2004). Patients with DLB were significantly

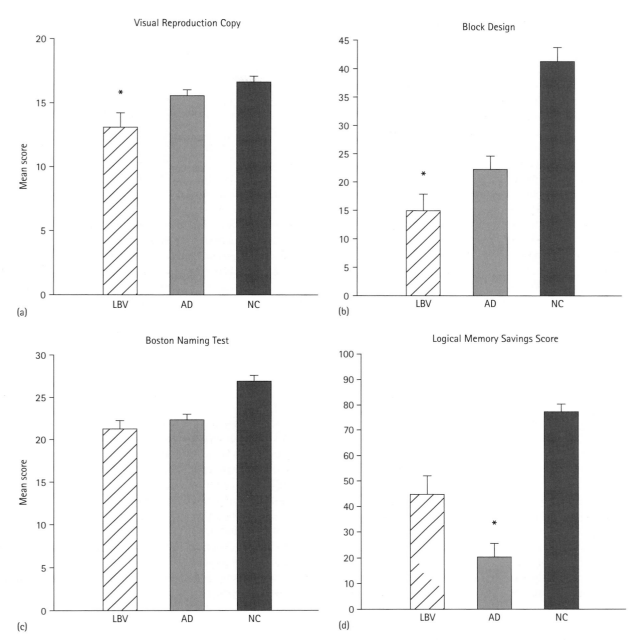

Figure 49.1(a–d)   *The average scores achieved by normal control (NC) subjects (n = 24), patients with Alzheimer's disease (AD; n = 24), and patients with dementia with Lewy bodies (DLB; all with the Lewy body variant of AD; n = 24) on several neuropsychological tests. Despite equivalent deficits on a test of confrontation naming (Boston Naming Test), the DLB patients were disproportionately impaired compared to the AD patients on tests of visuospatial ability (Visual Reproduction Copy and Block Design). (The opposite pattern was observed on a test of verbal memory [Logical Memory Savings Score]). (Adapted from Hamilton et al., 2004.)*

more impaired (relative to normal control subjects) on tests of visuoconstructive ability (i.e. WISC-R Block Design Test) than on tests of memory (i.e. Dementia Rating Scale [DRS] Memory Subtest), whereas the opposite pattern was true for patients with AD. These dissociable patterns of performance were apparent in both mild and moderate stages of dementia. Furthermore, there is some indication that distinct patterns of cognitive decline occur in patients with DLB and patients with AD. In a 1-year longitudinal study of 20 patients with autopsy-confirmed DLB (all with LBVAD) and 20 patients with autopsy-confirmed AD, Salmon and colleagues (1998) found that the two groups exhibited similar rates of decline on measures of confrontation naming (Boston Naming Test), general semantic knowledge (Number Information Test), and episodic memory (DRS Memory subtest), but the DLB patients declined more rapidly than those with AD on measures of verbal fluency (also see Ballard *et al.*, 1996) and visuospatial abilities (WISC-R Block Design Test).

The possible clinical utility of distinct cognitive profiles in patients with DLB and AD was examined in a study by Galasko and colleagues (1998). These investigators compared the neuropsychological test performances of 50 patients with autopsy-verified DLB (all with LBVAD) and 95 patients with autopsy-verified AD. As in the previous studies by this group of investigators (Hansen *et al.*, 1990; Hamilton *et al.*, 2004), the DLB patients performed significantly worse than the AD patients on tests of visuospatial ability, verbal fluency, and abstract reasoning, and exhibited greater psychomotor slowing than the AD patients. In contrast, the groups did not differ on tests of global cognitive functioning (i.e. the MMSE) or on specific tests of confrontation naming, general semantic knowledge, attention, or episodic memory (it should be noted that this study did not examine performance on the rigorous episodic memory tests used by Hamilton *et al.* [2004]).

Based upon these results, Galasko and colleagues (1998) developed a logistic regression model designed to differentiate between DLB and AD patients on the basis of their performances on tests of verbal fluency (Phonemic Fluency Test), visuospatial ability (WISC-R Block Design Test, Clock Drawing Test), psychomotor speed and attention (Part A of the Trail Making Test), and general semantic knowledge (Number Information Test). The resulting model was highly significant and correctly classified approximately 60 per cent of DLB patients and 88 per cent of AD patients, for an overall successful classification rate of 77 per cent.

The distinct patterns of neuropsychological deficits exhibited by DLB and AD patients on large batteries of rigorous cognitive tests are robust enough to be detected on relatively brief, standardized tests of mental status (Connor *et al.*, 1998; Ala *et al.*, 2002; Aarsland *et al.*, 2003). For example, when Connor and colleagues (1998) compared the Mattis DRS subscale scores of 23 autopsy-verified DLB (all with LBVAD) and 23 pure AD patients, they found that patients with DLB performed significantly worse than those with AD on the Initiation/Perseveration subscale, which is heavily weighted towards verbal fluency and other executive functions. In contrast, the AD patients performed significantly worse than those with DLB on the Memory subscale of the test (see Figure 49.2). When Connor *et al.* (1998) limited their analyses to mildly demented patients, the DLB patients also performed significantly worse than the AD patients on the Construction subtest. This pattern of results was recently replicated in a larger sample of 60 autopsy-verified patients with DLB whose performance was compared with 29 clinically diagnosed patients with AD (Aarsland *et al.*, 2003). Despite comparable dementia severity at the time of testing, Aarsland and colleagues (2003) found that the DLB patients had higher Memory subscale scores than patients with AD, but lower scores on the Initiation/Perseveration and Construction subscales. Interestingly, the subscale score profiles of patients with DLB were identical to those of patients who initially presented with idiopathic PD and developed concomitant dementia.

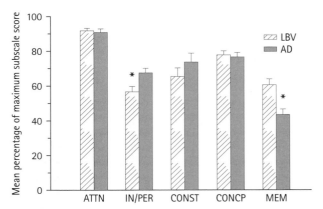

Figure 49.2 *The average percentage of the maximum possible score on each subtest of the Mattis Dementia Rating Scale achieved by patients with neuropathologically confirmed Alzheimer's disease (AD; solid bars) or dementia with Lewy bodies (DLB; striped bars). Patients with DLB scored significantly lower than patients with AD on the Initiation/Perseveration and Construction subtests but significantly higher on the Memory subtest. ATTN, Attention; IN/PER, Initiation/ Perseveration; CONST, Construction; CONCP, Conceptualization; MEM, Memory. (Adapted from Connor et al., 1998.)*

Reports of less impaired memory performance in patients with DLB than in patients with AD were recently confirmed by the results of a study that compared the two groups on rigorous tests of episodic memory (Hamilton *et al.*, 2004). Hamilton and colleagues (2004) compared the performances of 24 patients with autopsy-confirmed DLB (all with LBVAD) and 24 patients with autopsy-confirmed AD on the California Verbal Learning Test (CVLT) and the Logical Memory Test from the Wechsler Memory Scale – Revised. Although the DLB and AD patients were equally demented as shown by equivalent scores on the Mattis DRS, they exhibited distinct patterns of performance on various components of the episodic memory measures (see Figure 49.3). The two groups were equally impaired in their ability to learn new verbal information on these tests, but the DLB patients exhibited better retention and recognition memory than patients with pure AD. These results suggest that the episodic memory deficit associated with DLB is generally less severe than that of AD, substantiating previous studies that used less rigorous memory tests with smaller samples of autopsy-confirmed patients (Salmon *et al.*, 1996; Connor *et al.*, 1998; Heyman *et al.*, 1999) or that used clinically diagnosed patient groups (Ballard *et al.*, 1996; Graham *et al.*, 1997; Walker *et al.*, 1997; Shimomura *et al.*, 1998; Calderon *et al.*, 2001).

The differences exhibited by DLB and AD patients on the retention and recognition measures of the verbal memory tests suggest that specific memory processes may be differentially impaired in the two disorders. Consistent with previous studies (Delis *et al.*, 1991; Tröster *et al.*, 1993), the patients with AD exhibited a severe learning deficit, rapid forgetting

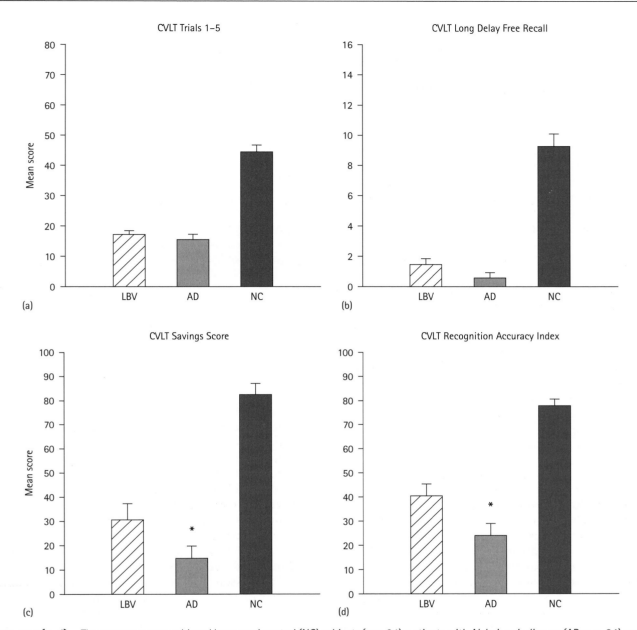

Figure 49.3(a–d)   *The average scores achieved by normal control (NC) subjects (n = 24), patients with Alzheimer's disease (AD; n = 24), and patients with dementia with Lewy bodies (DLB; all with the Lewy body variant of AD; n = 24) on various learning and memory measures from the California Verbal Learning Test (CVLT). Despite equivalent deficits in free recall, the DLB patients were less impaired than the AD patients on measures of retention (memory savings score) and recognition memory (recognition accuracy index). (Adapted from Hamilton et al., 2004.)*

of information over a delay interval (indicated by low Savings scores), and severely impaired recognition memory. This pattern of deficits suggests a primary impairment of encoding and storage in which information is unavailable even when retrieval support is provided by the recognition memory format (Delis *et al.*, 1991). Despite similarly severe impairment in the learning and delayed recall conditions when free recall was required, the patients with DLB had better savings over the delay interval than patients with AD, and performed better on the recognition memory component of the

CVLT. These differences in performance suggest that a deficit in retrieval plays a greater role in the memory impairment of patients with DLB than in that of patients with AD. While the pattern of deficits does not rule out the possibility that poor encoding contributes to memory impairment in the two disorders, it is clear that DLB patients have better retention than patients with AD when retrieval demands are reduced through the use of the recognition format.

The observed differences in the severity of impairment of specific memory processes in DLB and AD are consistent with the particular pathological changes that occur in the two disorders. As mentioned previously, a number of studies using neuropathologic (Lippa *et al.*, 1994, 1998) or magnetic resonance imaging (Hashimoto *et al.*, 1998; Barber *et al.*, 2000, 2001) procedures have shown that the medial temporal lobe structures important for memory (e.g. hippocampus, entorhinal cortex, parahippocampal gyrus) are more severely affected in AD than in DLB. The extensive damage to these structures that occurs in AD is thought to mediate the severe amnesia that characterizes the disorder (Hyman *et al.*, 1990). In contrast, damage to subcortical structures that are affected in Parkinson's disease and other disorders of the basal ganglia (e.g. Huntington's disease) is greater in DLB than in AD. Damage to these structures has been implicated in a memory disorder characterized by a general deficit in the ability to initiate and carry out the systematic retrieval of successfully stored information (Martone *et al.*, 1984; Butters *et al.*, 1985, 1986; Moss *et al.*, 1986; Delis *et al.*, 1991). Thus, the less severe retention deficit and the greater impact of deficient retrieval processes in DLB than in AD is consistent with the combination of moderate medial temporal lobe damage and frontostriatal dysfunction that occurs in the disease.

49.3 COGNITIVE DEFICITS IN PATIENTS WITH CLINICALLY DIAGNOSED DEMENTIA WITH LEWY BODIES

With the development of standardized criteria for the clinical diagnosis of probable DLB (e.g. McKeith *et al.*, 1996), a number of investigators have compared the cognitive deficits exhibited by clinically diagnosed DLB and AD patients who are relatively mildly demented. While these studies may be somewhat less reliable than studies of autopsy-verified patients because of the difficulty in clinically distinguishing between DLB and AD, they are informative and their results are generally consistent with those from autopsy series. In one such study, Shimomura and colleagues (1998) compared the performances of 26 patients with probable DLB and 52 patients with probable AD on items from the MMSE, the Alzheimer's Disease Assessment Scale (ADAS), the WAIS-R subtests, and the Raven Colored Progressive Matrices test. These investigators found that patients with probable DLB scored significantly worse than those with probable AD on the Raven Colored Progressive Matrices test and on the Picture Arrangement, Block Design, Object Assembly, and Digit Symbol Substitution subtests of the WAIS-R. In contrast, the patients with probable AD performed significantly better than those with probable DLB on measures of orientation and word recall. Consistent with the results from a study of autopsy-verified DLB and AD patients (Salmon *et al.*, 2002), a discriminant function analysis showed that the two groups could be most effectively differentiated by their scores on a word recall measure and the WAIS-R Block Design subtest. A similar discrepancy in the pattern of visuospatial and memory

deficits exhibited by patients with probable DLB and probable AD was reported by Walker and colleagues (1997).

A series of studies was carried out to compare the cognitive deficits exhibited by clinically diagnosed DLB and AD patients using a microcomputer-based testing paradigm (the CANTAB) that allowed a detailed assessment of memory, attention, and executive functions such as attentional set shifting, conditional pattern discrimination learning, and strategic thinking. In the first of these studies, Galloway and colleagues (1992) found that seven patients with probable DLB and 10 patients with probable AD were equally impaired on a recognition memory test, but DLB patients required significantly more trials than patients with AD to reach a learning criterion on a conditional pattern-location, paired-associates learning task. In a second study in this series, Sahgal and colleagues (1992a) showed that, while the same AD and DLB subjects from the Galloway *et al.* study were impaired on simultaneous and delayed matching to sample tasks, patients with probable DLB performed worse than those with probable AD only in the delayed condition. Sahgal and colleagues also showed in a third study (Sahgal *et al.*, 1992b) that these same DLB and AD patients were equally impaired on a complex set-shifting task that required both intradimensional (i.e. from one set of lines to another) and extradimensional (i.e. from lines to colours) shifts of attention, but only the patients with DLB were impaired (relative to normal control subjects) on a visual search task that assessed the ability to focus attention. In a final study in this series, Sahgal and colleagues (1995) compared the performance of DLB and AD patients on a spatial working memory task that assessed both spatial memory and the ability to use an efficient search strategy. In this task, subjects were required to search through a number of boxes presented on a computer screen in order to locate a hidden 'token'. They were not to re-examine an empty box before finding the token on the current trial (i.e. a within-search error), nor were they to search a box in which the token had been found on a previous trial (i.e. a between-search error). The results showed that patients with probable DLB made more within-search and between-search errors than those with probable AD, but the groups did not differ in the search strategies they used to complete the task.

Consistent with the disproportionately impaired visual attention and visuospatial working memory deficits exhibited by patients with DLB in the studies by Sahgal and colleagues, Calderon and colleagues (2001) found that 10 patients with probable DLB performed significantly worse than nine patients with probable AD on tests of fragmented letter identification, discrimination of 'real' objects from non-objects, and segregation of overlapping figures. These particularly severe deficits in visuospatial and visuoperceptual abilities were apparent even though the DLB patients performed significantly better than the patients with AD on a verbal memory test and at the same level on tests of semantic memory (also see Lambon Ralph *et al.*, 2001). Similar results were obtained by Mori and colleagues (2000) who found that

24 patients with probable DLB performed significantly worse than 48 equally demented patients with probable AD on tests of visual attention, size and form discrimination, and visual figure-ground segregation. Mori and colleagues noted that DLB patients with visual hallucinations were more impaired than those without hallucinations on the figure-ground segregation test. Simard *et al.* (2003) reported a similar finding in which patients with probable DLB with visual hallucinations performed worse than those without hallucinations on the Benton Judgement of Line Orientation task.

Several studies have reported that patients with DLB perform worse than those with AD on simple visuospatial tests such as the Clock Drawing Test, and suggest that such tasks might be useful for clinically differentiating between the two disorders (Gnanalingham *et al.*, 1996, 1997). While this possibility has some support, the utility of simple visuoconstructive tests for this purpose remains in question (Swanick *et al.*, 1996; Cahn-Weiner *et al.*, 2003).

Consistent with the results of studies that have compared groups of patients with clinically diagnosed probable DLB and probable AD, a number of studies have shown that AD patients with extrapyramidal motor signs (EPS; e.g. bradykinesia, rigidity, tremor) which may be indicative of DLB are more severely impaired on tests of visuospatial/visuoconstructive ability (e.g. Block Design, Figure Copying) and executive functions (e.g. Wisconsin Card Sorting Test, Trail Making Test, Verbal Fluency) than those without EPS, even though the groups exhibit comparable deficits on tests of long-term memory, naming, and verbal comprehension (Girling and Berrios, 1990; Richards *et al.*, 1993; Merello *et al.*, 1994). Furthermore, a 1-year longitudinal study showed that AD patients with EPS declined more rapidly than those without EPS on tests of reasoning and abstraction, visuospatial abilities, praxis, verbal fluency, and language processing (Soininen *et al.*, 1992). These differences in rate of decline occurred despite the two groups being equivalently impaired on all of these tests at their initial evaluation. This pattern of cognitive decline is consistent with the disproportionate decline in verbal fluency and visuospatial abilities displayed by autopsy-confirmed patients with DLB in the study by Salmon and colleagues (1998).

It is interesting to note that the cognitive abilities that appear to be disproportionately impaired in DLB are the same abilities that are mildly impaired in non-demented patients with PD. A number of studies have shown that compared with age-matched normal control subjects PD patients exhibit psychomotor slowing (Brown and Marsden, 1991) and have mild deficits in visuospatial abilities (Stern *et al.*, 1993; Jacobs *et al.*, 1995), verbal fluency (Jacobs *et al.*, 1995), and other executive functions that are necessary to perform tasks such as the Wisconsin Card Sorting Test (Lees and Smith, 1983; Brown and Marsden, 1988), the interference condition of the Stroop Test (Brown and Marsden, 1991), dual-processing tasks (Brown and Marsden, 1991; Dalrymple-Alford *et al.*, 1994), and tasks that require rapid shifts of attention (Filoteo *et al.*, 1997).

49.4 CONTRIBUTIONS OF LEWY BODY PATHOLOGY TO COGNITIVE DYSFUNCTION IN DEMENTIA WITH LEWY BODIES

While the studies described above suggest that the Lewy body pathology present in DLB contributes importantly to the severity and nature of the dementia associated with the disease, the presence of concomitant AD pathology in most DLB patients makes it difficult to determine the unique role this pathology plays in the disorder's clinical and neuropsychological manifestation. Fortunately, a number of clinicopathologic studies address this important question. Samuel and colleagues (1996), for example, compared quantitative measures of pathology and dementia severity in 14 patients with autopsy-verified DLB (all with LBVAD) and 12 patients with autopsy-verified pure AD. Despite being matched for disease duration and having similar scores on mental status tests when last evaluated prior to death, the DLB patients had fewer neurofibrillary tangles and total plaques than the AD patients, and were in a lower Braak stage (a rating system based upon severity of neurofibrillary tangle pathology in the medial temporal lobe and neocortex). Furthermore, the number of neurofibrillary tangles was correlated with level of dementia in the AD patients but not in the DLB patients, whereas the number of Lewy bodies was correlated with level of dementia in the DLB patients. These findings suggest that the additional Lewy body pathology in the DLB patients contributed to their dementia severity above and beyond the contribution of any AD pathology.

In a second study of 17 patients with autopsy-verified DLB (12 LBVAD, 5 DLBD), Samuel and colleagues (1997) found that the number of neocortical Lewy bodies, the number of neocortical neuritic plaques, Braak stage, and the severity of ChAT activity loss all correlated significantly with dementia severity as measured by the MMSE and the Information-Memory-Concentration Test of Blessed. In contrast to previous findings from patients with AD (e.g. Terry *et al.*, 1991), the severity of dementia in these DLB patients was not correlated with the number of neocortical neurofibrillary tangles or neocortical synaptic density. A strong relationship between ChAT activity and cognitive decline in patients with DLB was not supported by a subsequent study (Sabbagh *et al.*, 1999) of 41 patients with autopsy-verified DLB (all with LBVAD). In this study, Sabbagh and colleagues (1999) found only a weak correlation between ChAT activity and scores on the MMSE, and no significant relationship between ChAT activity and scores on the Information-Memory-Concentration Test of Blessed. The DLB patients in the study by Sabbagh and colleagues (1999) were more severely impaired than those studied by Samuel and colleagues (1997), but the strength of the correlations did not change appreciably when the most severely impaired patients were excluded from the analyses.

Further evidence for the role of Lewy body pathology in the dementia associated with DLB was provided by a study that retrospectively examined the neuropsychological test performance of five patients with DLBD (Salmon, *et al.*, 1996). All five of these patients initially presented with insidious cognitive decline that progressed to severe dementia. Sometime after the onset of cognitive decline, all of the patients developed mild extrapyramidal motor dysfunction, three developed visual, auditory or tactile hallucinations, and two developed delusions. All were clinically diagnosed with probable or possible AD or one of its variants (i.e. LBVAD, mixed AD and vascular dementia) at their initial evaluation. At autopsy, subcortical and diffusely distributed cortical Lewy bodies were observed in the brains of all five patients. AD pathology was absent in two of the cases and at a level comparable to that found in normal elderly individuals in the other three cases.

Despite only borderline to mild impairment on the MMSE (mean = 23.2; range = 22–26), detailed neuropsychological testing revealed deficits in memory, attention, language, executive functions, and visuospatial abilities in all five patients with DLBD. A comparison with five equally demented patients with autopsy-verified AD showed similar levels of impairment on tests of executive functions, language, and attention, but disproportionately severe deficits in the DLBD patients on tests of psychomotor speed (parts A and B of the Trail Making Test) and visuospatial/visuoconstructive ability (WISC-R Block Design Test, Clock Drawing Test). Indeed, four of the five DLBD patients were at floor performance on the WISC-R Block Design subtest and the fifth was severely impaired. A similarly severe deficit was evident in the performance of DLBD patients on the copy condition of the Clock Drawing test (see Figure 49.4).

All five of the DLBD patients scored two to three standard deviations below normal performance on key measures of the California Verbal Learning Tests (CVLT), but their performance differed somewhat from that typically observed in patients with AD. Mildly demented AD patients usually exhibit severe impairment on CVLT measures of immediate learning and recall, very poor retention over delay intervals (i.e. an average long delay savings score of 17 per cent), an increased propensity to produce intrusion errors in the cued recall condition, and very poor recognition discrimination (Delis *et al.*, 1991). In contrast to this typical AD pattern, four of the five DLBD patients did not show exceptionally poor retention and recognition discrimination, and three of the five did not show a strong propensity to produce intrusion errors. When the scores of the DLBD patients were subjected to discriminant function equations that have been previously shown to effectively distinguish between patients with cortical (e.g. AD) and subcortical (e.g. Huntington's disease) dementia using these key CVLT measures, four of the five DLBD patients were classified as 'subcortical' and one as 'cortical'.

The deficits exhibited by patients with DLBD in the study by Salmon and colleagues (1996) indicate that subcortical and diffusely distributed neocortical Lewy body pathology, in the absence of AD pathology, can produce a global dementia syndrome characterized by deficits in memory, attention,

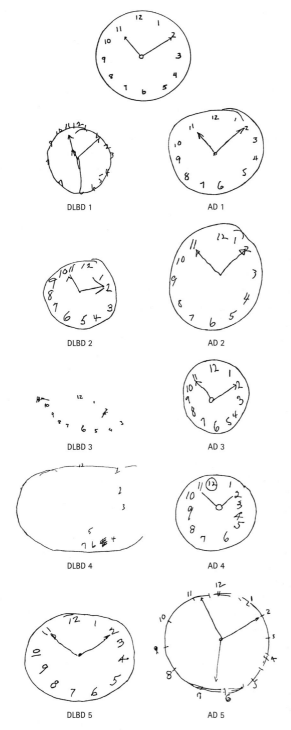

Figure 49.4 *Copies of clocks drawn by patients with diffuse Lewy body disease (DLBD) and Alzheimer's disease (AD) in the copy condition of the Clock Drawing Test. The clock on top illustrates the model that patients were asked to draw. Although each DLBD (cases 1–5) patient was matched in terms of overall severity of dementia to each AD (cases 1–5) patient, the patients with DLBD produced significantly worse copies than the patients with AD. (Reprinted by kind permission of Raven's Press from Salmon and Bondi, 1999 in Terry et al., Alzheimer's Disease 2E.)*

language, and executive functions, and strikingly severe deficiencies in visuospatial/visuoconstructive abilities and psychomotor speed. This pattern of neuropsychological deficits is consistent with the cortical and subcortical brain damage that occurs in the disease. DLBD results in neuropathological abnormalities in the neocortex of the temporal, frontal and parietal lobe, and these changes may be responsible for such cortical features of the dementia as impaired language, executive dysfunction, and impaired visuospatial abilities. Neuropathological changes in the substantia nigra of patients with DLBD, and the corresponding depletion of dopaminergic input to the striatum (Perry *et al.*, 1990), most likely contribute to the cognitive deficits typical of subcortical dysfunction, such as impaired learning, decreased attention, impaired visuoconstructive abilities, and psychomotor slowing (for review, see Cummings, 1990). The nature of the memory deficit associated with DLBD appears to reflect ineffective retrieval similar to that observed in other patients with striatal dysfunction (Butters *et al.*, 1986). Although ubiquitin-immunoreactive dystrophic neurites are often present in the CA2–3 region of the hippocampus in patients with DLBD (Dickson *et al.*, 1991, 1994), the hippocampus and related structures (e.g. entorhinal cortex, parahippocampal gyrus) that are thought to underlie memory storage are generally less damaged than in AD (Lippa *et al.*, 1994). This disparity leads to overall milder memory impairment in patients with DLBD than in those with AD.

49.5 CONCLUSIONS

A growing body of evidence indicates that DLB is a distinct clinicopathologic entity that can be differentiated from pure AD on the basis of specific clinical features. Neuropsychological studies indicate that distinct features of the cognitive decline associated with DLB might aid in this differentiation. Although both DLB and AD result in global cognitive impairment and often engender comparable impairments in new learning and language abilities, patients with DLB appear to have significantly greater deficits than patients with AD in visuospatial abilities, some executive functions, verbal fluency, some aspects of attention, and psychomotor speed. The nature of the memory deficits associated with DLB and AD may also differ, with DLB patients exhibiting milder deficits in retention and recognition memory than patients with AD.

The pattern of neuropsychological deficits exhibited by patients with DLB suggests that they are often as severely impaired as patients with AD in those cognitive abilities usually affected by AD pathology (e.g. episodic memory, language), but more impaired in those abilities thought to be additionally affected by subcortical (and possibly neocortical) Lewy body pathology (e.g. verbal fluency, psychomotor speed, visuospatial/constructional ability; Alexander *et al.*, 1986). This suggests that both AD and Lewy body pathology contribute importantly to the cognitive manifestations of

DLB. However, the specific neuropsychological processes and neuropathological factors that underlie the cognitive changes of DLB remain largely unknown. It is not known, for example, whether the disproportionately severe visuospatial and visuoconstructive deficits associated with DLB are due to:

- a primary visuoperceptual deficit that might arise from Lewy body pathology in the occipital cortex;
- an impaired ability to mentally manipulate information in space that might arise from concomitant AD and Lewy body pathology in parietal lobe cortex;
- an inability to plan constructions due to the interruption of frontostriatal circuits by pathology in the substantia nigra or frontal lobe cortex; or
- some combination of these or other factors.

Similar questions remain regarding the source of the severe deficits in attention, executive functions, verbal fluency, and psychomotor speed exhibited by patients with DLB. These questions can only be answered through additional systematic clinicopathologic studies of these patients.

REFERENCES

Aarsland D and Karlsen K. (1999) Neuropsychiatric aspects of Parkinson's disease. *Current Psychiatry Reports* **1**: 61–68

Aarsland D, Ballard C, Larsen JP, McKeith I. (2001) A comparative study of psychiatric symptoms in dementia with Lewy bodies and Parkinson's disease with and without dementia. *International Journal of Geriatric Psychiatry* **16**: 528–536

Aarsland D, Litvan I, Salmon D, Galasko D, Wentzel-Larsen T, Larsen JP. (2003) Performance on the dementia rating scale in Parkinson's disease with dementia and dementia with Lewy bodies: comparison with progressive supranuclear palsy and Alzheimer's disease. *Journal of Neurology, Neurosurgery, and Psychiatry* **74**: 1215–1220

Ala TA, Yang KH, Sung JH, Frey WH. (1997) Hallucinations and signs of parkinsonism help distinguish patients with dementia and cortical Lewy bodies from patients with Alzheimer's disease at presentation: a clinicopathological study. *Journal of Neurology, Neurosurgery, and Psychiatry* **62**: 16–21

Ala TA, Hughes LF, Kyrouac GA, Ghobrial MW, Elble RJ. (2002) The Mini-Mental State exam may help in the differentiation of dementia with Lewy bodies and Alzheimer's disease. *International Journal of Geriatric Psychiatry* **17**: 503–509

Albin RL, Minoshima S, D'Amato CJ, Frey KA, Kuhl DA, Sima AAF. (1996) Fluoro-deoxyglucose positron emission tomography in diffuse Lewy body disease. *Neurology* **47**: 462–466

Alexander GE, Delong MR, Strick PL. (1986) Parallel organization of functionally segregated circuits linking basal ganglia and cortex. *Annual Review of Neuroscience* **9**: 357–381

Armstrong RA, Cairns NJ, Lantos PL. (1998) The spatial patterns of Lewy bodies, senile plaques, and neurofibrillary tangles in dementia with Lewy bodies. *Experimental Neurology* **150**: 122–127

Ballard C, Patel A, Oyebode F, Wilcock G. (1996) Cognitive decline in patients with Alzheimer's disease, vascular dementia and senile dementia of the Lewy body type. *Age and Ageing* **25**: 209–213

Ballard C, Holmes C, McKeith I *et al.* (1999) Psychiatric morbidity in dementia with Lewy bodies: a prospective clinical and neuropathological comparative study with Alzheimer's disease. *American Journal of Psychiatry* **156**: 1039–1045

Ballard C, O'Brien J, Gray A *et al.* (2001) Attention and fluctuating attention in patients with dementia with Lewy bodies and Alzheimer disease. *Archives of Neurology* **58**: 977–982

Barber R, Ballard C, McKeith I, Gholkar A, O'Brien JT. (2000) MRI volumetric study of dementia with Lewy bodies: a comparison with AD and vascular dementia. *Neurology* **54**: 1304–1309

Barber R, McKeith IG, Ballard C, Gholkar A, O'Brien JT. (2001) A comparison of medial and lateral temporal lobe atrophy in dementia with Lewy bodies and Alzheimer's disease: magnetic resonance imaging volumetric study. *Dementia and Geriatric Cognitive Disorders*: **12**: 198–205

Beck BJ. (1995) Neuropsychiatric manifestations of diffuse Lewy body disease. *Journal of Geriatric Psychiatry and Neurology* **8**: 189–196

Boeve BF, Silber MH, Ferman TJ *et al.* (1998) REM sleep behavior disorder and degenerative dementia: an association likely reflecting Lewy body disease. *Neurology* **51**: 363–370

Brown RG and Marsden CD. (1988) An investigation of the phenomenon of 'set' in Parkinson's disease. *Movement Disorders* **3**: 152–161

Brown RG and Marsden CD. (1991) Dual task performance and processing resources in normal subjects and patients with Parkinson's disease. *Brain* **114**: 215–231

Brown DF, Risser RC, Bigio EH *et al.* (1998) Neocortical synapse density and Braak stage in the Lewy body variant of Alzheimer disease: a comparison with classic Alzheimer disease and normal aging. *Journal of Neuropathology and Experimental Neurology* **57**: 955–960

Butters N, Wolfe J, Martone M, Granholm E, Cermak L. (1985) Memory disorders associated with Huntington's Disease: verbal recall, verbal recognition and procedural memory. *Neuropsychologia* **23**: 729–743

Butters N, Wolfe J, Granholm E, Martone M. (1986) An assessment of verbal recall, recognition, and fluency abilities in patients with Huntington's disease. *Cortex* **22**: 11–32

Byrne EJ, Lennox G, Lowe J, Godwin-Austen RB. (1989) Diffuse Lewy body disease: clinical features in 15 cases. *Journal of Neurology, Neurosurgery, and Psychiatry* **52**: 709–717

Cahn-Weiner DA, Williams K, Grace J, Tremont G, Westervelt H, Stern RA. (2003) Discrimination of dementia with Lewy bodies from Alzheimer's disease and Parkinson disease using the Clock Drawing test. *Cognitive and Behavioral Neurology* **16**: 85–92

Calderon J, Perry RJ, Erzinclioglu SW, Berrios GE, Dening TR, Hodges JR. (2001) Perception, attention, and working memory are disproportionately impaired in dementia with Lewy bodies compared with Alzheimer's disease. *Journal of Neurology, Neurosurgery, and Psychiatry* **70**: 157–164

Cercy SP and Bylsma FW. (1997) Lewy body and progressive dementia: a critical review and meta-analysis. *Journal of the International Neuropsychological Society* **3**: 179–194

Connor DJ, Salmon DP, Sandy TJ, Galasko D, Hansen LA, Thal L. (1998) Cognitive profiles of autopsy-confirmed Lewy body variant versus pure Alzheimer's disease. *Archives of Neurology* **55**: 994–1000

Cummings JL. (1990) *Subcortical Dementia*. New York, Oxford University Press

Dalrymple-Alford JC, Kalders AS, Jones RD, Watson RW. (1994) A central executive deficit in patients with Parkinson's disease. *Journal of Neurology, Neurosurgery, and Psychiatry* **57**: 360–367

Del-Ser T, Munoz DG, Hachinski V. (1996) Temporal pattern of cognitive decline and incontinence is different in Alzheimer's disease and diffuse Lewy body disease. *Neurology* **46**: 682–686

Delis DC, Massman PJ, Butters N, Salmon DP, Kramer JH, Cermak L. (1991) Profiles of demented and amnesic patients on the California

Verbal Learning Test: implications for the assessment of memory disorders. *Psychological Assessment* **3**: 19–26

Dickson DW, Davies P, Mayeux R *et al.* (1987) Diffuse Lewy body disease: neuropathological and biochemical studies of six patients. *Acta Neuropathologica* **75**: 8–15

Dickson DW, Ruan D, Crystal H *et al.* (1991) Hippocampal degeneration differentiates diffuse Lewy body disease (DLBD) from Alzheimer's disease: light and electron microscopic immunocytochemistry of CA2–3 neurites specific to DLBD. *Neurology* **41**: 1402–1409

Dickson DW, Schmidt ML, Lee VM-Y, Zhao M-L, Yen S-H, Trojanowski JQ. (1994) Immunoreactivity profile of hippocampal CA2/3 neurites in diffuse Lewy body disease. *Acta Neuropathologica* **87**: 269–276

Double KL, Halliday GM, McRitchie DA *et al.* (1996) Regional brain atrophy in ideopathic Parkinson's disease and diffuse Lewy body disease. *Dementia* **7**: 304–313

Fenelon G, Mahieux F, Huon R, Ziegler M. (2000) Hallucinations in Parkinson's disease: prevalence, phenomenology and risk factors. *Brain* **123**: 733–745

Ferman TJ, Boeve BF, Smith GE *et al.* (2002) Dementia with Lewy bodies may present as dementia and REM sleep behavior disorder without parkinsonism or hallucinations. *Journal of the International Neuropsychological Society* **8**: 907–914

Filoteo JV, Delis DC, Salmon DP *et al.* (1997) An examination of the nature of attentional deficits in patients with Parkinson's disease: evidence from a spatial orienting task. *Journal of the International Neuropsychological Society* **3**: 337–347

Förstl H, Burns A, Luthert P, Cairns N, Levy R. (1993) The Lewy-body variant of Alzheimer's disease: clinical and pathological findings. *British Journal of Psychiatry* **162**: 385–392

Galasko D, Saitoh T, Xia Y *et al.* (1994) The apolipoprotein E e-4 allele is overrepresented in patients with the Lewy body variant of Alzheimer's disease. *Neurology* **44**: 1950–1951

Galasko D, Katzman R, Salmon DP, Thal LJ, Hansen L. (1996) Clinical and neuropathological findings in Lewy body dementias. *Brain and Cognition* **31**: 166–175

Galasko D, Salmon DP, Lineweaver T, Hansen L, Thal LJ. (1998) Neuropsychological measures distinguish patients with Lewy body variant from those with Alzheimer's disease. *Neurology* **50**: A181

Galloway PH, Sahgal A, McKeith IG *et al.* (1992) Visual pattern recognition memory and learning deficits in senile dementias of Alzheimer and Lewy body types. *Dementia* **3**: 101–107

Gearing M, Lynn M, Mirra SS. (1999) Neurofibrillary pathology in Alzheimer disease with Lewy bodies: two subgroups. *Archives of Neurology* **56**: 203–208

Gibb WRG, Esiri MM, Lees AJ. (1985) Clinical and pathological features of diffuse cortical Lewy body disease (Lewy body dementia). *Brain* **110**: 1131–1153

Gibb WRG, Luthert PJ, Janota I, Lantos PL. (1989) Cortical Lewy body dementia clinical features and classification. *Journal of Neurology, Neurosurgery, and Psychiatry* **52**: 185–192

Girling DM and Berrios GE. (1990) Extrapyramidal signs, primitive reflexes and frontal lobe function in senile dementia of the Alzheimer type. *British Journal of Psychiatry* **157**: 888–893

Gnanalingham KK, Byrne EJ, Thornton A. (1996) Clock-face drawing to differentiate Lewy body and Alzheimer type dementia syndromes. *Lancet* **347**: 696–697

Gnanalingham KK, Byrne EJ, Thornton A, Sambrook MA, Bannister P. (1997) Motor and cognitive function in Lewy body dementia comparison with Alzheimer's and Parkinson's diseases. *Journal of Neurology, Neurosurgery, and Psychiatry* **62**: 243–252

Gómez-Tortosa E, Newell K, Irizarry MC, Albert M, Growdon JH, Hyman BT. (1999) Clinical and quantitative pathologic correlates of dementia with Lewy bodies. *Neurology* 53: 1284–1291

Gómez-Tortosa E, Irizarry MC, Gómez-Isla T, Hyman BT. (2000) Clinical and neuropathological correlates of dementia with Lewy bodies. *Annals of the New York Academy of Sciences* 920: 9–15

Graham C, Ballard C, Saad K. (1997) Variables which distinguish patients fulfilling clinical criteria for dementia with Lewy bodies from those with Alzheimer's disease. *International Journal of Geriatric Psychiatry* 12: 314–318

Hamilton JM, Salmon DP, Galasko D, Hansen LA. (2004) Distinct memory deficits in dementia with Lewy bodies and Alzheimer's disease. *Journal of the International Neuropsychological Society* 10: 689–697

Hansen LA and Galasko D. (1992) Lewy body disease. *Current Opinion in Neurology and Neurosurgery* 5: 889–894

Hansen L, Salmon D, Galasko D *et al.* (1990) The Lewy body variant of Alzheimer's disease: a clinical and pathologic entity. *Neurology* 40: 1–8

Hansen LA, Galasko D, Samuel W, Xia Y, Chen X, Saitoh T. (1994) Apolipoprotein-E ε-4 is associated with increased neurofibrillary pathology in the Lewy body variant of Alzheimer's disease. *Neuroscience Letters* 182: 63–65

Harding AJ, Broe GA, Halliday GM. (2002) Visual hallucinations in Lewy body disease relate to Lewy bodies in the temporal lobe. *Brain* 125: 391–403

Haroutunian V, Serby M, Purohit DP *et al.* (2000) Contribution of Lewy body inclusions to dementia in patients with and without Alzheimer disease neuropathological conditions. *Archives of Neurology* 57: 1145–1150

Hashimoto M, Kitagaki H, Imamura T *et al.* (1998) Medial temporal and whole-brain atrophy in dementia with Lewy bodies. *Neurology* 51: 357–362

Hely MA, Reid W, Halliday GM *et al.* (1996) Diffuse Lewy body disease: clinical features in nine cases without coexistent Alzheimer's disease. *Journal of Neurology, Neurosurgery, and Psychiatry* 60: 531–538

Heyman A, Fillenbaum GG, Gearing M *et al.* (1999) Comparison of Lewy body variant of Alzheimer's disease with pure Alzheimer's disease: consortium to establish a registry for Alzheimer's disease, part XIX. *Neurology* 52: 1839–1844

Higuchi M, Tashiro M, Arai H *et al.* (2000) Glucose hypometabolism and neuropathological correlates in brains of dementia with Lewy bodies. *Experimental Neurology* 162: 247–256

Hohl U, Tiraboschi P, Hansen L, Thal LJ, Corey-Bloom J. (2002) Diagnostic accuracy of dementia with Lewy bodies. *Archives of Neurology* 57: 347–351

Hyman BT, Van Hoesen GW, Damasio AR. (1990) Memory-related neural systems in Alzheimer's disease: an anatomic study. *Neurology* 40: 1721–1730

Imamura T, Ishii K, Hirono N *et al.* (1999) Visual hallucinations and regional cerebral metabolism in dementia with Lewy bodies (DLB). *NeuroReport* 10: 1903–1907

Imamura T, Ishii K, Hirono N *et al.* (2001) Occipital glucose metabolism in dementia with Lewy bodies with and without parkinsonism: a study using positron emission tomography. *Dementia and Geriatric Cognitive Disorders*: 12: 194–197

Ince PG, Perry EK, Morris CM. (1998) Dementia with Lewy bodies: a distinct non-Alzheimer dementia syndrome? *Brain Pathology* 8: 299–324

Ishii K, Imamura T, Sasaki M *et al.* (1998) Regional cerebral glucose metabolism in dementia with Lewy bodies and Alzheimer's disease. *Neurology* 51: 125–130

Jacobs DM, Marder K, Cote LJ, Sano M, Stern Y, Mayeux R. (1995) Neuropsychological characteristics of preclinical dementia in Parkinson's disease. *Neurology* 45: 1691–1696

Katzman R, Galasko D, Saitoh T, Thal LJ, Hansen LA. (1995) Genetic evidence that the Lewy body variant is indeed a phenotypic variant of Alzheimer's disease. *Brain and Cognition* 28: 259–265

Khachaturian ZS. (1985) Diagnosis of Alzheimer's disease. *Archives of Neurology* 42: 1097–1105

Kosaka K. (1990) Diffuse Lewy body disease in Japan. *Journal of Neurology* 237: 197–204

Kosaka K and Iseki E. (1996) Dementia with Lewy bodies. *Current Opinion in Neurology* 9: 271–275

Kosaka K, Yoshimura M, Ikeda K, Budka H. (1984) Diffuse type of Lewy body disease: progressive dementia with abundant cortical Lewy bodies and senile changes of varying degree: a new disease? *Clinical Neuropathology* 3: 185–192

Lambon Ralph MA, Powell J, Howard D, Whitworth AB, Garrard P, Hodges JR. (2001) Semantic memory is impaired in both dementia with Lewy bodies and dementia of Alzheimer's type: a comparative neuropsychological study and literature review. *Journal of Neurology, Neurosurgery, and Psychiatry* 70: 149–156

Langlais PJ, Thal L, Hansen L, Galasko D, Alford M, Masliah E. (1993) Neurotransmitters in basal ganglia and cortex of Alzheimer's disease with and without Lewy bodies. *Neurology* 43: 1927–1934

Lees AJ and Smith E. (1983) Cognitive deficits in the early stages of Parkinson's disease. *Brain* 137: 221–224

Lennox G, Lowe J, Landon M *et al.* (1989) Diffuse Lewy body disease: correlative neuropathology using anti-ubiquitin immuno-cytochemistry. *Journal of Neurology, Neurosurgery, and Psychiatry* 52: 1236–1247

Levy R, Eagger S, Griffiths M. (1994) Lewy bodies and response to tacrine in Alzheimer's disease. *Lancet* 343: 176

Lippa CF, Smith TW, Swearer JM. (1994) Alzheimer's disease and Lewy body disease: a comparative clinicopathological study. *Annals of Neurology* 35: 81–88

Lippa CF, Johnson R, Smith TW. (1998) The medial temporal lobe in dementia with Lewy bodies: a comparative study with Alzheimer's disease. *Annals of Neurology* 43: 102–106

Lobotesis K, Fenwick JD, Phipps A *et al.* (2001) Occipital hypoperfusion on SPECT in dementia with Lewy bodies but not AD. *Neurology* 56: 643–649

Lopez OL, Hamilton RL, Becker JT, Wisniewski S, Kaufer DI, DeKosky ST. (2000) Severity of cognitive impairment and the clinical diagnosis of AD with Lewy bodies. *Neurology* 54: 1780–1787

McKeith IG, Perry RH, Fairbairn AF, Jabeen S, Perry EK. (1992) Operational criteria for senile dementia of Lewy body type (SDLT). *Psychological Medicine* 22: 911–922

McKeith IG, Fairbairn A, Harrison R. (1996a) Management of the non-cognitive symptoms of Lewy body dementia. In: R Perry, I McKeith, E Perry (eds), *Dementia with Lewy bodies.* New York, Cambridge University Press

McKeith IG, Galasko D, Kosaka K *et al.* (1996b) Clinical and pathological diagnosis of dementia with Lewy bodies (DLB): report of the Consortium on Dementia with Lewy Bodies (CDLB) International Workgroup. *Neurology* 47: 1113–1124

McKeith IG, Ballard CG, Perry RH *et al.* (2000) Prospective validation of consensus criteria for the diagnosis of dementia with Lewy bodies. *Neurology* 54: 1050–1058

McShane R, Gedling K, Reading M, McDonald B, Esiri MM, Hope T. (1995) Prospective study of relations between cortical Lewy bodies, poor eyesight, and hallucinations in Alzheimer's disease. *Journal of Neurology, Neurosurgery, and Psychiatry* **59**: 185–188

Martone M, Butters N, Payne M, Becker JT, Sax DS. (1984) Dissociations between skill learning and verbal recognition in amnesia and dementia. *Archives of Neurology* **41**: 965–970

Merdes AR, Hansen LA, Jeste DV *et al*. (2003) Influence of Alzheimer pathology on clinical diagnostic accuracy in dementia with Lewy bodies. *Neurology* **60**: 1586–1590

Merello M, Sabe L, Teson A *et al*. (1994) Extrapyramidalism in Alzheimer's disease: prevalence, psychiatric, and neuropsychological correlates. *Journal of Neurology, Neurosurgery, and Psychiatry* **57**: 1503–1509

Minoshima S, Foster NL, Sima A, Frey KA, Albin RL, Kuhl DE. (2001) Alzheimer's disease versus dementia with Lewy bodies: cerebral metabolic distinction with autopsy confirmation. *Annals of Neurology* **50**: 358–365

Mirra SS, Hart MN, Terry RD. (1993) Making the diagnosis of Alzheimer's disease. *Archives of Pathology and Laboratory Medicine* **117**: 132–144

Mori E, Shimomura T, Fujimori M *et al*. (2000) Visuoperceptual impairment in dementia with Lewy bodies. *Archives of Neurology* **57**: 489–493

Moss MB, Albert MS, Butters N, Payne M. (1986) Differential patterns of memory loss among patients with Alzheimer's disease, Huntington's disease, and alcoholic Korsakoff's syndrome. *Archives of Neurology* **43**: 239–246

Olichney JM, Hansen LA, Galasko D *et al*. (1996) The apolipoprotein E ε-4 allele is associated with increased neuritic plaques and cerebral amyloid angiopathy in Alzheimer's disease and Lewy body variant. *Neurology* **47**: 190–196

Olichney JM, Galasko D, Salmon DP *et al*. (1998) Cognitive decline is faster in Lewy body variant than in Alzheimer's disease. *Neurology* **51**: 351–357

Pellise A, Roig C, Barraquer-Bordas L, Ferrer I. (1996) Abnormal, ubiquitinated cortical neurites in patients with diffuse Lewy body disease. *Neuroscience Letters* **206**: 85–88

Perry EK, Marshall E, Perry RH *et al*. (1990) Cholinergic and dopaminergic activities in senile dementia of Lewy body type. *Alzheimer Disease and Associated Disorders* **4**: 87–95

Perry EK, Marshall E, Thompson P *et al*. (1993) Monoaminergic activities in Lewy body Dementia relation to hallucinosis and extrapyramidal features. *Journal of Neural Transmission* **6**: 167–177

Perry EK, McKeith I, Ballard C. (2003) Butyryl-cholinesterase and progression of cognitive deficits in dementia with Lewy bodies. *Neurology* **60**: 1852–1853

Perry RH, Irving D, Blessed G, Fairbairn A, Perry EK. (1990) Senile dementia of the Lewy body type: a clinically and neuropathologically distinct form of Lewy body dementia in the elderly. *Journal of the Neurological Sciences* **95**: 119–139

Perry RH, McKeith IG, Perry EK. (eds) (1996) *Dementia with Lewy Bodies*. Cambridge, Cambridge University Press

Reid RT, Sabbagh MN, Corey-Bloom J, Tiraboschi P, Thal LJ. (2000) Nicotinic receptor losses in dementia with Lewy bodies: comparisons with Alzheimer's disease. *Neurobiology of Aging*: **21**: 741–746

Rezaie P, Cairns NJ, Chadwick A, Lantos PL. (1996) Lewy bodies are located preferentially in limbic areas in diffuse Lewy body disease. *Neuroscience Letters* **212**: 111–114

Richards M, Bell K, Dooneief G *et al*. (1993) Patterns of neuropsychological performance in Alzheimer's disease patients with and without extrapyramidal signs. *Neurology* **43**: 1708–1711

Sabbagh MN, Corey-Bloom J, Tiraboschi P, Thomas R, Masliah E, Thal LJ. (1999) Neurochemical markers do not correlate with cognitive decline in the Lewy body variant of Alzheimer disease. *Archives of Neurology* **56**: 1458–1461

Sahgal A, Galloway PH, McKeith IG *et al*. (1992a) Matching-to-sample deficits in patients with senile dementias of the Alzheimer and Lewy body types. *Archives of Neurology* **49**: 1043–1046

Sahgal A, Galloway PH, McKeith IG, Edwardson JA, Lloyd S. (1992b) A comparative study of attentional deficits in senile dementias of Alzheimer and Lewy body types. *Dementia* **3**: 350–354

Sahgal A, McKeith IG, Galloway PH, Tasker N, Steckler T. (1995) Do differences in visuospatial ability between senile dementias of the Alzheimer and Lewy body types reflect differences solely in mnemonic function? *Journal of Clinical and Experimental Neuropsychology* **17**: 35–43

Salmon DP and Bondi MW. (1999) The neuropsychology of Alzheimer's disease. In: R Terry, R Katz, K Bick, S Sisodia (eds), *Alzheimer's Disease*, 2nd edition. New York, Raven's Press

Salmon DP, Galasko D, Hansen LA *et al*. (1996) Neuropsychological deficits associated with diffuse Lewy body disease. *Brain and Cognition* **31**: 148–165

Salmon DP, Lineweaver TT, Galasko D, Hansen L. (1998) Patterns of cognitive decline in patients with autopsy-verified Lewy body variant of Alzheimer's disease. *Journal of the International Neuropsychological Society* **4**: 228

Salmon DP, Galasko D, Hamilton J, Thal LJ, Hansen LA. (2002) Cognitive profiles differ across disease course in autopsy-proven dementia with Lewy bodies and Alzheimer's disease. *Neurobiology of Aging* **23**: S130. (Abstract)

Samuel W, Galasko D, Masliah E, Hansen LA. (1996) Neocortical Lewy body counts correlate with dementia in the Lewy body variant of Alzheimer's disease. *Journal of Neuropathology and Experimental Neurology* **55**: 44–52

Samuel W, Alford M, Hofstetter R, Hansen LA. (1997) Dementia with Lewy bodies versus pure Alzheimer's disease: differences in cognition, neuropathology, cholinergic dysfunction and synapse density. *Journal of Neuropathology and Experimental Neurology* **56**: 499–508

Shimomura T, Mori E, Yamashita H *et al*. (1998) Cognitive loss in dementia with Lewy bodies and Alzheimer disease. *Archives of Neurology* **55**: 1547–1552

Simard M, van Reekum R, Myran D. (2003) Visuospatial impairment in dementia with Lewy bodies and Alzheimer's disease: a process analysis approach. *International Journal of Geriatric Psychiatry* **18**: 387–391

Soininen H, Helkala EL, Laulumaa V, Soikkeli R, Hartikainen P, Riekkinen PJ. (1992) Cognitive profile of Alzheimer patients with extrapyramidal signs: a longitudinal study. *Journal of Neural Transmission* **4**: 241–254

Stern Y, Richards M, Sano M, Mayeux R. (1993) Comparison of cognitive changes in patients with Alzheimer's and Parkinson's disease. *Archives of Neurology* **50**: 1040–1045

Stern Y, Jacobs D, Goldman J *et al*. (2001) An investigation of clinical correlates of Lewy bodies in autopsy-proven Alzheimer disease. *Archives of Neurology* **58**: 460–465

Swanwick GR, Coen RF, Maguire CP, Coakley D, Lawlor BA. (1996) Clock-face drawing to differentiate dementia syndrome. *Lancet*: **347**: 696–697

Terry RD, Masliah E, Salmon DP *et al*. (1991) Physical basis of cognitive alterations in Alzheimer's disease: synapse loss is the major correlate of cognitive impairment. *Annals of Neurology* **30**: 572–580

Tiraboschi P, Hansen LA, Alford M, Masliah E, Thal LJ, Corey-Bloom J. (2000) The decline in synapses and cholinergic activity is asynchronous in Alzheimer's disease. *Neurology* **55**: 1278–1283

Tiraboschi P, Hansen LA, Alford M *et al.* (2002) Early and widespread cholinergic losses differentiate dementia with Lewy bodies from Alzheimer disease. *Archives of General Psychiatry* **59**: 946–951

Tröster AI, Butters N, Salmon DP *et al.* (1993) The diagnostic utility of savings scores: differentiating Alzheimer's and Huntington's diseases with Logical Memory and Visual Reproduction tests. *Journal of Clinical and Experimental Neuropsychology* **15**: 773–788

Turner RS, Chervin RD, Frey KA, Minoshima S, Kuhl DE. (1997) Probable diffuse Lewy body disease presenting as REM sleep behavior disorder. *Neurology* **49**: 523–527

Verghese J, Crystal HA, Dickson DW, Lipton RB. (1999) Validity of clinical criteria for the diagnosis of dementia with Lewy bodies. *Neurology* **53**: 1974–1982

Wagner MT and Bachman DL. (1996) Neuropsychological features of diffuse Lewy body disease. *Archives of Clinical Neuropsychology* **11**: 175–184

Walker Z, Allen R, Shergill S, Katona C. (1997) Neuropsychological performance in Lewy body dementia and Alzheimer's disease. *British Journal of Psychiatry* **170**: 156–158

Weiner MF, Risser RC, Cullum CM *et al.* (1996) Alzheimer's disease and its Lewy body variant: a clinical analysis of postmortem verified cases. *American Journal of Psychiatry* **153**: 1269–1273

Yeatman R, McLean CA, Ames D. (1994) The clinical manifestations of senile dementia of Lewy body type: a case report. *Australian and New Zealand Journal of Psychiatry* **28**: 512–515

The treatment of dementia with Lewy bodies

E JANE BYRNE

The treatment of dementia with Lewy bodies (DLB) presents the clinician with several challenges. The aetiology and nosology of the condition are unknown and some of the most persistent and troublesome symptoms may be made worse by 'conventional' therapies. Some treatments are empirical and there are a few controlled studies.

50.1 PRIMARY PREVENTION

In a condition whose nosological states is certain, it may seem premature to discuss therapies or strategies that may prevent or delay the onset of the condition. Whilst the pathological features of DLB are increasingly well described, the controversy lies in the interpretation of the histological features. Do they indicate a variety of Alzheimer's disease (AD), a variety of Parkinson's disease (PD), a separate distinct entity, the coexistence of the two, or a spectrum disorder? Some authors suggest that DLB is more similar to PD, especially in cases with dementia (Byrne, 1995). The recent proposal for the reclassification of neurodegenerative disorders into synucleinopathies or tauopathies may help clarify the nosological status of DLB. As described in Chapter 48, the pathology of DLB consists of Lewy bodies in brain stem and cortex together with varying degrees of Alzheimer-type histological change (Duda, 2004; Iseki, 2004). Clinically about 20 per cent of cases begin with a motor syndrome indistinguishable from idiopathic PD, 40 per cent with parkinsonism and dementia and 20 per cent with dementia alone (Lennox, 1992). The clinical presentation is influenced by the degree of concomitant AD histological change (Merdes et al., 2003).

So-called pure DLB cases (without significant Alzheimer histological change) are more likely to be young (under 70 years), male and with prominent early parkinsonian features (Kosaka, 1990; Hely et al., 1996; Byrne, 2003). A small number of familial cases have been described (Tsuang et al., 2004). The parasomnia rapid eye movement sleep behaviour disorder (RBD) is common in DLB and often precedes the development of the full syndrome by many years (Byrne, 1996, 2003; Boeve et al., 2003). Putative strategies to prevent motor or cognitive progression might be effective in such cases.

Exposure to pesticides has been postulated as a risk factor for the development of PD (Liou et al., 1997, Herishanu et al., 1998). Hubble et al. (1998) have reported a possible gene-toxin interaction as a putative risk factor for PD with dementia. They found that subjects who had exposure to pesticides and at least one copy of the CYP2D629B + allele had an 83 per cent predicted probability of the development of dementia in association with PD.

Apoptotic-like changes have been described in nigral cells in PD and DLB and in neurones containing LB in DLB (Tompkins et al., 1997; Katsuse et al., 2003). One mechanism whereby this may occur is through the actions of nitric oxide (NO) (Snyder, 1996). Nitric oxide is formed from arginine by NO synthase (NOs), which has three forms, each with different genetic derivation glutamate neurones from synapses with neuronal NOs (nNOs) neurones. Glutamate in excess causes a release of NO, which leads to cell death (Dawson et al., 1996). NO metabolites were found to be increased in the cerebrospinal fluid in 22 DLB patients compared with 13 normal controls in one study (Molina et al., 2002), and Xu et al. (2000) reported that the CCTTT polymorphism in the NOS2A gene was associated with DLB. The exon 22 inducible nitric oxide synthase (iNOs) genotype is protective against PD (Hague et al., 2004) and the expression of this gene was shown to be decreased in one study by the novel antioxidant EseroS-GS (Wei et al., 2003).

NOs inhibitors have been shown to prevent this NO-mediated cell death in MPTP treated baboons (Hantraye *et al.*, 1996). As NO has also been implicated as a cause of cell damage in AD (Molina *et al.*, 1998), the use of NOs inhibitors in DLB has some theoretical justification. This rationale might also suggest the potential of excitatory amino acid antagonists as putative treatments in DLB (Sandhu *et al.*, 2003). The aggregation of misfolded α-synuclein is postulated to be cytotoxic in PD and in DLB. One recent study reported that the molecular chaperone Hsp70 reduced the amount of misfolded, aggregated α-synuclein *in vivo*, in transgenic mice (Klucken *et al.*, 2004). Other neuroprotective or preventative strategies that might be applicable to DLB include antioxidants, anti-inflammatory drugs and oestrogen (Cummings, 1995; Beal, 2003; Di Matteo and Esposito, 2003; Fernandez-Espejo, 2004). The antioxidant vitamin E has been assessed as a therapeutic agent in both PD and AD. In PD the results are equivocal with both positive (de Rijk *et al.*, 1997) and negative results (Parkinson Study Group, 1993) reported. Negative results may have been due to too low a dose (Fariss and Zhang, 2003; Mandel *et al.*, 2003). In AD, recent research suggests that vitamin E in combination with vitamin C as dietary supplements may prevent the disease (Zandi *et al.*, 2004) and that vitamin E supplementation, only if given early in the course of the illness (at least in an animal model), may be beneficial (Sung *et al.*, 2004). In AD there is some, though limited, evidence that vitamin E slows the progression in established disease (Knopman, 1998). The free radical scavenger coenzyme Q10 (an antioxidant) reduces apoptosis, possibly independent of its antioxidant action (Papucci *et al.*, 2003). In a randomized controlled trial of coenzyme Q10 (at dosages of 300, 600 or 1200 mg/day) in 80 people with early PD, less disability developed in the treatment group compared with the placebo group, with the greatest effect in those receiving the highest dosage (Shults *et al.*, 2002).

There is also evidence from epidemiological studies that prior oestrogen use may delay the onset of AD (Henderson, 1997; Honjo *et al.*, 2003; Smith and Levin-Allerhand, 2003). In ovariectomized rats oestrogen administered concurrently with MPTP reduces the DA release induced by MPP + (Disshan and Dluzen, 1997). DLB certainly has a male preponderance and, in particular, pure DLB cases are predominantly male (Hely *et al.*, 1996). Oestrogen may be protective against PD as well as AD.

50.2 TREATMENT OF ESTABLISHED DEMENTIA WITH LEWY BODIES

There have been a number of reviews of the treatment of DLB (Byrne, 2002; Burn and McKeith, 2003; Fernandez *et al.*, 2003; Mosimann and McKeith, 2003; Wild *et al.*, 2003). Transmitter-related therapy and the treatment of prominent symptoms in DLB will now be reviewed.

50.2.1 Transmitter replacement therapy

50.2.1.1 ACETYLCHOLINESTERASE INHIBITORS

In DLB there is a severe cholineacetyltransferase (ChAT) deficiency, even more profound than that seen in AD (Dickson *et al.*, 1987; Perry *et al.*, 1990; Tiraboschi *et al.*, 2000). The Newcastle group were the first to suggest the use of acetylcholinesterase inhibitors (AChEIs) for the treatment of DLB. Evidence from the early placebo controlled trials of tacrine supported this suggestion when the first three responders in a London trial to reach autopsy were found to have cortical Lewy bodies (CLB) (Levy *et al.*, 1994). Others have found that response to tacrine was not limited to those AD cases with CLB (Wilcock and Scott, 1994). Lebert *et al.* (1998) studied the effects of tacrine (120 mg/day) in clinically diagnosed AD and DLB cases, using the McKhann *et al.* (1984) and the McKeith *et al.* (1996) criteria respectively. They found that whilst the ratio of AD and DLB cases did not differ between responders and non-responders, the pattern of response was different between the two groups. In the DLB group cognitive performance improved significantly on tests of attention (digit span and verbal initiation), while the AD group improved significantly on tests of conceptualization. In this study tacrine was apparently not associated with adverse effects on the mental state of DLB patients. However, in a smaller study of tacrine, and at a lower dose (80 mg/day), Querforth *et al.* (2000) found no clinical benefit in six DLB subjects. There is also a case report of possible adverse effects of tacrine in clinically diagnosed DLB (Witjeratne *et al.*, 1995).

Second generation AChEIs are beginning to be used in DLB. A recent Cochrane review of cholinesterase inhibitors (ChEIs) for DLB found only one randomized controlled trial (RCT) (McKeith *et al.*, 2000). The reviewers concluded that neuropsychiatric symptoms may be improved but that the evidence is modest (Wild *et al.*, 2003). In this single RCT of DLB (McKeith *et al.*, 2000), 120 patients were entered into the study and randomized to placebo or to rivastigmine (up to 12 mg/day by individual titration to maximum tolerated dose) for 20 weeks. Significant differences in neuropsychiatric symptoms (as measured by the Neuropsychiatric Inventory 4 and 10 item subscales (NPI-4 and NPI-10)) were found in favour of rivastigmine over placebo at 20 weeks in the analysis of observed cases (OC), but smaller differences were seen with intention to treat (ITT) and last observation carried forward (LOCF) analysis. In an open-label follow up of the treated subjects in this trial, improvement in NPI scores were maintained up to 24 weeks, and at 96 weeks these scores were not significantly worse than at baseline (Grace *et al.*, 2001).

Table 50.1 summarizes the other case series and open-label trials of ChEIs in DLB. All studies show benefit of treatment, most especially in neuropsychiatric symptoms. Only one study (Shea *et al.*, 1998) reports worsening of extrapyramidal symptoms during treatment. Two of these studies reported the effects of cholinesterase inhibitors on sleep disorder in DLB. Catt and Kauffer (1998) found beneficial effects on

Table 50.1   *Summary of open label studies of cholinesterase inhibitors in dementia with Lewy bodies*

Study	n	Duration (weeks)	Drug	Results	Adverse effects
Catt and Kaufer, 1998	2	NR	Donepezil	Improved; somnolence and psychosis	None
Shea *et al.*, 1998	9	12	Donepezil	Improved; cognition* and visual hallucinations	Worse EPS
Lancetot *et al.*, 2000	7	8	Donepezil	Improved; cognition* and BPSD	NR
MacLean *et al.*, 2001	8	NR	Rivastigmine	Improved; cognition** and sleep	GI
Edwards *et al.*, 2004	25	24	Galantamine	Improved; BPSD	GI

*Mini-Mental state score
**Extended Mini-Mental state score
BPSD, behavioural and psychological symptoms of dementia; GI, gastrointestinal symptoms; NR, not reported; EPS, extrapyramidal symptoms

hypersomnolence and psychotic features in two clinically diagnosed cases treated with donepezil (dose not stated for either case). These beneficial effects persisted in both cases at 6 months follow up. MacLean *et al.* (2001) reported that seven out of the eight cases at baseline had sleep disruption (some of which clinically resembled RBD), six of these seven cases improved with rivastigmine and their neuropsychiatric symptoms (NPI scores) also improved. One recent study (Onofrj *et al.*, 2003) found beneficial effects of donepezil on fluctuating cognition in dementia. Similar beneficial effects on neuropsychiatric symptoms are reported in a number of case series of PD with dementia (PDD) treated with ChEIs (Reading *et al.*, 2001; Aarsland *et al.*, 2002; Bullock and Cameron, 2002; Giladi *et al.*, 2003; Leroi *et al.*, 2004).

As with many drug therapies trial doses often have to be modified when used in clinical practice. Some DLB cases clinically diagnosed who are unable (because of adverse effects, predominantly severe nausea and vomiting) to tolerate full dose rivastigmine 6–12 mg/day in divided doses have benefited from low dose therapy (1.5 mg b.i.d.). This dose level has successfully stopped troublesome visual hallucinations and improved attention in one case in South Manchester who was unresponsive to any other empirical treatment. In clinical practice slow titration of the ChEIs enhances tolerability. A diagnosis of either DLB or PDD were predictive of response to ChEIs in a study of routine clinical practice (Pakrasi *et al.*, 2003) and Minett *et al.* (2003) showed the benefit of donepezil in both DLB and PDD. Of importance was their observation that sudden withdrawal of the drug was usually detrimental.

Other putative therapeutic agents aimed at enhancing cholinergic function in DLB are muscarinic agonists (Harrison and McKeith, 1995) and nicotinic agonists (Perry and Perry, 1996). Xanomeline, an MI muscarinic receptor agonist, has been the subject of a controlled trial in AD. Whilst significant improvements in both cognitive function and behavioural abnormalities were found, in oral form the drug is poorly tolerated (Bodick *et al.*, 1997). Trials of transdermal administration of xanomeline are currently under way.

Loss of nicotinic receptors has been described in both AD and PD (Newhouse *et al.*, 1997). Two trials of transdermal administration of nicotine in AD found no improvement in cognitive function, though both were of short duration (up to 4 weeks) (Wilson *et al.*, 1995; Snaedal *et al.*, 1996). Sahakian *et al.* (1989) reported improvement of attention in AD patients treated with nicotine and nicotinic agonists improve motor function and arousal in PD (Fagerstrom *et al.*, 1994). Sagar *et al.* (1996) suggested that nicotinic agonists may be an alternative to L-dopa for the treatment of DLB.

50.2.1.2 DOPAMINERGIC THERAPIES

Although dopamine levels are reduced in post-mortem studies in DLB (Perry *et al.*, 1990) and CSF homovanillic acid levels are reduced in autopsy-confirmed cases of DLB (Weiner *et al.*, 1996), there has been little systematic enquiry into the effects of L-dopa therapy in DLB. Some early studies found little or no L-dopa response in those who were treated (Hansen *et al.*, 1990; Perry *et al.*, 1990; Mark *et al.*, 1992).

Other early studies reported a variable response (Byrne *et al.*, 1989; Gibb *et al.*, 1989; Kosaka 1990). In eight autopsy diagnosed cases of DLB reported by Louis *et al.* (1995) four had been treated with L-dopa during life and all responded. In nine pure DLB cases described by Hely *et al.* (1996) six had received L-dopa. In four cases there was response and in two cases little or no response. In post-mortem diagnosed cases of DLB (Lippa *et al.*, 1994), three of six with prominent motor symptoms had responded to L-dopa or benztropine with no apparent worsening of mental state. Of 10 clinically diagnosed cases of DLB (Geroldi *et al.*, 1997), eight received L-dopa (or other antiparkinsonian therapy). Six showed a moderate to good response with no or only mild adverse effects. In clinically diagnosed cases of DLB reported by Gnanalingham *et al.* (1997), 12 of 15 received L-dopa and all responded to treatment. The case of DLB reported by Kato *et al.* (2002) showed improvement in motor and psychotic symptoms when treated with both L-dopa (300–750 mg/day) and risperidone (1 mg/day).

One small open trial of L-dopa in DLB has been reported (Williams *et al.*, 1993). Five cases who fulfilled clinical criteria for DLB (Byrne *et al.*, 1991) were longitudinally assessed in terms of motor function, cognitive function and activities of daily living (ADL), during an open trial of L-dopa and selegiline. The dose of L-dopa (with carbidopa) was commenced at a low level and slowly titrated upwards to reach best response (defined as a 2-week plateau in motor response). Three cases showed considerable improvement in motor function and two cases modest improvement. In no case was there an adverse effect on mental state.

Acute confusional states (delirium) and other adverse effects are not uncommon with L-dopa therapy. This may (together with the perception that parkinsonian symptoms are atypical or mild and not so responsive to treatment) lead to a lack of enthusiasm for using these drugs in DLB. In my clinical experience, and as Williams *et al.* (1993) have shown, some cases with DLB may benefit from L-dopa therapy. A pragmatic strategy is to start with low doses and titrate upwards having made a careful record of the mental state (non-cognitive and cognitive features) and the range of fluctuation in symptoms both before and during treatment. Only then can one assess whether the treatment is beneficial or harmful. This pragmatic approach has been advocated by others (McKeith *et al.*, 1995a; Mosimann and McKeith, 2003). Another strategy to treat motor symptoms in DLB has been beneficial in one reported case (Moutoussis and Orrell, 1996). This case fulfilled International Consensus Criteria (McKeith *et al.*, 1996) for DLB. Severe rigidity was ' markedly improved' by using baclofen 15 mg t.i.d., a γ-aminobutyric acid (GABA) mimetic. However, baclofen was found to be ineffective in treating a severe case of neuroleptic sensitivity in DLB (McKeith *et al.*, 1992).

50.2.1.3 OTHER TREATMENTS FOR NEUROPSYCHIATRIC SYMPTOMS

Psychiatric symptoms especially visual hallucinations are common and troublesome in DLB. The Newcastle group were the first to draw attention to the phenomenon of neuroleptic sensitivity in DLB (McKeith *et al.*, 1992). They noted a high rate of adverse responses (over 50 per cent of which were severe) in 16 of 20 autopsy-confirmed DLB cases. In contrast, only one of 21 AD cases showed a severe adverse reaction. The nature of the adverse response comprised worsening motor function, aggravation or precipitation of cognitive dysfunction or non-cognitive features and drowsiness, together with some features suggestive of neuroleptic malignant syndrome (NMS) with fever, generalized rigidity and raised serum creatinine kinase. In some cases the neuroleptic sensitivity response was life-threatening. Survival analysis of the seven cases with severe reactions showed increased mortality compared with those with no or mild neuroleptic sensitivity.

The most recent report from the same group (Ballard *et al.*, 1998) is of 80 longitudinally assessed autopsy-confirmed cases (40 AD, 40 DLB, matched for age and sex). Severe neuroleptic sensitivity only occurred in DLB and was seen in 29 per cent cases, in all instances occurring within 2 weeks of a new neuroleptic prescription or a dose change. In this series 47 per cent of the neuroleptics were the newer, atypical compounds compared with 16 per cent in the 1992 series (McKeith *et al.*, 1992). Although neuroleptic sensitivity is not an inevitable consequence of neuroleptic medication in DLB, it is certainly

common and commonly severe. Gnanalingham *et al.* (1997) found comparable rates of neuroleptic sensitivity, 33 per cent, in their clinical series though none was severe. This may have been related to the low doses of neuroleptics used. Of concern is the fact that no features have yet been identified that will distinguish those cases of DLB likely to develop neuroleptic sensitivity. Ballard *et al.* (1998) found no predictive value of age, sex, severity or clinical profile. Furthermore, of the six cases with severe reactions, four were on novel or atypical neuroleptics and all were on low doses. Two of these six cases died within 2 weeks of the prescription. The mechanism by which traditional antipsychotics induce neuroleptic sensitivity is not completely understood, Piggot *et al.* (1994) suggest it is due to a failure to up-regulate D_2 receptors. It is possible that other mechanisms may be involved with the atypical antipsychotics.

Adverse effects of neuroleptics are not confined to DLB. McShane *et al.* (1997), in a prospective clinical study of 71 people with dementia initially living at home who were followed to necropsy, found that the mean decline in cognitive score was twice as great in the 16 patients treated with neuroleptics compared with those who were not medicated. Forty-two of these subjects have undergone necropsy. Cortical Lewy body pathology did not make an independent contribution to more rapid decline. Those observations have been confirmed by Holmes *et al.* (1997) who studied 135 AD cases of whom 23 subjects took neuroleptics and 112 did not. Those who did had a significantly greater rate of cognitive decline than those who did not. They also found that apolipoprotein E ε4 allele carriers were most sensitive to the effects of neuroleptics.

Atypical neuroleptics have been reported as effective in treating psychotic symptoms in DLB. Risperidone has been used in DLB with benefit (remission of psychotic features) (Lee *et al.*, 1994; Allen *et al.*, 1995; Shiwach and Woods 1998; Kato *et al.*, 2002) However, adverse reactions including neuroleptic sensitivity are increasingly reported (McKeith *et al.*, 1995b; Ballard *et al.*, 1998; Morikawa and Kishimoto 2002). Although the case reported by Shiwach and Woods (1998) benefited from risperidone it was in an unusual way – this patient had severe withdrawal bruxism following cessation of traditional antipsychotic medication, which was reversed by risperidone. In some cases clozapine may be beneficial in treating psychotic symptoms in DLB (Ableskov and Tordahl, 1993; Chacko *et al.*, 1993) but others report worsening of cognition and behaviour with clozapine treatment in DLB (Burke *et al.*, 1998).

Olanzepine and quetiapine show similarly variable results in the treatment of DLB. In the case series reported by Walker *et al.* (1999), three of the eight cases were unable to tolerate even the lowest dose (2.5 mg/day); three showed minimal benefit and only two showed improvement in neuropsychiatric symptoms. In contrast, Cummings *et al.* (2002) found that olanzepine, 5–10 mg/day improved psychotic symptoms in DLB without worsening parkinsonism. Adverse effects (somnolence or orthostatic hypotension, worsening of parkinsonian symptoms) were reported in around 30 per cent of patients with DLB treated with quetiapine in two recent small case series (Fernandez et al., 2002; Takahashi et al., 2003). In both of these studies, those subjects who could tolerate the drug showed benefit in their troublesome psychotic symptoms.

Other empirical treatments of psychotic symptoms in DLB include chlormethiazole and carbamazepine. The use of chlormethiazole was suggested because of its effectiveness in delirium tremens and because some patients with DLB have delirious-like episodes. In addition there is some evidence that chlormethiazole has neuroprotective effects (Cross et al., 1991; Baldwin et al., 1993; Vaishnav and Lutsep, 2002). In clinical practice it may reduce or obviate visual hallucinations and is helpful in sleep disorders in DLB (McKeith et al., 1992; Byrne, 1995, 1997). Carbamazepine, an antiepileptic drug with antidepressant actions, has also been used empirically to treat psychotic features in DLB. Lebert et al. (1996) found great benefit in two cases of DLB treated with 100–400 mg/day. Both chlormethiazole and carbamazepine are GABAergic agents. GABA has been suggested as an important transmitter in delirium (Ross et al., 1991), and GABA has an important function in motor control.

50.3   TREATMENT OF SLEEP DISORDERS

Disturbance of sleep is common in dementia but have only recently been especially associated with DLB (Byrne, 1996; Grace et al., 2000; MacLean et al., 2001). Some case reports (Schenck et al., 1997; Turner et al., 1997) linked DLB with rapid eye movement (REM) sleep behaviour disorder (RBD). RBD is a 'parasomnia defined by intermittent loss of electromyographic atonia during REM sleep with emergence of complex and vigorous behaviours' (ICSD 1997; Schenck et al., 1997). Behaviours include kicking, punching and leaping from the bed. Boeve et al. (1998) found 37 patients with dementia and RBD confirmed by polysomnography; 34 per cent were male and 54 per cent had signs of parkinsonism; 92 per cent (32 cases) met criteria (McKeith et al., 1996) for DLB. Three patients underwent necropsy and all had limbic Lewy bodies with or without cortical Lewy bodies. More recent studies have suggested a specific relationship between RBD and the synucleinopathies (Olson et al., 2000; Boeve et al., 2001; MacLean et al., 2001) and, except in multisystem atrophy (MSA) the greater preponderance of male subjects (Olson et al., 2000); RBD may precede the onset of the full clinical syndrome of a synucleinopathy by many years (Boeve et al., 2001).

RBD can be successfully treated with clonazepam or desimipramine (Schenck et al., 1987; Massironi et al., 2003b). Potential problems with clonazepam (at a dose of 0.5 mg) are day-time sedation and loss of efficacy over time. In a study by Schenck et al. (1987), five patients did not experience these effects. Clonazepam is not always successful in treating RBD in established DLB (MacLean et al., 2001). Boeve et al. (2003b) report the use of melatonin (3–12 mg) in 14 people with RBD (including seven with a diagnosis of DLB). Eight of the 14 showed persistant benefit beyond 12 months of melatonin therapy. There is one case report of the successful treatment of RBD in DLB with L-dopa (Yamauchi et al., 2003). Hypersomnolence, which improved on donepezil, has also been reported in DLB (Catt and Kaufer, 1998). There is one case report of improvement in 'sundowning' (increased restlessness and agitation in dementia in the evening) in DLB with treatment with donepezil (Skjerve and Nygaard, 2000).

50.4   OTHER PUTATIVE TREATMENTS

A number of other putative treatments for DLB have been suggested. Ondansetron, a selective 5HT$_3$ antagonist, has been suggested as a treatment for DLB because of the relative serotonergic overactivity in the condition (Perry et al., 1993; Sagar et al., 1996). In PD, ondansetron at a dose of 12–24 mg daily reduced psychotic symptoms in the majority of 16 patients with severe disease in an open trial (Zoldan et al., 1993). Benzodiazepines have been reported as of use in the management of anxiety and restlessness in DLB (Lennox, 1992; McKeith et al., 1996). Neurotrophins, because of their neuroprotective effect, have been postulated as a therapy for AD and other neurodegenerative disorders. However, little is known about the role of neurotrophic factors in DLB (Wilcock, 1996).

50.5   CONCLUSION

The severity, persistance and adverse effects of the neuropsychiatric symptoms of DLB and their distressing consequences for both the person with dementia and for their carers, are familiar to all practising clinicians. The Committee on Safety of Medicines (CSM) recommendations (Committee on Safety of Medicines, 1994, and as noted by Ballard et al., 1998) to use caution in prescribing neuroleptic medication in dementia is warranted given the accumulating evidence cited above. However, it unfortunate that, at least in the UK, a risk aversion culture can dictate clinical practice at the expense of the very real and severe suffering of people with DLB. The recent prohibition of the prescription of risperidone and olanzapine for the treatment of behavioural and psychological symptoms in dementia because of increased stroke risk issued by the CSM in 2004, in the absence of an adequate risk/benefit calculation or of suggested alternative treatments, leaves clinicians to face the challenge of treating DLB deprived of an important part of their therapeutic armamentarium.

Whilst many of the treatments described in this chapter are empirical, some show great promise at least in producing symptomatic relief. Greater understanding of the neuropathological mechanisms underlying DLB will lead to treatments targeted at basic processes. Until that time the treatment of DLB presents great challenges to the physician in which art as much as science still plays a part.

REFERENCES

Aarsland D, Laake K, Larsen JP, Janvin C. (2002) Donepezil for cognitive impairment in Parkinson's disease:a randomised controlled study. *Journal of Neurology and Neurosurgery Psychiatry* **72**: 708–712

Abelskov KE and Tordahl P. (1993) Lewy body demens – en ny sygdomsenied. *Ugeskr Laeger* **155**: 457–459

Allen RL, Walter Z, D'ath PJ, Katona CLE. (1995) Risperidone for psychotic and behavioural symptoms in Lewy body dementia. *Lancet* **346**: 185

American Sleep Disorders Association. (1997) *ICSD – International Classification of Sleep Disorders, Revised: Diagnostic and Coding Manual*. Rochester, American Sleep Disorders Association

Baldwin HA, Jones JA, Cross AJ et al. (1993) Histological biochemical and behavioural evidence for the neuroprotective action of chlormethiazole following prolonged carotid artery occlusion. *Neurodegeneration* **2**: 139–146

Ballard C, Grace J, McKeith IG, Holmes C. (1998) Neuroleptic sensitivity in dementia with Lewy bodies and Alzheimer's disease. *Lancet* **351**: 1032–1033

Beal MF. (2003) Mitochondira oxidative damage and inflammation in Parkinson's disease. *Annals of the New York Academy of Science* **991**: 120–131

Bodick NC, Offen WW, Shannon AE et al. (1997) The selective muscarinic agonist xanomeline improves bath the cognitive deficits and behavioural symptoms of Alzheimer's disease. *Alzheimer Disease and Associated Disorders* **11** (Suppl. 4): 516–522

Boeve BF, Silber MH, Ferman TJ et al. (1998) REM sleep behaviour disorder and degenerative dementia: an association likely reflecting Lewy body disease. *Neurology* **51**: 363–370

Boeve BF, Silber MH, Ferman TJ, Lucas JA, Parisi JE. (2001) Association of REM sleep behaviour disorder and neurodegenerative disease may reflect an underlying synucleinopathy. *Movement Disorders* **16**: 622–630

Boeve BF, Silber MH, Parisi JE et al. (2003) Synucleinopathy pathology and REM sleep behaviour disorder, dementia or parkinsonism. *Neurology* **61**: 40–45

Bullock R and Cameron A. (2002) Rivastigmine for the treatment of dementia and visual hallucinations associated with Parkinson's disease. *Current Medical Research Opinion* **18**: 258–264

Burke WJ, Pfeipfer RF, McComb RD. (1998) Neuroleptic sensitivity to clozapine in dementia with Lewy bodies. *Journal of Neuropsychiatry Clinical Neurosciences* **10**: 227–229

Burn DJ and McKeith IG. (2003) Current treatment of dementia with Lewy bodies and dementia associated with Parkinson's disease. *Movement Disorders* **18** (Suppl. 6): S72–S79

Byrne EJ. (1995) Cortical Lewy body disease: an alternative view. In: R Howard and R Levy (eds), *Developments in Dementia and Functional Disorders in the Elderly*. Stroud, Wrightson, pp. 21–27

Byrne EJ. (1996) The nature of cognitive decline in Lewy body dementia. In: EK Perry, RH Perry, IG McKeith (eds), *Lewy Body Dementia*. Cambridge, Cambridge University Press, pp. 57–66

Byrne EJ. (1997) Lewy body dementia. *Journal of the Royal Society of Medicine* **90** (Suppl. 32): 14–15

Byrne EJ. (2002) The treatment of dementia with Lewy bodies. In: N Qizilbash, LS Schneider, H Chiu et al. (eds), *Evidence-based Dementia Practice*. Oxford, Oxford University Press, pp. 608–614

Byrne EJ. (2003) Clinical features of the synucleinopathies, the effects of age and gender. *International Psychogeriatrics* **15** (Suppl. 2): 115–116

Byrne EJ, Lennox G, Lowe J, Godwin-Austen RB. (1989) Diffuse Lewy body disease: clinical features in 15 cases. *Journal of Neurology, Neurosurgery, and Psychiatry* **52**: 709–717

Byrne EJ, Lennox GG, Godwin-Austen RB et al. (1991) Dementia associated with cortical Lewy bodies: proposed clinical diagnostic criteria. *Dementia* **2**: 283–284

Catt K and Kaufer D. (1998) Dementia with Lewy bodies: response of psychosis and hypersomnolence to Donepezil. *Journal of the American Geriatrics Society* **46**: (Suppl.): 581

Chacko RC, Hyrley RA, Jonkovic J. (1993) Clozapine use in diffuse Lewy body disease. *Journal of Neuropsychiatry and Clinical Neurosciences* **5**: 206–208

Committee on Safety of Medicines. (1994) Neuroleptic sensitively inpatients with dementia. *Current Problems in Pharmacovigilance* **20**: 6

Cross AJ, Jones JA, Baldwin HA, et al. (1991) Neuroprotective activity of chlormethiazole following transient forebrain ischaemic in the gerbil. *British Journal of Pharmacology* **104**: 406–411

Crystal HA, Hauser RA, Talavera F, Caselli RJ, Baker MJ, Lutsep HL. (2003) Dementia with Lewy bodies. www.emedicine.com/neuro/topic91.htm

Cummings JL. (1995) Lewy body diseases with dementia: pathophysiology and treatment. *Brain Cognition* **28**: 266–280

Cummings JL, Street J, Masterman D, Clark WS. (2002) Efficacy of olanzapine in the treatment of psychosis in dementia with Lewy bodies. *Dementia and Geriatric Cognitive Disorders* **13**: 67–73

Dawson VL, Kizushi VM, Huang PL, Synder SH, Dawson TM. (1996) Resistance to neurotoxicity in cortical cultures from neuronal nitric oxide synthase-deficient mice. *Journal of Neurosciences* **16**: 2479–2487

Duda JE. (2004) Pathology and neurotransmitter abnormalities of dementia with Lewy bodies. *Dementia and Geriatric Cognitive Disorders* **17** (Suppl. 1): 3–14

de Rijk MC, Breteler MM, den Bruijen JH et al. (1997) Dietary antioxidants and Parkinson disease: the Rotterdam study. *Archives of Neurology* **54**: 762–765

Di Matteo V and Esposito E. (2003) Biochemical and therapeutic effects of antioxidants in the treatment of Alzheimer's disease, Parkinson's disease and amyotrophic lateral sclerosis. *Current Drug Targets CNS Neurological Disorders* **2**: 95–107

Dickson DW, Davies P, Mayeux R et al. (1987) Diffuse Lewy body disease: neuropathological and biochemical studies in 6 patients. *Acta Neuropathologica* **75**: 8–15

Disshan KA and Dluzen DE. (1997) Oestrogen as a neuromodulater of MPTP-induced neurotoxicity: effects upon striatal dopamine release. *Brain Research* **764**: 9–16

Edwards K, Therriault O'Connor J, Gorman C. (2004) Switching from donepezil or rivastigmine to galantamine in clinical practice. *Journal of the American Geriatrics Society* **52**: 1965

Fagerstrom KO, Pomerleau O, Giodarni B, Stelson F. (1994) Nicotine may relieve symptoms of Parkinson's disease. *Psychopharmacology* **116**: 117–119

Fariss MW and Zhang JG. (2003) Vitamin E therapy in Parkinson's disease. *Toxicology* **189**: 129–146

Fernandez HH, Trieschmann ME, Burke MA, Friedman JH. (2002) Quetiapine for psychosis in Parkinson's disease versus dementia with Lewy bodies. *Journal of Clinical Psychiatry* **63**: 513–515

Fernandez HH, Wu CK, Ott BR. (2003) Pharmacotherapy of dementia with Lewy bodies. *Expert Opinion in Pharmacotherapy* **4**: 2027–2037

Fernandez-Espejo E. (2004) Pathogenesis of Parkinson's disease: prospects of neuroprotective and restorative therapies. *Molecular Neurobiology* **29**: 15–30

Geroldi C, Frisoni GB, Bianchetti A, Trabucchi M. (1997) Drug treatment in Lewy body dementia. *Dementia and Geriatric Cognitive Disorders* **8**: 188–197

Gibb WRG, Luthert PJ, Janota I, Lantos PL. (1989) Cortical Lewy body dementia: clinical features and classification. *Journal of Neurology, Neurosurgery, and Psychiatry* **52**: 185–192

Giladi N, Shabtai H, Gurevich T, Benbunan B, Anca M, Korczyn AD (2003) Rivastigmine (Exelon) for dementia in patients with Parkinson's disease. *Acta Neurologica Scandinavica* **108**: 368–373

Gnanalingham KK, Byrne EJ, Thornton A, Sambrook MA, Bannister P. (1997) Motor and cognitive function in Lewy body dementia: comparison with Alzheimer's and Parkinson's disease. *Journal of Neurology, Neurosurgery, and Psychiatry* **62**: 243–252

Grace JB, Walker MP, McKeith IG. (2000) A comparison of sleep profiles in patients with dementia with Lewy bodies and Alzheimer's disease. *International Journal of Geriatrics Psychiatry* **15**: 1028–1033

Grace J, Daniel S, Stevens T, Shankar KK et al. (2001) Long-term use of rivastigmine in patients with dementia with Lewy bodies: an open-label trial. *International Psychogeriatrics* **13**: 199–205

Hague S, Peuralinna T, Eeorola J et al. (2004) Confirmation of the protective effect of iNOS in an independent cohort of Parkinson disease. *Neurology* **62**: 635–636

Hansen I, Salmon D, Galasko D et al. (1990) The Lewy body variant of Alzheimer's disease: a clinical and pathologic entity. *Neurology* **40**: 1–8

Hantraye P, Brouillet E, Ferrante E et al. (1996) Inhibition of neuronal nitric oxide synthase prevents MPTP-induced parkinsonism in baboons. *Nature Medicine* **2**: 1017–1021

Harrison RWS and McKeith IG. (1995) Senile dementia of Lewy body type – a review of clinical and pathological features: Implications for treatment. *International Journal of Geriatric Psychiatry* **10**: 919–926

Hely MA, Reid WG, Halliday GM et al. (1996) Diffuse Lewy body disease: clinical features in nine cases without co-existent Alzheimer's disease. *Journal Neurology, Neurosurgery, and Psychiatry* **60**: 531–538

Henderson VW. (1997) Estrogen cognition and a woman's risk of Alzheimer's disease. *American Journal of Medicine* **103**: 115–185

Herishanu YO, Kordysh E, Goldmith JR. (1998) A case-referent study of extrapyramidal signs. (pre-parkinsonism) in rural communities of Israel. *Canadian Journal of Neurological Sciences* **25**: 127–133

Holmes C, Fortenza O, Powell J, Lovestone S. (1997) Do neuroleptic drugs hasten cognitive decline in dementia? Carriers of apolipoprotein E 4 allele seem particularly susceptible. *BMJ* **314**: 1411

Honjo H, Iwasa K, Fushiki S et al. (2003) Estrogen and non-feminizing estrogen for Alzheimer's disease. *Endocrinology Journal* **50**: 361–367

Hubble JP, Kurth JH, Glatt SL et al. (1998) Gene-toxin interaction as a putative risk factor for Parkinson's disease with dementia. *Neuroepidemiology* **17**: 96–104

Iseki E. (2004) Dementia with Lewy bodies: reclassification of pathological subtypes and boundary with Parkinson's disease or Alzheimer's disease. *Neuropathology* **24**: 72–78

Kato K, Wada T, Kawakatsu S, Otani K. (2002) Improvement of both psychotic symptoms and Parkinsonism case of dementia with Lewy bodies by the combination therapy risperidone and L-DOPA. *Progress in Neuropsychopharmacology and Biological Psychiatry* **26**: 201–203

Katsuse O, Iseki E, Kosaka K. (2003) Immunohistochemical study of the expression of cytokines and nitric oxide synthases in brains of patients with dementia with Lewy bodies. *Neuropathology* **23**: 9–15

Klucken J, Shin J, Masliah E, Hyman BT, McLean PJ. (2004) Hsp70 reduces alpha-synuclein aggregation and toxicity. *Journal of Biological Chemistry* **279**: 25497–25502

Knopman DS. (1998) Current pharmacotherapy's for Alzheimer's disease. *Geriatrics* **53**: (Suppl.): 531–534

Kosaka D. (1990) Diffuse Lewy body disease in Japan. *Journal of Neurology* **237**: 197–204

Lebert F, Souliez L, Pasquier F. (1996) Tacrine and symptomatic treatment. In: R Perry, I McKeith, E Perry (eds), *Dementia with Lewy Bodies*. Cambridge, Cambridge University Press, pp. 439–448

Lebert F, Pasquier F, Souliez L, Petit H. (1998) Tacrine efficacy in Lewy body dementia. *International Journal of Geriatric Psychiatry* **13**: 516–519

Lee H, Cooney JM, Lawlor BA. (1994) Case report: the use of risperidone an atypical neuroleptic in Lewy body disease. *International Journal of Geriatric Psychiatry* **9**: 415–417

Lennox G. (1992) Lewy body dementia. *Bailliere's Clinical Neurology* **1**: 653–676

Leroi I, Brandt J, Reich SG, Lyketsos CGL et al. (2004) Randomised placebo-controlled trial of donepezil in cognitive impairment in Parkinson's disease. *International Journal of Geriatric Psychiatry* **19**: 1–8

Levy R, Eagger S, Griffiths M et al. (1994) Lewy bodies and response to tacrine in Alzheimer's disease. *Lancet* **343**: 176

Liou HH, Tsai MC, Chen CJ et al. (1997) Environmental risk factors and Parkinson's disease: a case-control study in Taiwan. *Neurology* **48**: 1583–1588

Lippa CF, Smith TW, Swearer JM. (1994) Alzheimer's disease and Lewy body disease: a comparative clinicopathological study. *Annals of Neurology* **35**: 81–88

Louis ED, Goldman JE, Powers JM, Fahns S. (1995) Parkinsonian features of eight pathologically diagnosed cases of diffuse Lewy body disease. *Movement Disorders* **10**: 188–194

McKeith IG, Fairbairn A, Perry RH, Thompson P, Perry EK. (1992) Neuroleptic sensitivity in patients with senile dementia of Lewy body type. *BMJ* **305**: 673–678

McKeith IG, Galasko D, Wilcock GK, Byrne EJ. (1995a) Lewy body dementia – diagnosis and treatment. *British Journal of Psychiatry* **167**: 708–717

McKeith IG, Harrison RWS, Ballard CG. (1995b) Neuroleptic sensitivity to risperidone in Lewy body dementia. *Lancet* **346**: 699

McKeith IG, Galasko D, Kosaka K et al. (1996) Consensus guidelines for the clinical and pathologic diagnosis of dementia with Lewy bodies. (DLB): report of the consortium on DLB international workshop. *Neurology* **47**: 1113–1124

McKeith I, Del Ser T, Spano P et al. (2000) Efficacy of rivastigmine in dementia with Lewy bodies: a randomized, double-blind, placebo-contolled international study. *Lancet* **356**: 2031–2036

McKhann G, Drachman D, Folstein M, Katzman R, Price D, Stadlan EM. (1984) Clinical diagnosis of Alzheimer's disease. Report of the NINCDSS-ADRDA work group under the auspices of Department of Health and Human Services Task Force on Alzheimer's disease. *Neurology* **34**: 939–944

MacLean LE, Collins CC, Byrne EJ. (2001) Dementia with Lewy bodies treated with rivastigmine: effects cognition neuropsychiatric symptoms and sleep. *International Psychogeriatrics* **13**: 277–288

McShane R, Keene J, Gedling K, Fairburn C, Jacoby R, Hope T. (1997) Do neuroleptic drugs hasten cognitive decline in dementia? Prospective study with necropsy follow up. *BMJ* **314**: 266–270

Mandel S, Grunblatt E, Riederer P, Gerlach M, Levites Y, Youdim M. (2003) Neuroprotective strategies in Parkinson's disease: an update of progress. *CNS Drugs* **17**: 729–762

Mark MH, Sage JI, Dickson DW, Schwarz KO, Duvoision RC. (1992) Levodopa-non responsive Lewy body parkinsonism: clinicopathologic study of two cases. *Neurology* **42**: 1323–1327

Massironi G, Galluzzi S, Frisoni GB. (2003) Drug treatment of REM sleep behaviour disorders in dementia with Lewy bodies. *International Psychogeriatrics* **15**: 377–383

Merdes AR, Hansen LA, Jeste JV et al. (2003) Influence of Alzheimer pathology on clinical diagnostic accuracy in dementia with Lewy bodies. *Neurology* **60**: 1586–1590

Minett TS, Thomas A, Wilkinson LM et al. (2003) What happens when donepezil is suddenly withdrawn? An open label trial in dementia with Lewy bodies and Parkinson's disease with dementia. *International Journal of Geriatric Psychiatry* **18**: 988–993

Molina JA, Jiminez-Jiminez FJ, Orti-Pareja M, Navarino JA. (1998) The role of nitric oxide in neurodegeneration potential for pharmacological intervention. *Drugs and Ageing* **12**: 251–259

Molina JA, Leza JC, Ortiz S et al. (2002) Cerebrospinal fluid and plasma concentrations of nitric oxide metabolites are increased in dementia with Lewy bodies. *Neuroscience Letters* **333**: 151–153

Morikawa M and Kishimoto T. (2002) Probable dementia with Lewy bodies and Risperidone-induced delirium. *Canadian Journal of Psychiatry* **47**: 976

Mosimann UP and McKeith IG. (2003) Dementia with Lewy bodies – diagnosis and treatment. *Swiss Medical Weekly* **133**: 131–142

Moutoussis M and Orrell W. (1996) Baclofen therapy for rigidity associated with Lewy body dementia. *British Journal of Psychiatry* **169**: 795

Newhouse PA, Potter A, Levin ED. (1997) Loss of nicotinic receptors described in both Alzheimer's disease and Parkinson's disease. Implications for therapeutics. *Drugs and Ageing* **11**: 206–228

Olson EJ, Boeve BF, Silber MH. (2000) Rapid eye movement sleep behaviour disorder; demographic clinical and laboratory findings in 93 cases. *Brain* **123**: 331–339

Onofrj M, Thomas A, Iacono D, Luciano AL, Di Iorio A. (2003) The effects of a cholinesterase inhibitor are prominent in patients with fluctuating cognition: a part 3 study of the main mechanism of cholinesterase inhibitors in dementia. *Clinical Neuropharmacology* **26**: 239–251

Pakrasi S, Mukaetova-Ladinska EB, McKeith IG, O'Brien JT. (2003) Clinical predictors of response to Acetyl cholinesterase inhibitors: experience from routine clinical use in Newcastle. *International Journal of Geriatric Psychiatry* **18**: 879–886

Papucci L, Schiavone N, Witort E, Donnini M et al. (2003) Coenzyme Q10 prevents apoptosis by inhibiting mitochondrial depolarization independently of its free radical scavenging property. *Journal of Biological Chemistry* **278**: 28220–28228

Parkinson Study Group. (1993) Effects of tocopherol and deprenyl on the progression of disability in early Parkinson's disease. *New England Journal of Medicine* **328**: 176–183

Perry EK and Perry RH. (1996) Altered consciousness and transmitter signalling in Lewy body dementia. In: R Perry, I McKeith, E Perry (eds), *Dementia with Lewy Bodies.* Cambridge, University Press, pp. 397–413

Perry RH, Irvin D, Blessed G, Fairbairn A, Perry EK. (1990) Senile dementia of the Lewy body type: a clinically and neuropathologically distinct form of Lewy body dementia in the elderly. *Journal of the Neurological Sciences* **95**: 119–139

Perry EK, Irvin D, Kerwin JM et al. (1993) Cholinergic neurotransmitter and neurotrophic activities in Lewy body dementia. Similarity to Parkinson's and distinctions from Alzheimer's disease. *Alzheimer Disease and Associated Disorders* **7**: 62–79

Piggot MA, Perry EK, McKeith IG et al. (1994) Dopamine D_2 receptors in demented patients with severe neuroleptic sensitivity. *Lancet* **343**: 1044–1045

Querfurth HW, Allam GJ, Geffoy MA, Schiff HB, Kaplan RF. (2000) Acetylcholinesterase inhibition in dementia with Lewy bodies: results of a prospective pilot trial. *Dementia and Geriatric Cognitive Disorders* **11**: 314–321

Reading PJ, Luce AK, McKeith IG. (2001) Rivastigmine in the treatment of parkinsonian psychosis and cognitive impairment: preliminary findings from an open trial. *Movement Disorders* **16**: 1171–1195

Ross CA, Peyser CE, Shapiro I et al. (1991) Delirium: phenomenologic and etiologic subtypes. *International Psychogeriatrics* **3**: 135–147

Sagar HJ, Jonsen ENH, Perry EK. (1996) Resumé of treatment workshop sessions In: R Perry, I McKeith, E Perry (eds), *Dementia with Lewy Bodies.* Cambridge, Cambridge University Press, pp. 487–490

Sahakian B, Jones G, Levy R, Gray J, Warburton D. (1989) The effects of nicotine on attention information processing and short-term memory in patients with dementia of the Alzheimer type. *British Journal of Psychiatry* **154**: 797–800

Sandhu JK, Pandey S, Ribecco-Lutkiewicz M et al. (2003) Molecular mechanisms of glutamate neurotoxicity in mixed cultures of NT2-derived neurons and astrocytes: protective effects of coenzyme Q10.

Schenck CH, Bundle SR, Patterson AL, Mahowald NW. (1987) Rapid eye movement sleep behaviour disorder. *JAMA* **257**: 1786–1789

Schenck CH, Mahowald MW, Anderson ML, Silber MH, Boeve BF, Parisi JE. (1997) Lewy body variant of Alzheimer's disease (AD) identified by post-mortem ubiquitin staining in a previously reported case of AD associated with REM sleep behaviour disorder. *Biological Psychiatry* **42**: 527–528

Shea C, MacKnight C, Rockwood K. (1998) Donepezil for treatment of dementia with Lewy bodies; a case series of nine patients. *International Psychogeriatrics* **10**: 229–238

Shiwach RS and Woods S. (1998) Risperidone and withdrawal bruxism in Lewy body dementia. *International Journal of Geriatric Psychiatry* **13**: 64–67

Shults CW, Oakes D, Kieburtz K et al. (2002) Effects of coenzyme Q10 in early Parkinson disease: evidence slowing of the functional decline. *Archives of Neurology* **59**: 1541–1550

Skjerve A and Nygaard HA. (2000) Improvement in sundowning in dementia with Lewy bodies: a treatment with donepezil. *International Journal of Geriatrics Psychiatry* **15**: 1147–1151

Smith JD and Levin-Allerhand JA. (2003) Potential use of estrogen-like drugs for the prevention of Alzheimer's disease. *Journal of Molecular Neurological Science* **20**: 277–281

Snaedal J, Johannesson T, Jansson JE, Gottfries G. (1996) Nicotine in dermal plasters did not improve cognition in Alzheimer's disease. *Dementia* **7**: 47–52

Snyder SH. (1996) No NO prevents parkinsonism. *Nature Medicine* **2**: 965–966

Sung S, Yao Y, Uryu K et al. (2004) Early vitamin E supplementation in young but not aged mice reduces Abeta levels and amyloid deposition in a transgenic rate of Alzheimer's disease. *FASEB Journal* **18**: 323–325

Takahashi H, Yoshida K, Sugita T, Higuchi H, Shimizu T. (2003) Quetiapine treatment of psychotic symptoms and aggressive behaviour in patients with dementia with Lewy bodies: a case series. *Progress in Neuropsychopharmacology and Biological Psychiatry* **27**: 549–553

Tiraboschi P, Hansen LA, Alford M et al. (2000) Cholinergic dysfunction in diseases with Lewy bodies. *Neurology* **54**: 407–411

Tompkins MM, Basgall EJ, Zamrini E, Hill WD. (1997) Apoptotic-like changes in Lewy-body-associated disorders and normal ageing in substantia nigral neurons. *American Journal of Pathology* **150**: 119–131

Tsuang DW, DiGiacomo L, Bird TD. (2004) Familial occurrence of dementia with Lewy bodies. *American Journal of Geriatric Psychiatry* **12**: 179–188

Turner RS, Chervin RD, Frey KA, Minoshima S, Kuhl DE. (1997) Probable diffuse Lewy body disease presenting as REM sleep behaviour disorder. *Neurology* **49**: 523–527

Vaishnav A and Lutsep HL. (2002) GABA agonist: clomethiazole. *Current Medical Research Opinion* **18** (Suppl. 2): S5–S8

Walker Z, Grace J, Overshot R *et al.* (1999) Olanzapine in dementia with lewy bodies:a clinical study. *International Journal of Geriatric Psychology* **14**: 459–466

Wei T, Zhao X, Hou J *et al.* (2003) The antioxidant ESeroS-GS inhibits NO production and prevents oxidative stress in astrocytes. *Biochemical Pharmacology* **66**: 83–91

Weiner MF, Risser RC, Cullum M *et al.* (1996) Alzheimer's disease and its Lewy body variant: a clinical analysis of post-mortem verified cases. *American Journal of Psychiatry* **153**: 1269–1273

Wilcock GK. (1996) Neurotrophins and the cholinergic system in dementia In: R Perry, I McKeith, E Perry (eds), *Dementia with Lewy Bodies.* Cambridge, Cambridge University Press, pp. 486–496

Wilcock GK and Scott I. (1994) Tacrine for senile dementia of Alzheimer's or Lewy body type. *Lancet* **344**: 544

Wild R, Pettit T, Burns A. (2003) Cholinesterase inhibitors for dementia with Lewy bodies. (Cochrane review). *Cochrane Library* Issue 4

Williams SW, Byrne EJ, Stokes P. (1993) The treatment of diffuse Lewy body disease: a pilot study. *International Journal of Geriatric Psychiatry* **8:** 731–739

Wilson AL, Longley LK, Monley J *et al. (*1995) Nicotine patches in Alzheimer's disease: pilot study on learning memory and safety. *Pharmacological Biochemistry and Behaviour* **51**: 509–514

Witjeratne C, Bandyopadhyay D, Howard R. (1995) Failure of tacrine treatment in a case of cortical Lewy body dementia. *International Journal of Geriatric Psychiatry* **10**: 808

Xu W, Liu L, Emson P *et al.* (2000) The CCTTT polymorphism in the NOS2A gene is associated with dementia with Lewy bodies. *NeuroReport* **11**: 297–299

Yamauchi K, Takehisa M, Tsuno M *et al.* (2003) Levodopa improved rapid eye movement sleep behaviour disoder with diffuse Lewy body disease. *General Hospital Psychiatry* **25**: 140–142

Zandi PP, Anthony JC, Khachaturian AS *et al.* (2004) Reduced risk of Alzheimer disease in users of antioxidant vitamin supplements: the Cache County study. *Archives of Neurology* **61**: 82–88

Zoldan J, Freidberg G, Goldberg-Stern H, Melamed E. (1993) Ondansetron for hallucinosis in advanced Parkinson's disease. *Lancet* **341**: 562–563

51

Cognitive impairment and dementia in Parkinson's disease

DAG AARSLAND AND CARMEN JANVIN

Parkinson's disease (PD) is a common neurodegenerative disorder affecting about 1.5 per cent of people aged 65 or older (de Rijk et al., 1997). PD is defined pathologically as cell loss in the pigmented dopaminergic cells of substantia nigra, pars compacta and synuclein pathology (Lewy neurites and Lewy bodies) in the surviving cells. In addition, cholinergic forebrain nuclei and other brain stem nuclei including the serotonergic raphe nuclei and the noradrenergic locus caeruleus, are usually affected. The topographical progression subsequently involves the anteromedial temporal mesocortex, including the transentorhinal region, and reaches into adjoining high-order sensory association areas and important limbic structures such as amygdalae and hippocampus (Braak et al., 2003; Jellinger, 2003a). In addition, amyloid plaques and even neurofibrillary tangles, are found in most cases at autopsy (Mattila et al., 1999; Jellinger, 2002). The cardinal clinical features of PD are resting tremor, bradykinesia, rigidity and postural abnormalities. However, owing to the wide distribution of neurodegeneration, it is not surprising that a wide range of non-motor symptoms occur as well, including neuropsychiatric symptoms and autonomic dysfunction.

The treatment of PD involves dopamine replacement therapy with L-dopa, and several dopamine agonists including the selective dopamine D3 receptor agonists ropinirole and pramipexole. In addition, the monoamine oxidase inhibitor selegiline with a potential neuroprotective effect may slow disease progression. The use of anticholinergic agents has declined drastically owing to concerns relating to their risk of cognitive impairment and delirium, particularly in the elderly. Deep cerebral stimulation with implantation of electrodes can be very helpful for selected patients. A wide range of behavioural side effects can occur during drug and surgical treatments.

During the last decade a considerable literature has shown that cognitive impairment is common even in early PD, and that as the disease progresses, a substantial proportion develop dementia (Emre, 2003). In addition, other neuropsychiatric symptoms, such as visual hallucinations, depression and apathy, are also common (Aarsland et al., 1999). It is thus increasingly recognized that PD is a neuropsychiatric disorder and not merely a movement disorder. Independent of the motor symptoms of PD, dementia and other neuropsychiatric symptoms affect quality of life, contribute to caregiver distress and increased risk of nursing home placement, and is associated with more psychiatric symptoms such as depression and hallucinations, higher mortality and functional disability, and higher risk for drug toxicity. This chapter will discuss the epidemiology, pathophysiologic mechanism, clinical presentation and management of cognitive impairment and dementia in patients with PD.

51.1 MILD COGNITIVE IMPAIRMENT IN PARKINSON'S DISEASE

Cognitive impairment is present even at the earliest stages of PD. The prevalence of subjects with parkinsonism and mild cognitive impairment in the community is about 10 per cent (Waite et al., 2001), and cognitive impairment may be present even in young patients (Wermuth et al., 1996). In a series of 91 PD patients with a mean duration of PD of <2 years, impairment on a range of neuropsychological tests was found in 16 per cent of patients (Reid et al., 1996). Similarly, in a study of 10 high-functioning PD patients, identified on the basis of exceptional professional distinction who continued to function successfully in leadership positions, significant impairments on tests of episodic memory and visuospatial function were reported (Mohr *et al.*, 1990). In one of the few community-based studies, more than 50 per cent of the non-demented PD subjects had some form of cognitive impairment (Janvin *et al.*, 2003).

The cognitive profile in early PD varies. Executive impairment, including working memory and attention-shift, is the earliest cognitive manifestation in PD, but visuospatial functions, and even memory, may be impaired in some patients as well (Dubois and Pillon, 1997). In a study of 42 PD patients with mild cognitive impairment, 20 per cent exhibited predominantly memory deficits, 30 per cent a dominant executive impairment, whereas 50 per cent had a more global cognitive impairment (Janvin *et al.*, 2003). With advancing PD, there is an increase in severity and broadening of cognitive impairment (Owen *et al.*, 1992). Whereas mildly impaired subjects have reduced storage of new information and visuospatial impairment, reduced storage of old material was evident only in those with a more marked impairment (Huber *et al.*, 1990). Although variations occur, the cognitive impairment in early PD is of a fronto-subcortical type, with the superimposition of deficits typically associated with cortical dementia evolving later in course (Reid *et al.*, 1996; Aarsland *et al.*, 2003c).

51.1.1 Mechanisms underlying mild cognitive impairment in PD

The heterogeneous cognitive deficits in PD may reflect differing forms of neuropathological involvement. Executive impairment is related to the dopaminergic deficits, caused by either disruption of nigrostriatal circuitry with altered outflow of the caudate nuclei to frontal cortex via thalamus (Rinne *et al.*, 2000; Lewis *et al.*, 2003) or diminished dopamine activity in the frontal projections consequent to degeneration of mesocortical projections (Mattay *et al.*, 2002). This hypothesis is supported by the worsening of executive functioning, but not memory, after withdrawal of L-dopa (Lange *et al.*, 1995). Although the exact contribution of non-dopaminergic lesions to the cognitive impairments in PD is not known, there is some evidence linking the cortical noradrenergic system to extradimensional shift performance, whereas visual memory may be dependent on acetylcholine rather than DA (Robbins *et al.*, 2003).

The more global cognitive impairment in later disease stages suggests that cortical regions are becoming involved as well. In a study using single photon emission computed tomography, non-demented, but cognitively impaired PD patients with decrements in multiple spheres of cognition, had diminshed temporal perfusion relative to controls. A differential pattern of relationships between cortical perfusion and cognitive functions was observed, with temporal and parietal perfusion showing relationships to global cognitive impairment, while dorsolateral frontal perfusion was related to executive impairment (Jagust *et al.*, 1992). A positron emission tomography study revealed that non-demented PD patients had

widespread cortical glucose hypometabolism, involving mainly frontal, but also left temporal and parietal regions, compared with more a more marked and global reduction, including severe bilateral temporoparietal defects, in PD patients with dementia (Peppard *et al.*, 1992).

Thus, in early PD, heterogeneous cognitive impairments exist, ranging from executive dysfunction caused by degeneration of dopaminergic fronto-subcortical circuitry to a memory dominant impairment possibly related to cholinergic deficits. At least in some patients, the selective cognitive impairment progresses to a more global impairment secondary to involvement of medial temporal and parietal cortices. The aetiology of the cortical involvement is not yet clear, and Alzheimer-like changes, synuclein degeneration and cerebrovascular pathology may contribute.

51.1.2 Course of mild cognitive impairment in PD

Few prospective studies of mild cognitive impairment in PD exist. Overall, the annual decline on the Mini-Mental State Examination (MMSE) in PD is 1 point, but with wide interindividual variations (Aarsland *et al.*, 2004). Mild executive and memory impairments are predictors of subsequent dementia in PD, independent of age and stage of PD (Levy *et al.*, 2002a). In non-PD populations with mild cognitive impairment (MCI), the annual progression to dementia is about 15 per cent (Petersen *et al.*, 2001). In PD, this question has not been subject to systematic research yet. We reassessed 38 PD patients with MCI (six with amnestic, 17 with single non-memory, and 15 with multiple domains MCI) after 4 years, and found that 62 per cent had developed dementia, which is consistent with the conversion rate to dementia in non-PD MCI patients. The proportion that progressed to dementia did not differ between the three different MCI groups, but was higher than among cognitively intact patients (20 per cent) ($P < 0.05$) (unpublished results).

51.2 DEMENTIA

51.2.1 Epidemiology

51.2.1.1 CROSS–SECTIONAL STUDIES

In addition to the mild cognitive impairment discussed above, dementia develops in a considerable proportion of patients with a diagnosis of PD. Wide variation in prevalence estimates of dementia in PD have been reported, based on differences in selection and number of patients studied, diagnostic criteria for PD, assessment of cognition and diagnostic criteria for dementia. Studies using community-based samples of more than 100 patients, standardized cognitive assessment and DSM-IIIR criteria for dementia have yielded prevalences ranging from 23 to 41 per cent (Levy and Marder, 2003).

Since dementia is associated with increased mortality in PD (Levy *et al.*, 2002c); prevalence studies underestimate true frequency of dementia in PD, and longitudinal studies are thus required to accurately describe the frequency of dementia in PD.

51.2.1.2 LONGITUDINAL STUDIES

Few studies of the incidence of dementia in PD populations exist. Estimates vary from 42.6 (Hughes *et al.*, 2000) to 112.5 (Marder *et al.*, 1995) per 1000 patient years. In the two community-based studies, the incidence was 95.3 (Aarsland *et al.*, 2001) and 112.5 (Marder *et al.*, 1995), indicating that about 10 per cent of PD patients develop dementia per year. The risk for developing dementia in PD is nearly six times higher than in non-PD subjects (Aarsland *et al.*, 2001). Although little is known regarding the life-time risk of developing dementia in patients with a diagnosis of PD, the available evidence suggests that the risk is high. Only one study to date has prospectively followed *de novo* PD patients to assess the frequency of dementia. After 5 years a cumulative prevalence of dementia of 36 per cent could be estimated from the data presented (Reid *et al.*, 1996). We performed an 8-year prospective study of a community-based sample of 224 PD patients with a mean duration of disease of 9 years at baseline: 122 subjects received a diagnosis of dementia at baseline or at subsequent evaluations. After controlling for attrition due to death, the 8-year cumulative prevalence of dementia was calculated to be 78 per cent (Aarsland *et al.*, 2003a). Thus, it is clear that a substantial proportion of patients with PD develop dementia, which is usually diagnosed for the first time >10 years after the diagnosis of PD (Hughes *et al.*, 2000; Aarsland *et al.*, 2003a).

51.2.1.3 RISK FACTORS FOR DEMENTIA

Several factors have been reported to be associated with dementia in PD, including male sex, low education, depression, hallucinations, age, age at onset, mild cognitive impairment, family history of dementia and genetic factors (Emre, 2003). However, prospective studies that use multivariate statistical approach indicate that age, advanced parkinsonism and mild cognitive impairment are predictors of dementia in PD (Hughes *et al.*, 2000; Levy *et al.*, 2002b; Aarsland *et al.*, 2003a) With regard to parkinsonian symptoms, rigidity and symptoms mediated mainly by non-dopaminergic systems, such as speech, gait and postural disorders, are particularly related to subsequent development of dementia, whereas patients with a tremor-dominant pattern have a lower risk (Levy *et al.*, 2000). Although some studies suggest that patients with late onset of PD have a higher risk of dementia, the evidence suggests that it is age, and not age at onset, that is associated with incident dementia in PD (Hughes *et al.*, 2000; Levy *et al.*, 2002b; Aarsland *et al.*, 2003a). The relationship with age and severity of parkinsonism seems to be related to their combined effect rather than separate effects (Levy *et al.*, 2002b).

51.2.1.4 GENETICS AND DEMENTIA IN PD

Although PD was long thought of as a non-genetic disorder, over the past few years, several genes for the disorder have been cloned, including α-synuclein and parkin, both involved in the ubiquitin-dependent protein degradation pathway (Gwinn-Hardy, 2002). The relationship of these genes to dementia is not clear, but there are mutation carriers who have both PD and PD with dementia. (Muenter *et al.*, 1998). Several studies have explored the effect of apolipoprotein (ApoE) polymorphism, a risk factor for AD, on the risk for PD and dementia, with conflicting results. Increased risk of PD and, in particular, PD with dementia, in carriers of the ApoE ε2 allele has been reported (Harhangi *et al.*, 2000). An association between ApoE ε4 allele and Alzheimer pathology in PD patients has also been reported (Mattila *et al.*, 2000). Most studies have failed to find an association between ApoE polymorphism and dementia in PD, however.

51.2.2 Diagnosis of dementia in PD

The motor symptoms of PD, such as masked facies, bradykinesia, slow speech and apathy can make the diagnosis of cognitive impairment and dementia difficult, and both over- and underdiagnosis may occur (Litvan *et al.*, 1998). Cognitive rating scales should be used, taking into account the disabilities from motor symptoms. Screening tests such as the MMSE (Folstein *et al.*, 1975) may be employed, although instruments including executive dysfunction, such as the Dementia Rating Scale (Mattis, 1976) and the Cambridge Cognitive Examination (CAMCOG), the cognitive section of CAMDEX (Roth *et al.*, 1986), are more sensitive to the cognitive disorders in PD. Particular care should be taken to distinguish between dementia and confusional states from drug toxicity. There are no generally accepted clinical criteria for the dementia in PD. In research, the use of the dementia criteria of DSM-IV (American Psychiatric Association, 1994) is generally recommended, but it can be difficult to decide whether cognitive impairment adds to the social and occupational impairment caused by the motor symptoms of the disease. In addition to a careful history emphasizing the onset, course, profile and chronology of motor, cognitive and psychiatric symptoms, neuropsychological assessment is useful in the diagnosis of mildly affected cases.

Although subcortical clinical features, such as executive and visuospatial impairment, are typical in mildly impaired cases, some patients with more advanced PD exhibit more cortical features (see above). The cognitive profile is quite similar to the profile observed in DLB, and differs form the profile observed in patients with AD (less memory but more executive impairment) and a pure subcortical dementia such as progressive supranuclear palsy (more memory but less executive impairment) (Aarsland *et al.*, 2003c). A diagnosis of PDD should be made in patients who are diagnosed as PD and develop dementia >1 year later. If dementia develops before or within 1 year after the diagnosis of PD, a diagnosis of DLB should be made. However, this time-window is rather arbitrary. DLB and PDD overlap both clinically and neuropathologically, and there is debate whether they represent distinct diseases or rather two syndromes on a spectrum of Lewy body diseases.

51.2.2.1 IMAGING

Few studies have explored the dementia of PD using structural imaging techniques. Annual brain volume loss in non-demented PD patients correlated with cognitive decline (Hu et al., 2001). Reduced hippocampal volumes in PD patients have been shown, and in PDD patients, hippocampal volumes were even smaller than in AD patients (Laakso et al., 1996). Preliminary results from studies using modern techniques such as voxel-based morphometry, show volume loss in the temporal and frontal cortices, as well as hippocampus, in PDD compared with non-demented PD patients (Beyer et al., 2003), and frontal and temporal cortical loss in PDD compared with normal controls, indistinguishable from changes in DLB patients (Burton et al., 2003).

As discussed above, functional imaging studies have shown decreases in glucose metabolism of frontal, temporal and parietal cortices in patients with PDD (Peppard et al., 1992; Jagust et al., 1992; Vander Borght et al., 1997). In addition, and contrary to AD, occipital hyperfusion has been reported (Vander Borght et al., 1997), even in non-demented subjects (Abe et al., 2003), similar to findings in DLB. Although both structural and functional imaging techniques may assist in the diagnostic work-up of patients with parkinsonism and cognitive impairment, until longitudinal imaging studies with clinicopathological correlation are available, the final diagnosis must be based on the history and clinical examination including routine blood tests.

51.2.3 Mechanisms

The aetiology of dementia in PD is not yet clear. The heterogeneous cognitive profile of dementia in PD, with features of both subcortical and cortical dementia, is consistent with the various neuropathological and neurochemical involvements in PD. Cortical LBs are associated with dementia in PD (Hurtig et al., 2000), although LBs may occur in the cortex of non-demented PD patients (Colosimo et al., 2003). There is also evidence that Alzheimer-like changes contribute to dementia in PD (Jellinger, 2002). In elderly patients, vascular changes may contribute as well (Jellinger, 2003b), although the contribution of vascular factors to dementia in PD is not known. In a recent longitudinal study, an association of dementia with smoking, but not with hypertension or diabetes mellitus, nor with stroke or atrial fibrillation was found (Levy et al., 2002a).

As discussed above, neurochemical changes involving dopamine, noradrenaline and acetylcholine, may influence cognition in PD. In particular, much interest has focused on the relationship between cholinergic deficits and dementia in PDD. Selective loss of cells in the cholinergic nucleus basalis of Meynert and cortical cholinergic losses of similar degrees

as in AD have been reported, and these changes are more pronounced in PD patients with dementia compared with non-demented patients (Whitehouse et al., 1983; Perry et al., 1993; Kuhl et al., 1996; Tiraboschi et al., 2000).

51.3 TREATMENT

No pharmacological agents have been approved for treatment of dementia in PD. There are several pharmacological agents available to treat the various motor and psychiatric manifestations of PD, all of which have the potential to improve one symptom domain at the expense of exacerbating another. The only evidence-based treatment for neuropsychiatric symptoms in PD is the use of clozapine for hallucinations (Goetz, 2002). Non-specific measures such as reviewing and removing drugs that may cause worsening of cognition, such as anticholinergic agents, and treating comorbid conditions, are thus of importance. Informing the patient and family about the risk of progressive worsening of cognitive functioning in addition to motor symptoms are also important.

L-dopa treatment may improve some and impair other cognitive functions (see above), but has probably no effect on dementia. Other drugs frequently prescribed for PD patients may potentially improve cognition. In a placebo-controlled trial, neither selegiline nor vitamin E had a significant effect on cognitive functioning in non-demented PD patients (Kieburtz et al., 1994). An observational study suggested that post-menopausal oestrogen use was protective for the development of dementia within the setting of PD (Marder et al., 1998), but controlled studies supporting this promising result have not been performed.

The cholinergic loss in PDD, an increase of muscarinic receptor binding (Perry et al., 1993) and less neurodegenerative changes in neocortex compared with AD, indicate that cholinergic drugs may be particularly useful in PDD. This hypothesis received support from an early study showing remarkable improvements of cognition, hallucinations and even parkinsonism, during treatment with tacrine (Hutchinson and Fazzini, 1996). Subsequent uncontrolled case series have shown improved cognition in PDD during treatment with the more recently developed cholinesterase inhibitors, i.e. rivastigmine (Reading et al., 2001) and galantamine (Aarsland et al., 2003c), although the improvements were less dramatic than those reported with tacrine. These promising results were supported in one placebo-controlled cross-over trial with donepezil (Aarsland et al., 2002). Since there are clinical, neuropathological and neurochemical similarities between DLB and PDD, the improvement on rivastigmine in a large randomized trial with in DLB patients (McKeith et al., 2000) also supports the usefulness of cholinesterase inhibitors for PDD. Worsening of motor symptoms does occur in some patients, although most patients tolerate the drug well without increasing parkinsonism. A recent large-scale placebo-controlled trial provided strong evidence that the cholinesterase inhibitor rivastigmine can improve cognition, activities of daily living and neuropsychiatric symptoms in patients with PDD (Emre *et al.*, 2004).

The currently available cholinergic drugs differ in their pharmacodynamic profiles. It is currently not known whether these differences, such as the additional effect on butyryl cholinetransferase of rivastigmine and the modulating effect on nicotinic receptors of galantamine, have therapeutic relevance in the treatment of PDD. However, there is evidence that temporal cortex butyrylcholine esterase is associated with cognitive decline in DLB (Perry *et al.*, 2003); nicotine appears to have a beneficial effect on arousal, attention, and processing speed, and may even improve motor symptoms in PD (Rusted *et al.*, 2000), suggesting that these drugs may differ in their clinical effects in PDD. However, clinical trials are necessary to corroborate these hypotheses.

51.4 CONCLUSIONS

Cognitive impairment and dementia are very common in patients with PD, with important clinical consequences for patients and their caregivers. Clinicians need to focus on these and other neuropsychiatric symptoms in addition to the motor symptoms in order to provide optimal care for these patients. The underlying aetiology and the clinical presentation of cognitive impairment in PD are highly variable, and the nosological classification of PDD and its relationship to other dementias, in particular DLB, is not yet clarified. The complex clinical presentation in these frail and elderly individuals poses considerable challenges for the clinical management. Emerging evidence indicates that cholinesterase inhibitors are useful for patients with PDD.

REFERENCES

Aarsland D, Larsen JP, Lim NG *et al.* (1999) Range of neuropsychiatric disturbances in patients with Parkinson's disease. *Journal of Neurology, Neurosurgery, and Psychiatry* **67**: 492–496

Aarsland D, Andersen K, Larsen JP, Lolk A, Nielsen H, Kragh-Sorensen P. (2001) Risk of dementia in Parkinson's disease: a community-based, prospective study. *Neurology* **56**: 730–736

Aarsland D, Laake K, Larsen JP, Janvin C. (2002) Donepezil for cognitive impairment in Parkinson's disease: a randomised controlled study. *Journal of Neurology, Neurosurgery, and Psychiatry* **72**: 708–712

Aarsland D, Andersen K, Larsen JP, Lolk A, Kragh-Sorensen P. (2003a) Prevalence and characteristics of dementia in Parkinson disease: an 8-year prospective study. *Archives of Neurology* **60**: 387–392

Aarsland D, Hutchinson M, Larsen JP. (2003b) Cognitive, psychiatric and motor response to galantamine in Parkinson's disease with dementia. *International Journal of Geriatric Psychiatry* **18**: 937–941

Aarsland D, Litvan I, Salmon D, Galasko D, Wentzel-Larsen T, Larsen JP. (2003c) Performance on the dementia rating scale in Parkinson's disease with dementia and dementia with Lewy bodies: comparison with progressive supranuclear palsy and Alzheimer's disease. *Journal of Neurology, Neurosurgery, and Psychiatry* **74**: 1215–1220

Aarsland D, Andersen K, Larsen JP, Wentzel-Larsen T, Lolk A, Kragh-Sorensen P. (2004) The rate of cognitive decline in Parkinson's disease. *Archives of Neurology* **61**: 1906–1911

Abe Y, Kachi T, Kato T *et al.* (2003) Occipital hypoperfusion in Parkinson's disease without dementia: correlation to impaired cortical visual processing. *Journal of Neurology, Neurosurgery, and Psychiatry* **74**: 419–422

American Psychiatric Association. (1994) *Diagnostic and Statistical Manual of Mental Disorders (DSM IV)*. 4th edition, revised. Washington, DC, American Psychiatric Association

Beyer MK, Aarsland D, Burton EJ, Neckelmann G, Vossius C, Larsen JP. (2003) A voxel based morphometric study of patients with Parkinson's disease and cognitive impairment. 6th International AD/PD Conference, Sevilla, Spain, 8–12 May

Braak H, Del Tredici K, Rub U, de Vos RA, Jansen Steur EN, Braak E. (2003) Staging of brain pathology related to sporadic Parkinson's disease. *Neurobiological Aging* **24**: 197–211

Burton E, McKeith IG, Burn D, Williams ED, O'Brien JT. (2003) A voxel-based morphometric comparison of Parkinson's disease with and without dementia, Alzheimer's disease, dementia with Lewy bodies and elderly controls. In: *3rd International Workshop on Dementia with Lewy Bodies and Parkinson's Disease Dementia (DLB/PDD)*. Newcastle upon Tyne, UK

Colosimo C, Hughes AJ, Kilford L, Lees AJ. (2003) Lewy body cortical involvement may not always predict dementia in Parkinson's disease. *Journal of Neurology, Neurosurgery, and Psychiatry* **74**: 852–856

de Rijk MC, Tzourio C, Breteler MM *et al.* (1997) Prevalence of parkinsonism and Parkinson's disease in Europe: the EUROPARKINSON Collaborative Study. European Community Concerted Action on the Epidemiology of Parkinson's disease. *Journal of Neurology, Neurosurgery, and Psychiatry* **62**: 10–15

Dubois B and Pillon B. (1997) Cognitive deficits in Parkinson's disease. *Journal of Neurology* **244**: 2–8

Emre M. (2003) Dementia associated with Parkinson's disease. *Lancet Neurology* **2**: 229–237

Emre M, Aarsland D, Albanese A *et al.* (2004) Rivastigmine for dementia associated with Parkinson's disease. *New England Journal of Medicine* **351**: 2509–2518

Folstein MF, Folstein SE, McHugh PR. (1975) A practical method for grading the mental state of patients for the clinican. *Journal of Psychiatric Research* **12**: 189–198

Goetz CG *et al.* (2002) Management of Parkinson's disease. *Movement Disorders* **17** (Suppl. 4)

Gwinn-Hardy K. (2002) Genetics of parkinsonism. *Movement Disorders* **17**: 645–656

Harhangi BS, de Rijk MC, van Duijn CM, Van Broeckhoven C, Hofman A, Breteler MM. (2000) APOE and the risk of PD with or without dementia in a population-based study. *Neurology* **54**: 1272–1276

Hu MT, White SJ, Chaudhuri KR, Morris RG, Bydder GM, Brooks DJ. (2001) Correlating rates of cerebral atrophy in Parkinson's disease with measures of cognitive decline. *Journal of Neural Transmission* **108**: 571–580

Huber SJ, Chakeres DW, Paulson GW, Khanna R. (1990) Magnetic resonance imaging in Parkinson's disease. *Archives of Neurology* **47**: 735–737

Hughes TA, Ross HF, Musa S *et al.* (2000) A 10-year study of the incidence of and factors predicting dementia in Parkinson's disease. *Neurology* **54**: 1596–1602

Hurtig HI, Trojanowski JQ, Galvin J *et al.* (2000) Alpha-synuclein cortical Lewy bodies correlate with dementia in Parkinson's disease. *Neurology* **54**: 1916–1921

Hutchinson M and Fazzini E. (1996) Cholinesterase inhibition in Parkinson's disease. *Journal of Neurology, Neurosurgery, and Psychiatry* **61**: 324–325

Jagust WJ, Reed BR, Martin EM, Eberling JL, Nelson-Abbott RA. (1992) Cognitive function and regional cerebral blood flow in Parkinson's disease. *Brain* **115**: 521–537

Janvin C, Aarsland D, Larsen JP, Hugdahl K. (2003) Neuropsychological profile of patients with Parkinson's disease without dementia. *Dementia and Geriatric Cognitive Disorders* **15**: 126–131

Jellinger KA. (2002) Recent developments in the pathology of Parkinson's disease. *Journal of Neural Transmission* (Suppl.): 347–376

Jellinger KA. (2003a) Alpha-synuclein pathology in Parkinson's and Alzheimer's disease brain: incidence and topographic distribution – a pilot study. *Acta Neuropathologica (Berlin)* **106**: 191–201

Jellinger KA. (2003b) Prevalence of cerebrovascular lesions in Parkinson's disease. A postmortem study. *Acta Neuropathologica (Berlin)* **105**: 415–419

Kieburtz K, McDermott M, Como P *et al.* (1994) The effect of deprenyl and tocopherol on cognitive performance in early untreated Parkinson's disease. Parkinson Study Group. *Neurology* **44**: 1756–1759

Kuhl DE, Minoshima S, Fessler JA *et al.* (1996) In vivo mapping of cholinergic terminals in normal aging, Alzheimer's disease, and Parkinson's disease. *Annals of Neurology* **40**: 399–410

Laakso MP, Partanen K, Riekkinen P *et al.* (1996) Hippocampal volumes in Alzheimer's disease, Parkinson's disease with and without dementia, and in vascular dementia: an MRI study. *Neurology* **46**: 678–681

Lange KW, Paul GM, Naumann M, Gsell W. (1995) Dopaminergic effects on cognitive performance in patients with Parkinson's disease. *Journal of Neural Transmission* **46** (Suppl.): 423–432

Levy G and Marder K. (2003) Prevalence, incidence, and risk factors for dementia in Parkinson's disease. In: MA Bedard, Y Agid, S Chouinard, S Fahn, A Korczyn, P Lesperance (eds), *Mental and Behavioral Dysfunction in Movement Disorders*, Totowa, NJ, Humana Press, pp. 259–270

Levy G, Tang MX, Cote LJ *et al.* (2000) Motor impairment in PD: relationship to incident dementia and age. *Neurology* **55**: 539–544

Levy G, Jacobs DM, Tang MX *et al.* (2002a) Memory and executive function impairment predict dementia in Parkinson's disease. *Movement Disorders* **17**: 1221–1226

Levy G, Schupf N, Tang MX *et al.* (2002b) Combined effect of age and severity on the risk of dementia in Parkinson's disease. *Annals of Neurology* **51**: 722–729

Levy G, Tang MX, Louis ED *et al.* (2002c) The association of incident dementia with mortality in PD. *Neurology* **59**: 1708–1713

Lewis SJ, Dove A, Robbins TW, Barker RA, Owen AM. (2003) Cognitive impairments in early Parkinson's disease are accompanied by reductions in activity in frontostriatal neural circuitry. *Journal of Neuroscience* **23**: 6351–6356

Litvan I, MacIntyre A, Goetz CG *et al.* (1998) Accuracy of the clinical diagnoses of Lewy body disease, Parkinson disease, and dementia with Lewy bodies: a clinicopathologic study. *Archives of Neurology* **55**: 969–978

McKeith I, Del Ser T, Spano P *et al.* (2000) Efficacy of rivastigmine in dementia with Lewy bodies: a randomised, double-blind, placebo-controlled international study. *Lancet* **356**: 2031–2036

Marder K, Tang MX, Alfaro B *et al.* (1998) Postmenopausal estrogen use and Parkinson's disease with and without dementia. *Neurology* **50**: 1141–1143

Marder K, Tang MX, Cote L, Stern Y, Mayeux R. (1995) The frequency and associated risk factors for dementia in patients with Parkinson's disease. *Archives of Neurology* **52**: 695–701

Mattay VS, Tessitore A, Callicott JH *et al.* (2002) Dopaminergic modulation of cortical function in patients with Parkinson's disease. *Annals of Neurology* **51**: 156–164

Mattila PM, Rinne JO, Helenius H, Roytta M. (1999) Neuritic degeneration in the hippocampus and amygdala in Parkinson's disease in relation to Alzheimer pathology. *Acta Neuropathologica (Berlin)* **98**: 157–64

Mattila KM, Rinne JO, Roytta M *et al.* (2000) Dipeptidyl carboxypeptidase 1 (DCP1) and butyrylcholinesterase (BCHE) gene interactions with the apolipoprotein E epsilon 4 allele as risk factors in Alzheimer's disease and in Parkinson's disease with coexisting Alzheimer pathology. *Journal of Medical Genetics* **37**: 766–770

Mattis S. (1976) Dementia Rating Scale. In: L Bellak and TB Karasu (eds), *Geriatric Psychiatry. A Handbook for Psychiatrists and Primary Care Physicians.* New York, Grune and Stratton, pp. 108–121

Mohr E, Juncos J, Cox C, Litvan I, Fedio P, Chase TN. (1990) Selective deficits in cognition and memory in high-functioning parkinsonian patients. *Journal of Neurology, Neurosurgery, and Psychiatry* **53**: 603–606

Muenter MD, Forno LS, Hornykiewicz O *et al.* (1998) Hereditary form of parkinsonism–dementia. *Annals of Neurology* **43**: 768–781

Owen AM, James M, Leigh PN *et al.* (1992) Fronto-striatal cognitive deficits at different stages of Parkinson's disease. *Brain* **115**: 1727–1751

Peppard RF, Martin WR, Carr GD *et al.* (1992) Cerebral glucose metabolism in Parkinson's disease with and without dementia. *Archives of Neurology* **49**: 1262–1268

Perry EK, Irving D, Kerwin JM *et al.* (1993) Cholinergic transmitter and neurotrophic activities in Lewy body dementia: similarity to Parkinson's and distinction from Alzheimer disease. *Alzheimer Disease and Associated Disorders* **7**: 69–79

Perry E, McKeith I, Ballard C. (2003) Butyrylcholinesterase and progression of cognitive deficits in dementia with Lewy bodies. *Neurology* **60**: 1852–1853

Petersen RC, Stevens JC, Ganguli M, Tangalos EG, Cummings JL, DeKosky ST. (2001) Practice parameter: early detection of dementia: mild cognitive impairment (an evidence-based review). Report of the Quality Standards Subcommittee of the American Academy of Neurology. *Neurology* **56**: 1133–1142

Reading PJ, Luce AK, McKeith IG. (2001) Rivastigmine in the treatment of parkinsonian psychosis and cognitive impairment: preliminary findings from an open trial. *Movement Disorders* **16**: 1171–1174

Reid WG, Hely MA, Morris JG *et al.* (1996) A longitudinal study of Parkinson's disease: clinical and neuropsychological correlates of dementia. *Journal of Clinical Neuroscience* **3**: 327–333

Rinne JO, Portin R, Ruottinen H *et al.* (2000) Cognitive impairment and the brain dopaminergic system in Parkinson disease: [18F]fluorodopa positron emission tomographic study. *Archives of Neurology* **57**: 470–475

Robbins TW, Crofts HS, Cools R, Roberts AC. (2003) Evidence for DA-dependent neural dissociations in cognitive performance in PD. In: MA Bedard (ed.), *Mental and Behavioral Dysfunction in Movement Disorders.* Totowa, New Jersey, Humana Press, pp. 194–197

Roth M, Tym E, Mountjoy CQ *et al.* (1986) CAMDEX. A standardised instrument for the diagnosis of mental disorder in the elderly with special reference to the early detection of dementia. *British Journal of Psychiatry* **149**: 698–709

Rusted JM, Newhouse PA, Levin ED. (2000) Nicotinic treatment for degenerative neuropsychiatric disorders such as Alzheimer's disease and Parkinson's disease. *Behaviour and Brain Research* **113**: 121–129

Tiraboschi R, Hansen LA, Alford M *et al.* (2000) Cholinergic dysfunction in diseases with Lewy bodies. *Neurology* **54**: 407–411

Vander Borght T, Minoshima S, Giordani B *et al.* (1997) Cerebral metabolic differences in Parkinson's and Alzheimer's diseases matched for dementia severity. *Journal of Nuclear Medicine* **38**: 797–802

Waite LM, Broe GA, Grayson DA, Creasey H. (2001) Preclinical syndromes predict dementia: the Sydney older persons study. *Journal of Neurology, Neurosurgery, and Psychiatry* **71**: 296–302

Wermuth L, Knudsen L, Boldsen J. (1996) A study of cognitive functions in young Parkinsonian patients. *Acta Neurologica Scandinavica* **93**: 21–24

Whitehouse PJ, Hedreen JC, White CL 3rd, Price DL. (1983) Basal forebrain neurons in the dementia of Parkinson disease. *Annals of Neurology* **13**: 243–248

PART 6

Focal dementias

52

Frontotemporal dementia

DAVID NEARY

Frontotemporal dementia (FTD) is a focal degenerative disorder of the frontal and anterior temporal lobes, characterized by profound alteration in personality and social conduct and impaired frontal executive functions. The disorder is the most common of a spectrum of clinical syndromes that are associated with frontotemporal lobar degeneration and share a common non-Alzheimer pathology. Other related syndromes include progressive non-fluent aphasia and semantic dementia (Chapter 55). The distinct clinical syndromes reflect the distribution of pathological change within the anterior cerebral hemispheres. FTD involves bilateral and typically symmetrical atrophy of the prefrontal and anterior temporal lobes and the basal ganglia, whereas progressive aphasia involves the perisylvian regions of the left hemisphere and semantic dementia the anterior temporal neocortices.

52.1 HISTORICAL BACKGROUND

The earliest description of a progressive behavioural disorder associated with bilateral frontal lobe atrophy was by Pick (1906). The frontal lobe emphasis was noted in several subsequent reports of focal cerebral atrophy to which Pick's name was ascribed (Schneider, 1927; Lowenberg, 1935; Ferrano and Jervis, 1936; Neumann, 1949). Despite these early studies, by the second half of the twentieth century clinical reports of focal cerebral atrophy had dramatically diminished, reflecting the prevailing wisdom of dementia as a generalized and undifferentiated impairment of mental function.

Attention was revived by longitudinal clinical studies of patients in Lund, Sweden (Gustafson and Risberg, 1974; Gustafson et al., 1977; Gustafson, 1987, 1993) and Manchester, England (Neary et al., 1986, 1987, 1988; Snowden et al., 1996), who showed progressive alteration in personal and interpersonal behaviour in association with atrophy of the frontal and anterior temporal lobes. The histological changes were not uniform. In some brains microvacuolation was the prominent feature, whereas in others there was severe gliosis, sometimes with Pick cells and bodies (Brun, 1987, 1993; Mann and South, 1993; Mann et al., 1993). In some brains motor neurone disease-type pathological changes were present. The findings led to the publication of a consensus statement outlining the clinical and pathological characteristics (Lund and Manchester groups, 1994). The term frontotemporal dementia was introduced as a clinical descriptor of the behavioural syndrome, to avoid the pathological implications of the term Pick's disease and implicit assumptions of the aetiological equivalence of underlying histologies.

Reports of FTD have proliferated (e.g. Filley et al., 1994; Frisoni et al., 1995; Jagust et al., 1989; Knopman et al., 1990; Knopman, 1993; Miller et al., 1991, 1993; Starkstein et al., 1994; Stevens et al., 1998) and more detailed consensus diagnostic criteria have been produced (Neary et al., 1998) (Box 52.1). Moreover, in recognition of the need to draw the attention of non-specialists such as general practitioners to the existence of FTD, guidelines have been produced to aid its identification (McKhann et al., 2001).

in a first-degree relative is identified in about half of patients indicating a higher familial incidence than in Alzheimer's disease. The pattern of inheritance in some families with FTD clearly indicates the action of an autosomal dominant gene, whereas in other familial cases the mode of inheritance is less clearly defined. No environmental determinants have been identified. Patients come from all social classes and a wide range of occupational backgrounds and from different parts of the world. It has been estimated by some that FTD accounts for approximately a quarter of cases of early-onset degenerative dementia (Brun, 1987; Neary *et al.*, 1988), although other studies (Ratnavalli *et al.*, 2002) suggest the proportion may be even higher. The estimated prevalence in the Netherlands has been reported to be 3.6 per 100 000 (Rosso *et al.*, 2003) at age 50–59, increasing to 9.4 per 100 000 at age 60–69 and reducing to 3.8 per 100 000 at 70–79 years. A higher prevalence of 15 per 100 000 aged 45–64 years has been reported in the Cambridge area of the United Kingdom (Ratnavalli *et al.*, 2002). Differences in prevalence estimates may in part reflect natural geographical variation arising from the cluster effects that are common in highly familial disorders.

52.2 DEMOGRAPHIC FEATURES

Onset of symptoms is most commonly in the middle years of life (Box 52.2). However, there is a wide range. FTD can occur both in the elderly and in youth, the youngest recorded onset being 21 years (Lowenberg *et al.*, 1939; Snowden *et al.*, 2004). There is an equal incidence for men and women. The length of illness is variable. Very short duration is typically associated with the additional presence of motor neurone disease (MND) (see Section 52.9, p. 674). A family history of dementia

52.3 BEHAVIOUR AND AFFECT

52.3.1 Personal and social

The overriding presenting feature is of breakdown in the patient's personal and interpersonal conduct. Patients neglect personal responsibilities, leading to mismanagement of domestic and financial affairs and impaired occupational performance. Medical referral may occur following demotion or dismissal from work. Patients show a decline in their manners, social graces and decorum. Some patients are purposelessly overactive and may show frank social disinhibition, talking to strangers, or laughing or singing inappropriately. They may make social *faux-pas* or breaches of etiquette, such as drinking from the wine bottle in a restaurant. They may pace restlessly and wander. Other patients are apathetic and avolitional. In all cases there is a notable lack of insight into the mental changes.

Consistent with their general lack of concern patients may neglect personal hygiene and need to be encouraged, if not forced, to wash and change their clothes. Patients cease to show interest in their personal appearance. The tendency to put on the same clothes each day is one sign of patients' increasing inflexibility. Patients may adopt a fixed daily routine. They may be intransigent, having difficulty seeing another's point of view.

Behavioural disinhibition is commonly associated with overt distractibility and lack of attention to tasks. Both disinhibited and apathetic patients may show economy of effort and lack of persistence, so often abandon tasks unfinished.

52.3.2 Eating and oral behaviours

Changes in eating and drinking patterns are common, and may be an early symptom. Patients often become gluttonous, eating indiscriminately, cramming food and stealing food from the plates of others. Relatives may have to ration food to prevent obesity. Patients often develop a preference for sweet foods, which they may seek out and hoard. Excessive and indiscriminate eating may be superseded later in the disease by selective food fads, usually involving the favoured sweet foods. Hyperorality (Kluver–Bucy syndrome), involving the mouthing of inedible objects, is observed in some patients, although typically only in the late stages of disease. In some patients excessive eating or drinking appears attributable to gluttony, whereas in others it appears to be part of more general stimulus-boundedness and environmental dependency. Repetitive eating and drinking may constitute one aspect of utilization phenomena (Lhermitte, 1983), the tendency to use objects within reach, regardless of contextual inappropriateness (e.g. continued drinking from an empty cup; putting on another person's glasses on top of one's own).

52.3.3 Sleeping and sexual behaviour

Increased somnolence may occur, particularly in apathetic patients. Altered sexual behaviour is common. Usually this constitutes a loss of libido, particularly in apathetic, inert patients. Less commonly patients show some sexual disinhibition, making inappropriate sexual advances. This may reasonably be construed as secondary to the patients' behavioural disinhibition and lack of awareness of social mores. A smaller minority of patients do, however, exhibit a preoccupation with sex. Such patients may make increased sexual demands on their partner or acquire an interest in mild sexual perversions.

52.3.4 Repetitive behaviours, compulsions and rituals

Repetitive, stereotyped behaviours are common in FTD. They take different forms. They may comprise simple motor mannerisms, such as hand rubbing, foot tapping or grunting. Conversely they may constitute complex behavioural routines. Patients may clock-watch, carrying out a particular activity at precisely the same time each day. They may pace and wander a fixed route. They may produce verbal stereotypies, comprising a favoured word or phrase or a complete anecdote or repertoire, repeated verbatim on each occasion. They may repeatedly sing the same ditty, dance the same steps, produce the same puns, or clap a favoured rhythm.

Hygiene and dress and toileting may themselves be the source of stereotyped behaviours: the patient may carry out a set sequence of activities at precisely the same time each day. Occasionally patients adopt superstitious rituals such as not walking on the gaps between paving stones. Although many repetitive behaviours have a compulsive quality, they are not associated with the feelings of anxiety and relief from anxiety that are characteristic of obsessional–compulsive disorder. However, if rituals are interrupted or prevented by others, then irritability or aggression may be provoked.

One striking form of repetitive behaviour, present in a minority of patients, is that of forced-utilization. Objects that are within the patient's reach elicit the motor actions appropriate to those objects, even though the action may be contextually inappropriate: an empty cup elicits a drinking action; a comb results in the patient combing his or her hair. If the object remains in view the action may be repeated over and over again.

52.3.5 Affect

The onset of FTD is insidious and may sometimes be heralded by affective changes that include depression, anxiety and excessive sentimentality, as well as hypochondriasis and somatic preoccupation (Lund and Manchester groups, 1994). In some cases discrete episodes of mood disturbance, which can be treated effectively, may occur several months or even years before the emergence of gross behavioural change. Commonly, however, subtle mood disturbances are the precursor to the major alterations in personality and social conduct and profound blunting of affect that characterize the disease.

A salient feature of FTD is emotional unconcern. Affect is typically bland, shallow and indifferent. Patients show no frustration or distress at their own altered social and occupational circumstances. They demonstrate a lack of feelings of empathy, sympathy or compassion towards others and are described as selfish and self-centred. Indeed, relatives may be alerted to the fact that something is wrong by the patient's lack of demonstration of grief on the death of a close relative or callous response to a tragic incident. Patients no longer exhibit social emotions of shame or embarrassment, and may show a lack of personal modesty. Disinhibited patients may display a fatuous jocularity.

Loss of appropriate emotional responses may include a failure to respond to painful stimuli. Patients may respond with indifference to scalds and burns. However, sometimes the converse is seen: patients respond in an exaggerated, melodramatic way to neutral tactile stimuli, such as light touch. Paradoxically the two may co-occur in the same patient. The patient tolerates the pain of a needle without comment, yet withdraws in apparent agony as a person brushes past.

52.4 PHYSICAL FINDINGS

52.4.1 General physical examination

Patients typically are physically well. However, low and labile blood pressure may be noted. Incontinence is often an early feature.

52.4.2 Neurological signs

Typical patients remain remarkably free from neurological signs, even in the presence of gross behavioural and cognitive change. Signs generally are limited to the emergence of primitive reflexes, such as grasping, pouting, sucking and extensor plantar responses. Clinical signs of striatal disorder only become evident, in some cases, after many years, when akinesia, rigidity and tremor appear. The extrapyramidal signs reflect breakdowns in nigrostriatal dopaminergic function (Rinne et al., 2002). Myoclonus is not seen. Corticospinal weakness is not evident. Muscular wasting only occurs in a subgroup of patients who develop motor neurone disease. Ataxia does not occur.

52.5 INVESTIGATIONS

52.5.1 Electroencephalography (EEG)

Routine EEG typically remains normal even in the context of severe dementia, a feature that helps to distinguish FTD from Alzheimer's disease, in which there is slowing of wave forms.

52.5.2 Structural and functional brain imaging

Computed tomography (CT) reveals non-specific cerebral atrophy in the majority. Sometimes, however, pronounced widening of the interhemispheric and sylvian fissures suggests a frontotemporal distribution of atrophy. Emphasis of pathology in the frontal lobes is more reliably demonstrated on magnetic resonance imaging (MRI).

Single photon emission tomography (SPET) reveals reduced tracer activity in the frontal and temporal lobes (Plate 22). Abnormalities are typically bilateral, but may be symmetrical or asymmetrical. *Positron emission tomography (PET)* studies indicate ventromedial frontal cortex as the critical affected area (Salmon et al., 2003). The pattern of anterior hemisphere dysfunction contrasts with the prototypical pattern of posterior hemisphere dysfunction seen in Alzheimer's disease (Talbot et al., 1998). Functional MRI has shown loss of frontal activation even in early FTD cases in whom structural MRI imaging is normal (Rombouts et al., 2003).

In comparing the patterns of regional cerebral atrophy in FTD, Alzheimer's disease and vascular dementia, severe frontal atrophy (unilateral or bilateral) and/or asymmetrical atrophy on MRI is highly characteristic of FTD. By contrast milder or severe reductions in regional cerebral blood flow on SPET in the parietal lobes exclude FTD and is highly suggestive of Alzheimer's disease (Varma et al., 2002; Varrone et al., 2002).

52.6 NEUROPSYCHOLOGY

52.6.1 Historical reports

Features of personality and behavioural change are prominent, and outweigh specific cognitive symptoms. Nevertheless, some cognitive change may be reported. Relatives may comment on alterations in the patient's language, which may include a reduction in speech output, stereotyped usage of words or phrases, or preoccupation with certain themes. They may note a tendency to echo the speech of others. They may describe memory disturbances, although often feel that this is variable in the patient's favour (the patient remembers what they want to remember), suggesting absent-mindedness and faulty attention rather than a primary amnesia. Symptoms of visuospatial disorientation are, however, notably absent. Relatives may remark with surprise that the patient wanders several miles from the home, yet find their way back.

52.6.2 Quality of neuropsychological test performance

Some patients are markedly distractible and restless and a minority may wander and attempt to leave the room during a testing session, and compliance may be lost. Economy of mental effort and cursory, superficial responses characterize test performance in apathetic, inert patients. The lack of concerted application to tasks is an important feature, because it effectively impairs performance across a wide range of tests that are purportedly designed to evaluate a spectrum of psychological functions. Test scores taken at face value could lead to spurious interpretations of the nature of the patient's psychological deficit.

Other 'frontal' features that compromise test performance include perseveration and concreteness of thought. Response perseverations may occur on both verbal and motor tasks. They are a dominant characteristic of performance on traditional 'frontal-lobe' tests. However, they also may represent a major source of errors in naming tests, writing and drawing. In motor tasks, perseverations may occur at both an elementary (repetition of a single movement) and higher-order (repetition of a complete programme of actions) level. Concreteness of thought can compromise interpretation of verbal instructions, pictures and stories. Patients may fail to abstract an underlying narrative or draw inferences that go beyond the elements physically present.

52.6.3 Language

Speech output characteristically is reduced. Patients do not initiate conversation, and responses to questions are brief and unelaborated, with minimal application of mental effort. As noted above concreteness of thought is common, and is elicited most readily by the use of metaphors and proverbs. There may be increased reliance on irrelevant, stereotyped remarks, which contrast with the prevailing taciturnity. These may constitute favoured words or phrases, or sometimes an entire well rehearsed repertoire. Echolalia and verbal perseverations are common. Despite the economy of speech, utterances are fluent and effortless, without pronunciation difficulties. However, hypophonia and loss of prosody may become evident. Mutism invariably ensues in the final stages of the disease. The apparent lack of generative language or 'adynamia', which dominates the clinical picture, bears resemblance to the 'dynamic aphasia' described by Luria and Tsvetkova (1968).

The profound attenuation of conversational discourse stands in contrast to the relative preservation of overlearnt, 'automatic' aspects of language. Patients may repeat phrases, recite series such as the months of the year, complete nursery rhymes and join in songs at a time when spontaneous utterances are virtually absent.

There is typically little evidence of comprehension failure at a single word level. However, patients may have difficulty grasping complex syntax or following sequential commands. Performance on tests of comprehension is typically governed by the mental demands of the task.

Naming to confrontation is relatively well preserved, although may be compromised by response perseverations. Open-ended verbal fluency tasks, involving generation of words from a semantic category or beginning with a specified letter are usually disproportionately impaired compared with object naming.

Reading aloud is relatively preserved and free from linguistic errors. Indeed, patients may develop a habit of reading aloud road signs and advertising hoardings, even when their spontaneous conversation is minimal. In a test setting, virtually mute patients may read aloud test material accurately, much to the surprise of their relatives. Errors in reading typically arise secondary to patients' poor attention rather than to primary linguistic deficits. Reading for comprehension characteristically mirrors comprehension of spoken language. In reading a complete narrative, such as a fable-like short story, patients typically show poor abstractive and synthetic powers.

Written output usually is reduced and patients tend to write single words or brief phrases, rather than complete sentences. Spelling may be surprisingly accurate, although is sometimes erratic, reflecting lack of checking. Markedly perseverative responses characterize the writing of a proportion of patients.

The ability to communicate non-verbally by symbolic gesture, conveying actions such as waving, saluting or beckoning, may be preserved, at least initially. However, just as speech output decreases so too do the patient's body movements, and in late stage disease it may be impossible to elicit any gestures, either to command or by demonstration. Buccofacial movements typically fail to convey a range of facial expression: an inane or fatuous expression predominates.

52.6.4 Visual perception and spatial skills

Patients typically have no difficulty in the perceptual recognition of objects, do not make perceptual errors on naming tests involving pictorial material, and for the most part use objects appropriately. Moreover there is no convincing evidence of 'parietal'-type deficits, even with advanced disease. Clinical observation suggests that patients have no difficulty localizing objects, can manipulate and orientate clothing correctly, and negotiate their environment, without becoming lost. Even when patients become formally untestable and are mute, they may fixate and reach for objects without difficulty, and may show behaviours as part of a stereotypic repertoire, which demonstrate preserved spatial localization skills, such as repeated folding of a handkerchief or aligning of papers. It is noteworthy, however, that impairment often may be elicited on formal neuropsychological tests of perceptuospatial function as a secondary consequence of patients' poor mental application, failure to check responses, lack of concern for accuracy as well as their poor organizational and strategic skills. The notable preservation of spatial function in FTD patients contrasts with the severe impairment of spatial skills common in Alzheimer's disease.

52.6.5 Memory

Patients typically perform poorly on formal tests of memory, both recall and recognition. However, patients are not evidently clinically amnesic: they are typically orientated for time and place and can provide accurate information about current autobiographical events. Moreover, test performance can be improved under certain conditions. First, recall performance is enhanced by the use of specific, directed questions rather than broad open-ended questions. Second, memory performance benefits from cues and from the provision of multiple-choice alternative responses. These features suggest that patients have available to them information that they do not or are unable to generate spontaneously, and reinforce the notion that the patient's inefficient memorizing is not attributable to a primary failure of retention. This 'frontal' type of memory impairment contrasts with the classical amnesia typical of Alzheimer's disease. Memory performance in FTD patients may be compromised by failures of sustained and selective attention.

52.6.6 Motor skills

Patients have normal manual dexterity, and can manipulate objects, use feeding implements and carry out complex actions such as lighting a cigarette until relatively late in the disease. Some patients exhibit 'utilization behaviour', in which objects placed within reach of the patient elicits the motor actions appropriate to those objects even though those behaviours are contextually inappropriate. Despite the general preservation of motor skills, some abnormalities do occur on motor tasks, performance being compromised particularly by perseveration and motor impersistence.

With progression of disease it may become increasingly difficult to elicit motor responses in inert, apathetic patients. However, actions may be more easily evoked by imitation than through verbal command, and a minority of patients exhibit frank echopraxia, copying actions of the examiner without being requested to do so.

52.6.7 Frontal executive functions

Patients show impairments in a range of executive skills, including abstraction, planning, organizational and strategic functioning, sustained, selective and switching of attention. 'Frontal lobe' tests that are sensitive to such changes include the Wisconsin card sorting test, Weigls test, Stroop test, Trail Making test, verbal fluency, design fluency, Haylings and Brixton test and the Test of Everyday Attention. Details of test administration can be found in Lezak (2002).

52.6.8 Social cognition

There is accumulating evidence that FTD patients have impaired ability to infer the mental states of others, a capacity that has come to be known as 'theory of mind' (Lough *et al.*, 2001; Gregory *et al.*, 2002; Snowden *et al.*, 2003). These social inferential skills may be impaired even in patients who perform relatively well on standard executive tasks (Lough *et al.*, 2001), a factor likely to contribute to patients' severe breakdown in social, interpersonal conduct.

52.6.9 Performance on standard tests of intelligence

Some patients who present with disinhibition and overactivity may initially perform normally on standard test batteries, such as the Wechsler Adult Intelligence Scale, highlighting a dissociation between the profound alteration in personality and behaviour and breakdown in social competence, and relative preservation of cognitive skills. Often, however, performance is impaired, and becomes so in all individuals with progression of disease. A pattern of test scores may be evident, which points to a predominant frontal lobe dysfunction: disproportionate impairment for the Comprehension, Similarities and Picture Arrangement subtests. A verbal performance discrepancy, occurring in a minority of patients, will tend to favour performance items. However, commonly, performance is impoverished across all subtests, with no clear pattern

---

Box 52.3 *Cognitive characteristics of FTD*

Language
- Economy of mental effort and output
- Perseveration, echolalia, stereotypy
- Concreteness
- Late mutism

Perceptuospatial function
- Preserved; errors on constructional tasks arise secondary to organizational deficits

Memory
- Variable, idiosyncratic day to day memory
- Preserved orientation in time and place
- Poor information retrieval
- Recall enhanced by cues and directed probes

Motor skills
- Poor temporal sequencing
- Perseveration

Abstraction and planning
- Concrete responses
- Poor set shifting
- Organizational and sequencing failure
- Perseveration

---

of deficits emerging across tasks. This profile, which appears to arise as a consequence of patients' lack of effortful application to tasks and cursory mode of responding, may misleadingly give rise to the interpretation of a 'generalized' dementia.

The principal cognitive characteristics are summarized in Box 52.3.

52.7 BEHAVIOURAL SUBTYPES

FTD patients are not entirely homogeneous. All share the major features of gross change in personality and social conduct and exhibit a picture suggestive of 'frontal lobe' disorder on neuropsychological testing; the behavioural disorder outweighs both primary cognitive and physical deficits. Nevertheless, the precise characteristics of the disorder are not uniform. Three broad prototypical behavioural patterns have been identified (Box 52.4).

52.7.1 Disinhibited type

Some patients present with features reminiscent of hypomania. They are overactive, restless, inattentive and distractible, rushing unproductively from one activity to another, with

---

Box 52.4   *Clinical sub-types of FTD*

Disinhibited
- Restless, overactive, disinhibited
- Fatuous, jocular, unconcerned
- Profound social breakdown
- Behavioural disorder more prominent than cognitive disorder

Apathetic
- Inert, aspontaneous, avolitional
- Bland, apathetic, unconcerned
- Mentally rigid and perseverative
- Severely impaired on frontal-lobe cognitive tests

Stereotypic
- Stereotypic, ritualistic, compulsive
- Bland, unconcerned
- Mentally rigid
- Behavioural disorder salient feature

---

marked lack of application and persistence. Their demeanour is fatuous, inappropriately jocular, disinhibited and socially inappropriate. Patients may perform surprisingly well on cognitive tasks at least in the early stages of disease. In such patients functional imaging with SPET typically reveals relatively circumscribed tracer deficits involving the orbitofrontal and anterior temporal lobes.

52.7.2 Apathetic type

Some patients exhibit a pattern of behaviour that is at opposite poles to that described above. They present with an apathetic, amotivational, pseudodepressed state. Their behaviour is characterized by loss of volition and inertia, so that, if left to their own devices, they would spend their day in bed or sitting unoccupied. All behaviours are economical, with minimal expenditure of mental effort. Response latencies to questions are often excessively prolonged, although once initiated, rate of execution of verbal or motor responses is unremarkable. With disease progression the patient becomes increasingly unresponsive, so that virtually no verbal or motor behaviour can be elicited. It is in these patients that perseverative behaviour, both verbal and motor, is the most pronounced, and that marked loss of speech prosody is liable to occur. These patients are particularly impaired on formal tests of executive function. In these patients there is typically widespread anterior hemisphere abnormalities on SPET, with involvement of dorsolateral convexity regions.

52.7.3 Stereotypic type

In some patients the dominant presenting characteristic is of repetitive, ritualistic and idiosyncratic behaviours. Patients adhere to a rigid routine and become agitated if their daily schedule is altered. They adopt personal rituals, which have a compulsive quality, although lack the accompanying feelings of anxiety and release from anxiety characteristic of obsessive–compulsive states. Such patients exhibit extrapyramidal signs at a relatively early stage of the illness. In patients with marked stereotypic behaviour, SPET imaging typically reveals the frontal and temporal lobes to be functionally disordered in a widespread fashion.

Behavioural differences reflect differences in distribution of pathology within frontotemporal structures. The apathetic type reflects the presence of dorsolateral-frontal atrophy, whereas the disinhibited type corresponds to orbitobasal frontal degeneration. The stereotypic type is strongly related to severe striatal disease with lesser involvement of frontal or temporal neocortex. In all subtypes the temporal poles are affected. To some extent behavioural differences reflect stage of disease: patients who are initially disinhibited and have relatively circumscribed atrophy of the orbital frontal lobes and temporal poles may become increasingly apathetic with disease progression and pathological spread into dorsal frontal regions. However, there are also significant clinical differences in the earliest stages of disease: some patients present initially with disinhibition and others with apathy, indicating that phenotypic differences exist that are not mere artefacts of disease severity.

52.8 FRONTOTEMPORAL DEMENTIA AND MOTOR NEURONE DISEASE

An association between dementia and motor neurone disease (MND) (amyotrophic lateral sclerosis) is well known and the pathology has been extensively described, especially in Japan (Mitsuyama and Takamiya, 1979; Morita *et al.*, 1987). The form of dementia is identical to that of FTD (Neary *et al.*, 1990).

Patients present with a rapidly progressive dementia of the frontal lobe type and subsequently develop motor neurone disease of the amyotrophic type. Personality change with disordered personal and social conduct and stereotyped behaviours are prominent. Reduced verbal output in superseded rapidly by mutism. Profound abnormalities are evident on tests of frontal lobe function. Visuospatial abilities are notably preserved.

Neurological examination reveals widespread muscular fasciculations in the tongue, limbs and trunk in addition to the finding of primitive reflexes and hyperreflexia. With disease progression muscular wasting increases and bulbar palsy emerges, with dysarthria and ineffective coughing. Patients do not develop a spastic increase in tone of the limbs. Death due to bulbar palsy occurs within 3 years.

The EEG is normal and remains so on serial investigation. Electrophysiological studies of neuromuscular function reveal normal nerve conduction studies, multifocal muscular fasciculations, reduced muscular firing rates and giant motor units, compatible with widespread muscular denervation due to anterior horn cell death.

52.9 NEUROPATHOLOGY

The principal atrophy in FTD involves the frontal and anterior temporal neocortices, the amygdala and basal ganglia (Brun, 1987,1993; Mann and South, 1993; Mann et al., 1993). Within the neocortex the histological changes principally involve layers II and III, the origin of corticocortical associational neurones, sparing layer V, the major source of cortico-subcortical neurones. Three distinct histological changes are associated with the cortical atrophy (Lund and Manchester groups, 1994):

- microvacuolation or spongiosus (FLD-type);
- gliosis with or without swollen neurones and inclusion bodies (Pick-type);
- degeneration of bulbar cranial nerve nuclei and anterior horn cells (MND-type).

The distribution of the first two histologies are identical and either may underlie the clinical syndrome of FTD in both familial and non-familial cases. In FTD and MND the cerebral histology is usually of the first type (microvacuolation), and the degree of cerebral atrophy is milder, presumably due to the short duration of illness associated with death from MND.

A more detailed description of the neuropathological changes seen in FTD is given in Chapter 54.

52.10 NEUROCHEMISTRY

The neurochemical changes in autopsied cases of FTD have been compared with those of Alzheimer's disease (Procter et al., 1999). In FTD there is no cholinergic deficit. Serotonin receptors are lost from frontal and temporal cortex in FTD whereas they are lost from temporal and parietal cortex in Alzheimer's disease. In FTD there is no loss of kainate receptors but loss of AMPA receptors from both temporal and frontal lobes. Loss of AMPA receptors differentiated FTD with Pick-type histology from FTD with FLD-type histology, suggesting selective loss of subpopulations of cortical pyramidal neurones.

52.11 MOLECULAR GENETICS

In familial forms of FTD the mode of inheritance is autosomal dominant and in some families missense and splice-site mutations have been identified in the tau sequencing gene on chromosome 17 (Hutton et al., 1998; Poorkaj et al., 1998; Janssen et al., 2002; Pickering-Brown et al., 2002). Linkage to

chromosome 3 has been reported in an extended Danish family (Brown et al., 1995; Gydesen et al., 2002) and to chromosome 9 in patients with FTD/MND (Hosler et al., 2000). See Chapter 54 for a detailed description of the genetics and molecular pathology of FTD.

52.12 TREATMENT AND MANAGEMENT

The severe behavioural disorder of FTD places great a burden on carers. The early onset of the disorder entails breakdown in families where children may still be relatively young. The altered personality leads the patient to be regarded as a stranger and alien within the home and therefore social and psychiatric intervention with daycare provision and facilities for respite and relatively early potential hospitalization are even more desirable than in Alzheimer's disease. Unfortunately the youth and overactivity of many patients makes their placement in homes and hospitals largely dedicated to the elderly both inappropriate and distressing to carers. Facilities for the care of patients with presenile dementia are urgently required.

Tranquilizers may be effective in reducing overactive disinhibited behaviour and serotonin reuptake inhibitors (Swartz et al., 1997; Moretti et al., 2003) can sometimes diminish the repetitive behaviours that can dominate the patient's activities and place severe stress on carers.

Within the setting of a hospital environment the repetitive behaviours can sometimes be turned to the advantage of the group by harnessing the stereotypic activity to socially useful ends.

52.13 DIFFERENTIAL DIAGNOSIS

Features that distinguish FTD from Alzheimer's disease are summarized in Table 52.1. However, in the very early stages patients with both FTD and Alzheimer's disease may show few neurological symptoms or signs. Moreover, disinhibited FTD patients may perform relatively well on standard neuropsychological tests, including 'frontal lobe' tests (Gregory et al., 1999), so that neuropsychological assessment is not invariably informative. Neuroimaging techniques are not available in all centres. Differential diagnosis is therefore crucially dependent on the evaluation of the patient's behaviour and affect, hence the emphasis on behavioural features in current diagnostic criteria. Informant-based behavioural interviews can elicit information that is highly discriminating (Bozeat et al., 2000; Bathgate et al., 2001; Ikeda et al., 2002). In a comparative study of FTD and Alzheimer's disease (Bozeat et al., 2000) behavioural stereotypies, altered eating habits and loss of social awareness best discriminated the two groups. Similarly, in a comparative study of FTD, Alzheimer's disease and vascular dementia (Bathgate et al., 2001), the best discriminators included changes in eating habits, especially

Table 52.1   *Comparison of clinical features in FTD and AD*

Clinical features	FTD	AD
Demographics	Typically early onset	Typically late onset
History	Early personality change	Memory loss
	Social breakdown	Spatial disorientation
	Altered eating habits	Aphasia
Affect	Blunted, fatuous	Concerned, anxious
Neurology	Early primitive reflexes	Akinesia and rigidity, myoclonus
Language	Adynamic speech, mutism	Aphasia
Visuospatial skills	Preserved	Impaired
Memory	'Frontal-type' amnesia	'Limbic-type' amnesia
EEG	Normal	Abnormal, slow
SPECT	Anterior cerebral abnormality	Posterior cerebral abnormality

overeating and the presence of repetitive, stereotyped behaviours. Particularly discriminating also was the reduced capacity of FTD patients to demonstrate both primary and social emotions (e.g. sadness, fear, sympathy, embarrassment), and the loss of emotional insight (i.e. a lack of distress or concern when confronted by deficits). Informant-based interviews have been found to have discriminatory value even when carried out retrospectively several years after the patient's death (Barber *et al.*, 1995).

52.14   CONCLUSION

Frontotemporal dementia, arising from progressive degeneration of the frontal and temporal lobes, is a relatively common form of early-onset dementia. It is characterized by profound alteration in personality and social conduct, and by cognitive defects in attention, abstraction planning, judgement, organization and strategic functioning. In contrast, instrumental tools of cognition, particularly spatial navigational skills, are relatively preserved. The neuropsychological disorder, indicative of anterior hemisphere dysfunction, is the converse of that seen in Alzheimer's disease, in which profound breakdown in the tools of cognition: memory, language and perceptuospatial abilities, occur in the context of remarkably well preserved social skills. The paucity of neurological signs in FTD and in particular the absence of myoclonus, the normal EEG and the selective anterior hemisphere abnormalities seen on functional brain imaging also help to separate FTD from the relatively more common dementia of Alzheimer's disease. FTD is not clinically uniform. Distinct behavioural patterns mirror differences in the topographical distribution of pathological change within frontal and temporal structures, but are not determined by the precise histopathological features that are of frontotemporal lobar degeneration, Pick or MND-type. Molecular genetic advances already have distinguished mutations responsible for FTD in

some familial cases and are likely in the future to clarify nosological issues relating the status of the different histologies underlying FTD and its relationship to other clinical syndromes that share those same histopathologies. Genetic advancement also holds the prospect of future treatment for this devastating form of dementia.

REFERENCES

Barber RA, Snowden JS, Craufurd D. (1995) Retrospective differentiation of frontotemporal dementia and Alzheimer's disease using information from informants. *Journal of Neurology, Neurosurgery, and Psychiatry* **59**: 61–70

Bathgate D, Snowden JS, Varma A, Blackshaw A, Neary D. (2001) Behaviour in frontotemporal dementia, Alzheimer's disease and vascular dementia. *Acta Neurologica Scandinavica* **103**: 367–378

Bozeat S, Gregory CA, Lambon Ralph MA, Hodges JR. (2000) Which neuropsychiatric and behavioural features best distinguish frontal and temporal variants of frontotemporal dementia from Alzheimer's disease? *Journal of Neurology, Neurosurgery, and Psychiatry* **69**: 178–186

Brown J, Ashworth A, Gydesen S. (1995) Familial nonspecific dementia maps to chromosome 3. *Human Molecular Genetics* **4**: 1625–1628

Brun A. (1987) Frontal lobe degeneration of non-Alzheimer type. I. Neuropathology. *Archives of Gerontolology and Geriatrics* **6**: 193–208

Brun A. (1993) Frontal lobe degeneration of non-Alzheimer type revisited. *Dementia* **4**: 126–131

Ferrano A and Jervis GA. (1936) Pick's disease. *Archives of Neurology and Psychiatry* **36**: 739–767

Filley CM, Kleinschmidt-De Masters BK, Gross KF. (1994) Non-Alzheimer frontotemporal degenerative dementia. A neurobehavioural and pathologic study. *Clinical Neuropathology* **13**: 109–116

Frisoni GB, Pizzolato G, Geroldi C, Rossato A, Bianchetti A, Trabucchi M. (1995) Dementia of the frontal lobe type: neuropsychological and 99Tc-HM-PAO SPET features. *Journal of Geriatric Psychiatry and Neurology* **8**: 42–48

Gregory CA, Serra-Mestres J, Hodges JR. (1999) Early diagnosis of the frontal variant of frontotemporal dementia how sensitive are standard neuroimaging and neuropsychologic tests? *Neuropsychiatry Neuropsychology and Behavioural Neurology* **12**: 128–135

Gregory C, Lough S, Stone V *et al.* (2002) Theory of mind in patients with frontal variant frontotemporal dementia and Alzheimer's disease: theoretical and practical implications. *Brain* **125**: 752–764

Gustafson L. (1987) Frontal lobe degeneration of non-Alzheimer type. II. Clinical picture and differential diagnosis. *Archives of Gerontology and Geriatrics* **6**: 209–223

Gustafson L. (1993) Clinical picture of frontal lobe degeneration of non-Alzheimer type. *Dementia* **4**: 143–148

Gustafson L and Risberg J. (1974) Regional cerebral blood flow related to psychiatric symptoms in dementia with onset in the presenile period. *Acta Psychiatrica Scandanavica* **50** (Suppl.): 516–538

Gustafson L, Brun A, Ingvar DH. (1977) Presenile dementia clinical symptoms, pathoanatomical findings and cerebral blood flow. In: JS Meyer, H Lechner, M Reivich (eds), *Cerebral Vascular Disease.* Amsterdam, Excerpta Medica

Gydesen S, Brown JM, Brun A *et al.* (2002) Chromosome 3 linked frontotemporal dementia (FTD-3). *Neurology* **59**: 1585–1594

Hosler BA, Siddique T, Sapp PC et al. (2000) Linkage of familial amyotrophic lateral sclerosis with frontotemporal dementia to chromosome 9q21–q22. Journal of the American Neurological Association 284: 1664–1669

Hutton M, Lendon CL, Rizzu P et al. (1998) Association of missense and 5'-splice-site mutations in tau with the inherited dementia FTDP-17. Nature 393: 702–705

Ikeda M, Brown J, Holland AJ, Fukuhara R, Hodges JR. (2002) Changes in appetite, food preference and eating habits in frontotemporal dementia and Alzheimer's disease. Journal of Neurology, Neurosurgery, and Psychiatry 73: 371–376

Jagust WJ, Reed BR, Seab JP, Kramer JH, Budinger TF. (1989) Clinical-physiologic correlates of Alzheimer's disease and frontal lobe dementia. American Journal of Physiological Imaging 4: 89–96

Janssen JC, Warrington EK, Morris HR et al. (2002) Clinical features of frontotemporal dementia due to the intronic tau 10^{+16} mutation. Neurology 58: 1161–1168

Knopman DS. (1993) Overview of dementia lacking distinctive histology: pathological designation of a progressive dementia. Dementia 4: 132–136

Knopman DS, Mastri AR, Frey WH, Sung JH, Rustan T. (1990) Dementia lacking distinctive histologic features: a common non-Alzheimer degenerative dementia. Neurology 40: 251–256

Lezak MD. (2002) Neuropsychological Assessment. 4th edition. Oxford, Oxford University Press

Lhermitte F. (1983) Utilization behaviour and its relation to lesions of the frontal lobes. Brain 106: 237–255

Lough S, Gregory C, Hodges JR. (2001) Dissociation of social cognition and executive function in frontal variant frontotemporal dementia. Neurocase 7: 123–130

Lowenberg K. (1935) Pick's disease. Archives of Neurology and Psychiatry 36: 768–789

Lowenberg K, Boyd DA, Salon DD. (1939) Occurrence of Pick's disease in early adult years. Archives of Neurology and Psychiatry 41: 1004–1020

Lund and Manchester groups (1994) Consensus Statement. Clinical and neuropathological criteria for fronto-temporal dementia. Journal of Neurology, Neurosurgery, and Psychiatry 4: 416–418

Luria AR and Tsvetkova LS. (1968) The mechanism of 'dynamic aphasia'. Foundations of Language 4: 296–307

McKhann GM, Albert MS, Grossman M, Miller B, Dickson, Trojanowski JQ. (2001) Clinical and pathological diagnosis of frontotemporal dementia report of the Work Group on frontotemporal dementia and Pick's disease. Archives of Neurology 58: 1803–1809

Mann MA and South PW. (1993) The topographic distribution of brain atrophy in frontal lobe dementia. Acta Neuropathologica 85: 334–340

Mann DMA, South PW, Snowden JS, Neary D. (1993) Dementia of frontal lobe type; neuropathology and immunohistochemistry. Journal of Neurology, Neurosurgery, and Psychiatry 56: 605–614

Miller BL, Cummings JL, Villanueva-Meyer J et al. (1991) Frontal lobe degeneration: clinical, neuropsychological and SPECT characteristics. Neurology 41: 1374–1382

Miller BL, Chang L, Mena I, Boone K, Lesser IM. (1993) Progressive right frontotemporal degeneration: clinical, neuropsychological and SPECT characteristics. Dementia 4: 204–213

Mitsuyama Y and Takamiya S. (1979) Presenile dementia with motor neuron disease in Japan. A new entity? Archives of Neurology 36: 592–593

Moretti R, Torre P, Antonello RM, Cazzato G, Bava A. (2003) Frontotemporal dementia paroxetine as a possible treatment for behavior symptoms. A randomised, controlled open 14-month study. European Neurology 49: 13–19

Morita K, Kaiya H, Ikeda T, Namba M. (1987) Presenile dementia combined with amyotrophy: a review of 34 Japanese cases. Archives of Gerontology and Geriatrics 6: 263–277

Neary D, Snowden JS, Bowen DM et al. (1986) Neuropsychological syndromes in presenile dementia due to cerebral atrophy. Journal of Neurology, Neurosurgery, and Psychiatry 49: 163–174

Neary D, Snowden JS, Shields RA et al. (1987) Single photon emission tomography using 99mTc-HM-PAO in the investigation of dementia. Journal of Neurology, Neurosurgery, and Psychiatry 50: 1101–1109

Neary D, Snowden JS, Northen B, Goulding PJ. (1988) Dementia of frontal lobe type. Journal of Neurology, Neurosurgery, and Psychiatry 51: 353–361

Neary D, Snowden JS, Mann DMA, Northen B, Goulding PJ, Mcdermott N. (1990) Frontal lobe dementia and motor neuron disease. Journal of Neurology, Neurosurgery, and Psychiatry 53: 23–32

Neary D, Snowden JS, Gustafson L et al. (1998) Frontotemporal lobar degeneration. A consensus on clinical diagnostic criteria. Neurology 51: 1546–1554

Neumann MA. (1949) Pick's disease. Journal of Neuropathology and Experimental Neurology 8: 255–282

Pick A. (1906) Uber einen weiteren symptomenkomplex in rahmen der dementia senilis, bedingt durch umschriebene starkere hirnatrophie (gemischte apraxie). Monatsschrift für Psychiatrie und Neurologie 19: 97–108

Pickering-Brown SM, Richardson AMT, Snowden JS et al. (2002) Inherited frontotemporal dementia in nine British families associated with intronic mutations in the tau gene. Brain 125: 732–751

Poorkaj P, Bird TD, Wijsman E et al. (1998) Tau is a candidate gene for chromosome 17 frontotemporal dementia. Annals of Neurology 43: 815–825

Procter AW, Qume M, Francis PT. (1999) Neurochemical features of frontotemporal dementia. Dementia and Geriatric Cognitive Disorders 10 (Suppl. 1): 80–84

Ratnavalli E, Brayne C, Dawson K, Hodges JR. (2002) The prevalence of frontotemporal dementia. Neurology 58: 1615–1621

Rinne JO, Laine M, Kaasinen V, Norvasuo-Heila MK, Nagren K, Helenius H. (2002) Striatal dopamine transporter and extrapyramidal symptoms in frontotemporal dementia. Neurology 58: 1489–1493

Rombouts SA, Van Swieten JC, Pijnenburg YA et al. (2003) Loss of frontal fMRI activation in early frontotemporal dementia compared to early AD. Neurology 60: 1904–1908

Rosso SM, Donker Kaat L, Baks T et al. (2003) Frontotemporal dementia in the Netherlands: patient characteristics and prevalence estimates from a population-based study. Brain 126: 2016–2022

Salmon E, Garraux G, Delbeuck X et al. (2003) Predominant ventromedial frontopolar metabolic impairment in frontotemporal dementia. Neuroimage 20: 435–440

Schneider C. (1927) Uber Picksche Krankheit. Monatsschrift für Psychiatrie und Neurologie 65: 230–275

Snowden JS, Neary D, Mann DMA. (1996) Frontotemporal Lobar Degeneration: Frontotemporal Dementia, Progressive Aphasia, Semantic Dementia. London, Churchill Livingstone

Snowden JS, Gibbons ZC, Blackshaw A et al. (2003) Social cognition in frontotemporal dementia and Huntington's disease. Neuropsychologia 41: 688–701

Snowden JS, Neary D, Mann DMA. (2004) Autopsy proven, sporadic frontotemporal dementia, due to microvacuolar histology, with onset at 21 years of age. Journal of Neurology, Neurosurgery, and Psychiatry 75: 1337–1339

Starkstein SE, Migliorelli R, Teson A *et al.* (1994) Specificity of changes in cerebral blood flow in patients with frontal lobe dementia. *Journal of Neurology, Neurosurgery, and Psychiatry* **57**: 790–796

Stevens M, Van Duijn CM, Kamphorst W, De Knijff P *et al.* (1998) Familial aggregation in frontotemporal dementia. *Neurology* **50**: 1541–1545

Swartz JR, Miller BL, Lesser IM, Darby AL. (1997) Frontotemporal dementia treatment response to serotonin selective reuptake inhibitors. *Journal of Clinical Psychiatry* **58**: 212–216

Talbot PR, Lloyd JJ, Snowden JS, Neary D, Testa HJ. (1998) A clinical role for 99mTc-HMPAO SPECT in the investigation of dementia? *Journal of Neurology, Neurosurgery, and Psychiatry* **64**: 306–313

Varma AR, Adams W, Lloyd JJ *et al.* (2002) Diagnostic patterns of regional atrophy on MRI and regional cerebral blood flow change on SPECT in young onset patients with Alzheimer's disease, frontotemporal dementia and vascular dementia. *Acta Neurologica Scandinavica* **105**: 261–269

Varrone A, Pappata S, Caraco C *et al.* (2002) Voxel-based comparison of rCBF SPET images in frontotemporal dementia and Alzheimer's disease highlights involvement of different cortical networks. *European Journal of Nuclear Medicine and Molecular Imaging* **29**: 1447–1454

53

Pick's disease: its relationship to progressive aphasia, semantic dementia and frontotemporal dementia

ANDREW GRAHAM AND JOHN HODGES

Considerable advances continue to be made in our understanding of the group of neurodegenerative diseases that present with focal cognitive deficits arising from circumscribed pathology of the frontal and/or temporal lobes, most commonly referred to collectively as Pick's disease (PiD) or frontotemporal dementia (FTD) However, the literature on these conditions is filled with a confusing plethora of terms, which can make these developments difficult to follow for the nonexpert in the field. Central to the problem is a lack of clarity as to the intended level of description (clinical syndrome versus clinicopathological entity versus specific histological diagnosis) and a lack of concordance between these levels. For example, while some labels denote a clinical syndrome without specific histological implications (e.g. progressive aphasia, semantic dementia, or dementia of frontal type), others denote specific neuropathological entities (e.g. PiD, or familial tauopathy), hybrid clinicopathological entities (e.g. FTD), or even specific genetic disorders (e.g. FTD with parkinsonism linked to chromosome 17). Recent differences in opinion over terminology are well illustrated by the titles of the following books, all published in the last decade: *Pick's Disease and Pick Complex* (Kertesz and Munoz, 1998), *Frontotemporal Dementia* (Pasquier *et al.*, 1996) and *Fronto-Temporal Lobar Degeneration: Fronto-Temporal Dementia, Progressive Aphasia, Semantic Dementia* (Snowden *et al.*, 1996). This lack of clarity is acknowledged, and efforts to rationalize terminology and

achieve clinicopathological and nosological consensus have been made (Brun *et al.*, 1994; Neary *et al.*, 1998; McKhann *et al.*, 2001). Even at a recent meeting of experts, agreement over terms was far from universal (Kertesz *et al.*, 2003b).

The aims of this chapter are to review the evolution of the terms used to describe this spectrum of disorders; to highlight recent advances; and examine areas of continuing controversy. Whilst our own bias within the Cambridge group is to prefer the term Pick's disease for this group of disorders – which is more readily understood by carers and parallels our use of the label Alzheimer's disease (AD) – the current tide of opinion is to use frontotemporal dementia as an umbrella term for the overall clinical syndrome.

53.1 WHAT DID PICK ACTUALLY DESCRIBE?

In 1892, Arnold Pick, working in Prague, reported a 71-year-old man with progressive mental deterioration and unusually severe aphasia who at post mortem had marked atrophy of the cortical gyri of the left temporal lobe (Pick, 1892; Girling and Berrios, 1994). Pick wanted to draw attention to the fact that local accentuation of progressive brain atrophy may lead to symptoms of local disturbance (in this instance aphasia). He also made specific and, as we will see below, highly perceptive predictions regarding the role of the mid-temporal region of the left hemisphere in the representation of word meaning. In subsequent papers, he described four further patients with left temporal atrophy (Pick, 1904; Girling and Berrios, 1997) or frontotemporal atrophy (Pick, 1901; Girling and Markova, 1995), again stressing their progressive language disturbance. It was only in his 1906 publication that Pick turned his attention to bilateral frontal atrophy with resultant behavioural disturbance. Spatt (2003) has reviewed Pick's approach to cognitive disorders and his concept of dementia.

Several points should be emphasized:

- Pick's primary interest in these patients was their language disorder, particularly the clinicoanatomical correlates of aphasia.
- He did not claim to have discovered a new disease, merely novel phenomena arising from asymmetric degeneration.
- He did not describe distinct neuropathological changes in his patients with focal atrophy.
- Both the major syndromes now included under the rubric of FTD (dementia of frontal type and semantic dementia) were clearly reported by Pick.

In view of these monumental contributions, it is sad that Pick has been relegated to a minor place in the modern terminology of FTD.

The histological abnormalities associated with PiD were, in fact, described a few years later by Alzheimer (1911) who recognized changes distinct from those found in the form of cerebral degeneration later associated with his name. Alzheimer recognized both argyrophilic intracytoplasmic inclusions (Pick bodies), and diffusely staining ballooned neurones (Pick cells) in association with focal lobar atrophy. It is interesting to note that a comprehensive review of 20 patients from the literature with aphasia owing to focal lobar atrophy written soon after Alzheimer's description (Mingazzini, 1914) did not use the label Pick's disease, which was introduced by Gans some 8 years later (Gans, 1922). The term was then taken up by Onari and Spatz (1926), but Carl Schneider (1927, 1929) is probably most responsible for its popularization.

Unfortunately, however, Schneider concentrated on the frontal lobe component of the syndrome and thus began the neglect of the temporal lobe syndromes. He distinguished three clinical phases, the first characterized by impaired judgement and behaviour, the second by local symptoms, and the third by generalized dementia. Many papers describing PiD then appeared in the 1930s and 1940s (Ferrano and Jervis, 1936; Lowenberg and Arbor, 1936; Nichols and Weigner, 1938; Lowenberg et al., 1939; Neumann, 1949), which again mainly focused on the frontal lobe aspects of the disorder.

After World War II, interest in PiD faded, together with a general waning of interest in the cognitive aspects of neurology in the English-speaking world. The focus of interest in English-language publications became the neuropathology, and latterly the genetics, of PiD. This resulted in a gradual change in the criteria for PiD, which evolved to include the necessity for specific pathological changes (i.e. focal atrophy with Pick cells and or Pick bodies). Indeed, many authors went as far as to claim that AD and PiD were clinically indistinguishable in life (Katzman, 1986; Kamo et al., 1987). In continental Europe, however, there remained a strong interest in the clinical phenomena of the dementias; PiD remained an in vivo diagnosis based on a combination of clinical features suggestive of frontal and/or temporal lobe dysfunction and focal lobar atrophy (Mansvelt, 1954; Tissot et al., 1975). This controversy continues and has contributed to the adoption of the many labels to describe patients with the clinical syndrome of progressive frontal or temporal lobe degeneration (Baldwin and Förstl, 1993).

53.2 REDISCOVERING PICK'S DISEASE: FROM DEMENTIA OF THE FRONTAL TYPE AND PROGRESSIVE APHASIA TO FRONTOTEMPORAL DEMENTIA

53.2.1 Dementia of frontal type

A renaissance of interest in the focal dementias occurred in the 1980s. Workers from Lund (Gustafson, 1987; Brun, 1987) reported on a large series of patients with dementia and found that of 158 patients studied prospectively, who came to post mortem, 26 had evidence of frontal lobe degeneration. Since only a small proportion had Pick cells and Pick bodies – the remainder had very similar findings but without specific inclusions (i.e. focal lobar atrophy with severe neuronal loss and spongiosis) – the Lund group preferred to adopt the term 'frontal degeneration of non-Alzheimer type'. At approximately the same time, Neary and co-workers (1986) in Manchester began a series of important clinicopathological studies of patients with presenile dementia. They, likewise, found a high proportion of cases with a progressive frontal lobe syndrome that had neither specific changes of AD (plaques and tangles) nor specific Pick pathology. They introduced the term 'dementia of frontal type'. Over the next few years other groups described very similar cases under the labels 'frontal lobe degeneration' (Miller et al., 1991) and 'dementia lacking distinct histological features' (Knopman et al., 1990). Our own preferred term for this group of patients is frontal variant FTD (FvFTD).

In the advanced stages of the disease, patients with this disorder present no diagnostic difficulty. They have the triad of:

- a profound change in personality and behaviour;
- neuropsychological impairments indicative of selective or disproportionate frontal pathology; and
- appropriate changes on structural and/or functional brain imaging.

Diagnosing early cases is by no means as easy and one of the challenges is to develop better methods of early, accurate detection (Gregory et al., 1999). Since patients are typically unaware of the insidious changes noted by others, we rely upon carer-based assessments. One undoubted advance in the area has, therefore, been the development of standardized carer interviews such as the Neuropsychiatric Inventory (Cummings et al., 1994), which appears to differentiate patients with FTD and AD (Levy et al., 1996). In an attempt to develop a local instrument capable of early diagnosis, we identified 15 key symptoms that occurred very commonly in a group of 12 patients with FvFTD (Gregory and Hodges, 1993, 1996). Kertesz and his group have developed a tool specifically aimed at frontal behaviours, the Frontal Behaviour Inventory, which appears to discriminate patients with FTD from those with AD or depression (Kertesz et al., 1997, 2000, 2003a). Recent work has focused on specific behaviours that can discriminate patients with FvFTD and semantic dementia from patients with AD, such as changes in appetite, food preferences and eating habits (Ikeda et al., 2002), or the presence of stereotypies (Nyatsanza et al., 2003).

Many patients with FvFTD present to psychiatrists and acquire a label of functional psychiatric disorder (including simple schizophrenia, depression and obsessive-compulsive disorder) because despite gross behavioural changes other aspects of cognition are typically preserved (Ames et al., 1994; Tonkonogy et al., 1994; Gregory and Hodges, 1996; Miller et al., 1997). This is understandable in terms of the site of pathology in FvFTD, the orbital and mesial frontal lobes, which are critically involved in social judgement, motivation, risk assessment and the pathophysiology of obsessive-compulsive behaviour (Cummings, 1999). By contrast, dorsolateral frontal regions, which have been the focus of classic neuropsychological studies, are spared in the early stages of the disease. The development of quantifiable tasks sensitive to orbital and mesial frontal function has begun with paradigms involving probability and gambling (Rogers et al., 1998; Rahman et al., 1999), emotion processing (Keane et al., 2002), and 'theory of mind' (ToM) tasks (Gregory et al., 2002), but much work remains to be done in this area.

53.2.2 Progressive aphasia and semantic dementia

The other strand of the story concerns the rediscovery of the syndrome of progressive aphasia in association with focal left perisylvian or temporal lobe atrophy. In 1982, Mesulam reported six patients with a long history of insidiously worsening aphasia in the absence of signs of more generalized cognitive failure. One of these patients underwent a brain biopsy, which revealed non-specific histology without specific markers of either AD or PiD. Following Mesulam's seminal paper, approximately 100 patients with progressive aphasia were reported over the next 15 years (for reviews see: Mesulam and Weintraub, 1992; Hodges and Patterson, 1996; Snowden et al., 1996; Garrard and Hodges, 1999). From this literature it is clear that, although the language impairment

in patients with progressive aphasia is heterogeneous, there are two identifiable and distinct aphasia syndromes: progressive non-fluent aphasia and progressive fluent aphasia. In the latter syndrome, speech remains fluent and well articulated but becomes progressively devoid of content words. The language and other non-verbal cognitive deficits observed in these patients reflect a breakdown in semantic memory that has led many authors to apply the label of 'semantic dementia' (Snowden et al., 1989; Hodges et al., 1992; Hodges et al., 1994; Saffran and Schwartz, 1994; Hodges and Patterson, 1996).

Although the term 'semantic dementia' is recent, the syndrome has, as discussed above, been recognized under different labels for many years. Pick (1892, 1904) and a number of other early authors (Rosenfeld, 1909; Mingazzini, 1914; Stertz, 1926; Schneider, 1927) recognized that the chief clinical manifestations of temporal lobe atrophy were 'amnesic aphasia' or 'transcortical sensory aphasia', together attributed to atrophy of the middle and inferior temporal gyri leaving Wernicke's area intact. These language impairments were typically associated with a type of dementia variously described as a reduction in categorical or abstract thinking, psychic blindness or sensory or 'associative agnosia' (Malamud and Boyd, 1940; Robertson et al., 1958). These features – amnesic aphasia and associative agnosia – can now be united by the concept of 'semantic memory loss'.

Warrington (1975) was the first clearly to delineate the syndrome of semantic memory impairment in three patients. Drawing on the work of Tulving (1972, 1983), Warrington recognized that the progressive anomia in her patients was not simply a linguistic deficit, but reflected a fundamental loss of semantic memory (or knowledge) about the items, which thereby affected naming, word comprehension, and object recognition. Semantic memory is the term applied to the component of long-term memory that contains the permanent representation of our knowledge about things in the world and their interrelationship, facts and concepts as well as words and their meaning (Hodges et al., 1992, 1998; Garrard et al., 1997; Hodges and Patterson, 1997). Cases of semantic dementia have also been recognized for many years in Japan as cases of 'gogi (word meaning) aphasia' (Imura et al., 1971; Sasanuma and Mondi, 1975; Morita et al., 1987; Tanabe, 1992; Tanabe et al., 1992).

Our original paper reported five cases with progressive loss of semantic memory and focal temporal atrophy (Hodges et al., 1992). All five presented with a fluent aphasia and all the characteristics of semantic memory loss: empty speech with word finding difficulty and occasional semantic paraphasias (mother for father), a severe reduction in the generation of exemplars on category fluency tests (in which subjects are asked to produce as many examples as possible from defined semantic categories, such as animals or musical instruments, within 1 minute), impaired single word comprehension on picture-pointing tests, a loss of fine-grained attribution knowledge about a range of items with preservation of broad superordinate information on verbal and pictorial tests of knowledge. By contrast, other aspects of language competency (phonology and syntax) were strikingly preserved. In contrast to AD, the patients also had good day-to-day (episodic) memory, although we have more recently shown that this sparing of autobiographical memory applies to fairly recent memories only (Graham and Hodges, 1997; Hodges and Graham, 1998). They also showed no impairment on tests of immediate (working) memory, visually based problem solving or visuoperceptual abilities. Four of the five patients showed severe and circumscribed temporal lobe atrophy on computed tomography (CT) or magnetic resonance imaging (MRI) scanning. Since 1992, we have studied many further such patients and have confirmed the association with focal atrophy of the temporal lobe – involving the temporal pole and inferolateral neocortex (particularly the perirhinal cortex and fusiform gyrus), with relative sparing of the hippocampal formation. In many cases the atrophy is strikingly asymmetric but always involves the left side (Hodges et al., 1998; Mummery et al., 1999; Garrard and Hodges, 1999; Galton et al., 2001).

This lateralization raises the issue of what are the cognitive and/or behavioural signatures of isolated right temporal atrophy. In 1994, we reported a patient, VH, with progressive prosopagnosia followed by a specific loss of knowledge about people (Evans et al., 1995). VH was unable to identify from face or name even very famous people, yet had intact general semantic and autobiographical memory (Kitchener and Hodges, 1999). In a more recent study, Thompson et al. (2004) reported a dissociation of person-specific from general semantic knowledge in two patients with contrasting patterns of temporal atrophy. Subject MA, with predominantly left temporal atrophy, showed impairment of general semantics with relative preservation of knowledge about people, while subject JP, with predominantly right temporal atrophy, showed the opposite pattern of impairments with severely impaired person-specific knowledge in the context of relatively preserved knowledge about objects and animals. The group led by Miller have also drawn attention to the bizarre behaviours (including irritability, impulsiveness, alterations in dress, limited and fixed ideas and decreased facial expression) exhibited by patients with predominantly right temporal lobe atrophy (Edwards Lee et al., 1997; Miller et al., 1997). A recent review of 47 patients with semantic dementia identified distinct behavioural and cognitive profiles associated with the left and right temporal variants of the disease (Thompson et al., 2003). Social awkwardness, job loss, lack of insight and difficulty with person identification were all more likely to be associated with major right temporal atrophy; while word-finding difficulties and reduced comprehension were all more likely to be associated with predominantly left-sided atrophy.

There are a number of compelling reasons to consider semantic dementia as part of the same disease spectrum as FvFTD. The first is pathological: in early clinicopathological studies of cases fulfilling criteria for semantic dementia, all had either classic PiD (i.e. Pick bodies and/or Pick cells) or non-specific spongiform change of the type found in the majority of cases with the frontal form of lobar atrophy (Wechsler, 1977;

Wechsler et al., 1982; Holland et al., 1985; Poeck and Luzzatti, 1988; Graff-Radford et al., 1990; Snowden et al., 1992; Scholten et al., 1995; Harasty et al., 1996; Hodges et al., 1998; Schwarz et al., 1998). More recently, a broader spread of pathology has been described, including FTD of the motor neurone disease (MND) type with tau-negative but ubiquitin-positive inclusions (Rossor et al., 2000; Hodges et al., 2004). Second is the evolution of the pattern of cognitive and behavioural changes over time: although semantic dementia patients present with progressive anomia and other linguistic deficits, on follow up the features that characterize the frontal form of FTD emerge (Hodges and Patterson, 1996; Edwards Lee et al., 1997). Indeed, sematic dementia and FvFTD may share many behavioural features on presentation (Bozeat et al., 2000). Third is the fact that modern neuroimaging techniques demonstrate subtle involvement of the orbitofrontal cortex in the majority of cases presenting with prominent temporal atrophy and semantic dementia (Mummery et al., 2000; Rosen et al., 2002a).

The status of patients with the non-fluent form of progressive aphasia within the spectrum of FTD is less certain. Clinically, such cases are clearly separable from cases of semantic dementia. Speech is faltering and distorted with frequent phonological substitutions and grammatical errors. Other non-language-based aspects of cognition remain well preserved, as do activities of daily living. Changes in behaviour and personality of the type that typify dementia of frontal type, and are seen in the later stages of semantic dementia, are rare, but after a number of years, global cognitive decline occurs (Green et al., 1990; Hodges and Patterson, 1996). In Cambridge, some patients with progressive non-fluent aphasia have had classic Alzheimer pathology at post mortem, albeit with an atypical distribution; that is to say, marked involvement of perisylvian language areas but sparing of medial temporal structures (Greene et al., 1996; Croot et al., 1997; Galton et al., 2000). Review of the published literature reveals that approximately equal numbers of cases with non-fluent aphasia have AD pathology whilst the remainder have Pick-like pathology but almost invariably without Pick bodies or Pick cells (Weintraub et al., 1990; Mesulam and Weintraub, 1992). Recent functional neuroimaging studies have implicated the anterior insula as the key abnormal region (Nestor et al., 2003).

53.2.3 Frontotemporal dementia and frontotemporal lobar degeneration

The final terms to be considered are those of FTD and frontotemporal lobar degeneration (FTLD). In 1994, the Lund and Manchester groups introduced the term FTD and suggested tentative criteria for the diagnosis (Brun et al., 1994). The term FTD was subsequently replaced by FTLD, and consensus clinical diagnostic criteria were published (Neary et al., 1998). The adoption of the terms FTD or FTLD has the advantage of avoiding specific pathological implications; it also brings to attention the fact that patients with the same disease may present with different clinical syndromes and that with time both types of deficit are likely to emerge. Three main clinical syndromes are recognized: FTD, progressive non-fluent aphasia and semantic aphasia and associative agnosia (Neary *et al.*, 1998; see Figure 53.1). However, disadvantages of the term FTLD are the blurring of levels of description and the amalgamation of distinct clinical syndromes. In particular, confusion may occur between FTD (now referring only to the frontal or behavioural variant of the disorder) and FTLD (the new term for the overall spectrum of presentations). Figure 53.2 presents the preferred Cambridge nomenclature.

It remains to be established which of the long list of phenomena listed as 'criteria' actually separate FTD and AD, although a study by Miller *et al.* (1997), using SPECT as the gold standard, suggested that loss of personal awareness (self-care), disordered eating, perseverative behaviour and reduction in speech most clearly differentiate FTD from AD. We have also looked at a wide range of neurobehavioural symptoms in a large group of patients with FTD (FvFTD and semantic dementia) and AD and identified four distinct clusters of symptoms by factor analysis:

- stereotypic and eating behaviours;
- executive function and self care;
- mood changes; and
- loss of social awareness (Bozeat *et al.*, 2000).

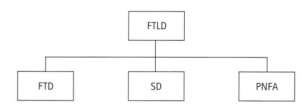

Figure 53.1   *Clinical classification of FTD according to the Lund–Manchester criteria. FTD, frontotemporal dementia; FTLD, frontotemporal lobar degeneration; PNFA, progressive non-fluent aphasia; SD, semantic dementia.*

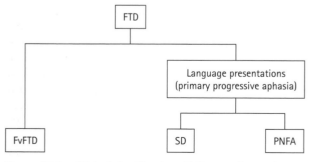

Figure 53.2   *Clinical classification of FTD according to the Cambridge group. FTD, frontotemporal dementia; FvFTD, frontal or behavioural variant of FTD; PNFA, progressive non-fluent aphasia; SD, semantic dementia.*

In this study, stereotypic and eating behaviours together with loss of social awareness reliably differentiated FTD from AD. At the level of individual symptoms, patients with semantic dementia showed increased rates of mental rigidity and depression compared with patients with FvFTD, while conversely, the latter group showed more disinhibition.

53.3 FAMILIAL CHROMOSOME 17-LINKED FRONTOTEMPORAL DEMENTIA AND THE DISCOVERY OF UNIQUE TAU PATHOLOGY

The term FTD increased in usage with the discovery of a specific gene mutation in familial cases. Linkage had been established in a number of families in which FTD was inherited as an autosomal dominant trait to chromosome 17q2 1–22, a region which contains the gene for the microtubule-associated protein tau (Wilhelmsen, 1997).

The story of the chromosome 17 linkage is extraordinary in a number of ways. Families around the world with what has become known as FTD with parkinsonism linked to chromosome 17 (Spillantini *et al.*, 1998a) had originally been reported under a range of headings including: disinhibition-dementia-parkinsonism–amyotrophy complex (DDPAC) (Wilhelmsen *et al.*, 1994); rapidly progressive autosomal dominant parkinsonism and dementia with pallidopontonigral degeneration (Wszolek *et al.*, 1992); familial progressive subclinical gliosis (Petersen *et al.*, 1995); hereditary dysphasic dementia (Morris *et al.*, 1984); hereditary FTD (Heutink *et al.*, 1997); multiple system tauopathy with presenile dementia (Spillantini *et al.*, 1997); familial presenile dementia with psychosis (Sumi *et al.*, 1992) and Pick's disease (Schenk, 1951). In 1996, a meeting of representatives from all of the groups identifying linkage to chromosome 17 was held in Ann Arbor, Michigan, USA (Foster *et al.*, 1997). Comparison of clinical and pathological data revealed a great deal of similarity between the families who all shared the characteristics of predominately frontotemporal distribution of pathology with marked behavioural changes. Extrapyramidal dysfunction was present in most. In some families psychotic symptoms were a major feature and a number had amyotrophy. It was recognized at that time that some of the families shared the common pathology with microtubule-associated protein tau-positive inclusions. Progress in the field was then rapid. It was soon discovered that most, if not all, families had tau inclusions with a distinctive morphological pattern leading to the coining of the term 'familial tauopathy' and the suggestion that the disease might reflect a mutation in the tau gene known to be located in the 17q21–22 region (Spillantini *et al.*, 1998a). Within 2 years of the Ann Arbor meeting, the first mutations were identified (Dumanchin *et al.*, 1998; Hutton *et al.*, 1998; Poorkaj *et al.*, 1998; Spillantini *et al.*, 1998b). Subsequent progress has been rapid: more than 25 different tau mutations have now been reported in association with familial FTD, differing according to their positions in the tau gene, their effects on tau mRNA and protein, and the type of tau pathology they cause (Ingram and Spillantini, 2002).

Not all cases of familial FTD are caused by tau mutations. In one large Danish family with autosomal dominant FTD, linkage has been established to chromosome 3 (Brown *et al.*, 1995; Brown, 1998) and, in some families with FTD-motor neurone disease, linkage has been established to chromosome 9. In a series of 22 cases of familial FTD, 11 (50 per cent) had tau mutations (Morris *et al.*, 2001). For 17 of the 22 families pathology was available, and three main pathological diagnoses were made: FTD with neuronal and glial tau deposition; FTD with ubiquitin inclusions; and FTD with neuronal loss and spongiosis but without intracellular inclusions. In this study, the families with neuronal and glial tau deposition all had a tau mutation, whereas no mutations were found in the other two pathological groups. A lack of tau deposition does not necessarily exclude an abnormality of tau processing: it has been suggested that a post-transcriptional deficit of brain tau may be the causative pathological process in cases FTD lacking distinctive histopathology (Zhukareva *et al.*, 2001, 2003).

53.4 CORTICOBASAL DEGENERATION, PROGRESSIVE SUPRANUCLEAR PALSY AND FRONTOTEMPORAL DEMENTIA

In 1967 Rebeiz, Kolodny and Richardson described three patients with a neurodegenerative illness affecting both cortex and basal ganglia (Rebeiz *et al.*, 1968). Each patient presented with a progressive asymmetrical akinetic-rigid syndrome and apraxia; on the basis of neuropathology findings Rebeiz *et al.* called the disorder 'corticodentatonigral degeneration with neuronal achromasia', later renamed to corticobasal degeneration (CBD). Initially CBD was conceptualized as a distinct clinicopathological entity, but in the early 1990s it was recognized that considerable clinical and pathological heterogeneity existed within the disorder. Clinically, cases of pathologically proven CBD were described presenting with the clinical syndromes of frontotemporal dementia (Mathuranath *et al.*, 2000) or progressive aphasia (Lippa *et al.*, 1991). Conversely, it was recognized that other pathologies might underlie the clinical syndrome of CBD; in a review of 32 consecutive cases of clinically diagnosed CBD (Boeve *et al.*, 1999), the underlying pathological diagnosis was CBD in 18; AD in three; PiD in two; progressive supranuclear palsy in six, and dementia lacking specific histology in two. A distinction has been drawn by some authors between the corticobasal syndrome (the constellation of clinical features characteristically associated with CBD) and corticobasal degeneration (the histopathological disorder itself). In our experience, there is considerable overlap between the clinical syndrome of CBD and progressive non-fluent aphasia (PNFA): many patients with PNFA develop apraxia and

parkinsonian features and conversely many CBD patients have subtle language production deficits that worsen as the disease progresses (Graham *et al.*, 2003).

The related disorder progressive supranuclear palsy (PSP), originally described by Steele, Richardson and Olszewski in 1964 is classically characterized by progressive axial rigidity, bradykinesia, vertical gaze palsy and dysarthria. Pathologically, tau-positive neurofibrillary tangles and threads are found in the substantia nigra, the subthalamic nucleus and the dentate nucleus. It is increasingly recognized that pathological PSP may present with the clinical features of CBD, or even progressive aphasia or a frontal lobe syndrome. Conversely, the PSP phenotype may result from tau gene mutations (Morris *et al.*, 2003; Soliveri *et al.*, 2003). Both CBD and PSP share an identified genetic risk factor, the H1 haplotype of the tau gene, and the tau deposits in both these diseases consist of the four-repeat isoforms of tau.

In their original case report, Rebeiz *et al.* (1968) recognized the similarity of the neuropathology in CBD to that seen in PiD. The Work Group on Frontotemporal Dementia and Pick's Disease (McKhann *et al.*, 2001) now includes both CBD and PSP among the pathological causes of the FTD syndromes.

53.5 FRONTOTEMPORAL DEMENTIA WITH MOTOR NEURONE DISEASE

Although MND has traditionally been regarded as a disorder which spares higher cognitive abilities, it has become clear since early reports from Japan (Mitsuyama and Takamiya, 1979) that the rate of dementia in MND is significantly greater than expected. Indeed, up to 10 per cent of patients with MND might show features of dementia and/or aphasia if such features are systematically elicited (Rakowicz and Hodges, 1998). Neuroimaging in MND with cognitive impairment demonstrates widespread frontal and temporal atrophy. Conversely, a significant minority of patients with FTD develop features of MND (Neary *et al.*, 1990; Caselli *et al.*, 1993; Rakowicz and Hodges, 1998; Bak and Hodges, 1999; Strong *et al.*, 2003). Most such patients present with cognitive symptoms, either FvFTD or progressive aphasia, which then progresses rapidly, followed by the emergence of bulbar features and mild limb amyotrophy. Such cases have a characteristic pattern of histological change with ubiquitin-positive, tau-negative, inclusions in cortical regions and the dentate gyrus. One interesting observation is that such patients almost invariably have disproportionately greater impairment of verb rather than noun processing, which affects both production and comprehension (Bak *et al.*, 2001).

From a practical perspective, this variant of FTD should be suspected in any cases with rapidly progressive disease or the emergence of bulbar symptoms. The overlap in clinical presentation between FTD and related disorders is illustrated schematically in Figure 53.3.

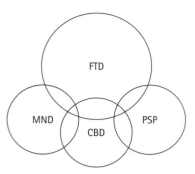

Figure 53.3 *Overlap in clinical presentation of FTD and related disorders. CBD, corticobasal degeneration; FTD, frontotemporal dementia; MND, motor neurone disease; PSP, progressive supranuclear palsy.*

53.6 CORRELATION BETWEEN CLINICAL SYNDROMES AND NEUROPATHOLOGY

The definitive diagnosis of FTD depends upon neuropathological examination. Unlike other dementia syndromes, notably AD, FTD encompasses considerable pathological heterogeneity. To summarize the preceding, three broad subdivisions have been recognized depending on the profile of immunohistochemical staining and the pattern of intracellular inclusions (Jackson and Lowe, 1996; Dickson, 1998; McKhann *et al.*, 2001; Hodges *et al.*, 2003). First, patients with tau-positive pathology, which in turn comprise a number of subvariants including those with classic argyrophilic, tau-positive, intraneuronal Pick bodies; those with tau gene mutations (FTDP-17) and diffuse tau-positive neuronal and astrocytic immunoreactivity; those characterized by tau-positive astrocytic plaques and ballooned achromatic neurones (CBD); and those with tau-positive argyrophilic grain disease (AGD). Second, cases with tau-negative, ubiquitin-positive inclusions in the dentate gyrus and brain stem motor nuclei (FTD with motor neurone disease or FTD-MND). Third, dementia lacking distinctive histology (DLDH).

The question as to whether distinct pathological subtypes map onto distinct clinical syndromes is of great interest. However, few clinicopathological series have been reported (Rosen *et al.*, 2002b; Rascovsky *et al.*, 2002). Munoz and

Ludwin (1984) studied, in detail, six patients whom they classified as either 'classical PiD' (i.e. marked focal neocortical atrophy with numerous Pick bodies) or 'atypical PiD' (i.e. those with predominant caudate atrophy and scarce inclusions). The ultrastructural changes in the two groups differed, and there was also a suggestion of a younger age of onset in the subcortical cases. A similar classification was proposed by Neumann in 1949. In the studies by Brun (Brun, 1987; Brun *et al.*, 1994), patients with frontal lobe atrophy and with Pick bodies were compared with those without specific histological changes. There were no demographic, clinical or neuropsychological differences, although the latter group had much less prominent cortical atrophy and involvement of the frontal convexity rather than the basal surface.

As discussed above, the majority of familial cases linked to chromosome 17 have lacked Pick bodies despite having abundant tau-positive inclusions, suggesting that classic Pick's disease cases are rarely familial.

A multicentre European initiative has pooled clinical and pathological data on 50 cases with classic PiD (i.e. with Pick bodies) and has proposed criteria that stress the marked asymmetry of atrophy found in many cases and the lack of family history. These criteria are currently being tested prospectively (Rossor, 1998). In a recent large series of 61 patients from Cambridge and Sydney (Hodges *et al.*, 2004), FvFTD was associated with a range of underlying pathologies. By contrast, motor neurone disease predicted ubiquitinated inclusions; parkinsonism and apraxia predicted corticobasal pathology; in progressive non-fluent aphasia there was a preponderance of tau-positive pathology while semantic dementia was generally associated with ubiquitin-positive (MND-type) inclusions. An attempted, and preliminary synthesis of the available clinicopathological data is illustrated in Figure 53.4.

53.7 HOW COMMON IS FRONTOTEMPORAL DEMENTIA?

Historically, it has long been recognized that FTD is less common than AD. Until recently, however, most estimates of the prevalence of FTD were based on reports from specialist units where FTD tended to be over-represented as a diagnosis. This

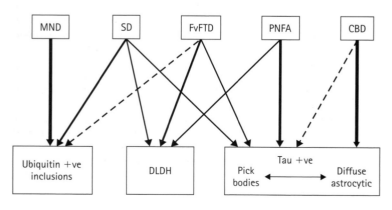

Figure 53.4 *Relationship between clinical syndrome and underlying pathology for FTD and related disorders. MND, motor neurone disease; SD, semantic dementia; fvFTD, frontal or behavioural variant of FTD; PNFA, progressive non-fluent aphasia; CBD, corticobasal degeneration; DLDH, dementia lacking distinctive histology. Thickness of arrow lines denotes the relative strengths of relationships between clinical syndromes and pathology.*

has changed with the publication of a number of community-based studies that give a clearer picture of the true prevalence of FTD.

Ratnavalli *et al.* (2002) conducted a prevalence survey aiming to ascertain all cases of early-onset dementia (age of onset less than 65 years) in a UK region with a total population of 326 000. The overall prevalence for early-onset dementia was 81 per 100 000 for patients aged 45–64 years, with equivalent prevalences of AD and FTD at 15 per 100 000. Of 185 cases seen by the study group, 23 (12 per cent) fulfilled the Lund–Manchester criteria for FTD, suggesting that, although FTD is by no means rare, it still represents only a minority of cases of dementia in the under-65s. (For comparison, AD was diagnosed in 34 per cent, vascular dementia in 18 per cent, alcohol-related dementia in 10 per cent and dementia with Lewy bodies in 7 per cent.)

Similar figures were obtained by Harvey *et al.* (2003), who surveyed three London boroughs with a total population of 567 500 people and calculated an overall prevalence for early onset-dementia of 98 per 100 000 for patients aged 45–64 years.

The prevalence of FTD in the over-65s is largely unknown. In a recent prospective investigation of 451 85-year-olds in Sweden, 86 (19 per cent) fulfilled the criteria for a frontal lobe syndrome and 14 (3 per cent) fulfilled the Lund–Manchester criteria for fvFTD (Gislason *et al.*, 2003).

53.8 CONCLUSIONS

It is clear that this is a rapidly evolving field but that further detailed clinicopathological studies are required to address the many outstanding questions. Kertesz (2003) suggests that the disorders of PiD, FTD, primary progressive aphasia, CBD, PSP and FTD-MND should be regarded as part of a clinically and biologically cohesive spectrum and subsumed by the umbrella term 'Pick's complex'. However, we continue to prefer the use of separate clinical syndromic labels, which avoid specific pathological connotations.

REFERENCES

Alzheimer A. (1911) Über eigenartige Krankheitsfälle des späteren Alters (About peculiar cases of disease in old age). *Zeitschrift für die gesamte Neurologie und Psychiatrie* **4**: 356–385

Ames D, Cummings JL, Wirshing WC *et al.* (1994) Repetitive and compulsive behavior in frontal lobe degenerations. *Journal of Neuropsychiatry and Clinical Neurosciences* **6**: 100–113

Bak T and Hodges JR. (1999) Cognition, language and behaviour in motor neurone disease: evidence of frontotemporal dementia. *Dementia and Geriatric Cognitive Disorders* **10**: 29–32

Bak TH, O'Donovan DG, Xuereb JH *et al.* (2001) Selective impairment of verb processing associated with pathological changes in the Brodman areas 44 and 45 in the motor neurone disease/dementia/aphasia syndrome. *Brain* **124**: 103–124

Baldwin B and Förstl H. (1993) Pick's disease – 101 years. Still there but in need of reform. *British Journal of Psychiatry* **163**: 100–105

Boeve BF, Maraganore DM, Parisi JE *et al.* (1999) Pathologic heterogeneity in clinically diagnosed corticobasal degeneration. *Neurology* **53**: 795–800

Bozeat S, Gregory CA, Lambon Ralph MA *et al.* (2000) Which neuropsychiatric and behavioural features distinguish frontal and temporal variants of frontotemporal dementia from Alzheimer's disease? *Journal of Neurology, Neurosurgery, and Psychiatry* **69**: 178–186

Brown J. (1998) Chromosome 3-linked frontotemporal dementia. *Cellular and Molecular Life Sciences* **54**: 925–927

Brown J, Ashworth A, Gydesen S *et al.* (1995) Familial nonspecific dementia maps to chromosome 3. *Human Molecular Genetics* **4**: 1625–1628

Brun A. (1987) Frontal lobe degeneration of non-Alzheimer's type. I. Neuropathology. *Archives of Gerontology and Geriatrics* **6**: 209–233

Brun A, Englund B, Gustafson L *et al.* (1994) Clinical and neuropathological criteria for frontotemporal dementia. *Journal of Neurology, Neurosurgery, and Psychiatry* **57**: 416–418

Caselli RJ, Windebank AJ, Petersen RC *et al.* (1993) Rapidly progressive aphasic dementia and motor neuron disease. *Annals of Neurology* **33**: 200–207

Croot K, Patterson K, Hodges JR. (1997) Phonological disruption in atypical dementia of the Alzheimer's type. *Brain and Cognition* **32**: 186–190

Cummings JL. (1999) Principles of neuropsychiatry: towards a neuropsychiatric epistemology. *Neurocase* **5**: 181–188

Cummings JL, Mega M, Gray K *et al.* (1994) The neuropsychiatric inventory: comprehensive assessment of psychopathology in dementia. *Neurology* **44**: 2308–2314

Dickson DW. (1998) Pick's disease: a modern approach. *Brain Pathology* **8**: 339–354

Dumanchin C, Camuzat A, Campion D *et al.* (1998) Segregation of a missense mutation in the microtubule-associated protein tau gene with familial frontotemporal dementia and parkinsonism. *Human Molecular Genetics* **7**: 1825–1829

Edwards Lee T, Miller B, Benson F *et al.* (1997) The temporal variant of frontotemporal dementia. *Brain* **120**: 1027–1040

Evans JJ, Heggs AJ, Antoun N *et al.* (1995) Progressive prosopagnosia associated with selective right temporal lobe atrophy: a new syndrome? *Brain* **118**: 1–13

Ferrano A and Jervis GA. (1936) Pick's disease. *Archives of Neurology and Psychiatry* **36**: 739–767

Foster NL, Wilhelmsen K, Sima AAF *et al.* (1997) Frontotemporal dementia and parkinsonism linked to chromosome 17: a consensus conference. *Annals of Neurology* **41**: 706–715

Galton CJ, Patterson K, Xuereb JH *et al.* (2000) Atypical and typical presentations of Alzheimer's disease: a clinical, neuropsychological, neuroimaging and pathological study of 13 cases. *Brain* **123**: 484–498

Galton CJ, Patterson K, Graham KS *et al.* (2001) Differing patterns of temporal atrophy in Alzheimer's disease and semantic dementia. *Neurology* **57**: 216–225

Gans A. (1922) Betrachtungen über Art und Ausbreitung des krankhaften Prozesses in einem fall von Picksher Atrophie des Stirhirns *Zeitschrift für die gesamte Neurologie und Psychiatrie* **80**: 10–28

Garrard P and Hodges JR. (1999) Semantic dementia: implications for the neural basis of language and meaning. *Aphasiology* **13**: 609–623

Garrard P, Perry R, Hodges JR. (1997) Disorders of semantic memory. *Journal of Neurology, Neurosurgery, and Psychiatry* **62**: 431–435

Girling DM and Berrios GE. (1994) On the relationship between senile cerebral atrophy and aphasia (translation of Pick A. Über die Beziehungen der senilen Atrophie zur Aphasie. *Prager Medizinische Wochenschrift* 1892 **17**: 165–7). *History of Psychiatry* **8**: 542–547

Girling DM and Berrios GE. (1997) On the symptomatology of left-sided temporal lobe atrophy (translation of Pick, A. Zur Symptomatologie der linksseitigen Schäfenlappenatrophie. *Monatschrift für Psychiatrie und Neurologie* 1904 **16**: 378–88). *History of Psychiatry* **8**: 149–159

Girling DM and Markova IS. (1995) Senile atrophy as the basis for focal symptoms (translation of Pick A. Senile Hirnatrophie als Grundlage für Herderscheinungen. *Wiener Klinische Wochenschrift* 1901 **14**: 403–404). *History of Psychiatry* **6**: 533–537

Gislason TB, Sjogren M, Larsson L *et al.* (2003) The prevalence of frontal variant frontotemporal dementia and the frontal lobe syndrome in a population based sample of 85 year olds. *Journal of Neurology, Neurosurgery, and Psychiatry* **74**: 867–871

Graff-Radford NR, Damasio AR, Hyman BT *et al.* (1990) Progressive aphasia in a patient with Pick's disease: a neuropsychological, radiologic, and anatomic study. *Neurology* **40**: 620–626

Graham KS and Hodges JR. (1997) Differentiating the roles of the hippocampal complex and the neocortex in long-term memory storage: evidence from the study of semantic dementia and Alzheimer's disease. *Neuropsychology* **11**: 77–89

Graham NL, Bak TH, Hodges JR. (2003) Corticobasal degeneration as a cognitive disorder. *Movement Disorders* **18**: 1224–1232

Green J, Morris JC, Sandson J *et al.* (1990) Progressive aphasia: a precursor of global dementia? *Neurology* **40**: 423–429

Greene JDW, Patterson K, Xuereb J *et al.* (1996) Alzheimer disease and nonfluent progressive aphasia. *Archives of Neurology* **53**: 1072–1078

Gregory C, Lough S, Stone V *et al.* (2002) Theory of mind in patients with frontal variant frontotemporal dementia and Alzheimer's disease: theoretical and practical implications. *Brain* **125**: 752–764

Gregory CA and Hodges JR. (1993) Dementia of frontal type and the focal lobar atrophies. *International Review of Psychiatry* **5**: 397–406

Gregory CA and Hodges JR. (1996) Frontotemporal dementia use of consensus criteria and prevalence of psychiatric features. *Neuropsychiatry, Neuropsychology and Behavioural Neurology* **9**: 145–153

Gregory CA, Serra-Mestres J, Hodges JR. (1999) Early diagnosis of the frontal variant of frontotemporal dementia: how sensitive are standard neuroimaging and neuropsychologic tests? *Neuropsychiatry, Neuropsychology and Behavioral Neurology* **12**: 128–135

Gustafson L. (1987) Frontal lobe degeneration of non-Alzheimer's type II: clinical picture and differential diagnosis. *Archives of Gerontology and Geriatrics* **6**: 209–223

Harasty JA, Halliday GM, Code C *et al.* (1996) Quantification of cortical atrophy in a case of progressive fluent aphasia. *Brain* **119**: 181–190

Harvey RJ, Skelton-Robinson M, Rossor MN. (2003) The prevalence and causes of dementia in people under the age of 65 years. *Journal of Neurology, Neurosurgery, and Psychiatry* **74**: 1206–1209

Heutink P, Stevens M, Rizzu P *et al.* (1997) Hereditary frontotemporal dementia is linked to chromosome 17q21-q22: a genetic and clinicopathological study of three Dutch families. *Annals of Neurology* **41**: 150–159

Hodges JR and Graham KS. (1998) A reversal of the temporal gradient for famous person knowledge in semantic dementia Implications for the neural organization of long-term memory. *Neuropsychologia* **36**: 803–825

Hodges JR and Patterson K. (1996) Non-fluent progressive aphasia and semantic dementia a comparative neuropsychological study. *Journal of the International Neuropsychological Society* **2**: 511–524

Hodges JR and Patterson KE. (1997) Semantic memory disorders. *Trends in Cognitive Science* **1**: 67–72

Hodges JR, Patterson K, Oxbury S *et al.* (1992) Semantic dementia progressive fluent aphasia with temporal lobe atrophy. *Brain* **115**: 1783–1806

Hodges JR, Patterson K, Tyler LK. (1994) Loss of semantic memory: implications for the modularity of mind. *Cognitive Neuropsychology* **11**: 505–542

Hodges JR, Garrard P, Patterson K. (1998) Semantic dementia. In: A Kertesz and DG Munoz (eds), *Pick's Disease and Pick Complex*. New York, Wiley-Liss Inc, pp. 83–104

Hodges JR, Davies R, Xuereb J *et al.* (2003) Survival in frontotemporal dementia. *Neurology* **61**: 349–354

Hodges JR, Davies RR, Xuereb J *et al.* (2004) Clinicopathological correlates in frontotemporal dementia. *Annals of Neurology* **56**: 399–406

Holland AL, McBurney DH, Moossy J *et al.* (1985) The dissolution of language in Pick's disease with neurofibrillary tangles: a case study. *Brain and Language* **24**: 36–58

Hutton M, Lendon CL, Rizzu P *et al.* (1998) Association of missense and 5'-splice-site mutations in tau with the inherited dementia FTDP-17. *Nature* **18**: 702–705

Ikeda M, Brown J, Holland AJ *et al.* (2002) Changes in appetite, food preference, and eating habits in frontotemporal dementia and Alzheimer's disease. *Journal of Neurology, Neurosurgery, and Psychiatry* **73**: 371–376

Imura T, Nogami Y, Asakawa K. (1971) Aphasia in Japanese Language. *Nihon University Journal of Medicine* **13**: 69–90

Ingram EM and Spillantini MG. (2002) Tau gene mutations: dissecting the pathogenesis of FTDP-17. *Trends in Molecular Medicine* **8**: 555–562

Jackson M and Lowe J. (1996) The new neuropathology of degenerative frontotemporal dementias. *Acta Neuropathologica* **91**: 127–134

Kamo H, McGeer PL, Harrop R *et al.* (1987) Positron emission tomography and histopathology in Pick's disease. *Neurology* **37**: 439–445

Katzman R. (1986) Differential diagnosis of dementing illnesses. *Neurologic Clinics* **4**: 329–340

Keane J, Calder AJ, Hodges JR *et al.* (2002) Face and emotion processing in frontal variant frontotemporal dementia. *Neuropsychologia* **40**: 655–665

Kertesz A. (2003) Pick's complex and FTDP-17. *Movement Disorders* **18** (Suppl. 6): S57–S62

Kertesz A and Munoz DG. (1998) *Pick's disease and Pick Complex*. New York, Wiley-Liss Inc

Kertesz A, Davidson W, Fox H. (1997) Frontal behavioral inventory: diagnostic criteria for frontal lobe dementia. *Canadian Journal of Neurological Sciences* **24**: 29–36

Kertesz A, Nadkarni N, Davidson W *et al.* (2000) The frontal behavioral inventory in the differential diagnosis of frontotemporal dementia. *Journal of the International Neuropsychological Society* **6**: 460–468

Kertesz A, Davidson W, McCabe P *et al.* (2003a) Behavioral quantitation is more sensitive than cognitive testing in frontotemporal dementia. *Alzheimer Disease and Associated Disorders* **17**: 223–229

Kertesz A, Munoz DG, Hillis A. (2003b) Preferred terminology. *Annals of Neurology* **54** (Suppl. 5): S3–S6

Kitchener E and Hodges JR. (1999) Impaired knowledge of famous people and events and intact autobiographical knowledge in a case of progressive right temporal lobe degeneration: implications for the organization of remote memory. *Cognitive Neuropsychology* **16**: 589–607

Knopman DS, Mastri AR, Frey WH *et al.* (1990) Dementia lacking distinctive histological features: a common non-Alzheimer degenerative disease. *Neurology* **40**: 251–256

Levy ML, Miller BL, Cummings JL *et al.* (1996) Alzheimer disease and frontotemporal dementias: behavioral distinctions. *Archives of Neurology* **53**: 687–690

Lippa CF, Cohen R, Smith TW *et al.* (1991) Primary progressive aphasia with focal neuronal achromasia. *Neurology* **41**: 882–886

Lowenberg K and Arbor A. (1936) Pick's disease: a clinicopathologic contribution. *Archives of Neurology and Psychiatry* **36**: 768–789

Lowenberg K, Boyd DA, Salon DD *et al.* (1939) Occurence of Pick's disease in early adult years. *Archives of Neurology and Psychiatry* **41**: 1004–1020

McKhann GM, Albert MS, Grossman M *et al.* (2001) Clinical and pathological diagnosis of frontotemporal dementia report of the Work Group on Frontotemporal Dementia and Pick's Disease. *Archives of Neurology* **58**: 1803–1809

Malamud N and Boyd DA. (1940) Pick's disease with atrophy of the temporal lobes: a clinicopathologic study. *Archives of Neurology and Psychiatry* **43**: 210–221

Mansvelt JV. (1954) Pick's disease: a syndrome of lobar cerebral atrophy, its clinico-anatomical and histopathological types. Utrecht University, Thèse

Mathuranath PS, Xuereb JH, Bak T *et al.* (2000) Corticobasal ganglionic degeneration and/or frontotemporal dementia? A report of two overlap cases and review of literature. *Journal of Neurology, Neurosurgery, and Psychiatry* **68**: 304–312

Mesulam MM. (1982) Slowly progressive aphasia without generalised dementia. *Annals of Neurology* **11**: 592–598

Mesulam MM and Weintraub S. (1992) Primary progressive aphasia. In F Boller (ed.), *Heterogeneity of Alzheimer's Disease*. Berlin, Springer-Verlag, pp. 43–66

Miller BL, Cummings JL, Villanueva-Meyer J *et al.* (1991) Frontal lobe degeneration: clinical, neuropsychological, and SPECT characteristics. *Neurology* **41**: 1374–1382

Miller BL, Darby A, Benson DF *et al.* (1997) Aggressive, socially disruptive and antisocial behaviour associated with frontotemporal dementia. *British Journal of Psychiatry* **170**: 150–155

Mingazzini G. (1914) On aphasia due to atrophy of the cerebral convolutions. *Brain* **36**: 493–524

Mitsuyama Y and Takamiya S. (1979) Presenile dementia with motor neuron in Japan. *Archives of Neurology* **36**: 592–593

Morita K, Kaiya H, Ikeda T *et al.* (1987) Presenile dementia combined with amyotrophy: a review of 34 Japanese cases. *Archives of Gerontology and Geriatrics* **6**: 263–277

Morris JC, Cole M, Banker BQ *et al.* (1984) Hereditary dysphasic dementia and the Pick-Alzheimer spectrum. *Annals of Neurology* **16**: 455–466

Morris HR, Khan MN, Janssen JC *et al.* (2001) The genetic and pathological classification of familial frontotemporal dementia. *Archives of Neurology* **58**: 1813–1816

Morris HR, Osaki Y, Holton J *et al.* (2003) Tau exon 10 + 16 mutation FTDP-17 presenting clinically as sporadic young onset PSP. *Neurology* **61**: 102–104

Mummery CJ, Patterson K, Wise RJS *et al.* (1999) Disrupted temporal lobe connections in semantic dementia. *Brain* **122**: 61–73

Mummery CJ, Patterson K, Price CJ *et al.* (2000) A voxel based morphometry study of semantic dementia. The relationship between temporal lobe atrophy and semantic dementia. *Annals of Neurology* **47**: 36–45

Munoz DG and Ludwin SK. (1984) Classic and generalized variants of Pick's disease: a clinicopathological, ultrastructural and immunocytochemical comparative study. *Annals of Neurology* **16**: 467–480

Neary D, Snowden JS, Bowen DM *et al.* (1986) Neuropsychological syndromes in presenile dementia due to cerebral atrophy. *Journal of Neurology, Neurosurgery, and Psychiatry* **49**: 163–174

Neary D, Snowdon JS, Mann DMA *et al.* (1990) Frontal lobe dementia and motor neuron disease. *Journal of Neurology, Neurosurgery, and Psychiatry* **53**: 23–32

Neary D, Snowden JS, Gustafson L *et al.* (1998) Frontotemporal lobar degeneration: a consensus on clinical diagnostic criteria. *Neurology* **51**: 1546–1554

Nestor PJ, Graham NL, Fryer TD *et al.* (2003) Progressive non-fluent aphasia is associated with hypometabolism centred on the left anterior insula. *Brain* **126**: 2406–2418

Neumann MA. (1949) Pick's disease. *Journal of Neuropathology and Experimental Neurology* **8**: 255–282

Nichols IC and Weigner WC. (1938) Pick's disease – a specific type of dementia. *Brain* **3**: 237–249

Nyatsanza S, Shetty T, Gregory C *et al.* (2003) A study of stereotypic behaviours in Alzheimer's disease and frontal and temporal variant frontotemporal dementia. *Journal of Neurology, Neurosurgery, and Psychiatry* **74**: 1398–1402

Onari K and Spatz H. (1926) Anatomische Beitrage zur Lehre von der Pickschen umschriebenen Grosshirnrindenatrophie (Piscksche Krankheit). *Zeitschrift für die gesamte Neurologie und Psychiatrie* **101**: 470–511

Pasquier F, Lebert F, Scheltens P. (1996) *Frontotemporal Dementia*. The Netherlands, ICG Publications

Petersen RB, Tabaton M, Chen SG *et al.* (1995) Familial progressive subcortical gliosis: presence of prions and linkage to chromosome 17. *Neurology* **45**: 1062–1067

Pick A. (1892) Über die Beziehungen der senilen Atrophie zur Aphasie. *Prager Medizinische Wochenschrift* **17**: 165–167

Pick A. (1901) Senile Hirnatrophie als Grundlage für Hernderscheinungen. *Wiener Klinische Wochenschrift* **14**: 403–404

Pick A. (1904) Zur symptomatologie der linksseitigen Schläfenlappenatrophie. *Monatschrift für Psychiatrie und Neurologie* **16**: 378–388

Pick A. (1906) Über einen weiteren symptomenkomplex im Rahmen der Dementia senilis, bedingt durch umschriebene starkere Hirnatrophie. *Monatschrift für Psychiatrie und Neurologie* **19**: 97–108

Poeck K and Luzzatti C. (1988) Slowly progressive aphasia in three patients: the problem of accompanying neuropsychological deficit. *Brain* **111**: 151–168

Poorkaj P, Bird TD, Wijsman E *et al.* (1998) Tau is a candidate gene for chromosome 17 frontotemporal dementia. *Annals of Neurology* **43**: 815–825

Rahman S, Sahakian BJ, Hodges JR *et al.* (1999) Specific cognitive deficits in mild frontal variant frontotemporal dementia. *Brain* **122**: 1469–1493

Rakowicz Z and Hodges JR. (1998) Dementia and aphasia in motor neurone disease: an under recognised association. *Journal of Neurology, Neurosurgery, and Psychiatry* **65**: 881–889

Rascovsky K, Salmon DP, Ho GJ *et al.* (2002) Cognitive profiles differ in autopsy-confirmed frontotemporal dementia and AD. *Neurology* **58**: 1801–1808

Ratnavalli E, Brayne C, Dawson K et al. (2002) The prevalence of frontotemporal dementia. Neurology 58: 1615–1621

Rebeiz JJ, Kolodny EH, Richardson EP. (1968) Corticodentatonigral degeneration with neuronal achromasia. Archives of Neurology 18: 20–33

Robertson EE, Le Roux A, Brown JH. (1958) The clinical differentiation of Pick's disease. Journal of Mental Science 104: 1000–1024

Rogers RD, Sahakian BJ, Hodges JR et al. (1998) Dissociating executive mechanisms of task control following frontal lobe damage and Parkinson's disease. Brain 121: 815–842

Rosen HJ, Gorno-Tempini ML, Goldman WP et al. (2002a) Patterns of brain atrophy in frontotemporal dementia and semantic dementia. Neurology 58: 198–208

Rosen HJ, Hartikainen KM, Jagust W et al. (2002b) Utility of clinical criteria in differentiating frontotemporal lobar degeneration (FTLD) from AD. Neurology 58: 1608–1615

Rosenfeld M. (1909) Die partielle Grosshirnatrophie. Journal für Psychologie und Neurologie 14: 115–130

Rossor MN. (1998) Provisional clinical and neuroradiological criteria for the diagnosis of Pick's disease: European Concerted Action on Pick's Disease (ECAPD) Consortium. European Journal of Neurology 5: 519–520

Rossor MN, Revesz T, Lantos PL et al. (2000) Semantic dementia with ubiquitin-positive tau-negative inclusion bodies. Brain 123: 267–276

Saffran EM and Schwartz MF. (1994) Of cabbages and things: semantic memory from a neuropsychological perspective – a tutorial review. In: C Umilta and M Moscovitch (eds), Attention and Performance XV. Hove and London, Lawrence Erlbaum, pp. 507–536

Sasanuma S and Mondi H. (1975) The syndrome of Gogi (word meaning) aphasia. Neurology 25: 627–632

Schenk VWS. (1951) Maladie de Pick: etude anatomo-clinique de 8 cas. Annales Medico-Psychologiques (Paris) 109: 574–587

Schneider C. (1927) Über Picksche Krankheit. Monatschrift für Psychologie und Neurologie 65: 230–275

Schneider C. (1929) Weitere Beitrage zur Lehre von der Pickschen Krankheit. Zeitschrift für die gesamte Neurologie und Psychiatrie 120: 340–384

Scholten IM, Kneebone AC, Denson LA et al. (1995) Primary progressive aphasia: serial linguistic, neuropsychological and radiological findings with neuropathological results. Aphasiology 9: 495–516

Schwarz M, De Bleser R, Poeck K et al. (1998) A case of primary progressive aphasia: a 14-year follow-up study with neuropathological findings. Brain 121: 115–126

Snowden JS, Goulding PJ, Neary D. (1989) Semantic dementia a form of circumscribed cerebral atrophy. Behavioural Neurology 2: 167–182

Snowden JS, Neary D, Mann DMA et al. (1992) Progressive language disorder due to lobar atrophy. Annals of Neurology 31: 174–183

Snowden JS, Neary D, Mann DMA. (1996) Fronto-temporal Lobar Degeneration: Fronto-temporal Dementia, Progressive Aphasia, Semantic Dementia. New York, Churchill Livingstone

Soliveri P, Rossi G, Monza D et al. (2003) A case of dementia parkinsonism resembling progressive supranuclear palsy due to mutation in the tau protein gene. Archives of Neurology 60: 1454–1456

Spatt J. (2003) Arnold Pick's concept of dementia. Cortex 39: 525–531

Spillantini MG, Goedert M, Crowther RA et al. (1997) Familial multiple system tauopathy with presenile dementia a disease with abundant neuronal and glial tau filaments. Proceedings of the National Academy of Sciences of the United States of America 94: 4113–4118

Spillantini MG, Bird TD, Ghetti B. (1998a) Frontotemporal dementia and parkinsonism linked to chromosome 17. A new group of tauopathies. Brain Pathology 8: 387–402

Spillantini MG, Murrell JR, Goedert M et al. (1998b) Mutation in the tau gene in familial multiple system tauopathy with presenile dementia. Proceedings of the National Academy of Sciences of the United States of America 95: 7737–7741

Steele JC, Richardson JC, Olszewski J. (1964) Progressive supranuclear palsy. a heterogeneous degeneration involving the brain stem, basal ganglia and cerebellum with vertical gaze and pseudobulbar palsy, nuchal dystonia and dementia. Archives of Neurology 10: 333–359

Stertz G. (1926) Über die Picksche atrophie. Zeitschrift für die gesamte Neurologie und Psychiatrie 101: 729–747

Strong MJ, Lomen-Hoerth C, Caselli RJ et al. (2003) Cognitive impairment, frontotemporal dementia, and the motor neuron diseases. Annals of Neurology 54 (Suppl. 5): S20–S23

Sumi SM, Bird TD, Nochlin D et al. (1992) Familial presenile dementia with psychosis associated with cortical neurofibrillary tangles and degeneration of the amygdala. Neurology 42: 120–127

Tanabe H. (1992) Personality of typical Gogi (word meaning) aphasics. Japanese Journal of Neuropsychology 8: 34–42

Tanabe H, Ikeda M, Nakagawa Y et al. (1992) Gogi (word meaning) aphasia and semantic memory for words. Higher Brain Function Research 12: 153–169

Thompson SA, Patterson K, Hodges JR. (2003) Left/right asymmetry of atrophy in semantic dementia behavioral-cognitive implications. Neurology 61: 1196–1203

Thompson SA, Graham KS, Williams G et al. (2004) Dissociating person-specific from general semantic knowledge: roles of the left and right temporal lobes. Neuropsychologia 42: 359–370

Tissot R, Constantinidis J, Richard J. (1975) La maladie de Pick. Paris, Masson

Tonkonogy JM, Smith TW, Barreira PJ. (1994) Obsessive-compulsive disorders in Pick's disease. Journal of Neuropsychiatry and Clinical Neurosciences 6: 176–180

Tulving E. (1972) Episodic and semantic memory. In: E Tulving and W Donaldson (eds), Organization of Memory. New York, Academic Press, pp. 381–403

Tulving E. (1983) Elements of Episodic Memory. New York, Oxford University Press

Warrington EK. (1975) Selective impairment of semantic memory. Quarterly Journal of Experimental Psychology 27: 635–657

Wechsler A. (1977) Presenile dementia presenting as aphasia. Journal of Neurology, Neurosurgery, and Psychiatry 40: 303–305

Wechsler AF, Verity MA, Rosenscheim S et al. (1982) Pick's disease: a clinical, computed tomographic and histological study with Golgi impregnation observations. Archives of Neurology 39: 3287–3290

Weintraub S, Rubin NP, Mesulam M-M. (1990) Primary progressive aphasia: longitudinal course, profile, and language features. Archives of Neurology 47: 1329–1335

Wilhelmsen KC. (1997) Frontotemporal dementia is on the MAP. Annals of Neurology 41: 139–140

Wilhelmsen KC, Lynch T, Pavlou E et al. (1994) Localization of disinhibition-dementia-parkinsonism-amyotrophy complex to 17q21–22. American Journal of Human Genetics 55: 1159–1165

Wszolek ZK, Pfeiffer RF, Bhatt MH et al. (1992) Rapidly progressive autosomal dominant parkinsonism and dementia with pallido-ponto-nigral degeneration. Annals of Neurology 32: 312–320

Zhukareva V, Vogelsberg-Ragaglia V, Van Deerlin VM et al. (2001) Loss of brain tau defines novel sporadic and familial tauopathies with frontotemporal dementia. Annals of Neurology 49: 165–175

Zhukareva V, Sundarraj S, Mann D et al. (2003) Selective reduction of soluble tau proteins in sporadic and familial frontotemporal dementias: an international follow-up study. Acta Neuropathologica (Berlin) 105: 469–476

54

The genetics and molecular pathology of frontotemporal lobar degeneration

DAVID M A MANN

Frontotemporal lobar degeneration (FTLD) refers to a clinically and pathologically heterogeneous group of early onset, non-Alzheimer forms of dementia. Although relatively rare when compared with Alzheimer's disease (AD) over all ages, FTLD is actually the second most common cause of dementia within the presenium, there being one case of FTLD for every four of AD with disease onset before 65 years of age (Snowden *et al.*, 1996). Historically, many of the various forms of FTLD were originally described under the rubric of 'Pick's disease' and its variants, though within the past 10–15 years there has been a great resurgence of interest in the disorder, largely because of the longitudinal clinical and pathological studies carried out in Lund and Manchester during the late 1980s and early 1990s from which the spectrum of disease has come to be recognized (see Snowden *et al.*, 1996), and with that consensus diagnostic criteria for the various clinical forms of FTLD have emerged (Neary *et al.*, 1998).

The prototypical, and most common, clinical syndrome within FTLD is frontotemporal dementia (FTD). This manifests as behavioural and personality changes involving disinhibition, stereotypy, antisocial acts and language disorders, and leads to apathy, mutism and late neurological (frontal release or extrapyramidal) signs. However, the breadth of illnesses can extend far wider and involve cases where a parkinsonian-type movement disorder or a progressive apraxia (PAX), with relatively mild dementia, is the major disabling feature, or others in which a language disorder of a fluent or non-fluent aphasia, known as semantic dementia (SD) or progressive aphasia (PA), respectively, predominate. Moreover, cases of FTD may be complicated both clinically, but more usually pathologically, by changes associated with motor neurone disease (MND), and in these instances the disorder

has been termed frontotemporal dementia with MND (FTD-MND), or recognizing the presence of MND-type pathology in the absence of MND clinical phenotype, motor neurone disease inclusion dementia (MNDID). The clinical and neuropsychological features of these disorders are described by David Neary in Chapter 52.

As described in this present chapter, molecular genetics has now begun to rationalize classification of FTLD, though major nosological uncertainties remain. Clinical diversity remains an obstacle and the pathological heterogeneity within this group of disorders remains largely unexplained. Here, the genetics and molecular pathology of FTLD associated with mutations in tau and other possible mutations on chromosome 17 and elsewhere, as well as that in other cases of FTLD, where no such chromosomal associations are present or at least known, is reviewed. It is recognized that FTLD is unlikely to have a single unifying cause to clinical symptomatology and underlying pathological change.

54.1 THE GENETICS OF FRONTOTEMPORAL LOBAR DEGENERATION

A previous family history of a similar disorder occurs in about half of patients with FTLD (Snowden *et al.*, 1996). It was this degree of inheritability that triggered much of the current upsurge in interest among research scientists into the biology of FTLD, by leading to the crucial identification that certain inherited forms of FTLD were genetically linked to a locus on chromosome 17 (this form of the disorder then became known as 'frontotemporal dementia with parkinsonism linked to chromosome 17' [FTDP-17] and was associated with mutations in the tau gene, tau [Hutton *et al.*, 1998; Poorkaj *et al.*, 1998; Spillantini *et al.*, 1998]). Since then there has been an explosion of data concerning the genetics and biochemistry of FTLD.

Although the occurrence of tau mutations within FTLD is relatively rare – prevalence rates vary from about 6 to 18 per cent (Houlden *et al.*, 1999a; Poorkaj *et al.*, 2001; Rosso *et al.*, 2003) – their identification has been of paramount importance, providing crucial insight through the ability to 'model' the disorder in cell systems and animals. This has greatly increased our knowledge not only of the pathogenesis of FTLD, but also how the production and function of tau protein is normally regulated. Moreover, the characterizing neuropathological feature of FTLD due to tau mutations is the presence of insoluble aggregates of tau protein in the absence of deposits of amyloid β protein (Aβ). This proves that tau pathology can lead to neurodegenerative disease in its own right and has focused attention once again upon the key role that neurofibrillary degeneration may play in AD.

54.1.1　Genetics of FTLD associated with tau mutations

54.1.1.1　THE STRUCTURE OF TAU AND THE FUNCTION OF TAU PROTEINS

Tau has 15 coding regions (exons), and transcripts of this gene are alternatively spliced to produce different isoforms within the brain and peripheral nervous system. In the central nervous system, the precise tau isoform expression pattern is under developmental regulatory control. In fetal brain only a single isoform containing exons 1, 4, 5, 7, 9 and 11–13 is expressed. However, in adult brain five additional isoforms are produced by the alternative inclusions of exons 2, 3 and 10, these ranging from 352 to 441 amino acids in length and differing according to the (alternatively spliced) inclusion of three or four (when exon 10 is included) imperfect repeat domains of 31 or 32 amino acids within the carboxy terminal region of the molecule, and also according to the absence or presence of one or two, 29 or 58 amino acid inserts (encoded by exons 2 and 3, respectively) in the amino terminal region. The conditional inclusion of exon 10 therefore generates three tau isoforms each with four microtubule binding domains compared with tau isoforms without exon 10 that have only three microtubule binding domains (known as 4-repeat tau, 4R, and 3-repeat tau, 3R, respectively). The six tau isoforms are designated 3R0N, 3R1N, 3R2N, 4R0N, 4R1N, 4R2N, respectively according to inclusion or otherwise of exons 2, 3 and 10. The carboxy-terminal domains, along with some adjoining sections of the molecule, act as the microtubule-binding region; the function of those sequences encoded by exons 2 and 3 remains unknown.

Splicing of exon 10 is regulated in a complex hierarchical way involving a variety of *cis*-acting sequences within exon 10, and within the intron to exon 11, which collectively modulate the function of a putative stem loop structure to determine the degree to which splicing of exon 10 is permitted (Hutton *et al.*, 1998; D'Souza and Schellenberg, 2002). In this way a strict stoichiometric balance between 3R and 4R tau isoforms is maintained, since it is both the presence and proportion of 3R and 4R tau isoforms that is critical to the proper functioning of tau. Slightly more than half the tau molecules normally produced are 3R forms.

Tau protein is localized in neuronal axons and is involved in the regulation of microtubule assembly/disassembly and the axonal transport of proteins and organelles. All six isoforms play a precise role in this maintenance of microtubular structure and if one or more of the various isoforms fails to function, or if there is a stoichiometric imbalance in the different variants, microtubule formation will become more difficult or the stability of microtubules formed will become compromised. Any excess of unused tau (of any isoform composition) can be bundled into indigestible residues that choke the cell. Hence, a neuropathological aggregation of tau within the somatodendritic compartment of the neurone occurs in several neurodegenerative diseases, including FTLD, but also in AD and certain parkinsonian disorders such as progressive supranuclear palsy (PSP) and corticobasal degeneration (CBD). The formation and accumulation of these insoluble tau aggregates within neurones (and sometimes glial cells) is widely believed to be critical to the neurodegenerative cascade that leads to nerve cell dysfunction and death in these disorders, possibly involving a toxic action of the filaments formed from the tau aggregates.

54.1.1.2　TAU MUTATIONS IN FTLD

To date, about 30 tau mutations in around 70 families with an FTLD phenotype have now been identified. Many of the tau mutations exist as missense, deletion or silent mutations within coding regions of exon 1 (R5H, R5L), exon 9 (K257T, I260V, L266V, G272V), exon 11 (L315R, S320F), exon 12 (Q336R, V337M, E342V, K369I) and exon 13 (G389R, R406W) (Hutton *et al.*, 1998; Poorkaj *et al.*, 1998, 2001; Rizzu *et al.*, 1999; Murrell *et al.*, 1999; Pickering-Brown *et al.*, 2000a, b; Rizzini *et al.*, 2000; Lippa *et al.*, 2000; Neumann *et al.*, 2001; Hayashi *et al.*, 2002; Saito *et al.*, 2002; Rosso *et al.*, 2002, 2003; Grover *et al.*, 2003; Hogg *et al.*, 2003; Kobayashi *et al.*, 2003b; van Herpen *et al.*, 2003). These tau mutations are located outside exon 10 and therefore affect all six tau isoforms. They generate mutated tau molecules that, *in vitro*, (variably) lose their ability to interact with α and β tubulin molecules in the promotion of microtubule assembly and axonal transport (Hasegawa *et al.*, 1998; Hong *et al.*, 1998). Some of the mutations also increase, but again variably, the propensity of the mutated tau to self-aggregate into the fibrils (Hasegawa *et al.*, 1998; Goedert *et al.*, 1999a; Nacharaju *et al.*, 1999) that form the characterizing pathological structures within the brain. Nonetheless, even those mutations that cause only a modest effect on microtubule binding or promote only mild or slow tau aggregation may over many years course of illness build sufficiently to cause FTLD.

Other tau mutations (N279K, ΔK280, L284L, ΔN296, N296H, N296N, P301L, P301S, S305S and S305N – the last two also being known as –1 and –2 splice site mutations) occur within the alternatively spliced exon 10, or lie close to the splice donor site of the intron that follows exon 10 within a regulatory region of tau that determines the alternative spliced inclusion of exon 10 during gene transcription (these being known as +3, +11, +12, +13, +14 and +16 splice site mutations) (Clark et al., 1998; Dumanchin et al., 1998; Hong et al., 1998; Hutton et al., 1998; Poorkaj et al., 1998; Spillantini et al., 1998, 2000; Delisle et al., 1999; D'Souza et al., 1999; Goedert et al., 1999b; Hasegawa et al., 1999; Iijima et al., 1999; Mirra et al., 1999; Morris et al., 1999; Nasreddine et al., 1999; Rizzu et al., 1999; Sperfeld et al., 1999; Yasuda et al., 1999, 2000a, b; Stanford et al., 2000, 2003; Tolnay et al., 2000; Iseki et al., 2001; Miyamoto et al., 2001; Pastor et al., 2001; Kowalska et al., 2002; Pickering-Brown et al., 2002; Kobayashi et al., 2003a; Werber et al., 2003). These mutations affect only that part of the tau protein sequence encoded by exon 10, and so affect only 4R tau isoforms.

The S305S (−1), S305N (−2), +3, +11, +12, +13, +14 and +16 splice mutations lie close to or within the predicted regulatory stem loop structure of a splice acceptor domain. These mutations may destabilize this stem loop, and disrupt its function, interfering with the binding of U1snRNP splice regulatory elements. Their effect is to increase the use of this particular splicing mechanism, thereby increasing the proportion of tau mRNA transcripts containing exon 10, and the amount of 4-repeat tau protein, such that the ratio between 4R and 3R tau isoforms becomes increased 2–3-fold (Hutton et al., 1998; Spillantini et al., 1998). With exception of S305N mutation, which changes the consensus sequence for 4-repeat tau isoforms, none of these regulatory mutations alter the primary amino acid structure of the tau proteins transcribed and therefore do not per se impair microtubule binding (Hong et al., 1998; Hasegawa et al., 1999).

The N279K mutation also increases the splicing of transcripts containing exon 10 by strengthening an exon-splicing-enhancing element in the 5′ region of exon 10, but likewise does not impair microtubule binding (D'Souza et al., 1999; Hasegawa et al., 1999). The L284L silent mutation likewise strengthens exon 10 splicing by destroying the function of a splice-silencing element, and as a consequence no tau transcripts without exon 10 (i.e. 3R tau isoforms) are produced (D'Souza et al., 1999). Conversely, the ΔK280 mutation destroys the function of the splice-enhancing region and results in the abolition of transcripts containing exon 10, i.e. only 3R tau isoforms are produced (D'Souza et al., 1999). Interestingly, this mutation also affects microtubule binding and may therefore possess a dual pathogenicity.

The coding P301L and P301S mutations do not affect the splicing of exon 10 (Hutton et al., 1998; D'Souza et al., 1999) but induce conformational changes in tau molecules containing exon 10 alone that interfere with microtubule function, and lead to the specific aggregation of the mutant 4-repeat tau into fibrils (Miyasaka et al., 2001). Mutational events at

codon 296 (N296H, N296N, ΔN296) (Spillantini et al., 2000; Stanford et al., 2000; Iseki et al., 2001; Pastor et al., 2001) also lead to impaired ability of mutated (4-repeat) tau to interact with microtubules and promote fibrillogenesis (Spillantini et al., 2000; Grover et al., 2002; Yoshida et al., 2002), though both N296H and N296N mutations increase splicing of exon 10 (Spillantini et al., 2000; Grover et al., 2002; Yoshida et al., 2002), perhaps by disrupting the exon-splicing-silencing sequence (Spillantini et al., 2000) or creating an exon-splicing-enhancing sequence (Grover et al., 2002). The ΔN296 mutation has been reported to lead to an increase (Yoshida et al., 2002) or no change (Grover et al., 2002) in exon 10 splicing.

There are also cis-acting intron splicing silencer (ISS) and intron splicing modulator (ISM) sequences extending downsteam from the 5′ splice site, encompassing nucleotides +11 to +18, and nucleotides +19 to +26 following the stem loop structure (D'Souza and Schellenberg, 2002). These act in conjunction with the splice-enhancing and splice-silencing sequences within exon 10 to collectively regulate exon 10 splicing. Damage to these ISS and ISM sequences should mimic the action of +12, +13, +14 and +16 point mutations (D'Souza and Schellenberg, 2002). Indeed, two Australian families with FTD have recently been described (Stanford et al., 2003) with mutations at positions +19 and +29 in the 5′ splice donor region of exon 10 which have been claimed to destroy the function of the ISM sequence, leading to the abolition of exon 10 splicing and thereby reducing splicing of exon 10, decreasing the proportion of 4R tau isoforms (Stanford et al., 2003), analogous to ΔK280 mutation (D'Souza et al., 1999). However, the +29 change has also been reported in controls (D'Souza et al., 1999; Poorkaj et al., 2001; Stanford et al., 2003; Hutton, personal communication) and may be a rare (coincidental) polymorphism. The +19 variant has not been reported in controls and may be pathogenic.

54.1.1.3 FOUNDER EFFECTS OF TAU MUTATIONS

Other than the above mutational events associated with FTLD, tau is 'naturally' subject to multiple polymorphic changes in exons 1, 2, 3, 7, 9 and 11 (Baker et al., 1999). These natural variations are usually in complete linkage dysequilibrium, being co-inherited as two common haplotypes H1 and H2; H1 has a frequency of 78.4 per cent in the normal Caucasian population. The P301L tau mutation is the most common FTLD mutation to date, being present worldwide in many families with French or Dutch ancestry (Hutton et al., 1998; Houlden et al., 1999a; Rizzu et al., 1999; Rosso et al., 2003; Sobrido et al., 2003). Because many of these families share the less common H2 haplotype on the disease gene, it is likely that they might share a common founder. However, Japanese families with P301L tau mutation share the extended H1 haplotype, implying separate founders. The presence of other varying tau polymorphisms under H1 haplotype unique to the Japanese population within P301L subjects suggests multiple founders. The P301S mutation has been reported in German (Sperfeld et al., 1999), Jewish-Algerian (Werber et al.,

2003) and Japanese (Yasuda *et al.*, 2000a) patients, but these are unlikely to be all related to a common founder. Hence, P301L and P301S tau mutations have probably arisen separately on multiple occasions, this particular codon being especially susceptible to mutagenesis.

The N279K mutation has been described in American (Clark *et al.*, 1998; Tsuboi *et al.*, 2002), French (Delisle *et al.*, 1998) and Japanese (Yasuda *et al.*, 1999) families but it is unlikely that any of these kindreds are related (Tsuboi *et al.*, 2002) with this particular mutation also having arisen independently on at least three occasions.

Haplotype analysis (Pickering-Brown *et al.*, 2004a) has shown a likely common founder for British, North American and Australian families with +16 splice site mutation. Indeed, even today, many of the British families with this mutation live in, or have originated from, North Wales, a rural and relatively remote region of United Kingdom. It is therefore quite likely that the founder with this mutation lived in this part of United Kingdom with 'spread' of the mutation into industrialized regions of the country during the Industrial Revolution.

54.1.2 Other genetic changes in FTLD

54.1.2.1 OTHER AUTOSOMAL DOMINANT MUTATIONS

Tau mutations only account for about 10–20 per cent cases of FTLD (Houlden *et al.*, 1999a; Rizzu *et al.*, 1999; Poorkaj *et al.*, 2001; Rosso *et al.*, 2003), but the frequency of these remains around 40 per cent when only cases with previous family history of similar disease consistent with autosomal dominance are considered (Rizzu *et al.*, 1999). Hence, other genetic loci may be associated with FTLD.

Indeed, there are at least five well described, definitely chromosome 17-linked, families in which no mutational event within tau has as yet been determined (Basun *et al.*, 1997; Froelich *et al.*, 1997; Lendon *et al.*, 1998; Rosso *et al.*, 2001; Rademakers *et al.*, 2002; Froelich Fabre *et al.*, 2003). Interestingly, in these families no insoluble aggregates of tau are seen either biochemically or histopathologically though ubiquitin positive inclusions may be variably present in some family members of at least three of these families (Rosso *et al.*, 2001; Rademakers *et al.*, 2002; Froelich Fabre *et al.*, 2003). Although intensive candidate gene investigations within the chromosome 17-linked region, including tau, has been performed in at least two of these families (Rademakers *et al.*, 2002; Froelich Fabre *et al.*, 2003), no disease-associated mutations have yet been detected. It remains possible therefore that in these particular families changes within promoter or regulatory elements within tau may be causal. Indeed, there may be (many) other 'tau-negative' FTLD families, with or without ubiquitin pathology, that share this presently unknown change on chromosome 17.

Alternatively, there may be genetic loci associated with autosomal dominant FTLD on chromosomes other than 17. In this latter respect linkage to chromosome 9 in several families clinically sharing an FTD and MND phenotype (also

known as frontotemporal dementia with ubiquitin inclusions) has been claimed (Hosler *et al.*, 2000) but not confirmed (Ostojic *et al.*, 2003). In one family with pathologically typical FTD and MND no definite linkage to chromosome 9q21–22 (or to chromosomes 17 or 3) was detected (Savioz *et al.*, 2003). Similarly, no linkage to chromosome 17 was found in another family with FTD and MND pathological phenotype (Kertesz *et al.*, 2000), but it is not known whether this family is linked to chromosome 9 or not.

Linkage to chromosome 3p11–12 has been reported in a Danish family showing FTD with frontotemporal atrophy, neuronal loss and gliosis, with a few tau immunoreactive neurofibrillary tangles in the absence of senile (amyloid) plaques (Gydesen *et al.*, 2002; Yancopoulou *et al.*, 2003). The significance of this particular family to the pathogenesis of FTD in general remains unknown, and it is possible that this family might represent a genetic change private to this geographically isolated kindred. Similarly, in a large Calabrian family with FTD phenotype, linkage studies excluded the above loci on chromosomes 3 and 9 but gave indeterminate data for chromosome 17 (Curcio *et al.*, 2002). Complicating matters is the finding of linkage to a different region of chromosome 9 in four families with hereditary inclusion body myopathy, Paget disease and frontotemporal dementia (Kovach *et al.*, 2001), but in these the brain pathology description is limited and does not appear to conform to FTLD.

Given the shortage of families of this kind for linkage and the lack of obvious candidate genes, this represents a difficult, but evolving, area of research that will be important in furthering our understanding of FTLD, providing insight into the pathogenetic mechanism underpinning the pathology in those cases where aggregation and accumulation of insoluble tau proteins are not the cardinal features.

54.1.2.2 TAU HAPLOTYPES AS GENETIC RISK FACTORS FOR FTLD

Possession of the H1 tau haplotype been associated with other neurodegenerative disorders characterized by tau pathology such as PSP and CBD. However, it is not clear whether this haplotype is acting simply as a marker for a more relevant change in a nearby gene or defining pathogenic changes in tau with which this is in linkage dysequilibrium. While the H1 tau haplotype and the H1H1 tau genotype may be overall increased in patients with clinically diagnosed FTD (Verpillat *et al.*, 2002, but see Sobrido *et al.*, 2003), other studies suggest this increase may be accentuated in patients with apolipoprotein E (ApoE) ε4 allele (Short *et al.*, 2002) or microvacuolar-type, rather than Pick-type, histology (Hughes *et al.*, 2003). An increase in the frequency of H2H2 tau genotype in cases with Pick-histology has been claimed (Russ *et al.*, 2001), but not confirmed (Morris *et al.*, 2002; Hughes *et al.*, 2003). Similarly, an increase in H2 tau haplotype frequency in SD, but not in PA or FTD, has been reported (Short *et al.*, 2002) but not confirmed (Hughes *et al.*, 2003). It is likely that differences in patient cohort size and ethnicity, and the use of clinically diagnosed, as opposed to autopsy verified, cases of FTLD with possible mixing of clinical and pathological sub-types have all contributed to the present lack of clear vision as to the role of tau haplotypes in FTLD. Further studies on carefully chosen clinical and pathological subgroups are therefore needed to define the association between tau hap-lotypes and FTLD.

While the tau H1H1 genotype may play a role in promot-ing, or at least predisposing towards the tau pathology of PSP and CBD in the form of NFT predominantly composed of 4R tau, the possible increase in H1H1 tau genotype in FTD from microvacuolar-histology is interesting, since in this particular pathological form of FTLD no insoluble tau species are present. This suggests therefore that, in this instance, the H1 haplotype is operating via a different mechanism, or that it is merely serving as a marker for an (as yet) unidentified susceptibility locus that is either present on the tau H1 hap-lotype itself, or on a nearby gene.

54.1.2.3 APOLIPOPROTEIN E (ApoE) ε4 ALLELE AS A RISK FACTOR

Although it is well known that the ApoE ε4 allele is a risk fac-tor for late onset sporadic and familial AD, the consensus seems to indicate that possession of this does not overall increase the risk of FTLD (Pickering-Brown et al., 2000b; Short et al., 2002; Verpillat et al., 2002). Nonetheless, within FTLD it is possible that ApoE ε4 allele frequency is raised in certain clinical subgroups. Short et al. (2002) reported ApoE ε4 allele frequency to be increased in patients with SD, com-pared with those with FTD and PA, though Pickering-Brown et al. (2000b) found this to be normal in FTD and SD, but tended to be increased in PA. Interactions between the tau haplotypes and ApoE ε4 allele have been variously claimed (Ingelson et al., 2001; Short et al., 2002) but not always con-firmed (Hughes et al., 2003). Further studies are needed to validate any such putative interactions.

In contrast to AD, possession of ApoE ε4 allele does not affect age at onset of disease (or duration of illness) in either sporadic FTLD (Pickering-Brown et al., 2000b; Short et al., 2002) or FTDP-17 (Houlden et al., 1999b; Pickering-Brown et al., 2002; Tsuboi et al., 2003). Hence it seems unlikely that ApoE ε4 allele acts either as a risk factor or disease modifier in FTLD generally or FTDP-17 specifically, but it remains possible that this may play a part in other clinical subtypes such as SD or PA.

Results from small series of FTLD patients have suggested ApoE ε2 allele might act as a risk factor (Lehmann et al., 2000; Verpillat et al., 2002), but again this remains to be sub-stantiated (Pickering-Brown et al., 2000b).

54.2 THE PATHOLOGY OF FRONTOTEMPORAL LOBAR DEGENERATION

Within FTLD, there are wide variations in the gross patho-logical appearance of the brain and in the underlying histological changes. To a large extent, the gross anatomical changes can be correlated with the clinical phenotype, though at tissue level variations in histological appearance do not necessarily correlate with, nor predict, the clinical or genetic phenotype.

54.2.1 The gross pathology of FTD

There is nothing distinctive to distinguish the pattern of brain atrophy in cases of FTD with tau mutations from those of FTD without such mutations. Indeed, despite the large range of mutations, and the differing underlying pathogenetic mechanisms and histopathological changes associated with coding or splice site mutations, the gross pathological changes within the brain in patients with FTD with tau mutations are also remarkably consistent. Furthermore, is it not possible to distinguish cases of 'sporadic' FTD owing to microvacuolar-type histology from those with Pick-type histology, either on the basis of brain weight or pattern of cerebral atrophy (Mann and South, 1993; Schofield et al., 2003). Hence, on external inspection alone, it cannot be predicted whether tau mutation will be present, nor whether Pick- or microvacuolar-type histology will occur.

Most patients with FTLD have a brain weight ranging within 1000–1250 g, though instances where this falls (well) below 1000 g are not uncommon (Lantos et al., 2002). Weight loss is due to atrophy involving mostly the frontal, anterior parietal, cingulate, insular and temporal regions of the cere-bral cortex, sometimes so severe as to produce 'knife-edge' atrophy (Plates 23 and 24). Usually the frontal and temporal lobes are equivalently affected, though the temporal lobes can be more affected in FTDP-17 cases when Pick-type pathology is involved (Rizzini et al., 2000; Neumann et al., 2001; Rosso et al., 2002; Pickering-Brown et al., 2004b). The pattern of cerebral atrophy generally appears symmetrical, or some-times displays a slightly greater involvement of the left cere-bral hemisphere. Even in extreme cases, motor, sensorimotor and posterior cerebral cortical regions, and the cerebellum and brain stem, are largely unaffected. Conspicuously, the super-ior temporal gyrus is often spared (Plate 24). The distinction between grey and white matter in atrophic areas is usually well maintained, although in severe cases there can be a great loss of axons and myelin, and the white matter becomes brown-ish in colour and soft and 'rubbery' in texture. The hippocam-pus and amygdala are frequently atrophic, as is the caudate nucleus, though the putamen, globus pallidus and thalamus are less affected. The corpus callosum is usually thinned, par-ticularly anteriorly. The lateral ventricles are much enlarged though the temporal horns are little changed, except in severe cases. In most instances the substantia nigra, and sometimes also the locus caeruleus, are noticeably underpigmented. The cerebellum usually appears normal. This typical pattern of brain atrophy is illustrated diagrammatically in Plate 25.

Nonetheless, when the disorder is terminated early, or in FTD cases where disinhibition remains the principal clinical symptom, even terminally, a preferential atrophy of the inferior frontal and anterior temporal gyri is seen (Snowden *et al.*, 1996). When stereotypic behaviours dominate in FTD, a marked striatal atrophy, particularly of the caudate nucleus, is present with lesser neocortical involvement, which in turn can be focused either on frontal or temporal lobes or involve both (Snowden *et al.*, 1996).

Cases of FTD and MND share a similar topography of brain atrophy to those with FTD alone though the severity of the atrophy is often less (Mann and South, 1993), possibly reflecting the shorter disease duration common among such cases. In most instances brain weight is reduced only little, to around 1250 g. Typically, the substantia nigra is underpigmented (Snowden *et al.*, 1996).

Cases of FTLD with a progressive language disorder of either a fluent aphasia (SD) or a non-fluent aphasia (PPA) may show preferential, bilateral atrophy of the temporal lobes or a grossly asymmetrical left hemispheric involvement, respectively (Snowden *et al.*, 1996). In PAX there is preferential involvement of the motor and premotor cortices.

These differing clinical syndromes reflect the topographical distribution of the brain pathology rather than the underlying histological nature.

54.2.2   The histopathology of FTLD

Histopathological changes underlying FTLD can vary widely and several patterns of histological change have been identified. In some instances the histological changes are tightly associated with a particular clinical form of FTLD, and indeed may be taken as the specific diagnostic features of that condition (e.g. some forms of FTLD with tau mutations and cases of MNDID), whereas in other instances the underlying histological changes cross over into more than one of the clinical phenotypes. These histological profiles are:

- tau mutation (FTDP-17)-type
- Pick-type
- microvacuolar type (DLDH-type)
- ubiquitin-type (MNDID-type).

54.2.2.1   HISTOLOGY OF FTD WITH *TAU* MUTATIONS

By conventional neurohistology, many cases of FTD owing to tau mutations show a microvacuolar type of histology with spongiosis of the outer cortical laminae (Lantos *et al.*, 2002; Pickering-Brown *et al.*, 2002), from shrinkage and severe loss of pyramidal nerve cell bodies and their processes (dendrites) from cortical layers II and III. Astrocytosis is usually mild and largely subpial. Loss of nerve cells from deeper laminae is less pronounced with many neurones being shrunken. Occasional swollen, chromatolytic (ballooned) neurones are seen, especially in layers V and VI. Conversely, other cases display a more severe and widespread neuronal loss with florid transcortical astrocytosis. Intraneuronal inclusion bodies can be seen and ballooned neurones are widely present.

However, it is by immunohistochemistry using antibodies to phosphorylated forms of tau protein that FTD in patients with tau mutations can be best distinguished both from other forms of FTLD and from each other according to the particular tau mutation they bear. Although all cases show a deposition of insoluble, aggregated tau proteins within neurones and (sometimes) glial cells of the cerebral cortex and other brain regions, there are nevertheless distinctive features to the tau pathology that fall into two histological patterns according to mutation type:

- FTDP-17 cases with microvacuolar histological changes are generally associated with mutations in and around the exon 10 splice site (i.e. S305S, S305N, +3, +11, +12, +13, +14 and +16 splice site mutations) and in these neurofibrillary tangle (NFT)-like structures within large and smaller pyramidal cells of cortical layers III and V (Plate 26a), and prominently within glial cells in the deep white matter, globus pallidus and internal capsule (Plate 26b) are seen (Lantos *et al.*, 2002; Pickering-Brown *et al.*, 2002). Typically, these NFT-like structures are 'classically' stained with phospho-dependent antibodies (e.g. AT8) against residues Ser202/Thr205 but not antibodies (e.g. 12E8) against Ser262 (Pickering-Brown *et al.*, 2002). Neurones within subcortical structures, such as corpus striatum, medial thalamus, nucleus basalis of Meynert, dorsal raphe, pontine and dentate nuclei, locus caeruleus and substantia nigra, can also be affected by neurofibrillary degeneration, but less severely so, and are similarly immunoreactive (for tau) as cortical neurones (Lantos *et al.*, 2002; Pickering-Brown *et al.*, 2002). However, in one patient with S305N mutation, Pick-type bodies not NFT were present within neurones (Kobayashi *et al.*, 2003b). Cases with P301L mutation show more neuronal than glial tau pathology (Mirra *et al.*, 1999) and N296H mutation more glial than neuronal pathology (Iseki *et al.*, 2001).

- Conversely, most cases associated with missense mutations in exons 9, 11, 12 and 13 show florid astrocytosis with swollen nerve cells (Plate 26c) and neuronal inclusions (Plates 26d and 26e). Here, the insoluble tau aggregates appear as rounded structures, reminiscent of Pick bodies (Plates 26d and 26e) (Pickering-Brown *et al.*, 2000; Rizzini *et al.*, 2000; Neumann *et al.*, 2001; Rosso *et al.*, 2002) as in some sporadic forms of FTLD (Plate 26f). These are mainly present within large and small pyramidal neurones, often scattered widely throughout affected cortical regions without laminar predilection. Pick bodies are also numerous within the pyramidal cells and the granule cells of the dentate gyrus of the hippocampus (Plate 26e). Again, these structures are strongly immunoreactive with AT8 but weakly, if at all, with 1268. The swollen cells are particularly immunoreactive to AT270 (Plate 24) as well as AT8 antibody. Similar Pick body-like structures are also widely seen throughout subcortical areas, particularly the corpus striatum. Tau-positive tufted astrocytes reminiscent of those seen in PSP, neuropil threads and coiled bodies are also sometimes widely seen within the cerebral cortex in some cases (Hogg *et al.*, 2003; Kobayashi *et al.*, 2003a).

Nevertheless, other mutations in exons 12 and 13 (V337M and R406W) are associated with NFT, similar both in appearance and in pattern of tau immunostaining (i.e. both AT8 and 12E8 immunoreactive) to those in AD, within nerve cells, but not glial cells, of the cerebral cortex (Van Swieten *et al.*, 1999; Saito *et al.*, 2002). Conversely, the exon 1 mutation, R5H displays a tau neurofibrillary pathology principally affecting oligodendroglial cells and, to a lesser extent, astrocytes (Hayashi *et al.*, 2002), but here the tangles are AT8, but not 12E8, immunoreactive.

Why certain tau mutations produce a (wholly) neuronal pathology (as in V337M and R406W mutations) and others both neuronal and glial pathology (as in splice site mutations) is not clear. It may reflect differing patterns of cellular expression of tau with neurones expressing all six isoforms whereas glial cells express only, or predominantly, 4R tau, and so are only involved when the mutation affects exon 10 splicing or function.

54.2.2.2 PICK–TYPE HISTOLOGY

About 25 per cent cases with FTLD not associated with tau mutations display Pick-type of histology similar to that seen in cases of FTD with tau mutations, where pyramidal cell loss in the cerebral cortex and hippocampus is accompanied by a florid transcortical astrocytosis (Mann *et al.*, 1993; Schofield *et al.*, 2003) and intraneuronal inclusions (Pick bodies) and swollen (Pick) cells (Taniguchi *et al.*, 2004). However, in contrast to cases of FTD with tau mutations, the Pick bodies in sporadic FTLD are distributed in laminar fashion, mostly in cortical layers II and VI (Taniguchi *et al.*, 2004). Nonetheless, the Pick bodies in these (presumed) sporadic cases of FTLD display the same tau immunohistochemical features as those in cases of FTD with tau mutations (Taniguchi *et al.*, 2004).

54.2.2.3 MICROVACUOLAR–TYPE HISTOLOGY

This is perhaps the most common histology present in FTLD, occurring in about 75 per cent of FTLD patients, including some of those cases of FTD with tau mutations (see above) as well as clinical cases of FTD, SD or PA (Taniguchi *et al.*, 2004). In these, a microvacuolar type of histology in outer cortical laminae, mainly in layer II and upper layer III, is present. Cases of FTLD with this form of histology have also in the past been known as having dementia lacking distinctive histological features (DLDH), recognizing the lack of 'specific' pathologies like plaques, tangles, Pick or Lewy bodies in this histopathological appearance. However, it is now accepted that this pattern of change is so characteristic and consistent between cases as to make it of diagnostic relevance. The

severity of tissue damage matches closely the topographic distribution of the atrophy. Astroglial reaction is less severe, usually being confined to subpial regions or occurring at the border between grey and white matter (Mann *et al.*, 1993; Schofield *et al.*, 2003). Loss of myelin and axons is often inconspicuous, except in severely atrophic areas, and white matter astrogliosis is mild. Microglial cell reaction is confined to white matter (Schofield *et al.*, 2003).

The hippocampus is usually quite normal, although sometimes a severe loss of nerve cells from area CA1 occurs in the absence of neurofibrillary degeneration. On occasions some NFTs are present among the stellate cells of layer II of the entorhinal cortex. Despite the widespread atrophy frequently seen within the basal ganglia and amygdala, no specific histopathological changes are evident microscopically in such regions except for a variable degree of astrocytosis. In some instances, particularly in cases where stereotypic behaviours are prominent, this can be more severe and obvious neuronal loss will also have taken place. Some cases show pronounced cell loss from the substantia nigra, with residual pigment free within the neuropil or in macrophages, and grumose bodies occur when neuronal cell loss is heavy. The locus caeruleus can be affected, though is usually spared, sometimes even when nigral involvement is severe. Occasionally, scattered ubiquitinated inclusions of the type more frequently seen in FTD and MND, are present within granule cells of the dentate gyrus (Tolnay and Probst, 1995; Taniguchi *et al.*, 2004) (see below).

54.2.2.4 UBIQUITIN–TYPE (MNDID) HISTOLOGY

In many, and perhaps up to two-thirds of, patients with FTLD with microvacuolar-type histology (Taniguchi *et al.*, 2004), and indeed in some with SD (Rossor *et al.*, 2000) and PPA (Caselli *et al.*, 1993), the pathological (and sometimes clinical) features of MND have also been recorded. Here, along with the microvacuolation and mild subpial astrocytosis, ubiquitin-, but not tau-, immunoreactive intraneuronal inclusions are characteristically seen in pyramidal cells of layer II of the frontal and temporal cortex, less commonly in layers III and V. This histology has been termed MND-type (Jackson *et al.*, 1996), and such cases referred variously as ones of FTD-MND as here, MNDID, inclusions, tau and synuclein negative, ubiquitinated (ITSNU) or frontotemporal dementia with ubiquitin-positive, tau-negative inclusions.

Similar ubiquitinated inclusions are (characteristically) present in granule cells of the dentate gyrus of the hippocampus (Jackson *et al.*, 1996; Woulfe *et al.*, 2001), less commonly so in the amygdala (Anderson *et al.*, 1995). Interestingly, some cases also show ubiquitinated inclusions within the nuclei of cortical pyramidal neurones, dentate gyrus granule cells and striatal neurones (Woulfe *et al.*, 2001). The substantia nigra is nearly always damaged, often severely so showing subtotal nerve cell loss but without inclusions (Jackson *et al.*, 1996; Snowden *et al.*, 1996). A profound astrocytosis is seen and grumose bodies are frequent.

Like classic MND, the characteristic skein or rounded ubiquitin inclusions within the motor neurones of the anterior horns of the spinal cord and brain stem cranial nerve nuclei can be seen in FTD-MND, and the pattern of nerve cell loss is similar though usually milder than that of classic MND.

54.2.2.5 OTHER PATHOLOGICAL CHANGES

Senile (neuritic) plaques are generally not seen in cases of FTLD with, or without, tau mutations. However, diffuse deposits of Aβ may sometimes occur mostly within the otherwise undamaged posterior cerebral cortex. Numerically, these are not usually beyond that which might be expected for age, and are commonly associated with possession of ApoE ε4 allele (Mann et al., 2001; Lantos et al., 2002; Pickering-Brown et al., 2002).

54.2.3 Clinicopathological correlations

It is important to recognize that any one of these four histological profiles can occur in patients with FTLD, and generally it is not immediately predictable from the clinical symptomatology which pattern will underlie the clinical changes. Similarly, an underlying microvacuolar- (Snowden et al., 1996) or Pick-type (Graff-Radford et al., 1990) histopathology can occur in cases of SD and PA, though most commonly this is microvacuolar-type. The fundamental pathological process behind these latter disorders is likely to be the same as in FTD, the differing topography of change dictating the clinical symptoms present. FTD-MND in conjunction with a Pick-type histology appears to be much less common (Sam et al., 1991). However, all cases of PAX to date appear to have Pick-type histology (Snowden et al., 1996) and this condition may therefore represent a parietal lobe manifestation of a pathological process that more usually afflicts frontal and temporal lobes. Although patients with progressive anomia and progressive proposagnosia have been described clinically (Snowden and Neary, 2003) pathological analysis remains incomplete, though one patient with progressive anomia showed underlying pathology of microvacuolar-type with ubiquitin inclusions in frontal cortex and hippocampus (Mann, unpublished data).

54.3 TAU BIOCHEMISTRY IN FRONTOTEMPORAL LOBAR DEMENTIA

54.3.1 Tau biochemistry in FTD with tau mutations

By Western blotting, the insoluble tau aggregates that accumulate in the brain as Pick-like bodies in neurones, and sometimes within glial cells and neuropil threads, in cases with missense mutations in exons 9 (K257T, L266V, G272V), 11 (S309N, L315P), 12 (G336R, G342V) and 13 (K369I, G389R)

are composed of variable mixtures of 3R and 4R tau species, sometimes with a preponderance of 4R species (Murrell et al., 1999; Lippa et al., 2000; Neumann et al., 2001; Pickering-Brown et al., 2001; Kobayashi et al., 2003a), but on other occasions more 3R is present (Rizzini et al., 2000; Hogg et al., 2003). The reasons for these differences in tau isoform composition remain unclear but may relate to the particular conformational properties to the tau molecules that each mutation imposes.

On the other hand, mutations in and around the stem loop structure at the exon 10 splice site (N279K, L284L, P301L, P301S and S305N plus +3, +11, +12, +13, +14 and +16 form insoluble tau aggregates) contain mostly 4R tau (Pickering-Brown et al., 2002), as do R5H and R5L mutations (Poorkaj et al., 2001; Hayashi et al., 2002).

In V337M and R406W, the insoluble tau aggregates are composed of an equal mixture of 3R and 4R tau (Hong et al., 1998; Hutton et al., 1998; Poorkaj et al., 1998; Rizzu et al., 1999; Van Swieten et al., 1999), similar to the paired helical filaments of AD.

54.3.2 Tau biochemistry in FTLD not associated with tau mutations

As in cases of FTD with tau mutations and Pick bodies, cases of sporadic FTLD with Pick histology show variable patterns of tau isoform by both western blotting and immunohistochemistry. In many instances, western blotting shows the insoluble tau is composed mostly, or even exclusively, of 3R tau isoforms (Delacourte et al., 1998), although on other occasions substantial quantities of 4R tau are present (Arai et al., 2001; Ikeda et al., 2002; Zhukareva et al., 2002; Taniguchi et al., 1994). As in some cases of FTD with tau mutations with Pick bodies (Hogg et al., 2003; Pickering-Brown et al., 2004b) the Pick bodies in such sporadic FTLD cases are in fact immunoreactive only with 3R, and not 4R, tau-specific antibodies (even though both 3R and 4R tau isoforms are detectable on western blotting (Arai et al., 2001; Ikeda et al., 2002), because of the presence of 4R tau isoforms in glial cells and neuropil threads, which show up on western blot. However, other immunohistochemical studies on cases showing 4R tau isoforms by western blot have revealed the Pick bodies also to contain 4R tau (Zhukareva et al., 2002). Hence, as in FTD with tau mutations, the precise tau isoform composition of Pick bodies in sporadic FTLD can vary greatly; why this biochemical heterogeneity of tau should occur remains unclear.

Cases of FTD, FTD and MND, SD and PPA not due to mutations in tau, but showing microvacuolar histology, display either no, or only trace amounts of, insoluble tau on western blot (Zhukareva et al., 2001, 2003; Taniguchi et al., 2004). When present, this tau is comprised of all six tau isoforms, consistent with the presence of rare (age-related) NFTs seen on immunohistochemistry (Taniguchi et al., 2004). However, there is considerable loss of soluble tau proteins

(Zhukareva *et al.*, 2000, 2003; Adamec *et al.*, 2001; Taniguchi *et al.*, 2004), both in microvacuolar- and Pick-type histological cases. Because this loss of soluble tau is paralleled by loss of other soluble neuronal perikaryal markers, and because similar losses of soluble tau are seen in severe cases of AD, Huntington's disease and FTD with tau mutations (Taniguchi *et al.*, 2004), it is more likely that this loss of soluble tau in FTLD reflects a broad neurodegeneration that carries tau proteins in its wake along with many other cellular proteins.

54.4 DIAGNOSTIC CONSIDERATIONS

54.4.1 How far does the FTLD phenotype extend?

A chromosome 3-linked family with FTD (Gydesen *et al.*, 2002) shows similar 'non-specific' features of FTLD, like neuronal loss and gliosis, sometimes with (a few) neurofibrillary changes in the absence of neuritic plaques (Yancopoulou *et al.*, 2003). Indeed, most recently, Josephs *et al.* (2003) reported four cases of FTD with microvacuolar histology and ubiquitin inclusions, the latter also, and atypically so for FTD/FTD and MND, being reactive with antibodies against heavy and light chain neurofilament proteins, which they termed neurofilament inclusion body disease; a similar case was also reported by Bigio *et al.* (2003). Whether these potentially related conditions should be included under FTLD is, for the present, uncertain – future molecular genetic analyses may define their nosological position.

Moreover, it can be asked whether the tauopathy of FTLD can, or even should, be extended to include other non-Alzheimer forms of dementia such as PSP and CBD. The increased frequency of the tau H1 haplotype may be a genetic pointer to such inclusion. Moreover, the tangles of PSP and CBD appear as flat ribbons of 4R tau (Sergeant *et al.*, 1999), and affect both nerve cells and glial cells. Such changes are strongly reminiscent of those FTD cases associated with (splicing) changes in exon 10 of tau (Pickering-Brown *et al.*, 2002), thereby further strengthening the case for including such disorders under FTLD.

54.4.2 Diagnostic relevance of *tau* mutations

Currently, there are no clear cut family history, clinical, radiological or gross histopathological distinctions that can distinguish cases of FTD owing to tau mutations from those without such (or other) mutations, nor is it possible to predict which cases of FTD might be associated with Pick bodies and which with a microvacuolar type change. Only direct tau gene analysis can determine which cases of FTLD are due to such mutations. Yet, as we have already seen, these account for less than 10 per cent of all cases of FTD. Clearly cases of FTD with tau mutations account for a minority of FTLD, and the expectation of detecting such cases by genetic analysis

is low. This is not only of practical histopathological diagnostic relevance, but also has implications for genetic testing, not only in actual patients with FTLD, but also in (unaffected) relatives who may be at risk and concerned about predictive testing. For a successful and meaningful genetic testing service that will be of benefit to patients and relatives in terms of the knowledge or reassurance it may provide and the potential for appropriate (future) therapeutic or clinical management, it is necessary to know the full extent of the association of the tau gene with disease phenotype, and questions relating to the degree of penetrance of mutations be fully answerable. As regards the former, it is likely that the full range of mutations within coding and associated splicing regions in tau will soon become known as research into the biology of FTLD continues apace. However, there may still be many cases of FTLD where causative changes in tau are less clear cut, affecting, for example, promoter or other regulatory elements leading to (variably) increased risk of disease. As with ApoE ε4 allele in AD, the diagnostic or predictive value of such risk factors may be limited. Second, there are issues of incomplete or delayed penetrance, even within presently known tau mutations associated with FTD (Murrell *et al.*, 1999; Pickering-Brown *et al.*, 2000a, 2002; van Herpen *et al.*, 2003). There may well also be several other causative genes for FTLD, each carrying its own particular load of questions relating to association and penetrance. All of these issues (presently) reduce the utility of clinical testing for FTLD by genetics. Nonetheless, there is current, albeit low, interest in genetic testing for early onset familial dementia, including FTD (Steinbart *et al.*, 2001). Whether this demand will increase with future knowledge regarding the genetics of FTLD is uncertain. Even in genetically 'well-understood' disorders such as Huntington's disease where genetic testing within a genetic counselling service has been widely available now for many years, and clear-cut advice can be given to the benefit of patients and relatives, take-up rates of genetic testing are still relatively low.

54.4.3 Ubiquitinopathy or tauopathy?

In the absence of any laboratory test based on the levels of pathological (i.e. phosphorylated) tau in blood, serum or cerebrospinal fluid that can unequivocally distinguish cases of FTLD from healthy controls, or from cases with other tauopathies such as AD, neuropathology remains the 'gold standard' for diagnosis. Nonetheless, here too there are pathological heterogeneity and nosological uncertainties that cloud diagnostic precision. Evaluations of autopsy-based series (Rosso *et al.*, 2003; Taniguchi *et al.*, 2004) show that cases with tau-based pathology (tauopathy) within FTLD only account for up to about 45 per cent cases. Of those with tau-positive inclusions, about half will have Pick bodies, but not be associated with a mutation in tau, with the remainder being associated with tau mutations displaying either a Pick-type histology or a NFT-type histology depending upon the mutation in question. Of the 55 per cent or more cases with non-tau (microvacuolar) histology, as many as half to two-thirds of these will have also ubiquitin-positive inclusions, seemingly making this the most common pathological form underlying FTLD.

However, the diagnostic relevance of these ubiquitin inclusions is not clear, nor is it certain that they are indexing the same cellular change in all instances. Apart from their widespread presence within frontal and hippocampal neurones in cases which have now become classed as FTD and MND (MNDID, ITSNU or frontotemporal dementia with ubiquitin inclusions), they are also present in these same brain regions (but less severely so) in cases of FTD without MND (see above), as well as in cases of MND alone (Kawashima et al., 2001; Mackenzie and Feldman, 2003). This suggests patients with FTD, but not MND, and MND alone, may represent polar points on an evolving pathological continuum, which eventually leads from either direction into the 'merging' pathology of FTD and MND. A cognitive change (perhaps eventually evolving into dementia) within classic MND may go thus unrecognized in many instances. Indeed frontal and temporal lobe deficits by SPECT in many cognitively normal patients with MND suggest the presence of preclinical changes in the frontal lobes, possibly commensurate with the (early) presence of ubiquitin inclusions.

54.5 OUTSTANDING ISSUES

Within the putative entity of FTLD, a spectrum of clinical and pathological phenotypes can be entered, all of which share, to a greater or lesser extent, a non-Alzheimer-type of histological profile characterized by cerebral cortical neuronal loss, gliosis and microvacuolar change, with or without intraneuronal tau or ubiquitin inclusions, along with subcortical glial and neuronal tau pathology and a (severe) degeneration of the substantia nigra. Such overlaps argue strongly for aetiopathogenetic interrelationships. Nonetheless, it remains to be established how much of the FTLD spectrum relates to a 'tau pathology' of some kind or other. For example, are cases of sporadic FTLD where no tau inclusions are present related to deleterious imbalances in regulatory elements of tau gene, which detrimentally disturb the normal levels, or stoichiometric composition, of tau proteins? Furthermore, how do disorders like MND-FTD, PA and SD, where ubiquitin inclusions are commonplace, relate genetically and biochemically to FTLD with tau inclusions? To date, no mutations in tau have been identified in patients with these particular disease phenotypes. What is the significance of the ubiquitin inclusions in FTD (SD/PA) + MND, and what is the key protein present within such inclusions that is being 'tagged' by the ubiquitin? Answers here will be critical to our understanding of the causative mechanism behind this form of FTLD, and will help to pin-point responsible genetic changes,

and clarify nosology with respect to cases of FTLD associated with tau inclusions.

The challenge to define and classify these non-Alzheimer forms of dementia, some of which manifest as FTLD, others as differing neuropsychological syndromes, remains to be completed. To date at least three major clinical syndromes, FTD, SD and PA, each combined or not with MND, can be included under FTLD, as well as less common disorders such as PAX, progressive anomia and progressive prosopagnosia. Maybe PSP and CBD should also be included under FTLD? Pathologically, there is also great heterogeneity underpinning each of these clinical syndromes, with microvacuolar-type or Pick-type histologies being present, the former often being associated with ubiquitin inclusions but on other occasions not or minimally so. Some cases of FTD with microvacuolar changes are associated with mutations in tau, which translate into distinctive tau pathology, but these are relatively rare within FTLD and may represent a minority cause of inherited FTLD. To what extent do other risk factors in tau, or other genes, contribute to 'sporadic' FTLD? The huge advances gained in the past 5 years through molecular genetics and biochemistry will no doubt continue to be built upon, and it will not be long before the many of the present mysteries surrounding the causes and mechanics of FTLD that confound attempts at nosology are ultimately yielded up and a proper and rational means of chemically and genetically defining these disorders becomes closer.

REFERENCES

Adamec E, Chang HT, Stopa EG et al. (2001) Tau protein expression in frontotemporal dementias. Neuroscience Letters 315: 21–24

Anderson VER, Cairns NJ, Leigh PN. (1995) Involvement of the amygala, dentate and hippocampus in motor neuron disease. Journal of the Neurological Sciences 129: 75–78

Arai T, Ikeda K, Akiyama H et al. (2001) Distinct isoforms of tau aggregated in neurones and glial cells in brains of patients with Pick's disease, corticobasal degeneration and progressive supranuclear palsy. Acta Neuropathologica 101: 167–173

Baker M, Litvan I, Houlden H et al. (1999) Association of an extended haplotype in the tau gene with progressive supranuclear palsy. Human Molecular Genetics 8: 711–715

Basun H, Almkvist O, Axelman K et al. (1997) Clinical characteristics of a chromosome 17-linked rapidly progressive familial frontotemporal dementia. Archives of Neurology 54: 539–544

Bigio EH, Lipton AM, White CL et al. (2003) Frontotemporal and motor neurone degeneration with neurofilament inclusion bodies: additional evidence for overlap between FTD and ALS. Neuropathology and Applied Neurobiology 29: 239–253

Caselli RJ, Windebank AJ, Petersen RC et al. (1993) Rapidly progressive aphasic dementia and motor neuron disease. Annals of Neurology 33: 200–207

Clark LN, Poorkaj P, Wzsolek Z et al. (1998) Pathogenic implications of mutations in the tau gene in pallido-ponto-nigral degeneration and related neurodegenerative disorders linked to chromosome 17. Proceedings of the National Academy of Sciences of the United States of America 95: 13103–13107

Curcio SAM, Kawarai T, Paterson AD *et al.* (2002) A large Calabrian kindred segregating frontotemporal dementia. *Journal of Neurology* **249**: 911–922

Delacourte A, Sergeant N, Wattez A *et al.* (1998) Vulnerable neuronal subsets in Alzheimer's and Pick's disease are distinguished by their tau isoform distribution and phosphorylation. *Annals of Neurology* **43**: 193–204

Delisle MB, Murrell JR, Richardson R *et al.* (1999) A mutation at codon 279 (N279K) in exon 10 of *Tau* gene causes a tauopathy with dementia and supranuclear palsy. *Acta Neuropathologica* **98**: 62–77

D'Souza I and Schellenberg GD. (2002) *Tau* exon 10 expression involves a bipartite intron 10 regulatory sequence and weak 5' and 3' splice sites. *Journal of Biological Chemistry* **277**: 26587–26599

D'Souza I, Poorkaj P, Hong M *et al.* (1999) Missense and silent *tau* gene mutations cause frontotemporal dementia with parkinsonism-chromosome 17 type, by affecting multiple alternative splicing regulatory elements. *Proceedings of the National Academy of Sciences of the United States of America* **96**: 5598–5603

Dumanchin C, Camuzat C, Campion D *et al.* (1998) Segregation of a missense mutation in the microtubule-associated protein *tau* gene with familial frontotemporal dementia with parkinsonism. *Human Molecular Genetics* **7**: 1825–1829

Froelich S, Basun H, Forsel C *et al.* (1997) Mapping of a disease locus for familial rapidly progressive frontotemporal dementia to chromosome 17q 20–21. *American Journal of Medical Genetics* **74**: 380–385

Froelich Fabre S, Axelman P, Almkvist A *et al.* (2003) Extended investigation of *tau* and mutation screening of other candidate genes on chromosome 17q21 in a Swedish FTDP-17 family. *American Journal of Medical Genetics Part B (Neuropsychiatric Genetics)* **121B**: 112–118

Goedert M, Jakes R, Crowther RA. (1999a) Effects of frontotemporal dementia FTDP-17 mutations on heparin-induced assembly of tau filaments. *FEBS Letters* **450**: 306–311

Goedert M, Spillantini MG, Crowther RA *et al.* (1999b) *Tau* gene mutation in familial progressive subcortical gliosis. *Nature Medicine* **5**: 454–457

Graff-Radford NR, Damasio AR, Hyman BT *et al.* (1990) Progressive aphasia in a patient with Pick's disease: a neuropsychological, radiologic and anatomic study. *Neurology* **40**: 620–626

Grover A, De Ture M, Yen S-H, Hutton M. (2002) Effects on splicing and protein function of three mutations in codon N296 of tau in vitro. *Neuroscience Letters* **323**: 33–36

Grover A, Englund E, Baker M *et al.* (2003) A novel *tau* mutation in exon 9 (I260V) causes a 4-repeat tauopathy. *Experimental Neurology* **184**: 131–140

Gydesen S, Brown JM, Brun A *et al.* (2002) Chromosome 3 linked frontotemporal dementia (FTD-3). *Neurology* **59**: 1585–1594

Hasegawa M, Smith MJ, Goedert M. (1998) Tau proteins with FTDP-17 mutations have a reduced ability to promote microtubule assembly. *FEBS Letters* **437**: 207–210

Hasegawa M, Smith MJ, Iijima M *et al.* (1999) FTDP-17 mutations N279K and S305N in tau produce increased splicing of exon 10. *FEBS Letters* **443**: 93–96

Hayashi S, Toyoshima Y, Hasegawa M *et al.* (2002) Late-onset frontotemporal dementia with a novel exon 1 (Arg5His) *tau* gene mutation. *Annals of Neurology* **51**: 525–530

Hogg M, Grujic ZM, Baker M *et al.* (2003) The L266V tau mutation is associated with frontotemporal dementia and Pick-like 3R and 4R tauopathy. *Acta Neuropathologica* **106**: 323–336

Hong M, Zhukareva V, Vogelsberg-Ragaglia V *et al.* (1998) Mutation-specific functional impairments in distinct *tau* isoforms of hereditary FTDP-17. *Science* **282**: 1914–1917

Hosler B, Siddique T, Sapp PC *et al.* (2000) Linkage of familial amyotrophic lateral sclerosis with frontotemporal dementia to chromosome 9q21–22. *JAMA* **284**: 1664–1669

Houlden H, Baker M, Adamson J *et al.* (1999a) Frequency of *tau* mutations in three series of non-Alzheimer's degenerative dementia. *Annals of Neurology* **46**: 243–248

Houlden H, Rizzu P, Stevens M *et al.* (1999b) Apolipoprotein E genotype does not affect age at onset of dementia in families with defined *tau* mutations. *Neuroscience Letters* **260**: 193–195

Hughes A, Mann D, Pickering-Brown SM. (2003) *Tau* haplotype frequency in frontotemporal lobar degeneration and amyotrophic lateral sclerosis. *Experimental Neurology* **181**: 12–16

Hutton M, Lendon CL, Rizzu P *et al.* (1998) Association of missense and 5'-splice-site mutations in *tau* with the inherited dementia FTDP-17. *Nature* **393**: 702–705

Iijima M, Tabira T, Poorkaj P *et al.* (1999) A distinct familial presenile dementia with a novel missense mutation in the *tau* gene. *NeuroReport* **10**: 497–501

Ikeda K, Akiyama H, Arai T, Tsuchiya K. (2002) Pick-body-like inclusions in corticobasal degeneration differ from Pick bodies in Pick's disease. *Acta Neuropathologica* **103**: 115–118

Ingelson M, Fabre SF, Lilius L *et al.* (2001) Increased risk for frontotemporal dementia through interaction between tau polymorphisms and apolipoprotein E epsilon4. *NeuroReport* **12**: 905–909

Iseki E, Matsumura T, Marui W *et al.* (2001) Familial frontotemporal dementia and parkinsonismwith a novel N296H mutation in exon 10 of the *tau* gene and a widespread tau accumulation in glial cells. *Acta Neuropathologica* **102**: 285–292

Jackson M, Lennox G, Lowe J. (1996) Motor neurone disease-inclusion dementia. *Neurodegeneration* **5**: 339–350

Josephs KA, Holton JL, Rossor MN *et al.* (2003) Neurofilament inclusion body disease: a new proteinopathy? *Brain* **126**: 2291–2303

Kawashima T, Doh-ura K, Kikuchi H, Iwaki T. (2001) Cognitive dysfunction in patients with amyotrohic lateral sclerosis is associated with spherical or crescent-shaped ubiquitinated intraneuronal inclusions in the parahippocampal gyrus and amygdala, but not in the neostriatum. *Acta Neuropathologica* **102**: 467–472

Kertesz A, Kawarai T, Rogaeva E *et al.* (2000) Familial frontotemporal dementia with ubiquitin-positive, tau-negative inclusions. *Neurology* **54**: 818–827

Kobayashi K, Kidani T, Ujike H *et al.* (2003a) Another phenotype of frontotemporal dementia and parkinsonism linked to chromosome-17 (FTDP-17) with a missense mutation of S305N closely resembling Pick's disease. *Journal of Neurology* **250**: 990–992

Kobayashi T, Ota S, Tanaka K *et al.* (2003b) A novel L266V mutation of the *tau* gene causes frontotemporal dementia with unique tau pathology. *Annals of Neurology* **53**: 133–137

Kovach MJ, Waggoner B, Leal SM *et al.* (2001) Clinical delineation and localisation to chromosome 9p13.3-p12 of a unique dominant disorder in four families: Hereditary inclusion body myopathy, Paget disease of bone, and frontotemporal dementia. *Molecular Genetics and Metabolism* **74**: 458–475

Kowalska A, Hasegawa M, Miyamoto K *et al.* (2002) A novel mutation at position +11 in the intron following exon 10 of the *tau* gene in FTDP-17. *Journal of Applied Genetics* **43**: 535–543

Lantos PL, Cairns NJ, Khan MN *et al.* (2002) Neuropathologic variation in frontotemporal dementia due to the intronic *tau* 10^{+16} mutation. *Neurology* **58**: 1169–1175

Lehmann DJ, Smith AD, Combrinck M et al. (2000) Apolipoprotein E ε2 may be a risk factor for sporadic frontotemporal dementia. *Journal of Neurology, Neurosurgery, and Psychiatry* **69**: 404–405

Lendon CL, Lynch T, Norton J et al. (1998) Hereditary dysphasic disinhibition dementia a frontotemporal dementia linked to 17q21–22. *Neurology* **50**: 1546–1555

Lippa CF, Zhukareva V, Kawarai T et al. (2000) Frontotemporal dementia with novel tau pathology and a Glu342Val mutation. *Annals of Neurology* **48**: 850–858

Mackenzie IRA and Feldman H. (2003) The relationship between extramotor ubiquitin-immunoreactive neuronal inclusions and dementia in motor neurone disease. *Acta Neuropathologica* **105**: 98–102

Mann DMA and South PW. (1993) The topographic distribution of brain atrophy in frontal lobe dementia. *Acta Neuropathologica* **85**: 335–340

Mann DMA, South PW, Snowden JS, Neary D. (1993) Dementia of frontal lobe type: neuropathology and immunohistochemistry. *Journal of Neurology, Neurosurgery, and Psychiatry* **56**: 605–614

Mann DMA, McDonagh AM, Pickering-Brown SM et al. (2001) Amyloid β protein deposition in patients with frontotemporal lobar degeneration: relationship to age and apolipoprotein E genotype. *Neuroscience Letters* **304**: 161–164

Mirra SS, Murrell JR, Gearing M et al. (1999) Tau pathology in a family with dementia and a P301L mutation in *tau*. *Journal of Neuropathology and Experimental Neurology* **58**: 335–345

Miyamoto K, Kowalska A, Hasegawa M et al. (2001) Familial frontotemporal dementia and parkinsonism with a novel mutation at intron 10 + 11 splice site in the *tau* gene. *Annals of Neurology* **50**: 117–120

Miyasaka T, Morishima-Kawashima M, Ravid R et al. (2001a) Selective deposition of mutant *tau* in the FTDP-17 brain affected by P301L mutation. *Journal of Neuropathology and Experimental Neurology* **60**: 872–884

Morris HR, Perez-Tur J, Janssen JC et al. (1999) Mutation in the tau exon 10 splice site region in familial frontotemporal dementia. *Annals of Neurology* **45**: 270–271

Morris HR, Baker M, Yasojima K et al. (2002) Analysis of *tau* haplotypes in Pick's disease. *Neurology* **59**: 443–445

Murrell JR, Spillantini MG, Zolo P et al. (1999) *Tau* gene mutation G389R causes a tauopathy with abundant pick body-like inclusions and axonal deposits. *Journal of Neuropathology and Experimental Neurology* **58**: 1207–1226

Nacharaju P, Lewis J, Easson C et al. (1999) Accelerated filament formation from tau protein with specific FTDP-17 missense mutations. *FEBS Letters* **447**: 195–199

Nasreddine ZS, Loginov M, Clark LN et al. (1999) From genotype to phenotype: a clinical, pathological and biochemical investigation of frontotemporal dementia and parkinsonism (FTDP-17) caused by the P301L *tau* gene mutation. *Annals of Neurology* **45**: 704–715

Neary D, Snowden JS, Gustafson L et al. (1998) Frontotemporal lobar degeneration: A consensus on clinical diagnostic criteria. *Neurology* **51**: 1546–1554

Neumann M, Schulz-Schaeffer W, Crowther RA et al. (2001) Pick's disease associated with the novel *tau* gene mutation K369I. *Annals of Neurology* **50**: 503–513

Ostojic J, Axelman K, Lannfelt L, Froelich-Fabre S. (2003) No evidence of linkage to chromosome 9q21–22 in a Swedish family with frontotemporal dementia and amyotrophic lateral sclerosis. *Neuroscience Letters* **340**: 245–247

Pastor P, Pastor E, Carnero C et al. (2001) Familial atypical progressive supranuclear palsy associated with homozygosity for the delN296 mutation in the *tau* gene. *Annals of Neurology* **49**: 263–267

Pickering-Brown SM, Baker M, Yen S-H et al. (2000a) Pick's disease is associated with mutations in the *tau* gene. *Annals of Neurology* **48**: 859–867

Pickering-Brown SM, Owen F, Snowden JS et al. (2000b) Apolipoprotein E ε4 allele has no effect on age at onset or duration of disease in cases of frontotemporal dementia with Pick- or microvacuolar-type histology. *Experimental Neurology* **163**: 452–456

Pickering-Brown SM, Richardson AMT, Snowden JS et al. (2002) Inherited frontotemporal dementia in nine British families associated with intronic mutations in the *tau* gene. *Brain* **125**: 732–751

Pickering-Brown SM, Baker M, Bird T et al. (2004a) Evidence of a founder effect in families with frontotemporal dementia that harbour the *tau* +16 splice mutation. *American Journal of Medical Genetics Part B Neuropsychiatric Genetics* **125B**: 79–82

Pickering-Brown SM, Baker M, Nonaka T et al. (2004b) Frontotemporal dementia with Pick-type histology associated with Q336R mutation in tau gene. *Brain* **127**: 1415–1426

Poorkaj P, Bird Th, Wijsman E et al. (1998) *Tau* is a candidate gene for chromosome 17 frontotemporal dementia. *Annals of Neurology* **43**: 815–825

Poorkaj P, Grossman M, Steinbart E et al. (2001) Frequency of *tau* gene mutations in familial and sporadic cases of non-Alzheimer dementia. *Archives of Neurology* **58**: 383–387

Rademakers R, Cruts M, Dermaut B et al. (2002) Tau-negative frontal lobe dementia at 17q21: significant finemapping of the candidate region to a 4.8-cm interval. *Molecular Psychiatry* **7**: 1064–1074

Rizzini C, Goedert M, Hodges J et al. (2000) *Tau* gene mutation K257T causes a tauopathy similar to Pick's disease. *Journal of Neuropathology and Experimental Neurology* **59**: 990–1001

Rizzu P, Van Swieten JC, Joosse M et al. (1999) High prevalence of mutations in the microtubule-associated protein tau in a population study of frontotemporal dementia in the Netherlands. *American Journal of Human Genetics* **64**: 414–421

Rosso SM, Kamphorst W, de Graaf B et al. (2001) Familial frontotemporal dementia with ubiquitin positive inclusions is linked to chromosome 17q21–22. *Brain* **124**: 1948–1957

Rosso SM, van Herpen E, Deelen W et al. (2002) A novel *tau* mutation, S320F, causes a tauopathy with inclusions similar to those in Pick's disease. *Annals of Neurology* **51**: 373–376

Rosso SM, Donker Kaat L, Baks T et al. (2003) Frontotemporal dementia in the Netherlands: patient characteristics and prevalence estimates from a population based study. *Brain* **126**: 2016–2022

Rossor MN, Revesz T, Lantos PL, Warrington EK. (2000) Semantic dementia with ubiquitin-positive tau-negative inclusion bodies. *Brain* **123**: 267–276

Russ C, Lovestone S, Baker M et al. (2001) The extended haplotype of the microtubule associated protein *tau* gene is not associated with Pick's disease. *Neuroscience Letters* **299**: 156–158

Saito Y, Geyer A, Sasaki R et al. (2002) Early-onset, rapidly progressive familial tauopathy with R406W mutation. *Neurology* **58**: 811–813

Sam M, Gutmann L, Doshi H, Schochet SS. (1991) Pick's disease: A case clinically resembling amyotrophic lateral sclerosis. *Neurology* **41**: 1831–1833

Savioz A, Riederer BM, Heutink P et al. (2003) Tau and neurofilaments in a family with frontotemporal dementia unlinked to chromosome 17q21–22. *Neurobiology of Disease* **12**: 46–55

Schofield E, Kersaitis C, Shepherd CE *et al.* (2003) Severity of gliosis in Pick's disease and frontotemporal lobar degeneration: tau-positive glia differentiate these disorders. *Brain* **126**: 827–840

Sergeant N, Wattez A, Delacourte A. (1999) Neurofibrillary degeneration in progressive supranuclear palsy and corticobasal degeneration: tau pathologies with exclusively 'exon 10' isoforms. *Journal of Neurochemistry* **72**: 1243–1249

Short RA, Graff-Radford NR, Adamson J *et al.* (2002) Differences in tau and Apolipoprotein E polymorphism frequencies in sporadic frontotemporal lobar degeneration syndromes. *Archives of Neurology* **59**: 611–615

Snowden JS and Neary D. (2003) Progressive anomia with preserved oral spelling and automatic speech. *Neurocase* **9**: 27–33

Snowden JS, Neary D, Mann DMA. (1996) *Fronto-Temporal Lobar Degeneration: Fronto-Temporal Dementia, Progressive Aphasia, Semantic Dementia.* Edinburgh, Churchill Livingstone, pp. 1–227

Sobrido M-J, Miller BL, Havlioglu N *et al.* (2003) Novel *tau* polymorphisms, *tau* haplotypes and splicing in familial and sporadic frontotemporal dementia. *Archives of Neurology* **60**: 698–702

Sperfeld AD, Collatz MB, Baier H *et al.* (1999) FTDP-17: an early onset phenotype and parkinsonism and epileptic seizures caused by a novel mutation. *Annals of Neurology* **46**: 708–715

Spillantini MG, Murrell JR, Goedert M *et al.* (1998) Mutation in the *tau* gene in familial multiple system tauopathy with presenile dementia. *Proceedings of the National Academy of Sciences of the United States of America* **95**: 7737–7741

Spillantini MG, Yoshida H, Rizzini C *et al.* (2000) A novel *tau* mutation (N296N) in familial dementia with swollen achromatic neurones and corticobasal inclusion bodies. *Annals of Neurology* **48**: 850–858

Stanford PM, Halliday GM, Brooks WS *et al.* (2000) Progressive supranuclear palsy pathology caused by a novel silent mutation in exon 10 of the *tau* gene: expansion of the disease phenotype caused by *tau* gene mutations. *Brain* **123**: 880–893

Stanford PM, Shepherd CE, Halliday GM *et al.* (2003) Mutations in the *tau* gene that cause an increase in three repeat tau and frontotemporal dementia. *Brain* **126**: 814–826

Steinbart EJ, Smith CO, Poorkaj P, Bird TD. (2001) Impact of DNA testing for early-onset familial Alzheimer's disease and frontotemporal dementia. *Archives of Neurology* **58**: 1828–1831

Taniguchi S, McDonagh AM, Pickering-Brown SM *et al.* (2004) The neuropathology of frontotemporal lobar degeneration with respect to the cytological and biochemical characteristics of tau protein. *Neuropathology and Applied Neurobiology* **30**: 1–18

Tolnay M and Probst A. (1995) Frontal lobe degeneration: novel ubiquitin-immunoreactive neurites within frontotemporal cortex. *Neuropathology and Applied Neurobiology* **21**: 492–497

Tolnay M, Spillantini MG, Rizzini C *et al.* (2000) A new case of frontotemporal dementia and parkinsonism resulting from an intron 10 + 3-splice site mutation in the *tau* gene: clinical and pathological features. *Neuropathology and Applied Neurobiology* **26**: 368–378

Tsuboi Y, Uitti RJ, Delisle M-B *et al.* (2002) Clinical features and disease haplotypes of individuals with the N279K *tau* gene mutation. *Archives of Neurology* **59**: 943–950

Tsuboi Y, Uitti RJ, Baker M *et al.* (2003) Clinical features of frontotemporal dementia due to the intronic *tau* 10^{+16} mutation. *Neurology* **60**: 525–526

Van Herpen E, Rosso SM, Severijnen LA *et al.* (2003) Variable phenotypic expression and extensive tau pathology in two families with the novel *tau* mutation L315R. *Annals of Neurology* **54**: 573–581

Van Swieten JC, Stevens M, Rosso SM *et al.* (1999) Phenotypic variation in hereditary frontotemporal dementia with tau mutations. *Annals of Neurology* **46**: 617–626

Verpillat P, Camuzat A, Hannequin D *et al.* (2002) Association between the extended *tau* haplotype and frontotemporal dementia. *Archives of Neurology* **59**: 935–939

Werber E, Klein C, Grunfeld J, Rabey JM. (2003) Phenotypic presentation of frontotemporal dementia with parkinsonism-chromosome 17 type P301S in a patient of Jewish-Algerian origin. *Movement Disorders* **18**: 595–598

Woulfe J, Kertesz A, Munoz D. (2001) Frontotemporal dementia with ubiquitinated cytoplasmic and intranuclear inclusions. *Acta Neuropathologica* **102**: 94–102

Yancopoulou D, Crowther A, Chakrabarti L *et al.* (2003) Tau protein in frontotemporal dementia linked to chromosome 3 (FTD-3). *Journal of Neuropathology and Experimental Neurology* **62**: 878–882

Yasuda M, Kawamata T, Komure O *et al.* (1999) A mutation in the microtubule-associated protein tau in pallido-nigral-luysian degeneration. *Neurology* **53**: 864–868

Yasuda M, Yokoyama K, Nakayasu T *et al.* (2000a) A Japanese patient with frontotemporal dementia and parkinsonism by a *Tau* P301S mutation. *Neurology* **55**: 1224–1227

Yasuda M, Takamatsu J, D'Souza I *et al.* (2000b) A novel mutation at position +12 in the intron following exon 10 of the *tau* gene in familial frontotemporal dementia (FTD-Kumamoto). *Annals of Neurology* **47**: 422–429

Yoshida H, Crowther AR, Goedert M. (2002) Functional effects of *tau* gene mutations ΔN296 and N296H. *Journal of Neurochemistry* **80**: 548–551

Zhukareva V, Vogelsberg-Ragaglia V, Van Deerlin VMD *et al.* (2001) Loss of brain tau defines novel sporadic and familial tauopathies with frontotemporal dementia. *Annals of Neurology* **49**:165–175

Zhukareva V, Mann D, Pickering-Brown SM *et al.* (2002) Sporadic Pick's disease: a tauopathy characterised by a spectrum of pathological τ isoforms in gray and white matter. *Annals of Neurology* **51**: 730–739

Zhukareva V, Sundarraj S, Mann D *et al.* (2003) Selective reduction of soluble tau proteins in sporadic and familial frontotemporal dementia an international follow-up study. *Acta Neuropathologica* **105**: 469–476

55

Semantic dementia

JULIE S SNOWDEN

Semantic dementia is a distinctive clinical syndrome that arises from circumscribed degeneration of the temporal lobes. It is one of a number of distinct syndromes, which include frontotemporal dementia and primary progressive non-fluent aphasia, encompassed within the pathological rubric of frontotemporal lobar degeneration. The disorder is characterized by a progressive loss of semantic (conceptual) knowledge about the world. This includes loss of the ability to understand the meaning of words, to recognize faces, and to understand the significance of objects, non-verbal sounds, tastes and smells. Despite the wide-ranging nature of this loss of 'meaning', the disorder is remarkably circumscribed in the sense that non-semantic aspects of cognitive functioning remain well preserved. Patients have normal sensory perception: the problem lies in ascribing meaning (connotative associations) to stimuli that are perceived normally. Moreover, day-to-day memory is well preserved. As a consequence patients are able to retain a high degree of functional independence well into the course of disease. It is the dramatic, yet selective nature of the semantic disorder, together with characteristic accompanying behavioural changes, that distinguishes this non-Alzheimer focal temporal lobe degeneration clinically from Alzheimer's disease. Although relatively rare, recognition of the disorder is important because of its distinct implications for management and treatment. Moreover, in recent years it has attracted considerable academic interest because of its potential to shed light on the organization of semantic memory and its neural basis.

55.1 HISTORICAL BACKGROUND

The term semantic dementia is relatively new. It was introduced (Snowden et al., 1989) to encapsulate the multimodal loss of semantic knowledge that occurs in the face of relatively preserved non-semantic cognitive skills and has since been widely adopted (e.g. Hodges et al., 1992a; Breedin et al., 1994; Graham et al., 1997; Lauro-Grotto et al., 1997). Clinical criteria have been published to aid its identification (Neary et al., 1998) and are summarized in Box 55.1.

Clinical cases of semantic dementia undoubtedly existed prior to the introduction of contemporary classifications. There are seminal reports in the literature of patients with circumscribed impairments of semantic memory occurring in association with a unspecified degenerative brain disease who would now be recognized as having semantic dementia (Warrington, 1975; Schwartz et al., 1979, 1980). Moreover, some patients, described as having a fluent form of primary progressive aphasia (Basso et al., 1988; Poeck and Luzzatti, 1988; Tyrrell et al., 1990a; Snowden et al., 1992), in fact have a disorder of semantics that extends beyond the domain of language and would fulfil criteria for semantic dementia. Similarly, patients with progressive prosopagnosia (Tyrrell et al., 1990b; Evans et al., 1995) may be examples of semantic dementia presenting in the visual domain. In the classical neurological and psychiatric literature there are reports of patients with lexical-semantic impairment occurring in association with

Box 55.1   *Clinical diagnostic features of semantic dementia.*

I Core diagnostic features

A. Insidious onset and gradual progression

B. Language disorder characterized by :

- i) progressive, fluent, empty spontaneous speech
- ii) loss of word meaning, manifest by impaired naming *and* comprehension
- iii) semantic paraphasias

and/or

C. Perceptual disorder characterised by:

- i) prosopagnosia: impaired recognition of identity of familiar faces

and/or

- ii) associative agnosia: impaired recognition of object identity

D. Preserved perceptual matching and drawing reproduction

E. Preserved single word repetition

F. Preserved ability to read aloud and write to dictation orthographically regular words

II Supportive diagnostic features

A. Speech and language

- i) pressure of speech
- ii) idiosyncratic word usage
- iii) absence of phonemic paraphasias
- iv) surface dyslexia and dysgraphia
- v) preserved calculation

B. Behaviour

- i) loss of sympathy and empathy
- ii) narrowed preoccupations
- iii) parsimony

C. Physical signs

- i) absent or late primitive reflexes
- ii) akinesia, rigidity and tremor

D. Neuropsychological testing

- i) profound semantic loss, manifest in failure of word comprehension and naming and/or face and object recognition
- ii) preserved phonology and syntax, elementary perceptual processing, spatial skills and day-to-day memorizing

E. Electrophysiology

- normal

F. Brain Imaging (structural and/or functional)

- predominant anterior temporal abnormality (symmetric or asymmetric)

Reproduced with kind permission from Lippincott, Williams & Wilkins from Neary *et al.* (Frontotemporal lobar degeneration. A consensus on clinical diagnostic criteria. *Neurology* [1998] **51**: 1546–1554)

focal temporal lobe atrophy (Pick, 1892; Rosenfeld, 1909), whose clinical description appears prototypical of semantic dementia (Snowden, 2001). The neurological term 'transcortical sensory aphasia' has historically been applied to the form of language disorder.

Aside from such cases it is likely that there are many patients with semantic dementia who, in the past, were not recognized as clinically distinct and were subsumed under the broad rubric of degenerative dementia or were wrongly classified as Alzheimer's disease. Alzheimer's disease continues to be the main misdiagnosis.

55.2 DEMOGRAPHIC FEATURES

Semantic dementia most commonly presents between the ages of 50 and 65 and affects both men and women. The time course of the illness is variable, the median illness duration being approximately 8 years, ranging from about 3 to 15 years. Most cases appear to occur sporadically. A history of dementia in a first-degree relative is documented in approximately 25 per cent of cases, although it is difficult to determine, in view of the retrospective nature of family history data, whether the form of dementia in affected relatives is similar. Nevertheless, the established clinical and pathological link between semantic dementia and the highly familial frontotemporal dementia (see below) suggests that genetic factors are likely to play an important role. There are no known geographical or socioeconomic factors that affect incidence. Accurate incidence and prevalence data are not currently available. However, the disorder would appear to be relatively rare. In an analysis of patient referrals to a specialist dementia clinic in a neurological department in Manchester, patients with prototypical, 'pure' semantic dementia accounted for approximately 10 per cent of cases of focal cortical degeneration (frontotemporal lobe degeneration), which in turn accounted for 20–25 per cent of cases of primary degenerative dementia presenting in the presenium.

55.3 PRESENTING COMPLAINTS

Patients' own complaints, often supported by reports from relatives, are often that they 'can't remember things'. However, careful history-taking will reveal that the problem is not one of memory loss in the traditional sense. Patients are able to remember day-to-day events, keep track of time, remember appointments, find their way around without becoming lost, and retain a degree of functional independence that would be incompatible with a classical amnesia. The problem lies in the realm of semantic memory: in remembering what words mean, who people are and what objects are for. The presenting symptoms are most often in the verbal domain, manifest by patients' difficulty in the understanding and use of words. Semantic errors occur in speech (for example, a rabbit is referred to as a 'cat') and patients may express perplexity and lack of understanding of words previously known to them. However, in some patients the earliest symptoms are in the visual realm, manifest particularly by a difficulty recognizing faces. Relatives may also report a failure of object recognition: patients may, for example, no longer recognize fruits and vegetables in the supermarket. Medical referral may sometimes be precipitated by behavioural alterations. Patients are typically physically well, without neurological symptoms.

55.4 COGNITIVE CHARACTERISTICS

55.4.1 Language

Patients speak fluently and effortlessly, with normal articulation and grammar and without phonological (sound-based) errors, giving the superficial impression of normal output. Indeed, patients are often garrulous (Box 55.2). Nevertheless, there is typically a reduction in content words, and patients' reliance on broad generic terms, stereotyped usage of words and phrases and in particular the presence of within-category

---

Box 55.2 *Characteristics of language disorder in semantic dementia*

Spontaneous speech
- Fluent, effortless, often garrulous
- Empty content, reduced nominal terms
- Semantic paraphasias
- Substitution of generic terms
- Verbal stereotypies
- Preserved use of syntax
- Preserved phonology
- Normal articulation and prosody

Comprehension
- Impaired word understanding
- Good understanding of syntax

Repetition
- Relatively preserved

Naming
- Profound anomia
- Semantic errors present (e.g. 'dog' for elephant)
- No benefit from phonemic cues

Reading
- Fluent reading aloud
- Accurate reading of regular words
- Regularization of irregular words (surface dyslexia)
- Impaired comprehension of written material

Writing
- Fluent, effortless execution
- Regularization of irregular words (e.g. 'cort' for caught) (surface dysgraphia)

---

errors such as 'sock' for glove may provide the clue to the underlying semantic impairment.

The semantic impairment, which may be scarcely apparent at clinical interview, becomes strikingly evident on formal testing of naming and word comprehension. Patients commonly exhibit difficulty naming even common objects and derive no benefit from first-letter cues. They may also show difficulty selecting the correct name when given semantically related alternatives, reflecting the fact that the naming problem is not simply one of word retrieval but represents a central breakdown of knowledge of the word itself. Word comprehension is affected. Expressions of lack of understanding of previously familiar words (e.g. 'Tiger, tiger, what's a tiger? I don't know what that is') commonly occur and are a revealing demonstration of the loss of word meaning. There is a tendency for vocabulary relating to patients' daily life to be better preserved than non-personally relevant vocabulary (Snowden *et al.*, 1994, 1995). Word comprehension and naming tests should therefore not be restricted to the common objects and body parts typically used in bedside testing, but should include names of animals, foods and objects, such as 'sheep', 'plum', 'violin' which are unlikely to relate directly to the patient's daily routine. Loss of knowledge about a word's meaning may not be absolute. The patient may, for example, know that a lemon is a food rather than an animal, but not know how it differs from an apple or banana. Assessment of word understanding should therefore probe knowledge of attributes as well as broad category knowledge.

Language comprehension problems arise principally at the single word level. Comprehension of syntactic rules of language is typically relatively well preserved. Thus, a patient may respond with ease to the question 'If the tiger is killed by the lion which animal is dead?', while failing the apparently simpler question 'Is a tiger bigger than a mouse?'. The former depends on understanding of grammatical relationships, whereas the latter on understanding of the lexical terms tiger and mouse.

Patients' ability to repeat what is said, to read aloud and write to dictation is relatively well preserved, although not entirely normal by virtue of the semantic deficit. Inevitably it is more difficult to repeat a meaningless sentence than one that carries meaning. In reading, patients read phonetically rather than for meaning, and produce regular pronunciations of words with irregular spelling-to-sound correspondences, consistent with surface dyslexia (Patterson *et al.*, 1985). Thus, 'glove' may be pronounced to rhyme with 'rove' and 'stove'; 'pint' to rhyme with 'mint'. Similar regularization errors occur also in writing: the word 'caught' written as 'cort'.

With progression of disease, speech content is increasingly empty and stereotyped in nature. Favoured terms may be adopted and used in a generic sense (e.g. 'twisting' to refer to all actions; 'plate' to refer to all objects). There is a gradual contraction in the themes of conversation, which centre exclusively on autobiographically relevant topics. At no time is speech non-fluent or effortful in production: conversational repertoire simply becomes progressively reduced until only a few verbal stereotypies remain.

55.4.2 Face recognition

Problems in recognizing familiar faces occur early in the course of disease. Difficulties are most profound for impersonal faces, such as those of current and past celebrities, and least marked for family and friends with whom the patient maintains daily contact. The problem in face recognition lies at a semantic level: in assigning an identity to faces. That patients are able to perceive and discriminate faces adequately is demonstrated by their ability to carry out matching tasks of unfamiliar faces.

55.4.3 Object recognition

Object recognition difficulties represent one component of the insidious breakdown in semantics. Such difficulties may not be evident early in the course, but emerge with disease progression. Recognition failure, like that for words, is not all or none. Patients may, for example, be able to sort objects into those which are edible and those non-edible, but be unable to distinguish foods that are normally cooked (e.g. potatoes) and those normally eaten uncooked (e.g. lettuce). Patients may recognize a picture of a camel as depicting an animal, but have no idea how it differs from a dog. Moreover, they may recognize and use entirely appropriately their own belongings while failing to recognize other examples of those same objects or pictures of those objects (Snowden et al., 1994; Bozeat et al., 2002). This latter feature helps to explain the clinical observation that the degree of functional independence maintained by patients in daily life belies the magnitude of their underlying semantic disorder: patients are able to function reasonably well within the narrow confines of their familiar environment and repertoire of daily activities at a time when abstract semantic knowledge is profoundly impaired. With progression of disease even highly familiar objects may no longer be recognized.

Non-semantic aspects of object perception are well preserved. Patients can copy drawings normally, sometimes to a strikingly proficient level (Snowden et al., 1996a). They also have no difficulty carrying out perceptual matching tasks, which are not dependent upon recognition of object meaning.

55.4.4 Numeracy

Understanding of number concepts and the ability to carry out arithmetical procedures are often remarkably well preserved (Cappelletti et al., 2001, 2002; Crutch and Warrington, 2002). Patients are able to count money and reckon change despite major difficulties in word comprehension and naming. Perhaps because of this preserved ability patients often enjoy number puzzles and television quiz shows involving manipulation of numbers. Eventually, however, arithmetical skills too become compromised by patients' semantic

disorder: patients may cease to recognize coins and no longer understand the meaning of spoken and written numerals.

55.4.5 Spatial skills

Spatial and navigational skills are generally excellent. Patients are able to find their way without becoming lost and may use spatial cues to compensate for object recognition difficulties (for example, by recalling the spatial location of food items on a supermarket shelf). On neuropsychological testing, patients perform well on traditional spatial tests such as line orientation (Benton et al., 1978), dot counting, position discrimination, and cube estimation (Warrington and James, 1991).

The preservation of spatial skills is an important feature in distinguishing semantic dementia from Alzheimer's disease. It is worth recognizing, however, that performance on putative spatial tasks may be compromised secondarily by failures of perceptual recognition or verbal skills. A patient who, for example, fails to 'locate' their comb or toothbrush, may do so because of impaired recognition of object identity and not because of a problem in spatial localization per se. A patient who, in late stage disease, fails a simple dot counting task may have difficulty recalling the names of numbers.

Evidence that spatial skills are indeed well preserved throughout the course of disease is suggested by qualitative characteristics of patients' behaviour. Patients with semantic dementia even in advanced disease negotiate their environment skilfully, have no difficulty orientating themselves with respect to furniture when sitting or lying down, recall the location of their chair or bed on a hospital ward, localize and manipulate with ease objects in the environment and spatially align objects perfectly.

55.4.6 Memory

A feature that is striking on clinical grounds and that helps to distinguish semantic dementia from other forms of dementia is the apparent preservation of patients' current autobiographical memory. Patients remember appointments and personally relevant events and keep track of time. They negotiate the environment without becoming lost. If they move home, they have no difficulty learning their new surroundings. In contrast, they show a gross breakdown in impersonal, factual (semantic) knowledge about the world, including knowledge about public figures and important world events. The preservation of autobiographical memory is not easily captured by standard memory tests, which typically involve lists of words, faces or line drawings that may have little meaning for the patient. Moreover, routine bedside questions, designed to probe orientation, such as 'What town are we in?' demand naming skills and thus may be compromised in semantic dementia. Bedside testing needs to include questions regarding the patient's own daily life, and formal neuropsychological testing should include recognition memory tests using perceptually distinct pictures. Also worthy of note is that semantic dementia patients commonly answer time orientation questions better than those relating to place orientation, reflecting the fact that number-related vocabulary is better preserved than the names of places.

55.4.7 Praxis

Motor actions are carried out adeptly, dextrously and effortlessly. Activities with high motor executive demands, such as painting, sewing or playing golf, may continue to be pursued with a high level of proficiency, a feature that is both clinically dramatic and important in distinguishing semantic dementia from Alzheimer's disease. Practical skills are inevitably compromised to some extent by patients' semantic loss: for example, a difficulty in cooking arises because of patients' inability to recognize ingredients or understand the words of a recipe.

55.4.8 Touch, taste, smell and hearing

Primary sensory abilities are well preserved, so patients have no difficulty detecting the presence of tactile, gustatory, olfactory and auditory stimuli and discriminating whether two stimuli are the same or different. However, the disorder of meaning may extend to all sensory modalities. Patients may have difficulty recognizing the identity of textures, tastes, smells, and non-verbal sounds such as the ringing of a telephone or doorbell, despite perceiving those stimuli normally.

55.5 BEHAVIOURAL CHANGES

Although the semantic deficits are the defining characteristic of the disorder, there are also accompanying behavioural changes. Some are included as supporting features in clinical diagnostic criteria (Box 55.1, p. 703). Others are summarized in Box 55.3. Recognition of behavioural changes is important because their highly characteristic nature is valuable in differential diagnosis. Moreover, behavioural changes may represent the most problematic aspect of the condition from the

---

Box 55.3 *Behavioural changes in semantic dementia*

- Self-centredness (narrowed world view)
- Inflexibility and intransigence
- Hyperreactivity to sensory stimuli
- Loss of awareness of danger
- Food fads
- Preference for sweet foods
- Preference for routine, clockwatching
- Stereotypies, rituals and compulsions

---

management point of view and the greatest source of burden to carers.

Patients are commonly described as self-centred and lacking in their former sympathy and empathy for others. They may be inflexible and intransigent and have difficulty seeing others' point of view. They may appear mean and lacking in their former generosity. Their behavioural repertoire becomes narrowed and they frequently become preoccupied with one or two activities, which they pursue relentlessly to the exclusion of all else. Moreover, they may become mentally preoccupied by one or two themes, which they repeat incessantly to the increasing exasperation of family members.

Patients may show hypersensitivity to sensory stimuli and overact to light touch or to ostensibly innocuous environmental sounds such as bird-song. Patients may be oblivious to danger, a feature that is probably linked to their loss of conceptual understanding of the world. Patients commonly show narrowed food preferences and usually favour sweet foods.

Perhaps the most striking change, however, is the presence of behaviours that have a compulsive quality. Patients commonly adopt a fixed routine and have a preference for order. They will clock-watch, carrying out specific activities at precisely the same time each day. They may align objects, straighten out folds in the curtains and plump up the cushions as soon as a person rises from an armchair. They may develop meaningless rituals, such as avoiding standing on a particular carpet tile, or playing the same few notes on the piano each time they enter the room where the piano is located. Nevertheless, the affective responses of anxiety and release from anxiety that are associated with obsessional-compulsive disorder are typically absent.

55.5.1 Insight

Patients are aware of and may become preoccupied by their difficulties. However, they frequently provide trivial explanations for them, such as being 'out of practice with talking' by virtue of being alone all day, and they demonstrate little real distress or concern. A possible reason is that they have no internal 'model' of their former conceptual knowledge for comparison and thus have no mechanism by which to appreciate the magnitude of what they have lost.

55.6 NEUROLOGICAL SIGNS

Patients are generally physically well and free from neurological signs until late in the disease. Extrapyramidal signs of akinesia and rigidity, and frontal release phenomena may emerge in advanced disease. Neurological signs of motor neurone disease may emerge in a small minority of patients. Myoclonus does not occur.

55.7 INVESTIGATIONS

55.7.1 Electroencephalography

This is usually normal, with minor slowing of wave forms occurring only in late stage disease.

55.7.2 Structural brain imaging

Magnetic resonance imaging reveals cerebral atrophy, particularly marked in the anterior temporal lobes (Mummery

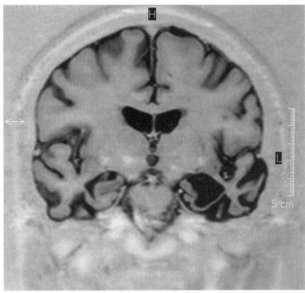

(a)

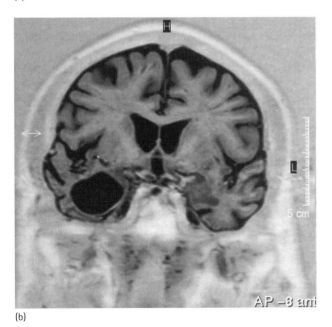

(b)

Figure 55.1 *MR scans of two patients with semantic dementia showing severe temporal lobe atrophy. In one case atrophy is more marked on the left side (a) and in the other case on the right (b).*

et al., 2000; Chan *et al.*, 2001). Temporal atrophy is typically bilateral, although may be asymmetrical (Figure 55.1), the left or right predominance being associated with a clinical presentation emphasizing word meaning or face recognition disorder respectively. The inferolateral parts of the temporal lobe are most affected. The hippocampi are often relatively spared.

55.7.3 Functional brain imaging

Positron emission tomography (PET) and single photon emission computed tomography (SPECT) show abnormalities in the anterior cerebral hemispheres, particularly the temporal regions (Plate 27). Appearances may be bilateral and symmetrical or markedly asymmetrical, affecting disproportionately the left or right hemisphere.

55.8 NEUROPATHOLOGY

Temporal lobe atrophy, usually bilateral but asymmetrical, is typically evident on gross examination of the brain. Histological changes chiefly affect the middle and inferior temporal gyri, with some involvement also of frontal cortex and relative sparing of the superior temporal gyrus, hippocampi, parietal and occipital cortex. The major histopathological feature is typically of a microvacuolar degeneration of the cortex, referred to as frontolobar degeneration (FLD)-type histology according to the Lund–Manchester consensus statement on frontotemporal dementia (Lund and Manchester Groups, 1994; see also Chapter 54). There is loss of large pyramidal nerve cells from affected areas of temporal and frontal cortex and a spongiform (microvacuolar) change due to neuronal fallout. Reactive astrocytosis is mild. Histopathogical features of Alzheimer's disease are absent. No deposits of Aβ4 amyloid protein are present in any cortical region, nor are there cells containing neurofibrillary tangles or Lewy-body-type inclusions. Pick-type inclusion bodies are also usually absent from surviving cortical nerve cells. Nevertheless, occasionally Pick-type (Lund and Manchester Groups, 1994) histological changes may occur, with severe astrocytic gliosis, and the presence of ballooned neurones and inclusion bodies. Semantic dementia has also been reported in association with ubiquitin-positive tau-negative inclusions, consistent with motor neurone disease (Rossor *et al.*, 2000).

55.9 NEUROCHEMISTRY

Neurochemical study of semantic dementia is limited. However, the evidence available indicates an absence of cholinergic deficits and similarities (A Procter, personal communication) with the findings of frontotemporal dementia (Francis *et al.*, 1993).

55.10 RELATIONSHIP BETWEEN SEMANTIC DEMENTIA AND OTHER FORMS OF FOCAL CEREBRAL DEGENERATION

The patterns of histology seen in semantic dementia are identical to those of the more common clinical syndrome of frontotemporal dementia, in which there is profound character change and breakdown in social conduct (see Chapters 52 and 54). Similar histological changes are also seen in progressive non-fluent aphasia (Snowden *et al.*, 1996a), in which the salient feature is a disorder of language expression and breakdown in phonological and syntactic aspects of language. These three distinct clinical syndromes appear to represent discrete clinical manifestations of a common underlying pathology, the clinical syndrome being determined by the anatomical distribution of pathological change within the frontal and temporal lobes. In the case of semantic dementia the pathology is dominant within the inferior and middle temporal lobes, whereas the frontal lobes and the traditional language areas of the superior temporal lobes (Wernicke's area) are relatively well preserved. By contrast, in frontotemporal dementia the frontal lobes and temporal poles are markedly affected, and in progressive non-fluent aphasia the perisylvian areas of the left hemisphere are preferentially involved. The link between the clinical syndromes of semantic dementia, frontotemporal dementia and progressive non-fluent aphasia is reinforced

- by clinical overlap between the syndromes in some patients;
- the presence of different syndromes in affected members of the same family, and
- by the co-occurrence of motor neurone disease in association with the prototypical syndromes (Neary *et al.*, 1990; Caselli *et al.*, 1993).

In prototypical semantic dementia patients do not show notable 'frontal lobe' behaviour. Nevertheless, an overlap between the clinical phenotypes of FTD and semantic dementia has been demonstrated in FTD patients who show mutations in the tau gene (Pickering-Brown *et al.*, 2002).

55.11 DIFFERENTIATION FROM FRONTOTEMPORAL DEMENTIA

Semantic dementia is unlikely to be confused with FTD on cognitive grounds (see Chapter 52). The problems in word and object recognition are quite distinct from the frontal executive failures of FTD. Nevertheless, both disorders involve behavioural change, which may appear superficially similar, leading to diagnostic confusion. Closer examination does, however, reveal differences between the 'temporal' behaviours of semantic dementia and the 'frontal' behaviours of FTD (Snowden *et al.*, 1996a, 2001) (Table 55.1).

Table 55.1 *Behavioural differences between semantic dementia and frontotemporal dementia*

Behaviour	Semantic dementia	Frontotemporal dementia
Affect	Restricted impairment, especially loss of fear	Pervasive loss of emotions
	Concern for illness	Unconcern
Social behaviour	May show exaggerated sociability	Reduced sociability common
Interest and motivation	Narrowed interests	General loss of interest
Response to sensory stimuli	Exaggerated	Diminished
Eating	Food fads	Gluttony, indiscriminate eating
Wandering	No wandering	Wandering common
Pacing fixed route	Absent	May be present
Repetitive behaviours	Complex routines common	Simple motor stereotypies more likely
	Repetitive themes	No repetitive themes
	Clockwatches	Unconcerned by time
	Compulsive quality	No compulsive quality

- In FTD behaviour tends to be unproductive and lacking in goal-direction, whereas in semantic dementia behavioural routines may be remarkably complex.
- In FTD there is poor mental application and impersistence whereas patients with semantic dementia frequently show dogged persistence, albeit on a narrowed range of activities.
- Patients with FTD show a lack of concern with personal appearance and hygiene, whereas the latter may become a source of preoccupation in patients with semantic dementia.
- FTD patients show generalized blunting of emotions, including a failure to show happiness, sadness and disgust. In semantic dementia affective changes are more selective, typically affecting particularly the capacity to show fear.
- FTD patients may show reduced sensitivity to pain, whereas semantic dementia patients are more likely to show an exaggerated response to sensory stimuli.
- FTD patients commonly exhibit gluttony and indiscriminate eating, whereas semantic dementia patients are more likely to show food fads.
- Perhaps the most striking difference is that repetitive behaviours have a much more compulsive quality in semantic dementia than FTD, suggesting an important role of the temporal lobes in obsessive-compulsive-type behaviour. The differences are most marked between semantic dementia and the apathetic form of FTD. Disinhibited FTD patients with more circumscribed atrophy of the orbitofrontal lobes and temporal pole may show some overlap with semantic dementia.

55.12 DIFFERENTIATION FROM ALZHEIMER'S DISEASE

Semantic dementia is most commonly misdiagnosed as Alzheimer's disease. This is unsurprising in view of the greater prevalence of Alzheimer's disease, the fact that presenting symptoms in both conditions are commonly of 'memory' problems and signs of semantic disorder may not be obvious at initial interview (Box 55.4). Nevertheless, the two conditions can be readily distinguished on clinical grounds (Table 55.2).

- In semantic dementia, 'memory loss' refers to loss of impersonal, conceptual knowledge about the world. Personal, autobiographical memories remain relatively well preserved. In Alzheimer's disease the converse is true. Memory is impaired predominantly for day-to-day events.
- Spatial abilities are well preserved in semantic dementia, whereas their breakdown is a frequent feature of Alzheimer's disease, manifest clinically by impaired localization of objects, inability to orientate clothing and objects correctly, and loss of topographical orientation within a familiar environment.
- Patients with both semantic dementia and Alzheimer's disease may have object recognition problems, yet the nature of the perceptual disorder is qualitatively different. In semantic dementia the difficulty lies in assigning meaning to objects that are perceived normally ('associative agnosia'). Patients can match stimuli on the basis of perceptual similarity, yet deny recognition of those stimuli, or make semantic errors (e.g. a camel identified as a 'dog'). They can copy accurately drawings of objects that they cannot recognize. In Alzheimer's disease, perceptual breakdown lies at the level of achieving an integrated percept ('apperceptive agnosia'). Misidentifications occur on the basis of interpretation of elements of a figure instead of the overall outline (e.g. a pair of scissors identified as a bowl on the basis of the circular handle). Patients have difficulty carrying out perceptual matching tasks, and are unable to reproduce line drawings, their copies often being fragmented with loss of the spatial relationships between elements of the figure.
- Language breakdown is a common feature of Alzheimer's disease, but is qualitatively distinct from that of semantic dementia. Whereas in semantic dementia speech is entirely effortless, in Alzheimer's disease speech it is typically hesitant and patients show evidence of actively searching for words, suggesting a difficulty in retrieval of words potentially within their vocabulary. Phonological errors may also occur. In Alzheimer's disease, moreover, sentences are unfinished and content broken, reflecting loss of train of thought and a reduced immediate memory span. Logoclonia, the festinating repetition of individual phonemes, may occur in moderate and advanced Alzheimer's disease, along with extrapyramidal

Box 55.4   *Factors affecting poor recognition of semantic dementia*

- Rare disorder
- Historical reports of 'memory' disorder
- Semantic disorder may not be evident at clinical interview
- Semantic impairments may be misinterpreted as classical amnesia
- Need explicit tests of word comprehension and naming, face and object recognition

Table 55.2   *Clinical differences between semantic dementia and Alzheimer's disease*

Characteristic	Semantic dementia	Alzheimer's disease
Age of onset	Most common in middle age	Most common in elderly
Language	Selective semantic disorder	No selective semantic disorder
	Impaired single word comprehension	Impaired sentence comprehension
Perception	Associative agnosia	Apperceptive agnosia
Calculation	Preserved early in course	Impaired early in course
Spatial orientation	Preserved	Impaired early in course
Constructional skills	Preserved	Impaired early in course
Memory	Day-to-day memory preserved	Day-to-day memory impaired
Neurological signs	Akinesia and rigidity relatively late	Akinesia and rigidity relatively early
	Myoclonus absent	Myoclonus may be present
Electroen-cephalography	Normal	Slowing of wave forms
Structural brain imaging	Focal temporal lobe atrophy typical	Focal atrophy rare
	Hippocampi relatively preserved	Hippocampi atrophic
	Marked hemispheric asymmetry common	Marked asymmetry rare
Functional brain imaging	Anterior hemisphere abnormalities	Posterior hemisphere abnormalities
	Marked hemispheric asymmetry common	Marked asymmetry rare

neurological signs and myoclonus, suggestive of increasing basal ganglia involvement. It is not a feature of semantic dementia.

- In AD comprehension is better preserved for single nominal terms than for complex syntax, whereas in semantic dementia the reverse is the case. Although patients with Alzheimer's disease may acquire difficulties in reading, writing and spelling they do not show the characteristic surface dyslexia and surface dysgraphia of semantic dementia.

- The presence of semantic impairment in Alzheimer's disease has been highlighted by a number of authors. However, whether this reflects a fundamental loss of knowledge (Hodges et al., 1992b; Martin, 1992; Hodges and Patterson, 1995; Salmon et al., 1999) as in semantic dementia or faulty access to information (Nebes, 1992; Nebes and Halligan, 1999; Ober and Shenaut, 1999) is controversial. In any event, in Alzheimer's disease semantic impairment is never a circumscribed deficit. It occurs typically as one component of a multifaceted disorder of language and invariably in the context of a demonstrable amnesia.

- Calculation difficulties are an early feature of Alzheimer's disease, whereas in semantic dementia preservation of numerical skills contrasts with the disorder of word meaning.

55.13   TREATMENT AND MANAGEMENT

Novel pharmacological therapies for Alzheimer's disease do not have a rational role in semantic dementia, because there is no demonstrated evidence of abnormalities in the cholinergic system. In patients with problematic behavioural changes, symptomatic treatment may be warranted. Repetitive, stereotypic behaviours may respond to serotonin reuptake inhibitors.

With regard to practical management of the disorder, it is of note that concepts (words, objects, etc.), relevant to the patient's daily life appear to be better retained than those which have no personal relevance (Snowden et al., 1994, 1995; Westmacott et al., 2003). Thus, for example, the word 'postman' may be understood better than the word 'milkman' if the patient has personal daily experience of the postman delivering letters to the home, but purchases milk from the supermarket. It has been argued that this feature results from patients' preserved autobiographical memory: concepts, which would otherwise be lost in their abstract sense, have some meaning to the patient if they are framed within the context of the patient's ongoing daily experience. By implication, input from speech therapists is more likely to be beneficial if this takes place in the patient's own surroundings using as referents patients' own belongings, than in the abstract setting of a clinical consulting room using standard pictorial materials.

There is clinical evidence in semantic dementia that some learning is possible. Patients may, for example, effectively learn the names of new acquaintances and the names of medicines prescribed to them. They may also succeed in relearning lost vocabulary (Graham et al., 1999; Snowden and Neary, 2002). However, such reacquired knowledge is tenuous and vocabulary can be maintained only so long as those words are used regularly and are linked to patients' ongoing daily experience.

55.14   THEORETICAL ISSUES

Semantic dementia has attracted considerable theoretical interest from neuropsychologists in recent years. Because of its circumscribed nature it is a natural experimental model for understanding how the brain represents 'meaning'. Experimental studies are motivated by the fact that semantic knowledge does not break down in an all-or-none fashion. At any one stage of the disease patients knows some words but not others, and recognize some objects and faces. Unearthing the factors that govern what is lost and retained ought to shed light on the cerebral representation of semantic knowledge. Contemporary issues include:

- *The role of the two hemispheres in meaning representation.* The traditional view has been that semantic memory is particularly dependent on the left hemisphere. However, patients with semantic dementia provide evidence that both hemispheres contribute and may have different roles (Thompson et al., 2003, 2004; Snowden et al., 2004). The left hemisphere appears to have a greater role in the knowledge of words and the right hemisphere in visual knowledge such as face recognition.

- *The representation of different categories of information.* Patients with semantic dementia may show disproportionate impairment in their knowledge of some categories (e.g. animals and vegetables) compared with others (e.g. household objects) (Basso et al., 1988; Cardebat et al., 1996). Such findings have been interpreted by some in terms of a distributed model of semantic memory, in which different properties of objects (e.g. sensory features, particularly important for discriminating between animals, and functional attributes, particularly important for discriminating between household objects) are represented separately (Warrington and Shallice, 1984; Warrington and McCarthy, 1987). It is assumed that cortical areas that have contributed to the development of various categories are also implicated in their representation (Gainotti, 2004). Other authors (Caramazza and Shelton, 1998) have argued that conceptual knowledge is truly organized by category.

- *The relationship between semantic memory and episodic memory.* Semantic memory is regarded as abstract knowledge independent of experience. However, findings in semantic dementia patients (Snowden et al., 1994, 1995,1996b; Westamacott et al., 2003) suggest a closer relationship between knowledge and personal experience and interdependence between memory systems than generally recognized.

55.15   CONCLUSION

Semantic dementia is a striking disorder, clinically distinct from Alzheimer's disease and other forms of dementia.

Patients exhibit unique patterns of cognitive and behavioural symptomatology, which demand novel approaches to treatment and management. Neuropsychological studies are likely to further understanding of the cognitive characteristics of the disorder. Meanwhile, advances in molecular biological research ought to shed light on the underlying aetiology of this and other clinical manifestations of frontotemporal lobar degeneration.

REFERENCES

Basso A, Capitani E, Laiacona M. (1988) Progressive language impairment without dementia a case with isolated category specific semantic defect. *Journal of Neurology, Neurosurgery, and Psychiatry* **51**: 1201–1207

Benton AL, Varney NR, Hamsher K de S. (1978) Visuo-spatial judgement: a clinical test. *Archives of Neurology* **35**: 364–367

Bozeat S, Lambon Ralph MA, Patterson K, Hodges J. (2002) The influence of personal familiarity and context on object use in semantic dementia. *Neurocase* **8**: 127–134

Breedin SD, Saffran EM, Coslett HB. (1994) Reversal of the concreteness effect in a patient with semantic dementia. *Cognitive Neuropsychology* **11**: 617–660

Cappelletti M, Butterworth B, Kopelman M. (2001) Spared numerical abilities in a case of semantic dementia. *Neuropsychologia* **39**: 1224–1239

Cappelletti M, Kopelman M, Butterworth B. (2002) Why semantic dementia drives you to the dogs (but not to the horses): a thoeretical account. *Cognitive Neuropsychology* **19**: 483–503

Caramazza A and Shelton J. (1998) Domain-specific knowledge in the brain the animate-inanimate distinction. *Journal of Cognitive Neuroscience* **10**: 1–34

Cardebat D, Demonet JF, Celsis P, Puel M. (1996) Living/non-living dissociation in a case of semantic dementia A SPECT activation study. *Neuropsychologia* **34**: 1175–1179

Caselli RJ, Windebank AJ, Petersen RC *et al.* (1993) Rapidly progressive aphasic dementia with motor neuron disease. *Annals of Neurology* **33**: 200–207

Chan D, Fox NC, Scahill RI *et al.* (2001) Patterns of temporal lobe atrophy in semantic dementia and Alzheimer's disease. *Annals of Neurology* **49**: 433–442

Crutch SJ and Warrington EK. (2002) Preserved calculation skills in a case of semantic dementia. *Cortex* **38**: 389–399

Evans JJ, Heggs AJ, Antoun N, Hodges JR. (1995) Progressive prosopagnosia associated with selective right temporal lobe atrophy: a new syndrome? *Brain* **118**: 1–13

Francis PT, Holmes C, Webster M-T *et al.* (1993) Preliminary neurochemical findings in non-Alzheimer dementia due to lobar atrophy. *Dementia* **4**: 172–177

Gainotti G. (2004) A metanalysis of impaired and spared naming for different categories of knowledge in patients with a visuo-verbal disconnection. *Neuropsychologia* **42**: 299–319

Graham KS, Becker JT, Hodges JR. (1997) On the relationship between knowledge and memory for pictures: evidence from the study of patients with semantic dementia and Alzheimer's disease. *Journal of the International Neuropsychological Society* **3**: 534–544

Graham KS, Patterson K, Pratt KH, Hodges JR. (1999) Relearning and subsequent forgetting of semantic category exemplars in a case of semantic dementia. *Neuropsychology* **13**: 359–380

Hodges JR and Patterson K. (1995) Is semantic memory consistently impaired early in the course of Alzheimer's disease? Neuroanatomical and diagnostic implications. *Neuropsychologia* **33**: 441–459

Hodges JR, Patterson K, Oxbury S, Funnell E. (1992a) Semantic dementia. Progressive fluent aphasia with temporal lobe atrophy. *Brain* **115**: 1783–1806

Hodges JR, Salmon DP, Butters N. (1992b) Semantic memory impairment in Alzheimer's disease: failure of access or degraded knowledge. *Neuropsychologia* **30**: 301–314

Lauro-Grotto R, Piccini C, Shallice T. (1997) Modality-specific operations in semantic dementia. *Cortex* **33**: 593–622

Lund and Manchester Groups. (1994) Consensus Statement. Clinical and neuropathological criteria for fronto-temporal dementia. *Journal of Neurology, Neurosurgery, and Psychiatry* **4**: 416–418

Martin A. (1992) Degraded knowledge representations in patients with Alzheimer's disease: implications for models of semantic and repetition priming. In: LR Squire and N Butters (eds), *Neuropsychology of Memory.* New York, Guilford Press, pp. 220–232

Mummery CJ, Patterson K, Price CJ *et al.* (2000) A voxel-based morphometry study of semantic dementia relationship between temporal lobe atrophy and semantic memory. *Annals of Neurology* **47**: 36–45

Neary D, Snowden JS, Mann DMA *et al.* (1990) Frontal lobe dementia and motor neuron disease. *Journal of Neurology, Neurosurgery, and Psychiatry* **53**: 23–32

Neary D, Snowden JS, Gustafson L *et al.* (1998) Frontotemporal lobar degeneration. A consensus on clinical diagnostic criteria. *Neurology* **51**: 1546–1554

Nebes RD. (1992) Semantic memory dysfunction in Alzheimer's disease: disruption of semantic knowledge or information processing limitation? In: LR Squire and N Butters (eds), *Neuropsychology of Memory.* New York, Guilford Press, pp. 233–340

Nebes RD and Halligan EM. (1999) Instantiation of semantic categories in sentence comprehension by Alzheimer patients. *Journal of the International Neuropsychological Society* **5**: 685–691

Ober BA and Shenaut GK. (1999) Well-organized conceptual domains in Alzheimer's disease. *Journal of the International Neuropsychological Society* **5**: 676–684

Patterson KE, Marshall JC, Coltheart M. (1985) *Surface Dyslexia: Neuropsychological and Cognitive Studies of Phonological Reading.* Hove, Erlbaum

Pick A. (1892) Uber die Beziehungen der senilen Hirnatrophie zur Aphasie. *Prager Medizinische Wochenschrift* **17**: 165–167

Pickering-Brown SM, Richardson AM, Snowden JS *et al.* (2002) Inherited frontotemporal dementia in nine British families associated with intronic mutations in the *tau* gene. *Brain* **125**: 732–751

Poeck K and Luzzatti C. (1988) Slowly progressive aphasia in three patients. The problem of accompanying neuropsychological deficit. *Brain* **111**: 151–168

Rosenfeld M. (1909) Die partielle Grosshirnatrophie. *Zeitschrift für Psychologie und Neurologie* **14**: 115–130

Rossor MN, Revesz T, Lantos PL, Warrington EK. (2000) Semantic dementia with ubiquitin-positive tau-negative inclusion bodies. *Brain* **123**: 267–276

Salmon DP, Heindel WC, Lange KL. (1999) Differential decline in word generation from phonemic and semantic categories during the course of Alzheimer's disease: implications for the integrity of semantic memory. *Journal of the Neuropsychological Society* **5**: 692–703

Schwartz MF, Marin OSM, Saffran EM. (1979) Dissociations of language function in dementia a case study. *Brain and Language* **7**: 277–306

Schwartz MF, Saffran EM, Marin OSM. (1980) Fractionating the reading process in dementia evidence for word-specific print-to-sound associations. In: M Coltheart, K Patterson, JC Marshall (eds), *Deep Dyslexia*. London, Routledge and Paul

Snowden JS. (2001) Commentary on Liepmann 1908 and Rosenfeld 1909. *Cortex* **37**: 563–571

Snowden JS and Neary D. (2002) Relearning of verbal labels in semantic dementia. *Neuropsychologia* **40**: 1715–1728

Snowden JS, Goulding PJ, Neary D. (1989) Semantic dementia a form of circumscribed atrophy. *Behavioural Neurology* **2**: 167–182

Snowden JS, Neary D, Mann DMA *et al.* (1992) Progressive language disorder due to lobar atrophy. *Annals of Neurology* **31**: 174–183

Snowden JS, Griffiths H, Neary D. (1994) Semantic dementia autobiographical contribution to preservation of meaning. *Cognitive Neuropsychology* **11**: 265–288

Snowden JS, Griffiths HL, Neary D. (1995) Autobiographical experience and word meaning. *Memory* **3**: 225–246

Snowden JS, Neary D, Mann DMA. (1996a) *Frontotemporal Lobar Degeneration: Frontotemporal Dementia, Progressive Aphasia, Semantic Dementia*. London, Churchill Livingstone

Snowden JS, Griffiths HL, Neary D. (1996b) Semantic-episodic memory interactions in semantic dementia implications for retrograde memory function. *Cognitive Neuropsychology* **13**: 1101–1137

Snowden JS, Bathgate D, Varma A *et al.* (2001) Distinct behavioural profiles in frontotemporal dementia and semantic dementia. *Journal of Neurology, Neurosurgery, and Psychiatry* **70**: 323–332

Snowden JS, Thompson JC, Neary D. (2004) Knowledge of famous faces and names in semantic dementia. *Brain* **127**: 860–872

Thompson SA, Patterson K, Hodges JR. (2003) Left/right asymmetry of atrophy in semantic dementia behavioural-cognitive implications. *Neurology* **61**: 1196–1203

Thompson SA, Graham KS, Williams G *et al.* (2004) Dissociating person-specific from general semantic knowledge: roles of the left and right temporal lobes. *Neuropsychologia* **42**: 359–370

Tyrrell PJ, Warrington EK, Frackowiak RSJ, Rossor MN. (1990a) Heterogeneity in progressive aphasia due to focal cortical atrophy. A clinical and PET study. *Brain* **113**: 1321–1336

Tyrrell PJ, Warrington EK, Frackowiak RSJ, Rossor MN. (1990b) Progressive degeneration of the right temporal lobe studied with positron emission tomography. *Journal of Neurology, Neurosurgery, and Psychiatry* **53**: 1046–1050

Warrington EK. (1975) The selective impairment of semantic memory. *Quarterly Journal of Experimental Psychology* **27**: 635–637

Warrington EK and James M. (1991) *The Visual Object and Space Perception Battery*. Bury St Edmonds, Thames Valley Test Company

Warrington EK and McCarthy RA. (1987) Categories of knowledge: further fractionations and an attempted integration. *Brain* **110**: 1273–1296

Warrington EK and Shallice T. (1984) Category specific semantic impairments. *Brain* **107**: 829–854

Westmacott R, Black SE, Freedman M, Moscovitch M. (2003) The contribution of autobiographical significance to semantic memory: evidence from Alzheimer's disease, semantic dementia and amnesia. *Neuropsychologia* **42**: 25–48

56

The cerebellum and cognitive impairment

ELSDON STOREY

The motor features of the cerebellar syndrome were crystallized by the great English neurologist Gordon Holmes soon after World War I. He did not ascribe any cognitive function to the cerebellum and, until the last decade or two, this view held general sway. However, a confluence of evidence from new neuroanatomical tracing techniques, functional neuro-imaging experiments and careful clinical studies now points strongly to a significant role for the cerebellum in cognition, of which the clinician should be aware. This chapter aims to distil some of the important studies supporting a non-motor role for the cerebellum. The reader interested in a detailed exposition is referred to *The Cerebellum and Cognition*, edited by Jeremy Schmahmann (1997), while several shorter reviews have also been published (e.g. Leiner *et al.*, 1993; Fiez, 1996; Diamond, 2000; Rapoport *et al.*, 2000).

56.1 THE NEUROANATOMICAL BASIS OF CEREBELLAR COGNITIVE FUNCTION

The cerebellum, which contains more neurones than the entire remainder of the brain, has a regular and relatively simple modular structure. The 'corticonuclear microcomplex' is essentially a positive loop through the deep cerebellar nuclei, modulated by a variable negative side loop through the cerebellar cortex (Ito, 1993). The degree of inhibitory influence of the cerebellar cortical Purkinje cells on the deep cerebellar nuclei is governed by the development of long-term depression (LTD) at the excitatory parallel fibre-Purkinje dendrite synapses (Ito, 1993). LTD itself develops in response to near-simultaneous Purkinje cell activation by parallel fibres, and by climbing fibres from the inferior olive. It may thus be considered to be analogous to associative long-term potentiation in the hippocampus. In the influential Marr–Albus–Ito model of cerebellar function, the climbing fibres are regarded as carrying the 'error signals' responsible for adaptive motor learning.

While there is no universally accepted model of the mechanism whereby LTD in the corticonuclear microcomplex might result in motor learning at the whole animal level, it is clear from its stereotyped modular structure that the cerebellum performs the same type of basic computation on whatever inputs it receives, and informs all its various efferent targets of the results of such computation. If different areas of the cerebellum differ in function, therefore, they do so by virtue of their differing inputs and outputs.

With this in mind, the evidence for cerebellar input from, and output to, non-motor areas can be considered. Such evidence is both indirect and direct. The former consists of the observation that, in primate phylogeny, and especially in hominids, the prefrontal portion of the frontal lobes and the lateral neocerebellum with its associated ventral macrogyric region of the dentate nucleus have undergone massive parallel selective enlargement, out of proportion to other brain areas (e.g. Matano, 2001; MacLeod *et al.*, 2003). More direct evidence has had to await the development of anterograde and retrograde trans-synaptic (viral) tracers (Middleton and Strick, 1997). Such tracers are necessary because cerebral cortical input to the cerebellum proceeds via corticopontine fibres synapsing on the pontine nuclei, which in turn project to the deep cerebellar nuclei and cerebellar cortex, while cerebellar output to the cortex proceeds via synaptic relays in the thalamus (Schmahmann and Pandya, 1997). Studies using such tracers in primates have shown that a series of anatomically discrete parallel cortico-ponto-cerebello-thalamo-cortical loops exist, with prefrontal input predominantly to the ventral, macrogyric portion of the dentate nucleus and associated lateral neocerebellar cortex, and output via the ventrolateral and medial dorsal thalamic nuclei (Middleton and Strick, 2000, 2001). Motor and premotor cortex, in contrast, are reciprocally connected to the phylogenetically older dorsolateral, microgyric portion of the dentate nucleus (Middleton and Strick, 2000, 2001). The analogy with separate, parallel corticobasal ganglionic circuits subserving motor and non-motor functions, as conceptualized by Alexander *et al.* (1986), is readily drawn (Middleton and Strick, 2000).

56.2 FUNCTIONAL NEUROIMAGING STUDIES

A large number of functional neuroimaging studies of cerebellar activation during tests of various cognitive domains have been reported over the last 15 years, using positron emission tomography (PET) or functional magnetic resonance imaging (fMRI). The typical design compares patterns of cerebellar activation on a cognitive task with that on what is thought to be a relevant control 'motor' and/or perceptual task. This section includes a broadly representative sample of such studies across various cognitive domains.

The cerebellum appears to play a role in language function. One of the earliest reports was that of Petersen *et al.* (1989), who used PET to study a verb association task (e.g. responding with 'bark' if shown the word 'dog'). The control tasks were reading aloud, and silently. Broca's area and the right lateral cerebellum were both activated. Hubrich-Ungureanu *et al.* (2002) extended these findings with an fMRI study of a silent verbal fluency task in left- and right-handed subjects. Fullbright *et al.* (1999) asked subjects to read silently. Their fMRI study showed that semantic comparison and judgement of non-word rhyming activated posterolateral (and especially right posterolateral) cerebellar cortex, compared with the control conditions of line orientation judgement, upper versus lower case print judgement, or judgement of real word rhyming. Xiang *et al.* (2003) recently confirmed the role of the right posterolateral cerebellum in semantic discrimination divorced from articulation. Such studies have led to the concept of the 'lateralized linguistic cerebellum', recently reviewed by Marien *et al.* (2001).

The cerebellum also appears to be involved in executive functioning and working memory. Cognitive processing during attempted solution of a pegboard puzzle task compared with simple peg movement was studied using fMRI estimation of dentate activation by Kim *et al.* (1994). The cognitively demanding task produced increased, and bilateral, dentate activation compared with the contralateral (to the moving hand) activation seen with simple peg movement. In as much as this task tapped visuospatial working memory, it is conceptually similar to the working memory fMRI study of Desmond *et al.* (1997), who found that delayed matching

of letter strings but not the control task activated the right inferolateral cerebellar hemisphere. The Wisconsin Card Sorting Test (WCST), a complex task often used to assess aspects of executive functioning, has also been found to activate the lateral cerebellum (e.g. Nagahama *et al.*, 1996).

An aspect of episodic memory was addressed by Andreasen *et al.* (1999) in a 'pure thought' PET experiment. Subjects were asked to recall a personal memory silently. The right lateral cerebellum was activated, in addition to several relevant supratentorial areas.

A further area of recent active study has been the role(s) of the cerebellum in attention. Allen *et al.* (1997) showed an anatomical double dissociation in cerebellar regional activation; a visual attention task activated the lateral cerebellum while the motor task activated more medial regions. Attention is, however, a multifaceted concept, placing a variety of different demands on the subject (e.g. sustained/directed attention, divided attention, attentional switching). Le *et al.* (1998) showed that shifting attention between stimulus dimensions (colour/shape) activated the right lateral cerebellum, while sustained attention did not. More recently, Bischoff-Grethe *et al.* (2002) have demonstrated that the lateral cerebellum's role in this paradigm may actually be in reassignment of a given motor response (e.g. pushing a button) to the new stimulus dimension, rather than in shifting attention *per se*.

It is clear that the weight of evidence from functional neuroimaging studies in favour of lateral cerebellar contributions to cognition is strong, as illustrated by the selected studies cited above. However, it is also clear that the exact role(s) of the lateral cerebellum in complex aspects of cognition such as language and attentional shifting still requires considerable clarification.

56.3 DIFFICULTIES IN STUDYING COGNITIVE FUNCTION IN SUBJECTS WITH CEREBELLAR DYSFUNCTION

The results of functional neuroimaging studies in normal people notwithstanding, the practising clinician is understandably primarily concerned with the potential impact of cerebellar disease or dysfunction on cognition. Unfortunately, several confounding factors must be borne in mind when interpreting such studies. The first problem is that performance on the neuropsychological tests used may be adversely affected by requirements for rapid verbal output, motor accuracy and speed, or by dependence on rapid visual scanning. A correlation between test results and ataxia severity will not necessarily indicate that such requirements are confounding the results, however; motor and cognitive function would be expected to decline in parallel in diffuse cerebellar degenerations, whether the observed cognitive dysfunction was secondary to the cerebellar disorder or was merely secondary to the resultant motor impairment.

Several types of neuropsychological task would be expected *a priori* to limit the potential for confounding of results. Some tests are untimed, and do not require motoric or visual speed or accuracy. In the executive domain, these include the WCST, Raven's Progressive Matrices, and the Zoo Map subtest (of planning) from the Behavioural Assessment of the Dysexecutive Syndrome (BADS) battery. Most measures of verbal anterograde episodic memory also fall into this category, provided that dysarthria is not so severe as to compromise intelligibility. Other tests include a timed internal control condition involving similar scanning and output to the test condition. The effects of visual, verbal and motor dysfunction can therefore be subtracted out. Such tests within the executive function cognitive domain would include Trails B (versus A) and the Stroop test. Yet other tests requiring verbal output are timed, but empirical observation suggests that speed of articulation is not the rate-limiting factor. The controlled oral word association test (COWAT, FAS) appears to fall into this category (Storey et al., 1999).

An indirect way of exploring the possibility that motor dysfunction might secondarily affect performance on cognitive tests is to study patients with Friedreich's ataxia (FA), whose motoric deficit is partly consequent upon disruption of afferent cerebellar input rather than direct disruption of the cerebellar microcorticonuclear units, although the deep cerebellar nuclei are also affected (Koeppen, 2002). While FA patients display impairments in a number of domains (Wollmann et al., 2002), they have been shown to be less impaired on verbal working memory and visuospatial reasoning tasks than patients with assorted other cerebellar degenerations (Botez-Marquard and Botez, 1997). Indeed, White et al. (2000) demonstrated slowed processing speed and decreased cognitive inhibition on the Stroop test, but preserved planning, verbal fluency, and WCST performance.

The potential confounding factor of motor deficit has recently been explicitly addressed by Timmann et al. (2002), who correctly pointed out that even ataxic patients who cope well with the motor demands of a test may do so at the cost of attentional resources not required by control patients. These authors reported that subjects with pure cerebellar cortical atrophies (spinocerebellar ataxia [SCA] 6, other pure cerebellar dominant ataxias, or idiopathic cerebellar cortical atrophy) demonstrated impairments of visual association learning independent of the separately manipulated motor output requirements of the task.

The second problem affecting patient studies is that of choice of patient type. The ideal patient group for such a study would have widespread/diffuse involvement of cerebellar corticonuclear microcomplex units, with complete sparing of all other central nervous system structures. Unfortunately, such patients probably do not exist, at least to the extent of satisfying those sceptical of the idea of cerebellar contributions to cognition. Even relatively 'pure' cerebellar ataxias such as SCA 6 often have mild non-cerebellar features (e.g. pyramidal signs). Other degenerative cerebellar diseases studied in this context, such as SCAs 1, 2 and 3, are even more problematic, as they are known to manifest extracerebellar involvement of structures potentially or actually contributing

to cognition, such as the cerebral cortex, the striatum and the substantia nigra (Koeppen, 2002). On the other hand, focal cerebellar lesions such as infarcts and resected tumours may be 'pure', but there is no guarantee that cerebellar region(s) potentially important for cognition will be involved, unless a range of lesions in different locations are studied. Pooled results may then conceal regional differences in cognitive contribution unless sufficient subjects are available in each group for comparison. While this is difficult, such studies do perhaps provide the most convincing clinical evidence, as outlined in the next section.

56.4 ALTERED COGNITION IN ADULTS WITH FOCAL CEREBELLAR LESIONS

In a seminal report, Schmahmann and Sherman (1998) described the features of an entity that they named the 'cerebellar cognitive affective syndrome' in 20 adults with isolated cerebellar lesions: strokes, resected tumours not treated with radiotherapy, and post-viral cerebellitis. Posterior (roughly equivalent to lateral neocerebellar) lobe lesions produced executive dysfunction, with impairments of planning, set-shifting, verbal fluency by semantic category and abstract reasoning. There was also impairment of spatial cognition, including visual organization and visual memory. Lesions of the posterior vermis tended to produce personality change with blunting or disinhibition, while anterior lobe lesions resulted only in motor deficit.

Similar findings were reported by Malm et al. (1998) in 24 consecutive young adult patients with cerebellar infarcts who were compared with 14 age-matched controls. The patients performed less well on working memory and cognitive flexibility tasks, while intelligence (Weschler Adult Intelligence Scale–Revised [WAIS-R] scores) and episodic memory were unaffected. Interestingly, while most made a good motor recovery, only half returned to work.

The broad conclusions of these studies have since been confirmed by Neau et al. (2000), who reported the neuropsychological profile of 15 consecutive patients with recent, isolated cerebellar infarcts, compared with 15 demographically matched controls. A further assessment was undertaken 1 year after the infarcts. These authors demonstrated impairments on a range of tasks tapping aspects of executive functioning, such as verbal fluency, working memory on the Paced Serial Addition Test (PASAT), and the Stroop colour/word interference test. These abnormalities were not accompanied by a clinically apparent 'frontal' neuropsychiatric syndrome. Block design was also affected; this deficit the authors likened to a mild parietal syndrome, although problems with block design can also be a feature of executive dysfunction (Lezak, 1995). Of interest is that infarcts in any of the three cerebellar arterial territories produced similar deficits, although the numbers in each group were small. As might be expected with infarcts, the deficits tended to have improved at the 1-year assessment.

The authors plausibly suggest that this improvement may have been partly responsible for the failure of Beldarrain et al. (1997) to demonstrate consistent deficits in a patient population including subjects with old cerebellar infarcts.

The specific role of the right lateral cerebellum in language, outlined in the section on functional neuroimaging above, was studied in control subjects and subjects with left lateral or right lateral cerebellar infarcts (Gebhart et al., 2002). Those with right lateral cerebellar damage were impaired only on antonym generation, and not on semantic (category) noun fluency or verb selection. This argues in favour of a cerebellar role in producing word associations, and not just in 'imaging' verb action to a noun cue. Helmuth et al. (1997) also failed to demonstrate impaired noun-triggered verb generation in subjects with right cerebellar lesions, in contrast to the evidence from earlier functional neuroimaging studies.

Various attentional processes have also been studied in subjects with cerebellar lesions. Orienting of visuospatial attention has been found to be markedly delayed in such subjects, independent of motor responses (Townsend et al., 1999). Most recently, Gottwald et al. (2003) compared 16 subjects with cerebellar tumours or haematomas to 11 matched control subjects and to demographically adjusted results from normative studies, and detected deficits in working memory and divided attention, but not in sustained directed attention. However, Helmuth et al. (1997) did not demonstrate deficits in spatial attention shifting or in intra- or interdimensional non-spatial attentional shifting, again failing to confirm functional neuroimaging studies in a clinical population. Moreover, Ravizza and Ivry (2001) found that, while patient groups with Parkinson's disease and with cerebellar lesions each showed impairment of attentional shifting, reducing the motor demands of the task improved the performance of the cerebellar patients only. It is obvious that the question of a cerebellar contribution to various forms of attention has generated conflicting results, and remains to be settled conclusively.

Studies in children with resected cerebellar tumours have produced similar results to those in adults (e.g. Levisohn et al., 2000).

56.5 EVIDENCE FOR COGNITIVE IMPAIRMENT IN DEGENERATIVE CEREBELLAR DISEASE

Evidence for cognitive impairment in degenerative cerebellar disease comes from both neurophysiological and clinical neuropsychological studies. The best-known neurophysiological method of studying cognition involves measuring the latency of the P_{300} event related cerebral potential. This occurs with conscious registration of an unusual stimulus, such as an occasional ('oddball') high-pitched tone inserted into a series of usual stimuli, such as many low-pitched tones. It may be regarded as a neurophysiological measure of selective attention and processing speed, and is delayed in various forms of dementia (reviewed by Goodin, 2003).

Tachibana et al. (1999) measured the P_{300} during a visual discrimination task, and found it to be delayed in 15 subjects with idiopathic late-onset cerebellar ataxia, when compared with 10 controls. Single photon emission computed tomography (SPECT) scanning in the ataxic subjects showed correlated cerebellar/frontal cortex hypoperfusion (that is, reversed cerebellar/frontal diaschisis). Tanaka et al. (2003) did not find any differences in P_{300} timing or scalp distribution to the classical auditory 'oddball' paradigm in 13 subjects with cerebellar cortical atrophy when compared with 13 demographically matched controls. However, P_{300} latency was prolonged, and its peak attenuated frontally, in the 'No Go' condition of the 'Go/No Go' paradigm. The authors suggested that the cerebellum contributes to the frontal inhibitory system.

The neuropsychological consequences of degenerative cerebellar disease have been studied extensively. In one early study, Grafman et al. (1992) compared nine patients with 'pure cortical cerebellar atrophy' with 12 controls. There were no differences on paired associate learning, verbal fluency, or procedural (skill) learning. However, the ataxic subjects performed significantly less well on the Tower of Hanoi planning task, which is conceptually similar to the Tower of London test. Botez-Marquard and Botez (1997) showed that cerebellar degenerations resulted in impaired executive functioning, visuospatial organization, working memory, and spontaneous retrieval of episodic memories. Cerebellar strokes produced similar patterns of impairment, but these cognitive deficits resolved in 2–5 months. In both types of subjects, SPECT scanning showed reverse cerebellar/frontoparietal diaschisis.

Drepper et al. (1999) studied nine subjects with 'isolated' cerebellar degeneration, and 10 controls. The ataxic subjects showed a significant impairment in novel associative learning (colours with numbers) that did not correlate with either simple reaction time or visual scanning time.

Kish et al. (1994) studied the performance of 43 subjects with undefined dominant cerebellar degenerations of varying ataxia severity on a number of neuropsychological measures. Impaired performance on the WCST correlated with ataxia severity; none of those with mild ataxia showed deficits, while all of those with severe ataxia were impaired. Some of the latter also showed evidence of mild generalized cognitive deficit. The authors concluded that the dominant ataxias are not homogeneous with respect to cognitive involvement, and indeed the topography of extracerebral neuropathological involvement does vary considerably between these disorders (Koeppen, 2002).

Trojano et al. (1998) also studied a mixed population of subjects with dominant ataxias of varying severity, although 15 of their 22 subjects had SCA 2. They attempted to avoid confounding effects of motor impairment on performance by restricting their investigation to tests with untimed verbal response modes. The domains examined were predominantly verbal memory, and non-verbal reasoning (Raven's Progressive Matrices). None of the four genetically confirmed but asymptomatic subjects performed poorly on any of the tests, while most of the symptomatic subjects showed impairment on at least one measure, most commonly the progressive matrices. Some showed more widespread deficits, but there was no correlation with ataxia severity. This might have reflected the small sample size, and the contaminating effects of inclusion of several SCA subtypes.

Several studies have assessed subjects with different SCA types singly or separately, thereby avoiding this particular confounding factor. Maruff *et al.* (1996) compared six patients with SCA 3 (Machado-Joseph disease) with 15 matched controls using a touch-screen testing system: the Cambridge Neuropsychological Test Automated Battery (CANTAB). Learning and visual memory were unaffected, but SCA 3 subjects displayed impaired visual information processing speed on high-demand tasks, and impaired attentional switching between visual stimulus dimensions. Executive dysfunction in SCA 3 was confirmed by Zawacki *et al.* (2002). Ishikawa *et al.* (2002) reported dementia with features of delirium including hallucinations in four young SCA 3 patients with severe disease, in the absence of MRI or pathological evidence of cortical neuronal loss.

SCA 2 may be associated with cortical atrophy and clinically obvious dementia in some pedigrees (Dürr *et al.*, 1995; Geschwind *et al.*, 1997). Although it is therefore not ideal for the purpose, it has been studied by several groups. Gambardella *et al.* (1998) and Storey *et al.* (1999) demonstrated impairments of executive function on the WCST and the Stroop test. Bürk *et al.* (1999) found that 25 per cent of their subjects were demented, while the others showed impairments of executive function and verbal memory that were independent of the severity of motor impairment. In contrast, Le Pira *et al.* (2002) reported that the impairments of executive function, attention and verbal memory in their SCA 2 patients were partly related to ataxia severity.

The pattern of neuropsychological impairment in SCA 1 patients compared with matched controls was reported by Bürk *et al.* (2001). Evidence of executive and verbal memory dysfunction was found, while visuospatial memory and attention were unaffected. The deficits did not correlate with CAG repeat length or with disease duration, which may be regarded as surrogate markers of disease severity in different dimensions.

While the studies on SCAs 1, 2 and 3 cited above paint a fairly consistent picture of executive dysfunction and verbal memory impairment, the effects of differences in the pattern and extent of extracerebellar neuropathological involvement, if any, can only be addressed adequately by direct comparison. This was undertaken by Bürk *et al.* (2003), who found that executive dysfunction was more marked in SCA 1 than in SCAs 2 or 3, while mild verbal memory impairment was present in all. On the basis of these findings, the authors suggested that the cognitive deficits were likely to result from disruption of cerebrocerebellar circuitry at the pontine rather than at the cerebellar level. Given that SCA 2 causes more severe pontine atrophy than SCA 1, the reasons for this conclusion are unclear. A problem with this study is the lack of control for ataxia severity.

Perhaps the best way of clarifying the relative contributions of cerebellar and extracerebellar pathology to cognitive dysfunction in the SCAs would be to study those disorders characterized by relatively pure cerebellar involvement, such as SCA 6. To the author's knowledge, at least two such studies on SCA 6 are planned or in progress, but neither have been published as yet. Failing this, the conclusion that cerebellar degeneration itself is responsible for at least some of the cognitive changes observed in SCAs 1, 2 and 3 will remain contentious, although this conclusion is consonant with the results of functional neuroimaging and focal lesion studies.

56.6 CONCLUSION

There is now converging evidence from neuroanatomical, neuroimaging, and neurophysiological and neuropsychological patient studies that the lateral cerebellum is involved in network(s) subserving a range of cognitive functions, including aspects of language and executive functioning. The exact nature of the cerebellar contributions to cognition, and especially to attention (if any) are still being debated and elucidated. Nevertheless, the broad picture is well enough established that clinicians should consider the possibility of cognitive dysfunction in patients with overt cerebellar disorders. In this context, executive dysfunction is both the most likely to be overlooked in the structured clinical setting, and potentially the most disruptive to the patients' ability to compensate for impaired motor functioning. Clinicians should also bear in mind that obvious cognitive dysfunction may result from cerebellar disease, and that such dysfunction does not necessarily signify that a second, supratentorial disorder has been overlooked.

REFERENCES

Alexander GE, DeLong PL, Strick PL. (1986) Parallel organization of functionally segregated circuits linking basal ganglia and cortex. *Annual Review of Neuroscience* 9: 357–381

Allen G, Buxton RB, Wong EC *et al.* (1997) Attentional activation of the cerebellum independent of motor involvement. *Science* 275: 1940–1943

Andreasen NC, O'Leary DS, Paradiso S *et al.* (1999) The cerebellum plays a role in conscious episodic memory retrieval. *Human Brain Mapping* 8: 226–234

Beldarrain MG, Garcia-Monco JC, Quintana JM *et al.* (1997) Diaschisis and neuropsychological performance after cerebellar stroke. *European Neurology* 37: 82–89

Bischoff-Grethe A, Ivry RB, Grafton ST. (2002) Cerebellar involvement in response reassignment rather than attention. *Journal of Neuroscience* 22: 546–553

Botez-Marquard T and Botez MI. (1997) Olivopontocerebellar atrophy and Friedreich's ataxia: neuropsychological consequences of bilateral versus unilateral cerebellar lesions. *International Review of Neurobiology* 41: 387–410

Bürk K, Globas C, Bösch S et al. (1999) Cognitive deficits in spinocerebellar ataxia 2. *Brain* **122**: 769–777

Bürk K, Bösch S, Globas C et al. (2001) Executive dysfunction in spinocerebellar ataxia type 1. *European Neurology* **46**: 43–48

Bürk K, Globas C, Bösch S et al. (2003) Cognitive deficits in spinocerebellar ataxia type 1, 2, and 3. *Journal of Neurology* **250**: 207–211

Desmond JE, Gabrieli J, Wagner A et al. (1997) Lobular patterns of cerebellar activation in verbal working-memory and finger-tapping tasks as revealed by functional MRI. *Journal of Neuroscience* **17**: 9675–9685

Diamond A. (2000) Close interrelation of motor development and cognitive development and of the cerebellum and prefrontal cortex. *Child Development* **71**: 44–56

Drepper J, Timmann D, Kolb FP, Diener HC. (1999) Non-motor associative learning in patients with isolated degenerative cerebellar disease. *Brain* **122**: 87–97

Dürr A, Smadja D, Cancel G et al. (1995) Autosomal dominant cerebellar ataxia type I in Martinique (French West Indies): clinical and neuropathological analysis of 53 patients from three unrelated SCA 2 families. *Brain* **118**: 1573–1581

Fiez JA. (1996) Cerebellar contributions to cognition. *Neuron* **16**: 13–15

Fullbright RK, Jenner AR, Mencl WE et al. (1999) The cerebellum's role in reading: a functional MR imaging study. *American Journal of Neuroradiology* **20**: 1925–1930

Gambardella A, Annesi G, Bono F et al. (1998) CAG repeat length and clinical features in three Italian families with spinocerebellar ataxia type 2 (SCA 2): early impairment of Wisconsin Card Sorting Test and saccade velocity. *Journal of Neurology* **245**: 647–652

Gebhart AL, Petersen SE, Thach WT. (2002) Role of the posterolateral cerebellum in language. *Annals of the New York Academy of Sciences* **978**: 318–333

Geschwind DH, Perlman S, Figueroa CP et al. (1997) The prevalence and wide clinical spectrum of the spinocerebellar ataxia type 2 trinucleotide repeat in patients with autosomal dominant cerebellar ataxia. *American Journal of Human Genetics* **60**: 842–850

Goodin DS. (2003) Long-latency event-related potentials. In: JS Ebersole and TA Pedley (eds), *Current Practice of Clinical Electroencephalography*, 3rd edition. Philadelphia, Lippincott Williams and Wilkins, pp. 923–935

Gottwald B, Mihajlovic Z, Wilde B, Mehdorn HM. (2003) Does the cerebellum contribute to specific aspects of attention? *Neuropsychologia* **41**: 1452–1460

Grafman J, Litvan I, Massaquoi S et al. (1992) Cognitive planning deficit in patients with cerebellar atrophy. *Neurology* **42**:1493–1496

Helmuth LL, Ivry RB, Shimizu N. (1997) Preserved performance by cerebellar patients on tests of word generation, discrimination learning, and attention. *Learning and Memory* **3**: 456–474

Hubrich-Ungureanu P, Kaemmerer N, Henn FA, Braus DF. (2002) Lateralized organization of the cerebellum in a silent verbal fluency task: a functional magnetic resonance imaging study in healthy volunteers. *Neuroscience Letters* **319**: 91–94

Ishikawa A, Yamada M, Makino K et al. (2002) Dementia and delirium in 4 patients with Machado-Joseph disease. *Archives of Neurology* **59**: 1804–1808

Ito M. (1993) Movement and thought: identical control mechanisms by the cerebellum. *Trends in Neuroscience* **16**: 448–450

Kim S, Ugurbil K, Strick P. (1994) Activation of a cerebellar output nucleus during cognitive processing. *Science* **265**: 949–951

Kish SJ, el-Awar M, Stuss D et al. (1994) Neuropsychological test performance in patients with dominantly inherited spinocerebellar ataxia: relationship to ataxia severity *Neurology* **44**: 1738–1746

Koeppen AH. (2002) Neuropathology of the inherited ataxias. In: MU Manto and M Pandolfo (eds), *The Cerebellum and its Disorders*. Cambridge, Cambridge University Press, pp. 387–405

Le Pira F, Zappala G, Saponara R et al. (2002) Cognitive findings in spinocerebellar ataxia type 2: relationship to genetic and clinical variables. *Journal of the Neurological Sciences* **201**: 53–57

Le TH, Pardo JV, Hu X. (1998) 4 T-fMRI study of nonspatial shifting of selective attention: cerebellar and parietal contributions. *Journal of Neurophysiology* **79**: 1535–1548

Leiner HC, Leiner AL, Dow RS. (1993) Cognitive and language functions of the human cerebellum. *Trends in Neuroscience* **16**: 444–447

Levisohn L, Cronin-Golomb A, Schmahmann JD. (2000) Neuropsychological consequences of cerebellar tumour resection in children: cerebellar cognitive affective syndrome in a paediatric population. *Brain* **123**: 1041–1050

Lezak M. (1995) *Neuropsychological Assessment*, 3rd edition. New York, Oxford University Press

MacLeod CE, Zilles K, Schleicher A et al. (2003) Expansion of the neocerebellum in Hominoidea. *Journal of Human Evolution* **44**: 401–429

Malm J, Kristensen B, Karlsson T et al. (1998) Cognitive impairment in young adults with infratentorial infarcts. *Neurology* **51**: 433–440

Marien P, Engelborghs S, Fabbro F, De Deyn PP. (2001) The lateralized linguistic cerebellum: a review and a new hypothesis. *Brain and Language* **79**: 580–600

Maruff P, Tyler P, Burt T et al. (1996) Cognitive deficits in Machado-Joseph disease. *Annals of Neurology* **40**: 421–427

Matano S. (2001) Brief communication: proportions of the ventral half of the cerebellar dentate nucleus in humans and great apes. *American Journal of Physical Anthropology* **114**: 163–165

Middleton FA and Strick PL. (1997) Cerebellar output channels. In: JD Schmahmann (ed.), *The Cerebellum and Cognition*. International Review of Neurobiology Vol. 41. San Diego, Academic Press, pp. 61–82

Middleton FA and Strick PL. (2000) Basal ganglia and cerebellar loops: motor and cognitive circuits. *Brain Research Reviews* **31**: 236–250

Middleton FA and Strick PL. (2001) Cerebellar projections to the prefrontal cortex of the primate. *Journal of Neuroscience* **21**: 700–712

Nagahama Y, Fukuyama H, Yamauchi H et al. (1996) Cerebral activation during performance of a card sorting test. *Brain* **119**: 1667–1675

Neau J-Ph, Arroyo-Anllo E, Bonnaud V et al. (2000) Neuropsychological disturbances in cerebellar infarcts. *Acta Neurologica Scandinavica* **102**: 363–370

Petersen SE, Fox PT, Posner MI et al. (1989) Positron emission tomographic studies of the processing of single words. *Journal of Cognitive Neuroscience* **1**: 153–170

Rapoport M, ven Reekum R, Mayberg H. (2000) The role of the cerebellum in cognition and behavior: a selective review. *Journal of Neuropsychiatry and Clinical Neurosciences* **12**: 193–198

Ravizza SM and Ivry RB. (2001) Comparison of the basal ganglia and cerebellum in shifting attention. *Journal of Cognitive Neuroscience* **13**: 285–297

Schmahmann JD (ed.) (1997) *The Cerebellum and Cognition*. International Review of Neurobiology Vol. 41. San Diego, Academic Press

Schmahmann JD and Pandya DN. (1997) The cerebrocerebellar system. In JD Schmahmann (ed.), *The Cerebellum and Cognition*. International Review of Neurobiology Vol. 41. San Diego, Academic Press, pp. 31–60

Schmahmann JD and Sherman JC. (1998) The cerebellar affective cognitive syndrome. *Brain* **121**: 561–579

Storey E, Forrest SM, Shaw JH *et al.* (1999) Spinocerebellar ataxia type 2: Clinical features of a pedigree displaying prominent frontal-executive dysfunction. *Archives of Neurology* **56**: 43–50

Tachibana H, Kawabata K, Tomino Y, Sugita M. (1999) Prolonged P$_3$ latency and decreased brain perfusion in cerebellar degeneration. *Acta Neurologica Scandinavica* **100**: 310–316

Tanaka H, Harada M, Arai M, Hirata K. (2003) Cognitive dysfunction in cortical cerebellar atrophy correlates with impairment of the inhibitory system. *Neuropsychobiology* **47**: 206–211

Timmann D, Drepper J, Maschke M *et al.* (2002) Motor deficits cannot explain impaired cognitive associative learning in cerebellar patients. *Neuropsychologia* **40**: 788–800

Townsend J, Courchesne E, Covington J *et al.* (1999) Spatial attention deficits in patients with acquired or developmental cerebellar abnormality. *Journal of Neuroscience* **19**: 5632–5643

Trojano L, Chiacchio L, Grossi D *et al.* (1998) Determinants of cognitive disorders in autosomal dominant cerebellar ataxia type 1. *Journal of the Neurological Sciences* **157**: 162–167

White M, Lalonde R, Botez-Marquard T. (2000) Neuropsychologic and neuropsychiatric characteristics of patients with Friedreich's ataxia. *Acta Neurologica Scandinavica* **102**: 222–226

Wollmann T, Barroso J, Monton F, Nieto A. (2002) Neuropsychological test performance of patients with Friedreich's ataxia. *Journal of Clinical and Experimental Neuropsychology* **24**: 677–686

Xiang H, Lin C, Ma X *et al.* (2003) Involvement of the cerebellum in semantic discrimination: an fMRI study. *Human Brain Mapping* **18**: 208–214

Zawacki TM, Grace J, Friedman JH, Sudarsky L. (2002) Executive and emotional dysfunction in Machado-Joseph disease. *Movement Disorders* **17**: 1004–1010

57

Progressive aphasia and other focal syndromes

JASON D WARREN, RICHARD J HARVEY AND MARTIN N ROSSOR

Progressive cognitive syndromes with circumscribed deficits and preserved intellect have been recognized for many years (e.g. Serieux, 1893) and have attracted much recent interest. These focal forms of dementia (variously termed 'focal cortical atrophies', 'lobar atrophies' or 'asymmetric cortical degenerations') manifest in diverse cognitive domains including language, praxis, specific categories of knowledge and cortical visual functions. Many patients with focal presentations will ultimately suffer a generalized intellectual decline; however, this is not inevitable and is often delayed for a number of years (Mesulam, 1982).

The focal dementias pose considerable nosological and neurobiological difficulties. While circumscribed lobar atrophy on structural brain imaging (especially magnetic resonance imaging, [MRI]) can support the impression of a focal cognitive syndrome, diagnosis remains essentially clinical. In this chapter, the focal dementias are classified according to clinical presentation and the various radiological and pathological correlates of each syndrome are outlined (see Table 57.1). The syndrome of semantic dementia, characterized by an early selective impairment of semantic memory, is discussed in Chapter 55.

57.1 PROGRESSIVE SPEECH AND LANGUAGE SYNDROMES

57.1.1 Primary progressive aphasia

Primary progressive aphasia (PPA) is a clinical syndrome of progressive language impairment with relative sparing of nonverbal cognitive and behavioural functions until late in the course. It may be the most common of the focal dementia syndromes. Although cases of the syndrome have been described for over a century (Luzzatti and Poeck, 1991) the first comprehensive modern account was Mesulam's (1982) series of six patients, five of whom had a progressive anomic aphasia. Diagnostic criteria have since been proposed (Mesulam, 2001). Non-fluent and fluent subtypes of PPA have been proposed on both clinical and anatomical grounds (Mesulam et al., 2003); these subtypes are represented with approximately equal overall frequency in the literature (Mesulam and Weintraub, 1992; Black, 1996), however, 'mixed' forms are common (Grossmann, 2002; Mesulam et al., 2003). The nosological status of fluent PPA is controversial: it is unclear whether this subtype should be considered a primary language disturbance, or rather subsumed within the semantic dementia spectrum. The heterogeneity of PPA reflects the distributed neuroanatomical networks and multiple cognitive operations that support language production and comprehension.

57.1.1.1 CLINICAL FEATURES

Difficulties in word-finding, naming or spelling and impoverished conversation are common presenting complaints; however, diagnosis is based on the form and content of the patient's spontaneous speech. Non-fluent PPA is characterized by effortful, sparse or 'telegraphic' speech with grammatical and phonemic errors. Comprehension is generally retained until late in the course of the condition, although an early selective deficit in comprehending verbs and grammatical relations may be evident on neuropsychometry (Grossman, 2002). Stuttering and articulatory errors may occur, and associated features may include orofacial apraxia, dysphonia, and dysphagia (Mesulam and Weintraub, 1992; Kertesz and Orange, 2000; Mesulam, 2001). In contrast, fluent PPA is characterized by circumlocutory, 'empty' but grammatically correct speech, with relatively normal articulation, rate and phrase length (Mesulam, 2001);

Table 57.1 Clinical, imaging and pathological features of the focal dementias

Syndrome	Clinical Features	Structural brain imaging (CT/MRI)	Functional brain imaging (SPECT/PET)	Pathology
Progressive aphasia				
Non-fluent	Anomia, sparse, effortful, telegraphic speech; phonemic paraphasias, agrammatism; may have orofacial apraxia, dysarthria, dysprosody, dysphagia	L perisylvian/inferior frontal atrophy	L > R frontal/ anterior temporal/ anterior insula hypometabolism/ perfusion	Predominantly non-AD (varies between series) including non-specific histology, PD, CBD, PSP, MND; AD may be more frequent (unclear)
Fluent*	Anomia, circumlocutory, 'empty' speech, impaired comprehension, may have word-finding pauses	L anterolateral temporal atrophy	L > R temporal/parietal hypometabolism/perfusion	
Other progressive speech/language syndromes*				
Orofacial apraxia	Severe early impairment of volitional facial, tongue, respiratory movements; associated speech production defect, dysarthria, dysgraphia; may have features MND	L > R frontotemporal atrophy	L > R frontal/anterior temporal hypometabolism/perfusion	PD, CBD
Anarthria	Prominent dysarthria; associated speech apraxia, dysprosody; late dysgraphia, dysphagia	L > R frontal opercular atrophy	L > R posterior-inferior frontal hypometabolism/perfusion	Non-specific histology
Aprosodia/amusia	Selective impairment of intonation and/or singing	R > L frontal/ anterior temporal atrophy	R > L frontal/ anterior temporal hypoperfusion	Uncertain
Conduction aphasia	Prominent difficulty with repetition; phonemic paraphasias	?L parietal atrophy	L parietotemporal hypometabolism/ perfusion	Uncertain
Word deafness	Early impairment of auditory comprehension, acoustic processing; dysprosody, phonemic paraphasias	L superior temporal atrophy	L temporal hypoperfusion	CBD (limited information)
Dynamic aphasia	Selective impairment of propositional speech		Uncertain	Uncertain
Agraphia	Early prominent impairment of writing; spelling variable; often associated apraxia, visuospatial deficits	L > R frontal atrophy; Bilateral parietal atrophy	L > R parieto-occipital hypoperfusion	AD (limited information)
Progressive prosopagnosia	Facial recognition defect; may be associated with other defects of person-specific knowledge, impaired facial emotion processing and expression	R > L anterior temporal atrophy	R > L temporal/orbitofrontal hypometabolism/perfusion	Non-AD pathology (limited information)
Progressive apraxia	Selective impairment of volitional movements of limbs (often asymmetric), trunk; may have selective gait disturbance; may be associated orofacial apraxia, speech production defect	Asymmetric parietal atrophy	Posterior frontal/inferior parietal hypometabolism/perfusion; mesial frontal hypometabolism with gait apraxia	PD, AD, CBD
Progressive visual syndromes				
Visuospatial	Visual disorientation, impaired visually guided movements; often associated agraphia, other parietal signs	Bilateral parietal atrophy	Bilateral (often asymmetric) parieto-occipital hypometabolism/ perfusion	Predominantly AD; also CJD, CBD, subcortical gliosis
Visual agnosia	Defective recognition of objects, written words, topography (apperceptive); alexia (without agraphia) for words or music	Bilateral parieto-temporo-occipital atrophy		
Primary visual dysfunction	Early impairments in colour and shape perception, visual fields, acuity	Bilateral posterior occipital atrophy		

* Nature of primary cognitive dysfunction uncertain.

AD, Alzheimer's disease; CBD, corticobasal degeneration; CJD, Creutzfeldt–Jakob disease; CT, computed tomography; L, left; MND, motor neurone disease; MRI, magnetic resonance imaging; PD, Pick's disease; PET, positron emission tomography; PSP, progressive supranuclear palsy; R, right; SPECT, single photon emission computed tomography impaired comprehension is an early feature, not uncommonly ascribed to 'deafness' by the patient's family. Patients with prolonged word-finding pauses may represent a 'logopenic' subgroup (Mesulam and Weintraub, 1992). Repetition is often abnormal in non-fluent PPA, but may be relatively accurate in fluent PPA (Mesulam, 2001; Grossman, 2002). Although both fluent and non-fluent PPA typically manifest initially as a deterioration in spoken language, other language channels (reading, writing and gesture) generally show analogous deficits as the illness progresses (Snowden et al., 1992; Mesulam, 2001). Mutism is an end-stage feature of both subtypes of PPA (Kertesz and Orange, 2000).

Relative preservation of memory, non-verbal cognitive domains and personality are core features distinguishing PPA from Alzheimer's disease and related dementias. Neuropsychometry has an important role to play in the clinical assessment, particularly in the evaluation of non-verbal cognitive domains; however, many neuropsychological tests and bedside instruments such as the Mini-Mental State Examination depend on verbal responses, and the extent of cognitive impairment in PPA should therefore always be interpreted with caution. Indeed, many patients remain able to care for themselves at home, to manage their financial affairs, and to drive safely, even as their language disintegrates, typically over the course of a decade or more. Eventually, non-verbal cognitive deficits such as executive dysfunction, limb apraxia, and dyscalculia may develop, and asymmetric (predominantly right-sided) pyramidal and extrapyramidal signs are not uncommon (Mesulam and Weintraub, 1992; Mesulam et al., 2003). Few patients suffer a significant personality change, although frontal features (obsessionality, aggression, abulia or disinhibition) may emerge (Snowden et al., 1992).

The age at onset of PPA ranges from the fifth to the eighth decade; males predominate among reported cases, and a variety of European and non-European languages are represented (Mesulam and Weintraub, 1992; Westbury and Bub, 1997). Patients with PPA not uncommonly have a personal or family history of developmental stuttering, dyslexia or other specific learning impairments (Mesulam and Weintraub, 1992), suggesting an underlying genetic or acquired vulnerability of brain language networks. Rarely, PPA is familial; an uncertain proportion of such families fall within the spectrum of dementia linked to chromosome 17, however relatively pure familial forms of PPA (with undetermined inheritance) have been described (Chapman et al., 1997; Krefft et al., 2003).

57.1.1.2 NEUROIMAGING

In PPA as in all the progressive focal syndromes, brain imaging should always be undertaken to exclude non-degenerative processes such as a cerebral tumour. Regional brain atrophy involving the posterior frontal/perisylvian region or temporal lobe can be identified on structural MRI in many cases of PPA (Westbury and Bub, 1997), however this is by no means invariable (Turner et al., 1996; Catani et al., 2003; Nestor et al., 2003a). Atrophy may be restricted to the left hemisphere or it may be bilateral. Focal changes frequently occur on a background of more diffuse atrophy, predominantly involving the frontal lobes. Patients with non-fluent presentations tend to have more severe inferior frontal/perisylvian atrophy (Figure 57.1a and b), while those with fluent presentations have predominantly anterolateral temporal involvement; however, a clear distinction has not been found in all series (Abe et al., 1997; Sonty et al., 2003). Proton magnetic resonance spectroscopy has documented asymmetric axonal injury within the arcuate fasciculus in PPA (Catani et al., 2003), consistent with the focal involvement of white matter tracts linking cortical language areas.

Functional brain imaging techniques (single photon emission computed tomography [SPECT]; positron emission tomography [PET]; and functional MRI) have demonstrated dysfunction of left hemisphere language networks (Turner et al., 1996; Westbury and Bub, 1997; Mesulam, 2001) that appears to pre-date the development of atrophy on structural imaging. The functional disturbance is more widespread than suggested by the distribution of structural changes, and there may be abnormal (possibly compensatory) activation beyond the classical language areas (Mesulam, 2001; Sonty et al., 2003). Functional changes may be confined to the left hemisphere or they may be bihemispheric (Westbury and Bub, 1997; Soriani-Lefèvre et al., 2003). Non-fluent phenotypes are associated with hypometabolism and decreased perfusion of frontal perisylvian language areas, while fluent phenotypes are associated with predominant temporal or temporoparietal dysfunction (Tyrrell et al., 1990a; Snowden et al., 1992; Abe et al., 1997; Mesulam, 2001; Soriani-Lefèvre et al., 2003). Involvement of the left anterior insula may disrupt speech production in non-fluent PPA (Nestor et al., 2003a). These patterns (though non-diagnostic) are not typical of other frontotemporal dementia phenotypes or Alzheimer's disease (Westbury and Bub, 1997; Nestor et al., 2003a) and correlate with neuropsychological profiles and clinical evolution (Tyrrell et al., 1990a; Nestor et al., 2003a). Selective right hemisphere hypometabolism has been documented in left-handed patients with PPA (Drzezga et al., 2002).

57.1.1.3 OTHER INVESTIGATIONS

Other investigations are of limited clinical usefulness in PPA, but may assist in differential diagnosis. Electroencephalography (EEG) is generally unremarkable, but may show excess slow activity in the left frontotemporal region; the presence of diffuse abnormalities or loss of α rhythm suggests a generalized process such as Alzheimer's disease. Lumbar puncture may be indicated to exclude an inflammatory or other reversible process (for example, in younger patients or cases where disease evolution has been relatively rapid); the routine cerebrospinal fluid examination is normal. Electromyography may be useful in confirming a motor neurone disease-aphasia syndrome. No pathogenetic mutations have been identified in hereditary PPA (Krefft et al., 2003); however, genetic screening may be indicated in younger patients to exclude atypical presentations of familial Alzheimer's disease or a familial tauopathy.

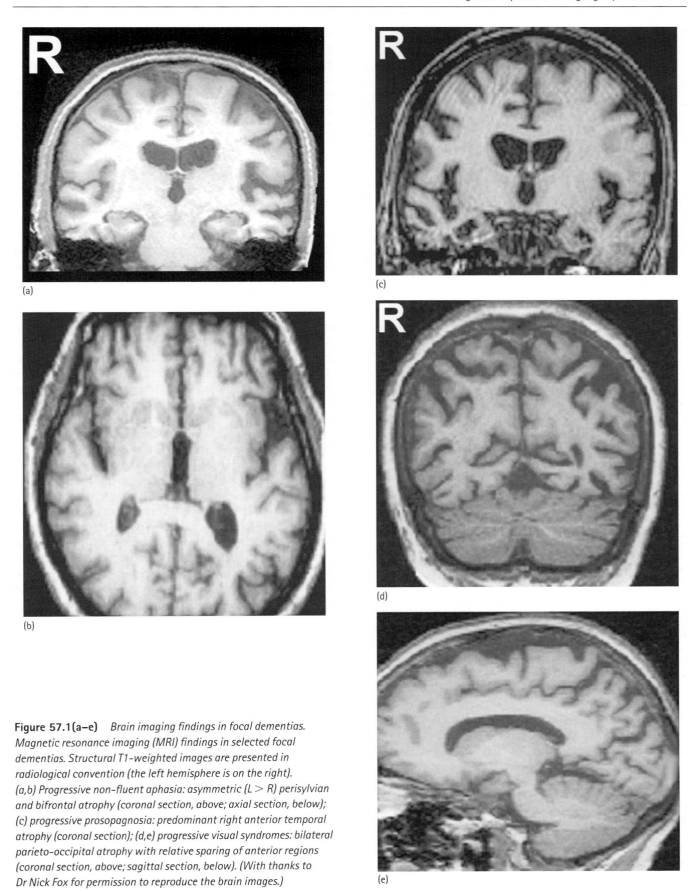

Figure 57.1(a–e) *Brain imaging findings in focal dementias.*
Magnetic resonance imaging (MRI) findings in selected focal
dementias. Structural T1-weighted images are presented in
radiological convention (the left hemisphere is on the right).
(a,b) Progressive non-fluent aphasia: asymmetric (L > R) perisylvian
and bifrontal atrophy (coronal section, above; axial section, below);
(c) progressive prosopagnosia: predominant right anterior temporal
atrophy (coronal section); (d,e) progressive visual syndromes: bilateral
parieto-occipital atrophy with relative sparing of anterior regions
(coronal section, above; sagittal section, below). (With thanks to
Dr Nick Fox for permission to reproduce the brain images.)

57.1.1.4 DISEASE BIOLOGY

A variety of neuropathological findings have been described in the relatively few patients with PPA who have come to post mortem or cerebral biopsy. In one review (Mesulam *et al.*, 2003), the most commonly reported pattern (approximately 60 per cent of cases) was a focal degeneration of the left frontal perisylvian and temporal cortex with neuronal loss, gliosis and mild spongifom changes within superficial cortical layers: 'dementia lacking distinctive histology'. Classical Pick's or Alzheimer's changes were less common (each approximately 20 per cent of cases). Other pathologies have been described infrequently: these include corticobasal degeneration (Ikeda *et al.*, 1996), progressive supranuclear palsy (Mochizuki *et al.*, 2003), and probable Creutzfeldt–Jakob disease (Mandell *et al.*, 1989), as well as less well characterized findings including glial cytoplasmic inclusions (Molina *et al.*, 1998). Cases of motor neurone disease-aphasia syndrome (Bak *et al.*, 2001) constitute a distinct subgroup.

Clinicopathological correlation in PPA remains problematic. There is general consensus that non-fluent PPA is rarely due to Alzheimer's disease (Snowden *et al.*, 1992; Kertesz *et al.*, 1994; Black, 1996; Turner *et al.*, 1996; Kramer and Miller, 2000; Mesulam *et al.*, 2003); however, this is not universally accepted (Hodges, 2001) and counter-examples are well documented (Galton *et al.*, 2000; Nestor *et al.*, 2003a). The situation is equally unclear for the fluent syndromes. Indeed, the pathological heterogeneity of PPA appears more in keeping with an anatomically determined neurolinguistic syndrome than a unitary disease. According to this view, the clinical and radiological features reflect the direction of spread of pathology from the dominant perisylvian region: if anteriorly, a predominantly non-fluent aphasia results; if posteriorly, a predominantly fluent syndrome with semantic disintegration (Kramer and Miller, 2000). Alternatively, PPA may represent a distinct anatomical variant of a common 'Pick's disease-tauopathy' spectrum of frontotemporal lobar degeneration (Kertesz *et al.*, 1994; Mesulam *et al.*, 2003). This concept could be extended to patients with corticobasal degeneration and motor neurone disease pathology (Kertesz *et al.*, 1994). The existence of familial forms of PPA, the apparent association between sporadic PPA and the *tau* H1/H1 genotype (Sobrido *et al.*, 2003) and the lack of association between PPA and the ε4 allele of apolipoprotein E (Mesulam *et al.*, 2003) are consistent with a distinct molecular pathogenesis; however, the significance of these observations remains uncertain. The recent discovery of the genetic basis for a developmental speech and language disorder (Vargha-Khadem *et al.*, 1998) raises the exciting prospect that a similar approach in familial PPA may transform our understanding of this condition.

57.1.2 Unusual syndromes

A number of progressive speech and language impairments that would not fulfil strict diagnostic criteria for PPA have been described. The extensive clinical and pathological overlap within this group and the tendency of fragmentary syndromes to evolve over time and to develop features more typical of PPA suggest that these syndromes represent a neuroanatomical continuum reflecting the topography of pathological involvement, rather than discrete disease entities (Mesulam, 2001). Patients presenting with progressive orofacial apraxia and speech production impairment represent a clinically well defined (though pathologically heterogeneous) group (Tyrrell *et al.*, 1991; Cappa *et al.*, 1993; Chapman *et al.*, 1997). Orofacial apraxia manifests as an inability to cough, yawn or take a deep breath to command, although these actions are normal when performed spontaneously. The illness may evolve over several years into a frontotemporal dementia-motor neurone syndrome accompanied by prominent dysphagia, fasciculations (especially involving triceps and deltoids) and muscle wasting, and electrophysiological evidence of denervation (Tyrrell *et al.*, 1991). Other non-fluent syndromes include progressive aphemia (a severe apraxia of speech; Cohen *et al.*, 1993), cortical anarthria (the anterior opercular syndrome: Broussolle *et al.*, 1996; Silveri *et al.*, 2003), aprosodia ('prosoplegia'; Ghacibeh and Heilman, 2003) and expressive amusia (a selective impairment of singing; Confavreux *et al.*, 1992). Progressive agraphia (Grossman *et al.*, 2001; O'Dowd and de Zubicaray, 2003) and adynamic aphasia (Warren *et al.*, 2003) have also been reported. Uncommon fluent syndromes include progressive pure word deafness and auditory agnosia (Ikeda *et al.*, 1996; Otsuki *et al.*, 1998), and conduction aphasia (Hachisuka *et al.*, 1999). Atrophy tends to be predominantly anterior in the non-fluent syndromes and superior temporal or parietotemporal in the fluent syndromes. Progressive aprosodia and amusia appear to localize to the right frontal or anterior temporal lobes; these syndromes may be accompanied by a loss of facial expressivity, difficulty in comprehending facial or vocal emotion, and later development of a speech production deficit (Confavreux *et al.*, 1992; Ghacibeh and Heilman, 2003). Presentations dominated by progressive agraphia appear to correlate with dominant or bilateral parietal involvement (Grossman *et al.*, 2001; O'Dowd and de Zubicaray, 2003). For unknown reasons, certain phenotypes (for example, jargon aphasia and agraphia; Östberg *et al.*, 2001) occur much less commonly in degenerative than in vascular disease. Neuropathological studies indicate that the majority of patients presenting with unusual PPA variants (in particular, the non-fluent syndromes) have non-Alzheimer pathology, including Pick's disease, corticobasal degeneration and non-specific histology (Cappa *et al.*, 1993; Broussolle *et al.*, 1996; Chapman *et al.*, 1997).

57.2 PROGRESSIVE PROSOPAGNOSIA

In contrast to the well-characterized impairments of language and semantic memory that accompany focal degenerations of the left temporal lobe, the correlates of selective right temporal atrophy remain poorly defined. The apparent rarity of focal right temporal degenerations may be due at least in part to the clinical silence of this region relative to the eloquent left temporal lobe, and indeed patients may not present to the neurologist until bilateral temporal lobe involvement produces a disturbance of semantic memory (Tyrrell *et al.*, 1990b). The best established clinical phenotype of right temporal lobe pathology is the syndrome of progressive prosopagnosia (Tyrrell *et al.*, 1990b; Evans *et al.*, 1995; Gainotti *et al.*, 2003). Patients present with a progressive inability to recognize faces; as the illness progresses, even famous and highly familiar faces (such as family members) may not be recognized, and generalization to other modalities (such as voices) may occur. Perceptual analysis of faces is generally normal (Tyrrell *et al.*, 1990b; Evans *et al.*, 1995; Gainotti *et al.*, 2003), and general semantic and autobiographical knowledge is typically preserved. These observations suggest that the core defect is loss of access to person-specific knowledge (Gainotti *et al.*, 2003). Focal right anterior temporal atrophy is observed on MRI (Figure 57.1c; p. 723); right temporal and orbitofrontal hypometabolism or hypoperfusion may be detected on functional imaging prior to the onset of structural change (Edwards-Lee *et al.*, 1997). Atrophy predominantly involving the right fusiform and parahippocampal gyri has been correlated with a variant prosopagnosia phenotype in which the core defect is an inability to form global perceptual representations of faces (Joubert *et al.*, 2003).

Some patients with selective right temporal atrophy have associated affective disturbances, personality change and sociopathy which may be due in part to an inability to interpret facial expressions, and the patient's own facial expressions frequently become blunted (Edwards-Lee *et al.*, 1997). Amygdala atrophy is often marked in these cases. Typical frontal behavioural features may develop. Associations between facial identity and emotion processing deficits and between prosopagnosia and other categories of perceptual deficit are variable (Evans *et al.*, 1995; Gentileschi *et al.*, 1999). Associative olfactory agnosia may accompany prosopagnosia (Mendez and Ghajarnia, 2001), perhaps illustrating a common mechanism of disconnection of right temporal cortex from mesial limbic structures. Based on limited evidence (Edwards-Lee *et al.*, 1997), the neuropathological correlates of progressive prosopagnosia may be similar to those of left temporal atrophy-semantic dementia and other frontotemporal dementias in the 'Pick-tauopathy' spectrum.

57.3 PROGRESSIVE APRAXIA

Primary progressive apraxia has been described only infrequently. Patients may complain initially of 'clumsiness' involving one hand (more commonly the left), and asymmetrical involvement is common as the illness evolves (Azouvi *et al.*, 1993). On examination, difficulty imitating gestures and meaningless hand positions, in pantomime and in the use of

objects may be evident; alien limb behaviour has been described (Ball *et al.*, 1993). Limb apraxia is often accompanied by deficits of buccofacial or truncal praxis. Aphasic and other cognitive deficits may develop later in the course. Structural MRI may demonstrate asymmetric parietal atrophy (Azouvi *et al.*, 1993; Kareken *et al.*, 1998), and PET has shown asymmetric posterior frontal and inferior parietal hypometabolism (Kareken *et al.*, 1998). Presentations dominated by a progressive frontal gait disorder ('gait apraxia') and fear of falling constitute a distinct clinical variant (Rossor *et al.*, 1999). There may be associated rigidity with the features of *gegenhalten* and initially few other signs; however, upper limb apraxia and more widespread cognitive dysfunction may develop later in the course. Structural brain imaging may be unremarkable; however, medial frontal hypometabolism may be evident on PET.

Progressive apraxia is a feature of corticobasal degeneration, in which limb apraxia is typically accompanied by asymmetric rigidity and other extrapyramidal or cortical sensory signs, and biparietal presentations of Alzheimer's disease, in which visuospatial impairments and other cognitive deficits are generally evident (Ball *et al.*, 1993; Mackenzie Ross *et al.*, 1996; Galton *et al.*, 2000). However, diagnostic and nosologic difficulties are posed by patients who have progressive apraxia with a paucity of associated neurological signs (Azouvi *et al.*, 1993; Kareken *et al.*, 1998). In support of a metabolic distinction from corticobasal degeneration, ^{18}F-DOPA PET in such patients has demonstrated normal presynaptic dopaminergic uptake (Kareken *et al.*, 1998; Rossor *et al.*, 1999), suggesting that the dopaminergic nigrostriatal system is intact in at least a proportion of cases. However, neuropathological evidence remains limited and inconclusive. In patients with progressive apraxia and parietal dysfunction, Pick's disease (Cambier *et al.*, 1981) and Alzheimer's disease (Ball *et al.*, 1993) have been demonstrated at post mortem. A patient with complex limb apraxia associated with language disturbance and orofacial apraxia had focal atrophy involving the left frontal operculum and lower precentral gyrus with histological features of Pick's disease and typical inclusion bodies (Fukui *et al.*, 1996). In one case of progressive gait disturbance, mixed features of corticobasal degeneration and Alzheimer's disease were found at post mortem (Rossor *et al.*, 1999). By analogy with the progressive aphasias, progressive apraxia is likely to represent a clinical syndrome produced by a spectrum of pathological processes.

57.4 PROGRESSIVE VISUAL SYNDROMES

Three focal syndromes of progressive visual disturbance have been described (Galton *et al.*, 2000; Tang-Wai *et al.*, 2004): progressive visuospatial impairment, progressive visual agnosia and progressive primary visual dysfunction. Clinically and anatomically, these disorders fall within the broad group of posterior cortical atrophies (Benson *et al.*, 1988); this group overlaps with progressive syndromes in which parietal dysfunction is prominent, including progressive apraxia, some fluent presentations of PPA, and biparietal presentations of Alzheimer's disease (Galton *et al.*, 2000). The progressive visual syndromes are likely to reflect differential involvement of the visual processing pathways of the posterior hemispheres (Mackenzie Ross *et al.*, 1996), and mixed features commonly appear as the illness evolves (Benson *et al.*, 1988; Attig *et al.*, 1993; Ardila *et al.*, 1997). Early involvement of the dorsal 'where' processing stream accounts for the majority of case reports (Attig *et al.*, 1993; Mackenzie Ross *et al.*, 1996; Goethals and Santens, 2001; Nestor *et al.*, 2003b). Patients with this syndrome typically present with difficulties in locating objects, planning visually-guided movements and reading lines of text. On examination, visual disorientation and/or optic ataxia, apraxia, agraphia and other parietal signs are frequent, and there may be difficulties in identifying fragmented figures; however, visual fields and early visual processing are intact. Initial disruption of the ventral 'what' processing stream (DeRenzi, 1986; Ardila *et al.*, 1997) produces impairments in the recognition of objects, written words and topographical features; on examination, features of visual apperceptive agnosia are present. Variant syndromes include progressive pure alexia for words or music (Beversdorf and Heilman, 1998) and hemiachromatopsia (Freedman and Costa, 1992). Rarely, early involvement of primary visual cortex produces impairments of early visual processing, which may include deficits or distortions of colour or shape perception, hallucinations or abnormal after-images (Levine *et al.*, 1993; Galton *et al.*, 2000; Chan *et al.*, 2001); visual field defects may develop, and visual acuity may be reduced. These different clinical syndromes broadly correspond to predominantly dorsal parietal, ventral parieto-temporo-occipital and posterior occipital patterns of atrophy on structural imaging (Figure 57.1d and e, p. 723) and pathological examination. Functional imaging generally shows bilateral (often asymmetric) parieto-occipital hypometabolism or hypoperfusion rather than the parieto-temporal pattern typical of Alzheimer's disease (Attig *et al.*, 1993; Victoroff *et al.*, 1994; Beversdorf and Heilman, 1998; Goethals and Santens, 2001; Nestor *et al.*, 2003b).

The majority of progressive visual cases that have been studied pathologically have histological features of Alzheimer's disease (Pantel and Schroder, 1996; Galton *et al.*, 2000; Nestor *et al.*, 2003b; Tang-Wai *et al.*, 2004), suggesting that these syndromes should be regarded principally as variant Alzheimer phenotypes; this generalization may apply particularly to patients with prominent dorsal stream involvement (Nestor *et al.*, 2003b). More typical impairments of memory and other cognitive functions not uncommonly develop later in the course, though visual features may dominate for a number of years. Loss of α rhythm on EEG and evidence of hippocampal atrophy on MRI support the diagnosis of Alzheimer's disease, however routine investigations may be normal. Non-Alzheimer degenerative pathologies including corticobasal degeneration (Tang-Wai *et al.*, 2003), Creutzfeldt–Jakob disease (Victoroff *et al.*, 1994) and subcortical gliosis (Victoroff *et al.*, 1994) have been described in a small number of cases.

57.5 MANAGEMENT

No specific disease-modifying therapies are currently available for any of the focal dementias. After exclusion of reversible disease processes, the main priorities of management are the provision of information and the mobilization of support services for patients and their carers. The social and occupational consequences of these diseases are often profound; appropriate counselling may allow patients and families to plan for the future, and disease support groups may be helpful for some. Pharmacotherapy has a limited role. Concomitant depression should be treated; however, no additional cognitive benefit has been established for neuro-modulatory agents such as the serotonin reuptake inhibitors (Litvan, 2001; Deakin *et al.*, 2003; Pasquier *et al.*, 2003). Patients with frontotemporal lobar degenerations may be particularly vulnerable to dopaminergic blockade and neuroleptics should be avoided in this group (Pijnenburg *et al.*, 2003). Patients with posterior cortical atrophy who fulfil diagnostic criteria for Alzheimer's disease may derive symptomatic benefit from acetylcholinesterase inhibitors such as donepezil; however, anecdotal evidence suggests that these agents may worsen behavioural symptoms in the non-Alzheimer dementias and appropriate controlled trials are awaited. Specific cognitive rehabilitation programmes have been proposed in PPA (Louis *et al.*, 2001), however, their use has not been widely evaluated.

57.6 CONCLUSIONS

The focal dementias present challenges for clinicians and neurobiologists alike. Patients are often disabled by their deficits and stand in need of considerable clinical and social support; yet accurate diagnosis is difficult, and focal cognitive symptoms are not infrequently misinterpreted as non-organic. The clinical syndromes generally represent topographical signatures of the distribution of pathology rather than markers of specific diseases. Histopathological information remains limited: further detailed clinicopathological studies are needed in order to define the spectrum of pathological changes that may be associated with particular clinical phenotypes and to identify features that distinguish these unusual focal variants from the more common diffuse degenerations. Diagnostic and terminological inconsistencies and the conflation of clinical, anatomical and pathological levels of description have given rise to much confusion in the literature of these disorders. Ultimately, this confusion may be resolved only through an improved understanding of the neurobiological and molecular mechanisms whereby regional vulnerabilities of neuronal function are translated into clinical deficits. Such an approach will be essential for the development of rational therapies in these often devastating diseases. Current classification schemes (for example, the distinction between 'fluent' and 'non-fluent' PPA) may be refined as more complete accounts of cognitive information processing become available. It is likely in turn that these rare disorders will provide fresh perspectives on human brain function (in particular, the operation of distributed neural networks) in both health and disease.

REFERENCES

Abe K, Ukita H, Yanagihara T. (1997) Imaging in primary progressive aphasia. *Neuroradiology* **39**: 556–559

Ardila A, Rosselli M, Arvizu L, Kuljis RO. (1997) Alexia and agraphia in posterior cortical atrophy. *Neuropsychiatry, Neuropsychology and Behavioral Neurology* **10**: 52–59

Attig E, Jacquy J, Uytdenhoef P, Roland H. (1993) Progressive focal degenerative disease of the posterior associative cortex. *Canadian Journal of Neurological Science* **20**: 154–157

Azouvi P, Bergego C, Robel L *et al.* (1993) Slowly progressive apraxia: two case studies. *Journal of Neurology* **240**: 347–350

Bak TH, O'Donnan DG, Xuereb JH, Boniface S, Hodges JR. (2001) Selective impairment of verb processing associated with pathological changes in Brodmann areas 44 and 45 in the motor neurone disease-dementia-aphasia syndrome. *Brain* **124**: 103–120

Ball JA, Lantos PL, Jackson M, Marsden CD, Scadding JW, Rossor MN. (1993) Alien hand sign in association with Alzheimer's histopathology. *Journal of Neurology, Neurosurgery, and Psychiatry* **56**: 1020–1023

Benson F, Davis J, Snyder BD. (1988) Posterior cortical atrophy. *Archives of Neurology* **45**: 789–793

Beversdorf DQ and Heilman KM. (1998) Progressive ventral posterior cortical degeneration presenting as alexia for music and words. *Neurology* **50**: 657–659

Black SE. (1996) Focal cortical atrophy syndromes. *Brain and Cognition* **31**: 188–229

Broussolle E, Bakchine S, Tommasi M *et al.* (1996) Slowly progressive anarthria with late anterior opercular syndrome: a variant form of frontal cortical atrophy syndromes. *Journal of the Neurological Sciences* **144**: 44–58

Cambier J, Masson M, Dairou R, Henin D. (1981) Etude anatomo-clinique d'une forme pareitale de maladie de Pick. *Revue Neurologique* **137**: 33–38

Cappa SF, De Fanti CA, De Marco R, Magni E, Messa C, Fazio F. (1993) Progressive dysphasic dementia with bucco-facial apraxia: a case report. *Behavioral Neurology* **6**: 159–163

Catani M, Piccirilli M, Cherubini A *et al.* (2003) Axonal injury within language network in primary progressive aphasia. *Annals of Neurology* **53**: 242–247

Chan D, Crutch SJ, Warrington EK. (2001) A disorder of colour perception associated with abnormal colour after-images: a defect of the primary visual cortex. *Journal of Neurology, Neurosurgery, and Psychiatry* **71**: 515–517

Chapman SB, Rosenberg RN, Weiner MF, Shobe A. (1997) Autosomal dominant progressive syndrome of motor-speech loss without dementia. *Neurology* **49**: 1298–1306

Cohen L, Benoit N, Van EP, Ducarne B, Brunet P. (1993) Pure progressive aphemia. *Journal of Neurology, Neurosurgery, and Psychiatry* **56**: 923–924

Confavreux C, Croisile B, Garassus P, Aimard G, Trillet M. (1992) Progressive amusia and aprosody. *Archives of Neurology* **49**: 971–976

Deakin JB, Rahman S, Nestor PJ, Hodges JR, Sahakian BJ. (2003) Paroxetine does not improve symptoms and impairs cognition in frontotemporal dementia: a double-blind randomized controlled trial. *Psychopharmacology* **172**: 400–408

De Renzi E. (1986) Slowly progressive visual agnosia or apraxia without dementia. *Cortex* **22**: 171–180

Drzezga A, Grimmer T, Siebner H, Minoshima S, Schwaiger M, Kurz A. (2002) Prominent hypometabolism of the right temporoparietal and frontal cortex in two left-handed patients with primary progressive aphasia. *Journal of Neurology* **249**: 1263–1267

Edwards-Lee T, Miller BL, Benson DF *et al.* (1997) The temporal variant of frontotemporal dementia. *Brain* **120**: 1027–1040

Evans JJ, Heggs AJ, Antoun N, Hodges JR. (1995) Progressive prosopagnosia associated with selective right temporal lobe atrophy. A new syndrome? *Brain* **118**: 1–13

Freedman L and Costa L. (1992) Pure alexia and right hemiachromatopsia in posterior dementia. *Journal of Neurology, Neurosurgery, and Psychiatry* **55**: 500–502

Fukui T, Sugita K, Kawamura M, Shiota J, Nakano I. (1996) Primary progressive apraxia in Pick's disease: a clinicopathologic study. *Neurology* **47**: 467–473

Gainotti G, Barbier A, Marra C. (2003) Slowly progressive defect in recognition of familiar people in a patient with right anterior temporal atrophy. *Brain* **126**: 792–803

Galton CJ, Patterson K, Xuereb JH, Hodges JR. (2000) Atypical and typical presentations of Alzheimer's disease: a clinical, neuropsychological, neuroimaging and pathological study of 13 cases. *Brain* **123**: 484–498

Gentileschi V, Sperber S, Spinnler H. (1999) Progressive defective recognition of familiar people. *Neurocase* **5**: 407–424

Ghacibeh GA and Heilman KM. (2003) Progressive affective aprosodia and prosoplegia. *Neurology* **60**: 1192–1194

Goethals M and Santens P. (2001) Posterior cortical atrophy: two case reports and a review of the literature. *Clinical Neurology and Neurosurgery* **103**: 115–119

Grossman M. (2002) Progressive aphasic syndromes: clinical and theoretical advances. *Current Opinion in Neurology* **15**: 409–413

Grossman M, Libon DJ, Ding XS *et al.* (2001) Progressive peripheral agraphia. *Neurocase* **7**: 339–349

Hachisuka K, Uchida M, Nozaki Y, Hashiguchi S, Sasaki M. (1999) Primary progressive aphasia presenting as conduction aphasia. *Journal of the Neurological Sciences* **167**: 137–141

Hodges JR. (2001) Frontotemporal dementia (Pick's disease): clinical features and assessment. *Neurology* **56**: S6–S10

Ikeda K, Akiyama H, Iritani S *et al.* (1996) Corticobasal degeneration with primary progressive aphasia and accentuated cortical lesion in superior temporal gyrus: case report and review. *Acta Neuropathologica* **92**: 534–539

Joubert S, Felician O, Barbeau E *et al.* (2003) Impaired configurational processing in a case of progressive prosopagnosia associated with predominant right temporal atrophy. *Brain* **126**: 2537–2550

Kareken DA, Unverzagt F, Caldemeyer K, Farlow MR, Hutchins GD. (1998) Functional brain imaging in apraxia. *Archives of Neurology* **55**: 107–113

Kertesz A and Orange JB. (2000) Primary progressive aphasia – the future of neurolinguistic and biologic characterization. *Brain and Language* **71**: 116–119

Kertesz A, Hudson L, Mackenzie IRA, Munoz DG. (1994) The pathology and nosology of primary progressive aphasia. *Neurology* **44**: 2065–2072

Kramer JH and Miller BL. (2000) Alzheimer's disease and its focal variants. *Seminars in Neurology* **20**: 447–454

Krefft TA, Graff-Radford NR, Dickson DW, Baker M, Castellani RJ. (2003) Familial primary progressive aphasia. *Alzheimer Disease and Associated Disorders* **17**: 106–112

Levine DN, Lee JM, Fisher CM. (1993) The visual variant of Alzheimer's disease. *Neurology* **43**: 305–313

Litvan I. (2001) Therapy and management of frontal lobe dementia patients. *Neurology* **56**: S41–S45

Louis M, Espesser R, Rey V, Daffaure V, Di Cristo A, Habib M. (2001) Intensive training of phonological skills in progressive aphasia: a model of brain plasticity in neurodegenerative disease. *Brain and Cognition* **46**: 197–201

Luzzatti C and Poeck K. (1991) An early description of slowly progressive aphasia. *Archives of Neurology* **48**: 228–229

Mackenzie Ross SJ, Graham N, Stuart-Green L et al. (1996) Progressive biparietal atrophy: an atypical presentation of Alzheimer's disease. *Journal of Neurology, Neurosurgery, and Psychiatry* **61**: 388–395

Mandell AM, Alexander MP, Carpenter S. (1989) Creutzfeldt–Jakob disease presenting as isolated aphasia. *Neurology* **39**: 55–58

Mendez MF and Ghajarnia M. (2001) Agnosia for familiar faces and odors in a patient with right temporal lobe dysfunction. *Neurology* **57**: 519–521

Mesulam MM. (1982) Slowly progressive aphasia without generalized dementia. *Annals of Neurology* **11**: 592–598

Mesulam MM. (2001) Primary progressive aphasia. *Annals of Neurology* **49**: 425–432

Mesulam MM and Weintraub S. (1992) Spectrum of primary progressive aphasia. In: MN Rossor (ed.), *Ballière's Clinical Neurology, Vol 1. Unusual Dementias*. London, Baillière Tindall, pp. 583–609

Mesulam MM, Grossman M, Hillis A, Kertesz A, Weintraub S. (2003) The core and halo of primary progressive aphasia and semantic dementia. *Annals of Neurology* **54** (Suppl. 5), S11–S14

Mochizuki A, Ueda Y, Komatsuzaki Y, Tuchiya K, Arai T, Shoji S. (2003) Progressive supranuclear palsy presenting with primary progressive aphasia – clinicopathological report of an autopsy case. *Acta Neuropathologica* **105**: 610–614 (abstract)

Molina JA, Probst A, Villanueva C et al. (1998) Primary progressive aphasia with glial cytoplasmic inclusions. *European Neurology* **40**: 71–77

Nestor PJ, Graham NL, Fryer TD, Williams GB, Patterson K, Hodges JR. (2003a) Progressive non-fluent aphasia is associated with hypometabolism centred on the left anterior insula. *Brain* **126**: 1–13

Nestor PJ, Caine D, Fryer TD, Clarke J, Hodges JR. (2003b) The topography of metabolic deficits in posterior cortical atrophy (the visual variant of Alzheimer's disease) with FDG-PET. *Journal of Neurology, Neurosurgery, and Psychiatry* **74**: 1521–1529

O'Dowd BS and de Zubicaray GI. (2003) Progressive dysgraphia in a case of posterior cortical atrophy. *Neurocase* **9**: 251–260

Östberg P, Bogdanovic N, Fernaeus SE, Wahlund LO. (2001) Jargonagraphia in a case of frontotemporal dementia. *Brain and Language* **79**: 333–339

Otsuki M, Soma Y, Sato M, Homma A, Tsuji S. (1998) Slowly progressive pure word deafness. *European Neurology* **39**: 135–140

Pantel J and Schroder J. (1996) Posterior cortical atrophy – a new dementia syndrome or Alzheimer's disease? *Fortschrift Neurologie Psychiatrie* **64**: 492–508

Pasquier F, Fukui T, Sarazin M, Pijnenburg Y et al. (2003) Laboratory investigations and treatment in frontotemporal dementia. *Annals of Neurology* **54**: S32–S35

Pijnenburg YAL, Sampson EL, Harvey RJ, Fox NC, Rossor MN. (2003) Vulnerability to neuroleptic side effects in frontotemporal lobar degeneration. *International Journal of Geriatric Psychiatry* **18**: 67–72

Rossor MN, Tyrrell PJ, Warrington EK et al. (1999) Progressive frontal gait disturbance with atypical Alzheimer's disease and corticobasal degeneration. *Journal of Neurology, Neurosurgery, and Psychiatry* **67**: 345–352

Serieux P. (1893) Sur un cas de surdite verbale pure. *Revue de Medicine, Paris* **13**: 733–750

Silveri MC, Cappa A, Salvigni BL. (2003) Speech and language in primary progressive anarthria. *Neurocase* **9**: 213–220

Snowden JS, Neary D, Mann DMA, Goulding PJ, Testa HJ. (1992) Progressive language disorder due to lobar atrophy. *Annals of Neurology* **31**: 174–183

Sobrido MJ, Abu-Khalil A, Weintraub S et al. (2003) Possible association of the tau H1/H1 genotype with primary progressive aphasia. *Neurology* **60**: 862–864

Sonty SP, Mesulam MM, Thompson CK et al. (2003) Primary progressive aphasia: PPA and the language network. *Annals of Neurology* **53**: 35–49

Soriani-Lefèvre MH, Hannequin D, Bakchine S et al. (2003) Evidence of bilateral temporal lobe involvement in primary progressive aphasia: a SPECT study. *Journal of Nuclear Medicine* **44**: 1013–1022

Tang-Wai DF, Josephs KA, Boeve BF, Dickson DW, Parisi JE, Petersen RC. (2003) Pathologically confirmed corticobasal degeneration presenting with visuospatial dysfunction. *Neurology* **61**: 1134–1135

Tang-Wai DF, Graff-Radford NR, Boeve BF et al. (2004) Clinical, genetic, and neuropathologic characteristics of posterior cortical atrophy. *Neurology* **63**: 1168–1174

Turner RS, Kenyon LC, Trojanowski JQ, Gonatas N, Grossman M. (1996) Clinical, neuroimaging and pathologic features of progressive nonfluent aphasia. *Annals of Neurology* **39**: 166–173

Tyrrell PJ, Warrington EK, Frackowiak RSJ, Rossor MN. (1990a) Heterogeneity in progressive aphasia due to focal cortical atrophy: a clinical and PET study. *Brain* **113**: 1321–1336

Tyrrell PJ, Warrington EK, Frackowiak RSJ, Rossor MN. (1990b) Progressive degeneration of the right temporal lobe studied with positron emission tomography. *Journal of Neurology, Neurosurgery, and Psychiatry* **53**: 1046–1050

Tyrrell PJ, Kartsounis LD, Frackowiak RS, Findley LJ, Rossor MN. (1991) Progressive loss of speech output and orofacial dyspraxia associated with frontal lobe hypometabolism. *Journal of Neurology, Neurosurgery, and Psychiatry* **54**: 351–357

Vargha-Khadem F, Watkins KE, Price CJ et al. (1998) Neural basis of an inherited speech and language disorder. *Proceedings of the National Academy of Sciences of the United States of America* **95**: 12695–12700

Victoroff J, Ross GW, Benson DF, Verity MA, Vinters HV. (1994) Posterior cortical atrophy: neuropathologic correlations. *Archives of Neurology* **51**: 269–274

Warren JD, Warren JE, Fox NC, Warrington EK. (2003) Nothing to say, something to sing: primary progressive dynamic aphasia. *Neurocase* **9**: 140–155

Westbury C and Bub D. (1997) Primary progressive aphasia: a review of 112 cases. *Brain and Language* **60**: 381–406

Dementia and neuropsychiatric disorders

58

Depression with cognitive impairment

BINDU SHANMUGHAM AND GEORGE ALEXOPOULOS

Depressed elders often have cognitive impairment. The number of community residents with both depressive symptoms and impaired cognition doubles at each 5-year interval after the age of 70 years. Depression accompanied by cognitive dysfunction occurs in 25 per cent of 85-year-old subjects (Arve et al., 1999). Even non-demented depressed elders often have impairments in speed of processing and executive function (Kindermann et al., 2000; Lockwood et al., 2000). About 18–57 per cent of depressed elderly patients may present with dementia that resolves with remission of depression (Emery, 1988). Finally, dementing disorders are often complicated by depressive symptoms.

58.1 COGNITIVE IMPAIRMENT IN NON-DEMENTED DEPRESSED PATIENTS

A variety of neuropsychological impairments have been reported in late-life depression (Lockwood et al., 2000, 2002). These include impairment in recall (Hart et al., 1987), recognition memory, visuospatial skills (Boone et al., 1995; Lesser et al., 1996), verbal fluency, psychomotor speed (Hart et al., 1987) and executive functions such as impaired planning, organizing, initiating, sequencing and attentional set shifting (Beats et al., 1996; Lesser et al., 1996; Butters et al., 2000). Even moderately depressed middle-aged patients have deficits in planning, strategy development, spatial working memory, and verbal fluency despite unimpaired psychomotor speed (Elliot et al., 1996). While tasks requiring development of performance strategies suffer in depressed patients,

automatic processes appear relatively preserved (Channon and Green, 1999).

Although focal deficits or even severe global impairment are observed in some depressed elderly patients, the cognitive functioning of others remains intact. Studies of cognitive response to psychopharmacological treatment of late-life depression indicate that a substantial number of patients continue to experience residual symptoms and neuropsychological deficits. Processing speed and working memory impairment persist after remission of geriatric depression (Butters et al., 2000; Nebes et al., 2000).

The neuropsychological dysfunctions of depression are consistent with frontal lobe abnormalities demonstrated by neuroimaging studies (Abrams and Taylor, 1987; Coffey, 1987; Sackeim and Steif, 1988; Deptula et al., 1991; Lodewyk and Wong, 1993). Structural abnormalities have been identified in the frontal lobes (Krishnan et al., 1993), the caudate (Krishnan et al., 1992), and the putamen (Husain et al., 1991). Hypometabolism has been reported in the dorsolateral prefrontal cortex (Baxter et al., 1985; Martinot et al., 1990; Bench et al., 1992), inferior temporal areas (Lesser et al., 1994), anterior cingulate (de Asis et al., 1997; Drevets et al., 1997; Mayberg et al., 1997) and basal ganglia (Buchsbaum et al., 1986). Notably, reduced metabolism of the rostral anterior cingulate may be associated with resistance to antidepressants in younger depressed patients (Mayberg et al., 1997). In contrast, an increase in frontal hypometabolism has been reported following successful treatment with antidepressant medications (Mayberg et al., 1999; Drevets, 2000). It has been proposed that abnormal function of the right dorsolateral prefrontal cortex is the biological substrate of poor sustained attention noted in depressed patients, while metabolic abnormalities of the anterior cingulate cortex account for impaired selective attention of these patients (Liotti and Mayberg, 2001).

58.2 DEPRESSION IN PATIENTS WITH DEMENTING DISORDERS

Depressive symptoms are common among demented patients. Major depression or clinically significant depressive symptoms can be found in approximately 17 per cent of Alzheimer's patients (Wragg and Jeste, 1989). Patients with subcortical dementias, including vascular dementia, and Parkinson's disease, are more likely to experience depression than patients with Alzheimer's disease (Sobin and Sackeim, 1997).

Late-onset depression is often a prodrome of dementing disorders. Depressed mood was associated with an increased risk of incident dementia during a 5-year follow up of elderly community residents (Devanand et al., 1996). Depressive symptoms predicted cognitive decline of elderly women during a 4-year follow up (Yaffe et al., 1999). Among elderly individuals with subclinical cognitive dysfunction, those who developed dementia 3 years later had more depressive symptoms at baseline (Ritchie et al., 1999). As subjects progressed to dementia, they exhibited fewer affective symptoms and more agitation and psychomotor slowing. These changes paralleled reduction of cerebral blood flow in the left temporal region. Finally, there is evidence that late-onset depression is associated with increased incidence of dementia in individuals without an apolipoprotein E (ApoE) ε4 allele (Steffens et al., 1997).

Recently, the National Institute of Mental Health's Provisional Diagnostic Criteria for Depression of Alzheimer's Disease were developed with the goal to promote research on the mechanisms and treatment of this disorder (Olin et al., 2002). The criteria require the presence of Alzheimer's disease diagnosis and 'clinically significant' depressive symptoms. Symptoms due to a medical condition other than Alzheimer's disease, or which are deemed to be a direct result of non-mood-related dementia symptoms (e.g. loss of weight due to difficulties with food intake) should not be used in making the diagnosis of depression of Alzheimer's disease.

58.3 DEPRESSION AS A RISK FACTOR FOR DEMENTIA

There is weak evidence that depression occurring in early life may be a risk factor for the later development of dementing disorders. In a meta-analytic study a past history of depression was associated with onset of Alzheimer's disease after the age of 70 years only when depressive symptoms had appeared within 10 years before the onset of dementia (Jorm et al., 1991). Depressive symptoms occurring more than 10 years from the onset of dementia were found to be a risk factor

for Alzheimer's disease (Speck et al., 1995). Lifetime history of depression may increase the risk of Alzheimer's disease, in patients with or without a family history of dementing disorders (van Duijn et al., 1994).

Depression may promote the clinical expression of dementia in patients with Alzheimer's disease. Lifetime duration of depression was observed to correlate with hippocampal volume reduction, although some disagreement exists (Sheline et al., 1999; Davidson et al., 2002). Excessive secretion of stress-related hormones (glucocorticoids) may contribute to hippocampal atrophy. These hormones can reduce the secretion of neurotrophic factors, inhibit neurogenesis and render neurones vulnerable to the toxic effect of amyloid, thus compounding the neuropathological changes of Alzheimer's disease and accelerating the clinical expression of dementia. Once depression develops as part of these brain changes, it may accelerate the progression of Alzheimer's neuropathological changes. Several antidepressants elevate brain-derived neurotrophic factor (BDNF) in the rat hippocampus. Through this action, antidepressants may prevent stress-induced inhibition of neurogenesis and increase dendritic branching (Duman et al., 1997). It remains to be investigated whether antidepressants delay the onset and inhibit the progression of Alzheimer's disease.

58.4 COGNITIVE IMPAIRMENT AND THE COURSE OF GERIATRIC DEPRESSION

Multiple pathways may lead to depression and cognitive impairment. Clinical as well as structural and functional neuroimaging studies suggest that depressive symptoms and executive impairment originate from related brain dysfunctions (Alexopoulos, 2001), at least in a subgroup of elderly patients. We described a 'depression-executive dysfunction syndrome' (DED), which is characterized by psychomotor retardation, reduced interest in activities, a rather mild vegetative syndrome, and pronounced functional disability disproportionate to the severity of the depression (Alexopoulos et al., 1996; Kiosses et al., 2000; Lockwood et al., 2000). DED patients have impaired verbal fluency and visual naming, as well as poor performance on tasks of initiation and perseveration (Alexopoulos et al., 1996). Psychomotor retardation, apathy and fluency deficits are symptoms often observed in frontal lobe syndromes. Yet, unlike patients with frontal lobe syndromes, patients with DED meet criteria for major depression, and have depressive symptomatology of comparable severity to that of geriatric major depression patients with unimpaired executive functions (Alexopoulos et al., 2000).

There is evidence that impaired performance in some tests of executive function is associated with poor and/or slow antidepressant response (Alexopoulos, 2002a). In younger women, abnormal executive functions were associated with poor response to fluoxetine (Dunkin et al., 2000). Abnormal scores in tests of initiation and perseveration were shown to predict poor antidepressant response and low remission rate in non-demented elderly patients with major depression treated with 'adequate' dosages of various antidepressants (Kalayam and Alexopoulos, 1999). Furthermore, other studies demonstrated that the efficacy of antidepressants is not compromised by broad cognitive dysfunction (Alexopoulos, 1995; Nyth *et al.*, 1992; Katona *et al.*, 1998) or medical comorbidity (Small *et al.*, 1996). Along with slow and poor response to antidepressants, abnormal scores of initiation and perseveration have been shown to predict early relapse and recurrence of late-life depression in elderly patients treated with nortriptyline (Alexopoulos *et al.*, 2000), while neither memory impairment, nor disability, medical burden, social support, nor number of previous episodes influenced the long-term outcomes of late-life depression.

Magnetic resonance imaging (MRI) studies have shown that white matter hyperintensities are associated both with executive dysfunction (Boone *et al.*, 1992; Lesser *et al.*, 1996) and with chronicity of geriatric depression (Coffey *et al.*, 1988; Hickie *et al.*, 1995). Severe hyperintensities in subcortical grey matter regions were associated with poor response of depressed elderly patients to electroconvulsive therapy (Steffens *et al.*, 2001). An electrical tomography analysis study suggests that anterior cingulate activity is a predictor of the extent of treatment response in depression (Pizzagalli *et al.*, 2001); functional integrity of the anterior cingulate cortex is required for the performance of executive functions.

Functional imaging studies of younger adults suggest that remission of depression is associated with metabolic increases in dorsal cortical regions (Mayberg *et al.*, 1999; Drevets, 2000) and metabolic decreases in ventral limbic and paralimbic structures (Mayberg *et al.*, 1999; Smith *et al.*, 1999; Liotti and Mayberg, 2001). Persistently elevated metabolism of the amygdala during remission of depression was associated with a high risk for relapse of depression in younger adults (Drevets, 1999). Reduced metabolism of the emotional subdivision of the anterior cingulate is associated with treatment resistance in depressed younger adults, while increased cingulate metabolism is a predictor of a good treatment response (Mayberg *et al.*, 1997). A diffusion tensor imaging study noted that microstructural abnormalities of the white matter lateral to the anterior cingulate are associated with poor or slow response of geriatric depression to citalopram (Alexopoulos *et al.*, 2002b). Disruption of white matter in this area may interfere with the dorsal cortical-ventral limbic reciprocal regulation and may contribute to adverse outcomes of geriatric depression.

58.5 'PSEUDODEMENTIA'

The concept of reversible dementia was introduced in the mid-nineteenth century (Berrios, 1985; Emery, 1988) and became the focus of clinical attention in the early 1960s when the term 'pseudodementia' was used to describe a broad range of reversible cognitive impairments associated with psychiatric syndromes (Kiloh, 1961). The current concept of 'pseudodementia' is that of an initially reversible cognitive impairment that occurs in the context of diverse psychiatric disorders, which influence its course.

The clinical presentation of depression with cognitive impairment is heterogeneous. The signs and symptoms are principally influenced by the patients' ages and underlying psychiatric disorders (Kiloh, 1961; Wells, 1979; Rabins *et al.*, 1984; Alexopoulos, 1990; Emery and Oxman, 1992). In a non-geriatric series, 'pseudodementia' was reported in patients with Ganser syndrome, personality disorders, melancholic depression, hypomania, atypical psychosis, paraphrenia, catatonia, depersonalization and malingering (Kiloh, 1961, 1981; Wells, 1971). Non-geriatric patients with 'pseudodementia' often had a history of prior psychiatric disorders, a recent and abrupt onset of current illness, complained about their cognitive loss, experienced distress, and were able to both precisely identify the onset and describe in detail the course of their illness (Kiloh, 1961; Wells, 1979). On cognitive tests, these patients often said they did not know the correct answers even though the tasks were within their abilities. Performance on tasks of similar difficulty was markedly variable and accompanied by an overdramatization of their failures.

As many younger patients with 'pseudodementia' have psychiatric syndromes other than depression, their clinical presentation is dissimilar to that of geriatric patients with 'pseudodementia' in whom depression is the most common diagnosis. Depressed elders with 'pseudodementia' usually have a severe depression syndrome and a mild dementia. The clinical profile of major depression accompanying 'pseudodementia' of older adults is characterized by motor retardation, depressive delusions, hopelessness and helplessness (Alexopoulos and Abrams, 1991). Geriatric inpatients with major depression and 'pseudodementia' had a later age of onset of illness than patients who only had major depression (Alexopoulos *et al.*, 1993a). A study of elderly inpatients and outpatients noted that those with depression and 'pseudodementia' had more psychic and somatic anxiety, early morning awakening, and loss of libido than patients with Alzheimer's disease complicated by depression (Reynolds *et al.*, 1988). Unlike younger adults, depressed elders with 'pseudodementia' express limited cognitive complaints or 'I don't know' responses (Young *et al.*, 1985; Meyers, 1987; Emery, 1988). As a rule, the symptoms of depression preceded those of cognitive dysfunction in patients with depressive 'pseudodementia'.

58.6 PROGNOSIS OF DEPRESSION WITH COGNITIVE IMPAIRMENT

As a rule, cognitive impairment improves after amelioration of geriatric depression. However, this improvement is partial in most cases (Abas *et al.*, 1990; Nebes *et al.*, 2000, 2001).

Follow-up studies suggest that geriatric patients with depression and an initially reversible dementia ('pseudodementia') are at high risk for developing irreversible dementia (Reynolds *et al.*, 1986; Kral and Emery, 1989; Copeland *et al.*, 1992; Alexopoulos *et al.*, 1993a). Taken together, these studies suggest that 9–25 per cent of elderly patients with depression and an initially reversible dementia develop irreversible dementia each year. However, many such patients do not meet criteria for irreversible dementia for a period of 2 years after the initial episode of depression with 'pseudodementia' (Alexopoulos *et al.*, 1993b). However, some studies observed that there exists a population of elderly depressed people with reversible dementia who remain cognitively intact at least for a few years after resolution of the dementia syndrome (Rabins *et al.*, 1984; Pearlson *et al.*, 1989).

Differences in the course of cognitive dysfunction in depressed patients with an initially reversible dementia suggest that this syndrome is heterogeneous (Alexopoulos, 2002b). Some depressed people with an initially reversible dementia may already have an early dementing disorder. This view is supported by recent studies suggesting that depression is a prodrome of dementing disorders. Several explanations may account for depressed elderly patients with reversible dementia who remain cognitively intact on follow up. Disturbances in attention and motivation may interfere with the examination of higher intellectual functions in severely depressed elderly patients. Another possibility is that the cognitive dysfunction of depression may be prominent in patients with asymptomatic non-progressive brain lesions, e.g. silent stroke. Such patients may develop a dementia syndrome only during depression but not develop dementia during follow up. Such depression–lesion interaction is supported by the observation that neurological symptoms and signs are exacerbated when patients become depressed (Fogel and Sparadeo, 1985). Another possibility may be that severe cognitive dysfunction is an integral part of severe geriatric depression. There is evidence suggesting that cognitive dysfunction is an expression of the functional brain changes occurring during depression rather than a behavioural consequence of the affective symptoms. Memory and executive dysfunction often occur in depressed elderly patients (Butters *et al.*, 2000; Kindermann *et al.*, 2000; Lockwood *et al.*, 2000; Nebes *et al.*, 2001) who sometimes do not completely recover (Butters *et al.*, 2000; Nebes *et al.*, 2001). Dysnomia has been noted in depressed elderly patients compared with controls (Speedie *et al.*, 1990). Functional neuroimaging studies showed reduced glucose metabolism in the basal ganglia and the prefrontal areas (Drevets, 2000) of depressed patients, while structural neuroimaging studies documented reduced volumes of the putamen (Husain *et al.*, 1991) and the caudate (Krishnan *et al.*, 1992) in depressed patients compared with normal controls. These observations suggest that the spectrum of clinical manifestations of depression includes a wide range of cognitive impairments that may account for some of the subjects with reversible dementia who did not deteriorate on follow up.

58.7 DIAGNOSTIC ASSESSMENT AND TREATMENT PLANNING

Depressed elderly patients with cognitive impairment should have an evaluation both of their psychiatric symptoms and signs as well as their cognitive impairment. Since depression and cognitive impairment have a complex association, the diagnosis of depression and cognitive dysfunction or dementia should be made independently of each other. In some cases the syndromes of depression and dementia are caused by the same disorders, e.g. vascular dementias, Parkinson's disease, Alzheimer's disease, hypothyroidism, autoimmune diseases or steroid-induced depression with cognitive impairment. In other cases, depression and dementia simply may coexist.

Identifying and characterizing cognitive impairment of depressed elderly patients has important clinical implications. Depressed elders often develop delirium in response to drug side effects, dehydration, infections and other factors. Therefore, cognitive examination should focus on manifestations of delirium, including inattention, fluctuating state of consciousness and sleep-wake disturbances. Of course, making the diagnosis of delirium does not exclude the diagnosis of dementia. As dementing disorders predispose to delirium, delirious patients should be re-examined for an underlying dementing disorder after the resolution of delirium. Identifying treatable causes of dementia, e.g. dementia owing to drug intoxication, organ failure, endocrinopathies, B_{12} deficiency, and space-occupying lesion is important as treatment of these conditions may reverse or arrest the progress of dementia.

When dementia is identified, the clinical characterization of the dementia syndrome can guide treatment. Among the dementia syndromes, subcortical dementia is the syndrome most likely to be complicated by depression. Subcortical dementia is characterized by significant memory impairment, executive dysfunction and psychomotor retardation. Disorders causing subcortical dementias include mixed Alzheimer's and vascular dementia, vascular dementia, Parkinson's disease, and dementia with Lewy bodies. These disorders require rather specific treatments, e.g. vascular dementia often is treated with aspirin and antioxidants, Parkinson's disease with dopamine acting agents, and dementia with Lewy bodies with cholinesterase inhibitors and anticonvulsants for behavioural control rather than antipsychotics. Unlike subcortical dementias, cortical dementias manifest broader impairment of cognitive functions, including memory impairment, apraxia, aphasia with paraphasic errors and graphomotor construction problems.

The most common cause of cortical dementia is Alzheimer's disease, a condition treated with cholinesterase inhibitors at least during the early and middle phase and with memantine during the advanced phase. Frontal lobe dementias are characterized by rather mild memory impairment and pronounced personality changes (apathy, socially inappropriate behaviour and disinhibition) often resulting in irritability. Frontal lobe dementia may be due to frontotemporal dementia, head trauma and stroke, disorders for which there are no specific treatments.

Identification of executive dysfunction is important even in non-demented depressed elderly patients. Depressed patients with psychomotor retardation, reduced interest in activities, suspiciousness and disability are likely to have executive dysfunction (Alexopoulos et al., 2002a). Depression with executive dysfunction may have a poor and unstable response to antidepressants (Kalayam and Alexopoulos, 1999; Alexopoulos et al., 2000). For this reason, patients with the depression-executive dysfunction syndrome of late life require a carefully planned psychopharmacological treatment and vigilant follow up since they are at high risk for relapse or recurrence (Alexopoulos et al., 2000). Non-pharmacological interventions need to be added, including problem-solving therapy aimed at remedying their behavioural deficits (Alexopoulos et al., 2003).

Evaluation of depressive syndromes in cognitively impaired patients is complicated by the symptomatologic overlap with dementia, the instability of depressive manifestations over time and the poor ability of elderly patients to report their symptoms. If criteria for one of the depressive syndromes are met, an antidepressant treatment trial should be offered. Beyond the benefits of alleviating the problems and the complications of depression, remission of the depressive syndrome can increase the clinician's ability to evaluate the severity of the remaining cognitive impairment and plan for further treatment and follow up. The Expert Consensus Guideline recommends antidepressant drug therapy combined with a psychosocial intervention as the treatment of choice for geriatric depression (Alexopoulos et al., 2001).

Variability in the course of elders with depressive 'pseudo-dementia' suggests the need for careful follow up. About 40 per cent of these patients are expected to receive the diagnosis of a dementing disorder within two years after the diagnosis of 'pseudodementia.' Prompt identification and treatment of the dementing disorder may increase the time during which the patient can function independently.

REFERENCES

Abas MA, Sahakian BJ, Levy R. (1990) Neuropsychological deficits and CT scan changes in elderly depressives. *Psychological Medicine* **20**: 507–520

Abrams and Taylor MA. (1987) Cognitive dysfunction in melancholia. *Psychological Medicine* **17**: 359–362

Alexopoulos GS. (1990) Clinical and biological findings in late-onset depression. In: A Tasman, SM Goldfinger, CA Kaufmann (eds), *American Psychiatric Press Review of Psychiatry Vol.* 9, 249–262

Alexopoulos GS. (1995) Methodology of treatment studies in geriatric depression. *American Journal of Geriatric Psychiatry* **3**: 280–289

Alexopoulos GS. (2001) The depression-executive dysfunction syndrome of late life: a target for D3 receptor agonists. *American Journal of Geriatric Psychiatry* **9**: 1–8

Alexopoulos GS. (2002a) Frontostriatal and limbic dysfunction in late-life depression. *American Journal of Geriatric Psychiatry* **10**: 687–695

Alexopoulos GS. (2002b) Depressive dementia: cognitive and behavioral correlates and course of illness. In: OB Emery and TE Oxman (eds), *Dementia: Presentations, Differential Diagnosis, and Nosology.* Baltimore, Johns Hopkins University Press, 398–416

Alexopoulos GS and Abrams RC. (1991) Depression in Alzheimer's disease. *Psychiatric Clinics of North America* **14**: 327–340

Alexopoulos G, Young R, Meyers B. (1993a) Geriatric depression: age of onset and dementia. *Biological Psychiatry* **34**: 141–145

Alexopoulos GS, Meyers BS, Young RC et al. (1993b) The course of geriatric depression with 'reversible dementia': a controlled study. *American Journal of Psychiatry* **150**: 1693–1699

Alexopoulos GS, Vrontou C, Kakuma T et al. (1996) Disability in geriatric depression. *American Journal of Psychiatry* **153**: 877–885

Alexopoulos GS, Meyers BS, Young RC et al. (2000) Executive dysfunction and long-term outcomes of geriatric depression. *Archives of General Psychiatry* **57**: 285–290

Alexopoulos GS, Katz IR, Reynolds CF et al. (2001) The Expert Consensus Guideline Series. Pharmacotherapy of Geriatric Depression. *Postgraduate Medicine (Special Report)*, October

Alexopoulos GS, Kiosses DN, Klimstra S et al. (2002a) Clinical presentation of the 'depression-executive dysfunction syndrome' of late life. *American Journal of Geriatric Psychiatry* **10**: 98–102

Alexopoulos GS, Kiosses DN, Choi SJ et al. (2002b) Frontal white matter microstructure and treatment response of late-life depression: a preliminary study. *American Journal of Psychiatry* **159**: 1929–1932

Alexopoulos GS, Raue P, Arean P. (2003) Problem-solving therapy versus supportive therapy in geriatric major depression with executive dysfunction. *American Journal of Geriatric Psychiatry* **11**: 46–52

Arve S, Tilvis RS, Lehtonen A et al. (1999) Coexistence of lowered mood and cognitive impairment of elderly people in five birth cohorts. *Aging (Milano)* **11**: 90–95

Baxter LR, Phelps ME, Mazziota JC et al. (1985) Cerebral metabolic rates for glucose in mood disorders. *Archives of General Psychiatry* **42**: 441–447

Beats BC, Sahakian BJ, Levy R. (1996) Cognitive performance in tests sensitive to frontal lobe dysfunction in the elderly depressed. *Psychological Medicine* **26**: 591–603

Bench CJ, Friston KJ, Brown RG et al. (1992) The anatomy of melancholia: focal abnormalities of cerebral blood flow in major depression. *Psychological Medicine* **22**: 607–615

Berrios GE. (1985) 'Depressive pseudodementia' or 'melancholic dementia': a 19th century view. *Journal of Neurology, Neurosurgery, and Psychiatry* **48**: 393–400

Boone KB, Miller BL, Lesser IM et al. (1992) Neuropsychological correlates of white matter lesions in healthy elderly subjects. *Archives of Neurology* **49**: 549–554

Boone KB, Lesser IM, Miller BL et al. (1995) Cognitive functioning in older depressed outpatients: relationship of presence and severity of depression to neuropsychological test scores. *Neuropsychology* **9**: 390–398

Buchsbaum MS, Wu J, DeLisi LE et al. (1986) Frontal cortex and basal ganglia metabolic rates assessed by positron emission tomography with [18F]2-deoxyglucose in affective illness. *Journal of Affective Disorders* **10**: 137–152

Butters MA, Becker JT, Nebes RD et al. (2000) Changes in cognitive functioning following treatment of late-life depression. *American Journal of Psychiatry* **157**: 1949–1954

Channon S and Green PS. (1999) Executive function in depression: the role of performance strategies in aiding depressed and non-depressed participants. *Journal of Neurology, Neurosurgery, and Psychiatry* **66**: 162–171

Coffey CE. (1987) Cerebral laterality and emotion: the neurology of depression. *Comparative Psychiatry* **28**: 197–219

Coffey CE, Figiel GS, Djang WT *et al.* (1988) Leukoencephalopathy in elderly depressed patients referred for ECT. *Biological Psychiatry* **24**: 143–161

Copeland JRM, Davidson IA, Dewey ME *et al.* (1992) Alzheimer's disease, other dementias, depression and pseudodementia: prevalence, incidence and three year outcome in Liverpool. *British Journal of Psychiatry* **161**: 230–239

Davidson RJ, Pizzagalli D, Nitschke JB, Putnam K. (2002) Depression: perspectives from affective neuroscience. *Annual Review of Psychology* **53**: 545–574

de Asis J, Silbersweig D, Blumberg H *et al.* (1997) *Lateralized Fronto-striatal Dysfunction in Geriatric Depression: a PET study.* Kona, Hawaii, ACNP

Deptula D, Manevitz A, Yozawitz A. (1991) Asymmetry of recall in depression. *Journal of Clinical and Experimental Neuropsychology* **13**: 854–870

Devanand DP, Sano M, Tang MX *et al.* (1996) Depressed mood and the incidence of Alzheimer's disease in the elderly living in the community. *Archives of General Psychiatry* **53**: 175–182

Drevets WC. (1999) Prefrontal cortical-amygdala metabolism in major depression. *Annals of the New York Academy of Sciences* **877**: 614–637

Drevets WC. (2000) Neuroimaging studies of mood disorders. *Biological Psychiatry* **48**: 813–819

Drevets WC, Price JL, Simpson JR *et al.* (1997) Subgenual prefrontal cortex abnormalities in mood disorders. *Nature* **386**: 824–827

Duman RS, Heninger GR, Nestler EJ. (1997) A molecular and cellular theory of depression. *Archives of General Psychiatry* **54**: 597–606

Dunkin JJ, Leuchter AF, Cook IA *et al.* (2000) Executive dysfunction predicts nonresponse to fluoxetine in major depression. *Journal of Affective Disorders* **60**: 13–23

Elliot R, Sahakian BJ, McKay AP *et al.* (1996) Neuropsychological impairments in unipolar depression: the influence of perceived failure on subsequent performance. *Psychological Medicine* **26**: 975–989

Emery VOB. (1988) *Pseudodementia: A Theoretical and Empirical Discussion. Western Reserve Geriatric Education Center Interdisciplinary Monograph Series.* Cleveland, Case Western Reserve University School of Medicine

Emery VO and Oxman TE. (1992) Update on the dementia spectrum of depression. *American Journal of Psychiatry* **149**: 305–317

Fogel BS and Sparadeo FR. (1985) Focal cognitive deficits accentuated by depression. *Journal of Nervous and Mental Disease* **173**: 120–124

Hart RP, Kwentus JA, Taylor JR, Harkins SW. (1987) Rate of forgetting in dementia and depression. *Journal of Consulting and Clinical Psychology* **55**: 101–105

Hickie I, Scott E, Mitchell P *et al.* (1995) Subcortical hyperintensities on magnetic resonance imaging: clinical correlates and prognostic significance in patients with severe depression. *Biological Psychiatry* **37**: 151–160

Husain MM, McDonald WM, Doraiswamy PM *et al.* (1991) A magnetic resonance imaging study of putamen nuclei in major depression. *Psychiatry Research: Neuroimaging* **40**: 95–99

Jorm AF, van Duijn CM, Chandra V *et al.* (1991) Psychiatric history and related exposures as risk factors for Alzheimer's disease: a collaborative re-analysis of case–control studies. *International Journal of Epidemiology* **20** (Suppl. 2): S43–S47

Kalayam B and Alexopoulos GS. (1999) Prefrontal dysfunction and treatment response in geriatric depression. *Archives of General Psychiatry* **56**: 713–718

Katona CL, Hunter BN, Bray J. (1998) A double-blind comparison of the efficacy and safely of paroxetine and imipramine in the treatment of depression with dementia. *International Journal of Geriatric Psychiatry* **13**: 100–108

Kiloh L. (1961) Pseudo-dementia. *Acta Psychiatrica Scandinavica* **37**: 336–351

Kiloh L. (1981) Depressive illness masquerading as dementia in the elderly. *Medical Journal of Australia* **2**: 550–553

Kindermann SS, Kalayam B, Brown GG *et al.* (2000) Executive functions and P300 latency in elderly depressed patients and control subjects. *American Journal of Geriatric Psychiatry* **8**: 57–65

Kiosses DN, Alexopoulos GS, Murphy C. (2000) Symptoms of striatofrontal dysfunction contribute to disability in geriatric depression. *International Journal of Geriatric Psychiatry* **15**: 992–999

Kral VA and Emery OB. (1989) Long-term follow up of depressive pseudodementia of the aged. *Canadian Journal of Psychiatry* **34**: 445–446

Krishnan KR, McDonald WM, Escalona PR *et al.* (1992) Magnetic imaging of the caudate nuclei in depression. Preliminary observations. *Archives of General Psychiatry* **49**: 553–557

Krishnan KR, McDonald WM, Doraiswamy PM *et al.* (1993) Neuroanatomical substrates of depression in the elderly. *European Archives of Psychiatry and Clinical Neuroscience* **243**: 41–46

Lesser IM, Mena I, Boone KB *et al.* (1994) Reduction of cerebral blood flow in older depressed adults. *Archives of General Psychiatry* **51**: 677–686

Lesser IM, Boone KB, Mehringer CM *et al.* (1996) Cognition and white matter hyperintensities in older depressed adults. *American Journal of Psychiatry* **153**: 1280–1287

Liotti M and Mayberg HS. (2001) The role of functional neuroimaging in the neuropsychology of depression. *Journal of Clinical and Experimental Neuropsychology* **23**: 121–136

Lockwood KA, Alexopoulos GS, Kakuma T, van Gorp WG. (2000) Subtypes of cognitive impairment in depressed older adults. *American Journal of Geriatric Psychiatry* **8**: 201–208

Lockwood CA, Alexopoulos GS, van Gorp WG. (2002) Executive dysfunction in geriatric depression. *American Journal of Psychiatry* **159**: 1119–1126

Lodewyk KS and Wong TN. (1993) Neuropsychological test performance in depression. *Journal of Clinical and Experimental Neuropsychology* **15**: 80

Martinot JL, Hardy P, Feline A. (1990) Left prefrontal glucose hypometabolism in the depressed state: a confirmation study. *American Journal of Psychiatry* **147**: 1313–1317

Mayberg HS, Brannan SK, Mahurin RK *et al.* (1997) Cingulate function in depression: a potential predictor of treatment response. *NeuroReport* **8**: 1057–1061

Mayberg HS, Liotti M, Brannan SK *et al.* (1999) Reciprocal limbic-cortical function and negative mood: converging PET findings in depression and normal sadness. *American Journal of Psychiatry* **156**: 675–682

Meyers BS. (1987) Adverse cognitive effects of tricyclic antidepressants in the treatment of geriatric depression: fact or fiction? In: CA Shamoian (ed.), *Psychopharmacological Treatment Complications in the Elderly.* Washington DC, American Psychiatric Press, pp. 1–16

Nebes RD, Butters MA, Mulsant BH *et al.* (2000) Decreased working memory and processing speed mediate cognitive impairment in geriatric depression. *Psychological Medicine* **30**: 679–691

Nebes RD, Butters MA, Houck PR *et al.* (2001) Dual-task performance in depressed geriatric patients. *Psychiatry Research* **102**: 139–151

Nyth AL, Gottfries CG, Lyby K *et al.* (1992) A controlled multicenter clinical study of citalopram and placebo in elderly depressed patients with and without concomitant dementia. *Acta Psychiatrica Scandinavica* **86**: 138–145

Olin JT, Schneider LS, Katz IR *et al.* (2002) National Institute of Mental Health – Provisional Diagnostic Criteria for Depression of Alzheimer Disease. *American Journal of Geriatric Psychiatry* **10**: 125–128

Pearlson GD, Rabins PV, Kim WS *et al.* (1989) Structural brain CT changes and cognitive deficits in elderly depressives with and without reversible dementia ('pseudodementia') *Psychological Medicine* **19**: 573–584

Pizzagalli D, Pascual-Marqui RD, Nitschke JB *et al.* (2001) Anterior cingulate activity as a predictor of degree of treatment response in major depression: evidence from brain electrical tomography analysis. *American Journal of Psychiatry* **158**: 405–415

Rabins P, Merchant A, Nestadt G. (1984) Criteria for diagnosing reversible dementia caused by depression: validation by 2-year follow up. *British Journal of Psychiatry* **144**: 488–492

Reynolds CF III, Kupfer DJ, Hoch CC *et al.* (1986) Two year follow up of elderly patients with mixed depression and dementia: clinical and electroencephalographic sleep findings. *Journal of the American Geriatrics Society* **34**: 793–799

Reynolds CF III, Hoch CC, Kupfer DJ *et al.* (1988) Bedside differentiation of depressive pseudodementia from dementia. *American Journal of Psychiatry* **145**: 1099–1103

Ritchie K, Gilham C, Ledesert B *et al.* (1999) Depressive illness, depressive symptomatology and regional cerebral blood flow in elderly people with sub-clinical cognitive impairment. *Age and Ageing* **28**: 385–391

Sackeim H and Steif B. (1988) Neuropsychology of depression and mania. In: A Georgotas and R Cancro (ed.), *Depression and Mania.* New York, Elsevier, pp. 265–289

Sheline YI, Sanghavi M, Mintun MA, Gado MH. (1999) Depression duration but not age predicts hippocampal volume loss in medically healthy women with recurrent major depression. *Journal of Neuroscience* **19**: 5034–5043

Small GW, Birkett M, Meyers BS *et al.* (1996) Impact of physical illness on quality of life and antidepressant response in geriatric major depression. Fluoxetine Collaborative Study Group. *Journal of the American Geriatrics Society* **44**: 1220–1225

Smith GS, Reynolds CF 3rd, Pollock B *et al.* (1999) Cerebral metabolic response to combined total sleep deprivation and antidepressant response in geriatric depression. *American Journal of Psychiatry* **156**: 683–689

Sobin C and Sackeim HA. (1997) Psychomotor symptoms of depression. *American Journal of Psychiatry* **154**: 4–17

Speck CE, Kukull WA, Brenner DE *et al.* (1995) History of depression as a risk factor for Alzheimer's disease. *Epidemiology* **6**: 366–369

Speedie L, Rabins P, Pearlson G, Moberg P. (1990) Confrontation naming deficit in dementia of depression. *Journal of Neuropsychiatry and Clinical Neuroscience* **2**: 59–63

Steffens DC, Plassman BL, Helms MJ *et al.* (1997) A twin study of late-onset depression and apolipoprotein E ε4 as risk factors for Alzheimer's disease. *Biological Psychiatry* **41**: 851–856

Steffens DC, Conway CR, Dombeck CB *et al.* (2001) Severity of subcortical gray matter hyperintensity predicts ECT response in geriatric depression. *Journal of ECT* **17**: 45–49

van Duijn CM, Clayton DG, Chandra V *et al.* (1994) Interaction between genetic and environmental risk factors for Alzheimer's disease: a reanalysis of case–control studies. *Genetic Epidemiology* **11**: 539–551

Wells CE. (1971) The symptoms and behavioral manifestations of dementia. *Contemporary Neurology Series* **9**: 1–11

Wells CE. (1979) Pseudodementia. *American Journal of Psychiatry* **136**: 895–900

Wragg RE and Jeste DV. (1989) Overview of depression and psychosis in Alzheimer's disease. *American Journal of Psychiatry* **146**: 577–589

Yaffe K, Blackwell T, Gore R *et al.* (1999) Depressive symptoms and cognitive decline in nondemented elderly women: a prospective study. *Archives of General Psychiatry* **56**: 425–430

Young RC, Manley M, Alexopoulos GS. (1985) 'I don't know' responses in elderly depressives and in dementia. *Journal of the American Geriatrics Society* **33**: 253–257

59

Alcohol-related dementia and the clinical spectrum of Wernicke–Korsakoff syndrome

STEPHEN C BOWDEN AND ALISON J RITTER

Dementia associated with alcohol dependence has seen a dramatic increase in the number of clinical and experimental studies undertaken but also a plurality of views regarding aetiology, clinical course and optimal treatment modalities (Victor, 1994). When Butters and Cermak (1980) wrote their landmark work on the neuropsychology of the 'alcoholic Korsakoff's syndrome' there were relatively few controlled studies of cognitive impairment associated with a diagnosis of alcohol dependence. The intervening period has seen a dramatic increase in our understanding of the prevalence of cognitive problems associated with long-term, and excessive, alcohol use that, in severe forms, is frequently interpreted as alcohol-related dementia. However, we have also witnessed a consonant increase in our understanding of the clinical spectrum of Wernicke–Korsakoff syndrome. While there is strong evidence that Wernicke–Korsakoff syndrome is caused by thiamin deficiency, it is most commonly reported in people with an associated diagnosis of alcohol dependence. The potential for Wernicke–Korsakoff syndrome to present as a dementia of fluctuating course and variable severity remains a concept unfamiliar to many clinicians. In this chapter, a diagnostic framework will be outlined for understanding dementia associated with alcohol dependence and important treatment and management considerations will be identified.

59.1 COGNITIVE IMPAIRMENT ASSOCIATED WITH ALCOHOL DEPENDENCE

Excessive alcohol consumption is a serious health problem in many countries with multiple direct and indirect social and health costs (Gordis, 2000; Royal College of Physicians, 2001). As part of a wider perspective addressing health effects of alcohol dependence, there has been great interest in the hypothesis that excessive alcohol intake may affect the brain. Interest in this ethanol neurotoxicity hypothesis has spanned the spectrum of beverage alcohol intake from levels of alcohol consumption commonly regarded as 'moderate' or socially acceptable, up to levels of regular intake associated with disruption of occupational and social function and the multiple health risks of alcohol dependence (American Psychiatric Association, 1994).

Most studies reporting tangible effects on cognitive and broader psychological function have focused on levels of intake reported from individuals seeking professional help for their alcohol dependence (Bowden, 1987; Grant, 1987; Parsons, 1998). In general terms, reliably identifiable cognitive impairment associated with ethanol consumption is reported from samples of people whose alcohol dependence became established in late teenage years or early adulthood, and who have been consuming in excess of 80–100 mL of pure ethanol on a regular daily basis for some, usually many, years. By the time they seek professional help, many people with alcohol dependence have alcohol-induced multiple organ disease, and other complicating conditions such as poor nutrition and head injuries. In such samples, the prevalence of cognitive impairment has been estimated at a substantial minority or perhaps a majority (Parsons, 1994; Rourke and Loberg, 1996; Bates et al., 2002).

In milder forms, this pattern of cognitive impairment was termed 'subclinical psychological deterioration' (Cutting, 1985), so named because in individual cases it may not be apparent until elicited with objective assessment of cognition (Parsons, 1994). In more severe forms this clinical picture has been termed alcohol-induced persisting dementia (American Psychiatric Association, 1994: Code 291.2) or alcohol-related dementia (Oslin *et al.*, 1998).

Several reviews have provided a comprehensive overview of the many cognitive, neuroimaging, neurochemical, neurophysiological observations in alcohol-dependent patients (Lishman, 1998; Bates *et al.*, 2002; Harper *et al.*, 2003). Aetiological processes considered in the explanation of alcohol-related dementia include pre-existing learning disabilities, family history of alcohol dependence both as an early environmental and as genetic risk factors, childhood behaviour problems and comorbid psychopathology (Rourke and Loberg, 1996; Adams *et al.*, 1998; Lishman, 1998; Oslin *et al.*, 1998; Bates *et al.*, 2002; Oscar-Berman and Marinkovic, 2004). Medical risk factors that may predispose to cognitive impairment include multiple organ disease, particularly liver disease, head injury and multiple nutritional deficiencies (Parsons, 1994; Bates *et al.*, 2002; Harper *et al.*, 2003). Despite the complexity of the pathophysiological issues many authors have clearly favoured the concept of an alcohol-*induced* dementia. The most important caveat on this nosological inference is the fact that some neurological conditions may be relatively asymptomatic, the only important sign being cognitive impairment (Victor, 1994; Oslin *et al.*, 1998). These nosological issues will be discussed in detail below.

Many studies have examined parameters of alcohol intake with the view to identifying a dose–response relationship underlying alcohol-related dementia. In general the search for a clear dose–response relationship has been disappointing, with only occasional reports of correlations between parameters of intake and behavioural or neurophysiological outcome measures (Rourke and Loberg, 1996; Walton and Bowden, 1997; Oslin *et al.*, 1998). In terms of the specific pattern of cognitive impairment in alcohol-related dementia, some studies have focused on the deficits in core cognitive abilities such as working memory and fluid intelligence (sometimes labelled executive functions); other studies have reported deficits in most or all aspects of cognitive function including additional deficits in crystallized intelligence and anterograde memory or long-term retrieval (see Rourke and Loberg, 1996; Leckliter and Matarazzo, 1998; Bates *et al.*, 2002; Oscar-Berman and Marinkovic, 2004). Also there have been some interesting attempts to provide a characterization of cognitive impairment in alcohol-related dementia as a means by which to provide a differential diagnosis from other dementias (e.g. Saxton *et al.*, 2000). However, the variable pattern of cognitive function across individuals in all conditions, particularly in less severe forms, does not promise useful diagnostic efficiency.

An important issue in clinical management of patients suspected of alcohol-related dementia relates to stabilization of cognitive status and the timing of assessment of cognition after cessation of drinking. For this purpose, many neuropsychologists recommend refraining from assessment of cognitive status until several weeks after withdrawal from alcohol (Goldman, 1985; Rourke and Loberg, 1996). However, this strategy may not always be practical and some evidence suggests that it may be possible to obtain a reasonable indication of cognitive function within a few days of cessation of drinking (Unkenstein and Bowden, 1990; Bowden *et al.*, 1995). Nevertheless, it is important to recognize that cognitive status may slowly improve after cessation of drinking, over a period of months or years, or worsen with resumption of alcohol abuse (Victor *et al.*, 1971; Sullivan *et al.*, 2000; Bates *et al.*, 2002; Oslin and Carey, 2003). Therefore, any assessment of cognitive status in detoxified alcohol-dependent persons, even in those patients showing a severe alcohol-related dementia, should be formulated on the assumption that cognitive status may evolve or resolve and may need to be reviewed regularly.

59.2 DIAGNOSTIC CRITERIA FOR ALCOHOL-RELATED DEMENTIA

A few years ago, Oslin and colleagues described provisional criteria for the diagnosis of alcohol-related dementia (Oslin *et al.*, 1998). Emulating consensus criteria for other dementias, Oslin and colleagues distinguished *possible*, *probable* and *definite* subcategories of alcohol-related dementia (*cf.* American Psychiatric Association, 1994: Code 291.2). The crux of their *probable* definition was a persisting dementia, not obviously attributable to any other condition, in the context of significant alcohol use defined as at least 35 standard drinks per week. Oslin and colleagues outlined a variety of inclusion and exclusion criteria for the various subcategories, and readily acknowledged that many of the diagnostic criteria were arbitrary and intended to stimulate debate and research. They also acknowledged that variants of Wernicke–Korsakoff syndrome or other unrecognized conditions may be the primary diagnosis in many cases of alcohol-related dementia.

Oslin and colleagues also acknowledged that there were no acceptable criteria for a *definite* diagnosis of alcohol-related dementia, in other words, no known neuropathological entity corresponding to the hypothesized clinical condition. This anomaly contrasts with other consensus criteria where, for example, a specific neuropathological condition provides the basis for a definite diagnosis of Alzheimer's disease (McKhann *et al.*, 1984). Despite the great interest, over recent decades, in identifying the pathophysiology, the anomaly persists, a specific neuropathological entity corresponding to alcohol-related dementia remains to be identified (Harper *et al.*, 2003; Oslin and Carey, 2003). In view of the ambiguities in diagnosis, it is not surprising that good prevalence figures are difficult to obtain. Nevertheless, clinical surveys suggest that alcohol dependence may be one of the most common apparent causes of dementia, after Alzheimer's and vascular dementia (Lishman, 1998; Oslin and Carey, 2003). In contrast many years ago Torvik and colleagues (Torvik *et al.*, 1982) inferred from their large post-mortem surveys that most patients diagnosed clinically as having alcohol-related dementia usually will be found to have Wernicke–Korsakoff syndrome at post mortem.

Other conditions can give rise to cognitive deterioration in association with alcohol dependence, for example, pellagra, Marchiafava–Bignami disease, or hepatic encephalopathy (Victor, 1994; Lishman, 1998). Most interesting is the observation that, apart from Wernicke–Korsakoff syndrome, other pathological conditions are infrequently observed in the brains of patients who had a clinical diagnosis of dementia associated with alcohol dependence (Torvik et al., 1982; Victor, 1994; Harper et al., 2003). In addition, there is increasing evidence that many physiological derangements, worsened by excessive alcohol intake, may interact to diminish intracellular thiamin in the brain, even in the context of an adequate diet (Cook et al., 1998; Crews et al., 2000; Thomson et al., 2002). The primary danger in giving a different name, for example alcohol-related dementia, to unrecognized clinical variants of known conditions, for example Wernicke–Korsakoff syndrome, is that appropriate treatment opportunities may be missed (Victor, 1994; Lishman, 1998; Thomson et al., 2002).

59.3 BROADENING THE DEFINITION OF WERNICKE–KORSAKOFF SYNDROME

Wernicke–Korsakoff syndrome is reported with a prevalence of approximately 0.6–2 per cent of post-mortem studies and an incidence of approximately 1 per cent, making it one of the more common neurological diseases (Victor et al., 1989; Torvik, 1991; Harper et al., 2003; Thomson et al., 2002). In addition, the classical diagnostic triad of neurological signs, namely eye signs, ataxia and cognitive impairment, is recognized as having high diagnostic specificity, but relatively low sensitivity, perhaps below 20 per cent, in the context of a disease that may have an acute onset, but also may be insidious and progressive with multiple episodes (Torvik et al., 1982; Harper, 1983; Lishman, 1986; Victor et al., 1989). While nystagmus and ataxia together have high specificity in the context of a history of alcohol dependence (Harper et al., 1986; Victor et al., 1989; Torvik, 1991), the one clinical sign that appears to have highest sensitivity, perhaps in excess of 80 per cent, is mental impairment observed on mental status examination (Torvik et al., 1982; Harper et al., 1986). As a consequence, it was recommended that any alcohol-dependent person showing signs of an organic brain syndrome, should be treated with parenteral thiamin (Schroeder et al., 1991).

A few years ago Harper's group provided a reformulation of diagnostic criteria for Wernicke–Korsakoff syndrome, which included post-mortem confirmation with replication in a separate subsample using a quasi-prospective method (Caine et al., 1997). On the basis of their results Caine and colleagues suggested that a diagnosis of Wernicke–Korsakoff syndrome should be made in any alcohol-dependent person

who shows any two of the following signs: ataxia, eye signs, nutritional deficiency or cognitive impairment (with or without selective amnesia). These clinical criteria were shown to have very high sensitivity and specificity (well in excess of 90 per cent in both cases), for the identification of both the acute and chronic phases of Wernicke–Korsakoff syndrome diagnosed at post mortem. On this basis, many of the patients conforming to the criteria for *probable* alcohol-related dementia (Oslin et al., 1998), might be diagnosed instead with Wernicke–Korsakoff syndrome.

In addition, the variable course and clinical spectrum of Wernicke–Korsakoff syndrome are still not widely appreciated, although this disorder is a major confound regarding the diagnosis of alcohol-related dementia (Reuler et al., 1985; Torvik, 1991; Thomson et al., 2002). One of the major impediments to understanding the spectrum of cognitive manifestations of Wernicke–Korsakoff syndrome was the way in which a neuropsychological research strategy, used to identify patients with Wernicke–Korsakoff syndrome *and* a severe selective amnesia, was promulgated as a diagnostic criterion (for review see Bowden, 1990; Victor, 1994). The resulting diagnostic criterion assumed that a discrepancy between relatively preserved general intellectual function versus relatively impaired anterograde memory, operationalized as a large discrepancy between a Wechsler Scale Intelligence Quotient (IQ) versus Memory Quotient (MQ) in favour of IQ, had high diagnostic sensitivity to Wernicke–Korsakoff syndrome (Butters and Cermak, 1980; American Psychiatric Association, 1994). This restrictive definition of severe, selective memory impairment should not be confused with the apparently high sensitivity of *any* mental impairment, cited above.

The restrictive diagnostic criterion of selective memory impairment became widely accepted even though the criterion was never based on a study of either the epidemiology of the thiamin deficiency disorder, or representative samples of patients with the clinical diagnosis (see Bowden, 1990), and is reiterated in numerous research studies and reviews as though it corresponds to a discrete behavioural category or neuropathological entity (e.g. Kopelman, 1995; Harding et al., 2000). Criticizing this narrow diagnostic focus on the IQ versus MQ discrepancy, Victor observed 'perhaps this notion of the Korsakoff amnesic syndrome is the conventional one, but if so, it is not consonant with the observed facts, clinical or pathologic' (Victor, 1994, p. 92). The narrow definition of the disorder, reinforced by the kind of patients often seen briefly in tertiary medical settings as an acute onset condition (the Wernicke's phase) with an apparently stable or slowly resolving chronic (Korsakoff's) phase, may be another example of what Cohen and Cohen termed the clinician's illusion (1984) and may be used inadvertently to exclude from consideration many patients with other variants of the thiamin deficiency disease (Homewood and Bond, 1999).

As a consequence of a failure to fully appreciate the variable clinical spectrum of Wernicke–Korsakoff syndrome, Torvik (1991) has inferred that perhaps only 1–20 per cent of patients with the disease are correctly diagnosed in life. Like

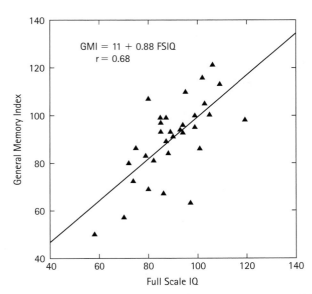

GMI = 11 + 0.88 FSIQ
r = 0.68

General Memory Index (y-axis)
Full Scale IQ (x-axis)

Figure 59.1 *WAIS-R Full Scale IQ (FSIQ) plotted against the WMS-R General Memory Index (GMI) for 32 cases showing two or more signs of Wernicke–Korsakoff syndrome. Also shown is the best-fitting line for the regression of FSIQ on the GMI (see text for details).*

Torvik (1982), Victor and colleagues (Victor *et al.*, 1989; Victor, 1994) were concerned to highlight the frequency with which patients with Wernicke–Korsakoff syndrome displayed a clinical profile of dementia. In a similar vein Reuler *et al.* (1985) concluded that most 'alcoholics that have been labelled demented will turn out to have inactive [chronic] Wernicke's encephalopathy' (p. 245).

To evaluate the hypothesis that a selective amnesia is a common accompaniment of Wernicke–Korsakoff syndrome (Butters and Cermak, 1980; American Psychiatric Association, 1994; Kopelman, 1995), we report in Figure 59.1 a consecutive series of 32 patients (30 male and 2 female) drawn from our clinical archive from a former State-run alcohol treatment centre. The average age of the patients was 44.6 years (SD = 11.9) with 9.0 years of education on average (SD = 2.9). All of these patients conformed to the clinical criterion shown to have high sensitivity and specificity to the neuropathology of Wernicke–Korsakoff syndrome (Victor *et al.*, 1989; Torvik, 1991; Caine *et al.*, 1997). Every patient had at least two of the requisite signs in addition to a history of alcohol dependence. Specifically, apart from their clinically obvious mental impairment, which was the motivation for referral, five (16 per cent) showed eye signs alone, 17 (53 per cent) showed ataxia alone, and 10 (31 per cent) showed eye signs and ataxia. Many also had poor diets, although this was not formally assessed. In this sample, mean duration of abstinence at testing was 20.3 days (SD = 12.0; range 8–60 days) and none of the patients were clinically confused or having delirium at the time of psychological assessment.

If the hypothesis of selective memory impairment (memory lower than intelligence) is correct then, the regression of intelligence on memory should produce a negative intercept,

that is, memory should be consistently poorer than intelligence. In the sample of 32 subjects (Figure 59.1), the Wechsler Memory Scale General Memory Index and Wechsler Full Scale IQ (Wechsler, 1981, 1987) were highly correlated (r = 0.68; $P < 0.01$) and the regression of Full Scale IQ on the General Memory Index produced a significant slope coefficient (slope = 0.88; standard error = 0.18; $P < 0.01$) but a non-significant intercept value (intercept = 11.17; standard error = 15.8; $P > 0.05$). There was no evidence of a non-linear component in this regression (quadratic term, $P > 0.1$). Despite a strong linear relationship, there was no evidence that memory was consistently poorer than intelligence.

A similar result was obtained when we regressed Full Scale IQ on the WMS-R Delayed Recall Index. These data have one important implication. In a sample of patients with clinical signs of Wernicke–Korsakoff syndrome known to have high sensitivity and specificity, the pattern of cognitive impairment is not one of selective amnesia, but rather a generalized cognitive impairment or dementia of variable severity. When memory is affected, intelligence is also. The present result is similar to that obtained by others (Talland, 1965; Jacobson and Lishman, 1987), although they tested similar hypotheses in patients selected for severe amnesia.

It might seem counter-intuitive to propose that Wernicke–Korsakoff syndrome be conceived as producing a dementia-like deterioration, in view of the striking amnesia seen in many patients. This inference may be better understood if it is appreciated that anterograde memory function is an instrumental daily-living skill, and deficits will be more striking than equivalent deficits in crystallized or fluid intellectual skills. We have seen many patients referred for assessment of a clinical amnesia who turn out, on objective assessment, to have equally severe intellectual impairment as well. This situation is not dissimilar to the pattern of intellectual impairment observed with irreversible degenerative conditions such as Alzheimer's disease. Although anterograde memory impairment is the clinical hallmark of Alzheimer's disease, broader intellectual impairment is often just as severe (e.g. Haxby *et al.*, 1992).

Two further points require special attention in broadening our understanding of Wernicke–Korsakoff syndrome. The first is the often overlooked potential for recovery. Current diagnostic guidelines suggest that 'once established the amnesia … usually persists indefinitely' (American Psychiatric Association, 1994, p. 162). However, this was not a view shared by Korsakoff who observed '*memory often improves … the intensity of the amnesia depends on the general course of the disease and on the depth of the affection, so that if the disease progresses toward improvement the amnesia diminishes and may entirely disappear; if the disease grows worse, however, the amnesia becomes deeper and deeper*' (Korsakoff, 1889, translated by Victor and Yakovlev, 1955, p. 398–399 – our emphasis added).

In addition, in the only large study of its type, Victor and colleagues (Victor *et al.*, 1971) reported that approximately three-quarters of a sample of 104 patients with an acute onset variant Wernicke–Korsakoff syndrome and severe post-acute phase were observed to recover to some extent over long-term follow up: 46 per cent showed substantial or complete recovery. Numerous other studies of patients admitted to hospitals with Wernicke–Korsakoff syndrome report recovery (for review see Bowden, 1990), although the relationship to refeeding and specific thiamin treatment remains little studied (Ambrose et al., 2001). Clinically, we have observed patients with Wernicke–Korsakoff syndrome who were severely demented, doubly incontinent, and dependent in all activities of daily living recover to independent living in a period of weeks.

A final aspect of Wernicke–Korsakoff syndrome that deserves further attention is the variable pattern of neuropathology, both in terms of local severity and distribution throughout the brain, including in the 'classic' periventricular and periaqueductal sites (Torvik, 1991; Harper et al., 2003). In experimental studies of thiamin deficiency Langlais and colleagues have shown rapidly developing and reversible changes in diffuse regions of the cerebrum (Langlais et al., 1996; Langlais and Zhang, 1997). Torvik (1991) discussed the potential clinical counterparts of the variable pattern of human pathology in cases of Wernicke–Korsakoff syndrome identified at post mortem, noting that, in view of the many mild and restricted lesions, the majority of patients exhibited much milder deficits than the Korsakoff's psychosis. Although there is continuing interest in the neuropathological basis of Korskoff's amnesia, it may be that accentuated histological abnormalities in certain structures are best viewed as one extreme of a clinicopathological spectrum rather than a discrete pathological subtype (e.g. Harding et al., 2000).

59.4 TREATMENT RECOMMENDATIONS

Behavioural management of cognitive impairment associated with alcohol dependence has been reviewed recently (Knight, 2001; Bates et al., 2002; Oslin and Carey, 2003). At the present time, identification of Wernicke–Korsakoff syndrome in all its variants, remains a clinical diagnosis because there is no satisfactory laboratory test routinely available (Thomson et al., 2002). Rather than waiting on some definitive diagnostic sign, it is more important to make a presumptive diagnosis and treat the patient as soon as possible (Cook et al., 1998). The need for a more pro-active approach to treatment of known or suspected Wernicke–Korsakoff syndrome has been argued strongly by Cook et al. (1998). Current medical management of acute Wernicke–Korsakoff syndrome, in particular with aggressive vitamin B therapy has been reviewed by Thomson et al. (2002). Although these authors focused on medical management in the accident and emergency setting, many of the same principles should apply to treatment of cognitive impairment, including apparent dementia, in association with alcohol dependence irrespective of the setting. As Thomson and colleagues (2002) show, the risks of parenteral B vitamin therapy are low, and the potential to minimize long-term

disability may be greatly enhanced by early and effective treatment.

In the light of the potential recovery of cognitive function with effective treatment and abstinence from alcohol, clinicians also should be encouraged to intervene with efficacious treatments for alcohol dependence. Research demonstrates the effectiveness of brief interventions in both emergency and general medical settings and should be encouraged as standard practice (Bien et al., 1993; Moyer et al., 2002). Developments in more specialized treatments for alcohol dependence include improvements in withdrawal management (Mayo-Smith, 1997), medications such as naltrexone and acamprosate for relapse prevention (Garbutt et al., 1999; Srisurapanont and Jarusuraisin, 2002) and cognitive behavioural interventions (Miller and Wilbourne, 2002). Every opportunity should be taken to actively treat any person with alcohol dependence.

59.5 CONCLUSIONS

Although Leevy (1982) invoked the term 'thiamin dementia' it may be simplest to retain the term Wernicke–Korsakoff syndrome to refer to all of the neurological and neuropsychological features of thiamin deficiency. The neurological usage of Wernicke–Korsakoff syndrome no longer applies only to those cases with the classical triad, but has broadened to encompass a highly variable neurological presentation (Torvik et al., 1982; Reuler et al., 1985; Victor et al., 1989). It may be that the neuropsychology of Wernicke–Korsakoff syndrome is best conceived as an example of a potentially reversible dementia. The value of a broader approach to diagnosis is to heighten sensitivity to the prevalence of the disorder in certain populations, particularly in association with alcohol dependence.

REFERENCES

Adams KM, Gilman S, Johnson-Green D et al. (1998) The significance of family history status in relation to neuropsychological test performance and cerebral glucose metabolism studied with positron emission tomography in older alcoholics. Alcoholism: Clinical and Experimental Research 22: 105–110

Ambrose ML, Bowden SC, Whelan G. (2001) Thiamin treatment and working memory function of alcohol-dependent people: preliminary findings. Alcoholism: Clinical and Experimental Research 25: 112–116

American Psychiatric Association. (1994) Diagnostic and Statistical Manual of Mental Disorders, 4th edition. Washington, DC, American Psychiatric Association

Bates ME, Bowden SC, Barry D. (2002) Neurocognitive impairment associated with alcohol use disorders: implications for treatment. Experimental and Clinical Psychopharmacology 10: 193–212

Bien T, Miller R, Tonigan J. (1993) Brief interventions for alcohol problems: a review. Addiction 88: 315–336

Bowden SC. (1987) Brain impairment in social drinkers? No cause for concern. *Alcoholism: Clinical and Experimental Research* 11: 407–410

Bowden SC. (1990) Separating cognitive impairment in neurologically asymptomatic alcoholism from Wernicke–Korsakoff syndrome: Is the neuropsychological distinction justified? *Psychological Bulletin* 107: 355–366

Bowden SC, Whelan G, Long C, Clifford C. (1995) The temporal stability of the WAIS-R and WMS-R in a heterogeneous sample of alcohol dependent clients. *Clinical Neuropsychologist* 9: 194–197

Butters N and Cermak LS. (1980) *Alcoholic Korsakoff's Syndrome: An Information–Processing Approach to Amnesia.* London, Academic Press

Caine D, Halliday GM, Kril JJ, Harper CG. (1997) Operational criteria for the classification of chronic alcoholics: identification of Wernicke's encephalopathy. *Journal of Neurology, Neurosurgery, and Psychiatry* 62: 51–60

Cohen P and Cohen J. (1984) The clinician's illusion. *Archives of General Psychiatry* 41: 1178–1182

Cook CCH, Hallwood PM, Thomson AD. (1998) B Vitamin deficiency and neuropsychiatric syndromes in alcohol misuse. *Alcohol and Alcoholism* 33: 317–336

Crews FT. (2000) Neurotoxicity of alcohol: excitotoxicity, oxidative stress, neurotrophic factors, apoptosis, and cell adhesion molecules. In: A Noronha, MJ Eckardt, K Warren (eds), *Review of NIAAA's Neuroscience and Behavioral Research Portfolio.* National Institute on Alcohol Abuse and Alcoholism (NIAAA) Research Monograph No. 34. Bethesda, MD, NIAAA, pp. 189–206

Cutting J. (1985) Korsakoff' syndrome. In: JAM Frederiks (ed.), *Handbook of Clinical Neurology: Vol. 45 (Revised) Series 1. Clinical Neuropsychology,* Amsterdam, Elsevier, pp. 193–204

Garbutt JC, West SL, Carey TS, Lohr KN, Crews FT. (1999) Pharmacological treatment of alcohol dependence: a review of the evidence. *JAMA* 281: 1318–1325

Goldman M. (1995) Recovery of cognitive functioning in alcoholics. *Alcohol Health and Research World* 19: 148–154

Gordis E. (2000) *Tenth Special Report to the US Congress on Alcohol and Health.* Washington, DC, National Institute of Health

Grant I. (1987) Alcohol and the brain: neuropsychological correlates. *Journal of Consulting and Clinical Psychology* 55: 310–324

Harding A, Halliday G, Caine D, Kril J. (2000) Degeneration of anterior thalamic nuclei differentiates alcoholics with amnesia. *Brain* 123: 141–154

Harper C. (1983) The incidence of Wernicke's encephalopathy in Australia – a neuropathological study of 131 cases. *Journal of Neurology, Neurosurgery, and Psychiatry* 46: 593–598

Harper CG, Giles M, Finlay-Jones R. (1986) Clinical signs in the Wernicke–Korsakoff complex: a retrospective analysis of 131 cases diagnosed at autopsy. *Journal of Neurology, Neurosurgery, and Psychiatry* 49: 341–345

Harper CG, Dixon G, Sheedy D, Garrick T. (2003) Neuropathological alterations in alcoholic brains. Studies arising form the New South Wales Tissue Resource Centre. *Progress in Neuropharmacology and Biological Psychiatry* 27: 951–961

Haxby JV, Raffaele K, Gillette J, Shapiro MB, Rapoport SI. (1992) Individual trajectories in cognitive decline in patients with dementia of the Alzheimer type. *Journal of Clinical and Experimental Neuropsychology* 14: 575–592

Homewood J and Bond NW. (1999) Thiamin deficiency and Korsakoff's syndrome: failure to find memory impairments following non-alcoholic Wernicke's encephalopathy. *Alcohol and Alcoholism* 19: 75–84

Jacobson RR, Lishman WA. (1987) Selective memory loss and global intellectual deficits in alcoholic Korsakoff's syndrome. *Psychological Medicine* 17: 649–655

Knight RG. (2001) Neurological consequences of alcohol use. In: N Heather, TJ Peters (eds), *International Handbook of Alcohol Dependence and Problems.* New York, John Wiley and Sons Ltd, pp. 129–148

Kopelman MD. (1985) The Korsakoff syndrome. *British Journal of Psychiatry* 166: 154–173

Langlais PJ and Zhang SX. (1997) Cortical and subcortical white matter damage without Wernicke's encephalopathy after recovery from thiamine deficiency in the rat. *Alcohol: Clinical and Experimental Research* 19: 1073–1077

Langlais PJ, Zhang SX, Savage LM. (1996) Neuropathology of thiamine deficiency: an update on the comparative analysis of human disorders and experimental models. *Metabolic Brain Disease* 11: 19–37

Leevy CM. (1982) Thiamin deficiency and alcoholism. *Annals of the New York Academy of Sciences* 378: 316–326

Leckliter IN and Matarazzo JD. (1989) The influence of age, education, IQ, gender, and alcohol abuse on Halstead-Reitan Neuropsychological Test Battery performance. *Journal of Clinical Psychology* 45: 484–512

Lishman WA. (1986) Alcoholic dementia. A hypothesis. *Lancet* 8491: 1184–1186

Lishman WA. (1998) *Organic Psychiatry: The Psychological Consequences of Cerebral Disorder,* 3rd edition. Oxford, Blackwell Scientific Publications

McKhann G, Drachman D, Folstein M, Katzman R, Price D, Stadlan EM. (1984) Clinical diagnosis of Alzheimer's disease: report of the NINCDS-ADRDA Work Group under the auspices of Department of Health and Human Services Task Force on Alzheimer's Disease. *Neurology* 34: 939–944

Mayo-Smith MF. (1997) Pharmacological management of alcohol withdrawal: a meta-analysis and evidence-based practice guideline. *JAMA* 278: 144–151

Miller WR and Wilbourne PL. (2002) Mesa Grande: a methodological analysis of clinical trials of treatments for alcohol use disorders. *Addiction* 97: 265–277

Moyer A, Finney JW, Swearingnen CE, Vergun P. (2002) Brief interventions for alcohol problems: a meta-analytic review of controlled investigations in treatment seeking and non-treatment-seeking populations. *Addiction* 97: 279–292

Oscar-Berman M and Marinkovic K. (2003) Alcoholism and the Brain: An overview of techniques for assessing damage, and implications for treatment. *Alcohol Research and Health* 27: 125–133

Oslin D, Atkinson RM, Smith DM, Hendrie H. (1998) Alcohol-related dementia: Proposed clinical criteria. *International Journal of Geriatric Psychiatry* 13: 203–212

Oslin D and Carey MS. (2003) Alcohol-related dementia: Validation of diagnostic criteria. *American Journal of Geriatric Psychiatry* 11: 441–447

Parsons OA. (1994) Determinants of cognitive deficits in alcoholics: the search continues. *Clinical Neuropsychologist* 8: 39–58

Parsons OA. (1998) Neurocognitive deficits in alcoholics and social drinkers: a continuum? *Alcohol: Clinical and Experimental Research* 22: 954–961

Reuler JB, Girard DE, Cooney TG. (1985) Wernicke's encephalopathy. *New England Journal of Medicine* 312: 1035–1039

Rourke SB and Loberg T. (1996) The neurobehavioral correlates of alcoholism. In: I Grant and KM Adams (eds), *Neuropsychological Assessment of Neuropsychiatric Disorders.* New York, Oxford University Press, pp. 423–485

Royal College of Physicians. (2001) *Report of a Working Party: Alcohol – Can the NHS Afford It? Recommendations for a Coherent Alcohol Strategy for Hospitals.* London, Royal College of Physicians

Saxton J, Munro CA, Butters MA, Schramke C, McNeill MA. (2000) Alcohol, dementia, and Alzheimer's disease: comparison of neuropsychological profiles. *Journal of Geriatric Psychiatry and Neurology* **13**: 141–149

Schroeder SA, Krupp MA, Tierney LM, McPhee SJ. (1991) *Current Medical Diagnosis and Treatment 1991.* Norwalk, CT, Appleton and Lange

Srisurapanont M and Jarusuraisin N. (2002) Opioid antagonists for alcohol dependence (Cochrane Review). *Cochrane Library* **1**

Sullivan EV, Rosenbloom MJ, Lim KO, Pfefferbaum A. (2000) Longitudinal changes in cognition, gait, and balance in abstinent and relapsed alcoholic men: relationships to changes in brain structure. *Neuropsychology* **14**: 178–188

Talland GA. (1965) *Deranged Memory: A Psychonomic Study of the Amnesic Syndrome.* New York, Academic Press

Thomson AD. Cook CC, Touquet R, Henry JA. (2002) The Royal College of Physicians report on alcohol: guidelines for managing Wernicke's encephalopathy in the accident and Emergency Department. *Alcohol and Alcoholism* **37**: 513–521

Torvik A. (1991) Wernicke's encephalopathy – prevalence and clinical spectrum. *Alcohol and Alcoholism* (Suppl. 1): 381–384

Torvik A, Lindboe CF, Rogde S. (1982) Brain lesions in alcoholics: a neuropathological study with clinical correlations. *Journal of the Neurological Sciences* **56**: 233–248

Unkenstein AE and Bowden SC. (1990) The individual course of neuropsychological recovery in recently abstinent alcoholics: a pilot study. *Clinical Neuropsychologist* **5**: 24–32

Victor M. (1994) Alcoholic dementia. *Canadian Journal of Neurological Science* **21**: 88–99

Victor M and Yakovlev PI. (1955) SS Korsakoff's psychic disorder in conjunction with peripheral neuritis. *Neurology* **5**: 394–406

Victor M, Adams RD, Collins GH. (1971) *The Wernicke–Korsakoff Syndrome.* Oxford, Basil Blackwell

Victor M, Adams RD, Collins GH. (1989) *The Wernicke–Korsakoff Syndrome and Related Neurological Disorders Due to Alcoholism and Malnutrition.* Philadelphia, FA Davis

Walton NH and Bowden SC. (1997) Does liver function explain neuropsychological status in recently detoxified alcohol-clients? *Alcohol and Alcoholism* **32**: 287–295

Wechsler D. (1981) *Wechsler Adult Intelligence Scale – Revised.* New York, Harcourt Brace Jovanovich

Wechsler D. (1987) *Wechsler Memory Scale – Revised Manual.* New York, The Psychological Corporation

Dementia and intellectual disability

JENNIFER TORR

60.1 DEMOGRAPHY OF DEMENTIA IN INTELLECTUAL DISABILITY

Early in the twentieth century children with intellectual disability (ID) in developed nations had a life expectancy of less than 20 years (Carter and Jancar, 1983). By the close of the twentieth century average life expectancy for people with ID had increased to 60 years. People with mild ID, few comorbid conditions and a protective life style have a life expectancy approaching and in some instances exceeding that of the general population (Patja *et al.*, 2000). People with Down syndrome (DS), cerebral palsy, greater levels of disability or comorbid physical conditions have lower life expectancies (Eyman *et al.*, 1989; Strauss and Eyman, 1996).

The number of people with ID aged 60 and over is expected to at least double and perhaps quadruple in the next two decades (Bigby *et al.*, 2001). The Edinburgh Principles promote the rights of people with ID and dementia to have access to the same standard of care provided to the general population and outline principles for the design of services to support people with ID with dementia and their carers (Wilkinson and Janicki, 2002). However, aged care and disability services have failed to develop coherent policy and programme responses to the rapidly increasing population of older people with ID.

60.2 DOWN'S SYNDROME AND ALZHEIMER'S DISEASE

The relationship between DS and the development of Alzheimer's disease (AD) in middle age is well established.

Post-mortem studies show neuropathological changes consistent with AD by 40 years of age (Wisniewski *et al.*, 1985). The average age of clinical diagnosis of dementia is about 50 years and prevalence may be as high as 75 per cent in those aged over 60 years (Holland, 1998).

DS, the commonest cause of ID, is due to trisomy 21 in 95 per cent of cases. The remainder are due to translocations, partial trisomies and mosaicism (Stoll *et al.*, 1998). Overexpression of a number of genes on chromosome 21 are implicated in the pathogenesis of AD in DS. Triplication of the amyloid precursor protein (APP) gene in trisomy 21, resulting in precocious and excessive amyloid production and cerebral deposition, is postulated to be the root cause of early onset AD in DS (Robakis *et al.*, 1987). Indeed, the expression of APP is 3–4 times higher than that expected from the 1.5 times increased gene load. Expression of APP is promoted by a transcriptional regulator that is also coded on chromosome 21 (Wolvetang *et al.*, 2003). A gene encoding for a β-secretase, located on chromosome 21, is overexpressed and cleaves APP to produce Aβ amyloid (Barbiero *et al.*, 2003). Serum levels of $A\beta_{1-40}$ and $A\beta_{1-42}$ are increased in DS and are associated with the development of dementia (Schupf *et al.*, 2001). Aβ amyloid contributes to neurofibrillary tangle formation as well as mediating inflammatory factors contributing to the rapid accumulation of neuropathology in the DS brain and may also trigger apoptotic pathways (Head *et al.*, 2001, 2002).

Overexpression of superoxide dismutase is thought to lead to excess free radical production and cell damage (Dickinson and Singh, 1993). In addition, at least 10 genes on chromosome 21 are involved in mitochondrial functioning (Hattori *et al.*, 2000). Mitochondrial dysfunction has been shown to increase oxidative stress that may lead to neuronal death and altered metabolism of APP (Arbuzova *et al.*, 2002; Busciglio *et al.*, 2002).

Other factors modulate the risk of developing AD in DS. The presence of one or two apolipoprotein E (ApoE) ε4 alleles increases the risk of earlier onset AD in people with DS whilst the presence of ApoE ε2 is protective (Schupf *et al.*, 1996; Rubinsztein *et al.*, 1999). Serum levels of $A\beta_{1-42}$ are increased in DS subjects with the ApoE ε4 allele (Schupf *et al.*, 2001). Women with DS have early menopause. The earlier the menopause the greater the risk of AD and the earlier it develops. The bioavailability of endogenous oestradiol is thought to be associated with dementia (Cosgrave *et al.*, 1999; Schupf *et al.*, 2003; Patel *et al.*, 2004).

60.3 PREVALENCE OF AND RISK FACTORS FOR DEMENTIA IN OTHER PEOPLE WITH INTELLECTUAL DISABILITY

Less attention has been focused on dementia in people with ID not due to DS. Prevalence rates of 22 per cent have been reported (Lund, 1985; Cooper, 1997a) in epidemiological samples of people with ID over the age of 65 years. However, other studies have found rates of dementia not significantly different from that expected in the general population (Evenhuis, 1997; Zigman *et al.*, 2004). This considerable variance in the reported prevalence of dementia in ID reflects diagnostic challenges, choice of diagnostic criteria, sample selection, and other methodological differences. 'Dementia' and 'Alzheimer's disease' are often used interchangeably (Zigman *et al.*, 2004) and few researchers attempt to subtype dementia. Evenhuis (1997) reports cases of vascular and mixed dementia. However, the possibility of vascular dementia generally is overlooked. The presence of cerebrovascular disease or other major medical disorders may confound and therefore preclude a research diagnosis of dementia (Evenhuis, 1997; Zigman *et al.*, 2004).

Risk factors for dementia in people with ID not due to DS have not been a major focus for investigators. A large postmortem series from an institutional population (Popovitch *et al.*, 1990) demonstrates the common presence of senile plaques and neurofibrillary tangles, increasing with age and correlated with a history of seizures, congenital malformations and head trauma. Neuropathological criteria for AD were fulfilled in 9.5 per cent of cases aged <50 years of age, increasing to 87 per cent for those >75 years. However, in most cases the plaques were not neuritic and substantial numbers of neurofibrillary tangles were found in the frontal lobes. Neither clinicopathological correlations nor the presence or absence of vascular pathology were reported.

In support of these findings Cooper (1997b) reported higher rates of poorly controlled epilepsy in those with dementia, raising questions about the cumulative effects of excitotoxic neurone death. Prevalence rates for epilepsy in people with ID are 30 per cent compared with 1 per cent for the general population (Ettinger and Steinberg, 2001). Head injury is also associated with dementia in the general population and in people with ID. Head injury may be the cause of ID and people with ID are at risk of head injury due to falls and self-injurious behaviour such as head banging.

Low intellectual quotient (IQ) and low educational status are frequently quoted as being risk factors for AD and a low reserve hypothesis is invoked. Prenatal exposure to toxins such as alcohol (Dumas and Rabe, 1994) and microcephaly (Lee and Rabe, 1992) predispose to early cognitive decline in animal models, although the mechanism for this has not been elucidated. Is it the greater impact of age-related neurone loss on an already compromised brain or do prenatal insults affect some basic processes resulting in premature ageing?

The potential for vascular dementia in people with ID is high. The identification and management of vascular risk factors in people with ID is often overlooked by generic health care and health promotion (Wallace, 2004). High rates of pathological lipid profiles, obesity (Rimmer *et al.*, 1994), smoking (Tracy and Hosken, 1997), hypertension, other cardiovascular disease and cerebrovascular disease (Cooper, 1999) have been reported in people with ID. Certain genetic syndromes also predispose to hypertension, diabetes mellitus, obesity, hyperhomocysteinaemia, hyperlipidaemia and abnormalities in vasculature increasing the risk of vascular disease (Wallace, 2004).

60.4 DIAGNOSIS OF DEMENTIA IN PEOPLE WITH INTELLECTUAL DISABILITY

Currently there are no internationally recognized gold standard instruments for the diagnosis of dementia in people with intellectual disability. Standard tools such as the Mini-Mental State Examination and general neuropsychological assessments are not valid for use in people with ID because of substantial floor effects. A range of instruments have been used in dementia in ID research including tools for adaptive functioning, diagnosis of dementia and for testing specific cognitive domains. Measures of adaptive functioning were not specifically developed for use in dementia studies. A modified version of the CAMDEX informant interview has been shown to be a valid and reliable tool for use in the diagnosis of dementia in adults with DS (Ball *et al.*, 2004a). The Dementia Questionnaire for Persons with Mental Retardation (DMR; Evenhuis, 1996), an informant rated instrument and the Down Syndrome Dementia Scale (DSDS), completed by psychologist informant interview, both have good correlations with clinician diagnosis and correlate well with each other (Deb and Braganza, 1999).

The pattern and progression of cognitive decline in AD in people with DS follows the pattern in the general population with early memory impairment followed by declines in visual spatial skills and dyspraxia (Dalton *et al.*, 1999; Devenny *et al.*, 2000; Krinsky-McHale *et al.*, 2002). There are modified versions of the selective reminding test (Krinsky-McHale *et al.*, 2002) and cued recall test (Devenny *et al.*, 2002). Parietal functioning can be tested by a dyspraxia scale (Dalton and Fedor, 1998).

Consensus diagnostic criteria for dementia for people with intellectual disability are given in Box 60.1. The clinical diagnosis of dementia in people with intellectual disability is complicated by the pre-existing impairments in intellectual and adaptive functioning. Decline from baseline functioning must be established. This is difficult if family members are not available for interview or when carers have not known the person over a sufficient period of time. In the clinical setting memory in people who are non-verbal can be tested by hiding three objects around the room and then testing delayed recall. Dyspraxia can be assessed by asking the person to take off and put back on shoes and jackets, but ability to complete these tasks needs to be measured against the person's baseline functioning. Comparison of current samples of writing and art work with earlier work is helpful in identifying decline in visuospatial skills.

Behavioural and psychological symptoms are common clinical features of dementia in people with intellectual disability. The onset of a variety of maladaptive behaviours may precede or coexist with the decline in adaptive functioning. Pre-existing levels of maladaptive behaviours tend to remain stable in the absence of a decline in functioning (Urv et al., 2003). Mood changes, poor emotional control, irritability, onset of or increase in aggression, withdrawal, loss of interest, anhedonia, sleep and appetite disturbances have all been reported (Moss and Patel, 1995; Cooper, 1997a; Urv et al., 2003). Psychotic symptoms include delusions of theft and persecution and visual hallucinations of strangers in the house (Cooper, 1997a). The earliest signs of AD in DS may be changes in executive functioning, behaviour and personality (Ball et al., 2004b). Depression may precede or occur with AD and DS (Burt et al., 1992; Sung et al., 1997).

Decline in cognitive and adaptive function may be due to or complicated by a multitude of factors. Comorbid sensory impairment, mobility problems and medical conditions are common in people with intellectual disability, increase with age and are more common in those with dementia (Cooper, 1997b) Conditions such as hypothyroidism are particularly common in people with DS. Delirium and depression, both common conditions, may present with cognitive and functional decline. Psychotropic polypharmacy is rife amongst people with intellectual disability, especially in the older group who are also prescribed greater amounts of anticholinergic medications (Pary, 1995). Psychotropic medications may result in significant cognitive impairment that could mimic dementia (Gedye, 1998).

Neuroimaging is important in establishing the presence of cerebrovascular disease or congenital abnormalities; however, its place in diagnosing AD in people with ID is less clear. Interpretation of neuroimages involves an understanding of the baseline differences in the brains of people with ID. People with DS and no AD have significantly smaller hippocampal volumes than cognitively normal adults even when smaller total brain volume is taken into account. In subjects with DS and AD, hippocampal and amygdala volumes decline (Aylward et al., 1999). Serial MRI examinations maybe useful in individual patients with DS in tracking the development of AD; however, a single individual scan may not be particularly useful in establishing a diagnosis of AD (Prasher et al., 1996). Cerebral single photon emission computed tomography (SPECT) scans of people with DS and clinical AD show reduced cerebral blood flow in the frontal, temporal, parietal and occipital regions of both hemispheres (Melamed et al., 1987).

60.5 MANAGEMENT AND CARE OF PEOPLE WITH INTELLECTUAL DISABILITY AND DEMENTIA

The principles of care of people with ID and dementia are essentially the same as for all people with dementia. This includes the identification and management of coexistent medical conditions, attention to sensory impairments, immobility and nutrition. Medications need to be reviewed and limited to essential medications at the lowest effective dose. Alternatives to the use of medications with significant anticholinergic effects should be found. Careful assessment of the person's accommodation and care needs, the physical environment, routines and programmes as well as the expectations of others, needs to be conducted. Simple concrete explanations and visual aids can help co-residents to understand what is happening to their housemate (Lynggaard and Alexander, 2004). Carer education and support are essential. Training for carers is offered by the Down Syndrome Society in the United Kingdom and Alzheimer's Australia.

There is a small but growing body of evidence of the potential benefits of treating people with DS and AD with cholinesterase inhibitors. A small randomized controlled trial of donepezil in people with DS and AD found nonsignificant improvements in the treatment group (Prasher et al., 2002). However, in an open label extension there was a

---

Box 60.1 *DC-LD category IIIB1.1 unspecified dementia (Royal College of Psychiatrists, 2001, with permission)*

A The symptoms/signs must be present for at least 6 months

B They must not be a direct consequence of other psychiatric or physical disorders

C The symptoms and signs must represent a change from the person's premorbid state

D Impaired memory must be present

E Impairment in other cognitive skills, judgement and thinking must be present

F Items D and E must not be solely attributed to clouding of consciousness as in delirium

G Reduced emotional control or motivation of change in social behaviour must be present

significant difference between the always-treated versus the never-treated group (Prasher *et al.*, 2003). A convenience sample of six patients with DS and AD treated with donepezil for 5 months showed significant improvement over nine closely matched historical control subjects (Lott *et al.*, 2002).

These studies found donepezil to be safe in people with DS, the main side effects being nausea, incontinence, agitation and listlessness. However, a case report of a person with DS and AD treated with donepezil 5 mg developing a bradycardia of 48 beats per minute and collapsing urges caution in the use of cholinesterase inhibitors in a population with high rates of major congenital cardiac defects. Relatively minor abnormalities such as generally low heart rates and conduction abnormalities may be overlooked (Torr, 2004).

There is no published guidance on the pharmacological treatments of behavioural and psychological symptoms of dementia (BPSD) in people with ID. However, it is known that people with ID are sensitive to psychotropic medications. In the absence of evidence to the contrary management of BPSD in people with ID should be the same as for the general population. Many older people with ID are already prescribed psychotropic medications that may not have been reviewed for many years. Psychotic disorders tend to be over-diagnosed and major mood disorders, especially bipolar disorder, are often unrecognized and untreated.

REFERENCES

Arbuzova S, Hutchin T, Cuckle H. (2002) Mitochondrial dysfunction and Down's syndrome. *Bioessays* **24**: 681–684

Aylward EH, Li Q, Honeycutt NA, Warren AC *et al.* (1999) MRI volumes of the hippocampus and amygdala in adults with Down's syndrome with and without dementia. *American Journal of Psychiatry* **156**: 564–568

Ball SL, Holland AJ, Huppert FA *et al.* (2004a) The modified CAMDEX informant interview is a valid and reliable tool for use in the diagnosis of dementia in adults with Down's syndrome. *Journal of Intellectual Disability Research* **48**: 611–620

Ball SL, Treppner P, Holland AJ, Huppert FA. (2004b) Alzheimer disease (AD) in people with Down syndrome (DS): are personality and behaviour changes an early indicator? In: Lifespan and Ageing. *Journal of Intellectual Disability Research* **48**: 437

Barbiero L, Benussi L, Ghidoni R *et al.* (2003) BACE-2 is overexpressed in Down's syndrome. *Experimental Neurology* **182**: 335–345

Bigby C, Fyffe C, Balandin S, McCubberty J, Gordon M. (2001) *Ensuring Successful Ageing: Report of a National Study of Day Support Service Options for Older Adults With a Disability.* Melbourne, Latrobe University, School of Social Work and Social Policy

Burt DB, Loveland KA, Lewis KR. (1992) Depression and the onset of dementia in adults with mental retardation. *American Journal of Mental Retardation* **96**: 502–511

Busciglio J, Pelsman A, Wong C *et al.* (2002) Altered metabolism of the amyloid beta precursor protein is associated with mitochondrial dysfunction in Down's syndrome. *Neuron* **33**: 677–688

Carter G and Jancar J. (1983) Mortality in the mentally handicapped: a 50 year survey at the Stoke Park group of hospitals (1930–1980) *Journal of Mental Deficiency Research* **27**: 143–156

Cooper S-A. (1997a) Psychiatric symptoms of dementia among elderly people with learning disabilities. *International Journal of Geriatric Psychiatry* **12**: 662–666

Cooper S-A. (1997b) High prevalence of dementia amongst people with learning disabilities not attributed to Down's syndrome. *Psychological Medicine* **27**: 609–616

Cooper S-A. (1999) The relationship between psychiatric and physical health in elderly people with intellectual disability. *Journal of Intellectual Disability Research* **43**: 54–60

Cosgrave MP, Tyrrell J, McCarron M, Gill M, Lawlor BA. (1999) Age at onset of dementia and age of menopause in women with Down's syndrome. *Journal of Intellectual Disability Research* **43**: 461–465

Dalton A, Mehta PD, Fedor BL, Patti PJ. (1999) Cognitive changes in memory precede those in praxis in aging persons with Down syndrome. *Journal of Intellectual and Developmental Disability* **24**: 169–187

Dalton AJ and Fedor BA. (1998) Onset of dyspraxia in aging persons with Down syndrome: longitudinal studies. *Journal of Intellectual and Developmental Disability* **23**: 13–24

Deb S and Braganza J (1999) Comparison of rating scales for the diagnosis of dementia in adults with Down's syndrome. *Journal of Intellectual Disability Research* **43**: 400–407

Devenny DA, Krinsky-McHale SJ, Sersen G, Silverman WP. (2000) Sequence of cognitive decline in dementia in adults with Down's syndrome. *Journal of Intellectual Disability Research* **44**: 654–665

Devenny DA, Zimmerli EJ, Kittler P, Krinsky-McHale SJ. (2002) Cued recall in early-stage dementia in adults with Down's syndrome. *Journal of Intellectual Disability Research* **46**: 472–483

Dickinson MJ and Singh I. (1993) Down's syndrome, dementia, and superoxide dismutase. *British Journal of Psychiatry* **162**: 811–817

Dumas RM and Rabe A. (1994) Augmented memory loss in aging mice after one embryonic exposure to alcohol. *Neurotoxicology and Teratology* **16**: 605–612

Ettinger AB and Steinberg AL. (2001) Psychiatric issues in patients with epilepsy and mental retardation. In: AB Ettinger and AM Kanner (eds), *Psychiatric Issues in Epilepsy: a Practical Guide to Diagnosis and Treatment.* Philadelphia, Lippincott Williams and Wilkins pp. 181–200

Evenhuis HM. (1996) Further evaluation of the Dementia Questionnaire for Persons with Mental Retardation (DMR). *Journal of Intellectual Disability Research* **40**: 369–373

Evenhuis HM. (1997) The natural history of dementia in ageing people with intellectual disability. *Journal of Intellectual Disability Research* **41**: 92–96

Eyman RK, Call TL, White JF. (1989) Mortality of elderly mentally retarded persons in California. *Journal of Applied Gerontology* **8**: 203–215

Gedye A. (1998) Neuroleptic-induced dementia documented in four adults with mental retardation. *Mental Retardation* **36**: 182–186 [Erratum appears in *Mental Retardation* **37**: 138]

Hattori M, Fujiyama A, Taylor TD, Watanabe H, Yada T, Park HS. (2000) The DNA sequence of human chromosome 21. *Nature* **405**: 311–319 [Erratum appears in *Nature* **407**: 110]

Head E, Azizeh BY, Lott IT, Tenner AJ, Cotman CW, Cribbs DH. (2001) Complement association with neurones and beta-amyloid deposition in the brains of aged individuals with Down Syndrome. *Neurobiology of Disease* **8**: 252–265

Head E, Lott IT, Cribbs DH, Cotman CW, Rohn TT. (2002) Beta-amyloid deposition and neurofibrillary tangle association with caspase activation in Down syndrome. *Neuroscience Letters* **330**: 99–103

Holland AJ. (1998) Down's syndrome. In: MP Janicki and AJ Dalton (eds), *Dementia, Aging and Intellectual Disabilities: A Handbook.* Philadelphia, Bunner/Mazel, pp. 183–193

Krinsky-McHale SJ, Devenny DA, Silverman WP. (2002) Changes in explicit memory associated with early dementia in adults with Down's syndrome. *Journal of Intellectual Disability Research* **46**: 198–208

Lee MH and Rabe A. (1992) Premature decline in Morris water maze performance of aging microencephalic rats. *Neurotoxicology and Teratology* **14**: 383–392

Lott IT, Osann K, Doran E, Nelson L. (2002) Down syndrome and Alzheimer disease: response to donepezil. *Archives of Neurology* **59**: 1133–1136

Lund J. (1985) Epilepsy and psychiatric disorder in the mentally retarded adult. *Acta Psychiatrica Scandinavica* **72**: 557–562

Lynggaard H and Alexander N. (2004) Why are my friends changing? Explaining dementia to people with learning disabilities. *British Journal of Learning Disabilities* **32**: 30–34

Melamed E, Mildworf B, Sharav T, Belenky L, Wertman E. (1987) Regional cerebral blood flow in Down's syndrome. *Annals of Neurology* **22**: 275–278

Moss S and Patel P. (1995) Psychiatric symptoms associated with dementia in older people with learning disability. *British Journal of Psychiatry* **167**: 663–667

Pary RJ. (1995) Discontinuation of neuroleptics in community-dwelling individuals with mental retardation and mental illness. *American Journal of Mental Retardation* **100**: 207–212

Patel BN, Pang D, Stern Y *et al.* (2004) Obesity enhances verbal memory in postmenopausal women with Down syndrome. *Neurobiology of Aging* **25**: 159–166

Patja K, Iivanainen M, Vesala H, Oksanen H, Ruoppila I. (2000) Life expectancy of people with intellectual disability: a 35-year follow-up study. *Journal of Intellectual Disability Research* **44**: 591–599

Popovitch ER, Wisniewski HM, Barcikowska M *et al.* (1990) Alzheimer neuropathology in non-Down's syndrome mentally retarded adults. *Acta Neuropathologica* **80**: 362–367

Prasher VP, Barber PC, West R, Glenholmes P. (1996) The role of magnetic resonance imaging in the diagnosis of Alzheimer disease in adults with Down syndrome. *Archives of Neurology* **53**: 1310–1313

Prasher VP, Huxley A, Haque MS for Down Syndrome Ageing Study Group. (2002) A 24-week, double-blind, placebo-controlled trial of donepezil in patients with Down syndrome and Alzheimer's disease–pilot study. *International Journal of Geriatric Psychiatry* **17**: 270–278

Prasher VP, Adams C, Holder R. (2003) Long term safety and efficacy of donepezil in the treatment of dementia in Alzheimer's disease in adults with Down syndrome: open label study. *International Journal of Geriatric Psychiatry* **18**: 549–551

Rimmer JH, Braddock D, Fujiura G. (1994) Cardiovascular risk factor levels in adults with mental retardation. *American Journal on Mental Retardation* **98**: 510–518

Robakis NK, Wisniewski HM, Jenkins EC *et al.* (1987) Chromosome 21q21 sublocalisation of gene encoding beta-amyloid peptide in cerebral vessels and neuritic (senile) plaques of people with Alzheimer disease and Down syndrome. *Lancet* **1**: 384–385

Royal College of Psychiatrists. (2001) *DC-LD: Diagnostic Criteria for Psychiatric Disorders for Use With Adults with Learning Disabilities/Mental Retardation.* London, Gaskell

Rubinsztein DC, Hon J, Stevens F *et al.* (1999) Apo E genotypes and risk of dementia in Down syndrome. *American Journal of Medical Genetics* **88**: 344–347

Schupf N, Kapell D, Lee JH *et al.* (1996) Onset of dementia is associated with apolipoprotein E ε4 in Down's syndrome. *Annals of Neurology* **40**: 799–801

Schupf N, Patel B, Silverman W *et al.* (2001) Elevated plasma amyloid beta-peptide 1–42 and onset of dementia in adults with Down syndrome. *Neuroscience Letters* **301**: 199–203

Schupf N, Pang D, Patel BN *et al.* (2003) Onset of dementia is associated with age at menopause in women with Down's Syndrome. *Annals of Neurology* **54**: 433–438

Stoll C, Alembik Y, Dott B, Roth MP. (1998) Study of Down syndrome in 238,942 consecutive births. *Annales de Genetique* **41**: 44–51

Strauss D and Eyman RK. (1996) Mortality of people with mental retardation in California with and without Down syndrome, 1986–1991. *American Journal of Mental Retardation* **100**: 643–653

Sung H, Hawkins BA, Eklund SJ *et al.* (1997) Depression and dementia in aging adults with Down syndrome: a case study approach. *Mental Retardation* **35**: 27–38

Torr J. (2004) Clinical assessment of Alzheimer's disease in Down syndrome and treatment with acetylcholinesterase inhibitors. In: IASSID 12th World Congress, Montpellier. Congress Abstracts. *Journal of Intellectual Disability Research* **48**: 439

Tracy J and Hosken R. (1997) The importance of smoking education and preventative health strategies for people with intellectual disability. *Journal of Intellectual Disability Research* **41**: 416–421

Urv TK, Zigman WB, Silverman W. (2003) Maladaptive behaviors related to adaptive decline in aging adults with mental retardation. *American Journal on Mental Retardation* **108**: 327–339

Wallace R. (2004) Risk factors for coronary artery disease among individuals with rare syndrome intellectual disabilities. *Journal of Policy and Practice in Intellectual Disabilities* **1**: 31–41

Wilkinson H and Janicki MP. (2002) The Edinburgh Principles with accompanying guidelines and recommendations. *Journal of Intellectual Disability Research* **46**: 279–284

Wisniewski KE, Dalton AJ, McLachlan C, Wen GY, Wisniewski HM. (1985) Alzheimer's disease in Down's syndrome: clinicopathologic studies. *Neurology* **35**: 957–961

Wolvetang EW, Bradfield OM, Tymms M *et al.* (2003) The chromosome 21 transcription factor ETS2 transactivates the beta-APP promoter: implications for Down syndrome. *Biochimica et Biophysica Acta* **1628**: 105–110

Zigman WB, Schupf N, Devenny DA *et al.* (2004) Incidence and prevalence of dementia in elderly adults with mental retardation without down syndrome. *American Journal of Mental Retardation* **109**: 126–141

61

Schizophrenia, cognitive impairment and dementia

OSVALDO P ALMEIDA AND ROBERT HOWARD

Kraepelin used the term 'dementia praecox' to describe what he believed to be two key features of what is now known as schizophrenia: functional and intellectual deterioration. Such a concept implies that people with schizophrenia experience some degree of functional and cognitive impairment, and that these deficits represent a decline from a previous level of function. Since Kraepelin's seminal description of the key features of schizophrenia, research has been carried out with the aim of clarifying whether:

- the onset of schizophrenia is associated with cognitive decline;
- schizophrenia is associated with a specific pattern of cognitive deficits; and
- the cognitive deficits of schizophrenia are progressive and ultimately lead to the development of dementia.

This chapter will selectively review currently available evidence covering these three areas of research.

61.1 IS THE ONSET OF SCHIZOPHRENIA ASSOCIATED WITH COGNITIVE DECLINE?

Data on this topic remain sparse and come mostly from studies of people presenting to health services with first-episode psychosis (Bilder et al., 2000). A recently published Canadian study exemplifies our current knowledge in this area (Addington et al., 2003). The investigators recruited 312 subjects who were admitted to the Calgary Early Psychosis Programme with their first ever psychotic episode. The subjects' mean age

was 24.7 years and 89.8 per cent were receiving treatment with atypical antipsychotic medication at the time of neuropsychological assessment. The most frequent diagnoses were schizophrenia (39.7 per cent), schizophreniform disorder (38.5 per cent), psychotic disorder not otherwise specified (14.1 per cent), brief psychotic disorder (3.9 per cent) and delusional disorder (1.6 per cent). Cognitive assessment included an estimate of premorbid cognitive abilities, verbal fluency, verbal and visual memory, working memory, attention, visual-constructional ability, visuomotor sequencing, psychomotor speed, and set-shifting ability. Subjects' performance was significantly worse than that of non-psychiatric controls in all of the tests and subscores examined. The authors highlighted that patients' performance was particularly poor on tests of verbal fluency and immediate and long delayed verbal recall (more than 1.5 standard deviations below the norm), but concluded that there was 'no evidence to support differences in cognition among the different schizophrenia spectrum diagnostic groups'. Of note, such findings cannot be explained by the use of antipsychotic medication, as demonstrated by Ho et al. (2003a).

However, do the cognitive deficits observed among patients with first-episode psychosis represent a decline from a previous level of function? The results of volumetric magnetic resonance imaging (MRI) studies indicate that some of the brain abnormalities associated with schizophrenia precede the onset of the illness (Pantelis et al., 2003), which suggests that cognitive deficits are also likely to be present prior to psychotic symptoms becoming apparent. Findings from the relatively small number of observational studies available to date are more or less consistent with such a hypothesis. Cannon et al.

(1999) used a nested case–control study design to investigate the premorbid elementary school performance of Finnish individuals born in Helsinki between 1951 and 1960. Subjects who received the diagnosis of schizophrenia up to the year 1991 (n = 400) did not have poorer academic performance in elementary school than controls (n = 408), but were significantly more likely to display difficulties in sports and handicrafts. In addition, a smaller number of subjects with schizophrenia than controls progressed to high school, which suggests that some level of premorbid dysfunction might already have been present before the onset of the illness.

A recent case–control study from Singapore (Ang and Tan, 2004) examined the academic progression of a sample of 30 young men with schizophrenia and 30 age- and sex-matched controls enlisted in the Singapore Armed Forces between January 1998 and December 2000. Subjects with schizophrenia showed objective evidence of academic decline 2–4 years before the onset of symptoms, as measured by differences in the results of the Primary School Leaving Examination (usually taken at around the age of 12 years) and the Cambridge General Certificate of Education Examination (usually taken at around the age of 16 years). Similar findings have been reported by others (Caspi *et al.*, 2003).

Taken together, these results suggest that cognitive deficits precede the onset of clinical symptoms in schizophrenia – i.e. the cognitive deficits are not triggered by the onset of the illness. They also indicate that such deficits represent a decline from a relatively normal previous level of function.

61.2 IS SCHIZOPHRENIA ASSOCIATED WITH A SPECIFIC PATTERN OF COGNITIVE IMPAIRMENT?

Schizophrenia is associated with pervasive cognitive deficits including memory, attention, set-shifting and visuospatial abilities, psychomotor speed and planning (Heinrichs and Zakzanis, 1998). Findings amongst young people presenting with a first-ever psychotic episode suggest that this pattern of generalized cognitive impairment is already present during the early stages of the illness, although some have chosen to highlight the potential clinical relevance of the executive dysfunction (Riley *et al.*, 2000; Weickert *et al.*, 2000; Joyce *et al.*, 2002). Emerging empirical data suggest that the parietal cortex and cerebellum, rather than the frontal lobes, are involved in the production of bizarre psychotic phenomena, such as delusions of control (Blakemore *et al.*, 2002, 2003).

Psychotic disorders with onset in later life are also associated with generalized cognitive impairment. For example, Almeida *et al.* (1995) examined a convenience sample of 47 non-demented older people with psychotic symptoms and 33 controls using a comprehensive neuropsychological battery of tests. Patients showed significantly lower scores than controls on general measures of cognitive functioning (Mini-Mental State Examination – MMSE, Cambridge Cognitive

Examination, Wechsler Adult Intelligence Scale [Revised] verbal and performance scores), as well as on tests of delayed recall, working memory and executive function. Such findings have been replicated and extended by other studies, which have also shown that the pattern of cognitive impairment in schizophrenia with late onset is indistinguishable from the deficits displayed by patients with early illness onset (Sachdev *et al.*, 1999).

The clinical and social relevance of the neuropsychological deficits of schizophrenia become apparent when one examines their association with the functional capacity of patients. Evans *et al.* (2003) assessed 93 patients with diagnosis of schizophrenia or schizoaffective disorder (mean age = 57.2 ± 9.1 years) and 73 controls (mean age = 59.2 ± 11.2 years). The mean age at the onset of illness was 29.9 ± 13.7 years. Functional capacity, as measured by the Direct Assessment of Functional Status, was significantly correlated with processing speed, attention, abstract thinking, learning, delayed recall, verbal and motor skills ($P < 0.001$ for all correlations). Of note, psychotic patients presenting with functional impairment are less likely to be living independently (Twamley *et al.*, 2002). In addition, the level of functional impairment of elderly institutionalized patients with schizophrenia has been shown to be directly correlated to the severity of the cognitive deficits (Kurtz *et al.*, 2001).

In summary, young and old adults with schizophrenia display a non-specific pattern of generalized cognitive impairment compared with normal controls. The more severe the cognitive deficits, the greater the functional impairment and disability experienced by patients.

61.3 HOW DO THE COGNITIVE DEFICITS OF SCHIZOPHRENIA EVOLVE OVER TIME?

61.3.1 Schizophrenia with early onset

A fascinating recent development in schizophrenia research has been the demonstration that the brains of patients change significantly over time. For example, Ho *et al.* (2003b) reported the results of a 3-year MRI follow-up study of 73 young adults with schizophrenia (mean age = 24.5 ± 4.7 years) and 23 controls (mean age = 26.9 ± 5.3 years). They found that, compared with controls, the brains of patients displayed accelerated enlargement of the cortical sulcal cerebrospinal fluid spaces, progressive reduction in frontal lobe white matter volume and corresponding enlargement of frontal lobe cerebrospinal fluid volume. Such findings would suggest that the cognitive deficits of people with schizophrenia might also increase over time. However, the results of most follow-up studies investigating the progression of cognitive deficits in schizophrenia available to date do not support this hypothesis.

Hoff *et al.* (1999) reported the results of a 5-year longitudinal study of 42 patients with first-episode schizophrenia and

16 normal controls – they found that the cognitive performance of patients on tasks assessing language, executive function, verbal memory, spatial memory, concentration/speed and sensory-perception had remained relatively stable 1–1.5 standard deviations below the baseline level of performance of controls over the follow-up period. Another study by Gold *et al.* (1999) confirmed that the cognitive performance of patients does not deteriorate during the first 5 years of illness – in fact, it may actually improve with treatment. Other small-scale studies have confirmed that the overall cognitive performance of patients with schizophrenia tends to remain relatively stable over time (Stirling *et al.*, 2003).

61.3.2 Schizophrenia with late onset

Few studies have attempted to follow up patients with late-onset schizophrenia. Hymas *et al.* (1989) reported that patients with 'late paraphrenia' experienced a statistically significant, but clinically irrelevant, deterioration on the Mental Test Score. More recently, Palmer *et al.* (2003) have shown that the cognitive changes observed amongst patients with late-onset schizophrenia over a 2-year period are similar to those seen in people with early-onset schizophrenia and controls, which suggests that schizophrenia starting in later life is not associated with progressive cognitive decline.

In contrast, Brodaty *et al.* (2003) have argued that their 19 patients with onset of schizophrenia after the age of 50 years showed greater deterioration on MMSE scores over a 5-year follow-up period than 24 controls. However, patients recruited into this study had significantly fewer years of education and had lower baseline MMSE scores than controls (mean MMSE = 25.5 ± 3.5 versus 29.7 ± 1.0) – this is likely to have biased the overall results of the study significantly in favour of the control group.

In summary, there is no obvious evidence, at present, that schizophrenia with either early or late onset is associated with progressive cognitive decline. However, information on this topic remains sparse and conclusions are limited by small sample size, lack of sensitivity of the tests to change over time, and relative short follow-up periods.

61.4 WHAT IS THE ASSOCIATION BETWEEN SCHIZOPHRENIA AND DEMENTIA?

Preliminary evidence suggests that the risk of functional decline in schizophrenia may increase with increasing age after the age of 70 years. Friedman *et al.* (2001) followed up for 6 years a sample of 107 patients with schizophrenia aged 20–80 years. Functional decline, as measured by the Clinical Dementia Rating increased at around age 70 years and reached the same level as seen amongst patients with Alzheimer's disease at the age of 80 years. The authors concluded that the cognitive and functional status of institutionalized patients with schizophrenia is very stable until later in life, when a

progressive rate of cognitive and functional decline becomes apparent.

Histopathological investigations of the brains of patients with schizophrenia, however, have failed to show any sign of Alzheimer's disease-related pathology. Purohit *et al.* (1998) found no evidence of an excessive number of senile plaques, neurofibrillary tangles or neuronal loss amongst 100 consecutive autopsy brain specimens of subjects with chronic schizophrenia aged 52–101 years. Similarly, Arnold *et al.* (1998), who used a steriological counting method to quantify the presence of neurofibrillary tangles, amyloid plaques and Lewy bodies, found that their 23 elderly patients with schizophrenia did not present a larger number of neurodegenerative lesions than the 14 normal controls – both groups differed significantly in that respect from the 10 subjects with Alzheimer's disease.

More recently, Religa *et al.* (2003) have used specific antibodies against $A\beta_{40}$ and $A\beta_{42}$ to assist with the examination of the brains of 10 patients with Alzheimer's disease, 11 controls and 26 patients with schizophrenia (β-amyloid is thought to be central to the pathogenetic process that leads to the development of Alzheimer's disease). As expected, the levels of β-amyloid were highest amongst patients with Alzheimer's disease, and the mean concentration of $A\beta_{42}$ amongst patients with schizophrenia was similar to that of controls.

Taken together, these findings indicate that the mechanisms that lead to cognitive impairment in schizophrenia are different from those observed in common neurodegenerative disorders such as Alzheimer's disease.

61.5 CONCLUSION

Schizophrenia is a debilitating disorder that is associated with marked generalized cognitive impairment. These deficits are already present at the time of the onset of the illness and seem to remain relatively stable over time, although a small number of patients may experience significant cognitive and functional deterioration at follow up. There is no evidence that schizophrenia is a neurodegenerative disorder – in fact, all available evidence to date indicates that schizophrenia is not associated with any form of neurodegeneration. The use of the label 'dementia' to describe the cognitive deficits of patients with schizophrenia is misleading and should be avoided.

REFERENCES

Addington J, Brooks BL, Addington D. (2003) Cognitive functioning in first episode psychosis: initial presentation. *Schizophrenia Research* **62**: 59–64
Almeida OP, Howard R, Levy R, David A, Morris R, Sahakian BJ. (1995) Cognitive features of psychotic states arising in late life (late paraphrenia). *Psychological Medicine* **25**: 685–698

Ang YG and Tan HY. (2004) Academic deterioration prior to first episode schizophrenia in young Singaporean males. *Psychiatry Research* **121**: 303–307

Arnold SE, Trojanowski JQ, Gur RE *et al.* (1998) Absence of neurodegeneration and neural injury in the cerebral cortex in a sample of elderly patients with schizophrenia. *Archives of General Psychiatry* **55**: 225–232

Bilder RM, Goldman RS, Robinson D *et al.* (2000) Neuropsychology of first-episoded schizophrenia: initial characterization and clinical correlates. *American Journal of Psychiatry* **157**: 549–559

Blakemore SJ, Wolpert DM, Frith CD. (2002) Abnormalities in the awareness of action. *Trends in Cognitive Sciences* **6**: 237–241

Blakemore SJ, Oakley DA, Frith CD. (2003) Delusions of alien control in the normal brain. *Neuropsychologia* **41**: 1058–1067

Brodaty H, Sachdev P, Koschera A, Monk D, Cullen B. (2003) Long-term outcome of late-onset schizophrenia: 5-year follow-up study. *British Journal of Psychiatry* **183**: 213–219

Cannon M, Jones P, Huttunen MO *et al.* (1999) School performance in Finnish children and later development of schizophrenia: a population-based longitudinal study. *Archives of General Psychiatry* **56**: 457–463

Caspi A, Reichenberg A, Weiser M *et al.* (2003) Cognitive performance in schizophrenia patients assessed before and following the first psychotic episode. *Schizophrenia Research* **65**: 87–94

Evans JD, Heaton RK, Paulsen JS, Palmer BW, Patterson T, Jeste DV. (2003) The relationship of neuropsychological abilities to specific domains of functional capacity in older schizophrenia patients. *Biological Psychiatry* **53**: 422–430

Friedman JI, Harvey PD, Coleman T *et al.* (2001) Six-year follow-up study of cognitive and functional status across the lifespan in schizophrenia: a comparison with Alzheimer's disease and normal aging. *American Journal of Psychiatry* **158**: 1441–1448

Gold S, Arndt S, Nopoulos P, O'Leary DS, Andreasen N. (1999) Longitudinal study of cognitive function in first-episode and recent-onset schizophrenia. *American Journal of Psychiatry* **156**: 1342–1348

Heinrichs RW and Zakzanis KK. (1998) Neurocognitive deficit in schizophrenia: a quantitative review of the evidence. *Neuropsychology* **12**: 426–445

Ho BC, Alicata D, Ward J *et al.* (2003a) Untreated initial psychosis: relation to cognitive deficits and brain morphology in first-episode schizophrenia. *American Journal of Psychiatry* **160**: 142–148

Ho BC, Andreasen NC, Nopoulos P, Arndt S, Magnotta V, Flaum M. (2003b) Progressive structural brain abnormalities and their relationship to clinical outcome: a longitudinal magnetic resonance imaging study early in schizophrenia. *Archives of General Psychiatry* **60**: 585–594

Hoff AL, Sakuma M, Wieneke M, Horon R, Kushner M, DeLisi LE. (1999) Longitudinal neuropsychological follow-up study of patients with first-episode schizophrenia. *American Journal of Psychiatry* **156**: 1336–1341

Hymas N, Naguib M, Levy R. (1989) Late paraphrenia: a follow-up study. *International Journal of Geriatric Psychiatry* **4**: 23–29

Joyce E, Hutton S, Mutsatsa S *et al.* (2002) Executive dysfunction in first-episode schizophrenia and relationship to duration of untreated psychosis: the West London Study. *British Journal of Psychiatry* **43** (Suppl.): 38–44

Kurtz MM, Moberg PJ, Mozely LH *et al.* (2001) Cognitive impairment and functional status in elderly institutionalized patients with schizophrenia. *International Journal of Geriatric Psychiatry* **16**: 631–638

Palmer BW, Bondi MW, Twamley EW, Thal L, Golshan S, Jeste DV. (2003) Are late-onset schizophrenia spectrum disorders neurodegenerative conditions? Annual rates of change on two dementia measures. *Journal of Neuropsychiatry and Clinical Neurosciences* **15**: 45–52

Pantelis C, Velakoulis D, McGorry PD *et al.* (2003) Neuroanatomical abnormalities before and after the onset of psychosis: a cross-sectional and longitudinal MRI comparison. *Lancet* **361**: 281–288

Purohit DP, Perl DP, Haroutunian V *et al.* (1998) Alzheimer disease and related neurodegenerative diseases in elderly patients with schizophrenia: a post-mortem neuropathologic study of 100 cases. *Archives of General Psychiatry* **55**: 205–211

Religa D, Laudon H, Styczynska M, Winblad B, Näslund J, Haroutunian V. (2003) Amyloid β pathology in Alzheimer's disease and schizophrenia. *American Journal of Psychiatry* **160**: 867–872

Riley EM, McGovern D, Mockeler D *et al.* (2000) Neuropsychological functioning in first-episode psychosis – evidence of specific deficits. *Schizophrenia Research* **43**: 47–55

Sachdev P, Brodaty H, Rose N, Cathcart S. (1999) Schizophrenia with onset after age 50 years: neurological, neuropsychological and MRI investigation. *British Journal of Psychiatry* **175**: 416–421

Stirling J, White C, Lewis S *et al.* (2003) Neurocognitive function and outcome in first-episode schizophrenia: a 10-year follow up of an epidemiological cohort. *Schizophrenia Research* **65**: 75–86

Twamley EW, Doshi RR, Nayak GV *et al.* (2002) Generalized cognitive impairments, ability to perform everyday tasks, and levels of independence in community living situations of old patients with psychosis. *American Journal of Psychiatry* **159**: 2013–2020

Weickert TW, Goldberg TE, Gold JM, Bigelow LB, Egan MF, Weinberger DR. (2000) Cognitive impairments in patients with schizophrenia displaying preserved and compromised intellect. *Archives of General Psychiatry* **57**: 907–913

Huntington's disease

PHYLLIS CHUA AND EDMOND CHIU

62.1 CLINICAL FEATURES

Huntington's disease (HD) is a hereditary progressive neuro-degenerative disorder beginning classically in mid-life with the characteristic features of abnormal involuntary movements, mental impairment, psychiatric disorder, with death from complications of immobilization such as aspiration pneumonia (SuttonBrown and Suchowersky, 2003), occurring some 20–30 years after onset. In her monograph on HD, Folstein (Folstein, 1989) referred to the 'triad of clinical features' – motor disorder, cognitive disorder and emotional disorder. Within this characteristic triad, there is variety in the clinical phenotype with respect to onset timing, symptoms and progression.

62.1.1 Onset

The age of onset usually refers to the onset of typical motor symptoms, with the mean previously being reported from the late thirties to the early forties. Kremer (2003) argues that the median age of onset which is in the late forties or early fifties is the more accurate measure of onset age rather than the mean, due the fact that the onset age is not normally distributed, and that the truncated intervals of observation in many studies biases the results towards the younger onset group. Penney *et al.* (1990) introduced the term 'zone of onset', referring to the insidious onset of symptoms over many years before the definitive appearance of extrapyramidal signs such as chorea.

Various studies have indicated that the length of the trinucleotide repeats in the HD gene accounts for 50–70 per cent of the statistical variance in onset age (Duyao *et al.*, 1993). The phenomenon of anticipation whereby the disease onset is earlier in successive generations has been observed in some families. In the majority of families, the age of onset has tended to be similar.

62.1.2 Motor disorder

Although chorea is usually the predominant feature, dystonia, athetosis, motor restlessness, myoclonus and voluntary movement abnormalities may also be present. The chorea consists typically of rapid, non-repetitive contractions involving the orofacial and truncal areas and the limbs, and worsens with anxiety. Common manifestations include lip pouting, twitching of the cheeks, irregular grimacing, alternate lifting of the eyebrows, head nodding from neck muscle involvement, irregular breathing, fingers and toes flexion and extension, crossing and uncrossing of the legs and truncal restlessness (Kremer, 2003). The choreoathetosis tends to be absent during sleep and present during the waking hours, when falling asleep or on wakening. The movements cannot be suppressed voluntarily, although early on the patient may be able to integrate some of these movements into purposeful actions or minimize them by holding onto a chair, for example. In this early stage, there is hypotonia with hyperreflexia (SuttonBrown and Suchowersky, 2003). In advanced cases, the diaphragm and vocal apparatus may be involved leading to dysarthria (SuttonBrown and Suchowersky, 2003).

Dystonia frequently accompanies chorea early in the illness or during the course of the condition but can be very severe in advanced cases, juvenile-onset patients or in the 'Westphal variant' of adult-onset cases. The dystonia may be manifest as abnormal posturing of the extremities and head, internal shoulder rotation, sustained fist clenching, excessive knee flexion and foot inversion (Kremer, 2003).

Abnormalities in saccadic eye movements, poor opto-kinetic nystagmus and slowness with refixation may also be found in the majority of patients. Saccadic abnormalities with an inability to suppress reflexive glances to sudden novel stimuli and delayed initiation of voluntary saccades and slow saccades, particularly in the vertical movements, are seen early in the majority of patients (Lasker and Zee, 1997).

As the condition progresses, voluntary movements are increasingly impaired by the occurrence of clumsiness, brady-kinesia, rigidity, inability to sustain complex voluntary movement patterns leading to gait abnormalities and dysarthria. There is difficulty with tandem walking, turning, falls; eventually the patient is confined to a wheelchair. The dysarthria starts off as reduced clarity, which becomes worse as the rate and rhythm of speech becomes affected. Towards the late stage of the disease, rigidity and akinesia frequently overtake other aspects of the motor disorder accompanied by dysphagia and urinary incontinence. Frontal release reflexes such as snouting, sucking or grasping are seen when there is significant cognitive decline.

62.1.3 Cognitive disorder

62.1.3.1 NEUROPSYCHOLOGICAL DEFICITS

The cognitive changes in HD primarily reflect a form of subcortical dementia characterized by memory deficit, psychomotor slowing, apathy and depression. Cognitive domains affected include executive, language, perceptual and spatial skills, and memory functions. Executive function refers to a collection of higher order cognitive functions including the ability to plan and organize, monitor one's performance and self-correct, mental flexibility, shift attention set as circumstances change, and inhibit impulsive behaviours. Psychomotor slowing is evident in timed tasks such as digit symbol substitution and trail-making.

Intact verbal recognition memory, word recognition and object naming allows the person with HD to continue communicating initially despite mild dysarthria and dysprosody being present. In the advanced stages, language may be impaired leading to a mute state. This is due to a combination of motor disorder affecting phonation leading to severe dysarthria, impairment of comprehension of both affective and propositional prosody leading to failure to appreciate rhythm and changes of tone in normal speech and other cognitive deficits such as reduced verbal fluency, psychomotor slowing and apathy.

Visuospatial disorder in HD is evident early during performance in object assembly and block design tests (Craufurd and Snowden, 2003), as well as deficits in tests of pattern and spatial recognition memory, simultaneous and delayed matching-to-sample and spatial, which are complex tasks (Lawrence et al., 2000) that also require planning and organization. Further studies are needed to determine whether these deficits represent 'true' deficits in visuospatial/visual object processing or reflect other processes such as deficits in context recognition/registration (Lawrence et al., 2000).

Memory problems are a common complaint of patients with HD with studies indicating an inefficient memory strategy for acquiring and retrieving memories rather than a primary disorder of retention (Craufurd and Snowden, 2003). Craufurd and Snowden suggested that the memory deficits reflect executive dysfunction leading to ineffective information retrieval strategies. Performance on paired associated learning improved when a strategy was suggested (Craufurd and Snowden, 2003).

These cognitive deficits appear early in the course of the illness and may predate the motor signs. The rate of decline and cognitive domains affected in each individual are variable. Correlation between the rate of cognitive decline and CAG repeat length have been inconsistent (Craufurd and Snowden, 2003). The neural basis for these cognitive deficits is believed to be involvement of the basal ganglia and fronto-striatal connections.

62.1.4 Psychiatric disorder

There is increasing awareness that the behavioural and psychological aspects of HD cause as much, if not more, distress to the person with HD and their carer as the motor and cognitive decline. Any treatments aiming to slow disease progression need to address all three aspects of Folstein's 'triad of clinical features'. Using DSM-III criteria, 30 per cent of the sample in Folstein's Maryland sample of 186 persons with HD were free from any psychiatric disorder, 33 per cent had affective disorder, and 30 per cent intermittent explosive disorder, 4.8 per cent had dysthymic disorder, 15.6 per cent alcoholism; 5.9 per cent antisocial personality and 5.9 per cent schizophrenia (Folstein, 1989). In a similar population based study, Watt and Seller (1993) reported on a higher prevalence of depression (54 per cent), schizophrenia (12 per cent) and behavioural and personality disorder (42 per cent). The latter consisted of aggressiveness, which was the most frequent reported, followed by suspiciousness and temper. The prevalence of bipolar disorder, mania and hypomania is less clear, with reports ranging up to 10 per cent (Folstein, 1989).

The aetiology of affective disorder in HD is likely to be multifactorial. Depression can precede the onset of motor symptoms of HD by many years and can occur in those who may not be aware of being at-risk for the disorder (Craufurd and Snowden, 2003). It has also been postulated that the underlying neurodegenerative process in the caudate nucleus may also be responsible for the depressive symptoms. Craufurd et al. (2001) did not find a correlation between affective symptoms and severity of motor and cognitive symptoms. Several studies have shown that specific psychiatric symptoms such as psychosis (Tsuang et al., 2000) and affective disorder (Folstein et al., 1983) tended to cluster in certain families suggesting that other familial factors such as genetic heterogeneity at the HD locus, or a gene predisposing to the psychiatric disorder and closely linked to the HD gene may be responsible.

Irritability is reported frequently by family members who find such personality changes most difficult to tolerate. The potential role of alcohol and benzodiazepine side effects in precipitating such symptoms should not be ignored. Irritability as part of the symptoms complex of depressive illness should also be considered.

Other psychiatric manifestations such as obsessive-compulsive symptoms (Anderson et al., 2001), excessive worrying and somatizations have been reported but often do not meet criteria to warrant a formal psychiatric diagnosis. The common obsessions reported have aggressive and contamination themes (Anderson et al., 2001). Checking rituals were the most commonly reported (Anderson et al., 2001). Psychotic symptoms in HD tend to be isolated and atypical rather than schizophreniform, with persecutory delusions being the most common. The psychotic symptoms are more common early on in the illness and decrease with the cognitive decline. Sleep disturbances of frequent nocturnal awakenings, reduced sleep efficiency and sleep phase disturbances have also been reported in HD (Nance and Westphal, 2002).

A high rate of suicide has been associated with HD in many studies (Di Maio et al., 1993) and may be partially explained by a high prevalence of major affective disorder in this population. Undiagnosed or inadequately treated major depressive disorder can be uncovered by clinical examination and suicide can be prevented by energetic treatment with antidepressants or electroconvulsive therapy. Other symptoms in HD may increase the likelihood of suicide, including irritability, emotional lability and impulsiveness.

62.1.5 Advanced stage

A recent study by Foroud et al. (1999) reported the median duration of the disease as 21.4 years with a range of 1.2–40.8 years. In the late stages, the person with HD is usually confined to a wheelchair and reliant on care in a nursing home. Clinically, the bradykinesia, dystonia and rigidity dominate the clinical picture. Choreiform movements may still be evident in the orobuccal region and the extremities. Communication and swallowing are severely impaired. Nasogastric or percutaneous endoscopic gastric (PEG) feeds may be necessary to prevent aspiration and to offset the weight loss commonly seen in the advanced stage. Increased muscle tone may result in joint contractures. Pressure sores occur secondary to the immobility. Cognition is impaired and slow. It may be difficult to assess for psychiatric symptoms because of the limited communication. Sleep disturbance and agitation may be a problem. Some are incontinent of faeces and urine. Cachexia despite adequate intake may be seen during the latter part of the illness. The leading causes of death are from pneumonia, choking, nutritional deficiencies, skin ulcers and heart disease.

62.1.6 Clinical variants

Clinical variants of HD include the juvenile-onset, adult-onset Westphal variant and late-onset disease (Kremer, 2003).

Juvenile onset refers to the 10 per cent of all patients with HD who have onset before 20 years of age. Children with juvenile-onset HD often present with a decline in school performance and non-specific behavioural problems, with the motor disorder appearing a few years later. Other features of the juvenile onset are prominent rigidity and bradykinesia early on and minimal chorea, a rapidly progressive dementia, cerebellar abnormalities, myoclonus, epilepsy and long CAG repeats. The adult-onset Westphal variant refers to the cases with prominent rigidity earlier on rather than chorea. These patients are usually young with onset in their twenties or rarely in their thirties. Late-onset HD patients have a slower, milder form of HD with onset usually after age 50 years. Motor and cognitive symptoms are present but less severe while psychiatric symptoms are less common. Despite a more benign course, the number of years of survival after disease onset may still be similar to earlier-onset cases (James et al., 1994).

62.2 EPIDEMIOLOGY

The prevalence of HD has been largely based on estimates of point prevalence and has shown wide variations between countries and studies due to differences in selection criteria, source population, and sampling methods. In the US most studies gave a rate between 5 and 7 per 100 000 of population (Folstein, 1989). The prevalence is much lower among non-European ethnic groups.

62.3 GENETICS

62.3.1 The HD gene

HD is transmitted as an autosomal dominant trait with high penetrance (Gusella et al., 1993). In 1983, the linkage of a marker probe G8 (D4 S10) on the short arm of chromosome 4 to the HD gene was established (Gusella et al., 1983). Presymptomatic testing of persons at risk of HD and prenatal diagnosis of at-risk pregnancies were thus first made available by the application of genetic linkage analysis.

Ten years later in March, 1993, the Huntington's Disease Collaborative Research Group (1993) announced the discovery of a novel gene, IT15 (interesting transcript), located at 4p16.3 (short arm of chromosome 4) which contains a polymorphic trinucleotide CAG repeat that is expanded and unstable. A (CAG)n repeat longer than the normal range was observed. The number of CAG repeats on normal chromosomes ranges from 11 to 34 (Gusella et al., 1993). The zone of reduced penetrance (ZRP) refers to the CAG size range where the majority of persons will manifest the disease within their expected lifetime but a few will remain asymptomatic. In HD, the ZRP range is 36–38 (Andrew et al., 1997). In the CAG size range 29–35 (intermediate alleles), individuals do not manifest signs of HD (Goldberg et al., 1993) but their offspring are at risk of inheriting an expanded CAG gene and therefore of developing HD (Andrew et al., 1997). The estimate risk of an expansion to 36 or more repeats in the offspring of male intermediate HD gene carriers is between 2 and 10 per cent (Goldberg et al., 1993). There is a bias towards increased number of CAG repeats especially in paternal transmission leading to anticipation (Duyao et al., 1993) – earlier onset and greater severity of disease in later generations.

Mutation rate is very low, and variously calculated to be between 0.07×10^{-6} and 9.6×10^{-6} (Harper, 1991). Since the discovery of the gene, many suspected cases with no clinically affected parents were found to have parents in the intermediate allele range.

Increased number of CAG repeats is associated with an earlier age of onset (Duyao et al., 1993; Illarioshkin et al., 1994; Kieburtz et al., 1994; Brandt et al., 1996). However, the correlation is not sufficiently strong enough to predict the age of onset for a given individual (Gusella et al., 1993). In the CAG repeat size range of 37–52 CAG units (88 per cent of all HD repeats), the variation around the predicted age of onset is ± 18 years (Gusella et al., 1993). Late-onset HD has less correlation with the CAG repeat size (Kremer et al., 1993) and increased likelihood of an intermediate CAG range (James et al., 1994). Other factors aside from the number of CAG repeats clearly also have a role in determining the age of onset (Andrew et al., 1997); possible contenders are modifying genes (Gusella et al., 1993), environmental factors (Gusella et al., 1993) or stochastic effects (Gusella et al., 1993).

Severity of brain pathology as assessed by various measures such as striatal atrophy (Penney et al., 1997) has been correlated with the size of the CAG repeat in the majority of studies. Some studies examining for correlation with regional brain atrophy have not found any correlation with the CAG repeat size (Sieradzan et al., 1997). The relationship between CAG repeat size and rate of disease progression is controversial, partly due to the different markers of disease progression used in different studies and partly due to the confounding factor of age of onset, which may be related to disease progression. Illarioshkin et al. (1994) reported on a significant positive correlation between the rate of progression of neurological and psychiatric symptoms and CAG repeat size. In a 2-year longitudinal follow up, Brandt et al. (1996) found there was a greater decline in neurological and cognitive functioning in those with CAG repeats greater than 47. In contrast, Kieburtz et al. (1994) failed to find such a correlation between clinical progression of disease and CAG size. Similarly, no relationship has been found between size of CAG repeat, symptoms at onset (Sieradzan et al., 1997) or psychiatric symptoms (Berrios et al., 2001).

62.3.2 Mouse genetic models

The mouse genome can now be altered to produce transgenic mice. The term transgenic mice refers to mice generated by pronuclear microinjection of recombinant DNA or modification of endogenous mouse genes. The three main models (Bates and Murphy, 2003) are:

- mice where transgenes expressing truncated or full length versions of the huntingtin in the form of genomic or cDNA constructs have been introduced into the mouse germline;
- 'knockouts'– transgenic animals where a specific gene has been deleted; and
- knock-ins – transgenic mice where the sequence in exon 1 of the Hdh gene (the mouse homologue for the IT15 gene) has been replaced with a CAG repeat that is pathogenic in humans (Bates and Murphy, 2003). In the knock-in mice, the Hdh gene in mice has been modified by inserting a pure mouse gene or a HD/Hdh chimera (SuttonBrown and Suchowersky, 2003).

There are several lines of transgenic mice with different phenotypes and ages of onset.

62.3.3 Huntingtin

The gene IT15 codes for huntingtin, a protein located in tissue throughout the body but which is concentrated in the brain (DiFiglia, 1997). The polymorphic CAG repeat encodes for glutamate. In HD, the increased number of CAG repeats in the IT15 gene results in an expanded polyglutamine tract at the N-terminus of the huntingtin protein. IT15 is expressed throughout the body and concentrated in the brain, ovaries, testes and lungs, and is not only present in the brain regions affected in HD (Gusella et al., 1993). In HD, the distribution of the normal and abnormal huntingtin protein is heterogeneous throughout the brain (Gourfinkel-An et al., 1997). The abnormal huntingtin is not limited to cerebral structures most affected by the neurodegenerative process (Sharp et al., 1995). Within the brain, huntingtin is predominantly found in the neurones and to a smaller extent in the glial cells (Sharp et al., 1995). It is present primarily in the cytoplasm and has been variably detected in the nucleus (Sharp et al., 1995).

The normal function of IT15 and the mechanism by which the HD gene leads to neuronal loss and causes the symptoms of HD still remain unclear but is postulated to be more likely a gain rather than a loss of function. Recent studies suggest that the formation and accumulation of huntingtin aggregates in neuronal cells is crucial in the pathogenesis of HD (Wanker and Droge, 2002).

62.4 NEUROPATHOLOGY

Macroscopically, the brain is smaller and lighter in HD than in age-matched controls (MacMillan and Quarrell, 1996). Autopsy of brains of advanced HD patients demonstrate atrophy of the frontal lobes, caudate nucleus, putamen and globus pallidus (MacMillan and Quarrell, 1996), thickened leptomeninges and white matter loss under the cortical mantel (Gutekunst et al., 2002). The ventricles are enlarged to a greater extent than can be explained by the striatal loss. Under light microscopy, there are diagnostic findings of neuronal loss and gliosis in the striatum (putamen and caudate; MacMillan and Quarrell, 1996). The neuronal loss in the striatum primarily involves the medium sized neurones that are the major cell type in the striatum and act as the inhibitory projection neurones from the striatum to the globus pallidus and substantia nigra. As these medium sized neurones degenerate, there is a decrease in the neurotransmitter gamma-aminobutyric acid (GABA) and other neurochemicals such as substance P, glutamic acid decarboxylase, enkephalin, calcineurin, calbindin, adenosine and dopamine receptors (Gutekunst et al., 2002). These neuropathological changes evolve with time with the major cell loss starting in the dorsomedial 'tail' of the caudate and dorsal putamen, progressing ventrally, posteriorly and laterally until there is widespread severe neuronal loss and gliosis in the caudate and putamen, and moderate loss in the nucleus accumbens.

62.5 NEUROIMAGING

62.5.1 Structural imaging studies in HD

Early computer-assisted tomography (CAT) imaging techniques and recent magnetic resonance imaging (MRI) have consistently revealed bicaudate atrophy. The bicaudate ratio (BCR) is the ratio CC/OTcc where CC is the bicaudate diameter, the shortest distance between the indentations of the caudate nucleus, and OTcc is the distance between the outer tables of the skull alone on the same plane as the bicaudate measurement. The BCR is increased in HD compared with normals. MRI studies have also demonstrated atrophy of the putamen, caudate and globus pallidus in HD patients (Aylward et al., 1996). Frontal lobe atrophy, involving primarily the white matter and total brain atrophy have been noted (Aylward et al., 1998). Age of onset of disease and CAG repeat length have been correlated with change in volume of caudate and total basal ganglia, even after controlling for length between scans, duration of illness and symptoms severity (Aylward et al., 1997). Similar findings of increased BCR, smaller basal ganglia volume and caudate hypometabolism have also been found in the gene-positive HD group who were asymptomatic or had early choreiform movements (Grafton et al., 1992).

62.5.2 Magnetic resonance spectroscopy (MRS) studies in HD

Studies using ^{1}H-MRS in HD have found decreased N-acetylaspartate (NAA)/Cr in the putamen (Davie et al., 1994),

lower concentration of NAA in the combined caudate head and anterior putamen (Sanchez-Pernaute et al., 1999), decreased NAA and increased choline relative to creatine in the basal ganglia (Jenkins et al., 1993), suggesting neuronal loss in these structures. Reduced creatine in the basal ganglia has also been reported (Sanchez-Pernaute et al., 1999). Elevated lactate levels in the basal ganglia and occipital region have been noted in symptomatic HD patients (Jenkins et al., 1993). Some of these findings have been extended to the presymptomatic gene-positive group.

62.5.3 Functional imaging

Single photon emission computed tomography (SPECT) studies of cerebral blood flow have consistently revealed reduced cerebral perfusion in the basal ganglia before evidence of atrophy on MRI (Sax et al., 1996). Hypoperfusion in the cortical areas such as the prefrontal cortex (Sax et al., 1996) has been reported although these findings have not always been replicable.

Initial positron emission tomography (PET) studies of cerebral glucose metabolism mirrored the hypoperfusion findings in SPECT studies. These findings were extended to some (Feigin et al., 2001) but not all (Young et al., 1987) considered at risk of developing HD. Cortical hypometabolism has been demonstrated in some (Kuwert et al., 1990) but not all studies (Young et al., 1986).

PET $H_2(15)O$ PET cerebral activation (Weeks et al., 1997) and 99mTc-HMPAO SPECT (Deckel et al., 2001) studies have examined the functional significance of the above findings. These results suggest that there is impairment of the output part of the basal ganglia-thalamo-cortical motor circuit and compensatory recruitment of additional accessory motor pathways in the cortex.

Decreased benzodiazepine receptor density in the caudate but not the putamen in early HD using ^{11}C-flumazenil PET has been reported (Holthoff et al., 1993). ^{11}C-SCH23390 PET and ^{11}C-raclopride PET are used to study dopamine D1 and D2 receptor binding respectively. D1 (Sedvall et al., 1994; Ginovart et al., 1997) and D2 (Ginovart et al., 1997) receptor binding is reduced in the striatum in symptomatic HD. Dopamine D1 receptors are reduced in the frontal (Sedvall et al., 1994) and the temporal (Ginovart et al., 1997) cortices in symptomatic HD subjects. Various studies have found some asymptomatic HD subjects with reduced dopamine D1 and D2 receptor binding in the putamen and caudate (Weeks et al., 1996).

There have been few studies to date using functional MRI (fMRI) to examine neural activity in patients with HD. Clark et al. (2002) reported reduced fMRI signal in the three patients relative to the three controls in occipital, parietal and somato-motor cortex and in the caudate, while increased signal was found in HD in the left post-central and right middle frontal gyri during performance of the Porteus maze task.

62.6 MANAGEMENT

The main management issues in patients with diagnosed HD are:

- movement disorders causing involuntary movements, gait disorder, dystonia and rigidity;
- oral motor disorder affecting speech and eating;
- cognitive disorder;
- behavioural and psychiatric disorder of depression, psychosis, anxiety, obsessive-compulsive behaviours, irritability, agitation in late stage;
- medical issues of weight loss, sleep disturbance, complications in late-stage HD from infections, regurgitation, cachexia, delirium;
- social issues of work, finances, care and placement, driving ability;
- support for the caregiver and families; and
- education of the patient, family and other healthcare professionals (Nance and Westphal, 2002).

62.6.1 Genetic counselling

Guidelines of the International Huntington Association (IHA) and the World Federation of Neurology for HD (WFN; International Huntington Association and World Federation of Neurology Research Group on Huntington's Chorea, 1994), developed soon after the HD gene testing became available, have provided the framework for presymptomatic, prenatal and confirmatory testing. The presymptomatic predictive testing programmes include:

- helping the individual and accompanying person understand the diagnosis, probable course and current management available for HD;
- helping appreciation of the hereditary contribution to the disorder;
- pedigree analysis, which allows the risk to the individual to be assessed and some insight into the family dynamics;
- discussion of their personal experiences, goals, financial and social resources, coping styles and other support;
- reason for testing;
- psychological assessment of their coping ability; and
- possible neurological assessment for symptom onset.

Approximately 20 per cent of at-risk individuals worldwide have taken the opportunity to confirm their gene status through tests (SuttonBrown and Suchowersky, 2003). Despite initial concerns, with the appropriate support from pretest counselling, the risk of suicide and other events such as suicide attempts or hospitalization for psychiatric reasons have been low, with a worldwide risk reported at 0.97 per cent (Almqvist et al., 1999). High risk factors include a positive gene test, psychiatric history <5 years prior to testing, and unemployment. All who committed suicide were symptomatic at the time of the suicide. Prenatal testing of the fetus has had low uptake. Preimplantation genetic testing combines assisted reproduction and genetic testing, so that only HD negative embryos are implanted. This has become available only in recent years.

62.6.2 Pharmacological treatments

Currently pharmacological treatment is aimed at symptomatic control of the motor and psychiatric aspects of the disorder. Neuroleptics such as haloperidol, a dopamine antagonist, are used to suppress abnormal movements. In later stages of the illness, as dopamine receptors are destroyed with the neurones containing them, medication will gradually be less useful and may aggravate dystonia, bradykinesia and dysphagia, gait and balance problems. Given this natural progression of the chorea to decrease with time, antichoreic agents should be given only if the involuntary movements are severe and disabling. Low doses of haloperidol (less than 10 mg/day) have been shown to be most effective. Atypical neuroleptics such as risperidone and olanzapine are now preferred as they have a lower incidence of side effects. Tetrabenazine, a presynaptic dopamine-depleting agent is effective but may cause depression as a side effect (Gimenez-Roldan and Mateo, 1989). Trials of clozapine (doses up to 150 mg/day) have shown modest antichoreic effects but the side effects outweigh the potential benefits in most cases (van Vugt et al., 1997). Benzodiazepines such as clonazepam may reduce anxiety and some of the motor symptoms (Peiris et al., 1976).

The depression responds to the same treatments as it does in the general population but persons with HD may be more sensitive to the side effects such as sedation (Craufurd and Snowden, 2003) and anticholinergic-induced cognitive decline (Leroi and Michalon, 1998). HD patients have been reported to be sensitive to lithium toxicity owing to their high risk of dehydration (Leroi and Michalon, 1998). Management of irritability or behavioural disturbance should focus initially on any possible underlying cause such as depression or psychosis. Psychotic symptoms, irritability or behavioural disturbance respond to neuroleptics. Propranolol, serotonin reuptake inhibitors, carbamazepine and sodium valproate can be helpful in the management of irritability (Ranen et al., 1996; Grove et al., 2000; Craufurd and Snowden, 2003).

Specific treatments such as antioxidants and other neuroprotective drugs, which theoretically target the disease process to slow functional decline in manifest disease, are under trial. Drugs shown to be tolerated and which may slow the progression or improve the chorea include coenzyme Q (Feigin et al., 1996), an antioxidant, and remacemide (Kieburtz et al., 1996), a non-competitive N-methyl-D-aspartate (NMDA) receptor antagonist. Other drug trials reporting beneficial effects on chorea include tiapride, a highly selective striatal adenylate cyclase-independent dopamine-2 receptor antagonist (Dose and Lange, 2000), apomorphine (Albanese et al., 1995), α-tocopherol (a free radical scavenger; Peyser *et al.*, 1995), lamotrigine (an antiepileptic drug that inhibits glutamate release; Kremer *et al.*, 1999), and riluzole (an antiglutamatergic agent; Rosas *et al.*, 1999).

62.6.3 Psychosocial and physical management

Supportive psychotherapy aims to deal with losses of health, work, independence for the individual, and their implications for the other family members. Cognitive assessment can assist in decision-making on employment, driving, self-care, and other legal and safety issues. As the disease progresses, assistance with personal care and other activities of daily living will become necessary. Day care and respite care programmes may need to be considered. Attention to nutrition is important as weight loss is an inherent feature of the disease. It may be compounded by dysphagia in the late stages of the disease, poor dentition, unusual food-related behaviours such as obsessive intake of sweet foods and food refusals, psychiatric disorders and medication side effects. The use of a gastrostomy feeding tube at the end stage of the disease should be discussed early on, when the patient is able to express his or her wishes on this matter. Local branches of the Huntington's Disease Association can provide valuable support, advice on local resources and educational material on HD. Finally, residential care may be needed for some HD patients.

62.6.4 Research into new therapies

Clinical research determining the early onset and progressive symptoms of HD are currently being undertaken by the Huntington Study Group, an international collaboration of researchers in HD. Restorative therapies that rejuven-ate or replace malfunctioning neurones in order to restore functions are also being developed. Since 1989, there have been over 50 cases of cell transplantation using fetal striatal tissues (Dunnett and Rosser, 2002). Most reports have shown no major adverse effect with evidence of improved function and striatal graft viability in the short follow up of 12–33 months postoperatively (Dunnett and Rosser, 2002). However, there are many issues related to fetal striatal tissue transplantation in the ethical and practical domains that are likely to limit its availability. Another alternative is stem cells, which have the potential for self-renewal and are capable of forming at least one, sometimes, many, specialized cell types. Currently, the task is to control the differentiation potential of these cells in the adult brain environment.

REFERENCES

Albanese A, Cassetta E, Carretta D *et al.* (1995) Acute challenge with apomorphine in Huntington's disease: a double-blind study. *Clinical Neuropharmacology* **18**: 427–434

Almqvist EW, Bloch M, Brinkman R *et al.* (1999) A worldwide assessment of the frequency of suicide, suicide attempts, or psychiatric hospitalisation after predictive testing for Huntington disease. *American Journal of Human Genetics* **64**: 1293–1304

Anderson KE, Louis ED, Stern Y, Marder KS. (2001) Cognitive correlates of obsessive and compulsive symptoms in Huntington's disease. *American Journal of Psychiatry* **158**: 799–801

Andrew SE, Goldberg YP, Hayden MR. (1997) Rethinking genotype and phenotype correlations in polyglutamine expansion disorders. *Human Molecular Genetics* **6**: 2005–2010

Aylward EH, Codori AM, Barta PE *et al.* (1996) Basal ganglia volume and proximity to onset in presymptomatic Huntington disease. *Archives of Neurology* **53**: 1293–1296

Aylward EH, Li Q, Stine OC *et al.* (1997) Longitudinal change in basal ganglia volume in patients with Huntington's disease. *Neurology* **48**: 394–399

Aylward EH, Andersen NB, Blysma FW *et al.* (1998) Frontal lobe volume in patients with Huntington's disease. *Neurology* **50**: 252–258

Bates GP and Murphy KPSJ. (2003) Mouse models of Huntington's disease. In: G Bates, PS Harper, L Jones (eds), *Huntington's Disease*, 3rd edition. Oxford, Oxford University Press, pp. 387–426

Berrios GE, Wagle AC, Markova IS *et al.* (2001) Psychiatric symptoms and CAG repeats in neurologically asymptomatic Huntington's disease gene carriers. *Psychiatry Research* **102**: 217–225

Brandt J, Bylsma FW, Gross R *et al.* (1996) Trinucleotide repeat length and clinical progression in Huntington's disease. *Neurology* **46**: 527–531

Clark VP, Lai S, Deckel AW. (2002) Altered functional MRI responses in Huntington's disease. *NeuroReport* **13**: 703–706

Craufurd D and Snowden JS. (2003) Neuropsychological and neuropsychiatric aspects of Huntington's disease. In: G Bates, PS Harper, L Jones (eds), *Huntington's Disease*, 3rd edition. Oxford, Oxford University Press, pp. 62–94

Craufurd D, Thompson J, Snowden JS. (2001) Behavioural changes in Huntington's disease. *Journal of Neuropsychiatry, Neuropsychology and Behavioral Neurology* **14**: 219–226

Davie CA, Barker GJ, Quinn N *et al.* (1994) Proton MRS in Huntington's disease. *Lancet* **343**: 1580

Deckel AW, Gordinier A, Nuttal D *et al.* (2001) Reduced activity and protein expression of NOS in R6/2 HD transgenic mice: effects of L-NAME on symptom progression. *Brain Research* **919**: 170–181

Di Maio L, Squitieri F, Napolitano G *et al.* (1993) Suicide risk in Huntington's disease. *Journal of Medical Genetics* **30**: 292–295

DiFiglia M. (1997) Huntington's disease: from the gene to pathophysiology. *American Journal of Psychiatry* **154**: 1046

Dose M and Lange HW. (2000) The benzamide tiapride: treatment of extrapyramidal motor and other clinical syndromes. *Pharmacopsychiatry* **33**: 19–27

Dunnett SB and Rosser AE. (2002) Cell and tissue transplantation. In: G Bates, PS Harper, L Jones (eds), *Huntington's Disease*, 3rd edition. Oxford, Oxford University Press, pp. 512–546

Duyao M, Ambrose C, Myers R *et al.* (1993) Trinucleotide repeat length instability and age of onset in Huntington's disease. *Nature Genetics* **4**: 387–392

Feigin A, Kieburtz K, Como P *et al.* (1996) Assessment of coenzyme Q10 tolerability in Huntington's disease. *Movement Disorders* **11**: 321–323

Feigin A, Leenders KL, Moeller JR *et al.* (2001) Metabolic network abnormalities in early Huntington's disease: an [(18)F]FDG PET study. *Journal of Nuclear Medicine* **42**: 1591–1595

Folstein SE. (1989) *Huntington's Disease: A Disorder of Families.* Baltimore, John Hopkins University Press

Folstein SE, Abbott MH, Chase GA *et al.* (1983) The association of affective disorder with Huntington's disease in a case series and in families. *Psychological Medicine* **13**: 537–542

Foroud T, Gray J, Ivashina J, Conneally PM. (1999) Differences in duration of Huntington's disease based on age at onset. *Journal of Neurology, Neurosurgery, and Psychiatry* **66**: 52–56

Gimenez-Roldan S and Mateo D. (1989) Huntington disease: tetrabenazine compared to haloperidol in the reduction of involuntary movements. *Neurologia* **4**: 282–287

Ginovart N, Lundin A, Farde L *et al.* (1997) PET study of the pre- and post-synaptic dopaminergic markers for the neurodegenerative process in Huntington's disease. *Brain* **1**: 503–514

Goldberg YP, Kremer B, Andrew SE *et al.* (1993) Molecular analysis of new mutations causing Huntington disease: intermediate alleles and sex of origin effects. *Nature Genetics* **5**: 174–179

Gourfinkel-An I, Cancel G, Trottier Y *et al.* (1997) Differential distribution of the normal and mutated forms of huntingtin in the human brain. *Annals of Neurology* **42**: 712–719

Grafton ST, Mazziotta JC, Pahl JJ *et al.* (1992) Serial changes of cerebral glucose metabolism and caudate size in persons at risk for Huntington's disease. *Archives of Neurology* **49**: 1161–1167

Grove VE Jr, Quintanilla J, DeVaney GT. (2000) Improvement of Huntington's disease with olanzapine and valproate. *New England Journal of Medicine* **343**: 973–974

Gusella J, Wexler NS, Conneally PM *et al.* (1983) A polymorphic DNA marker genetically linked to Huntington's disease. *Nature* **306**: 234–238

Gusella JF, MacDonald ME, Ambrose CM, Duyao MP. (1993) Molecular genetics of Huntington's disease. *Archives of Neurology* **50**: 1157–1163

Gutekunst CA, Norflus F, Hersch SM. (2002) The neuropathology of Huntington's disease. In: G Bates, PS Harper, L Jones (eds), *Huntington's Disease*, 3rd edition. Oxford, Oxford University Press, pp. 251–275

Harper PS. (1991) *Huntington's Disease.* London, WB Saunders Company Ltd

Holthoff VA, Koeppe RA, Frey KA *et al.* (1993) Positron emission tomography measures of benzodiazepine receptors in Huntington's disease. *Annals of Neurology* **34**: 76–81

Huntington's Disease Collaborative Research Group. (1993) A novel gene containing a trinucleotide repeat that is expanded and unstable on Huntington's disease chromosomes. *Cell* **72**: 971–983

Illarioshkin SN, Igarashi S, Onodera A *et al.* (1994) Trinucleotide repeat length and rate of progression of Huntington's disease. *Annals of Neurology* **36**: 630–635

International Huntington Association and World Federation of Neurology Research Group on Huntington's Chorea. (1994) Guidelines for the molecular genetics predictive test in Huntington's disease. *Journal of Medical Genetics* **31**: 555–559

James CM, Houlihan GD, Snell RG *et al.* (1994) Late-onset Huntington's disease: a clinical and molecular study. *Age Ageing* **23**: 445–448

Jenkins BG, Koroshetz WJ, Beal MF, Rosen BR. (1993) Evidence for impairment of energy metabolism in vivo in Huntington's disease using localised 1H NMR spectroscopy. *Neurology* **43**: 2689–2695

Kieburtz K, MacDonald M, Shih C *et al.* (1994) Trinucleotide repeat length and progression of illness in Huntington's disease. *Journal of Medical Genetics* **31**: 872–874

Kieburtz K, Feigin A, McDermott M *et al.* (1996) A controlled trial of remacemide hydrochloride in Huntington's disease. *Movement Disorders* **11**: 273–277

Kremer B. (2003) Clinical neurology of Huntington's disease. In: G Bates, P Harper, L Jones (eds), *Huntington's Disease*, 3rd edition. Oxford, Oxford University Press, pp. 28–61

Kremer B, Clark CM, Almqvist EW *et al.* (1999) Influence of lamotrigine on progression of early Huntington disease: a randomised clinical trial. *Neurology* **53**: 1000–1011

Kremer B, Squitieri F, Telenius H *et al.* (1993) Molecular analysis of late onset Huntington's disease. *Journal of Medical Genetics* **30**: 991–995

Kuwert T, Lange HW, Langen KJ *et al.* (1990) Cortical and subcortical glucose consumption measured by PET in patients with Huntington's disease. *Brain* **113**: 1405–1423

Lasker AG and Zee DS. (1997) Ocular motor abnormalities in Huntington's disease. *Vision Research* **37**: 3639–3645

Lawrence AD, Watkins LH, Sahakian BJ *et al.* (2000) Visual object and visuospatial cognition in Huntington's disease: implications for information processing in corticostriatal circuits. *Brain* **123**: 1349–1364

Leroi I and Michalon M. (1998) Treatment of the psychiatric manifestations of Huntington's disease: a review of the literature. *Canadian Journal of Psychiatry – Revue Canadienne de Psychiatrie* **43**: 933–940

MacMillan J and Quarrell O. (1996) The neurobiology of Huntington's disease. In: PS Harper (ed.), *Huntington's Disease*, 2nd edition. London, WB Saunders Company Ltd, pp. 317–357

Nance MA and Westphal B. (2002) Comprehensive care in Huntington's disease. In: G Bates, PS Harper, L Jones (eds), *Huntington's Disease*, 3rd edition. Oxford, Oxford University Press, pp. 475–500

Peiris JB, Boralessa H, Lionel ND. (1976) Clonazepam in the treatment of choreiform activity. *Medical Journal of Australia* **1**: 225–227

Penney JB, Young AB, Shoulson I. (1990) Huntington's disease in Venezuala: 7 years of follow-up on symptomatic and asymptomatic individuals. *Movement Disorders* **5**: 93–99

Penney JB Jr, Vonsattel JP, MacDonald ME *et al.* (1997) CAG repeat number governs the development rate of pathology in Huntington's disease. *Annals of Neurology* **41**: 689–692

Peyser CE, Folstein M, Chase GA *et al.* (1995) Trial of d-α-tocopherol in Huntington's disease. *American Journal of Psychiatry* **152**: 1771–1775

Ranen NG, Lipsey JR, Treisman G, Ross CA. (1996) Sertraline in the treatment of severe aggressiveness in Huntington's disease. *Journal of Neuropsychiatry and Clinical Neurosciences* **8**: 338–340

Rosas HD, Koroshetz WJ, Jenkins BG *et al.* (1999) Riluzole therapy in Huntington's disease (HD). *Movement Disorders* **14**: 326–330

Sanchez-Pernaute R, Garcia-Segura JM, del Barrio AA *et al.* (1999) Clinical correlation of striatal 1H MRS changes in Huntington's disease. *Neurology* **53**: 806–812

Sax DS, Powsner R, Kim A *et al.* (1996) Evidence of cortical metabolic dysfunction in early Huntington's disease by single-photon-emission computed tomography. *Movement Disorders* **11**: 671–677

Sedvall G, Karlsson P, Lundin A *et al.* (1994) Dopamine D1 receptor number – a sensitive PET marker for early brain degeneration in Huntington's disease. *European Archives of Psychiatry and Clinical Neuroscience* **243**: 249–255

Sharp AH, Loev SJ, Schilling G *et al.* (1995) Widespread expression of Huntington's disease gene (IT15) protein product. *Neuron* **14**: 1065–1074

Sieradzan K, Mann DMA, Dodge A. (1997) Clinical presentation and patterns of regional cerebral atrophy related to the length of trinucleotide repeat expansions in patients with adult onset Huntington's disease. *Neuroscience Letters* **225**: 45–48

SuttonBrown M and Suchowersky O. (2003) Clinical and research advances in Huntington's disease. *Canadian Journal of Neurological Sciences* **30** (Suppl. 1): S45–S52

Tsuang D, Almqvist EW, Lipe H *et al.* (2000) Familial aggregation of psychotic symptoms in Huntington's disease. *American Journal of Psychiatry* **157**: 1955–1959

van Vugt JP, Siesling S, Vergeer M *et al.* (1997) Clozapine versus placebo in Huntington's disease: a double blind randomised comparative study. *Journal of Neurology, Neurosurgery, and Psychiatry* **63**: 35–39

Wanker EE and Droge A. (2002) Structural biology of Huntington's disease. In: G Bates, PS Harper, L Jones (eds), *Huntington's Disease*, 3rd edition. Oxford, Oxford University Press, pp. 327–347

Watt DC and Seller A. (1993) A clinico-genetic study of psychiatric disorder in Huntington's chorea. *Psychological Medicine Monograph* (Suppl. 23): 1–46

Weeks RA, Piccini P, Harding AE, Brooks DJ. (1996) Striatal D1 and D2 dopamine receptor loss in asymptomatic mutation carriers of Huntington's disease. *Annals of Neurology* **40**: 49–54

Weeks RA, Ceballos-Baumann A, Piccini P *et al.* (1997) Cortical control of movement in Huntington's disease. A PET activation study. *Brain* **120**: 1569–1578

Young AB, Penney JB, Starosta-Rubinstein S *et al.* (1986) PET scan investigations of Huntington's disease: cerebral metabolic correlates of neurological features and functional decline. *Annals of Neurology* **20**: 296–303

Young AB, Penney JB, Starosta-Rubinstein S *et al.* (1987) Normal caudate glucose metabolism in persons at risk for Huntington's disease. *Archives of Neurology* **44**: 254–257

Creutzfeldt–Jakob disease and other prion diseases

JOHN COLLINGE

63.1 TRANSMISSION AND AETIOLOGY

The human prion diseases, also known as the transmissible spongiform encephalopathies, have been traditionally classified into Creutzfeldt–Jakob disease (CJD), Gerstmann–Sträussler syndrome (GSS; also known as Gerstmann–Sträussler–Scheinker disease) and kuru. Remarkable attention has been recently focused on these diseases because of the unique biology of the transmissible agent or prion, and also because of the epidemic of bovine spongiform encephalopathy (BSE) and the evidence that BSE prions have infected humans, causing the new human prion disease known as variant CJD (vCJD). Human prion infection can be associated with extremely long incubation periods, which may span decades, and considerable uncertainty remains as to the eventual epidemic size of BSE-related human prion disease and the risks of its secondary transmission via medical and surgical procedures.

The transmissibility of the human diseases was demonstrated with the transmission (by intracerebral inoculation with brain homogenates) to chimpanzees of kuru and CJD in 1966 and 1968 respectively (Gajdusek et al., 1966; Gibbs et al., 1968). Transmission of GSS followed in 1981. Scrapie is a naturally occurring disease of sheep and goats, recognized in Europe for over 200 years (McGowan, 1922) and present in the sheep flocks of many countries. Scrapie was demonstrated to be transmissible in 1936 (Cuillé and Chelle, 1936) and the recognition that kuru, and then CJD, resembled scrapie in its histopathological appearances led to the suggestion that these diseases may also be transmissible (Hadlow, 1959). Kuru reached epidemic proportions amongst the Fore in the Eastern Highlands of Papua New Guinea and was transmitted by ritual cannibalism. Since the cessation of cannibalism in the 1950s, the disease has declined but a few cases still occur as

a result of the long incubation periods in this condition. The term Creutzfeldt–Jakob disease was introduced by Spielmeyer in 1922 bringing together the case reports published by Creutzfeldt and Jakob. Several of these cases would not meet modern diagnostic criteria for CJD and it was not until the demonstration of transmissibility allowing diagnostic criteria to be reassessed and refined that a clear diagnostic entity developed. All these diseases share common histopathological features; the classical triad of spongiform vacuolation (affecting any part of the cerebral grey matter), astrocytic proliferation and neuronal loss, which may be accompanied by the deposition of amyloid plaques (Beck and Daniel, 1987).

Prion diseases are associated with the accumulation of an abnormal, partially protease-resistant, isoform of a host-encoded glycoprotein known as prion protein (PrP). This disease-related isoform, PrP^{Sc}, is derived from its normal cellular precursor, PrP^C, by a post-translational process and involves a conformational change. PrP^C is rich in α-helical structure while PrP^{Sc} is predominantly composed of β-sheet. According to the 'protein-only' hypothesis (Griffith, 1967), an abnormal PrP isoform (Prusnier, 1990) is the principal, and possibly the sole, constituent of the transmissible agent or prion. It is hypothesized that PrP^{Sc} acts as a conformational template, promoting the conversion of PrP^C to further PrP^{Sc}. PrP^C may be poised between two radically different folding states: α- and β-forms of PrP can be interconverted in suitable conditions (Jackson et al., 1999). Soluble β-PrP aggregates in physiological salt concentrations to form fibrils with morphological and biochemical characteristics similar to PrP^{Sc}. A molecular mechanism for prion propagation can now be proposed (Jackson et al., 1999). Prion replication, with recruitment of PrP^C into the aggregated PrP^{Sc} isoform, may be initiated by a pathogenic mutation (resulting in a PrP^C predisposed to form β-PrP) in inherited prion diseases, by exposure to a 'seed' of PrP^{Sc} in acquired cases, or as a result of the spontaneous conversion of PrP^C to β-PrP (and subsequent formation of aggregated material) as a rare stochastic event in sporadic prion disease.

The human PrP gene (designated PRNP) is located on chromosome 20p and was an obvious candidate for genetic linkage studies in the familial forms of CJD and GSS, which show an autosomal dominant pattern of disease segregation. A milestone in prion research was the identification of PRNP mutations in familial CJD and GSS in 1989. The first mutation to be identified in PRNP was in a family with CJD and consisted of a 144bp insertion (Owen et al., 1989). A second mutation was reported in two families with GSS and genetic linkage was confirmed between this missense variant at codon 102 and GSS, confirming that GSS is an autosomal dominant Mendelian disorder (Hsiao et al., 1989). These diseases are therefore both inherited and transmissible, a biologically unique feature. Approximately 15 per cent of prion diseases are inherited and around 30 coding mutations in PRNP are now recognized (Collinge 2001).

With the exception of rare iatrogenic CJD cases, most prion disease occurs as sporadic CJD where, by definition, there will not be a family history. However, PRNP mutations are seen in some apparently sporadic cases, since the family history may not be apparent, owing to late age of onset or non-paternity. Human prion diseases can therefore be subdivided into three aetiological categories: inherited, sporadic and acquired.

A common PrP polymorphism at residue 129, where either methionine or valine can be encoded, is, however, a key determinant of genetic susceptibility in acquired and sporadic forms of prion disease, the large majority of which occur in homozygotes (Collinge et al., 1991a; Palmer et al., 1991). This protective effect of PRNP codon 129 heterozygosity is also seen in some of the inherited prion diseases (Baker et al., 1991; Hsiao et al., 1992).

Sporadic CJD is thought to arise from somatic mutation of PRNP or spontaneous conversion of PrP^C to PrP^{Sc} as a rare stochastic event. The alternative hypothesis, that of exposure to an environmental source of either human or animal prions, is not supported by epidemiological studies to date (Brown et al., 1987) but it remains possible that a minority of patients have an as yet unidentified environmental exposure to human or animal prions.

The existence of multiple isolates or strains of prions with distinct biological properties has provided a challenge to the 'protein-only' model of prion replication. Indeed, understanding how a protein-only infectious agent could encode phenotypic information is of considerable biological interest. However, it is now clear that prion strains can be distinguished by differences in the biochemical properties of PrP^{Sc}. Prion strain diversity appears to encoded by differences in PrP conformation and pattern of glycosylation (Collinge et al., 1996b). Molecular strain typing is now possible and has allowed the identification of four main types in CJD, sporadic and iatrogenic CJD being of PrP^{Sc} types 1–3, while all vCJD cases are associated with a type 4 PrP^{Sc} type (Collinge et al., 1996b; Wadsworth et al., 1999). That a similar PrP^{Sc} type to that seen in vCJD is seen in BSE transmitted to several other species (Collinge et al., 1996b) strongly supported the hypothesis that vCJD was human BSE. This conclusion was strengthened by transmission studies of vCJD into both transgenic and conventional mice, which indicated that cattle BSE and vCJD were caused by the same prion strain (Bruce et al., 1997; Hill et al., 1997). Molecular classification of human prion diseases is now possible and it is likely that additional PrP^{Sc} types will be identified (Hill et al., 2003). Such studies, where patients are aetiologically classified by human prion strain, rather than by descriptive clinicopathological phenotype, allows re-evaluation of epidemiological risk factors and may provide new insights into causes of 'sporadic' CJD.

The ability of a protein to encode a disease phenotype has important implications in biology, as it represents a non-Mendelian form of transmission. It would be surprising if this mechanism had not been used more widely during evolution and may prove to be of wider relevance in pathobiology.

Transmission of prion diseases between different mammalian species is restricted by a 'species barrier' (Pattison, 1965). Early studies of the molecular basis of this barrier argued that it resided in differences in PrP primary structure between the species from which the inoculum was derived and the inoculated host. Transgenic mice expressing hamster PrP were, unlike wild type mice, highly susceptible to infection with hamster prions (Prusiner et al., 1990). That most sporadic and acquired CJD occurred in individuals homozygous at PRNP polymorphic codon 129 supported the view that prion propagation proceeded most efficiently when the interacting PrP^{Sc} and PrP^C were of identical primary structure (Palmer et al., 1991). However, prion strain type affects ease of transmission to another species. Interestingly, with BSE prions this strain component to the barrier seems to predominate, with BSE not only transmitting efficiently to a range of species, but maintaining its transmission characteristics even when passaged through an intermediate species with a distinct PrP gene (Bruce et al., 1994; Hill et al., 1997). The term 'species–strain barrier' or simply 'transmission barrier' may be preferable (Collinge, 1999). Both PrP amino acid sequence and strain type affect the 3D-structure of glycosylated PrP^{Sc} which will presumably affect the efficiency of the protein–protein interactions determining prion propagation. Other components to the species barrier are possible and may involve interacting cofactors, although no such factors have yet been identified.

The species barrier between cattle BSE and humans cannot be directly measured but can be modelled in transgenic mice expressing human PrP^C, which produce human PrP^{Sc} when challenged with human prions (Collinge et al., 1995b). While classical CJD prions transmit efficiently to such mice at around 200 days, only infrequent transmissions at over 500 days were seen with BSE (and vCJD) prions, consistent with a substantial species barrier for this human PRNP genotype (Hill et al., 1997). In transgenic mice expressing only human PrP methionine 129, while transmission assessed by onset of clinical disease was again inefficient, remarkably a large proportion of the inoculated animals were subclinically infected (Asante *et al.*, 2002b) suggesting a considerably lower barrier to infection in this genotype. To date vCJD has only been recognized in humans of PRNP codon 129 methionine homozygous genotype. Interestingly, transmissions of BSE to mice expressing human PrP methionine 129 resulted in the generation of two distinct pathological and molecular phenotypes in these animals: one closely resembling vCJD (with type 4 PrP^{Sc} and the characteristic neuropathology of vCJD) and the other sporadic CJD with type 2 PrP^{Sc}. This raises the possibility that BSE infection of humans may result in phenotypes resembling classical CJD as well as the distinctive phenotype of vCJD (Asante *et al.*, 2002b).

63.2 CLINICAL FEATURES AND DIAGNOSIS

The human prion diseases can be divided aetiologically into inherited, sporadic and acquired forms, with CJD, GSS and kuru now seen as clinicopathological syndromes within a wider spectrum of disease. Kindreds with inherited prion disease have been described with phenotypes of classical CJD, GSS and other syndromes including fatal familial insomnia (Medori *et al.*, 1992b). Some kindreds show remarkable phenotypic variability which can encompass both CJD- and GSS-like cases as well as other cases that do not conform to either phenotype (Collinge *et al.*, 1992). Atypical cases (diagnosed by PRNP analysis) have been reported which entirely lack the classical histological features (Collinge *et al.*, 1990). There is significant clinical overlap with familial Alzheimer's disease, Pick's disease, frontal lobe degeneration of non-Alzheimer type and amyotrophic lateral sclerosis with dementia. It now seems sensible to designate the familial illnesses as inherited prion diseases and to subclassify according to PRNP mutation. Acquired prion diseases include iatrogenic CJD, kuru and vCJD. Sporadic prion diseases at present consist of CJD and atypical variants of CJD. As there are at present no equivalent aetiological diagnostic markers for sporadic prion diseases to those for the inherited diseases, it cannot yet be excluded that more diverse phenotypic variants of sporadic prion disease exist.

63.2.1 Sporadic prion disease

63.2.1.1 CREUTZFELDT–JAKOB DISEASE

The core clinical syndrome of classical CJD is a rapidly progressive multifocal dementia, usually with myoclonus. Most have onset between ages 45 and 75, with peak between 60 and 65 and a clinical progression to akinetic mutism and death in <6 months. Around one-third of cases have prodromal features including fatigue, insomnia, depression, weight loss, headaches, general malaise and ill-defined pain sensations. Frequent additional neurological features include extrapyramidal signs, cerebellar ataxia, pyramidal signs and cortical blindness.

Routine haematological and biochemical investigations are normal (although occasional patients have raised serum transaminases or alkaline phosphatase). There are no immunological markers and acute phase proteins are not elevated. Cerebrospinal fluid is normal, although neuronal specific enolase (NSE), and S-100 are usually elevated. However, they are not specific for CJD and represent markers of neuronal injury (Jimi *et al.*, 1992; Zerr *et al.*, 1995; Otto *et al.*, 1997). Estimation of CSF 14-3-3 protein, while again not a specific disease marker, appears useful in the appropriate clinical context (Collinge, 1996; Hsich *et al.*, 1996). It is also positive in recent cerebral infarction or haemorrhage and in viral encephalitis, which are unlikely to present diagnostic confusion with CJD, but more recent studies have found 14-3-3 positive in other non-prion related conditions (Satoh *et al.*, 1999). While 14-3-3 is usually positive in typical CJD, its use in differential diagnosis in more challenging diagnostic contexts in less clear, as it may be negative in long duration atypical CJD and positive in patients with rapidly progressive Alzheimer's disease with myoclonus for example.

Neuroimaging with computed tomography (CT) is useful to exclude other causes of subacute neurological illness but there are no diagnostic features; cerebral and cerebellar atrophy may be present. However, magnetic resonance imaging (MRI) changes are increasingly recognized and may be extremely helpful diagnostically. Signal changes are frequently seen in the basal ganglia in T2-weighted images. More widespread signal changes may be seen in diffusion-weighted images, which appears more sensitive diagnostically and which may be present at an early clinical stage (Shiga *et al.*, 2004). The electroencephalogram (EEG) may show characteristic pseudoperiodic sharp wave activity, which is helpful in diagnosis but present only in around 70 per cent of cases. This finding may be intermittent and serial EEG is appropriate to try to demonstrate this appearance.

Neuropathological confirmation is by demonstration of spongiform change, neuronal loss and astrocytosis. PrP amyloid plaques are usually not present although PrP immunohistochemistry, with appropriate pretreatments (Budka *et al.*, 1995), will nearly always be positive. PrP^{Sc}, seen in all the currently recognized prion diseases, can be demonstrated by western blot. PRNP analysis is essential to exclude pathogenic mutations as a family history may not always be apparent. PRNP mutations should certainly be excluded prior to brain biopsy, which may be considered in some patients to exclude alternative, potentially treatable diagnoses. Tonsil biopsy (see below) is negative in sporadic CJD but may be considered in younger patients where a diagnosis of vCJD is being considered. Most cases of classical CJD are homozygous with respect to the codon 129 PRNP polymorphism (see the aetiology section above).

Sporadic CJD can now be subclassified by prion strain type using western blot analysis of brain tissue at biopsy or autopsy, although there is not as yet an international consensus on the number or nomenclature of these molecular types. Distinctive phenotypes are associated with different PrP^{Sc}

types (Parchi *et al.*, 1999; Hill *et al.*, 2003). For example, sub-acute patients whose illnesses have been of short clinical duration (several weeks) are associated with type 1 PrP^Sc in the brain (Wadsworth *et al.*, 1999; Hill *et al.*, 2003).

63.2.1.2 ATYPICAL CREUTZFELDT–JAKOB DISEASE

Atypical forms of CJD are well recognized. Around 10 per cent of CJD has a prolonged clinical course with duration of over 2 years (Brown *et al.*, 1984). Patients with a valine homozygous or methionine valine heterozygous genotype at PRNP codon 129 are more often atypical clinical forms than are methionine homozygotes (Collinge and Palmer, 1994) and may lack a characteristic EEG. It is unclear yet to what extent this represents propagation of different prion strains or a direct effect of the genotype on disease expression (Collinge, 2001). Approximately 10 per cent of CJD cases present with cerebellar ataxia rather than cognitive impairment – ataxic CJD (Gomori *et al.*, 1973). Heidenhain's variant refers to cases in which cortical blindness predominates, with severe involvement of the occipital lobes. In panencephalopathic CJD, predominately reported from Japan, there is extensive degeneration of the cerebral white matter in addition to spongiform vacuolation of the grey matter (Mizutani, 1981). Amyotrophic variants of CJD have been described with prominent early muscle wasting. However, most cases of dementia with amyotrophy are not experimentally transmissible (Salazar *et al.*, 1983) and their relationship with CJD is unclear. Most cases are probably variants of motor neurone disease with associated dementia. Amyotrophic features in CJD are usually seen in late disease when other features are well established. There are numerous individual case reports in the literature of other unusual presentations of CJD, mimicking many other neurological and psychiatric disorders.

63.2.2 Acquired prion diseases

While human prion diseases can be transmitted to experimental animals by inoculation, they are not contagious in humans. Documented case to case spread has only occurred by direct exposure to infected human tissues during ritual cannibalistic practices (kuru) or following accidental inoculation with prions during medical or surgical procedures (iatrogenic CJD).

63.2.2.1 KURU

Kuru reached epidemic proportions amongst a relatively isolated population (the Fore linguistic group and their neighbours with whom they intermarried) in the Eastern Highlands of Papua New Guinea. It predominantly affected women and children (of both sexes), with only 2 per cent of cases in adult males (Alpers, 1987) and was the commonest cause of death amongst women. It had been the practice in these communities to consume dead relatives, as a mark of respect and mourning. Women and children predominantly ate the brain

and internal organs, which is thought to explain the different age and sex incidence. Preparation of the cadaver was performed by the women and children such that other routes of exposure may also have been relevant. It is thought that the epidemic related to a single sporadic CJD case occurring in the region some decades earlier. Epidemiological studies provided no evidence for vertical transmission, since most of the children born after 1956 (when cannibalism had effectively ceased) and all of those born after 1959 of mothers affected with or incubating kuru were unaffected (Alpers, 1987). From the age of the youngest affected patient, the shortest incubation period is estimated as 4.5 years, although may have been shorter, since time of infection was usually unknown. Currently, two to three cases are occurring annually, all in individuals born prior to the cessation of cannibalism and indicating that incubation periods can be 40 years or more (Whitfield *et al.*, in preparation).

Onset of disease has ranged from age 5 to over 60 with a mean duration of 12 months (range 3 months to 3 years). The key clinical feature is progressive cerebellar ataxia. In sharp contrast to CJD, dementia is much less of a feature, even in the latter stages (Alpers, 1987).

Kuru typically begins with prodromal symptoms consisting of headache, aching of limbs and joint pains which can last for several months. Kuru was frequently self-diagnosed by patients at the earliest onset of unsteadiness in standing or walking, or of dysarthria or diplopia. At this stage there may be no objective signs of disease. Gait ataxia, however, worsens and patients develop a broad-based gait, truncal instability and titubation. A coarse postural tremor is usually present and accentuated by movement; patients characteristically hold their hands together in the mid-line to suppress this. Standing with feet together reveals clawing of toes to maintain posture. This marked clawing response is regarded as pathognomonic of kuru. Patients often become withdrawn at this stage and occasionally develop a severe reactive depression. Prodromal symptoms tend to disappear. Astasia and gait ataxia worsen and the patient requires a stick for walking. Intention tremor, dysmetria, hypotonia and dysdiadochokinesis develop. Strabismus, usually convergent, may occur particularly in children. Photophobia is common and there may be an abnormal cold sensitivity with shivering and piloerection even in a warm environment. Tendon reflexes are reduced or normal and plantar responses are flexor. Dysarthria usually occurs.

As ataxia progresses the patient passes from the first (ambulatory) stage to the second (sedentary) stage. At this stage patients are able to sit unsupported but cannot walk. Attempted walking with support leads to a high steppage, wide-based gait with reeling instability and flinging arm movements in an attempt to maintain posture. Hyperreflexia is seen, although plantar responses usually remain flexor with intact abdominal reflexes. Clonus is characteristically short lived. Athetoid and choreiform movements and parkinsonian tremors may occur. There is no paralysis, although muscle power is reduced. Obesity is common at this stage but may be present in early disease associated with bulimia.

Characteristically, there is emotional lability and bizarre uncontrollable laughter, which has led to the disease being referred to as 'laughing death'. There is no sensory impairment. In sharp contrast to CJD, myoclonic jerking is rarely seen. EEG is usually normal or may show non-specific changes. When truncal ataxia reaches the point where the patient is unable to sit unsupported, the third or tertiary stage is reached. Hypotonia and hyporeflexia develop and the terminal state is marked by flaccid muscle weakness. Plantar responses remain flexor and abdominal reflexes intact. Progressive dysphagia occurs and patients become incontinent of urine and faeces. Inanition and emaciation develop. Transient conjugate eye signs and dementia may occur. Primitive reflexes develop in occasional cases. Brain stem involvement and both bulbar and pseudobulbar signs occur. Respiratory failure and broncho-pneumonia eventually lead to death.

63.2.2.2 IATROGENIC CREUTZFELDT–JAKOB DISEASE

Iatrogenic transmission of CJD has occurred by inadvertent inoculation with human prions during medical procedures. Such iatrogenic routes include the use of inadequately steril-ized neurosurgical instruments, dura mater and corneal grafting, and use of human cadaveric pituitary-derived growth hormone or gonadotrophin. Cases arising from intracerebral or optic inoculation manifest typically as classical CJD, with a rapidly progressive dementia, while those resulting from peripheral inoculation (pituitary-derived growth hormone exposure) typically present with a progressive cerebellar syn-drome, and are in that respect reminiscent of kuru. Unsur-prisingly, the incubation period in intracerebral cases is short (19–46 months for dura mater grafts) compared with peri-pheral cases (typically 15 years or more). There is evidence for genetic susceptibility to iatrogenic CJD with an excess of codon 129 homozygotes; heterozygosity appears protective with a more prolonged incubation period (Collinge et al., 1991a; Brandel et al., 2003).

Epidemiological studies have not shown association of CJD with occupations that may expose people to human or animal prions, although individual cases in two histopath-ology technicians, a neuropathologist and a neurosurgeon, have been documented. Similarly, extensive epidemiological analysis in the UK has found no evidence that blood transfu-sion is a risk factor (Esmonde et al., 1993). It cannot be assumed that the same picture will hold for vCJD as this is caused by a distinct prion strain (Collinge et al., 1996b) from those causing classical CJD and has a distinct pathogenesis (Hill et al., 1999). Indeed, vCJD has now been reported in a recipient of blood from an infected donor (Llewelyn et al., 2004). In addition, prion infection has been demonstrated in a second recipient of blood from an infected donor who died of a unrelated cause (Peden et al., 2004). These early cases amongst a very small cohort of known exposed individuals is concerning, as the number of clinically silent individuals cur-rently incubating vCJD, a proportion of whom will be blood donors, is unknown but may be substantial (Collinge, 1999).

63.2.3 Variant CJD

In late 1995, two cases of sporadic CJD were reported in the UK in teenagers (Bateman et al., 1995; Britton et al., 1995). Only four cases of sporadic CJD had previously been recorded in teenagers, and none of these cases occurred in the UK. In addition, both were unusual in having kuru-type plaques, seen in only around 5 per cent of CJD cases. Soon afterwards a third very young sporadic CJD case occurred (Tabrizi et al., 1996). These cases caused considerable concern and the pos-sibility was raised that they were BSE-related. By March 1996, further extremely young onset cases were apparent and review of the histology of these cases showed a remarkably consistent and unique pattern. These cases were named 'new variant' CJD (Will et al., 1996). Review of neuropathological archives failed to demonstrate such cases. The statistical probability of such cases occurring by chance was vanish-ingly small and ascertainment bias seemed unlikely as an explanation. It was clear that a new risk factor for CJD had emerged and appeared to be specific to the UK. The UK Government Spongiform Encephalopathy Advisory Committee (SEAC) concluded that, while there was no direct evidence for a link with BSE, exposure to specified bovine offal (SBO) prior to the ban on its inclusion in human food-stuffs in 1989 was the most likely explanation. A case of vCJD was soon after reported in France (Chazot et al., 1996). Direct experimental evidence that vCJD is caused by BSE was pro-vided by molecular analysis of human prion strains and transmission studies in transgenic and wild type mice (see aetiology section above). While it is now clear that vCJD is the human counterpart of BSE, it is unclear why this particu-lar age group should be affected and why none of these cases had a pattern of unusual occupational or dietary exposure to BSE. However, very little was known about which foodstuffs contained high-titre bovine offal. It is possible that certain foods containing particularly high titres were eaten predom-inately by younger people. An alternative is that young people are more susceptible to BSE following dietary exposure or that they have shorter incubation periods. It is important to appreciate that BSE-contaminated feed was fed to sheep, pigs and poultry and that, although there is no evidence of natural transmission to these species, it would be prudent to remain open minded about other dietary exposure to novel animal prions.

There are considerable concerns that extensive human infection may have resulted from the widespread dietary expo-sure to BSE prions. Cattle BSE has now been reported, albeit at much lower levels than in the UK, in most member states of the EU, Switzerland, USA, Canada and Japan. Fortunately, the number of recognized cases of vCJD (up to 150 by early 2004) in the UK has been relatively small to date. Six patients have been identified in France and individual patients in Ireland, Italy, USA, Canada and Hong Kong. However, the number of infected individuals is unknown. Human prion disease incubation periods, as evidenced by kuru, are known to span decades. Furthermore, prion disease transmission from one species to another is invariably associated with a considerable prolongation of mean incubation periods – the so called 'species-barrier' effect (Collinge, 1999). Recent estimates, based on mathematical modelling and clinically recognized vCJD, suggest the total epidemic may be relatively small (Ghani et al., 2003) but key uncertainties, notably with respect to major genetic effects on incubation period (Lloyd et al., 2001) suggest the need for caution; also such models cannot estimate the number of infected individuals and it is these that are most relevant to assessing risks of secondary transmission. Also, the possibility of subclinical carrier states of prion infection in humans, as recognized in several animal models, must also be considered (Hill et al., 2000; Asante et al., 2002b).

A recent attempt to estimate prevalence of vCJD prion infection in the UK by anonymous screen of archival, largely appendix, tissue, necessarily using a method of unknown sensitivity, found three positives in around 12 000 samples (Hilton et al., 2004). The risk of secondary transmission via medical and surgical procedures is unquantifiable at present but continues to cause considerable concern. As discussed above, vCJD appears transmissible by blood transfusion; also prions are known to be resistant to conventional sterilization, and indeed iatrogenic transmission from neurosurgical instruments has long been documented (Bernoulli et al., 1977). The wider tissue distribution of infectivity in vCJD (Wadsworth et al., 2001), unknown prevalence of clinically silent infection, together with the recent experimental demonstration of the avid adherence to, and ease of transmission from, surgical steel surfaces (Flechsig et al., 2001) highlight these concerns. From a public health standpoint, it is prudent therefore to operate on the basis that the majority of variant CJD cases are yet to occur and may not present clinically for many years (Collinge, 1999). Furthermore, studies in transgenic mouse models of human susceptibility to BSE prion infection suggest that BSE may also induce propagation of a prion strain indistinguishable from the commonest type of sporadic CJD (Asante et al., 2002a), in addition to that causing variant CJD. Other novel prion disease phenotypes may be anticipated in alternative PRNP genotypes (Hill et al., 1997).

Presentation of vCJD is with behavioural and psychiatric disturbances and, in some cases, sensory disturbance (Will et al., 1996). Initial referral is often to a psychiatrist with depression, anxiety, withdrawal and behavioural change (Zeidler et al., 1997a). Suicidal ideation is, however, infrequent and response to antidepressants poor. Delusions, which are complex and unsustained, are common. Other features include emotional lability, aggression, insomnia, and auditory and visual hallucinations. Dysaesthesiae, or pain in the limbs or face, which was persistent rather than intermittent and unrelated to anxiety levels, is a frequent early feature, sometimes prompting referral to a rheumatologist. A minority of cases have early memory loss or gait ataxia but in most such overt neurological features are not apparent until some months later (Zeidler et al., 1997b). Typically, a progressive cerebellar syndrome then develops with gait and limb ataxia

followed with dementia and progression to akinetic mutism. Myoclonus is frequent, and may be preceded by chorea. Cortical blindness develops in a minority of patients in late disease. Upgaze paresis, an uncommon feature of classical CJD, has been noted in some patients (Zeidler et al., 1997b). The age at onset has widened since the initial descriptions but remains dominated by young adults: range 12–74 years (mean 28 years) and the clinical course is relatively prolonged when compared with typical sporadic CJD (9–35 months, median 14 months). The EEG is nearly always abnormal, most frequently showing generalized slow wave activity, but without the pseudoperiodic pattern seen in most sporadic CJD cases. Neuroimaging by CT is either normal or shows only mild atrophy. However, a high signal in the posterior thalamus on T2-weighted MRI is seen in the majority but not all recognized cases (Zeidler et al., 1997b; Hill et al., 1999).

Recently, cases of sporadic CJD mimicking vCJD both clinically and on MRI have been described, with high signal from the pulvinar on FLAIR and diffusion-weighted imaging (Martindale et al., 2003; Rossetti et al. 2004; Summers et al. 2004). Such a vCJD-like variant of sCJD appears to correlate with homozygosity for valine at codon 129 in the prion gene, or with methionine/valine heterozygosity. Cerebrospinal fluid (CSF) 14-3-3 protein may be elevated or normal.

No PRNP mutations are present in vCJD (Collinge et al., 1996a) and gene analysis is important to exclude pathogenic mutations, as inherited prion disease presents in this age group and a family history is not always apparent. The codon 129 genotype has uniformly been homozygous for methionine at PRNP codon 129 to date.

Clear ante-mortem tissue based diagnosis of vCJD can now be made by tonsil biopsy with detection of characteristic PrP immunostaining and PrP^{Sc} type (Hill et al., 1999). It has long been recognized that prion replication, in experimentally infected animals, is first detectable in the lymphoreticular system, considerably earlier than the onset of neurological symptoms. Importantly, PrP^{Sc} is only detectable in tonsil in vCJD, and not other forms of human prion disease studied. The PrP^{Sc} type detected on western blot in vCJD tonsil has a characteristic pattern designated type 4t (Hill et al., 1999). A positive tonsil biopsy obviates the need for brain biopsy, which may otherwise be considered in such a clinical context to exclude alternative, potentially treatable, diagnoses. To date, tonsil biopsy has proved 100 per cent specific and sensitive for vCJD diagnosis and is well tolerated.

The neuropathological appearances of vCJD are striking and consistent. In addition to widespread spongiform change, gliosis and neuronal loss (most severe in the basal ganglia and thalamus), there are abundant PrP amyloid plaques in cerebral and cerebellar cortex. These consisted of kuru-like, 'florid' (surrounded by spongiform vacuoles) and multicentric plaque types. The 'florid' plaques, seen previously only in scrapie, were a particularly unusual but highly consistent feature. There is abundant pericellular PrP deposition in the cerebral and cerebellar cortex and, unusually, extensive PrP immunoreactivity in the molecular layer of the cerebellum.

In some respects, vCJD resembles kuru, in which behavioural changes and progressive ataxia predominate. Peripheral sensory disturbances are well recognized in the kuru prodrome and kuru plaques are seen in around 70 per cent of cases (and are especially abundant in younger kuru cases). That iatrogenic prion disease related to peripheral exposure to human prions has a more kuru-like than CJD-like clinical picture may well be relevant and would be consistent with a peripheral prion exposure in vCJD also.

This relatively stereotyped clinical presentation and neuropathology of vCJD contrasts sharply with sporadic CJD. This may be because vCJD is caused by a single prion strain and/or because a relatively homogeneous, genetically susceptible, subgroup with short incubation periods to BSE has been infected to date. It will be important to be alert to different clinical presentations.

63.2.4 Inherited prion diseases

63.2.4.1 GERSTMANN–STRÄUSSLER–SCHEINKER (GSS) SYNDROME

The first case was described by Gerstmann in 1928 and was followed by a more detailed report of seven other affected members of the same family in 1936 (Gerstmann et al., 1936). The classical presentation is a chronic cerebellar ataxia accompanied by pyramidal features, with dementia occurring later. The histological hallmark is the presence of multicentric amyloid plaques. Numerous GSS kindreds from several countries have now been demonstrated to have PRNP mutations. GSS is an autosomal dominant disorder which can be classified within the spectrum of inherited prion disease.

63.2.4.2 INHERITED PRION DISEASES

The identification of a pathogenic PRNP mutation in a patient with neurodegenerative disease allows both diagnosis of inherited prion disease and its subclassification according to mutation. Around 30 pathogenic mutations in PRNP are described and consist of two groups:

- point mutations resulting in amino acid substitutions in PrP (or production of a stop codon);
- insertions encoding additional integral copies of an octapeptide repeat present in a tandem array of five copies in the normal protein.

An aetiological notation for these diseases (Collinge and Prusiner, 1992) is 'inherited prion disease (PrP mutation)'; for instance: inherited prion disease (PrP 144bp insertion) or inherited prion disease (PrP P102L). Phenotypic descriptions of some of these mutations follow:

1. **Missense mutations**
- *PrP P102L.* This was first reported in 1989 in a UK and US family and is now demonstrated in many kindreds worldwide. Progressive ataxia is the dominant clinical feature, with dementia and pyramidal features. However,

marked variability both at the clinical and neuropathological level is apparent in some families (Hainfellner et al., 1995). A family with marked amyotrophic features has also been reported (Kretzschmar et al., 1992). Cases with severe dementia in the absence of prominent ataxia are also recognized. Neuropathological examination reveals PrP immunoreactive plaques in the majority of cases. Transmissibility to experimental animals has been demonstrated.

- *PrP P105L.* Reported in three Japanese families (Kitamoto et al., 1993) with a history of spastic paraparesis and dementia, its clinical duration is around 5 years. There was no periodic synchronous discharge on EEG but MRI scans showed atrophy of the motor cortex. Neuropathological examination showed plaques in cerebral cortex (but not cerebellum) and neuronal loss but no spongiosis. Neurofibrillary tangles were variably present.

- *PrP A117V.* First described in a French family (Doh ura et al., 1989) and subsequently in a US family of German origin (Hsiao et al., 1991b), its clinical features are presenile dementia with pyramidal signs, parkinsonism, pseudobulbar features and cerebellar signs. Neuropathologically, PrP immunoreactive plaques are usually present. This mutation has also been identified in a large family in the UK (Mallucci et al., 1999).

- *PrP Y145STOP.* This mutation was detected in a Japanese patient with a clinical diagnosis of Alzheimer's disease. She developed memory disturbance at age 38 with a duration of illness of 21 years. Neuropathology revealed typical Alzheimer-like pathology without spongiform change (Kitamoto et al., 1993a). Many amyloid plaques were seen in the cortex along with paired helical filaments. However, plaques were PrP immunoreactive. βA_4 immunocytochemistry was negative. These clinicopathological findings emphasize the importance of PRNP analysis in the differential diagnosis of dementia.

- *PrP D178N.* This was originally described in two Finnish families with a CJD-like phenotype (although without typical EEG appearances) (Goldfarb et al., 1991b) and since demonstrated in CJD families in Hungary, Netherlands, Canada, Finland, France and UK. In the large Finnish kindred the mean onset was 47 and duration 27.5 months. Neuropathology showed spongiform change without amyloid plaques. This mutation was also reported in two families with fatal familial insomnia (FFI) (Lugaresi et al., 1986; Medori et al., 1992a). The first cases described had a rapidly progressive disease characterized clinically by untreatable insomnia, dysautonomia and motor signs, and neuropathologically by selective atrophy of the anterioventral and mediodorsal thalamic nuclei. There was marked thalamic astrocytosis. Mild spongiform change was seen in some cases and protease-resistant PrP demonstrated, albeit weakly, by immunoblotting. Proteinase-K treatment of extracted

PrP^{Sc} from FFI cases has shown a different sized PrP band on western blots than PrP^{Sc} from CJD cases (Monari *et al.*, 1994) suggesting that FFI may be caused by a distinct prion strain type. In a recent study Goldfarb *et al.* (1992) reported that, in all the codon 178 families studied with a CJD-like disease, the codon 178 mutation was encoded on a valine 129 allele, while all FFI kindreds encoded the same codon 178 mutation on a methionine 129 allele and suggested that the genotype at codon 129 determines phenotype. Recently an inherited case with the E200K mutation, which is normally associated with a CJD-like phenotype, has been reported with an FFI phenotype (Chapman *et al.*, 1996). An Australian family has also been reported with the FFI genotype but in which affected family members have a range of phenotypes encompassing typical CJD, FFI and an autosomal dominant cerebellar ataxia-like illness (McLean *et al.*, 1997). CJD-like codon 178 cases have frequently transmitted to experimental animals while the FFI type did not transmit to laboratory primates (Brown *et al.*, 1994). However, transmission of FFI to mice has been reported (Collinge *et al.*, 1995a; Tateishi *et al.*, 1995).

- *PrP V180I*. This was identified in two Japanese patients with subacute dementia and myoclonus (Kitamoto *et al.*, 1993b). The period from onset to akinetic mutism was 6–10 months. No family history was noted. EEG did not show pseudoperiodic sharp wave activity. Neuropathological examination demonstrated spongiform change, neuronal loss and astrocytosis. Interestingly, one of the patients with PrP Ile 180 also had PrP Arg 232.

- *PrP T183A*. This was reported in a single Brazilian family with frontotemporal dementia of mean onset 45 years and duration 4 years (Nitrini *et al.*, 1997). Parkinsonian features were also present in some patients. Neuropathological examination revealed severe spongiform change and neuronal loss in deep cortical layers and putamen with little gliosis. PrP immunoreactivity was demonstrated in putamen and cerebellum.

- *PrP F198S*. This was described in a single large Indiana kindred. Neuropathologically, there are widespread Alzheimer-like neurofibrillary tangles in cortex and subcortical nuclei in addition to PrP amyloid plaques (Dlouhy *et al.*, 1992). There is an apparent codon 129 effect with this mutation, in that individuals who were heterozygous at codon 129 had a later age of onset than homozygotes.

- *PrP E200K*. This was first described in families with CJD. Affected individuals develop a rapidly progressive dementia with myoclonus and pyramidal, cerebellar or extrapyramidal signs and a duration of illness usually <12 months. The average age of onset is 55. Neuropathological features are typical of CJD; plaques are absent but PrP^{Sc} can be demonstrated by immunoblotting. In marked contrast to other inherited prion diseases, the EEG usually shows pseudoperiodic activity. This mutation accounts for the three ethnogeographic clusters of CJD (amongst Libyan Jews and in regions of Slovakia and Chile; Goldfarb *et al.*, 1990; Hsiao *et al.*, 1991a; Brown *et al.*, 1992). Atypical forms have now been identified. Peripheral neuropathy can occur in this disease (Neufeld *et al.*, 1992). Elderly unaffected carriers of the mutation have been reported. Penetrance is age dependent and thought to approach 100 per cent by the age 80 (Chapman *et al.*, 1994). There also appears to be a separate UK focus for this inherited prion disease (Collinge *et al.*, 1993). The codon 129 genotype does not appear to affect age at onset of this disorder. Transmission to experimental animals has been demonstrated.

- *PrP R208H*. Although reported in a single patient with CJD, no details of the family history or phenotype are as yet published (Mastrianni *et al.*, 1995).

- *PrP V210I*. This was reported in a single case in France (Davies *et al.*, 1993) with a rapidly progressive dementia, cerebellar signs and myoclonus and age of onset of 63. EEG showed pseudoperiodic sharp wave activity. The clinical duration was 4 months and neuropathological examination showed spongiform change, neuronal loss and astrocytosis. No amyloid plaques were seen. Parents had died at ages of 60 and 66 without dementia. A sister with the mutation had died of colon cancer at age 67. It is possible that this mutation produces a very late onset disease or is incompletely penetrant.

- *PrP Q217R*. Reported to date only in a single Swedish family, the presentation is with dementia followed by gait ataxia, dysphagia and confusion (Hsiao *et al.*, 1992). As with inherited prion disease (PrP F198S) there are prominent neurofibrillary tangles.

- *PrP M232R*. First found on the opposite allele to V180I mutation in a Japanese patient with prion disease (Kitamoto *et al.*, 1993b), it was further demonstrated in two additional Japanese patients with progressive dementia, myoclonus and periodic synchronous discharges in the EEG but without an apparent family history of neurological disease. The mean duration of illness was 3 months. Neuropathology showed spongiform change, neuronal loss and astrocytosis. PrP immunostaining revealed diffuse grey matter staining, but no plaques.

2. Insertional mutations

- *PrP 24bp insertion (one extra repeat)*. Reported in a single French individual, the patient presented at age 73 with dizziness followed by visual agnosia, cerebellar ataxia and intellectual impairment with diffuse periodic activity on EEG. Myoclonus and cortical blindness developed and he progressed to akinetic mutism. Disease duration was 4 months. The patient's father had died at age 70 from an undiagnosed neurological disorder. No neuropathological information is available.

- *PrP 48bp insertion (two extra repeats)*. Reported in a single US family (Goldfarb *et al.*, 1993), the proband had a CJD-like phenotype both clinically and pathologically with a typical EEG and an age at onset of 58. However, the proband's mother had onset of cognitive decline at age 75 with a slow progression to a severe dementia over 13 years. The maternal grandfather had a similar late onset (at age 80) and slow progressive cognitive decline over 15 years.

- *PrP 96bp insertion (four extra repeats).* This was first reported in an individual who died aged 63 of hepatic cirrhosis (Goldfarb *et al.*, 1991a) with no history of neurological illness, but it is unclear if this finding indicates incomplete penetrance of this mutation. This is the only recorded case of a PRNP insertional mutation other than in an affected or an at-risk individual. Two separate four octapeptide repeat insertional mutations have been reported in affected individuals, each differing in the DNA sequence from the original four repeat insertion, although all three of the mutations encode the same PrP. Laplanche *et al.* reported a 96bp insertion in an 82-year-old French woman who developed progressive depression and behavioural changes (Laplanche *et al.*, 1995). She progressed over 3 months to akinetic mutism with pyramidal signs and myoclonus. EEG showed pseudoperiodic complexes. Duration of illness was 4 months. There was no known family history of neurological illness. Another 96bp insertional mutation was seen in a patient with classical clinical and pathological features of CJD with the exception of the unusual finding of pronounced PrP immunoreactivity in the molecular layer of the cerebellum (Campbell *et al.*, 1996).

- *PrP 120bp insertion (five extra repeats).* This was reported in a US family with an illness characterized by progressive dementia, abnormal behaviour, cerebellar signs, tremor, rigidity, hyperreflexia and myoclonus. The age at onset was 31–45 with a clinical duration of 5–15 years (Goldfarb *et al.*, 1991a). EEG showed diffuse slowing only. Histological features were of spongiosis, neuronal loss and gliosis. Transmission has been demonstrated.

- *PrP 144bp insertion (six extra repeats).* This was the first PrP mutation to be reported in a small UK family with familial CJD (Owen *et al.*, 1989). The diagnosis in the family had been based on an individual who died in the 1940s with a rapidly progressive illness characteristic of CJD (Meyer *et al.*, 1954). Pathologically there was gross status spongiosis and astrocytosis affecting the entire cerebral cortex. However, other family members had a much longer duration GSS-like illness. Histological features were also extremely variable. This observation led to screening of various case of neurodegenerative disease and to the identification of a case classified on clinical grounds as familial Alzheimer's disease (Collinge *et al.*, 1989). More extensive screening work identified further families with the same mutation, who were then demonstrated by genealogical studies to form part of an extremely large kindred (Collinge *et al.*, 1992; Poulter *et al.*, 1992). Clinical information has been collected on

around 50 affected individuals over seven generations. Affected individuals develop in the third to fourth decade onset of a progressive dementia associated with a varying combination of cerebellar ataxia and dysarthria, pyramidal signs, myoclonus and occasionally extrapyramidal signs, chorea and seizures. The dementia is often preceded by depression and aggressive behaviour. A number of cases have a long-standing personality disorder, characterized by aggression, irritability, antisocial and criminal activity, and hypersexuality, which may be present from early childhood, long before overt neurodegenerative disease develops. The histological features vary from those of classical spongiform encephalopathy (with or without PrP amyloid plaques) to cases lacking any specific features of these conditions (Collinge *et al.*, 1990). Age at onset in this condition can be predicted according to genotype at polymorphic codon 129. Since this pathogenic insertional mutation occurs on a methionine 129 PrP allele, there are two possible codon 129 genotypes for affected individuals, methionine 129 homozygotes or methionine 129/valine 129 heterozygotes. Heterozygotes have an age at onset that is about a decade later than homozygotes (Poulter *et al.*, 1992). Limited transmission studies to marmosets were unsuccessful. Transmission to transgenic mice expressing human prion protein has been achieved (Collinge *et al.*, in preparation). Further families with 144bp insertions, of different nucleotide sequence, have now been reported in the UK (Nicholl *et al.*, 1995) and Japan (Oda *et al.*, 1995).

- *PrP 168bp insertion (seven extra repeats).* This has been reported in a US family. Clinical features were mood change, abnormal behaviour, confusion, aphasia, cerebellar signs, involuntary movements, rigidity, dementia and myoclonus. The age at onset was 23–35 years and the clinical duration 10 to over 13 years. The EEG was atypical. Neuropathology showed spongiform change, neuronal loss and gliosis to varying degrees (Goldfarb *et al.*, 1991a). Experimental transmission has been demonstrated.

- *PrP 192bp insertion (eight extra repeats).* Reported in a French family with clinical features including abnormal behaviour, cerebellar signs, mutism, pyramidal signs, myoclonus, tremor, intellectual slowing and seizures, the disease duration ranged from 3 months to 13 years. The EEG findings include diffuse slowing, slow wave burst suppression and periodic triphasic complexes. Neuropathological examination revealed spongiform change, neuronal loss, gliosis and multicentric plaques in the cerebellum (Goldfarb *et al.*, 1991a; Guiroy *et al.*, 1993). Experimental transmission has been reported.

- *PrP 216bp insertion (nine extra repeats).* This was first reported in a single case from the UK (Owen *et al.*, 1992). The clinical onset was around 54 years with falls, axial rigidity, myoclonic jerks and progressive dementia. Although there was no clear family history of a similar illness, the mother had died at age 53 with a cerebrovascular event. The maternal grandmother had died at age 79 with senile dementia. EEG was atypical. Neuropathological examination showed no spongiform encephalopathy but marked deposition of plaques, which in the cerebellum and the basal ganglia showed immunoreactivity with PrP antisera (Duchen *et al.*, 1993). In the hippocampus there were neuritic plaques positive for both β-amyloid protein and tau. Some neurofibrillary tangles were also seen. In some respects therefore the pathology resembled Alzheimer's disease. Experimental transmission studies have not been attempted. A second, German, family with a nine octapeptide repeat insertion of different sequence has also been reported (Krasemann *et al.*, 1995).

- *PrP 48bp deletion.* While deletion of a single octapeptide repeat element is a well recognized polymorphic variant of human PrP (with a frequency of around 1 per cent in the UK population), which does not appear to be associated with disease (Palmer *et al.*, 1993), a two repeat deletion has been described in two individuals with CJD (Beck *et al.*, 2001; Capellari *et al.*, 2002).

63.2.4.3 GENETIC COUNSELLING AND PRESYMPTOMATIC TESTING

PRNP analysis allows unequivocal diagnosis in patients with inherited prion disease. This has also allowed presymptomatic testing of unaffected, but at-risk, family members, as well as antenatal testing following appropriate genetic counselling (Collinge *et al.*, 1991b). The effect of codon 129 genotype on the age of onset of disease associated with some mutations also means it is possible to determine within a family whether a carrier of a mutation will have an early or late onset of disease. Most of the well-recognized pathogenic PRNP mutations appear fully penetrant; however, experience with some mutations is extremely limited. In families with the E200K mutation there are examples of elderly unaffected gene carriers who appear to have escaped the disease.

63.2.4.4 SECONDARY PROPHYLAXIS AFTER ACCIDENTAL EXPOSURE

Certain occupational groups are at risk of exposure to human prions, for instance neurosurgeons and other operating theatre staff, pathologists and morticians, histology technicians, as well as an increasing number of laboratory workers. Because of the prolonged incubation periods to prions following administration to sites other than the central nervous system (CNS), which is associated with clinically silent prion replication in the lymphoreticular tissue (Aguzzi, 1997), treatments inhibiting prion replication in lymphoid organs may represent a viable strategy for rational secondary prophylaxis after accidental exposure. A preliminary suggested regimen is a short course of immunosuppression with oral corticosteroids in individuals with significant accidental exposure to human prions (Aguzzi and Collinge, 1997). Urgent surgical excision of the inoculum might also be considered in exceptional circumstances. There is hope that progress in the understanding of the peripheral pathogenesis will identify the precise cell types and molecules involved in colonization of the organism by prions. The ultimate goal will be to target the rate-limiting steps in prion spread with much more focused pharmacological approaches, which may eventually prove useful in preventing disease even after iatrogenic and alimentary exposure (Collinge and Hawke, 1998). A proof of principle of immunoprophylaxis by passive immunization using anti-PrP monoclonals has already been demonstrated in mouse models (White *et al.*, 2003).

63.2.4.5 PROGNOSIS AND POSSIBLE THERAPIES

All known forms of prion diseases are invariably fatal following a relentlessly progressive course and there is no effective therapy. The duration of illness in sporadic patients is very short with a mean duration of 3–4 months. However, in some of the inherited cases the duration can be 20 years or more (Collinge *et al.*, 1990). Symptomatic treatment of various neurological and psychiatric features can be provided and a range of supportive services are likely to be required in the later stages of the disease (see UK National Prion Clinic website for factsheets and specialist advice: http://www. nationalprionclinic.org).

While no effective treatment for the human disease is known, several drugs are currently being studied in patients. In the UK, a clinical trial protocol for evaluation of potential CJD therapeutics has been developed and is designated the MRC PRION-1 trial (http://www.ctu.mrc.ac.uk/studies/cjd.asp). Currently the drug quinacrine is being evaluated. Current agents are unlikely to stop prion propagation and may at best be expected to delay disease progression. Clearly, advances towards early diagnosis, to allow therapies to be used prior to extensive neuronal loss, will be important. While the challenge of interrupting this aggressive, non-focal and uniformly fatal neurodegenerative process is daunting, major advances are being made in understanding the basic processes of prion propagation and neurotoxicity. Considerable optimism is provided by the recent finding that onset of clinical disease in established neuroinvasive prion infection in a mouse model can be halted and indeed early pathology reversed (Mallucci *et al.*, 2003). A number of approaches to rational therapeutics are being studied in experimental models. Anti-PrP antibodies have been shown to block progression of peripheral prion propagation in mouse models and humanized versions of these antibodies could in principle be developed and used for both post-exposure prophylaxis or during established clinical disease. In the longer term, the development of drugs that selectively bind PrP^{Sc} or which bind to PrP^{C} to inhibit its conversion might be able to block prion propagation and allow natural clearance mechanisms to eradicate remaining PrP^{Sc} and so cure prion infection.

REFERENCES

Aguzzi A. (1997) Neuro-immune connection in spread of prions in the body. *Lancet* **349**: 742–743

Aguzzi A and Collinge J. (1997) Post-exposure prophylaxis after accidental prion inoculation [letter]. *Lancet* **350**: 1519–1520

Alpers MP. (1987) Epidemiology and clinical aspects of kuru. In: SB Prusiner and MP McKinley (eds), *Prions: Novel Infectious Pathogens Causing Scrapie and Creutzfeldt–Jakob Disease.* San Diego, Academic Press, pp. 451–465

Asante EA, Linehan JM, Desbruslais M *et al.* (2002) BSE prions propagate as either variant CJD-like or sporadic CJD-like prion strains in transgenic mice expressing human prion protein. *EMBO Journal* **21**: 6358–6366

Baker HE, Poulter M, Crow TJ *et al.* (1991) Amino acid polymorphism in human prion protein and age at death in inherited prion disease. *Lancet* **337**: 1286

Bateman D, Hilton D, Love S *et al.* (1995) Sporadic Creutzfeldt-Jakob disease in a 18-year old in the UK. *Lancet* **346**: 1155–1156

Beck E and Daniel PM. (1987) Neuropathology of transmissible spongiform encephalopathies. In: SB Prusiner and MP McKinley (eds), *Prions: Novel Infectious Pathogens Causing Scrapie and Creutzfeldt–Jakob Disease.* San Diego, Academic Press, pp. 331–385

Beck JA, Mead S, Campbell TA (2001) Two-octapeptide repeat deletion of prion protein associated with rapidly progressive dementia. *Neurology* **57**: 354–356

Bernoulli C, Siegfried J, Baumgartner G *et al.* (1977) Danger of accidental person-to-person transmission of Creutzfeldt–Jakob disease by surgery. *Lancet* **1**: 478–479

Brandel JP, Preece M, Brown PA *et al.* (2003) Distribution of codon 129 genotype in human growth hormone-treated CJD patients in France and the UK. *Lancet* **362**: 128–130

Britton TC, Al-Sarraj S, Shaw C, Campbell T, Collinge J. (1995) Sporadic Creutzfeldt–Jakob disease in a 16-year-old in the UK. *Lancet* **346**: 1155

Brown P, Rodgers-Johnson P, Cathala F, Gibbs CJ Jr, Gajdusek DC. (1984) Creutzfeldt–Jakob disease of long duration: clinicopathological characteristics, transmissibility, and differential diagnosis. *Annals of Neurology* **16**: 295–304

Brown P, Cathala F, Raubertas RF, Gajdusek DC, Castaigne P. (1987) The epidemiology of Creutzfeldt–Jakob disease: conclusion of a 15-year investigation in France and review of the world literature. *Neurology* **37**: 895–904

Brown P, Galvez S, Goldfarb LG *et al.* (1992) Familial Creutzfeldt–Jakob disease in Chile is associated with the codon 200 mutation of the PRNP amyloid precursor gene on chromosome 20. *Journal of the Neurological Sciences* **112**: 65–67

Brown P, Gibbs CJ Jr, Rodgers Johnson P *et al.* (1994) Human spongiform encephalopathy: the National Institutes of Health series of 300 cases of experimentally transmitted disease. *Annals of Neurology* **35**: 513–529

Bruce M, Chree A, McConnell I, Foster J, Pearson G, Fraser H. (1994) Transmission of bovine spongiform encephalopathy and scrapie to mice: Strain variation and the species barrier. *Philosophical Transactions of the Royal Society of London B: Biological Sciences* **343**: 405–411

Bruce ME, Will RG, Ironside JW *et al.* (1997) Transmissions to mice indicate that 'new variant' CJD is caused by the BSE agent. *Nature* **389**: 498–501

Budka H, Aguzzi A, Brown P *et al.* (1995) Neuropathological diagnostic criteria for Creutzfeldt–Jakob disease (CJD) and other human spongiform encephalopathies (Prion diseases). *Brain Pathology* **5**: 459–466

Campbell TA, Palmer MS, Will RG, Gibb WRG, Luthert P, Collinge J. (1996) A prion disease with a novel 96-base pair insertional mutation in the prion protein gene. *Neurology* **46**: 761–766

Capellari S, Parchi P, Wolff BD *et al.* (2002) Creutzfeldt–Jakob disease associated with a deletion of two repeats in the prion protein gene. *Neurology* **59**: 1628–1630

Chapman J, Arlazoroff A, Goldfarb LG *et al.* (1996) Fatal insomnia in a case of familial Creutzfeldt–Jakob disease with the codon 200^{Lys} mutation. *Neurology* **46**: 758–761

Chapman J, Ben-Israel J, Goldhammer Y, Korczyn AD. (1994) The risk of developing Creutzfeldt–Jakob disease in subjects with the *PRNP* gene codon 200 point mutation. *Neurology* **44**: 1683–1686

Chazot G, Broussolle E, Lapras CI, Blattler T, Aguzzi A, Kopp N. (1996) New variant of Creutzfeldt–Jakob disease in a 26-year-old French man. *Lancet* **347**: 1181

Collinge J. (1996) New diagnostic tests for prion diseases. *New England Journal of Medicine* **335**: 963–965

Collinge J. (1999) Variant Creutzfeldt–Jakob disease. *Lancet* **354**: 317–323

Collinge J. (2001) Prion diseases of humans and animals: their causes and molecular basis. *Annual Review of Neuroscience* **24**: 519–550

Collinge J and Hawke S. (1998) B lymphocytes in prion neuroinvasion: central or peripheral players. *Nature Medicine* **4**: 1369–1370

Collinge J and Palmer MS. (1994) Molecular genetics of human prion diseases. *Phil Trans R Soc Lond B* **343**: 371–378

Collinge J and Prusiner SB. (1992) Terminology of prion disease. In: SB Prusiner *et al.* (eds), *Prion Diseases of Humans and Animals*, 1st edition. London, Ellis Horwood, pp. 5–12

Collinge J, Harding AE, Owen F *et al.* (1989) Diagnosis of Gerstmann-Straussler syndrome in familial dementia with prion protein gene analysis. *Lancet* **2**: 15–17

Collinge J, Owen F, Poulter M *et al.* (1990) Prion dementia without characteristic pathology. *Lancet* **336**: 7–9

Collinge J, Palmer MS, Dryden AJ. (1991a) Genetic predisposition to iatrogenic Creutzfeldt–Jakob disease. *Lancet* **337**: 1441–1442

Collinge J, Poulter M, Davis MB *et al.* (1991b) Presymptomatic detection or exclusion of prion protein gene defects in families with inherited prion diseases. *American Journal of Human Genetics* **49**: 1351–1354

Collinge J, Brown J, Hardy J *et al.* (1992) Inherited prion disease with 144 base pair gene insertion. II: Clinical and pathological features. *Brain* **115**: 687–710

Collinge J, Palmer MS, Campbell TA, Sidle KCL, Carroll D, Harding AE. (1993) Inherited prion disease (PrP lysine 200) in Britain: two case reports. *BMJ* **306**: 301–302

Collinge J, Palmer MS, Sidle KCL *et al.* (1995a) Transmission of fatal familial insomnia to laboratory animals. *Lancet* **346**: 569–570

Collinge J, Palmer MS, Sidle KCL *et al.* (1995b) Unaltered susceptibility to BSE in transgenic mice expressing human prion protein. *Nature* **378**: 779–783

Collinge J, Beck J, Campbell T, Estibeiro K, Will RG. (1996a) Prion protein gene analysis in new variant cases of Creutzfeldt–Jakob disease. *Lancet* **348**: 56

Collinge J, Sidle KCL, Meads J, Ironside J, Hill AF. (1996b) Molecular analysis of prion strain variation and the aetiology of 'new variant' CJD. *Nature* **383**: 685–690

Collinge J, Hill AF, Ironside J, Zeidler M. (1997) Diagnosis of new variant Creutzfeldt–Jakob disease by tonsil biopsy – authors' reply to Arya and Evans. *Lancet* **349**: 1322–1323

Cuillé J and Chelle PL. (1936) La maladie dite tremblante du mouton est-elle inocuable?. *Compte Rendu de l'Academie des Sciences* **203**: 1552–1554

Davies PTG, Jahfar S, Ferguson IT, Windl O. (1993) Creutzfeldt–Jakob disease in individual occupationally exposed to BSE. *Lancet* **342**: 680

Dlouhy SR, Hsiao K, Farlow MR *et al.* (1992) Linkage of the Indiana kindred of Gerstmann-Straussler-Scheinker disease to the prion protein gene. *Nature Genetics* **1**: 64–67

Doh ura K, Tateishi J, Sasaki H, Kitamoto T, Sakaki Y. (1989) Pro–leu change at position 102 of prion protein is the most common but not the sole mutation related to Gerstmann-Straussler syndrome. *Biochemical and Biophysical Research Communications* **163**: 974–979

Duchen LW, Poulter M, Harding AE. (1993) Dementia associated with a 216 base pair insertion in the prion protein gene. Clinical and neuropathological features. *Brain* **116**: 555–567

Esmonde TFG, Will RG, Slattery JM *et al.* (1993) Creutzfeldt–Jakob disease and blood transfusion. *Lancet* **341**: 205–207

Flechsig E, Hegyi I, Enari M, Schwarz P, Collinge J, Weissmann C. (2001) Transmission of scrapie by steel-surface-bound prions. *Molecular Medicine* **7**: 679–684

Gajdusek DC, Gibbs CJ Jr, Alpers MP. (1966) Experimental transmission of a kuru-like syndrome to chimpanzees. *Nature* **209**: 794–796

Gerstmann J, Straussler E, Scheinker I. (1936) Über eine eigenartige hereditär-familiäre Erkrankung des Zentralnervensystems. Zugleich ein Beitrag zur Frage des vorzeitigen lakalen Alterns. *Zeitschrift für Neurologie* **154**: 736–762

Ghani AC, Donnelly CA, Ferguson NM, Anderson RM. (2003) Updated projections of future vCJD deaths in the UK. *BMC Infectious Diseases* **3**: 4

Gibbs CJ Jr, Gajdusek DC, Asher DM *et al.* (1968) Creutzfeldt–Jakob disease (spongiform encephalopathy): transmission to the chimpanzee. *Science* **161**: 388–389

Goldfarb LG, Korczyn AD, Brown P, Chapman J, Gajdusek DC. (1990) Mutation in codon 200 of scrapie amyloid precursor gene linked to Creutzfeldt–Jakob disease in Sephardic Jews of Libyan and non-Libyan origin. *Lancet* **336**: 637–638

Goldfarb LG, Brown P, McCombie WR *et al.* (1991a) Transmissible familial Creutzfeldt–Jakob disease associated with five, seven, and eight extra octapeptide coding repeats in the *PRNP* gene. *Proceedings of the National Academy of Sciences of the United States of America* **88**: 10926–10930

Goldfarb LG, Haltia M, Brown P *et al.* (1991b) New mutation in scrapie amyloid precursor gene (at codon 178) in Finnish Creutzfeldt–Jakob kindred. *Lancet* **337**: 425

Goldfarb LG, Petersen RB, Tabaton M *et al.* (1992) Fatal familial insomnia and familial Creutzfeldt–Jakob disease: disease phenotype determined by a DNA polymorphism. *Science* **258**: 806–808

Goldfarb LG, Brown P, Little BW *et al.* (1993) A new (two-repeat) octapeptide coding insert mutation in Creutzfeldt–Jakob disease. *Neurology* **43**: 2392–2394

Gomori AJ, Partnow MJ, Horoupian DS, Hirano A. (1973) The ataxic form of Creutzfeldt–Jakob disease. *Archives of Neurology* **29**: 318–323

Griffith JS. (1967) Self replication and scrapie. *Nature* **215**: 1043–1044

Guiroy DC, Marsh RF, Yanagihara R, Gajdusek DC. (1993) Immunolocalization of scrapie amyloid in non-congophilic, non-birefringent deposits in golden Syrian hamsters with experimental transmissible mink encephalopathy. *Neuroscience Letters* **155**: 112–115

Hadlow WJ. (1959) Scrapie and kuru. *Lancet* **ii**: 289–290

Hainfellner JA, Brantner-Inthaler S, Cervenáková L *et al.* (1995) The original Gerstmann-Straussler-Scheinker family of Austria: divergent clinicopathological phenotypes but constant PrP genotype. *Brain Pathology* **5**: 201–211

Hill AF, Desbruslais M, Joiner S, Sidle KCL, Gowland I, Collinge J. (1997) The same prion strain causes vCJD and BSE. *Nature* **389**: 448–450

Hill AF, Butterworth RJ, Joiner S *et al.* (1999) Investigation of variant Creutzfeldt–Jakob disease and other human prion diseases with tonsil biopsy samples. *Lancet* **353**: 183–189

Hill AF, Joiner S, Linehan J, Desbruslais M, Lantos PL, Collinge J. (2000) Species barrier independent prion replication in apparently resistant species. *Proceedings of the National Academy of Sciences of the United States of America* **97**: 10248–10253

Hill AF, Joiner S, Wadsworth JD *et al.* (2003) Molecular classification of sporadic Creutzfeldt–Jakob disease. *Brain* **126**: 1333–1346

Hilton DA, Ghani AC, Conyers L *et al.* (2004) Prevalence of lymphoreticular prion protein accumulation in UK tissue samples. *J Pathol* **203**(3): 733–739

Hsiao K, Baker HF, Crow TJ *et al.* (1989) Linkage of a prion protein missense variant to Gerstmann- Straussler syndrome. *Nature* **338**: 342–345

Hsiao K, Meiner Z, Kahana E *et al.* (1991a) Mutation of the prion protein in Libyan Jews with Creutzfeldt- Jakob disease. *New England Journal of Medicine* **324**: 1091–1097

Hsiao KK, Cass C, Schellenberg GD *et al.* (1991b) A prion protein variant in a family with the telencephalic form of Gerstmann-Straussler-Scheinker syndrome. *Neurology* **41**: 681–684

Hsiao K, Dlouhy SR, Farlow MR *et al.* (1992) Mutant prion proteins in Gerstmann-Straussler-Sheinker disease with neurofibrillary tangles. *Nature Genetics* **1**: 68–71

Hsich G, Kenney K, Gibbs CJ, Jr. *et al.* (1996) The 14-3-3 brain protein in cerebrospinal fluid as a marker for transmissible spongiform encephalopathies. *New England Journal of Medicine* **335**(13): 924–930

Jackson GS, Hosszu LLP, Power A *et al.* (1999) Reversible conversion of monomeric human prion protein between native and fibrilogenic conformations. *Science* **283**: 1935–1937

Jimi T, Wakayama Y, Shibuya S *et al.* (1992) High levels of nervous system-specific proteins in cerebrospinal fluid in patients with early stage Creutzfeldt–Jakob disease. *Clinica Chimica Acta* **211**: 37–46

Kitamoto T, Iizuka R, Tateishi J. (1993a) An amber mutation of prion protein in Gerstmann-Straussler syndrome with mutant PrP plaques. *Biochemical and Biophysical Research Communications* **192**: 525–531

Kitamoto T, Ohta M, Doh-ura K, Hitoshi S, Terao Y, Tateishi J. (1993b) Novel missense variants of prion protein in Creutzfeldt–Jakob disease or Gerstmann-Straussler syndrome. *Biochemical and Biophysical Research Communications* **191**: 709–714

Krasemann S, Zerr I, Weber T, Poser S, Kretzschmar H, Hunsmann G, Bodemer W. (1995) Prion disease associated with a novel nine octapeptide repeat insertion in the PRNP gene. *Molecular Brain Research* **34**: 173–176

Kretzschmar HA, Kufer P, Riethmuller G, DeArmond SJ, Prusiner SB, Schiffer D. (1992) Prion protein mutation at codon 102 in an Italian family with Gerstmann-Straussler-Scheinker syndrome. *Neurology* **42**: 809–810

Laplanche JL, Delasnerie Laupretre N, Brandel JP, Dussaucy M, Chatelain J, Launay JM. (1995) Two novel insertions in the prion protein gene in patients with late-onset dementia. *Human Molecular Genetics* **4**: 1109–1111

Llewelyn CA, Hewitt PE, Knight RSG et al. (2004) Possible transmission of variant Creutzfeldt-Jakob disease by blood transfusion. *Lancet* **363**: 417–421

Lloyd SE, Onwuazor ON, Beck JA et al. (2001) Identification of multiple quantitative trait loci linked to prion disease incubation period in mice. *Proceedings of the National Academy of Sciences of the United States of America* **98**: 6279–6283

Lugaresi E, Medori R, Baruzzi PM et al. (1986) Fatal familial insomnia and dysautonomia, with selective degeneration of thalamic nuclei. *New England Journal of Medicine* **315**: 997–1003

McGowan JP. (1922) Scrapie in sheep. *Scottish Journal of Agriculture* **5**: 365–375

McLean CA, Storey E, Gardner RJM, Tannenberg AEG, Cervenáková L, Brown P. (1997) The D178N (cis-129M) 'fatal familial insomnia' mutation associated with diverse clinicopathologic phenotypes in an Australian kindred. *Neurology* **49**: 552–558

Mallucci GR, Campbell TA, Dickinson A et al. (1999) Inherited prion disease with an alanine to valine mutation at codon 117 in the prion protein gene. *Brain* **122**: 1823–1837

Mallucci G, Dickinson A, Linehan J, Klohn PC, Brandner S, Collinge J. (2003) Depleting neuronal PrP in prion infection prevents disease and reverses spongiosis. *Science* **302**: 871–874

Martindale J, Geschwind MD, De Armond S et al. (2003) Sporadic Creutzfeldt-Jakob disease mimicking variant Creutzfeldt-Jakob disease. *Archives of Neurology* **60**: 767–770

Mastrianni JA, Iannicola C, Myers R, Prusiner SB. (1995) Identification of a new mutation of the prion protein gene at codon 208 in a patient with Creutzfeldt-Jakob disease. *Neurology* **45** (Suppl. 4): A201

Medori R, Montagna P, Tritschler HJ et al. (1992a) Fatal familial insomnia: a second kindred with mutation of prion protein gene at codon 178. *Neurology* **42**: 669–670

Medori R, Tritschler HJ, LeBlanc A et al. (1992b) Fatal familial insomnia, a prion disease with a mutation at codon 178 of the prion protein gene. *New England Journal of Medicine* **326**: 444–449

Meyer A, Leigh D, Bagg CE. (1954) A rare presenile dementia associated with cortical blindness (Heidenhain's syndrome). *Journal of Neurology, Neurosurgery, and Psychiatry* **17**: 129–133

Mizutani T. (1981) Neuropathology of Creutzfeldt-Jakob disease in Japan. With special reference to the panencephalopathic type. *Acta Pathologica Japonica* **31**: 903–922

Monari L, Chen SG, Brown P et al. (1994) Fatal familial insomnia and familial Creutzfeldt-Jakob disease: Different prion proteins determined by a DNA polymorphism. *Proceedings of the National Academy of Sciences of the United States of America* **91**: 2839–2842

Neufeld MY, Josiphov J, Korczyn AD. (1992) Demyelinating peripheral neuropathy in Creutzfeldt-Jakob disease. *Muscle Nerve* **15**: 1234–1239

Nicholl D, Windl O, De Silva R et al. (1995) Inherited Creutzfeldt-Jakob disease in a British family associated with a novel 144 base pair insertion of the prion protein gene. *Journal of Neurology, Neurosurgery, and Psychiatry* **58**: 65–69

Nitrini R, Rosemberg S, Passos-Bueno MR et al. (1997) Familial spongiform encephalopathy associated with a novel prion protein gene mutation. *Annals of Neurology* **42**: 138–146

Oda T, Kitamoto T, Tateishi J et al. (1995) Prion disease with 144 base pair insertion in a Japanese family line. *Acta Neuropathologica (Berlin)* **90**: 80–86

Otto M, Stein H, Szdura A et al. (1997) S-100 protein concentration in the cerebrospinal fluid of patients with Creutzfeldt-Jakob disease. *Journal of Neurology* **244**: 566–570

Owen F, Poulter M, Lofthouse R et al. (1989) Insertion in prion protein gene in familial Creutzfeldt-Jakob disease. *Lancet* i: 51–52

Owen F, Poulter M, Collinge J et al. (1992) A dementing illness associated with a novel insertion in the prion protein gene. *Molecular Brain Research* **13**: 155–157

Palmer MS, Dryden AJ, Hughes JT, Collinge J. (1991) Homozygous prion protein genotype predisposes to sporadic Creutzfeldt-Jakob disease. *Nature* **352**: 340–342

Palmer MS, Mahal SP, Campbell TA et al. (1993) Deletions in the prion protein gene are not associated with CJD. *Human Molecular Genetics* **2**: 541–544

Parchi P, Giese A, Capellari S et al. (1999) Classification of sporadic Creutzfeldt-Jakob Disease based on molecular and phenotypic analysis of 300 subjects. *Annals of Neurology* **46**: 224–233

Pattison IH. (1965) Experiments with scrapie with special reference to the nature of the agent and the pathology of the disease. In: CJ Gajdusek, CJ Gibbs, MP Alpers (eds), *Slow, Latent and Temperate Virus Infections, NINDB Monograph 2*. Washington DC, US Government Printing, pp. 249–257

Peden AH, Head MW, Ritchie DL, Bell JE, Ironside JW. (2004) Preclinical vCJD after blood transfusion in a PRNP codon 129 heterozygous patient. *Lancet* **364**: 527–529

Poulter M, Baker HF, Frith CD et al. (1992) Inherited prion disease with 144 base pair gene insertion. I: Genealogical and molecular studies. *Brain* **115**: 675–685

Prusiner SB, Scott M, Foster D et al. (1990) Transgenetic studies implicate interactions between homologous PrP isoforms in scrapie prion replication. *Cell* **63**: 673–686

Rossetti AO, Bogousslavsky J, Glatzel M, Aguzzi A. (2004) Mimicry of variant Creutzfeldt-Jakob disease by sporadic Creutzfeldt-Jakob disease: importance of the pulvinar sign. *Archives of Neurology* **61**: 445–446

Salazar AM, Masters CL, Gajdusek DC, Gibbs CJ Jr. (1983) Syndromes of amyotrophic lateral sclerosis and dementia: relation to transmissible Creutzfeldt-Jakob disease. *Annals of Neurology* **14**: 17–26

Satoh J-I, Kurohara K, Yukitake M et al. (1999) The 14-3-3 protein detectable in the cerebrospinal fluid of patients with prion-unrelated neurological diseases is expressed constitutively in neurons and glial cells in culture. *European Neurology* **41**: 216–225

Shiga Y, Miyazawa K, Sato S et al. (2004) Diffusion-weighted MRI abnormalities as an early diagnostic marker for Creutzfeldt-Jakob disease. *Neurology* **63**: 443–449

Summers DM, Collie DA, Zeidler M, Will RG. (2004) The pulvinar sign in variant Creutzfeldt-Jakob disease. *Archives of Neurology* **61**: 446–447

Tabrizi SJ, Scaravilli F, Howard RS, Collinge J, Rossor MN. (1996) GRAND ROUND. Creutzfeldt-Jakob disease in a young woman. Report of a Meeting of Physicians and Scientists, St. Thomas' Hospital, London. *Lancet* **347**: 945–948

Tagliavini F, Giaccone G, Prelli F et al. (1993) A68 is a component of paired helical filaments of Gerstmann-Straussler-Scheinker disease, Indiana kindred. *Brain Research* **616**: 325–328

Tateishi J, Brown P, Kitamoto T et al. (1995) First experimental transmission of fatal familial insomnia. *Nature* **376**: 434–435

Wadsworth JDF, Hill AF, Joiner S, Jackson GS, Clarke AR, Collinge J. (1999) Strain-specific prion-protein conformation determined by metal ions. *Nature Cell Biology* **1**: 55–59

Wadsworth JDF, Joiner S, Hill AF *et al.* (2001) Tissue distribution of protease resistant prion protein in variant CJD using a highly sensitive immunoblotting assay. *Lancet* **358**: 171–180

White AR, Enever P, Tayebi M *et al.* (2003) Monoclonal antibodies inhibit prion replication and delay the development of prion disease. *Nature* **422**: 80–83

Will RG, Ironside JW, Zeidler M *et al.* (1996) A new variant of Creutzfeldt–Jakob disease in the UK. *Lancet* **347**: 921–925

Zeidler M, Johnstone EC, Bamber RWK *et al.* (1997a) New variant Creutzfeldt–Jakob disease: psychiatric features. *Lancet* **350**: 908–910

Zeidler M, Stewart GE, Barraclough CR *et al.* (1997b) New variant Creutzfeldt–Jakob disease: neurological features and diagnostic tests. *Lancet* **350**: 903–907

Zerr I, Bodemer M, Räcker S *et al.* (1995) Cerebrospinal fluid concentration of neuron-specific enolase in diagnosis of Creutzfeldt–Jakob disease. *Lancet* **345**: 1609–1610

64

Human immunodeficiency virus type 1-associated dementia: pathology, clinical features and treatment

APSARA KANDANEARATCHI AND IAN PAUL EVERALL

The latest reports indicate that since the beginning of 1980s, 60 million people have been infected with HIV (UNAIDS-WHO, 2001). Today, in certain parts of the world such as Sub-Saharan Africa, it is the leading cause of death amongst its population. In 1983 the Centers for Disease Control (CDC) issued the first classification of acquired immunodeficiency syndrome (AIDS), which was then revised in 1987 (CDC, 1987) and again in 1993 (MMWR). The 1983 and 1987 classifications were clinical symptom based, consisting of four groups of disorders:

- *Group I*: Acute infection (seroconversion)
- *Group II*: Asymptomatic infection
- *Group III*: Persistent generalized lymphadenopathy
- *Group IV*: with subgroups:
    (A) constitutional disease with fever, weight loss, fatigue and night sweats
    (B) neurological disease
    (C) secondary infectious diseases
    (D) secondary cancers
    (E) other conditions.

In 1993 a second classification revision was accepted, which incorporated laboratory data and symptom-based classification as two parallel categories to rate the affected individual's condition (Table 64.1). The laboratory category is the CD4+ lymphocyte counts; this is the primary cell infected and destroyed by HIV and it is the loss of this population that results in severe immune suppression. For example, a person categorized as A3 will be clinically asymptomatic but has marked immunosuppression. The clinical

Table 64.1 *Classification of AIDS (1993), using a combination of clinical features and laboratory investigations*

Clinical features	Laboratory CD4+ counts (cells/mL)
Group A: asymptomatic	Group 1: 501–1000
Group B: constitutional symptoms	Group 2: 201–500
Group C: AIDS indicator illnesses	Group 3: <200

groups are progressive in that one proceeds from A through to C, but not back again. Thus, the category A3 means that this individual has never experienced any clinical symptoms. Since the mid-1990s the term HIV disease has tended to replace the term AIDS, which does not occur so frequently now that antiretroviral treatment is available.

Apart from CD4+ cells, the brain is a major target of infection resulting in cognitive dysfunction. The most severe neuropsychiatric manifestation is HIV dementia. In the last decade there has been significant progress in clarifying the brain pathology, clinical features, and more recently therapeutic strategies of this dementia. This chapter will cover these issues, including clarification of the range of brain pathology, correlation of which pathological events results in cognitive impairments, description of the clinical features and investigations, and finally the current treatment options for HIV dementia. This chapter will not address the secondary HIV-associated brain disorders that include opportunistic infections and neoplasms, which have been reviewed elsewhere (Everall and Lantos, 1991).

64.1 NEUROPATHOLOGICAL ABNORMALITIES ASSOCIATED WITH HIV

Since the mid-1980s a variety of virological, neuropathological and neuroscientific investigations have attempted to address: the characteristic features of the virus mediating cellular entry, the mechanism and timing of viral brain entry, which brain resident cells does HIV infect and replicate in, the spectrum of HIV-associated brain damage, the mechanism of neurotoxicity, and finally the relationship between this damage and the clinical onset of HIV-associated cognitive impairments. These will be discussed below.

64.1.1 Characteristics of HIV and the mechanism of cellular entry

HIV is a retrovirus and contains a single-stranded RNA genome with an RNA-dependent DNA polymerase, reverse transcriptase. When the viral genome enters the cell the reverse transcriptase synthesizes a double-stranded viral DNA copy. The DNA can remain unintegrated in the cytoplasm or enter the nucleus and become integrated with the host genome, a so-called provirus, which can replicate along with the host chromosomal DNA. The molecular structure of the HIV genome includes genes coding for structural, enzymatic and regulatory functions. The env gene codes for structural proteins of the viral envelope, such as gp120 and gp41. Gag codes for core structural viral proteins including matrix (p17), capsid (p24, p9 and p6). The enzymatic proteins are coded by the pol gene, and include reverse transcriptase, RNAase H, integrase and protease. The regulatory genes are tat, nef, rev, vif, vpr and vpu and their functions are gradually being elucidated. They are known to enhance every step of viral replication, including the early events of viral cellular entry, reverse transcription, nuclear transport and establishment of the provirus; or during the later events of provirus regulation during transcription, viral polyprotein processing and transport, and finally virion release and infectivity. Regulation of replication is also influenced by host factors such as cytokines and transcription factors. The regulation of viral replication is reviewed by Stevenson and O'Brien (1998).

HIV predominantly infects either CD4+ T lymphocytes or mononuclear phagocytes such as circulating monocytes or tissue macrophages. The ability to replicate in macrophages is due to genetic heterogeneity, which is greatest in the env gene (Hahn et al., 1986; Koyanagi et al., 1987; Saag et al., 1988; Hwang et al., 1991; Westervelt et al., 1991). The cellular determinant of viral entry are the expression of an appropriate cell surface receptor. Thus, for lymphocytic strains, cell entry is mediated by not only binding to the CD4+ receptor but also to a coreceptor, CXCR-4. By comparison in monocyte-/macrophage-tropic strains the β-chemokine receptors, such as CCR-1, CCR-3 and CCR-5, are important cell receptors. These chemokine receptors are known to selectively act as co-receptors to CD4 to mediate HIV binding and entry (Dimitrov,

1997). Broadly speaking the ability to use either CXCR4 or CCR5 defines the tropism of the HIV strain, i.e. lymphocyte or macrophage tropic respectively. In the brain, microglia and macrophages, neurones and astrocytes all possess chemokine receptors. CXCR-4 is expressed by neurones and microglia (Lavi et al., 1997), as well as reactive astrocytes (Miller and Meucci, 1999). CCR-1 has been reported in astrocytes, CCR-3 in microglia and CCR-5 in both microglia and neurones (Miller and Meucci, 1999). He et al. (1997) reported that both CCR3 and CCR5 are important for microglia infection, Ghorpade et al. (1998) found an essential role for only CCR5, while Shieh et al. (1998) observed that CCR5 was used for macrophage entry but failed to replicate the use of either CCR3 or CCR5 receptors for microglial infection. During recent years, a vast number of chemokine receptors have been discovered and the involvement of chemokine receptors in HIV is still being pursued. Attempts have also been made to identify viral features that would predict neurotropism. This is the property that facilitates entry into the nervous system. It has been suggested that the development of neurotropism is thought to be linked to alterations in the envelope glycoprotein gp120 (Cordonnier et al., 1989; Power et al., 1994; DiStefano et al., 1998). To date the results have been intriguing but inconsistent; thus, the notion of a readily identifiable neurotropic strain has not been substantiated.

64.1.2 The timing of viral brain entry

HIV antigen and antibody (Ho et al., 1985) can be identified in the cerebrospinal fluid during seroconversion but it remains unclear whether this represents a limited meningeal infection or indicative of widespread invasion of the central nervous system (CNS). Limited meningeal infection is most likely in the vast majority of individuals. Only a few isolated case reports have highlighted approximately three individuals who had documented fatal illnesses during seroconversion (for review see Gray et al., 1996). Following seroconversion there is a prolonged and variable time interval of asymptomatic infection. Examination of the brain during this period is rare, unless an individual dies of an unrelated cause. The few studies on asymptomatically infected individuals revealed only occasional detectable proviral DNA (Sinclair and Scaravilli, 1992; Donaldson et al., 1994). As the duration of HIV infection was not known, it is possible that where proviral DNA was found the individuals may have had more advanced infection and more likely to develop HIV disease in the near future if they had lived.

In order to gain entry to the brain the virus has to cross the blood–brain barrier (BBB). It is widely believed that is does this through the systemic circulation either as cell-free virus, or through infected monocytes, macrophages or lymphocytes or through the choroid plexus (Kalams and Walker, 1995; Nottet et al., 1996). The existence of the BBB and the low level of expression of major histocompatibility complex (MHC) molecules on cells within the brain, has led to the view that the brain is an immunologically privileged site. However, in HIV infection and other inflammatory diseases inducible, adhesion molecules, selectins, chemokines and cytokines are expressed by the immune system and BBB, which promote adhesion of immune cells to endothelial cells and then transmigration across the BBB.

64.1.3 Cellular localization of HIV in the brain

Demonstration of the virus within cells can be performed by detecting HIV DNA, messenger RNA (mRNA), or viral protein. Immunohistochemistry of viral proteins has demonstrated that macrophages, microglia and multinucleated giant cells are the major cellular reservoirs of HIV in the brain (Koenig et al., 1986; Wiley et al., 1986). However, recent application of in situ polymerase chain reaction (PCR) and reverse transcriptase-PCR has provided evidence that the DNA and RNA may be present in a wider variety of cell types, including oligodendrocytes (Albright et al., 1996) and even neurones (Nuovo et al., 1994; Bagasra et al., 1996). Evidence for a 'restrictive infection' in astrocytes is now emerging (Canki et al., 2001; Galey et al., 2003) in which regulatory proteins such as nef are produced (Saito et al., 1994). However, full replication of structural HIV proteins is absent. So, while there is evidence of HIV DNA and RNA in a wide population of brain cells, full replicative infection only occurs in microglia, macrophages and multinucleated giant cells.

64.1.4 Primary neuropathological damage associated with HIV

This is a consequence of HIV brain infection, and is distinct from the myriad of opportunistic infections and neoplasms that can arise secondarily to immune compromision (for review see Cohen and Berger, 1998). The primary damage consists of a range of neuropathologically recognized disorders, dendritic and synaptic damage, and neuronal loss. These can occur together, and are pathological phenomena, which can only be diagnosed by examination of the brain. The development of these events does not necessarily imply onset of clinical symptoms (Price et al., 1991). These disorders will be considered below.

64.1.4.1 NEUROPATHOLOGICALLY RECOGNIZED DISORDERS

These disorders are discrete inflammatory and degenerative disorders (Budka, 1991), whose frequencies are derived from several autopsy series from various European and North and South American countries (Budka, 1998; Table 64.2). These disorders are summarized below.

- *HIV encephalitis (HIVE)*. This is characterized histologically by inflammatory foci of microglia, macrophages and multinucleated giant cells. The latter are the histological hallmark of HIVE. These tend to be

Table 64.2 *HIV-related brain pathology, and their observed frequencies in several studies (data from Budka, 1998)*

Type of lesion	Frequency in several series (%)
HIV-specific lesions	21.5
HIV encephalitis (HIVE)	16
HIV leukoencephalopathy (HIVL)	12
HIVE combined with HIVL	14
HIV meningoventriculoencephalitis	0.6
HIV-associated lesions	46
Diffuse poliodystrophy (DPD)	44
Lymphocytic meningitis	4
Multifocal vacuolar leukoencephalopathy	1
Vacuolar myelopathy	8

widely distributed throughout the brain but may be more common in the deep grey structures (basal ganglia and thalamus), as well as the cortical white matter (Budka, 1991). Viral proteins can often be demonstrated. The clinical consequence of developing HIVE is not clear and potential clinicopathological correlations will be discussed in Section 64.3 (p. 781). Recently, Davies et al. (1998) examined the neuropathological findings of 1144 brains collected over a 10-year period from six centres throughout Europe and the United States. HIVE comprised 26 per cent of the overall observed pathology, which is similar to the 16 per cent estimated by Budka (1998). However, the frequency varied between centres, from 13 to 44 per cent, and between those cases collected before and after 1988. This date was the approximate general introduction date for zidovudine, after which the rate of HIVE declined. This has also been reported by Gray et al. (1994). In a UK national neuroepidemiological survey, Davies et al. (1997) similarly revealed that the frequency of HIVE was 25 per cent but, more importantly, that it varied among risk groups, with intravenous drug users having a rate over 50 per cent. This indicated that brain pathology can be influenced by risk group.

- *HIV leukoencephalopathy (HIVL)*. In this disorder there is diffuse damage to the white matter with myelin loss, reactive astrocytosis, macrophages and multinucleated giant cells (Kleihues et al., 1985). The white matter is usually affected symmetrically and the cerebellar white matter can also be affected. In addition to the myelin damage axonal shrinkage has also been reported (Kaus et al., 1991). While HIVE and HIVL are presented as two distinct entities they have inflammatory features in common and may represent a spectrum disorder. A rare variant of the leukoencephalopathy has been noted with numerous vacuolar myelin swellings and macrophages. This is called *vacuolar leukoencephalopathy*. Recently, a severe form of HIVL has been described by Langford et al. (2002) in AIDS patients who had undergone antiretroviral therapy prior to death. This may indicate the identification of a new form of neuropathology since the introduction of highly active antiretroviral therapy (HAART).

- *Diffuse poliodystrophy.* This refers to a picture diffuse reactive astrocytosis, gliosis, microglial activation and presumed neuronal loss in the grey matter of the cortex, basal ganglia and brain stem (Budka, 1990).
- *Lymphocytic meningitis.* The leptomeninges, including the perivascular spaces are infiltrated with lymphocytes. No opportunistic pathogens are ever identified, and clinically this is presumed to be associated with the aseptic meningitis that can occur during primary systemic infection.
- *Cerebral vasculitis.* Blood vessel walls are infiltrated with multinucleated giant cells and lymphocytes. There may be accompanying necrosis, and so clinically this may produce focal neurological deficits. Vascular lesions are more common in those with haemophilia (Davies *et al.*, 1997).

64.1.4.2 NEURONAL INJURY AND LOSS

This consists of the following:

- *Dendritic and synaptic damage.* There is significant dendritic and synaptic damage in the cortex of those who die of AIDS. There is a significant 10–40 per cent decrease in the microscopic area occupied by microtubule-associated protein-2 (MAP2) immunolabeled dendrites (Masliah *et al.*, 1992a), a decrease in the complexity of synaptophysin-immunoreactive presynaptic terminals (Wiley *et al.*, 1991; Masliah *et al.*, 1992a, 1996a), and a notable dendritic simplification with decreased dendritic length and loss of spines (Masliah *et al.*, 1992b). Ultrastructurally, there is dendritic vacuolization with disruption of the neuritic endomembrane system (Wiley *et al.*, 1991). The extent of dendritic and synaptic damage is closely correlated with the amount of envelope viral protein, gp41, in the brain (Masliah *et al.*, 1992a, 1997; Everall *et al.*, 1998). A transgenic mouse model over-expressing the HIV envelope protein gp120 (Toggas *et al.*, 1994) has similar dendritic alterations to those observed in HIV encephalitis. This indicates that active damage to synapses is a primary pathogenic event of this disorder, and that gp120 is involved in this process (Masliah *et al.*, 1996a, b).
- *Neuronal loss.* While the majority of neuronal loss studies have been on those who died of AIDS, a stereological study of a previously described French series of individuals who died while asymptomatically infected (Gray *et al.*, 1993) did not reveal neuronal loss (Everall *et al.*, 1992). This is consistent with the observation that there are low levels of provirus found in some but not all asymptomatic brains, compared with the high levels of provirus reported in brains from those who died of AIDS (Donaldson *et al.*, 1994; Sinclair *et al.*, 1994). In contrast,

those who died of AIDS have significant cortical neuronal loss, which disproportionately affects larger pyramidal neurones (Ketzler *et al.*, 1990; Wiley *et al.*, 1991; Weis *et al.*, 1993; Asare *et al.*, 1996). The frontal cortex, with nearly 40 per cent decrease in neuronal number, is more greatly affected than other cortical areas (Everall *et al.*, 1991, 1993). There is degeneration of the striatocortical, corticocortical and limbic intrinsic/inhibitory circuitries (Masliah *et al.*, 1996a, b). Neo-cortical width is reduced by approximately 20 per cent (Wiley *et al.*, 1991), and mean neuronal volume was also altered in the regions with the most marked neuronal loss (Everall *et al.*, 1993). Loss has also been observed in extracortical regions, including the putamen, globus pallidus and hippocampus (Spargo *et al.*, 1993; Masliah *et al.*, 1995, 1996a), substantia nigra (Reyes *et al.*, 1991), and cerebellum (Grauss *et al.*, 1990). These observations suggest that neuronal loss develops during symptomatic disease when viral load is increased.

64.2 POTENTIAL MECHANISM OF HIV-ASSOCIATED NEURONAL INJURY AND LOSS

There is evidence that the mechanism of neuronal damage and clinical onset of cognitive impairment probably involves two main groups of potential pathogenic factors: *viral proteins* and *cytokines*.

64.2.1 Viral proteins

A variety of the HIV proteins have been shown to be neuro-toxic. The envelope glycoprotein gp120 causes a toxic calcium influx by stimulating the glutamate N-methyl-D-aspartate (NMDA) receptors (Dreyer *et al.*, 1990), which *in vitro* results in cell death (Brenneman *et al.*, 1988). This can be prevented by applying either calcium channel antagonists (e.g. nimodipine) or NMDA antagonists (e.g. MK801 or memantine). Similarly, the viral regulatory protein tat affects membrane permeability causes depolarization (Sabatier *et al.*, 1991), and stimulates the α-amino-3-hydroxy-5-methyl-4-isoxazole propionic acid (AMPA) glutamate receptors. AMPA receptors are decreased in AIDS (Everall *et al.*, 1995). Interactions with the cellular surface of ion channels have been demonstrated for the envelope protein gp41 (Werner *et al.*, 1991) and the regulatory protein nef has recently been shown to be neurotoxic (Trillo-Pazos *et al.*, 1998).

64.2.2 Cytokines

A wide range of cytokines are involved in the immunological response to inflammatory disease. Microglia and macrophages are capable, for example, of producing tumour necrosis factor

(TNF)-α, interleukin-1 (IL-1) and transforming factor β (TGF-β; Wahl et al., 1991; Tyor et al., 1992). Both gp120 and gp41 are able to induce cytokine production, especially TNF-α and IL-1β (Merrill and Chen, 1991). A number of other cytokines have been demonstrated to be produced when HIV is present. Importantly, cytokines (TNF-α and IL-1β) activate gene expression and so induce productive infection (Swingler et al., 1992). Thus, a positive cycle is set up with viral products inducing cytokines, which in turn induce viral replication and therefore increase the viral load in the brain. In addition TNF-α can activate programmed cell death, also called apoptosis. Other cytokines that have been implicated are TGF-β, produced by mononuclear cells and found in areas of tissue pathology (Wahl et al., 1991) and IL-6 which affects HIV expression (Tesmer et al., 1993). Another cytokine CD23 expressed by astrocytes was found extensively in HIVE brains and additionally involved in the activation of nitric oxide pathway and IL-1β (Dugas et al., 2001).

64.2.3 Other potential factors

In the HIV-infected brain both the gp120-mediated NMDA-activated calcium influx and the excess cytokines can induce *oxidative stress*. For example, glutamate receptor activation can stimulate nitric oxide synthase production of nitric oxide (Dawson et al., 1994), and cytokines can induce macrophages and microglia to produce nitric oxide in more prolonged bursts. Nitric oxide and superoxide radicals produce the peroxynitrite radical, resulting in lipid peroxidation and demyelination. Brain antioxidant mechanisms include glutathione peroxidase, superoxide dismutase, ascorbic acid, vitamin E and glutathione. However, the brain is still susceptible to oxidative damage (Floyd and Carney, 1992), which is exacerbated by a 60 per cent reduction in the levels of ascorbic acid in the frontal cortex in HIV disease (Everall et al., 1997). Platelet-activating factor (PAF) and arachidonic acid may also contribute to the pathogenic mechanism (reviewed by Griffin, 1998). PAF receptors in the nervous system are present at synapses, and PAF's effects include upregulation of TNF-α synthesis, release of glutamate, increases in intracellular calcium and death of neurones in tissue culture.

64.3 CORRELATION OF PRIMARY NEUROPATHOLOGICAL DAMAGE WITH ONSET OF HIV-RELATED COGNITIVE DISORDERS AND DEMENTIA

The pathogenesis of HIV-related cognitive impairments is not clear. When HIVE was first recognized it was thought that this may underlie cognitive deficits. However, Glass et al. (1993) found that less than 50 per cent of cases with known HIV-associated dementia during life had HIVE. In fact multinucleated giant cells, which are regarded as the histological hallmark of HIVE are poor indicators for dementia. The number of

macrophages and microglia correlate more closely with cognitive abnormalities (Glass et al., 1993, 1995). *In vitro* soluble factors secreted from peripheral blood macrophages of individuals with HIV dementia are far more toxic than those from symptom-free or uninfected individuals (Pulliam et al., 1996). These observations support the notion that macrophages and microglia are the site of toxin production resulting in neuronal damage and death.

Subtle cognitive impairments are accompanied by dendritic and synaptic damage, and this damage is also related to rising brain viral load (Masliah et al., 1997; Everall et al., 1998). In those who are developing dementia the severity correlates with particular neuronal populations. In mild HIV-associated dementia there is loss affecting large pyramidal neurones, and in those who have progressed to severe dementia the loss also affects small interneurones (Asare et al., 1996). The relationship between cognitive impairments and selective neuronal damage and loss provides insight into the pathogenic mechanism. The pyramidal neurones are likely to bear glutamate receptors and have low levels of calcium-binding proteins (Everall et al., 1995; Masliah et al., 1995), while the interneurones often express cytokines receptors (Masliah et al., 1996a) and high levels of calcium-binding proteins (Masliah et al., 1995). There is a significant decrease in the calcium-binding protein calbindin-immunoreactive pyramidal neurones and interneurones in the neocortex, which correlates with viral burden, while calbindin-positive neurones in the basal ganglia and hippocampus are unaffected (Masliah et al., 1995). Similarly, neocortical parvalbumin containing interneurones are not lost, while those in CA3 region of the hippocampus showed marked loss (Masliah et al., 1992c). In the basal ganglia, the calbindin-positive cells that appear to be resistant to neurodegeneration are gamma-aminobutyric acid (GABA) containing spiny cells (Wilson, 1990). These regional differences in the patterns of selective damage to neurones in the HIV-infected brain suggest different pathogenic mechanisms may be operating. In the neocortex neurones may be more vulnerable to HIV-1-mediated damage, e.g. gp120, tat etc., while in the hippocampus and basal ganglia cytokines might play a significant role.

There is indirect evidence to support the role of viral proteins in the pathogenesis of HIV-associated dementia. Gp120 administered to neonatal rats causes cognitive and motor impairments, and pathologically dystrophic dendritic changes of pyramidal neurones in all cortical areas and the development of behavioural retardation (Hill et al., 1993). In the cerebrospinal fluid of patients with AIDS and cognitive and motor abnormalities there are elevated levels of quinolinic acid (Heyes et al., 1991), an endogenous NMDA agonist, suggesting it is involved in excitotoxic-mediated neuronal damage.

64.4 CLINICAL FEATURES OF HIV-ASSOCIATED COGNITIVE IMPAIRMENTS

A variety of cognitive impairments can occur in HIV-infected individuals. They can be classified as follows (for review see

---

Box 64.1   *HIV-1 minor cognitive motor disorder (MCMD) (data from American Academy of Neurology AIDS Taskforce, 1991)*

Probable – must have each of the following:

1. Acquired cognitive/motor/behavioural abnormalities, verified by clinical history, neurological and neuropsychological examination
2. Mild impairment of ability to work or other activities of daily living
3. Not of sufficient degree to meet the criteria for HIV dementia or HIV myelopathy
4. No other aetiology

Possible – must have one of the following:

1. Conditions 1, 2 and 3 above are present but an alternative aetiology is present and the cause of condition 1 is not certain
2. Conditions 1, 2 and 3 above are present but the aetiology of condition 1 cannot be determined because of incomplete clinical evaluation

---

Box 64.2   *HIV-1 associated mild neurocognitive disorder (data from Grant and Atkinson, 1995)*

1. Acquired impairment in cognitive functioning, involving at least two ability domains in which the performance is at least 1 standard deviation below the mean for age-educated-appropriate norms on standardized neuropsychological tests. The neuropsychological assessment must survey at least the following abilities: verbal/language, attention/speeded processing, abstraction/executive, memory, complex perceptual-motor performance, motor skills
2. The cognitive impairment results in at least mild interference in daily functioning (at least on the following):
   - self-report of reduced mental acuity, inefficiency in work, homemaking or social functioning
   - observation by knowledgeable others that the individual has undergone at least mild decline in mental acuity, with resultant inefficiency in work, homemaking or social functioning
3. The cognitive impairment has been present for at least 1 month
4. The cognitive impairment does not meet criteria for delirium or dementia
5. There is no other pre-existing cause of the mild neurocognitive disorder

---

McArthur and Grant, 1998):

- *Neuropsychological deficit.* There is an abnormality on one cognitive domain during neuropsychological testing.
- *Neuropsychological impairment (NPI).* Here an individual has underperformed on two or more cognitive domains during neuropsychological testing.
- *HIV minor cognitive/motor disorder (MCMD).* This differs from the previous two categories in that the neurocognitive impairment is sufficient to affect day-to-day functioning at least in a mild degree. Confusingly, there are currently two sets of criteria for the diagnosis of MCMD. The American Academy of Neurology AIDS Taskforce (1991) developed the first criteria to recognize the disorder (Box 64.1), while the latter by Grant and Atkinson (1995) has a more detailed specification (Box 64.2).
- *HIV dementia.* There is marked cognitive impairment of sufficient degree to interfere markedly with activities of daily living.

64.4.1   Stage of onset of cognitive impairment

There have been various studies investigating when cognitive impairment or the more disabling dementia occur. However, study design has varied between investigations, which has hampered comparisons. White *et al.* (1995) reviewed 57 neuropsychological studies and summarized that 35 per cent of asymptomatically infected individuals had neuropsychological impairment, compared with 12 per cent in seronegative controls, and concluded that the more detailed the test battery the more likely to find impairment. However, Heaton

et al. (1994) showed that these preclinical abnormalities probably had a subtle effect on an individual's daily performance, as almost 27 per cent of those with neurocognitive abnormalities were unemployed compared with just under 10 per cent of asymptomatically infected individuals without impairment.

It is unclear whether these impairments remain static or worsen over time. In the Multicentre AIDS Cohort Study (MACS) Sacktor *et al.* (1996) showed that transient changes in neuropsychological function were relatively frequent, whereas sustained abnormalities only affected 15 per cent of asymptomatic individuals. Newman *et al.* (1995), in a meta-analysis of neuropsychological studies, identified four previous longitudinal studies in which neurocognitive decline had been observed. The HIV Neurobehavioural Research Center (HNRC) showed that over a 1-year period 2 per cent of those who were cognitively normal had developed MCMD, while 11 per cent of those who had had previous neurocognitive impairment deteriorated to MCMD (McArthur and Grant, 1998). The HNRC data also revealed that a number of individuals with neuropsychological impairment improved: 47 per cent became cognitively normal, while of those with MCMD 36 per cent improved to only mild impairment and a further 21 per cent became cognitively normal. These observations highlight the fact that cognitive impairments are not necessarily permanent or progressive.

64.4.2 Diagnostic criteria for HIV dementia

As with other dementias, HIV dementia is primarily a disorder of cognition in which the functions involved in processing new information, recalling information, and being able to perform the activities of daily living are severely curtailed. Additionally, there may also be concurrent problems of motor function and behavioural problems including personality change. During the description and definition of this new disease, four classification systems have evolved, they are:

- AIDS dementia complex (ADC) – described by Navia *et al.* (1986);
- HIV-associated dementia complex (HAD) – formulated by the American AIDS Neurology Taskforce (1991);
- HIV dementia – defined by Grant and Atkinson (1995);
- HIV-1-associated dementia – defined by the World Health Organization (1990).

The first to be described was ADC by Navia *et al.* in 1986. Importantly, this classification described the dementia as a 'complex' thus recognizing the triad of cognitive, motor and behavioural features. The ADC system also provided a rating scale from mild to severe ADC (Box 64.3). However, there is apparently equal importance given to all three features, so theoretically an individual could be diagnosed as having severe ADC because of marked motor abnormalities, such as inability to walk or incontinence, and not because of cognitive changes (Catalan, 1991).

This potential problem may have provided the impetus for another classification system. The American AIDS Neurology Taskforce (1991) set forward operational criteria for HIV-1 Associated Dementia Complex (HAD). This system restated cognitive changes as the core feature. Prominent motor changes in the absence of cognitive changes are termed HIV myelopathy. Cognitive impairment was to be newly acquired,

not constitutional, and they could not be explained by alternative aetiologies such as systemic illness, effects of medications or other drugs, or even other brain infections. Thus, it was highlighted that HAD was a diagnosis of exclusion. To this end a diagnosis of *possible* HAD could be applied if it was not possible to exclude other causes, because of incomplete clinical or investigative evaluation; or *probable* HAD if other causes were ruled out by clinical investigations (Box 64.4). The definitive diagnosis could only be confirmed if the brain itself could be examined microscopically, which is not possible during life. Grant and Atkinson (1995) have attempted to refine these operational criteria by stipulating the assessment of cognitive abnormalities.

The World Health Organization (1990) proposed the concept of HIV-1 associated dementia derived from the ICD-10 classification of dementia. This is reviewed by Catalan and Burgess (1996) who remark that this definition encompassed three broad areas. The first was the presence of recorded decline in memory and cognitive function for at least 1 month duration, the second was evidence of HIV-1 infection, and the third was the absence of other potential causes of the dementia. With these various classification systems in existence it would seem prudent to use those which offer the most consistent operational criteria for diagnosis of HIV dementia. The American Academy of Neurology AIDS Taskforce (1991) definition is gaining acceptance, as are the modifications

---

Box 64.3 *Classification of AIDS dementia complex (data from Price and Brew, 1988)*

Stage 0 (Normal): Normal mental and motor function

Stage 0.5 (Subclinical): Minimal or equivocal neurocognitive symptoms without impairment of work or activities of daily living (ADL)

Stage 1 (Mild): Definite impairment present, but able to perform all, but the more demanding aspects of work or ADL

Stage 2 (Moderate): Unable to work, but can perform basic activities of self-care, ambulatory but may require some assistance

Stage 3 (Severe): Major intellectual or motor impairment, cannot follow commands or sustain complex conversation, unable to walk without support

Stage 4 (End-stage): Nearly vegetative, rudimentary intellectual function, nearly mute, paraplegic, incontinent

---

Box 64.4 *Classification of HIV associated dementia complex (data from American Academy of Neurology AIDS Taskforce, 1991)*

Probable – must have each of the following:
1. Acquired abnormality in two or more cognitive domains, which have been present for a minimum of 1 month's duration, AND cognitive dysfunction of sufficient degree to impair activities of daily living and/or ability to work. **N.B.** These symptoms must not be attributable to systemic illness or other factors
2. Acquired abnormality in motor function as verified by clinical examination and/or neuropsychological tests, AND/OR decline in motivation, emotional control or change in social behaviour
3. Absence of clouding of consciousness
4. Exclusion, by various clinical and laboratory investigations of other potential aetiological causes, e.g. opportunistic central nervous system infections or neoplasm, systemic illness, psychiatric illness, treatment side effects and substance misuse

Possible – must have one of the following:
1. Conditions 1, 2 and 3 above are present, but an alternative aetiology is present and so the actual cause of 1 is not clear
2. Conditions 1, 2 and 3 above are present, but the aetiology of 1 is not clear owing to an incomplete clinical and laboratory investigation

proposed by Grant and Atkinson (1995) based upon the work carried out by the HIV Neurobehavioural Research Center (Heaton *et al.*, 1995; Box 64.5).

The variety of motor and behavioural changes that can occur can be varied and progressive. Motor changes may start with minor alterations such as the patient becoming more clumsy, including being more likely to trip up while walking and dropping things, as well as deteriorating handwriting. More serious changes include difficulty walking without assistance and falling over, to loss of power in the legs, paraplegia, and urinary and faecal incontinence. Behavioural changes can also be varied and broadly include changes in behaviour and the person's previous personality. Thus, some may become socially withdrawn apathetic, talking less or even mute. In this situation the presence of *depression*, or other treatable psychiatric conditions must be excluded. Other individuals can become disinhibited resulting in behaviour that can put them in vulnerable and potentially dangerous situations. Such disinhibition can be accompanied with features seen in *mania* with elevated or irritable mood, grandiosity, pressure of speech, flight of ideas and inappropriate behaviour. It is now recognized that mania can be a presenting feature of HIV-associated dementia. However, this is not clear cut as those who have either a past personal or family history of manic illness may develop a coincidental manic illness. Those individuals without this history are more likely to be developing mania in the setting of dementia (Lyketsos *et al.*, 1993, 1997). It is beginning to be recognized that some individuals continue with a predominantly manic type illness that is often difficult to control. Whether HIV-related mania becomes

recognized as a discrete disorder will only become clear by future research.

64.4.3 Epidemiology of HIV dementia

As early as 1983, Snider *et al.* recognized that individuals with AIDS could develop frank cognitive deficits, a disorder that they labelled subacute encephalopathy. Navia *et al.* (1986) further described the clinical features, applied the term AIDS dementia complex, and also realized that the dementia can occur as a first presenting feature of AIDS (Navia *et al.*, 1987). It is now accepted that HIV dementia is very rare in those with asymptomatic HIV infection, affecting less than 1 per cent. In 3 per cent of those who develop AIDS, dementia is the first AIDS-defining illness. While those with symptomatic HIV disease have a prevalence of 7–10 per cent, and in those with advanced HIV disease (AIDS) this rises to 15–20 per cent (McArthur *et al.*, 1993). It has been reported that, when dementia develops in those with less advanced immunodeficiency, the course is less rapid than in those with advanced disease (Bouwman *et al.*, 1996). There is less consistency in reporting the incidence of HIV dementia. Day *et al.* (1992) observed an annual incidence of 14 per cent in symptomatically infected individuals, compared with 7 per cent by McArthur *et al.* (1993), and 9 per cent in a study from Edinburgh (Pretsell *et al.*, 1996). Dore *et al.* (1999) reported that, although AIDS dementia complex reduced with the introduction of HAART, the reduction was less marked compared with other AIDS-defining illnesses.

The incidence and prevalence of HIV dementia have been effected by the introduction of antiretroviral therapy. After the introduction of azidothymidine (AZT) a decline in the frequency of the dementia was reported (Portegies *et al.*, 1989; Chiesi *et al.*, 1990), while the MACS were not able to demonstrate an neuroprotective effect (Day *et al.*, 1992; McArthur *et al.*, 1993; Bacellar *et al.*, 1994). It is possible that this discrepancy is in part explained by a dose effect. Following its introduction AZT was used at a high dose of 1200–1500 mg/day, compared with the current daily dose of 500–600 mg. It is possible that this lower dose is suboptimal. However, this issue has now been complicated by the recent arrival within the last 2 years of the new generation of antiretroviral agents. The issue of treatment for HIV dementia will be discussed below. The introduction of HAART has resulted in a reduction of HIV-associated dementia; however, the prevalence rate is increasing as the number of HIV patients survive longer.

64.4.4 Risk factors for dementia

Wang *et al.* (1995) reported a higher risk of dementia in those of increasing age, following the diagnosis of AIDS, and intravenous drug use. Similarly data from the MACS (McArthur *et al.*, 1993) revealed several variables: lower haemoglobin up to 6 months prior to the onset of AIDS, lower body mass up to 6 months prior to the onset of AIDS, more constitutional

---

Box 64.5   *HIV-1-associated dementia (data from Heaton* et al.*, 1995)*

1. Marked acquired impairment in cognitive functioning, involving at least two ability domains (e.g. memory, attention): typically the impairment is in multiple domains, especially in learning of new information, slowed information processing, and defective attention/concentration. The cognitive impairment can be ascertained by history, mental status examination, or neuropsychological testing
2. The cognitive impairment produces marked interference with day-to-day functioning (work, home life, social activities)
3. The marked cognitive impairment has been present for at least 1 month. The pattern of cognitive impairment does not meet criteria for delirium (i.e. clouding of consciousness is not a prominent feature); or, if delirium is present, criteria for dementia had been met on a prior examination before delirium was present
4. There is no evidence of another pre-existing aetiology that could explain the dementia, e.g. CNS infection or neoplasm, cerebrovascular disease, coincidental neurological disease, substance misuse, etc.

symptoms up to 12 months before the onset of AIDS, and older age of onset of AIDS. However, specific AIDS indicator illnesses, use of AZT before AIDS, and CD4 count before AIDS were not significant indicators.

64.5 CLINICAL AND LABORATORY INVESTIGATION OF HIV DEMENTIA

As stated previously, HIV dementia is a diagnosis of exclusion, in which other potential aetiologies are ruled out. Typically, three groups of investigations can be performed: neuropsychological testing, neuroimaging, and examination of the CSF. These will be briefly outlined below.

64.5.1 Neuropsychological testing

This should be performed in conjunction with the neurological examination, and is useful in assessing both the severity and pattern of cognitive impairment. HIV dementia has the clinical features typical of a 'subcortical dementia' with abnormalities on information processing speed, motor speed, attentional set shifting and new information acquisition. By contrast the usual features of a 'cortical dementia', such as accelerated forgetting, intrusion errors, naming problems and constructional dyspraxia, are uncommon. It must be remembered that the division of 'subcortical' and 'cortical' dementias is descriptive of a constellation of clinical symptoms and does not mean that in the former there are no cortical neuropathological lesions and in the latter no subcortical pathology.

There is no correct approach to which battery of neuropsychological tests are performed. McArthur and Grant (1998) stated general guidelines that the tests should be sensitive to a wide range of impairments, robust to the effect of serial repetition, sensitive to known abnormalities in HIV dementia, and the length of the battery kept as short as is feasible. The confounding effects of age, years of education, and culture are beyond the scope of this chapter, but they add to the complexity of this area so that development and implementation of neuropsychological testing remains confined to expert neuropsychologists. Both the MACS (Selnes and Miller, 1994) and the HNRC (Heaton et al., 1995) study groups have comprehensive test batteries, with modified, shorter or 'step-down' versions for those who are too ill or cognitively impaired to complete the full test battery. The respective test batteries are outlined in Box 64.6 and Table 64.3.

In the absence of access to a psychologist to perform neuropsychological testing, quick and easy to apply bedside tests have been suggested. One of the most widely used bedside tests is the Mini-Mental State Examination (MMSE). However, it is limited in the assessment of HIV-infected individuals as it does not have timed tests, which is important in a disorder with motor/psychomotor slowing. This has recently been addressed by Power et al. (1995), who modified the MMSE to encompass timed tasks (Table 64.4). It can be administered in about 5 minutes.

Box 64.6 *Neuropsychological Battery of Multicentre AIDS Cohort Study (MACS)*

Trail Making Tests A and B
- Grooved Pegboard — Dominant and non-dominant hands
- Symbol Digit Modalities — Raw score and paired recall
- Rey Auditory Verbal Learning Test — Trails 1 to 5, interference, recall after interference, delayed recall, delayed recognition
- Rey–Osterreith Complex Figure Test Copy — Immediate recall
- Stroop Color Interference test — Delayed recall
- California Computerized Assessment Package — Simple reaction time
- Choice reaction time
- Serial pattern matching (sequential reaction time)

Table 64.3 *Neuropsychological Battery of the HNRC*

Neuropsychological test	Domain tested
Boston Naming Test	Verbal
Thurstone Word Fluency (written)	Verbal
Letter and Category Fluency (oral)	Verbal
Category Test	Executive function
Trail Making Test	Executive function
Story Memory Test	Learning, memory
California Verbal Learning Test	Learning, memory
Figure Memory Test	Learning, memory
WAIS-R Digit Span	Attention/information processing speed
WAIS-R Arithmetic	Attention/information processing speed
Paced Auditory	Attention/information processing speed
Serial Addition Test	Attention/information processing speed
WAIS-R Block Design	Complex perceptual motor skills
WAIS-R Digit Symbol	Complex perceptual motor skills
Grooved Pegboard	Motor skills
Finger Tapping	Motor skills
Sensory Perceptual Examination	Sensory-perceptual skills
Estimates of Premorbid IQ	
National Adult Reading Test	
WAIS-R Vocabulary	
Mood Scales	
Beck Depression Inventory	
Profile of Mood States	
Speilberger State-Trail Anxiety Inventory	
Assessment of Everyday Functioning	
Patient's Assessment of Own Functioning Inventory	
Employment Questionnaire	

Table 64.4   *HIV Dementia Rating Scale (data from Power et al., 1995)*

Maximum score on each test	Test score achieved	Domain tested
4		**Memory – Registration** Give four words to recall (dog, hat, green peach) – 1 second to say each. Then ask patient to repeat all four words after you have said them
6		**Attention** Antisaccadic eye movements:* 20 commands ____errors of 20 trials $\leqslant$3 errors = 4; 4 errors = 3; 5 errors = 2; 6 errors = 1; >6 errors = 0
4		**Psychomotor speed** Ask patient to write the alphabet (uppercase letters) horizontally across the page, and record the time taken: ____seconds $\leqslant$21 s = 6; 21.1–24 s = 5; 24.1–27 s = 4; 27.1–30 s = 3; 30.1–33 s = 2; 33.1–36 secs = 1; >36 s = 0
Give one point for each correct remembered word. For words not recalled, prompt with a 'semantic' clue, as follows: animal (dog), piece of clothing (hat), colour (green), fruit (peach). Give ½ point for each correct response after prompting		**Memory – Recall** Ask patient to repeat the four words from the **Memory – Registration** above
2		**Construction** Ask patient to copy the cube below, and record the time taken: ___seconds <25 s = 2; 5–35 s = 1; >35 s = 0
Total score: ___ /16		A score of <10 is used as the cut-off for indicating the presence of HIV-associated dementia

* Ask the patient to initially focus on the examiner's nose, and then to look to and from the examiner's moving index finger and nose. This is done with alternating hands, with the examiner's hands held at the patient's shoulder width and eye height. When the patient is comfortable looking at the finger that moved, he/she is asked to look at the index finger not moving. The task is practised until the patient is familiar with the task. The patient is then asked to perform 20 serial antisaccades. An error is noted if the patient looked towards the finger that moved

64.5.2 Neuroimaging investigations

Computed tomography (CT) and magnetic resonance imaging (MRI) scans can detect atrophy, which is more often ventricular but can affect sulci. MRI is the more sensitive imaging modality. T2-weighted images are sensitive to oedematous changes, such as the bilateral diffuse white matter hyperintensities that can be observed throughout the cortical white matter. While T1-weighted images can detect anatomical changes such as atrophy. These changes can occasionally be observed in asymptomatic individuals but are more common in those with symptomatic disease and dementia. Focal changes or mass effects are more consistent with the presence of opportunistic infections or a tumour.

Single photon emission computed tomography (SPECT) perfusion studies with HMPAO (Tc^{99}m-hexamethylpropyleneamine oxine) can show multiple scattered perfusion deficits, though the specificity of this observation is low as many conditions can produce a similar picture. Positron emission tomography (PET) have shown changes in regional metabolic rates for glucose, especially in the prefrontal area in asymptomatical infected individuals compared with seronegative individuals (Pascal *et al.*, 1991). In those with AIDS, hypermetabolism in the basal ganglia and thalamus has been reported (van Gorp *et al.*, 1992), and increasingly hypometabolism with worsening HIV dementia has been noted (van Gorp *et al.*, 1992). Interestingly an increase in regional cerebral blood volume in the basal ganglia in HIV-infected individuals has been observed using functional MRI (Gonzalez *et al.*, 1998).

Proton magnetic resonance spectroscopy (MRS) studies have demonstrated a global reduction in *N*-acetylaspartate (NAA), which is a neuronal marker (Salvan *et al.*, 1997), and an in increase in choline, a cell membrane component, in

HIV dementia (Chong *et al.*, 1993, 1994). Phosphorus-MRS has also revealed lower ATP/inorganic phosphate ratios in asymptomatical infected individuals (Deicken *et al.*, 1991). All of these findings support the notion of metabolic dysfunction during HIV infection, which worsens with deteriorating cognitive function. However, the specificity and sensitivity of these observations is still unclear.

64.5.3 Examination of the CSF

Assessment of the CSF is useful for excluding opportunistic infections and clarifying abnormalities associated with HIV infection. The latter include pleiocytosis, the presence of both viral antibodies and antigen (p24, a core protein), raised cytokine levels, such as TNF-α, IL-1β and -6; and the MHC I associated protein β$_2$-microglobulin. Our understanding of the relationship between these factors and disease progression is not clear, except that it has been reported that in the absence of opportunistic infections a raised β$_2$-microglobulin supports a diagnosis of HIV-associated dementia (Brew *et al.*, 1992).

In the last few years CSF viral RNA has also been assessed, allowing the relationship between viral load and cognitive performance to be examined. CSF viral RNA levels have been observed to rise over time in otherwise healthy infected individuals studied over a 3-year period (Gisslen *et al.*, 1998). This was not accompanied by a similar rise in serum levels, which appear to be associated with clinical disease progression. CSF viral RNA levels are influenced by the number of mononuclear cells in the CSF (Martin *et al.*, 1998). Furthermore, higher levels of CSF HIV-1 RNA are associated neuropathologically with the presence of HIV encephalitis. The severity of the encephalitis, as rated by increasing numbers of microglia, correlates with increasing viral load (Cinque *et al.*, 1998). However, no correlation was observed between CSF viral load and assumed HIV encephalitis in living patients using radiological and other laboratory markers (Bossi *et al.*, 1998). This may indicate the unreliability of these investigations in accurately predicting underlying brain pathology.

Generally it has been found that CSF viral load is high in patients with a range of AIDS-related neurological disorders (DiStefano *et al.*, 1998). Ellis *et al.* (1997) have found that in asymptomatical infected individuals the viral load in the CSF is correlated with plasma viral load, while in symptomatic disease the CSF viral load was noted to be higher in those with neuropsychological impairments. Similarly, the CSF viral load was found to be higher in individuals with dementia and to correlate with the severity of dementia (Brew and Portegies, 1997; McArthur *et al.*, 1997; McCutchan *et al.*, 1997).

64.6 TREATMENT OF HIV DEMENTIA

The synaptic and dendritic abnormalities, which occur before the onset of obvious neuronal loss and correlate with the onset of mild cognitive deficits, are potentially reversible.

Table 64.5 *Antiretroviral agents*

Initial designation	Drug name	Proprietary name
Nucleoside reverse transcriptase inhibitors		
Azidothymidine (AZT)	Zidovudine (ZDV)	Retrovir
3TC	Lamivudine	Epivir
ddI	Didanosine	Videx
ddC	Zalcitabine	Hivid
d4T	Stavudine	Zerit
AZT and 3Tc		Combivir
Adefovir*		
Non-nucleoside reverse transcriptase inhibitors		
DMP 266**	Efavirenz	Stocrin
	Nevaripine	Viramune
	Delavirdine**	Rescriptor
Protease inhibitors		
141W94*	Amprenavir	
	Nelfinavir	Viracept
	Saquinavir	Fortavase
	Ritonavir	Norvir
	Indinavir	Crixavan

* Currently undergoing Phase III Clinical Trials in UK
** Available on open-label expanded access

This has relevance to the advent of a new generation of antiretroviral agents, including the use of protease inhibitors, and the introduction of plasma viral load testing to monitor response to treatment. There are three group of agents: nucleoside reverse transcriptase inhibitors, non-nucleoside reverse transcriptase inhibitors, and protease inhibitors. A list of these agents is presented in Table 64.5. Ideally an antiretroviral agent will fully penetrate all tissue compartments of the body including the central nervous system, and be 100 per cent effective in suppressing viral replication, which in turn will alleviate viral persistence and the emergence of resistant strains. No single agent is totally effective, hence the establishment of combination therapy, which, if it incorporates a protease inhibitor or at least three agents, is termed HAART.

64.6.1 Central nervous system penetration of antiretrovirals

In animal models it has been shown that AZT can pass into the brain passively by diffusion (Thomas and Segal, 1997), and that both AZT and d4T (stavudine) rapidly distribute, probably passively, within the central nervous system following intravenous administration (Yang *et al.*, 1997). The ratio of brain to plasma concentrations was higher for d4T and the drugs did not interfere with one another. Nevirapine has been demonstrated to cross an experimental bovine blood–brain barrier model (Glynn and Yazdanian, 1997). In the human brain AZT has been demonstrated in individuals who died of AIDS (Artigas *et al.*, 1991). However, theoretical models to calculate drug levels in the human brain indicate that clinically effective doses may not be achieved (Groothius and Levy,

1997), although clinical response is apparently at variance with this.

More information is available with regard to CSF penetration, which is taken to be a marker for entry into the brain. Brew and Portegies (1997) and Portegies and Rosenberg (1998) have summarized information regarding a number of anti-retroviral agents. Of the nucleoside reverse transcriptase inhibitors, AZT has a steady state CSF level of 0.3 μM following an oral dose of 200 mg, although the CSF concentration of AZT is independent of dose (Burger et al., 1993); d4T has a concentration of 0.24 μM and 3TC 0.28 μM, while didanosine (ddI) and zalcitabine (ddC) are lower at 0.17 μM and 0.01 μM respectively. As no brain penetration data are available on these latter two agents, the low CSF levels suggest that they may not be as effective as AZT and d4T. In our own studies we assessed the direct effects of AZT, d4T and abacavir (ABC) on brain cells with the aid of a human brain aggregate model infected with an HIV-1 macrophage tropic strain. We observed neuroprotection and a reduction in astrocyte proliferation by all three agents, whereas the rate of decrease in viral replication was superior with d4T (Kandanearatchi et al., 2002a, b, 2004). Peripheral neuropathy is a dose-dependent complication of both d4T and ddC, especially in individuals with advanced HIV disease. The new agent ABC is also known to penetrate the CSF.

With regard to the non-nucleoside reverse transcriptase inhibitors no CSF concentrations are currently available though the CSF to serum ratio for nevaripine is stated to be 0.45. A protease inhibitor such as indinavir, even though highly protein bound, is present in the CSF at a level of 0.23 μM (Stahle et al., 1997). Saquinavir CSF concentrations are very low, and there are no reports for ritonavir. In a bovine microvascular model the permeability was highest for ampre-navir (141W94), followed by indinavir and then saquinavir (Glynn and Yazdanian, 1998). Saquinavir was a substrate for the p-glycoprotein efflux pump, which may explain the poor results seen with this drug, and possibly other protease inhibitors, in penetrating the central nervous system.

There are a number of antiretroviral drugs that are still at developmental stages or in clinical trials and their potential therapeutic effects in the central nervous system is yet to be evaluated. These include entry inhibitors (T20, PRO 542) targeted to prevent binding of gp120 to CD4 receptor (More and Doms, 2003). Other forms of treatment strategies include vaccines for the prevention of persistent infection or to control infection.

64.6.2 Antiviral therapy and CSF viral load

It is known that AZT reduces CSF levels of viral antigen and β_2-microglobulin levels (Royal et al., 1994). Now it is becoming clear that initiation of combination antiretroviral therapy can have a dramatic effect on viral RNA load in the CSF. HIV RNA was undetectable after approximately 5 months treatments in 10 patients, eight of whom were taking a protease inhibitor, and seven were taking AZT, and three d4T (Gisslen

et al., 1997). Sereni et al. (1998) have observed similar findings in nine individuals taking a combination of amprenavir, AZT and 3TC for up to 32 weeks. McArthur et al. (1998) assessed HAART in 36 HIV-infected individuals and found undetectable levels in the CSF at 3 months, but at 6 months 50 per cent of the subjects showed a rise in both plasma and CSF viral load, indicating 'escape' from therapeutic control of viral replication. Ellis et al. (1998) by serial examination of the CSF in five patients noted a decline in viral load but that it was slower than in the plasma. A one log drop in viral load took a mean of 4 days in plasma and 20 days in the CSF.

While combination therapy has a significant impact on viral load in the CSF, the issue of whether a protease inhibitor or which composition of the combination of antiretroviral agents is superior in terms of duration of the effective suppression of viral replication is still to be clarified. Nevertheless, as higher CSF viral loads are associated with deteriorating cognitive performance, the ability to reduce CSF viral replication is an important marker in preventing or treating HIV-related cognitive disorder.

64.6.3 Effect of therapy on cognitive symptoms

AZT is the only agent that has been assessed on its own. In individuals without neurological problems it was found that after 1 year's AZT 500 mg/day treatment electrophysiological event-related potentials (EVP) were maintained within normal limits, whereas in an untreated group they became prolonged (Evers et al., 1998). Prolongation of EVPs has been proposed as a possible early marker for HIV-associated dementia. There have been a few studies demonstrating that AZT protects against the development of HIV-associated dementia (Portegies et al., 1989; Chiesi et al., 1996). For the treatment of HIV-related cognitive dysfunction and dementia there have been a number of studies demonstrating the efficacy of AZT in improving neurological and cognitive status (Yarchoan et al., 1987; Schmitt et al., 1988; Portegies et al., 1993). However, reports are conflicting as to the optimal dose, with some investigators reporting greater improvement with high doses: 800–1200 mg/day in the Nordic Medical Research Council's HIV Therapy trial (1992), and 2000 mg/day in the Sidtis et al. study (1993), while others suggested that levels as low as 500 mg/day can be effective (Tozzi et al., 1993). Benefits of AZT are not permanent and symptoms tend to reappear after 6–12 months of therapy. There is little evidence available for other antiretroviral agents as monotherapy. Didanosine was not observed to have a significant effect in protecting against the development of HIV-related cognitive impairment (Darbyshire and Aboulker, 1992). Atervirdine, in a small pilot study of five individuals with HIV-associated dementia, produced improvement in four (Brew et al., 1996).

Attention is now on the effectiveness of combination antiretroviral therapy in preventing and treating HIV-associated cognitive impairments and dementia. Evidence is now being gathered that the inclusion of a protease inhibitor into the combination may be even more beneficial. Galgani *et al.* (1998) showed that individuals taking a protease inhibitor and two nucleoside analogues (AZT and ddI, AZT and ddC, AZT and d4T) had less neurological impairment than those just taking two nucleoside analogues. Tozzi *et al.* (1999) also reported that combination of two nucleoside analogue with one protease inhibitor improved minor cognitive motor disorder. Similarly, Sacktor *et al.* (1998) found that HAART was superior than combination therapy without a protease inhibitor in improving various measures of neuropsychological performance. Suarez *et al.* (2001) confirmed these results by reporting that HAART improved subcortical cognitive functions. A proton MRS study on HIV-infected patients with cognitive and motor dysfunctions showing cerebral metabolite abnormalities were found to improve following HAART treatment (Chang *et al.*, 1999). However, as stated previously Dore *et al.* (1999) reported that, although AIDS dementia complex declined with the introduction of HAART, this decline was less marked compared with other AIDS-defining illnesses. There was also an increase in CD4 cell count at diagnosis of ADC at the beginning of HAART. They concluded that HAART produced less protection against ADC compared with ADI. Combination therapies, including HAART, are exciting and powerful treatment options but studies have yet to establish which combinations are the most effectives. Factors such as brain and CSF penetration, the combined agents' ability to reduce viral load and the development of viral resistance and mutations will all have to be taken into account when therapeutic management is planned.

64.6.4 Adjunctive therapy

A variety of therapeutic strategies have been proposed in addition to antiretroviral therapy for treatment of HIV dementia. These are based on interfering with the known mechanism of HIV-related cellular brain pathology. For instance, calcium channel antagonist agents, such as nimodipine, can block the excitotoxic gp120-mediated calcium current *in vitro*, and similarly it has been proposed that memantine can be used to block the glutamate channel. Furthermore, pentoxifylline has been proposed as a TNF-α antagonist. However, to date clinical trials on memantine and pentoxifylline are either still in progress or the results are not widely known. Other forms of protection includes the blocking of signalling pathways such as the wnt signalling pathway with the regulation of GSK-3β. Both lithium and fibroblast growth factor 1 (FGF1) were observed to be neuroprotective against HIV-1 gp120 by regulating GSK-3β (Everall *et al.*, 2001, 2002).

64.7 TREATMENT OF MOTOR AND BEHAVIOURAL PROBLEMS

In assessing potential HIV-associated cognitive impairments, it is important to recognize and treat and comorbid psychiatric conditions such as hypomania, depression or anxiety.

64.7.1 Motor problems

These are often problems with mobility or incontinence, which may be important in planning a care package to maintain independence. Assisted care by providing a carer for a number of hours per week may be necessary, even if the person has a partner/carer, in order to relieve the burden of care. Similarly a buddy, a volunteer from a HIV voluntary agency, may be appropriate if the person is socially isolated. If high levels of care are needed then regular respite care at a residential unit may be useful, if acceptable to the person concerned. This will provide a break from care, and help prevent stress amongst carers, hopefully allowing community care to continue for longer.

64.7.2 Behavioural and psychological problems

As outlined above, behavioural and psychological problems can sometimes be the first presenting symptoms of a developing dementia and require thorough psychiatric and neurological evaluation. Hypomania will usually require medication with antipsychotic agents. As a general rule these should be given initially at low doses and titrated up as required to improve the mental state. Use of two or more antipsychotics should be avoided and vigilance for the development of side effects including extrapyramidal side effects should be maintained. The possibility of drug interactions may be increased as the patient is often taking multiple medications, and onset of neuroleptic malignant syndrome should be borne in mind if the patient's physical health deteriorates without other cause apparent. Depression can occasionally develop in individuals with cognitive impairments, especially if they have insight in to their condition. In this situation the depression requires a through assessment and appropriate management with antidepressant medication, supportive psychotherapy, or both.

Depending on symptom severity the patient may be cared for in the community or may require inpatient admission, including compulsory detention under (in the UK) the Mental Health Act 1983. Close liaison between medical and mental health teams with planning of nursing care plans should identify which is the optimal setting (medical or psychiatric) for assessment and treatment, and minimize the possibility of transfer between medical and psychiatric wards. This is often distressing to the patient and adversely affects their response to treatment.

64.8 PROGNOSIS OF HIV DEMENTIA

The prognosis is currently unclear. It is known that without treatment, as occurred in earlier years, the survival rate was very poor with progression from mild to severe dementia occurring within a few months, while those with severe dementia often died within weeks or a few months. However, the use of combination antiretroviral therapy appears to have significantly improved prognosis although, until longer term studies with the new therapies have been fully assessed, their full impact is difficult to determine.

REFERENCES

Albright AV, Strizki J, Harouse JM, Lavi E, O'Connor M, Gonzalez-Scarano F. (1996) HIV-1 infection of cultured human adult oligodendrocytes. *Virology* **217**: 211–219

American Academy of Neurology AIDS Taskforce. (1991) Nomenclature and research case definitions for neurologic manifestations of HIV-1 infection. *Neurology* **41**: 778–785

Artigas J, Arasteh K, Averdunk R *et al*. (1991) Hyaline globules reacting positively with zidovudine antibody in brain and spinal cord of AIDS patients. *Lancet* **337**: 1127–1128

Asare E, Dunn G, Glass J *et al*. (1996) Neuronal pattern correlates with the severity of human immunodeficiency virus-associated dementia complex. Usefulness of spatial pattern analysis in clinicopathological studies. *American Journal of Pathology* **148**: 31–38

Bacellar H, Munoz A, Miller E *et al*. (1994) Temporal trends in the incidence of HIV-1-related neurological diseases: multi-center AIDS cohort study. *Neurology* **44**: 1892–1900

Bagasra O, Lavi E, Bobroski L *et al*. (1996) Cellular reservoirs of HIV-1 in the central nervous system of infected individuals: identification by the combination of in situ polymerase chain reaction and immunohistochemistry. *AIDS* **10**: 573–585

Bossi P, Dupin N, Coutellier A *et al*. (1998) The level of human immunodeficiency virus (HIV) type 1 RNA in the cerebrospinal fluid as a marker of HIV encephalitis. *Clinical Infectious Diseases* **26**: 1072–1073

Bouwman F, Skolasky R, Dal Pan G, Glass J, Selnes OA, McArthur JC. (1996) Variation in clinical progression of HIV-associated dementia. XIth International Conference on AIDS, Vancouver, BC

Brenneman DE, Westbrook GL, Fitzgerald SP *et al*. (1988) Neuronal cell killing by the envelope protein of HIV and its prevention by vasoactive intestinal peptide. *Nature* **335**: 639–642

Brew B and Portegies P. (1997) *A Practical Guide to the Pathogenesis and Treatment of HIV CNS Infection*. London, International Medical Press

Brew BJ, Bhalla R, Paul M *et al*. (1992) Cerebrospinal fluid β2-microglobulin in patients with AIDS dementia complex: an expanded series, including response to zidovudine treatment. *AIDS* **6**: 461–465

Brew B, Dunbar N, Druett JA, Freun J, Ward P. (1996) Pilot study of the efficacy of atevirdine in the treatment of AIDS dementia. *AIDS* **10**: 1357–1360

Budka H. (1990) Human immunodeficiency virus (HIV)-induced disease of the central nervous system: pathology and implications for pathogenesis. *Acta Neuropathologica* **77**: 225–236

Budka H. (1991) Neuropathology of human immunodeficiency virus infection. *Brain Pathology* **1**: 163–175

Budka H. (1998) HIV-Associated neuropathology. In: HE Gendelman, SA Lipton, L Epstein, S Swindells (eds), *The Neurology of AIDS*. Chapman and Hall, New York, pp. 241–260

Burger DM, Kraaijeveld CL, Meenhorst PL *et al*. (1993) Penetration of zidovudine into the cerebrospinal fluid of patients with HIV. *AIDS* **7**: 1581–1587

Canki M, Thai JN, Chao W, Ghorparde A, Potash MJ, Volsky DJ. (2001) Highly productive infection with pseudotyped human immunodeficiency virus type 1 (HIV-1) indicates no intracellular restrictions to HIV-1 replication in primary human astrocytes. *Journal of Virology* **75**: 7925–7933

Catalan J. (1991) HIV-associated dementia: review of some conceptual and terminological problems. *International Review of Psychiatry* **3**: 321–330

Catalan J and Burgess A. (1996) HIV associated dementia and related disorders. *International Review of Psychiatry* **8**: 237–244

Centers for Disease Control. (1987) Revision of the CDC surveillance case definition for acquired immunodeficiency syndrome. *Morbidity and Mortality Weekly Reports* **36**: 3S–14S

Chang L, Ernst T, Leonido-Yee M *et al*. (1999) Highly active antiretroviral therapy reverses brain metabolite abnormalities in mild HIV dementia. *Neurology* **53**: 782–789

Chiesi A, Agresti MG, Dally LG *et al*. (1990) Decrease in notifications of AIDS dementia complex in 1989–1990 in Italy: possible role of the early treatment with zidovudine. *Medicina* **10**: 415–416

Chiesi A, Vella S, Dally LG *et al*. (1996) Epidemiology of AIDS dementia complex in Europe. AIDS in Europe Study Group. *Journal of Acquired-Immune-Deficiency Syndromes and Human Retrovirology* **11**: 39–44

Chong WK, Sweeny B, Wilkinson ID. (1993) Proton spectroscopy of the brain in HIV infections: correlation with clinical, immunologic and MRI findings. *Radiology* **188**: 119–124

Chong WK, Paley M, Wilkinson ID *et al*. (1994) Localized cerebral proton MR spectroscopy in HIV infection and AIDS. *American Journal of Neuroradiology* **15**: 21–25

Cinque P, Vago L, Ceresa D *et al*. (1998) Cerebrospinal fluid HIV-1 RNA levels: correlation with HIV encephalitis. *AIDS* **12**: 389–394

Cohen BA and Berger JR. (1998) Neurologic opportunistic infections in AIDS. In: HE Gendelman, SA Lipton, L Epstein, S Swindells (eds), *The Neurology of AIDS*. New York, Chapman and Hall, pp. 303–332

Cordonnier A, Montagnier L, Emerman M. (1989) Single amino-acid changes in HIV envelope affect viral tropism and receptor binding. *Nature* **340**: 571–574

Darbyshire JH and Aboulker J-P. (1992) Didanosine for zidovudine-intolerant patients with HIV disease. *Lancet* **340**: 1346–1347

Davies J, Everall IP, Weich S, McLaughlin J, Scaravilli F, Lantos PL. (1997) HIV-associated brain pathology in the United Kingdom: an epidemiological study. *AIDS* **11**: 1145–1150

Davies J, Everall IP, Weich S *et al*. (1998) HIV-associated brain pathology: a comparative international study. *Neuropathology and Applied Neurobiology* **24**: 118–124

Dawson TM, Dawson VL, Snyder SH. (1994) Molecular mechanisms of nitric oxide actions in the brain. *Annals of the New York Academy of Sciences* **738**: 76–85

Day JJ, Grant I, Atkinson JH *et al*. (1992) Incidence of AIDS dementia in a two-year follow-up of AIDS and ARC patients on an initial Phase II AZT placebo-controlled study: San Diego cohort. *Journal of Neuropsychiatry* **4**: 15–20

Deicken RF, Hubesch B, Jensen PC *et al*. (1991) Alterations in brain phosphate metabolic concentrations in patients with human immunodeficiency virus infection. *Archives of Neurology* **49**: 203–209

Dimitrov DS. (1997) How do viruses enter cells? The HIV coreceptors teach us a lesson of complexity. *Cell* **91**: 721–730

DiStefano M, Monno L, Fiore *et al*. (1998) Neurological disorders during HIV-1 infection correlate with viral load in cerebrospinal fluid but not with virus phenotype. *AIDS* **12**: 737–743

Donaldson YK, Bell JE, Ironside JW *et al.* (1994) Redistribution of HIV outside the lymphoid system with onset of AIDS. *Lancet* **343**: 382–385

Dore GJ, Correll PK, Li Y, Kaldor JM, Cooper DA, Brew BJ. (1999) Changes in AIDS dementia complex in the era of highly active antiretroviral therapy. *AIDS* **13**: 1249–1253

Dreyer EB, Kaiser PK, Offermann JT, Lipton SA. (1990) HIV-1 coat protein neurotoxicity prevented by calcium channel antagonists. *Science* **248**: 364–367

Dugas N, Lacroix C, Kilchherr E, Defraissy JF, Tardieu M. (2001) Role of CD23 in astrocytes inflammatory reaction during HIV-1 related encephalitis. *Cytokine* **15**: 96–107

Ellis RJ, Hsia K, Spector SA *et al.* (1997) Cerebrospinal fluid human immunodeficiency virus type 1 RNA levels are elevated in neurocognitively impaired individuals with acquired immunodeficiency syndrome. HIV Neurobehavioural Research Center Group. *Annals of Neurology* **42**: 679–688

Ellis RJ, Spector SA, Hsia K *et al.* for the HNRC Group. (1998) HIV-1 viral dynamics differ in cerebrospinal fluid and plasma. 5th Conference on Retroviruses and Opportunistic Infections, Chicago, Abstract 453

Everall IP. (1995) Neuropsychiatric aspects of HIV infection. *Journal of Neurology, Neurosurgery, and Psychiatry* **58**: 399–402

Everall IP and Lantos PL. (1991) The neuropathology of HIV disease. *International Review of Psychiatry* **3**: 307–320

Everall IP, Luthert PJ, Lantos PL. (1991) Neuronal loss in the frontal cortex in HIV infected individuals. *Lancet* **337**: 1119–1121

Everall I, Gray F, Barnes H, Durigon M, Luthert P, Lantos P. (1992) Neuronal loss in symptom-free HIV infection. *Lancet* **340**: 1413

Everall IP, Luthert PJ, Lantos PL. (1993) Neuronal number and volume alterations in the neocortex of HIV infected individuals. *Journal of Neurology, Neurosurgery, and Psychiatry* **56**: 481–486

Everall IP, Hudson L, Al-Sarraj S, Honavar M, Lantos P, Kerwin R. (1995) Decreased expression of AMPA receptor messenger RNA and protein in AIDS: a model for HIV-associated neurotoxicity. *Nature Medicine* **1**: 1174–1178

Everall IP, Hudson L, Kerwin RW. (1997) Decreased absolute levels of ascorbic acid and unaltered vasoactive intestinal polypeptide receptor binding in the frontal cortex in acquired immunodeficiency syndrome. *Neuroscience Letters* **224**: 119–122

Everall IP, Heaton RK, Marcotte TD *et al.* for the HNRC Group. (1998) Cortical synaptic density is reduced in mild to moderate human immunodeficiency virus neurocognitive disorder. *Brain Pathology* **9**: 209–217

Everall IP, Trillo-Pazos G, Bell C, Mallory M, Sanders V, Masliah E. (2001) Amelioration of neurotoxic effects of HIV envelope protein gp120 by fibroblast growth factor: a strategy for neuroprotection. *Journal Neuropathology and Experimental Neurology* **60**: 293–301

Everall P, Bell C, Mallory M *et al.* (2002) Lithium ameliorates HIV-gp120 mediated neurotoxicity. *Molecular and Cellular Neuroscience* **21**: 493–501

Evers S, Grotmeyer KH, Reichelt D, Luttmann S, Husstedt IW. (1998) Impact of antiretroviral treatment on AIDS dementia: a longitudinal prospective event-related potential study. *Journal of Acquired Immune Deficiency Syndromes and Human Retrovirology* **17**: 143–148

Floyd RA and Carney JM. (1992) Free radical damage to protein and DNA: mechanisms involved and relevant observations on brain undergoing oxidative stress. *Annals of Neurology* **32** (Suppl.): S22–S27

Galey D, Becker K, Haughey N *et al.* (2003) Differential transcriptional regulation by human immunodeficiency virus type 1 and gp120 in human astrocytes. *Journal of Neurovirology* **9**: 358–371

Galgani S, Balestra P, Tozzi V, Ferri F, D'Amato C. (1998) Comparison of efficacy of different antiretroviral regimens on neuropsychological performance in HIV-1 patients. Neuroscience of HIV infection, Chicago June 3–6, Abstract. *Journal of Neurovirology* **4**: 350

Gisslen M, Hagberg L, Svennerholm B, Norkrans G. (1997) HIV-1 RNA is not detectable in the cerebrospinal fluid during antiretroviral combination therapy. *AIDS* **11**: 1194

Gisslen M, Hagberg L, Fuchs D, Norkrans G, Svennerholm B. (1998) Cerebrospinal fluid viral load in HIV-1 infected patients without antiretroviral treatment. *Journal of Acquired Immune Deficiency Syndromes and Human Retrovirology* **17**: 291–295

Glass JD, Wesselingh SL, Selnes OA, McArthur JC. (1993) Clinical neuropathological correlation in HIV associated dementia. *Neurology* **43**: 2230–2237

Glass JD, Fedor H, Wesselingh SL, McArthur JC. (1995) Immunocytochemical quantitation of human immunodeficiency virus in the brain: correlations with dementia. *Annals of Neurology* **38**: 755–762

Glynn SL and Yazdanian M. (1998) In-vitro blood-brain barrier permeability of nevirapine compared to other HIV antiretroviral agents. *Journal of the Pharmaceutical Sciences* **87**: 306–310

Gonzalez RG, Ruiz A, Tracey I, McConnell J. (1998) Structural, functional and molecular neuroimaging in AIDS. In: HE Gendelman, SA Lipton, L Epstein, S Swindells (eds), *The Neurology of AIDS*. New York, Chapman and Hall pp 333–352

Grant I and Atkinson JH. (1995) Psychiatric aspects of acquired immune deficiency syndrome. In: HI Kaplan and BJ Sadock (eds), *Comprehensive Textbook of Psychiatry, Vol VI*. Baltimore, Williams and Wilkins, pp. 1644–1669

Grauss F, Ribalta T, Abbos J *et al.* (1990) Subacute cerebellar syndrome as the first manifestation of AIDS dementia complex. *Acta Neuropathologica* **81**: 118–120

Gray F, Hurtrel M, Hurtre IB. (1993) Early central nervous system changes in human immunodeficiency virus (HIV)-infection. *Neuropathology and Applied Neurobiology* **19**: 3–9

Gray F, Belec L, Keohane C *et al.* (1994) Zidovudine therapy and HIV encephalitis: a 10-year neuropathological survey. *AIDS* **8**: 489–493

Gray F, Scaravilli F, Everall IP *et al.* (1996) Neuropathology of early HIV-1 infection. *Brain Pathology* **6**: 1–15

Griffin DE. (1998) HIV Infection of the brain: viruses, cytokines, and immune regulatory factors associated with dementia. In: HE Gendelman, SA Lipton, L Epstein, S Swindells (eds), *The Neurology of AIDS*. New York, Chapman and Hall pp. 73–85

Groothius DR and Levy RM. (1997) The entry of antiviral and antiretroviral drugs into the central nervous system. *Journal of Neurovirology* **3**: 387–400

Hahn BH, Shaw GM, Tayor ME *et al.* (1986) Genetic variation in HTLV-III/LAV over time in patients with AIDS or at risk for AIDS. *Science* **232**: 1548–1553

He J, Chen Y, Farzan M *et al.* (1997) CCR3 and CCR5 are coreceptors for HIV-1 infection of microglia. *Nature* **385**: 645–649

Heaton RK, Velin RA, McCutchan JA *et al.* for the HNRC Group. (1994) Neuropsychological impairment in human immunodeficiency virus-infection: implications for employment. *Psychosomatic Medicine* **56**: 8–17

Heaton RK, Grant I, Butters N *et al.* for the HNRC Group. (1995) The HNRC 500 – Neuropsychology of HIV infection at different disease stages. *Journal of the International Neuropsychological Society* **1**: 231–251

Heyes MP, Brew BJ, Martin A *et al.* (1991) Quinolinic acid in cerebrospinal fluid and serum in HIV-1 infection: relationship to clinical and neurological status. *Annals of Neurology* **29**: 202–209

Hill JM, Mervis RF, Avidor R, Moody TW, Brenneman DE. (1993) HIV envelope protein-induced neuronal damage and retardation of behavioral development in rat neonates. *Brain Research* **603**: 222–233

Ho DD, Rota TR, Schooley RT *et al.* (1985) Isolation of HTLV-III from cerebrospinal fluid and neural tissues of patients with neurologic syndromes related to the acquired immunodeficiency syndrome. *New England Journal of Medicine* **313**: 1493–1497

Hwang SS, Boyle TJ, Lyerly HK, Cullen BR. (1991) Identification of envelope V3 loop as then primary determinant of cell tropism in HIV-1. *Science* **253**: 71–74

Kalams SA and Walker BD. (1995) Cytotoxic T lymphocytes and HIV-1 related neurologic disorders. *Current Topics in Microbial Immunology* **202**: 79–88

Kandanearatchi A, Zuckerman M, Smith M, Vyakarnam A, Everall IP. (2002a) Granulocyte – macrophage colony – stimulating factor enhances viral load in human brain tissue: amelioration with stavudine. *AIDS* **16**: 413–420

Kandanearatchi A, Trillo-Pazos G, Vyakarnam A, Everall IP. (2002b) Zidovudine and abacavir prevents neuronal loss in a HIV infected human brain aggregate system. 7th European Conference on Experimental AIDS Research. Genoa, Italy, 8–11 June

Kandanearatchi A, Vyakarnam A, Landau S, Everall I. (2004) Suppression of human immunodeficiency virus (HIV) replication in human brain tissue by nucleoside reverse transcriptase inhibitors. *Journal of Neurovirology* **10**:136–139

Kaus J, Zurlinden B, Schlote W. (1991) Axonal volume and myelin sheath thickness of the central nervous system myelinated fibres are reduced in HIV-encephalopathy. *Clinical Neuropathology* **10**: 38

Ketzler S, Weis S, Haug H, Budka H. (1990) Loss of neurons in the frontal cortex in AIDS brains. *Acta Neuropathologica* **80**: 92–94

Kleihues P, Lang W, Burger PC *et al.* (1985) Progressive diffuse leukoencephalopathy in patients with acquired immune deficiency syndrome. *Journal of Neuropathology and Experimental Neurology* **50**: 171–183

Koenig S, Gendelman HE, Orenstein JM *et al.* (1986) Detection of AIDS virus in macrophages in brain tissue from AIDS patients with encephalopathy. *Science* **233**: 1089–1093

Koyanagi Y, Miles S, Mituyasu RT *et al.* (1987) Dual infection of the central nervous system by AIDS viruses with distinct cellular tropisms. *Science* **236**: 819–822

Langford TD, Latendre SL, Marcotte TD *et al.* for the HNRC Group. (2002) Severe, demyelinating leukoencephalopathy in AIDS patients on antiretroviral therapy. *AIDS* **16**:1019–1029

Lavi E, Strizki JM, Ulrich AM *et al.* (1997) CXCR-4 (fusin), a co-receptor for the type 1 human immunodeficiency virus (HIV-1), is expressed in the human brain in a variety of cell types, including microglia and neurons. *American Journal of Pathology* **151**: 1035–1042

Lyketsos CG, Hanson AL, Fishman M, Rosenblatt A, McHugh PR, Treisman GJ. (1993) Manic syndrome early and late in the course of HIV. *American Journal of Psychiatry* **150**: 326–327

Lyketsos CG, Schwartz J, Fishman M, Treisman G. (1997) AIDS mania. *Journal of Neuropsychiatry and Clinical Neuroscience* **9**: 277–279

McArthur JC and Grant I. (1998) HIV neurocognitive disorders. In: HE Gendelman, SA Lipton, L Epstein, S Swindells (eds), *The Neurology of AIDS*. New York, Chapman and Hall, pp. 499–523

McArthur JC, Hoover DR, Bacellar H *et al.* (1993) Dementia in AIDS patients: incidence and risk factors. *Neurology* **43**: 2245–2252

McArthur JC, McClernon DR, Cronin MF *et al.* (1997) Relationship between human immunodeficiency virus-associated dementia and viral load in cerebrospinal fluid and brain. *Annals of Neurology* **42**: 689–698

McArthur JC, Nance-Sproson T, Childs E, Jackson JB, Lanier ER, McClernon D. (1998) Virologic response in cerebrospinal fluid after initiation of antiretroviral therapy. Neuroscience of HIV infection, Chicago June 3–6, Abstract. *Journal of Neurovirology* **4**: 359

McCutchan JA, Ellis R, Hsia K *et al.* (1997) Relationship of cerebrospinal fluid HIV RNA levels (CSF RNA) to plasma RNA, CSF pleiocytosis, stage of HIV infection and cognitive functioning. 4th Conference on Retroviruses and Opportunistic Infections. Washington DC, 22–26 January, Abstract 7

Martin C, Albert J, Hansson P, Pehrsson P, Link H, Sonnerborg A. (1998) Cerebrospinal fluid mononuclear cell counts influence CSF HIV-1 RNA levels. *Journal of Acquired Immune Deficiency Syndromes and Human Retrovirology* **17**: 214–219

Masliah E, Achim CL, Ge N, DeTeresa R, Terry RD, Wiley CA. (1992a) Spectrum of human immunodeficiency virus-associated neocortical damage. *Annals of Neurology* **32**: 321–329

Masliah E, Ge N, Morey M, DeTeresa R, Terry RD, Wiley CA. (1992b) Cortical dendritic pathology in human immunodeficiency virus encephalitis. *Laboratory Investigation* **66**: 285–291

Masliah E, Ge N, Achim C, Hansen LA, Wiley CA. (1992c) Selective neuronal vulnerability in HIV encephalitis. *Journal of Neuropathology and Experimental Neurology* **51**: 585–593

Masliah E, Ge N, Achim CL, Wiley CA. (1995) Differential vulnerability of calbindin-immunoreactive neurons in HIV encephalitis. *Journal of Neuropathology and Experimental Neurology* **54**: 350–357

Masliah E, Ge N, Achim CL, DeTeresa R, Wiley CA. (1996a) Patterns of neurodegeneration in HIV encephalitis. *NeuroAIDS* **1**: 161–173

Masliah E, Ge N, Mucke L. (1996b) Pathogenesis of HIV-1 associated neurodegeneration. *Critical Reviews in Neurobiology* **10**: 57–67

Masliah E, Heaton RK, Marcotte TD *et al.* (1997) Dendritic injury is a pathological substrate for human immunodeficiency virus-related cognitive disorders. HNRC group. The neurobehavioral research center. *Annals of Neurology* **42**: 963–972

Merrill JE and Chen ISY. (1991) HIV-1: macrophages, glial cells, and cytokines in AIDS nervous system disease. *FASEB Journal* **5**: 2391–2397

Miller RJ and Meucci O. (1999) AIDS and the brain: is there a chemokine connection. *Trends in Neurosciences* **22**: 471–476

More JP and Doms RW (2003) The entry of entry inhibitors: a fusion of science and medicine. *Proceedings of the National Academy of Sciences of the United States of America* **100**:10598–10602

Navia BA, Cho ES, Petito CK, Price RW. (1986) The AIDS dementia complex I: clinical features. *Annals of Neurology* **19**: 517–524

Navia BA and Price RW. (1987) The acquired immunodeficiency syndrome dementia complex as the presenting or sole manifestation of human immunodeficiency virus infection. *Archives of Neurology* **44**: 6569

Newman SP, Lunn S, Harrison MJG. (1995) Do asymptomatic HIV-seropositive individuals show cognitive deficit? *AIDS* **9**: 1211–1220

Nottet HSLM, Persidsky Y, Sasseville VG *et al.* (1996) Mechanisms for the transendothelial migration of HIV-1 infected monocytes into the brain. *Journal of Immunology* **156**: 1284–1295

Nuovo GJ, Gallery F, MacConnell P, Braun A. (1994) In situ detection of polymerase chain reaction-amplified HIV-1 nucleic acids and tumor necrosis factor-alpha RNA in the central nervous system. *American Journal of Pathology* **144**: 659–666

Pascal S, Resnick L, Barker WW *et al.* (1991) Metabolic asymmetries in asymptomatic HIV-1 seropositive subjects: relationship to disease onset and MRI findings. *Journal of Nuclear Medicine* **32**: 1725–1729

Portegies P, de-Gans J, Lange JM et al. (1989) Declining incidence of AIDS dementia complex after introduction of zidovudine treatment. BMJ 299: 819–821

Portegies P, Enting RH, de-Gans J et al. (1993) Presentation and course of AIDS dementia complex: 10 years of follow-up in Amsterdam, The Netherlands. AIDS 7: 669–675

Portegies P and Rosenberg NR. (1998) AIDS dementia complex. CNS Drugs 9: 31–40

Power C, McArthur JC, Johnson RT, Griffin DE, Glass JD, Perryman S, Chesebro B. (1994) Demented and nondemented patients with AIDS differ in bain-derived human immunodeficiency virus type 1 envelope sequences. Journal of Virology 68: 4643–4649

Power C, Selnes OA, Grim JA, McArthur JC. (1995) HIV Dementia Scale: a rapid screening test. Journal of Acquired Immune Deficiency Syndromes and Human Retrovirology 8: 273–278

Pretsell DO, Chiswick A, Egan VG, Brettle RP, Goodwin GM. (1996) HIV dementia in the Edinburgh cohort of IV-drug users. Journal of Neurovirology 2: 47

Price RW and Brew BJ. (1988) The AIDS dementia complex. Journal of Infectious Diseases 158: 1079–1083

Price RW, Sidtis JJ, Brew BJ. (1991) AIDS dementia complex and HIV-1 infection: a view from the clinic. Brain Pathology 1: 155–162

Pulliam L, Clarke JA, McGrath MS, Moore D, McGuire D. (1996) Monokine products as predictors of AIDS dementia. AIDS 10: 1495–1500

Reyes MG, Faraldi F, Senseng CS, Flowers C, Fariello R. (1991) Nigral degeneration in acquired immune deficiency syndrome (AIDS). Acta Neuropathologica 82: 39–44

Royal W 3rd, Selnes OA, Concha M, Nance-Sproson TE, McArthur JC. (1994) Cerebrospinal fluid human immunodeficiency virus type 1 (HIV-1) p24 antigen levels in HIV-1-related dementia. Annals of Neurology 36: 32–39

Saag MS, Hahn BH, Gibbons J et al. (1988) Extensive variation of human immunodeficiency virus type-1 in vivo. Nature 334: 440–444

Sabatier JM, Vives E, Mabrouk K et al. (1991) Evidence for neurotoxic activity of tat from human immunodeficiency virus type 1. Journal of Virology 65: 961–967

Sacktor NC, Bacellar H, Hoover DR et al. (1996) Psychomotor slowing in HIV infection: a predictor of dementia, AIDS and death. Journal of Neurovirology 6: 404–410

Sacktor NC, Skolasky RL, Lyles RH et al. (1998) Highly active antiretroviral therapy (HAART) improves cognitive impairment in HIV+ve homosexual men. Neuroscience of HIV infection, Chicago June 3–6, Abstract. Journal of Neurovirology 4: 365

Saito Y, Sharer L, Epstein L et al. (1994) Overexpression of nef as a marker for restricted HIV-1 infection of astrocytes in postmortem pediatric central nervous system tissues. Neurology 44: 474–480

Salvan A-M, Vion-Dury J, Confort-Gouny S, Nicoli F, Lamoureux S, Cozzone PJ. (1997) Brain proton magnetic resonance spectroscopy in HIV-related encephalopathy: identification of evolving metabolic patterns in relation to dementia and therapy. AIDS Research and Human Retroviruses 13: 1055–1066

Schmitt FA, Bigley JW, McKinnis R, Logue PE, Evans RW, Drucker JL. (1988) Neuropsychological outcome of zidovudine (AZT) treatment of patients with AIDS and AIDS-related complex. New England Journal of Medicine 319: 1573–1578

Selnes OA and Miller EN. (1994) Development of a screening battery for HIV related cognitive impairment: the MACS experience. In: I Grant and A Martin A (eds), Neuropsychology of HVI Infection. New York, Oxford University Press, pp. 176–187

Sereni D and the PROA1002 and PROA2002 International Study Groups. (1998) Antiretroviral activity of amprenavir in combination with zidovudine/3TC in plasma and CSF in patients with HIV infection. Neuroscience of HIV infection, Chicago June 3–6, Abstract. Journal of Neurovirology 4: 365

Shieh JT, Albright AV, Sharron M et al. (1998) Chemokine receptor utilization by human immunodeficiency virus type 1 isolates that replicate in microglia. Journal of Virology 72: 4243–4249

Sidtis JJ, Gatsonis C, Price RW et al. and the AIDS Clinical Trials Group. (1993) Zidovudine treatment of the AIDS dementia complex: results of a placebo-controlled trial. AIDS Clinical Trials Group. Annals of Neurology 33: 343–349

Sinclair E and Scaravilli F. (1992) Detection of HIV proviral DNA in cortex and white matter of AIDS brains by non-isotopic polymerase chain reaction: correlation with diffuse poliodystrophy. AIDS 6: 925–932

Sinclair E, Gray F, Ciardi A, Scaravilli F. (1994) Immunohistochemical changes and PCR detection of HIV provirus DNA in brains of asymptomatic HIV-positive patients. Journal of Neuropathology and Experimental Neurology 53: 43–50

Snider WD, Simpson DM, Nielsen S, Gold JWM, Metroka CE, Posner JB. (1983) Neurological complications of acquired immune deficiency syndrome: analysis of 50 patients. Annals of Neurology 14: 403–418

Spargo E, Everall IP, Lantos PL. (1993) Neuronal loss in the hippocampus in Huntington's disease: a comparison with HIV infection. Journal of Neurology, Neurosurgery, and Psychiatry 56: 487–491

Stahle L, Martin C, Svensson JO, Sonnerborg A. (1997) Indinavir in the cerebrospinal fluid of HIV-1 infected patients. Lancet 350: 1823

Stevenson M and O'Brien WA. (1998) Molecular biology of HIV-1. In: HE Gendelman, SA Lipton, L Epstein, S Swindells (eds), The Neurology of AIDS. New York, Chapman and Hall, pp. 13–35

Suarez S, Baril L, Stankoff B et al. (2001) Outcome of patients with HIV-1 related cognitive impairment on highly active antiretroviral therapy. AIDS 15: 195–200

Swingler S, Easton A, Morris A. (1992) Cytokine augmentation of HIV-1 LTR-driven gene expression in neural cells. AIDS-Research and Human Retroviruses 8: 487–493

Tesmer VM, Rajadhyaksha A, Babin J, Bina M. (1993) NF-IL6-mediated transcriptional activation of the long terminal repeat of the human immunodeficiency virus type 1. Proceedings of the National Academy of Sciences of the United States of America 90: 72298–72302

Thomas SA and Segal MB. (1997) The passage of azidodeoxythymidine into and within the central nervous system: does it follow the parent compound, thymidine? Journal of Pharmacology and Experimental Therapeutics 281: 1211–1218

Toggas SM, Masliah E, Rockenstein EM, Mucke L. (1994) Central nervous system damage produced by expression of the HIV-1 coat protein gp120 in transgenic mice. Nature 367: 188–193

Tozzi V, Narciso P, Galgani S et al. (1993) Effects of zidovudine in 30 patients with mild to end-stage AIDS dementia complex. AIDS 7: 683–692

Trillo-Pazos G, Pilkington GJ, Everall IP. (1998) Assessment of the neurotoxic effects of HIV's nef protein on the SK-N-SH human neuroblastoma cell line (Abstract). Journal of Neurovirology 4: 369

Tyor WR, Glass JD, Griffin JW et al. (1992) Cytokine expression in the brain during the acquired immunodeficiency syndrome. Annals of Neurology 31: 349–360

UNAIDS-WHO. (2001) AIDS epidemic update. Joint United Nations Programme on HIV/AIDS, pp. 1–22 van Gorp WG, Mandelkern MA, Gee M *et al.* (1992) Cerebral metabolic dysfunction in AIDS: findings in a sample with and without dementia. *Journal of Neuropsychiatry and Clinical Neuroscience* **4**: 280–287

Wahl SM, Allen JB, McCartney-Francis N *et al.* (1991) Macrophage- and astrocyte-derived transforming growth factor b as a mediator of central nervous system dysfunction in acquired immune deficiency syndrome. *Journal of Experimental Medicine* **173**: 981–991

Wang F, So Y, Vittinghoff E *et al.* (1995) Incidence proportion of and risk factors for AIDS patients diagnosed with HIV dementia, central nervous system toxoplasmosis, and cryptococcal meningitis. *Journal of Acquired Immune Deficiency Syndromes and Human Retrovirology* **8**: 75–82

Weis S, Haug H, Budka H. (1993) Neuronal damage in the cerebral cortex of AIDS brains: a morphometric study. *Acta Neuropathologica* **85**: 185–189

Werner T, Ferroni S, Saermark T *et al.* (1991) HIV-1 Nef protein exhibits structural and functional similarity to scorpion peptides interacting with K+ channels. *AIDS* **5**: 1301–1308

Westervelt P, Gendelman HE, Ratner L. (1991) Identification of a determinant within the HIV-1 surface envelope glycoprotein critical for productive infection of cultured primary monocytes. *Proceedings of the National Academy of Sciences of the United States of America* **88**: 3097–3101

White DA, Heaton RK, Monsch AU and The HNRC Group. (1995) Neuropsychological studies of asymptomatic human immunodeficiency virus-type-1 infected individuals. *Journal of the International Neuropsychological Society* **1**: 304–315

Wiley CA, Schrier RD, Nelson JA, Lampert PW, Oldstone MBA. (1986) Cellular localization of human immunodeficiency virus infection within the brains of acquired immune deficiency syndrome patients. *Proceedings of the National Academy of Sciences of the United States of America* **83**: 7089–7093

Wiley CA, Masliah E, Morey M *et al.* (1991) Neocortical damage during HIV infection. *Annals of Neurology* **29**: 651–657

Wilson CJ. (1990) Basal ganglia. In: GM Shepherd (ed.), *The Synaptic Organization of the Brain*. New York, Oxford University Press, pp. 279–316

World Health Organization. (1990) *Report of the Second Consultation on the Neuropsychiatric Aspects of HIV-1 Infection.* Geneva, WHO

Yang Z, Brundage RC, Barbhaiya RH, Sawchuk RJ. (1997) Microdialysis studies of the distribution of stavudine into the central nervous system in the freely-moving rat. *Pharmaceutical Research* **14**: 865–872

Yarchoan R, Berg G, Brouwers P *et al.* (1987) Response of human-immunodeficiency-virus-associated neurological disease to 3'-azido-3'-deoxythymidine. *Lancet* **1**: 132–135

Uncommon forms of dementia

ANOOP VARMA

The preceding chapters have discussed the common types of dementias including Alzheimer's disease (AD), vascular dementia (VaD), dementia with Lewy bodies (DLB), fronto-temporal dementia (FTD), etc. In 1–5 per cent of patients with dementia the underlying disorders are uncommon. Many of these patients develop dementia as part of a more prominent neurological syndrome (e.g. corticobasal degeneration). However, awareness of these disorders may lead to effective treatments (e.g. Whipple's disease), or lead to better care from the knowledge of evolution of the disease and its attendant symptoms and signs. Patients whose disorders have an underlying genetic basis may require genetic counselling. This chapter attempts to summarize the clinical, diagnostic and therapeutic aspects of these disorders.

65.1 DEMENTIAS ASSOCIATED WITH NEURODEGENERATIVE DISORDERS

65.1.1 Progressive supranuclear palsy (PSP; Steele–Richardson–Olszweski syndrome)

PSP is characterized by supranuclear ophthalmoplegia (especially downgaze), pseudobulbar palsy, dysarthria, retrocollis, parkinsonism and dementia (Steele et al., 1964; Steele, 1972). Patients are commonly affected in the seventh decade with no significant difference between the sexes (Maher and Lees, 1986). The disorder is often misdiagnosed (Osaki et al., 2004) and initial diagnoses include Parkinson's disease, balance disorders and stroke (Burn and Lees, 2002). Presenting complaints include abrupt falls, unsteadiness of gait, slurred speech or memory impairment. As the disease progresses, marked and relatively symmetrical rigidity (pronounced in the neck) and

the characteristic downgaze palsy emerge. Cerebellar and pyramidal signs and pseudobulbar palsy may be observed.

Although severe dementia is uncommon, subcortical cognitive impairment and depression are common. Mentation is slowed and difficulty in switching set, perseveration, apathy and poor abstraction are prominent neuropsychological features (Albert et al., 1974). Significant depression may occur in addition to emotional lability that often accompanies the pseudobulbar syndrome.

The diagnosis rests on clinical history and examination. Mid-brain atrophy on magnetic resonance imaging (MRI) and/or signal changes in the mid-brain, red nucleus or globus pallidus are supportive (Asato et al., 2000; Warmuth-Metz et al., 2001). Functional imaging studies including blood flow single photon emission computed tomography (SPECT), dopamine transporter and dopamine (D2) receptor imaging are not diagnostically specific to PSP (Brooks, 1993; Kim et al., 2002).

Treatment with levodopa, dopamine agonists, amantadine, tricyclic antidepressants and anticholinergics has proved disappointing.

Over a period of 5–7 years severe physical decline leads to loss of ambulation and eventually to death. Autopsy reveals tau positive neurofibrillary tangles, neuronal loss and tau-positive glial inclusions in the substantia nigra, globus pallidus, subthalamic nucleus and mid-brain (Jellinger and Blancher, 1992).

65.1.2 Corticobasal degeneration (CBD)

CBD is a striking parkinsonian syndrome characterized by grossly asymmetrical dystonia, alien limb phenomenon, apraxia and myoclonus (Ribeiz et al., 1968; Gibb et al., 1989; Stover and Watts, 2001).

Patients usually present in late middle life, often with a useless arm. The asymmetry is marked and eventually the disorder spreads contralaterally. The involved arm may be initially apraxic but rigidity and dystonia supervene. Myoclonus may be reported or elicited at action. Patients may describe alien limb phenomenon and intermanual conflict. Rigidity, corticospinal signs, cortical sensory loss, supranuclear gaze palsy and dysarthria may occur. Dementia is not severe but includes subcortical deficits, apraxia, constructional and spatial impairment (Gibb *et al.*, 1989; Stover and Watts, 2001).

MRI may show severe asymmetrical posterior frontal and parietal atrophy (Savoiardo, 2003). Regional cerebral blood flow (rCBF) SPECT shows reduced uptake in the affected posterior frontal, superior, anterior, inferior and posterior parietal cortices with less prominent changes in the thalamus and basal ganglia (Markus *et al.*, 1995). A recent study suggests a more widespread rCBF change (Hossain *et al.*, 2003).

The characteristically asymmetrical cortical (apraxia and myoclonus) and basal (dystonia, with akinesia and rigidity) signs are the hallmark of the syndrome. Even when a limb is severely rigid and postured due to dystonia, it is usually possible to elicit apraxia in the contralateral limb or orofacial musculature.

Sustained benefit with levodopa, dopamine agonists or amantadine is unusual. The disorder is relentlessly progressive leading to a severe akinetic-rigid syndrome with dysarthria, dysphagia and eventually a wheelchair and bed-bound state. The life span from the onset of symptoms ranges from 6 to 9 years.

Pathological features (Gibb *et al.*, 1989) include neuronal loss in the thalamus, basal ganglia, brain stem and the frontoparietal cortex. Swollen achromatic neurones in the frontoparietal region are pathologically characteristic. The nosology of corticobasal degeneration is debated between lumpers (Kertesz, 1997) and splitters (Neary, 1997). However, it seems an eminently sensible suggestion to carefully document the clinical, histopathological (Hachinski, 1997) and genetic features of all reported cases, regardless of one's position.

65.1.3 Multiple system atrophy (MSA)

The term MSA was proposed in 1969 (Graham and Oppenheimer, 1969) and has gained wide acceptance over the years (Quinn, 1989; Gilman *et al.*, 1999). The disorder affects both sexes in the sixth decade. The main features include autonomic dysfunction, parkinsonism, cerebellar ataxia and pyramidal signs in varying combinations (Wenning *et al.*, 2004). The two main subtypes are the parkinsonian (MSA-P) and the ataxic (MSA-C) variants, depending on the major motor feature. Patients may also develop inspiratory stridor or rapid eye movement (REM) sleep behaviour disorder. Dementia is usually mild and neuropsychological tests reveal deficits in tests sensitive to frontosubcortical dysfunction. Cognitive dysfunction is heterogeneous with some patients revealing no impairment even when severely physically disabled (Robbins *et al.*, 1992).

MRI may show putaminal or olivopontocerebellar atrophy, sometimes with hyperintensities in the pons and middle cerebellar peduncles (Schrag *et al.*, 2000). Hypointensities in the putamen with a hyperintense rim are thought to be characteristic of MSA (Kraft *et al.*, 1999). Denervation on sphincter electromyography (EMG) may be diagnostically helpful if other causes of sphincter denervation have been ruled out (Vodusek, 2001).

Most patients are levodopa unresponsive and symptomatic treatment centres around relief from dysautonomic symptoms. MSA progresses relentlessly and most patients are severely disabled in 5 years. Argyrophilic glial cytoplasmic inclusions are the pathological hallmark of MSA. The distribution of pathology varies with the predominance of parkinsonian or cerebellar features (Wenning *et al.*, 2004).

65.1.4 Autosomal dominant cerebellar ataxias (ADCAs)

ADCAs cause progressive ataxia of gait typically presenting in the third to fifth decades (Harding, 1982). The underlying genetic heterogeneity includes various different genetic loci with CAG/polyglutamine expansions (SCA – spinocerebellar ataxia) 1–13 genes (Durr and Brice, 2000). No clinical sign can be confidently attributed to a genotype in most forms of ADCA. Nonetheless several signs occur more commonly in one genotype than in another. SCA1 is associated with gait spasticity and a more aggressive course. SCA2 may present with slowed saccades and hyporeflexia with axonal neuropathy. These patients have prominent and early cognitive dysfunction (Burk *et al.*, 1999). Patients with SCA3 may have gaze-evoked nystagmus and parkinsonism. SCA7 uniquely causes reduced visual acuity owing to progressive macular degeneration (Durr and Brice, 2000).

Burk *et al.* (1999) found approximately 25 per cent of SCA2 patients to be clinically demented; the remaining patients had neuropsychological evidence of memory impairment and executive dysfunction. Another study has replicated these findings and additionally reported attentional deficits (Le Pira *et al.*, 2002). Cognitive dysfunctions have also been described in other varieties of ADCA, e.g. SCA1 (Trojano *et al.*, 1998), and there is some suggestion that these deficits are related to disease severity (Trojano *et al.*, 1998; Le Pira *et al.*, 2002). It is possible that cognitive impairment in these patients is due to dysfunction of less well-known cognitive functions of the cerebellum (Leiner *et al.*, 1993), and/or disruption of frontoponto-cerebellar pathways (Le Pira *et al.*, 2002).

MRI may reveal cerebellar hemispheric or vermien atrophy (especially in SCA6), or brain stem atrophy (especially in SCA2; Durr and Brice, 2000). Molecular analyses identify CAG/polyglutamine expansions in approximately 50–90 per cent of all cases with a demonstrable autosomal dominant pattern of inheritance. Conversely the diagnostic yield is very low in patients without family histories (Pujana *et al.*, 1999; Durr and Brice, 2000).

65.2 DEMENTIAS ASSOCIATED WITH INHERITED METABOLIC DISEASES

A wide variety of inherited metabolic diseases, usually thought to be limited to infancy or childhood, may manifest in adolescence or young adulthood (Coker, 1991). They may present with predominantly neurological disease or with associated systemic involvement (Box 65.1). Although the brunt of pathology may vary from dominant grey matter involvement (seizures, dementia) to white matter disease (motor weakness, spasticity, ataxia), most of these disorders, if untreated, eventually lead to severe mental and physical disability.

65.2.1 Metachromatic leukodystrophy (MLD)

MLD is an autosomal recessive disorder owing to arylsulphatase deficiency. Sulphatide accumulation, especially in the brain and peripheral nerves is accompanied with central and peripheral demyelination. Late infantile, juvenile and adult forms are recognized. The adult form usually presents in the second decade, although late onset cases in the sixth decade have been described (Duyff and Weinstein, 1996). These patients usually present with personality change and intellectual deterioration (Hageman et al., 1995), although mainly motor forms (pyramidal, extrapyramidal and cerebellar involvement with peripheral neuropathy) are also recognized (Baumann et al., 2002). Some of these patients may

---

Box 65.1 *Dementia associated with inherited metabolic diseases*

Predominantly neurological disease
- Predominantly white matter
  - metachromatic leukodystrophy
  - adrenoleukodystrophy
  - cerebrotendinous xanthomatosis
- Predominantly grey matter
  - GM2 gangliosidosis
  - Kufs' disease
  - Lafora body disease

Associated systemic disease
- Gaucher's disease
- Niemann–Pick disease type C
- Wilson's disease

Prominent extrapyramidal signs
- Wilson's disease
- Hallervorden–Spatz disease
- Metachromatic leukodystrophy
- Kufs' disease
- GM2 gangliosidosis
- Niemann–Pick disease type C
- Gaucher's disease

---

have psychotic features and could be misdiagnosed as schizophrenia (Hyde et al., 1992).

The disease progresses over 20+ years and in the terminal stages patients become quadriparetic and mute. The diagnosis is confirmed by demonstration of reduced arylsulphatase activity in peripheral blood white cells. Cerebrospinal fluid (CSF) studies reveal raised protein. T2-weighted MRI brain scans show bilaterally symmetrical, predominantly periventricular high signal changes in the deep white matter (Faerber et al., 1999). Stem cell gene therapy has met with limited success in mouse models (Matzner et al., 2002).

65.2.2 Adrenoleukodystrophy (ALD)

ALD is an X-linked disorder (gene locus on Xq28) characterized by impaired ability to oxidize very long chain fatty acids (VLCFA), leading to their accumulation in the brain and adrenal glands (Igarashi et al., 1976). Moser (1997) and colleagues (Moser et al., 1984) found that cerebral forms occur alone in 30 per cent, adrenomyeloneuropathy alone in 20 per cent and combined childhood cerebral and myelopathic forms in the remainder. Most cases present in the first decade with decline in intellect, change in personality with inappropriate laughter and crying. Unsteadiness, incoordination and intention tremor soon develop. Vomiting, circulatory collapse, oral mucosal and skin pigmentation may occur. In the late stage blindness, deafness, pseudobulbar paralysis and bilateral hemiplegia supervene. Adult patients usually present with mild cerebral symptoms and spastic myelopathy with neuropathy. Some patients may present with dementia, behavioural changes and/or psychosis (Kitchin et al., 1987).

Brain MRI shows widespread white matter changes with a predilection for the parieto-occipital white matter and may, therefore, be confused with multiple sclerosis. The diagnosis is confirmed by the demonstration of an excess of VLCFA in blood (plasma, red and white cells). Markers of adrenal insufficiency support the diagnosis. Dietary supplementation with monounsaturated fatty acids and bone marrow transplantation have been shown to stabilize disability (van Geel et al., 1997).

65.2.3 Cerebrotendinous xanthomatosis (CTX)

CTX is a rare autosomal recessive disorder with accumulation of cholestanol and cholesterol. Patients usually present in the second and third decades. Cataracts, diarrhoea and tendon xanthomas may be noted from an early age. With progression, intellectual deficit and inattentiveness give way to progressive dementia, spasticity, ataxia, pseudobulbar palsy and peripheral neuropathy (Moghadasian et al., 2002).

Computed tomography (CT) and MRI demonstrate diffuse brain and spinal cord atrophy, white matter changes and occasionally focal lesions (Kaye, 2001). Laboratory investigations reveal elevated levels of plasma and bile cholestanol (normally cholestanol is 0.1–0.2 per cent of total cholesterol;

in CTX there is a 10–100-fold rise) and increased urinary excretion of bile alcohol glucuronides (Koopman, et al., 1988). Treatment with chenodeoxycholic acid may reverse neurological deficits, especially when started in young patients (Berginer et al., 1984).

65.2.4 Adult GM2 gangliosidosis

GM2 gangliosidosis is due to deficiency of hexosaminidase A, which leads to accumulation of gangliosides in neurones (Argov and Navon, 1984). Partial deficiency of hexosaminidase A (<15 per cent) is associated with later (juvenile and adult) onset syndromes. Patients may present with slowly progressive motor neurone disorder, with or without pyramidal and cerebellar signs. Some patients have psychiatric disturbances, personality changes and intellectual deterioration. Dystonia, myoclonus, seizures and ocular motor disorders may also be observed (Hund et al., 1997).

The diagnosis is confirmed by enzyme assays in white cells. MRI shows generalized atrophy with particularly severe cerebellar involvement (Clarke, 2002). Electromyography reveals denervation even in patients without overt clinical signs.

65.2.5 Kufs' disease (neuronal ceroid lipofuscinosis, NCL)

Kufs' disease is the juvenile/adult form of NCL, a group of lysosomal storage disorders. Unlike the early onset forms, Kufs' disease develops later (15–25 years) and is unattended by retinal and visual changes (Berkovic et al., 1988). Most cases are autosomal recessive although autosomal dominant patterns have been described (Josephson et al., 2001). Varying combinations of progressive myoclonic epilepsy, generalized tonic clonic epilepsy, dysarthria, ataxia and dystonia may be observed. Some patients have prominent neuropsychiatric symptoms including behavioural changes, psychosis and dementia (Berkovic et al., 1988; Hinkebein and Callahan, 1997).

The diagnosis may prove difficult and involves demonstration of accumulation of autofluorescent ceroid and lipofuscin in nerve-containing tissue (Goebel and Braak, 1989). Skin biopsies can be positive and are easier to obtain than brain tissue. The disease is relentlessly progressive and results in death in 10–15 years.

65.2.6 Lafora body disease

Lafora body disease is autosomal recessive and one of the genes responsible has been mapped to chromosome 6q24 (Serratosa et al., 1995; Minassian et al., 1998). These patients usually present with intractable seizures in the second decade of life. Myoclonus and occipital seizures are characteristic. Dysarthria, ataxia, emotional disturbances, confusion and dementia develop gradually. Patients eventually become severely demented, mute, quadriparetic and bed-bound. Death occurs within 10 years of onset (Minassian, 2001).

The electroencephalogram (EEG) shows generalized epileptiform discharges with photomyoclonus. Background EEG is persistently slow. Skin, liver, muscle or brain biopsies may reveal the pathognomonic periodic-acid-Schiff (PAS) positive Lafora bodies. At pathology Lafora bodies, composed of polyglucosans, are present throughout the brain, especially in the cerebral and cerebellar cortices, basal ganglia, thalamus and the spinal cord. Similar accumulations are also found in skin, muscle, heart and liver.

65.2.7 Hallervorden–Spatz disease

The original description dates back to 1922 (Hallervorden and Spatz, 1922). Over the years deviations from the original description have been included within the term Hallervorden–Spatz syndrome. Halliday (1995) suggests reserving the term Hallervorden–Spatz disease for the paediatric neurodegenerative disorder and Hallervorden–Spatz syndrome to include disorders with the pallidal triad of iron deposition, axial spheroids and gliosis.

The onset is usually before the age of 10 years and death occurs in the early twenties (Dooling et al., 1974). Adult-onset cases (atypical disease) are reported and develop progressive dementia, quadriparesis and extrapyramidal features including parkinsonism, dystonia and/or chorea (Halliday, 1995); the course may be more prolonged over 15–40 years.

The disorder is autosomal recessive and many cases with the syndrome result from mutations in a gene called PANK2 (encoding the enzyme pantothenate kinase, which regulates biosynthesis of coenzyme A) on chromosome 20p13 (Hayflick et al., 2003). All patients with classical Hallervorden–Spatz syndrome and a third with atypical disease have PANK2 mutations. The atypical cases have prominent psychiatric features, palilalia, dysarthria, dystonia and cognitive decline including personality change, impulsivity and emotional lability. Patients with PANK2 mutations show bilateral hyperintensity surrounded by hypointensity in the medial globus pallidus on T2-weighted MRI scans ('eye of the tiger' sign).

The globus pallidus shows a rusty discoloration. Microscopy reveals axonal spheroids in the basal ganglia, cerebellum and brain stem. Neurofibrillary tangles and Lewy bodies may be seen in some patients with Hallervorden–Spatz syndrome (Halliday, 1995).

65.2.8 Gaucher's disease

Gaucher's disease is an autosomal recessive inherited lysosomal storage disorder owing to glucocerebrosidase deficiency. Glucocerebroside accumulates in visceral organs, reticuloendothelial tissue and the nervous system.

The clinical manifestations of Gaucher's disease vary enormously. Many patients remain asymptomatic all their lives; at the opposite end of the spectrum some patients with the rare acute neuronopathic form die by the age of 18 months.

Type I Gaucher's disease is without neurological manifestations and visceral manifestations include hepatosplenomegaly, anaemia, thrombocytopenia and skeletal abnormalities. The adult forms are stable and slowly progressive. Type II Gaucher's disease is characterized by early-onset neurological and visceral disease. Severe neck rigidity and arching, bulbar signs, appendicular rigidity, chorea and dystonia follow eye movement disorders and strabismus. Type III Gaucher's disease is the intermediate form with onset between 0.1 and 14 years (usually 1 year). Eye movement disorders, ataxia, spasticity, and slowly progressive dementia may be accompanied by visceral involvement (Balicki and Beutler, 1995).

Investigations show a rise in acid phosphatase, characteristic histiocytes (Gaucher cells) in marrow smears and liver or spleen biopsies. The diagnosis is confirmed by detecting reduced glucocerebrosidase activity in peripheral white cells. Type I Gaucher's disease responds to enzyme replacement therapy with recombinant glucocerebrosidase (Charrow et al., 2004).

65.2.9 Niemann–Pick disease type C (NPD–C)

NPD-C is a lipid storage disorder with hepatosplenomegaly and a variety of neurological and psychiatric symptoms and signs (Patterson, 2003). The diagnosis should be considered in any individual with unexplained dementia or psychiatric impairment, especially when accompanied by ataxia, dystonia or vertical supranuclear gaze palsy. The absence of organomegaly, normal imaging or bone marrow biopsy does not rule out the diagnosis.

NPD-C can present at any age. Psychiatric and cognitive dysfunction predominate later-onset presentations. Dysarthria, dementia and ataxia may be accompanied by vertical supranuclear gaze palsy. Psychosis may be the occasional presenting feature and rarely choreoathetosis may occur. A mixture of partial and generalized seizures may occur. Gelastic cataplexy (ranging from subtle head nodding to profound atonia, usually provoked by humorous situations) may be seen in approximately 20 per cent of patients (Shulman et al., 1995a, b).

Most patients with NPD-C have mutations in the NPC1 gene located on chromosome 18q11. Although genotyping may be helpful in diagnosis, the frequency of polymorphisms makes detection and interpretation of changes in the DNA sequence difficult in some cases. The diagnosis is strongly supported by detecting polymorphous cytoplasmic bodies on electron microscopic examination of skin, rectal or conjunctival biopsies (Patterson, 2003). There is no definitive therapy for NPD-C.

65.2.10 Wilson's disease

Wilson's disease is an autosomal recessive disorder of copper homeostasis. The responsible gene has been identified on chromosome 13. Most clinical manifestations can be directly attributed to copper accumulation, especially in the brain and liver (Jones and Weissenborn, 1997; Gitlin, 2003).

Thirty-five per cent of all patients may present with neurological Wilson's disease in the second or third decades of life, without overt liver disease. Incoordination, clumsiness, tremor, dysarthria, excess salivation, dysphagia and movement disorders (a variety of tremors, dystonia, bradykinesia, chorea) produce a prominent motor syndrome. Psychiatric symptoms may dominate the clinical picture in a third of all patients and include behavioural and personality changes, psychosis, depression and/or cognitive impairment (Jones and Weissenborn, 1997; Gitlin, 2003). T2-weighted MRI may reveal the 'face of the giant panda' sign consisting of high signal in the mid-brain tegmentum except the red nucleus, preservation of signal in the substantia nigra and hypointensity of the superior colliculus (Hitoshi et al., 1991). Slit lamp examination reveals Kayser–Fleischer rings and peripheral blood ceruloplasmin concentration is <20 mg/dl. Urinary copper excretion is >100 μg/24 hours (normal <40). Treatment requires lifelong chelation with D-penicillamine, trientine or tetrathiomolybdate. Advanced liver failure may require hepatic transplantation (Jones and Weissenborn, 1997; Gitlin, 2003).

65.3 OTHER UNCOMMON DEMENTIAS

65.3.1 Mitochondrial cytopathy (MC)

Mitochondrial encephalomyopathies (ME) are a group of multisystem disorders characterized by biochemical and genetic mitochondrial defects with a variable mode of inheritance. Oxidative phosphorylation (ATP synthesis by oxygen consuming respiratory chain [RC]) supplies most organs and tissues with energy. RC components originate from nuclear DNA and mitochondrial DNA. Patients with a defect of oxidative phosphorylation may present with:

- an unexplained combination of neuromuscular/non-neuromuscular symptoms;
- a progressive course;
- involvement of seemingly unrelated organs or tissues (Munnich and Rustin, 2001).

The central and/or peripheral nervous system may be involved. Patients may present with a range of manifestations, i.e. encephalopathy, brain stem involvement (ophthalmoplegia), cerebellar disorders (ataxia), myoclonus, seizures, pyramidal dysfunction, leukodystrophy, poliodystrophy or peripheral neuropathy and/or myopathy. MELAS (mitochondrial encephalomyopathy with lactic acidosis and stroke-like episodes), MERRF (myoclonic epilepsy with ragged red fibres), subacute necrotizing encephalomyopathy (Leigh syndrome), MNGIE (mitochondrial myopathy, peripheral neuropathy, encephalopathy and gastrointestinal disease) are commonly recognized ME, whereas progressive external ophthalmoplegia (PEO) and Kearns–Sayre syndrome (KSS) are mitochondrial myopathies (Rahman and Schapira, 1999).

Cognitive impairment and dementia are commonly recorded features of MC. However, the neuropsychological deficits in MC have not been studied in detail. Many reports of cognitive deficits in MC could be attributed to focal deficits from strokes (e.g. MELAS) or seizures. Turconi *et al.* (1999) reported memory and constructional impairment in MC (PEO, KSS and one patient with MERRF). Bosbach *et al.* (2003) studied similar patients (PEO and KSS) with rigorous neuropsychological assessment including executive functions. They reported executive dysfunction, constructional impairment and attentional difficulties suggesting fronto-subcortical dysfunction.

Combinations of clinical features like deafness, diabetes mellitus, cardiomyopathy, myopathy and encephalopathy are strongly suggestive of MC. Diagnostic approaches are tailored to the clinical presentation (for details see Finsterer, 2004). T2-weighted MRI may show high signal changes in the deep white matter or grey–white interface, especially posteriorly, in patients with MELAS. Electrophysiology may reveal neuropathy in a third of cases; electromyography may be normal, neurogenic and/or myogenic. EEG may be slow and reflect encephalopathy. CSF protein is raised in KSS; CSF lactate may be elevated e.g. in MELAS, MERRF or Leigh syndromes. Muscle biopsy may show ragged red fibres (MELAS, MERRF) on light microscopy; further immunohistochemical and electron microscopy studies may detail mitochondrial abnormalities. Negative genetic tests require cautious interpretation. Mitochondrial deletions are usually not detected in blood. Further DNA analysis from muscle tissue may be required (Rahman and Schapira, 1999; Munnich and Rustin, 2001; Finsterer, 2004). Treatment remains symptomatic.

65.3.2 Whipple's disease

Whipple's disease is a systemic infectious disorder usually presenting with weight loss, arthralgia, diarrhoea and abdominal pain. Small intestinal biopsy confirms the diagnosis by demonstrating PAS-positive inclusions in the lamina propria. These inclusions represent the causative bacteria, *Tropheryma whipplei* (Marth and Raoult, 2003). Neurological symptoms occur in approximately 15 per cent of patients and may present without prominent gastrointestinal disorder (Louis *et al.*, 1996; Marth and Raoult, 2003).

Eighty per cent of patients with central nervous system (CNS) Whipple's disease have systemic signs. Cognitive changes with or without neuropsychiatric manifestations are frequent. Patients may develop frank dementia. Supranuclear gaze palsy, myoclonus, oculomasticatory myorhythmia or oculofacial-skeletal myorhythmia are characteristically present in a third to half of all such patients. Ataxia and/or seizures are not infrequent (Louis *et al.*, 1996).

Tissue biopsy (small bowel, brain, lymph node or vitreous fluid) is positive in about 75 per cent of patients. Polymerization chain reaction (PCR) gene amplification may be positive for *T. whipplei* in gastric fluid, small bowel, synovial or saliva samples (Louis *et al.*, 1996; Delanty *et al.*, 1999).

Currently recommended treatment regimes include 2 weeks of parenteral ceftriaxone followed by long-term oral trimethoprim-sulfamethoxazole administration (Marth and Raoult, 2003).

65.3.3 Hashimoto's encephalopathy (HE)

HE characteristically presents with a fluctuating confusional state, tremor and myoclonus (Shaw *et al.*, 1991). Seizures, stroke like episodes, pyramidal weakness, extrapyramidal rigidity and ataxia may emerge over the ensuing weeks and months. The onset may be abrupt or insidious and the evolution is typically subacute (Kothbauer-Margreiter *et al.*, 1996).

The EEG is usually slow. MRI and SPECT scans may be normal or show non-specific changes. CSF protein is usually raised with a normal cell count. High titre of antithyroid antibodies with normal thyroid function clinches the diagnosis (Neary and Snowden, 2003).

The disorder responds to steroids and often prolonged courses are required. Remissions and relapses necessitate appropriate adjustments in steroid therapy. HE is most likely to be confused with fluctuating encephalopathies including DLB, Creutzfeldt–Jakob disease (CJD), metabolic encephalopathy, cerebral vasculitis and paraneoplastic limbic encephalitis (PLE) (Box 65.2).

65.3.4 Cerebral vasculitis

Cerebral vasculitis may occur as part of a systemic vasculitis, e.g. systemic lupus erythematosus (SLE). However, occasionally a neurological syndrome may be the presenting feature of systemic vasculitis or less commonly due to an isolated primary vasculitis of the central nervous system, i.e. without peripheral clinical or laboratory (absence of autoantibodies, normal erythrocyte sedimentation rate and C-reactive protein) markers of systemic vasculitis. The latter condition poses diagnostic difficulties and detection requires a high degree of clinical suspicion and experience. Patients may develop multifocal symptoms and signs with stepwise progression. Headache and confusion (subacute encephalopathy), usually with focal signs and myoclonus, may raise suspicion of an underlying cerebral vasculitis. Investigations including MRI, EEG and CSF studies may be normal. Cerebral angiography and leptomeningeal biopsies may also be falsely negative. The diagnosis is sometimes established after repeated investigations (vascular changes on MRI, CSF pleocytosis and raised

---

Box 65.2 *Fluctuating encephalopathies*

- Metabolic encephalopathy
- Dementia with Lewy bodies
- Creutzfeldt–Jakob disease
- Hashimoto's encephalopathy
- Cerebral vasculitis
- Paraneoplastic limbic encephalitis

protein, multifocal narrowing of blood vessels on angiography and vasculitic lesions on leptomeningeal biopsy). Treatment is aggressive with immunosuppression (cyclophosphamide) and steroids (Scolding, 1997; Joseph and Scolding, 2002).

65.3.5 Paraneoplastic limbic encephalitis (PLE)

Paraneoplastic syndromes represent remote effects of cancer rather than direct effects such as metastatic invasion. PLE is characterized by personality changes, behavioural changes including irritability and depression, seizures (complex partial, generalized or a combination), memory impairment and even frank dementia (Corsellis *et al.*, 1968; Gultekin *et al.*, 2000). Memory loss and confusion are the commonest presenting symptoms. Neurological dysfunction may develop 0.5–33 months (median 3.5 months) before tumour detection. Other parts of the nervous system may also be involved (sensory neuronopathy, cerebellar ataxia, brain stem diplopia and dizziness). The course is subacute and may fluctuate with progression over weeks or months (Newman *et al.*, 1990).

MRI shows unilateral/bilateral high signal changes in mesial temporal lobes on T2-weighted image that may enhance with contrast (Dirr *et al.*, 1990; Gultekin *et al.*, 2000). The CSF may show pleocytosis, raised protein or oligoclonal bands. Paraneoplastic antibodies are detected in 60 per cent of patients, most commonly anti-Hu (associated with small cell lung cancer) or anti-Ta (associated with testicular tumours). Seventy-eight per cent of patients have positive MRI findings and/or CSF abnormalities (Gultekin *et al.*, 2000).

It is thought that tumour expression triggers autoimmunity against the nervous system (Newman *et al.*, 1990; Gultekin *et al.*, 2000). Although a variety of treatments including steroids, intravenous immunoglobulins and plasma exchange have been tried, none is of proven value. Early identification of the tumour and prompt treatment appears to offer the greatest chance for neurological improvement (Gultekin *et al.*, 2000).

Box 65.3   *Myoclonic dementias*

- Alzheimer's disease
- Dementia with Lewy bodies
- Creutzfeldt–Jakob disease
- Metabolic encephalopathy
- Hashimoto's encephalopathy
- Cerebral vasculitis
- Whipple's disease
- Mitochondrial encephalomyopathy
- Paraneoplastic limbic encephalitis
- Corticobasal degeneration
- Lafora body disease
- Kufs' disease
- GM2 gangliosidosis
- HIV encephalopathy

65.4 CONCLUSION

An awareness of the clinical syndromes (Boxes 65.1–65.3) and a high index of suspicion make accurate diagnosis of uncommon dementias possible. Some of these disorders can be conclusively diagnosed with the help of biological markers (biochemical or genetic) or radiological findings. Since effective treatments are available for some conditions (Wilson's disease, Hashimoto's encephalopathy, Whipple's disease, etc.), knowledge of these dementias, though uncommon, is essential.

REFERENCES

Albert ML, Feldman RG, Day J *et al.* (1974) The 'subcortical dementia' of progressive supranuclear palsy. *Journal of Neurology, Neurosurgery, and Psychiatry* **37**: 121–230

Argov Z and Navon R. (1984) Clinical and genetic variations in the syndrome of adult GM2 gangliosidosis resulting from hexosaminidase A deficiency. *Annals of Neurology* **16**: 14–20

Asato R, Akiguchi I, Masunaga S, Hashimoto N. (2000) Magnetic resonance imaging distinguishes progressive supranuclear palsy from multiple system atrophy. *Journal of Neural Transmission* **107**: 1427–1436

Balicki D and Beutler E. (1995) Gaucher disease. *Medicine (Baltimore)* **74**: 305–323

Baumann N, Turpin J-C, Lefevre M, Colsch B. (2002) Motor and psycho-cognitive clinical types in adult metachromatic leukodystrophy: genotype/phenotype relationships? *Journal of Physiology – Paris* **96**: 301–306

Berginer VM, Salen G, Shefer S. (1984) Long term treatment of cerebrotendinous xanthomatosis with chenodeoxycholic acid. *New England Journal of Medicine* **311**: 1649–1652

Berkovic SF, Carpenter S, Andermann F, Andermann E, Wolfe LS. (1988) Kufs' disease: a critical appraisal. *Brain* **111**: 27–62

Bosbach S, Kornblum C, Schroder R, Wagner M. (2003) Executive and visuospatial deficits in patients with chronic progressive external ophthalmoplegia and Kearns–Sayre syndrome. *Brain* **126**: 1231–1240

Brooks DJ. (1993) Functional imaging in relation to Parkinsonian syndromes. *Journal of the Neurological Sciences* **115**: 1–17

Burk K, Globas C, Bosch S *et al.* (1999) Cognitive deficits in spinocerebellar ataxia 2. *Brain* **122**: 769–777

Burn DJ and Lees AJ. (2002) Progressive supranuclear palsy: where are we now? *Lancet Neurology* **1**: 359–369

Charrow J, Andersson HC, Kaplan P *et al.* (2004) Enzyme replacement therapy and monitoring for children with Type 1 Gaucher disease: consensus recommendations. *Journal of Paediatrics* **144**: 112–120

Clarke JTR. (2002) *A Clinical Guide to Inherited Metabolic Diseases*, 2nd edition. Cambridge, Cambridge University Press, pp. 18–64

Coker SB. (1991) The diagnosis of childhood neurodegenerative disorders presenting as dementia in adults. *Neurology* **41**: 794–798

Corsellis JA, Goldberg GJ, Norton AR. (1968) 'Limbic encephalitis' and its association with carcinoma. *Brain* **91**: 481–496

Delanty N, Georgescu L, Lynch T, Paget S, Stubgen J-P. (1999) Synovial fluid polymerase chain reaction as an aid to the diagnosis of central nervous system Whipple's disease. *Annals of Neurology* **45**: 137–138

Dirr LY, Elster AD, Donofrio PD, Smith M. (1990) Evolution of brain MRI abnormalities in limbic encephalitis. *Neurology* **40**: 1304–1306

Dooling EC, Schoene WC, Richardson EP. (1974) Hallervorden–Spatz syndrome. *Archives of Neurology* **30**: 70–83

Durr A and Brice A. (2000) Clinical and genetic aspects of spinocerebellar degeneration. *Current Opinion in Neurology* **13**: 407–413

Duyff RF and Weinstein HC. (1996) Late-presenting metachromatic leukodystrophy. *Lancet* **348**: 1382–1383

Faerber EN, Melvin J, Smergel EM. (1999) MRI appearances of metachromatic leukodystrophy. *Pediatric Radiology* **29**: 669–672

Finsterer J. (2004) Mitochondriopathies. *European Journal of Neurology* **11**: 163–186

Gibb WRG, Luthert PJ, Marsden CD. (1989) Corticobasal degeneration. *Brain* **112**: 1171–1192

Gilman S, Low P, Quinn N *et al.* (1999) Consensus statement on the diagnosis of multiple system atrophy. *Journal of the Neurological Sciences* **163**: 94–98

Gitlin JA. (2003) Wilson disease. *Gastroenterology* **125**: 1868–1877

Goebel HH and Braak H. (1989) Adult neuronal ceroid-lipofuscinosis. *Clinical Neuropathology* **8**: 109–119

Graham J and Oppenheimer DR. (1969) Orthostatic hypotension and nicotine sensitivity in a case of multiple system atrophy. *Journal of Neurology, Neurosurgery, and Psychiatry* **32**: 28–34

Gultekin HS, Rosenfeld MR, Voltz R, Eichen J, Posner JB, Dalmau J. (2000) Paraneoplastic limbic encephalitis: neurological symptoms, immunological findings and tumour association in 50 patients. *Brain* **123**: 1481–1494

Hachinski V. (1997) Frontotemporal degeneration, Pick disease, and corticobasal degeneration: one entity or three? *Archives of Neurology* **54**: 1429

Hageman ATM, Gabreel FJM, De Jong JGN *et al.* (1995) Clinical symptoms of adult metachromatic leukodystrophy and arylsulphatase A pseudodeficiency. *Archives of Neurology* **52**: 408–413

Hallervorden J and Spatz H. (1922) Eigenartige erkrankung im extrapyramidalen system mit besonderer beteiligung des globus pallidus und der substantia nigra. *Zeitschrift für die Gesamte Neurologie und Psychiatrie.* **79**: 254–302

Halliday W. (1995) The nosology of Hallervorden–Spatz disease. *Journal of the Neurological Sciences* **134** (Suppl.): 84–91

Harding AE. (1982) The clinical features and classification of late onset autosomal dominant cerebellar ataxias: a study of eleven families, including descendants of the 'Drew family of Walworth'. *Brain* **105**: 1–28

Hayflick SJ, Westaway SK, Levinson B *et al.* (2003) Genetic, clinical, and radiographic delineation of Hallervorden-Spatz syndrome. *New England Journal of Medicine* **348**: 33–40

Hinkebein JH and Callahan CD. (1997) The neuropsychology of Kufs' disease: a case of atypical early onset dementia. *Archives of Clinical Neuropsychology* **12**: 81–89

Hitoshi S, Iwata M, Yoshikawa K. (1991) Mid-brain pathology of Wilson's disease: MRI analysis of three cases. *Journal of Neurology, Neurosurgery, and Psychiatry* **54**: 624–626

Hossain AK, Murata Y, Zhang L *et al.* (2003) Brain perfusion SPECT in patients with corticobasal degeneration: analysis using statistical parametric mapping. *Movement Disorders* **18**: 697–703

Hund E, Grau A, Fogel W *et al.* (1997) Progressive cerebellar ataxia, proximal neurogenic weakness and ocular motor disturbances: hexosaminidase A deficiency with late clinical onset in four siblings. *Journal of the Neurological Sciences* **145**: 25–31

Hyde TM, Ziegler JC, Weinberger DR *et al.* (1992) Psychiatric disturbances in metachromatic leukodystrophy: insight into the neurobiology of psychosis. *Archives of Neurology* **49**: 401–406

Igarashi M, Schaumburg HH, Powers J *et al.* (1976) Fatty acid abnormality in adrenoleukodystrophy. *Journal of Neurochemistry* **26**: 851–860

Jellinger KA and Blancher C. (1992) Neuropathology: In: I Litvan and Y Agid (eds), *Progressive Supranuclear Palsy: Clinical and Research Approaches.* Oxford, Oxford University Press, pp. 44–88

Jones EA and Weissenborn K. (1997) Neurology and the liver. *Journal of Neurology, Neurosurgery, and Psychiatry* **63**: 279–293

Joseph FG and Scolding NJ. (2002) Cerebral vasculitis a practical approach. *Practical Neurology* **2**: 80–93

Josephson SA, Schmidt RE, Millsap P, McManus DQ, Morris JC. (2001) Autosomal dominant Kufs' disease: a cause of early onset dementia. *Journal of the Neurological Sciences* **188**: 51–60

Kaye EM. (2001) Update on genetic disorders affecting white matter. *Pediatric Neurology* **24**: 11–24

Kertesz A. (1997) Frontotemporal degeneration, Pick disease, and corticobasal degeneration: one entity or three? 1. *Archives of Neurology* **54**: 1427–1429

Kim YJ, Ichise M, Ballinger JR *et al.* (2002) Combination of dopamine transporter and D2 receptor SPECT in the diagnostic evaluation of PD, MSA and PSP. *Movement Disorders* **17**: 45–53

Kitchin W, Cohen-Cole SA, Mickel SF. (1987) Adrenoleukodystrophy: frequency of presentation as a psychiatric disorder. *Biological Psychiatry* **22**: 1375–1387

Koopman BJ, Wolthers BG, van der Slik W, Wattereus RJ, van Spereeken A. (1988) Cerebrotendinous xanthomatosis: a review of biochemical findings of the patient population in the Netherlands. *Journal of Inherited Metabolic Diseases.* **11**: 56–75

Kothbauer-Margreiter I, Sturzenegger M, Komor J, Baumgartner R, Hess CW. (1996) Encephalopathy associated with Hashimoto thyroiditis: diagnosis and treatment. *Journal of Neurology* **243**: 585–593

Kraft E, Schwarz J, Trenkwalder C, Vogl T, Pfluger T, Oertel WH. (1999) The combination of hypointense and hyperintense signal changes on T2 weighted magnetic resonance imaging sequences: a specific marker of multiple system atrophy? *Archives of Neurology* **56**: 225–228

Le Pira F, Zappala G, Saponara R *et al.* (2002) Cognitive findings in spinocerebellar ataxia type 2: relationship to genetic and clinical variables. *Journal of the Neurological Sciences* **201**: 53–57

Leiner HC, Leiner AL, Dow RS. (1993) Cognitive and language functions of the cerebellum. *Trends in Neurosciences* **16**: 444–447

Louis ED, Lynch T, Kaufmann P, Fahn S, Odel J. (1996) Diagnostic guidelines in central nervous system Whipple's disease. *Annals of Neurology* **40**: 561–568

Maher ER and Lees AJ. (1986) The clinical features and natural history of Steele-Richardson-Olszweski syndrome (progressive supranuclear palsy) *Neurology* **36**: 1005–1008

Markus HS. Lees AJ, Lennox G, Marsden CD, Costa DC. (1995) Patterns of regional cerebral blood flow in corticobasal degeneration studied using HMPAO SPECT; comparison with Parkinson's disease and normal controls. *Movement Disorders* **10**: 179–187

Marth T and Raoult D. (2003) Whipple's disease. *Lancet* **361**: 239–246

Matzner U, Hartmann D, Lullman-Rauch R *et al.* (2002) Bone marrow stem cell-based gene transfer in a mouse model for metachromatic leukodystrophy: effects on visceral and nervous system disease manifestations. *Gene Therapy* **9**: 53–63

Minassian BA, Lee JR, Herbrick JA *et al.* (1998) Mutations in a gene encoding a novel protein tyrosine phosphatase cause progressive myoclonus epilepsy. *Nature Genetics* 171–174

Minassian BA. (2001) Lafora's disease: towards a clinical, pathologic and molecular synthesis. *Pediatric Neurology* **25**: 21–29

Moghadasian MH, Salen G, Frohlich JJ, Scudamore CH. (2002) Cerebrotendinous xanthomatosis, a rare disease with diverse manifestations. *Archives of Neurology* **59**: 527–529

Moser HW. (1997) Adrenoleukodystrophy: phenotype, genetics, pathogenesis and therapy. *Brain* **120**: 1485–1508

Moser HW, Moser AW, Singh I *et al.* (1984) Adrenoleukodystrophy: survey of 303 cases: biochemistry, diagnosis, therapy. *Annals of Neurology* **16**: 628–641

Munnich A and Rustin P. (2001) Clinical spectrum and diagnosis of mitochondrial disorders. *American Journal of Medical Genetics (Seminars in Medical Genetics)* **106**: 4–17

Neary D. (1997) Frontotemporal degeneration, Pick disease, and corticobasal degeneration One entity or three? 3. *Archives of Neurology* **54**: 1425–1427

Neary D and Snowden JS. (2003) Sorting out subacute encephalopathy. *Practical Neurology* **3**: 268–281

Newman NJ, Bell IR, McKee AC. (1990) Paraneoplastic limbic encephalitis: neuropsychiatric presentation. *Biological Psychiatry* **27**: 529–542

Osaki Y, Ben-Shlomo Y, Lees AJ *et al.* (2004) Accuracy of clinical diagnosis of progressive supranuclear palsy. *Movement Disorders* **19**: 181–189

Patterson MC. (2003) A riddle wrapped in a mystery: understanding Niemann-Pick disease, type C. *Neurologist* **9**: 301–310

Pujana MA, Corral J, Gratacos M *et al.* (1999) Spinocerebellar ataxias in Spanish patients: genetic analysis of familial and sporadic cases. The Ataxia Study Group. *Human Genetics* **104**: 516–522

Quinn N. (1989) Multiple system atrophy: the nature of the beast. *Journal of Neurology, Neurosurgery, and Psychiatry* **52** (Suppl.): 78–89

Rahman S and Schapira AHV. (1999) Mitochondrial myopathies: clinical features, molecular genetics, investigation and management. In: AHV Schapira and RC Griggs (eds), *Muscle Diseases, Blue Books of Practical Neurology (24)*. Woburn, MA, Butterworth-Heinemann, pp. 177–223

Ribeiz JJ, Kolodny EH, Richardson EP. (1968) Corticodentatonigral degeneration with neuronal achromasia. *Archives of Neurology* **18**: 20–33

Robbins TW, James M, Lange KW, Owen AM, Quinn NP, Marsden CD. (1992) Cognitive performances in multiple system atrophy. *Brain* **115**: 271–291

Savoiardo M. (2003) Differential diagnosis of Parkinson's disease and atypical parkinsonian disorders by magnetic resonance imaging. *Neurological Sciences* **24** (Suppl. 1): S35–S37

Schrag A, Good CD, Miszkiel K *et al.* (2000) Differentiation of atypical parkinsonian syndromes with routine MRI. *Neurology* **54**: 697–702

Scolding NJ, Jayne DR, Zajicek JP, Meyer PAR, Wraight EP, Lockwood CM. (1997) The syndrome of cerebral vasculitis: recognition, diagnosis and management. *Quarterly Journal of Medicine* **90**: 61–73

Serratosa JM, Delgado-Escueta AV, Posada I *et al.* (1995) The gene for progressive myoclonus epilepsy of the Lafora type maps to chromosome 6q. *Human Molecular Genetics* **4**: 1657–1663

Shaw PJ, Walls TJ, Newman PK, Cleland PG, Cartlidge NE. (1991) Hashimoto's encephalopathy: a steroid responsive disorder associated with high antithyroid antibody titres – report of five cases. *Neurology* **41**: 228–233

Shulman LM, David NJ, Weiner WJ. (1995a) Psychosis as the initial manifestation of adult-onset Niemann Pick disease type C. *Neurology* **45**: 1739–1743

Shulman LM, Lang AE, Jankovic J *et al.* (1995b) Case 1: 1995: psychosis, dementia, chorea, ataxia, and supranuclear gaze dysfunction. *Movement Disorders* **10**: 257–262

Steele JC. (1972) Progressive supranuclear palsy. *Brain* **95**: 693–704

Steele JC, Richardson JC, Olszweski J. (1964) Progressive supranuclear palsy. *Archives of Neurology* **10**: 333–359

Stover NP and Watts RL. (2001) Corticobasal degeneration. *Seminars in Neurology* **21**: 49–58

Trojano L, Chiacchio L, Grossi D *et al.* (1998) Determinants of cognitive disorders in autosomal dominant cerebellar ataxia type 1. *Journal of the Neurological Sciences* **157**: 162–167

Turconi AC, Benti R, Castelli E *et al.* (1999) Focal cognitive impairment in mitochondrial encephalomyopathies: a neuropsychological and neuroimaging study. *Journal of the Neurological Sciences* **170**: 57–63

van Geel MB, Assies J, Wanders RJ, Barth P'G. (1997) X linked adrenoleukodystrophy: clinical presentation, diagnosis and therapy. *Journal of Neurology, Neurosurgery, and Psychiatry* **63**: 4–14

Vodusek B. (2001) Sphincter EMG and differential diagnosis of multiple system atrophy. *Movement Disorders* **16**: 600–607

Warmuth-Metz M, Naumann M, Csoti I, Solymosi I. (2001) Measurement of the midbrain diameter on routine magnetic resonance imaging: a simple and accurate method of differentiating between Parkinson disease and progressive supranuclear palsy. *Archives of Neurology* **58**: 1076–1079

Wenning GK, Colosimo C, Geser F, Poewe W. (2004) Multiple system atrophy. *Lancet Neurology* **3**: 93–103

Appendix: national Alzheimer's associations

Argentina
Asociación de Lucha contra el Mal de Alzheimer
Lacarra No 78, 1407 Capital Federal, Buenos Aires,
Argentina
Tel/Fax: +54 11 4671 1187
Email: alma@satlink.com
Web: www.alma-alzheimer.org.ar

Australia
Alzheimer's Australia
P.O. Box 108, Higgins, ACT 2615, Australia
Tel: +61 2 6254 4233
Helpline: 1800 639 331
Fax: +61 2 6254 2522
Email: glenn@alzheimers.org.au
Web: www.alzheimers.org.au

Austria
Alzheimer Angehorige Austria
Obere Augartenstrasse 26–28, 1020 Vienna, Austria
Tel: +43 1 332 5166
Fax: +43 1 334 2141
Email: alzheimeraustria@via.at
Web: www.alzheimer-selbsthilfe.at

Belgium
Ligue Alzheimer
Clinique Le Perî, 4B Rue Montagne, Sainte Walburge
Belgium, B-4000 Liège
Tel: +32 4 225 8793
Helpline: 0800 15 225
Fax: +32 4 225 8693
Email: henry.sabine@skynet.be
Web: www.alzheimer.be

Brazil
FEBRAZ – Federação Brasileira de Associaçãoes de
Alzheimer
c/o ABRAZ – Associação Brasileira de Alzheimer
Caixa Postal 3913, Sao Paulo – SP – Brazil, 01160-970
Tel/Fax: +55 11 270 8791
Helpline: 0 800 55 1906
Email: abraz@abraz.org.br
Web: www.abraz.com.br

Canada
Alzheimer Society of Canada
20 Eglinton Avenue, W., Suite 1200, Toronto,
Ontario M4R 1K8, Canada
Tel: +1 416 488 8772
Helpline: 1800 616 8816
Fax: +1 416 488 3778
Email: info@alzheimer.ca
Web: www.alzheimer.ca

Chile
Corporación Alzheimer Chile
Desiderio Lemus 0143, Recoleta, Santiago, Chile
Tel: +56 2 236 0846
Fax: +56 2 777 7431
Email: alzchile@adsl.tie.cl
Web: www.alzheimer.cl

China
Chinese Association of Alzheimer's Disease and Related
Disorders
Department of Neurology, Beijing Hospital
Ministry of Health
#1 Da Hua Road, Dong Dan, Beijing 100730, China
Tel: +8610 6521 2012
Fax: +8610 6521 2386
Email: xuxh@public.bta.net.cn

Colombia
Asociacion Colombiana de Alzheimer y Desordenes
Relacionados
Calle 69 A No. 10–16, Santafe deBogota D.C., Colombia
Tel: +57 1 348 1997
Fax: +57 1 321 7691
Email: alzheimercolombia@hotmail.com

Costa Rica
Asociación Costarricense de Alzheimer y otras Demecias
Asociadas
Los Lagos de Heredia, House 58C, San Francisco,
03004 Heredia, Costa Rica
Tel: +506 237 7527
Fax: +506 260 1716
Email: ascada@msn.com

Cuba
Cuban Section of Alzheimer's Disease and Related Disorders
Calle 146 No 2504 e/ 25 y 31
Cubanacan Playa, Ciudad de la Habana, Cuba
Tel: +537 220974
Fax: +537 336857
Email: inmo@teleda.get.tur.cu
Web: www.scual.sld.cu

Cyprus
Pancyprian Association of Alzheimer's Disease
31A Stadiou, 6020 Larnaca, Cyprus
Tel: +357 24 627 104
Fax: +357 24 627 106
Email: alzhcyprus@yahoo.com

Czech Republic
Ceska Alzheimerovska Spolecnost
Centre of Gerontology
Simunkova 1600, 18200 Praha 8, Czech Republic
Tel: +420 2 88 36 76
Fax: +420 2 88 27 88
Email: Petr.Veleta@gerontocentrum.cz
Web: www.gerontocentrum.cz/cals/framepage.htm

Denmark
Alzheimerforeningen
Sankt Lukas Vej 6, 1, DK 2900 Hellerup, Denmark
Tel: +45 39 40 04 88
Fax: +45 39 61 66 69
Email: post@alzheimer.dk
Web: www.alzheimer.dk

Dominican Republic
Asociacion Dominicana de Alzheimer
Apartado Postal # 3321, Santo Domingo
Republica Dominicana
Tel: +1 809 544 1711
Fax: +1 809 544 1731
Email: dr.pedro@codetel.net.do

Ecuador
Fundacion Alzheimer Ecuador
Avenida de la Prensa #5204 y Avenida de Maestro,
Quito, Ecuador
Tel: +593 2 2594 997
Fax: +593 2 2594 997
Email: gustavomatute@andinanet.net

Egypt
Egyptian Alzheimer Group
c/o Professor A Ashour
1 Gawad Hosni Street, Abdeen, Cairo 11111, Egypt
Tel: +202 392 0074
Fax: +202 302 3270
Email: amashour2002@yahoo.com

El Salvador
Asociacion de Familiares Alzheimer de El Salvador
Asilo Sara Zaldivar, Colonia Costa Rica,
Avenida Irazu, San Salvador, El Salvador
Tel: +503 237 0787
Email: ricardolopez@vianet.com.sv

Finland
Alzheimer Society of Finland
Luotsikatu 4E, 00160 Helsinki, Finland
Tel: +358 9 6226 200
Fax: +358 9 6226 2020
Email: tarja.tapaninen@alzheimer.fi
Web: www.alzheimer.fi

France
France Alzheimer et Maladies Apparentées
21 Boulevard Montmartre, 75002 Paris, France
Tel: +33 1 42 97 52 41
Fax: +33 1 42 96 04 70
Email: contact@francealzheimer.com
Web: www.francealzheimer.com

Germany
Deutsche Alzheimer Gesellschaft
Friedrichstr. 236, 10969 Berlin, Germany
Tel: +49 30 315 057 33
Helpline: 01803 171 017
Fax: +49 30 315 057 35
Email: deutsche.alzheimer.ges@t-online.de
Web: www.deutsche-alzheimer.de

Greece
Greek Association of AD and Related Disorders
Charisio Old People's Home
Terma Dimitriou Charisi
Ano Toumba 543 52, Thessaloniki, Greece
Tel/Fax : +30 2310 925802
Helpline: +30 2310 909000
Email: alzheimer@hellasnet.gr
Web: www.alzheimer-hellas.gr

Guatemala
Asociación Grupo ERMITA
10a. Calle 11–63, Zona 1, Apto B,
P O Box 2978, 01901 Guatemala
Tel: +502 2 381122
Fax: +502 2 381122
Email: alzguate@quetzal.net
Web: www.alzheimer-guatemala.org.gt

Hong Kong SAR
Hong Kong Alzheimer's Disease Association
c/o GF Wang Lai House
Wang Tau Hom Estate, Kowloon, Hong Kong SAR, China
Tel: +852 27943010
Carer Hotline: +(852) 2338 2277
Fax: +852 23384820
Email: info@hkada.org.hk
Web: www.hkada.org.hk

Iceland
FAAS
Austurburn 31, 104 Reyjkjavik, Iceland
Tel: +354 533 1088
Fax: +354 533 1086
Email: faas@alzheimer.is
Web: www.alzheimer.is

India
Alzheimer's & Related Disorders Society of India
Guruvayoor Road, PO Box 53, Kunnamkulam
Kerala 680 503, India
Tel: +91 4885 223801
Fax: +91 4885 223801/ 222347
Email: alzheimr@md2.vsnl.net.in
Web: www.alzheimerindia.org

Indonesia
IAzA Secretariat
c/o Wahyudi Nugroho
Sasana Tresna Werda "Yayasan Karya Bakti Ria
Pembangunan"
jl. Pusdika RT 008 RW 07, KM 17 Cibubur
Jakarta 13720, Indonesia
Tel: +62 21 8730179
Fax: +62 21 39899128
Email: nasrun@indosat.net.id

Ireland
The Alzheimer Society of Ireland
Alzheimer's House
43 Northumberland Avenue,
Dunlaoghaire, Co Dublin, Ireland
Tel: +353 1 284 6616
Helpline: 1800 341 341
Fax: +353 1 284 6030
Email: info@alzheimer.ie
Web: www.alzheimer.ie

Iran
Iran Alzheimer Association
Shahid Ghaffari Health Clinic
Shahrak Ekbatan, Phase II, Tehran 13969, Iran
Tel: +98 21 4651122
Fax: +98 21 4651122
Email: info@alzheimer.ir
Web: www.alzheimer.ir

Israel
Alzheimer's Association of Israel
P O Box 8261, Ramat Gan, Israel 52181
Tel: +972 3 578 7660
Fax: +972 3 578 7661
Email: a-a-i@zahav.net.il
Web: www.alz-il.net

Italy
Federazione Alzheimer Italia
Via Tommaso Marino 7, 20121 Milano, Italy
Tel: +39 02 809767
Fax: +39 02 875781
Email: alzit@tin.it
Web: www.alzheimer.it

Japan
Alzheimer's Association Japan
c/o Kyoto Social Welfare Hall
Horikawa-Marutamachi, Kamigyo-Ku, Kyoto
Japan 602-8143
Tel: +81 75 811 8195
Fax: +81 75 811 8188
Email: office@alzheimer.or.jp
Web: www.alzheimer.or.jp

Korea
Alzheimer's Association, Korea
#52, Machon 2-Dong, Songpa-ku, Seoul 138-122, Korea
Tel: +82 2 431 9963
Helpline: +82 2 431 9993
Fax: +82 2 431 9964
Email: afcde01@unitel.co.kr
Web: www.alzza.or.kr

Lebanon
Alzheimer's Association Lebanon
La Palma Bldg. 1st floor, Aoukar, Lebanon
Tel: +961 3 245606
Email: d.mansour@alzlebanon.org
Web: www.alzlebanon.org

Luxembourg
Association Luxembourg Alzheimer
45, rue Nicolas Hein, BP 5021, L 1050 Luxembourg
Tel: +352 42 16 76 1
Fax: +352 42 16 76 30
Email: info@alzheimer.lu
Web: www.alzheimer.lu

Malaysia

Alzheimer's Disease Foundation Malaysia
9a, Lorong Bukit Raja, Taman Seputeh
58000 Kuala Lumpur, Malaysia
Tel: +603 2260 3158/ 2274 9060
Fax: +603 2273 8493
Email: alzheimers@pd.jaring.my

Mexico

Federación Mexicana de Alzheimer
Carretera Cubitos La Paz # 122
Lomas Residencial Pachuca, Pachuca, Hgo. 42094,
Mexico
Tel/Fax: +771 71 9 47 52/ 71 902 97
Email: fedma2002@hotmail.com
Web: www.fedma.net

Netherlands

Alzheimer Nederland
Post Bus 183, 3980 CD BUNNIK, The Netherlands
Tel: +31 30 659 6900
Helpline: 030 656 7511
Fax: +31 30 659 6901
Email: info@alzheimer-nederland.nl
Web: www.alzheimer-nederland.nl

New Zealand

Alzheimer's New Zealand
Level 2, Magnum Mac House, 5-7 Vivian Street
PO Box 3643, Wellington, New Zealand
Tel: +64 4 381 2361
Helpline: 0800 004 001
Fax: +64 4 381 2365
Email: alzheimers@alzheimers.org.nz
Web: www.alzheimers.org.nz

Nigeria

Alzheimer's Disease Association of Nigeria
c/o Dept. of Psychiatry
Nnamdi Azikiwe University Teaching Hospital
Nnewi, Anambra State, Nigeria
Tel: +234 46 463663
Fax: +234 46 462496
Email: tifine@infoweb.abs.net

Norway

Nasjonalforeningen Demensforbundet
Oscarsgt 36 A, Postboks
7139 Majorstua, N 0307 Oslo, Norway
Tel: +47 23 12 00 00
Helpline: +47 815 33 032
Fax: +47 23 12 00 01
Email: post@nasjonalforeningen.no
Web: www.nasjonalforeningen.no

Pakistan

Alzheimer's Pakistan
146/1 Shadman Jail Road, Lahore 54000, Pakistan
Tel: +92 42 759 6589
Fax: +92 42 757 3911
Email: info@alz.org.pk
Web: www.alz.org.pk

Panama

AFA PADEA
PO Box 6-6839, El Dorado, Panama
Email: hopemil@sinfo.net

Peru

Asociacion Peruana de Enfermedad de Alzheimer y Otras
Demencias
Los Galeanos # 976, Urb. Higuereta, Surco, Lima, Peru
Tel: +511 448 2237 / 272 1365
Fax: +511 442 8046
Email: asociacion@alzheimerperu.org
Web: www.alzheimerperu.org

Philippines

Alzheimer's Disease Association of the Philippines
St Luke's Medical Center, Medical Arts Bldg, Rm 410
E Rodriguez Sr Avenue, Quezon City, Philippines
Tel/fax: +632 723 1039
Email: adap@alzphilippines.com
Web: www.alzphilippines.com

Poland

Polish Alzheimer's Association
ul. Hoza 54/1, 00-682 Warszawa, Poland
Tel/Fax: +48 22 622 11 22
Email: alzheimer_pl@hotmail.com
Web: www.alzheimer.pl

Portugal

Associação Portuguesa de Familiares e Amigos de Doentes
de Alzheimer
Avenida de Ceuta Norte
Lote 1 – Lojas 1 e 2 – Quinta do Loureiro,
1350-410 Lisboa, Portugal
Tel: +351 21 361 0460
Fax: +351 21 361 0469
Email: alzheimer@netcabo.pt
Web: www.alzheimerportugal.org

Puerto Rico

Asociación de Alzheimer y Desórdenes Relacionados de
Puerto Rico
Apartado 362026, San Juan, Puerto Rico 00936-2026
Tel: +1 787 727 4151
Fax: +1 787 727 4890
Email: alzheimerpr@alzheimerpr.org
Web: www.alzheimerpr.org

Romania
Romanian Alzheimer Society
Bd. Mihail Kogalniceanu, nr 49A (fost 95 A)
Sc.A, Ap.8, Sector 5, 050108 Bucharest, Romania
Tel: +402 1 334 8940
Fax: +402 1 334 8940
Email: contact@alz.ro
Web: www.alz.ro

Russia
Association for Support of Alzheimer's Disease Victims
34 Kashirskoye shosse, 115522 Moscow, Russia
Tel: +7 095 324 9615
Fax: +7 095 114 4925
Email: gavrilova@mail.tascom.ru

Scotland
Alzheimer Scotland – Action on Dementia
22 Drumsheugh Gardens, Edinburgh, EH3 7RN, Scotland
Tel: +44 131 243 1453
Helpline: 0808 808 3000
Fax: +44 131 243 1450
Email: alzheimer@alzscot.org
Web: www.alzscot.org

Serbia and Montenegro
Alzheimer Society of Serbia and Montenegro
Dr Suhotica 6, Institute of Neurology
Belgrade 11000, Serbia and Montenegro
Tel: +381 11 361 4122
Fax: +381 11 684 577
Email: dpavlovic@drenik.net

Singapore
Alzheimer's Disease Association
Blk 157, Toa Payoh Lorong 1, #01- 1195,
Singapore 310157
Tel: +65 353 8734
Fax: +65 353 8518
Email: alzheimers.tp@pacific.net.sg
Web: www.alzheimers.org.sg

Slovak Republic
Slovak Alzheimer's Society
Dúbravaká 9, Bratislava 84246, Slovak Republic
Tel: +421 7 594 13353
Fax: +421 7 547 74276
Email: nilunova@savba.sk

South Africa
Alzheimer's South Africa
P O Box 81183, Parkhurst, Johannesburg 2120, South Africa
Tel: +27 11 478 2234/5/6
Fax: +27 11 478 2251
Email: info@alzheimers.org.za
Web: www.alzheimers.org.za

Spain
Confederación Española de Familiares de Enfermos de Alzheimer
C/ Pedro Miguel Alcatarena nº 3
31014 Pamplona (Navarra), Spain
Tel: +34 948 174517
Fax: +34 948 265739
Email: alzheimer@cin.es
Web: www.ceafa.org

Sri Lanka
Lanka Alzheimer's Foundation
19 Havelock Road, Colombo 5, Sri Lanka
Tel: +94 1 583488
Fax: +94 1 732745
Email: alzheimers_foundation@serendib.ws

Sweden
Alzheimerföreningen i Sverige
Sunnanväg 14 S, 222 26 Lund, Sweden
Tel: +46 46 14 73 18
Fax: +46 46 18 89 76
Email: info@alzheimerforeningen.se
Web: www.alzheimerforeningen.se

Switzerland
Association Alzheimer Suisse
8 Rue des Pêcheurs, CH-1400 Yverdon-les-Bains, Switzerland
Tel: +41 24 426 2000
Fax: +41 24 426 2167
Email: alz@bluewin.ch
Web: www.alz.ch

Thailand
Alzheimer's and Related Disorders Association of Thailand
114 Pinakorn 4, Boramratchachunee Road
Talingchan, Bangkok 10170, Thailand
Tel: +66 2 880 8542/7539
Fax: +66 2 880 7244
Web: www.geocities.com/alzheimerasso

Trinidad and Tobago
Alzheimer's Association of Trinidad and Tobago
c/o Soroptimist International Port of Spain
15 Nepaul Street, St James, Port of Spain
Republic of Trinidad and Tobago
Tel: +1 868 622 6134
Fax: +1 868 627 6731
Email: norinniss@wow.net

Turkey
Turkish Alzheimer Society
Halaskargazi Cad. No: 115 Da: 4 Harbiye, Istanbul, Turkey
Tel: +90 212 224 41 89
Helpline: 0800 211 8024
Fax: +90 212 296 05 79
Email: alzheimervakfi@ttnet.net.tr
Web: www.alz.org.tr

Uganda

Alzheimer's and Dementia Awareness Society
c/o Eng. Chris Ntegakarija
PO Box 8371, Kampala, Uganda
Tel/Fax: +256 486 22290
Email: adasuga@talk21.com

Ukraine

The Association for the Problems of Alzheimer's Disease
Institute of Gerontology
67 Vyshgorodskaya Street, 04114 Kiev, Ukraine
Tel: +380 44 431 0526
Fax: +380 44 432 9956
Email: bachinskaya@geront.kiev.ua

United Kingdom (except Scotland)

Alzheimer's Society
Gordon House, 10 Greencoat Place
London, SW1P 1PH, United Kingdom
Tel: +44 20 7306 0606
Helpline: 0845 300 0336
Fax: +44 20 7306 0808
Email: enquiries@alzheimers.org.uk
Web: www.alzheimers.org.uk

United States of America

Alzheimer's Association
225 N Michigan Avenue, Suite 1700
Chicago, Illinois 60601, United States of America
Tel: +1 312 335 8700
Helpline: 0800 272 3900
Fax: +1 312 335 1110
Email: info@alz.org
Web: www.alz.org

Uruguay

Asociación Uruguaya de Alzheimer y Similares
Casilla de Correo 5092, Magallanes 1320
11200 Montevideo – Uruguay
Tel: +598 2 400 8797
Fax: +598 2 400 8797
Email: audasur@adinet.com.uy

Venezuela

Fundación Alzheimer de Venezuela
Calle El Limon, Qta Mi Muñe, El Cafetal
Caracas, Venezuela
Tel: +58 212 4146129
Fax: +58 212 9859183
Email: alzven@cantv.net
Web: www.gentiuno.com/seccion.asp?seccion=53

Zimbabwe

Zimbabwe Alzheimer's and Related Disorders Association
PO Box CH 336, Chisipite, Harare, Zimbabwe
Tel: +263 4 703 423/7
Fax: +263 4 704 487
Email: coxsu@renniestravel.co.zw

REGIONAL ASSOCIATIONS

Europe

Alzheimer Europe
145 rte de Thionville, L-2611, Luxembourg
Web: www.alzheimer-europe.org

Latin America

Alzheimer Iberoamerica
Calle El Limon, Qta Mi Muñe, El Cafetal
Caracas, Venezuela
Tel: +58 212 9859183
Fax: +58 212 4146129
Web: aib.alzheimer-online.org

Index